HUMAN PRION DISEASES

HANDBOOK OF CLINICAL NEUROLOGY

Series Editors

MICHAEL J. AMINOFF, FRANÇOIS BOLLER, AND DICK F. SWAAB

VOLUME 153

ELSEVIER

HUMAN PRION DISEASES

Series Editors

MICHAEL J. AMINOFF, FRANÇOIS BOLLER, AND DICK F. SWAAB

Volume Editors

MAURIZIO POCCHIARI AND JEAN MANSON

VOLUME 153

3rd Series

ELSEVIER

ELSEVIER
Radarweg 29, PO Box 211, 1000 AE Amsterdam, Netherlands
The Boulevard, Langford Lane, Kidlington, Oxford OX5 1GB, United Kingdom
50 Hampshire Street, 5th Floor, Cambridge, MA 02139, United States

British Library Cataloguing-in-Publication Data
A catalogue record for this book is available from the British Library

Library of Congress Cataloging-in-Publication Data
A catalog record for this book is available from the Library of Congress

ISBN: 978-0-444-63945-5

Publisher: Nikki Levy
Editorial Project Manager: Kristi Anderson
Production Project Manager: Sujatha Thirugnana Sambandam
Cover Designer: Alan Studholme

Typeset by SPi Global, India

Handbook of Clinical Neurology 3rd Series

Available titles

Vol. 79, The human hypothalamus: basic and clinical aspects, Part I, D.F. Swaab, ed. ISBN 9780444513571
Vol. 80, The human hypothalamus: basic and clinical aspects, Part II, D.F. Swaab, ed. ISBN 9780444514905
Vol. 81, Pain, F. Cervero and T.S. Jensen, eds. ISBN 9780444519016
Vol. 82, Motor neurone disorders and related diseases, A.A. Eisen and P.J. Shaw, eds. ISBN 9780444518941
Vol. 83, Parkinson's disease and related disorders, Part I, W.C. Koller and E. Melamed, eds. ISBN 9780444519009
Vol. 84, Parkinson's disease and related disorders, Part II, W.C. Koller and E. Melamed, eds. ISBN 9780444528933
Vol. 85, HIV/AIDS and the nervous system, P. Portegies and J. Berger, eds. ISBN 9780444520104
Vol. 86, Myopathies, F.L. Mastaglia and D. Hilton Jones, eds. ISBN 9780444518996
Vol. 87, Malformations of the nervous system, H.B. Sarnat and P. Curatolo, eds. ISBN 9780444518965
Vol. 88, Neuropsychology and behavioural neurology, G. Goldenberg and B.C. Miller, eds. ISBN 9780444518972
Vol. 89, Dementias, C. Duyckaerts and I. Litvan, eds. ISBN 9780444518989
Vol. 90, Disorders of consciousness, G.B. Young and E.F.M. Wijdicks, eds. ISBN 9780444518958
Vol. 91, Neuromuscular junction disorders, A.G. Engel, ed. ISBN 9780444520081
Vol. 92, Stroke – Part I: Basic and epidemiological aspects, M. Fisher, ed. ISBN 9780444520036
Vol. 93, Stroke – Part II: Clinical manifestations and pathogenesis, M. Fisher, ed. ISBN 9780444520043
Vol. 94, Stroke – Part III: Investigations and management, M. Fisher, ed. ISBN 9780444520050
Vol. 95, History of neurology, S. Finger, F. Boller and K.L. Tyler, eds. ISBN 9780444520081
Vol. 96, Bacterial infections of the central nervous system, K.L. Roos and A.R. Tunkel, eds. ISBN 9780444520159
Vol. 97, Headache, G. Nappi and M.A. Moskowitz, eds. ISBN 9780444521392
Vol. 98, Sleep disorders Part I, P. Montagna and S. Chokroverty, eds. ISBN 9780444520067
Vol. 99, Sleep disorders Part II, P. Montagna and S. Chokroverty, eds. ISBN 9780444520074
Vol. 100, Hyperkinetic movement disorders, W.J. Weiner and E. Tolosa, eds. ISBN 9780444520142
Vol. 101, Muscular dystrophies, A. Amato and R.C. Griggs, eds. ISBN 9780080450315
Vol. 102, Neuro-ophthalmology, C. Kennard and R.J. Leigh, eds. ISBN 9780444529039
Vol. 103, Ataxic disorders, S.H. Subramony and A. Durr, eds. ISBN 9780444518927
Vol. 104, Neuro-oncology Part I, W. Grisold and R. Sofietti, eds. ISBN 9780444521385
Vol. 105, Neuro-oncology Part II, W. Grisold and R. Sofietti, eds. ISBN 9780444535023
Vol. 106, Neurobiology of psychiatric disorders, T. Schlaepfer and C.B. Nemeroff, eds. ISBN 9780444520029
Vol. 107, Epilepsy Part I, H. Stefan and W.H. Theodore, eds. ISBN 9780444528988
Vol. 108, Epilepsy Part II, H. Stefan and W.H. Theodore, eds. ISBN 9780444528995
Vol. 109, Spinal cord injury, J. Verhaagen and J.W. McDonald III, eds. ISBN 9780444521378
Vol. 110, Neurological rehabilitation, M. Barnes and D.C. Good, eds. ISBN 9780444529015
Vol. 111, Pediatric neurology Part I, O. Dulac, M. Lassonde and H.B. Sarnat, eds. ISBN 9780444528919
Vol. 112, Pediatric neurology Part II, O. Dulac, M. Lassonde and H.B. Sarnat, eds. ISBN 9780444529107
Vol. 113, Pediatric neurology Part III, O. Dulac, M. Lassonde and H.B. Sarnat, eds. ISBN 9780444595652
Vol. 114, Neuroparasitology and tropical neurology, H.H. Garcia, H.B. Tanowitz and O.H. Del Brutto, eds. ISBN 9780444534903
Vol. 115, Peripheral nerve disorders, G. Said and C. Krarup, eds. ISBN 9780444529022
Vol. 116, Brain stimulation, A.M. Lozano and M. Hallett, eds. ISBN 9780444534972
Vol. 117, Autonomic nervous system, R.M. Buijs and D.F. Swaab, eds. ISBN 9780444534910
Vol. 118, Ethical and legal issues in neurology, J.L. Bernat and H.R. Beresford, eds. ISBN 9780444535016
Vol. 119, Neurologic aspects of systemic disease Part I, J. Biller and J.M. Ferro, eds. ISBN 9780702040863
Vol. 120, Neurologic aspects of systemic disease Part II, J. Biller and J.M. Ferro, eds. ISBN 9780702040870
Vol. 121, Neurologic aspects of systemic disease Part III, J. Biller and J.M. Ferro, eds. ISBN 9780702040887
Vol. 122, Multiple sclerosis and related disorders, D.S. Goodin, ed. ISBN 9780444520012
Vol. 123, Neurovirology, A.C. Tselis and J. Booss, eds. ISBN 9780444534880

Vol. 124, Clinical neuroendocrinology, E. Fliers, M. Korbonits and J.A. Romijn, eds. ISBN 9780444596024
Vol. 125, Alcohol and the nervous system, E.V. Sullivan and A. Pfefferbaum, eds. ISBN 9780444626196
Vol. 126, Diabetes and the nervous system, D.W. Zochodne and R.A. Malik, eds. ISBN 9780444534804
Vol. 127, Traumatic brain injury Part I, J.H. Grafman and A.M. Salazar, eds. ISBN 9780444528926
Vol. 128, Traumatic brain injury Part II, J.H. Grafman and A.M. Salazar, eds. ISBN 9780444635211
Vol. 129, The human auditory system: Fundamental organization and clinical disorders, G.G. Celesia and G. Hickok, eds. ISBN 9780444626301
Vol. 130, Neurology of sexual and bladder disorders, D.B. Vodušek and F. Boller, eds. ISBN 9780444632470
Vol. 131, Occupational neurology, M. Lotti and M.L. Bleecker, eds. ISBN 9780444626271
Vol. 132, Neurocutaneous syndromes, M.P. Islam and E.S. Roach, eds. ISBN 9780444627025
Vol. 133, Autoimmune neurology, S.J. Pittock and A. Vincent, eds. ISBN 9780444634320
Vol. 134, Gliomas, M.S. Berger and M. Weller, eds. ISBN 9780128029978
Vol. 135, Neuroimaging Part I, J.C. Masdeu and R.G. González, eds. ISBN 9780444534859
Vol. 136, Neuroimaging Part II, J.C. Masdeu and R.G. González, eds. ISBN 9780444534866
Vol. 137, Neuro-otology, J.M. Furman and T. Lempert, eds. ISBN 9780444634375
Vol. 138, Neuroepidemiology, C. Rosano, M.A. Ikram and M. Ganguli, eds. ISBN 9780128029732
Vol. 139, Functional neurologic disorders, M. Hallett, J. Stone and A. Carson, eds. ISBN 9780128017722
Vol. 140, Critical care neurology Part I, E.F.M. Wijdicks and A.H. Kramer, eds. ISBN 9780444636003
Vol. 141, Critical care neurology Part II, E.F.M. Wijdicks and A.H. Kramer, eds. ISBN 9780444635990
Vol. 142, Wilson disease, A. Członkowska and M.L. Schilsky, eds. ISBN 9780444636003
Vol. 143, Arteriovenous and cavernous malformations, R.F. Spetzler, K. Moon and R.O. Almefty, eds. ISBN 9780444636409
Vol. 144, Huntington disease, A.S. Feigin and K.E. Anderson, eds. ISBN 9780128018934
Vol. 145, Neuropathology, G.G. Kovacs and I. Alafuzoff, eds. ISBN 9780128023952
Vol. 146, Cerebrospinal fluid in neurologic disorders, F. Deisenhammer, C.E. Teunissen and H. Tumani, eds. ISBN 9780128042793
Vol. 147, Neurogenetics Part I, D.H. Geschwind, H.L. Paulson and C. Klein, eds. ISBN 9780444632333
Vol. 148, Neurogenetics Part II, D.H. Geschwind, H.L. Paulson and C. Klein, eds. ISBN 9780444640765
Vol. 149, Metastatic diseases of the nervous system, D. Schiff and M.J. van den Bent, eds. ISBN 9780128111611
Vol. 150, Brain banking in neurologic and psychiatric diseases, I. Huitinga and M.J. Webster, eds. ISBN 9780444636393
Vol. 151, The parietal lobe, G. Vallar and H.B. Coslett, eds. ISBN 9780444636225
Vol. 152, The neurology of HIV infection, B.J. Brew, ed. ISBN 9780444638496

All volumes in the 3rd Series of the **Handbook of Clinical Neurology** are published electronically, on Science Direct: http://www.sciencedirect.com/science/handbooks/00729752.

Foreword

We are delighted to present the first volume in the *Handbook of Clinical Neurology* (HCN) series devoted entirely to prion diseases, after 60 years of tremendous progress in this field.

The topic of human transmissible spongiform encephalopathies has a relatively short but very exciting history, as described vividly in the first chapter of this volume. Kuru, a disease caused by ritual cannibalism, was discovered in New Guinea, where it took an epidemic form in the middle of the 20th century. In 1959, Igor Klatzo remarked that Creutzfeldt–Jakob disease showed histopathologically a close resemblance to kuru, and William J. Hadlow was struck by the histopathologic similarities between kuru and scrapie, a progressive degenerative neurologic disease that affects sheep and goats. Injection of brain suspensions into the brains of chimpanzees confirmed that Creutzfeldt–Jakob disease, like scrapie and kuru, was transmissible. Carleton Gajdusek's investigation of the possibility that not only kuru but also other progressive degenerative neurologic diseases of humans might be caused by infectious agents – thought at the time to be viruses – led to his being awarded the Nobel Prize in 1976. Stanley Prusiner rejected the viral hypothesis and subsequently coined the term "prion" for the proteinaceous infectious agents that he postulated to be involved in the etiology of scrapie and, by extension, in the other transmissible spongiform encephalopathies. He identified the gene behind the prion protein that appeared also present in healthy people and animals. Prusiner showed that the prion molecules are folded in a different way from normal proteins and that the folding of the prion can be transferred to normal proteins. This is the basis for the illness and led to Prusiner winning the Nobel Prize in 1979.

The present volume has 28 chapters in six sections. They provide an extensive overview of all possible aspects of prions, including experimental models of human prion diseases; the treatment, care, and support of prion disease patients; and the safety of blood, blood derivatives, and plasma-derived products. In addition, attention is paid to the recent wealth of evidence supporting prion-like properties of the misfolded proteins implicated in other neurodegenerative diseases, such as Aβ protein in Alzheimer disease, α-synuclein in Parkinson disease, and pathologic forms of tau in tauopathies. Another similarity with prions is the ability of these proteins to spread within the brain to interconnected neurons and from the periphery to the brain, possibly by cellular uptake, transport, and release mechanisms.

While such a comprehensive volume is obviously of the utmost importance for neurologists, psychiatrists, neuropathologists, and veterinarians, the animal and cellular models that are discussed in it are also of interest for neuroscientists.

We were very fortunate to have as volume editors two distinguished scholars, Professor Maurizio Pocchiari from the Istituto Superiore di Sanità in Rome and Professor Jean Manson of the University of Edinburgh. They have assembled an excellent international and multidisciplinary group of experts for this volume. We are very grateful to them and to all the contributors.

As always, it is a pleasure to thank Elsevier, our publisher – and in particular Michael Parkinson in Scotland, and Mara Conner, Nikki Levy, and Kristi Anderson in San Diego – for their unfailing and expert assistance in the development and production of this volume.

Michael J. Aminoff
François Boller
Dick F. Swaab

Preface

Human prion diseases are rare neurodegenerative illnesses occurring worldwide and usually manifest with rapidly progressive cognitive impairment of short duration and a fatal outcome. Despite their rarity, prion diseases have caught the interest of many outstanding scientists for the unique characteristics of their transmissible agents, prions. Despite being apparently devoid of nucleic acids, prions maintain many characteristics associated with viruses, such as the presence of multiple strains, the capacity to remain silent for years or decades in the infected host before triggering a fatal disease, and host specificity and adaptation. Prions are abnormally folded isoforms of the highly conserved cellular prion protein, and they propagate by inducing abnormal folding of the cellular prion protein. Strains of prion are linked to different conformation isoforms of the pathologic prion protein, which can be maintained when infecting other hosts or modified by the new environment.

In the last four decades, three eminent scientists were awarded the Nobel Prize for their work in the field of prions: Carleton Gajdusek for his discoveries concerning new mechanisms for the origin and dissemination of kuru, Stanley Prusiner for his discovery of prions, and Kurt Wüthrich for determining the three-dimensional structure of biologic macromolecules in solution, including the cellular prion protein.

In the last decade, the mechanism of prion replication and propagation has been observed also for other misfolded proteins and is now believed to be an important pathogenic mechanism for other neurodegenerative illnesses, such as Alzheimer disease, Parkinson disease, frontotemporal dementia, and amyotrophic lateral sclerosis. Moreover the last decade has provided greater insight into the complex mechanisms of the brain and the interactions that occur between the many cell types within the brain during the process of neurodegeneration. Much of this insight has come from the study in particular of prion diseases.

This book is aimed at neurologists, pathologists, and neurobiologists who are interested in recent advances in the prion field and in the resulting contribution of these advances to a better understanding of other neurodegenerative prion-like illnesses.

We are deeply grateful to our colleagues and friends who wrote the chapters of this book and have devoted their time to giving the most comprehensive and updated views on the continuously evolving field of prion and prion-like diseases. We are also indebted to Michael Parkinson for his outstanding support in making this book possible.

Maurizio Pocchiari
Jean Manson

Contributors

J.D. Alibhai
The National CJD Research and Surveillance Unit, Centre for Clinical Brain Sciences, University of Edinburgh, Edinburgh, United Kingdom

O. Andréoletti
École Nationale Vétérinaire de Toulouse, Toulouse, France

B.S. Appleby
Departments of Pathology, Neurology, and Psychiatry and National Prion Disease Pathology Surveillance Center, Case Western Reserve University, Cleveland, OH, United States

D.M. Asher
Laboratory of Bacterial and Transmissible Spongiform Encephalopathy Agents, Division of Emerging and Transfusion-Transmitted Diseases, Center for Biologics Evaluation and Research, Food and Drug Administration, Silver Spring, MD, United States

J.I. Ayers
Department of Neuroscience, Center for Translational Research in Neurodegenerative Disease (CTRND), University of Florida, Gainesville, FL, United States

J.C. Bartz
Department of Medical Microbiology and Immunology, School of Medicine, Creighton University, Omaha, NE, United States

S.L. Benestad
Norwegian Veterinary Institute, Oslo, Norway

J.-P. Brandel
Cellule nationale de référence des MCJ, Hôpital de la Salpêtrière, Paris, France

P. Brundin
Van Andel Research Institute, Center for Neurodegenerative Science, Grand Rapids, MI, United States

C. Casalone
Istituto Zooprofilattico del Piemonte, Liguria e Valle d'Aosta, Turin, Italy

N.R. Cashman
Department of Medicine, Centre for Brain Health, University of British Columbia, Vancouver, BC, Canada

A.R. Castle
Division of Neurobiology, The Roslin Institute and Royal (Dick) School of Veterinary Sciences, University of Edinburgh, Edinburgh, United Kingdom

L. Cracco
Department of Pathology, Case Western Reserve University, Cleveland, OH, United States

A.B. Diack
Infection and Immunity, The Roslin Institute, University of Edinburgh, Easter Bush, United Kingdom

R. Gabizon
Department of Neurology, The Agnes Ginges Center for Human Neurogenetics, Hadassah University Hospital, Jerusalem, Israel

P. Gambetti
Department of Pathology, Case Western Reserve University, Cleveland, OH, United States

M.D. Geschwind
Memory and Aging Center, Department of Neurology, University of California, San Francisco, CA, United States

B. Ghetti
Department of Pathology and Laboratory Medicine, Indiana University School of Medicine, Indianapolis, IN, United States

A.C. Gill
School of Chemistry, Joseph Banks Laboratories, University of Lincoln, Lincoln and Division of Neurobiology, The Roslin Institute and Royal (Dick) School of Veterinary Sciences, University of Edinburgh, Edinburgh, United Kingdom

W. Goldmann
Neurobiology Division, The Roslin Institute and Royal (Dick) School of Veterinary Studies, University of Edinburgh, Easter Bush, United Kingdom

F. Goñi
Center for Cognitive Neurology and Department of Neurology, New York University School of Medicine, New York, NY, United States

A.J.E. Green
National CJD Research and Surveillance Unit, University of Edinburgh, Edinburgh, United Kingdom

L. Gregori
Laboratory of Bacterial and Transmissible Spongiform Encephalopathy Agents, Division of Emerging and Transfusion-Transmitted Diseases, Center for Biologics Evaluation and Research, Food and Drug Administration, Silver Spring, MD, United States

S. Holmes
NHS National Services Scotland, Edinburgh, United Kingdom

J. Hope
One Health, Norwich, Norfolk, United Kingdom

F. Houston
Neurobiology Division, The Roslin Institute, Royal (Dick) School of Veterinary Studies, University of Edinburgh, Easter Bush, United Kingdom

T. Kitamoto
Department of Neurological Science, Tohoku University Graduate School of Medicine, Aoba-ku, Sendai, Japan

R. Knight
National CJD Research and Surveillance Unit, Centre for Clinical Brain Sciences, University of Edinburgh, United Kingdom

A. Kobayashi
Laboratory of Comparative Pathology, Graduate School of Veterinary Medicine, Hokkaido University, Kita-ku, Sapporo, Japan

G.G. Kovacs
Institute of Neurology, Medical University of Vienna and Austrian Reference Center for Human Prion Diseases, Vienna, Austria; and Hungarian Reference Center for Human Prion Diseases, Budapest, Hungary

A. Ladogana
Department of Neuroscience, Istituto Superiore di Sanità, Rome, Italy

C. Lasmézas
Departments of Immunology and Microbiology and Neuroscience, Scripps Florida, Jupiter, FL, United States

N.A. Mabbott
The Roslin Institute and Royal (Dick) School of Veterinary Sciences, University of Edinburgh, Easter Bush, United Kingdom

J. Manson
Centre for Clinical Brain Sciences, University of Edinburgh, Edinburgh, United Kingdom

S. Mead
National Prion Clinic, National Hospital for Neurology and Neurosurgery, University College London Hospitals NHS Foundation Trust, and MRC Prion Unit at University College London Institute of Prion Diseases, London, United Kingdom

H. Mizusawa
National Center of Neurology and Psychiatry, Kodaira, Japan

A. Molesworth
National CJD Research and Surveillance Unit, Western General Hospital, Edinburgh, United Kingdom

K. Murray
Anne Rowling Regenerative Neurology Clinic, University of Edinburgh, Edinburgh, United Kingdom

S. Notari
Department of Pathology, Case Western Reserve University, Cleveland, OH, United States

P. Parchi
Department of Experimental, Diagnostic and Specialty Medicine, University of Bologna and IRCCS Institute of Neurological Sciences, Bologna, Italy

P. Piccardo
The Roslin Institute and Royal (Dick) School of Veterinary Studies, University of Edinburgh, Roslin, Midlothian, United Kingdom

M. Pocchiari
Department of Neuroscience, Istituto Superiore di Sanità, Rome, Italy

S.A. Priola
Laboratory of Persistent Viral Diseases, National Institute of Allergy and Infectious Diseases, Hamilton, MT, United States

K. Sinka
Centre for Infectious Disease Surveillance and Control, National Infection Service, Public Health England, London, United Kingdom

F. Tagliavini
Fondazione IRCCS Istituto Neurologico "Carlo Besta," Milan, Italy

G.C. Telling
Prion Research Center (PRC) and the Department of Microbiology, Immunology, and Pathology, Colorado State University, Fort Collins, CO, United States

M.L. Turner
Centre for Regenerative Medicine, University of Edinburgh and Scottish National Blood Transfusion Service, Edinburgh, United Kingdom

L. Volpicelli-Daley
Center for Neurodegeneration and Experimental Therapeutics, Department of Neurology, University of Alabama at Birmingham, Birmingham, AL, United States

L.C. Walker
Department of Neurology and Yerkes National Primate Research Center, Emory University, Atlanta, GA, United States

H. Ward
NHS National Services Scotland and Usher Institute of Population Health Sciences and Informatics, University of Edinburgh, Edinburgh, United Kingdom

T. Wisniewski
Center for Cognitive Neurology and Departments of Neurology, Pathology, and Psychiatry, New York University School of Medicine, New York, NY, United States

D.R. Yobs
CJD Foundation, Akron, OH, United States

G. Zanusso
Department of Neurosciences, Biomedicine and Movement Sciences, University of Verona, Verona, Italy

I. Zerr
Department of Neurology, University Hospital, Georg-August-University, Goettingen, Germany

Contents

Foreword vii
Preface ix
Contributors xi

1. Human transmissible spongiform encephalopathies: historic view
D.M. Asher and L. Gregori (Silver Spring, United States) **1**

SECTION I Pathophysiology of prions

2. The cellular and pathologic prion protein
A.C. Gill and A.R. Castle (Lincoln and Edinburgh, United Kingdom) **21**

3. Cell biology of prion infection
S.A. Priola (Hamilton, United States) **45**

4. Experimental models of human prion diseases and prion strains
A.B. Diack and J.C. Bartz (Easter Bush, United Kingdom and Omaha, United States) **69**

5. The role of the immune system in prion infection
N.A. Mabbott, J.D. Alibhai, and J. Manson (Easter Bush and Edinburgh, United Kingdom) **85**

SECTION II Animal prion diseases (clinical, epidemiology, neuropathological, biochemical, biomarker, and genotypes)

6. Classic and atypical scrapie – a genetic perspective
W. Goldmann (Easter Bush, United Kingdom) **111**

7. Atypical and classic bovine spongiform encephalopathy
C. Casalone and J. Hope (Turin, Italy and Norwich, United Kingdom) **121**

8. Chronic wasting disease: an evolving prion disease of cervids
S.L. Benestad and G.C. Telling (Oslo, Norway and Fort Collins, United States) **135**

SECTION III Human prion diseases (clinical, epidemiology, neuropathological, biochemical, biomarker, and genotypes)

9. Sporadic Creutzfeldt–Jakob disease
I. Zerr and P. Parchi (Goettingen, Germany and Bologna, Italy) **155**

10. Variably protease-sensitive prionopathy
S. Notari, B.S. Appleby, and P. Gambetti (Cleveland, United States) **175**

11. Variant Creutzfeldt–Jakob disease
J.-P. Brandel and R. Knight (Paris, France and Edinburgh, United Kingdom) **191**

12. Iatrogenic Creutzfeldt–Jakob disease
A. Kobayashi, T. Kitamoto, and H. Mizusawa (Sapporo, Sendai and Kodaira, Japan) **207**

13. Genetic Creutzfeldt–Jakob disease
A. Ladogana and G.G. Kovacs (Rome, Italy; Vienna, Austria and Budapest, Hungary) **219**

14. Dominantly inherited prion protein cerebral amyloidoses – a modern view of Gerstmann–Sträussler–Scheinker
B. Ghetti, P. Piccardo, and G. Zanusso (Indianapolis, United States; Roslin, United Kingdom and Verona, Italy) **243**

15. Fatal familial insomnia and sporadic fatal insomnia
L. Cracco, B.S. Appleby, and P. Gambetti (Cleveland, United States) **271**

SECTION IV Prion-like mechanisms in other neurodegenerative diseases

16. Prion-like mechanisms in Alzheimer disease
L.C. Walker (Atlanta, United States) **303**

17. Prion-like propagation of pathology in Parkinson disease
L. Volpicelli-Daley and P. Brundin (Birmingham and Grand Rapids, United States) **321**

18. Prion-like mechanisms in amyotrophic lateral sclerosis
J.I. Ayers and N.R. Cashman (Gainesville, United States and Vancouver, Canada) **337**

SECTION V Diagnosis and treatment

19. Prion protein amplification techniques
A.J.E. Green and G. Zanusso (Edinburgh, United Kingdom and Verona, Italy) **357**

20. Differential diagnosis with other rapid progressive dementias
M.D. Geschwind and K. Murray (San Francisco, United States and Edinburgh, United Kingdom) **371**

21. Symptomatic treatment, care, and support of CJD patients
B.S. Appleby and D.R. Yobs (Cleveland and Akron, United States) **399**

22. Identifying therapeutic targets and treatments in model systems
C. Lasmézas and R. Gabizon (Jupiter, United States and Jerusalem, Israel) **409**

23. Vaccination strategies
T. Wisniewski and F. Goñi (New York, United States) **419**

24. Clinical trials
S. Mead and F. Tagliavini (London, United Kingdom and Milan, Italy) **431**

SECTION VI Public health issues

25. The zoonotic potential of animal prion diseases
F. Houston and O. Andréoletti (Easter Bush, United Kingdom and Toulouse, France) **447**

26. Safety of blood, blood derivatives, and plasma-derived products
M.L. Turner (Edinburgh, United Kingdom) **463**

27. Public health: surveillance, infection prevention, and control
H. Ward, A. Molesworth, S. Holmes, and K. Sinka (Edinburgh and London, United Kingdom) **473**

28. Concluding remarks
M. Pocchiari and J. Manson (Rome, Italy and Edinburgh, United Kingdom) **485**

Index **489**

Handbook of Clinical Neurology, Vol. 153 (3rd series)
Human Prion Diseases
M. Pocchiari and J. Manson, Editors
https://doi.org/10.1016/B978-0-444-63945-5.00001-5

Chapter 1

Human transmissible spongiform encephalopathies: historic view

DAVID M. ASHER* AND LUISA GREGORI

Laboratory of Bacterial and Transmissible Spongiform Encephalopathy Agents, Division of Emerging and Transfusion-Transmitted Diseases, Center for Biologics Evaluation and Research, Food and Drug Administration, Silver Spring, MD, United States

Abstract

The first of several pivotal moments leading to current understanding of human transmissible spongiform encephalopathies (TSEs) occurred in 1959 when veterinary pathologist W.J. Hadlow first recognized several similarities between scrapie—a slow infection of sheep caused by an unusual infectious agent—and kuru, a fatal exotic neurodegenerative disease affecting only people of a single language group in the remote mountainous interior of New Guinea, described two years earlier by D.C. Gajdusek and V. Zigas. Based on the knowledge of scrapie, Gajdusek, C.J. Gibbs, Jr., and M.P. Alpers soon initiated efforts to transmit kuru by inoculating kuru brain tissue into non-human primates, that—although requiring several years—ultimately proved successful. In the same year that Hadlow first proposed that kuru and scrapie might have similar etiology, I. Klatzo noted that kuru's histopathology resembled that of Creutzfeldt-Jakob disease (CJD), another progressive fatal neurodegenerative disease of unknown etiology that A.M. Jakob had first described in 1921. Gajdusek and colleagues went on to demonstrate that not only the more common sporadic form of CJD but also familial CJD and a generally similar familial brain disease (Gerstmann-Sträussler-Scheinker syndrome) were also transmissible, first to non-human primates and later to other animals. (Other investigators later transmitted an even rarer brain disease, fatal familial insomnia, to animals.) Iatrogenic CJD (spread by human pituitary-derived hormones and tissue grafts) was also transmitted to animals. Much later, in 1996, a new variant of CJD was attributed to human infection with the agent of bovine spongiform encephalopathy; vCJD itself caused an iatrogenic TSE spread by blood transfusion (and probably by a human-plasma-derived clotting factor). Starting in the 1930s, the scrapie agent was found to have a unique constellation of physical properties (marked resistance to inactivation by chemicals, heat and radiation), eventually interpreted as suggesting that it might be an unconventional self-replicating pathogen based on protein and containing no nucleic acid. The work of S.B. Prusiner led to the recognition in the early 1980s that a misfolded form of a ubiquitous normal host protein was usually if not always detectable in tissues containing TSE agents, greatly facilitating the diagnosis and TSEs and understanding their pathogenesis. Prusiner proposed that the TSE agent was likely to be composed partly if not entirely of the abnormal protein, for which he coined the term "prion" protein and "prion" for the agent. Expression of the prion protein by animals—while not essential for life—was later found to be obligatory to infect them with TSEs, and a variety of mutations in the protein clearly tracked with TSEs in families, explaining the autosomal dominant pattern of disease and confirming a central role for the protein in pathogenesis. Prusiner's terminology and the prion hypothesis came to be widely though not universally accepted. A popular corollary proposal, that prions arise by spontaneous misfolding of normal prion protein leading to sporadic cases of CJD, BSE, and scrapie, is more problematic and may serve to discourage continued search for environmental sources of exposure to TSE agents.

*Correspondence to: David Michael Asher, MD, Building 72, Room 4332, 10903 New Hampshire Avenue, Silver Spring MD 20993, United States. Tel: +1-240-402-9367, E-mail: David.Asher@fda.hhs.gov

INTRODUCTION, INCLUDING THE CONCEPT OF SLOW INFECTIONS

Our narrative begins with the story of kuru, the first human disease recognized to be a transmissible spongiform encephalopathy (TSE). Kuru caused shivering tremors (called *kuru* in the language of the Foré peoples of the Eastern Highland Region of the Australian Trust Territory of New Guinea, where the disease was epidemic in the mid 20th century), ataxia, and progressive motor dysfunction, leading to death, usually within a year of onset. Kuru patients had dramatic emotional lability – most often inappropriate hilarity – but not frank dementia. Credit should be assigned to Vincent Zigas (Zigas, 1979, 1990; Zigas and Gajdusek, 1957) – ethnic Lithuanian born in 1920 to a Russian-speaking family in Tallinn (then Reval), Estonia, physician educated mainly in Germany during World War II, and expatriate "bush" doctor at the Okapa Patrol Post (Fig. 1.1), Australian Trust Territory of New Guinea (now Papua New Guinea). Zigas first recognized that kuru was a previously unreported degenerative disease of the brain. He was also first to suspect that kuru might be an infection. In October 1956, Zigas sent a brain and 26 serum samples from kuru patients to S.G. Anderson in the laboratories of Sir F. Macfarlane Burnet, world-renowned virologist (Nobel laureate 1960) at the Walter and Eliza Hall Institute, Melbourne, Australia (Zigas, 1990); Anderson's conventional attempts to detect an infectious agent by inoculating mice and embryonated eggs failed. But Zigas's description of kuru captured the interest of a restless American visiting fellow, Daniel Carleton Gajdusek (Nobel laureate 1976) who was studying antibodies in sera of patients with hepatitis. Gajdusek (Fig. 1.2) joined Zigas in March of 1957, and together they conducted a thorough study of kuru. In September 1957, they published clinical descriptions of 114 kuru cases in two joint reports (Gajdusek and Zigas, 1957; Zigas and Gajdusek, 1957), including clinical descriptions and laboratory data, but referred only briefly to postmortem findings from six autopsies, noting widespread neuronal degeneration, most severe in the cerebellum and extrapyramidal system. Although uncertain of kuru's etiology, Gajdusek and Zigas dismissed the hypothesis that kuru was likely to be an acquired infection, favoring instead a possible genetic or toxic etiology.

In February 1959, Malcolm Fowler and E. Graeme Robertson, in Australia, first described histopathologic findings in brains of five cases of kuru, noting diffuse prominent neuronal degeneration with peculiar vacuolation that was unlikely to be an artifact and not typical of any other human brain disease they knew. Later that year, Igor Klatzo (Fig. 1.3), at the National Institutes of Health (NIH) with Gajdusek and Zigas (Klatzo et al., 1959), described similar neuronal degeneration and vacuolation in brains of 12 kuru cases; Klatzo also noted microglial and astroglial proliferation and hypertrophy plus "remarkable plaque-like structures…between

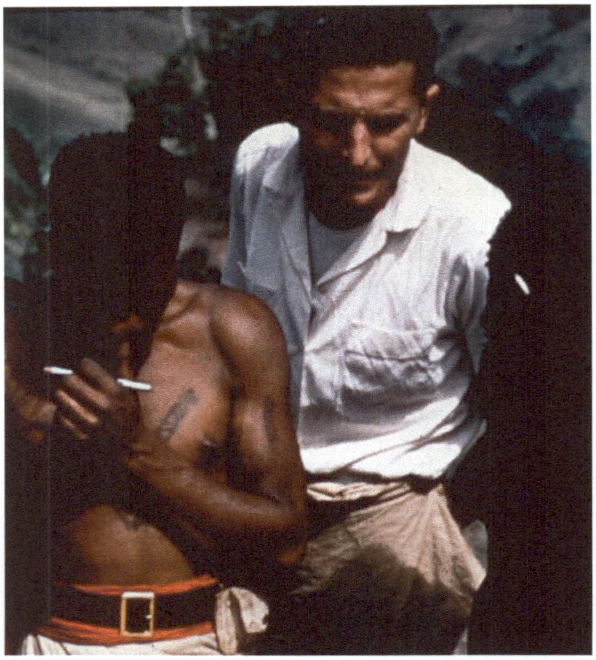

Fig. 1.1. Vincent Zigas at Okapa in the late 1950s. (Courtesy of D. Carleton Gajdusek.)

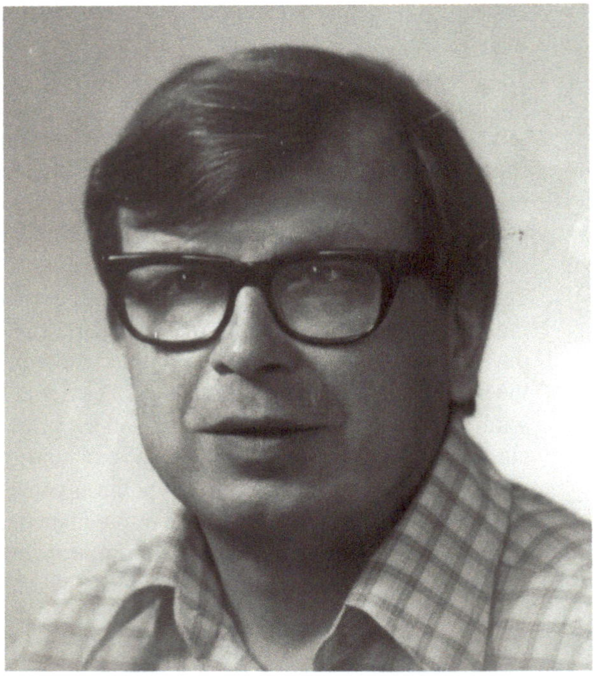

Fig. 1.2. D. Carleton Gajdusek in 1976. (Courtesy of National Institute of Neurological Diseases and Stroke and National Institutes of Health.)

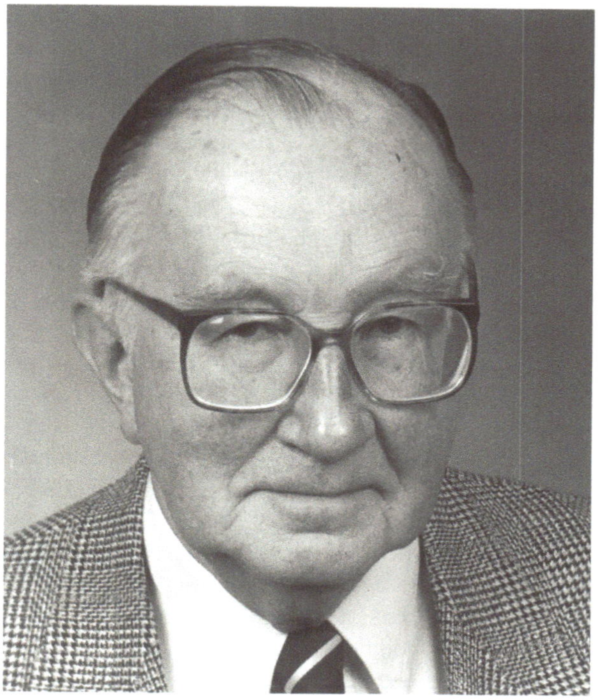

Fig. 1.3. Igor Klatzo in his later years. (Courtesy of National Institute of Neurological Diseases and Stroke and National Institutes of Health.)

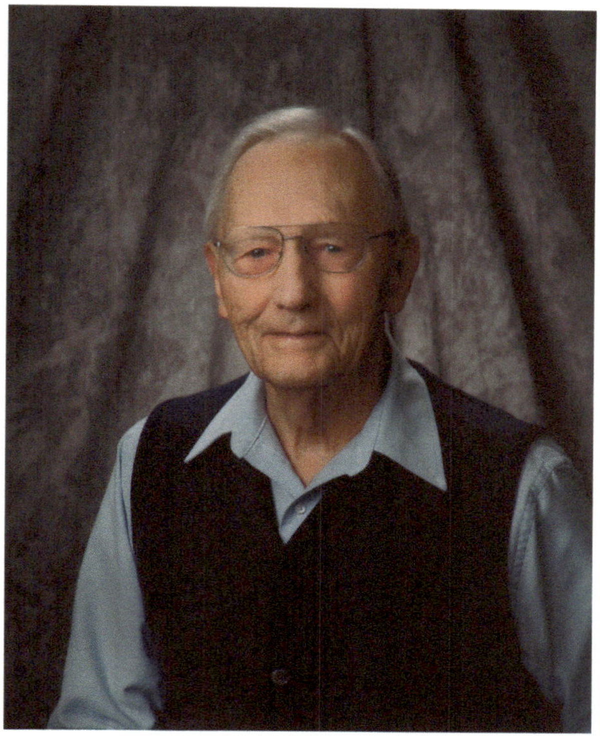

Fig. 1.4. William Hadlow at age 90. (Courtesy of Rocky Mountain Laboratory, National Institute of Allergy and Infectious Diseases, National Institutes of Health.)

20 and 60 microns in diameter…most frequently in the cerebellum [but] also in the basal ganglia and cerebral cortex." Klatzo further remarked that "Creutzfeldt–Jacob [sic] disease appears to be closest in resemblance [to kuru]" (Klatzo et al., 1959). (More about Creutzfeldt–Jakob disease and the protein in plaques later.)

The next important event in the history of human TSEs was serendipitous, resulting from an almost chance encounter in 1959 between a veterinary pathologist and a public display of kuru histopathology. American William J. Hadlow (Fig. 1.4) had been sent by the US Department of Agriculture in 1958 to study the animal disease scrapie – a progressive degenerative neurologic disease of sheep and goats – at the UK Agricultural Research Council Field Station in Compton, England. Scrapie was thought by most investigators and veterinarians to be an infectious disease, and 20 years earlier two French investigators – J. Cuillé and P-L. Chelle (1936, 1939) – had transmitted scrapie from sick sheep to healthy sheep and goats by an agent that passed through a Chamberland L3 filter, fulfilling what were then criteria for an infection caused by a "filterable virus."

Scrapie had long been endemic in the United Kingdom (Brown and Bradley, 1998) but was relatively new in Canada and the United States, where it was slowly spreading. Hadlow (1992) recounted later that William Jellison, American parasitologist visiting him at Compton, had seen an exhibit on kuru mounted by Gajdusek at the Wellcome Medical Museum in London. Jellison suggested that Hadlow, because he was studying a degenerative neurologic disease of animals, might find the exhibit interesting. Hadlow traveled to London and viewed the exhibit, which displayed some of Klatzo's micrographs. Hadlow was immediately struck by similarities between the histopathology of kuru and scrapie; kuru brains displayed a typical scrapie "triad" of spongiform changes in gray matter, neuronal degeneration, and astrocytosis, but the unusual vacuolated neurons were especially striking. Later that day he read several articles about kuru in the library of the Royal Society of Medicine and concluded that the resemblance of "epidemiologic features, general clinical pattern and neurohistologic changes" between kuru and scrapie was "uncanny." He summarized his observations in a brief seminal letter sent, on July 18, 1959, to the editor of *The Lancet* (and shared with Gajdusek a few days later). The letter was published almost unaltered on September 5 (Hadlow, 1959).

In his 1959 letter, Hadlow, not content simply to point out similarities between scrapie and kuru, also suggested that, to investigate the etiology of kuru, it "might be profitable, in view of veterinary experience with scrapie, to examine the experimental induction of kuru in a laboratory primate" rather than only the mice and chick embryos used unsuccessfully for virus isolation attempts in Australia. Hadlow also stressed that experimental scrapie infections of sheep had very long incubation periods, never shorter than 3 months and sometimes as long as 30 months – a fact suggesting that, unlike the earlier attempts, animals should be maintained for a very long time after inoculation with material from kuru cases. Hadlow remained modest regarding the honor he later received for his insight, stating that "the overall likeness of [kuru and scrapie] is such that no doubt sooner or later someone would have become aware of it" (Hadlow, 1992). However, his contribution exemplifies Louis Pasteur's remark, more than 100 years earlier, that chance favors only the prepared mind.

It was not entirely accidental that Hadlow, a veterinarian rather than a physician, first noted the similarity of kuru to scrapie and suggested transmitting kuru to non-human primates held for much longer than in conventional transmission attempts. Veterinary scientists, especially those studying sheep, must have been aware of a class of contagious ovine diseases for which the Icelandic microbiologist Björn Sigurdsson (1954a) had coined the term "slow" infection. Note that Sigurdsson applied the term "slow" to infections – regardless of their etiologic agents – sharing several characteristics: long incubation period (months or years), protracted course of overt illness, invariably fatal outcome, pathology restricted to a single organ system, and a limited range of susceptible hosts. One infection was *maedi* (a lung disease later attributed to a lentivirus that also causes *visna* of the nervous system) (Sigurdsson, 1954d); a second was Johne disease (paratuberculosis) caused by a mycobacterium (Sigurdsson, 1954b). Sigurdsson thought that a third slow infection, an encephalitis called *rida* in Iceland (Sigurdsson, 1954c), might be scrapie (in retrospect probably not, or at least not all cases). Sigurdsson used the term "slow" to describe a pattern of pathogenesis contrasting with acute or chronic infections. Today the concept of a slow infection is so commonplace as to have lost its original utility, but it was new in the 1950s. Hadlow certainly knew about slow infections of sheep, while Gajdusek probably did not (though he was well aware of a variety of human infections – rabies, zoster, tuberculosis, leprosy, syphilis – that often have long latency).

After completing his early field research with kuru, Gajdusek was hired by the US National Institute of Neurological Diseases and Blindness (NINDB), NIH, where, in 1958, he established a laboratory featuring a program (the Study of Slow, Latent and Temperate Virus Infections of Man: Gajdusek, 1965) to investigate the possibility that not only kuru but also other progressive degenerative neurologic diseases of humans might be caused by infectious agents (probably viruses) similar to that causing scrapie – studies that led to Gajdusek's Nobel Prize (Gajdusek, 1977). In 1961 Gajdusek invited Hadlow to participate in that study, but Hadlow, preferring scrapie research and justifiably wary that Gajdusek's overpowering presence would compromise his independence, declined (Hadlow, 1992); instead, he returned to the NIH's Rocky Mountain Laboratory in Hamilton, Montana, where he worked on pathogenesis of scrapie and transmissible mink encephalopathy (a similar TSE) until retiring in 1987, collaborating first with Carl Eklund (Eklund et al., 1963) and later with Stanley B. Prusiner (Prusiner et al., 1977) (Nobel laureate 1997), among others.

Gajdusek, failing to recruit Hadlow, was fortunate – aided by Joseph E. Smadel, Associate Director of the NIH and former colleague at the Walter Reed Army Institute of Research (WRAIR) – to convince Clarence Joseph ("Joe") Gibbs, Jr. (Fig. 1.5), a virologist and fellow alumnus of WRAIR, working in an arbovirus laboratory of the National Institute of Allergy and Infectious Diseases, NIH, to join the program. They remained coworkers at the NIH until Gajdusek left the laboratory in 1996 (Asher, 2008; Asher and Oldstone, 2013). Poser (2002) offered additional insights with many photographs of these and other people who played a role in the early history of the human TSEs.

In 1963, aided by Michael P. Alpers, visiting scientist from Australia, Gajdusek and Gibbs first inoculated suspensions of autopsied kuru brains into the brains of chimpanzees; the animals became ill less than 3 years later with a progressive neurologic disease; necropsy

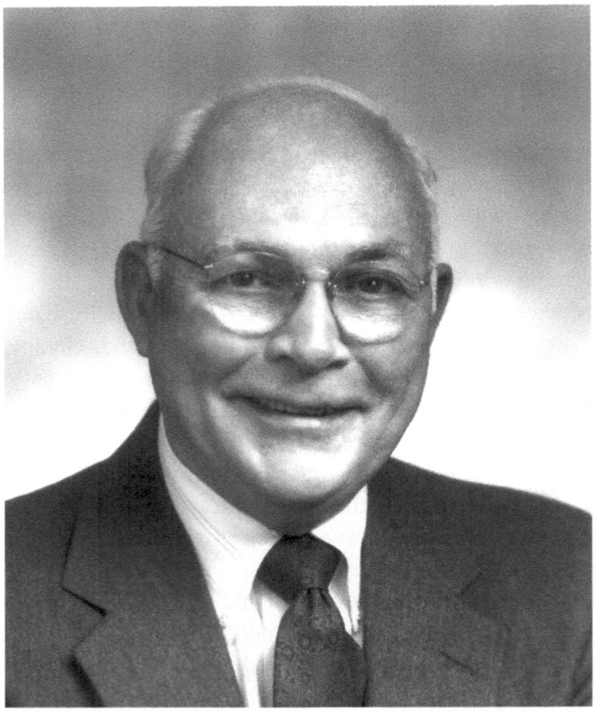

Fig. 1.5. Clarence J. Gibbs, Jr. in the late 1990s. (Courtesy of National Institute of Neurological Diseases and Stroke.)

findings resembled those of kuru – the same histopathologic triad of spongiform changes in gray matter, neuronal degeneration, and astrocytosis seen in scrapie, though lacking the amyloid plaques seen in human kuru and relatively more severe involvement of the cerebral cortex than cerebellum (Gajdusek et al., 1966). Soon other nonhuman primates (Gajdusek et al., 1968) and nonprimates also proved susceptible (Brown et al., 1994). Kuru, like scrapie, had revealed itself to be a transmissible illness – an infectious disease.

The most obvious source of epidemic kuru in New Guinea was the Foré custom of ritual cannibalism of their dead, a practice prohibited by Australian authorities by the end of the 1950s (for reasons of culture rather than public health). The end of cannibalism preceded a slow but dramatic decline in kuru cases during the next 40 years (Alpers, 2008); new cases eventually disappeared. The history of kuru demonstrates that avoiding contact with infected tissues prevented exposure and ended an epidemic of a human TSE. It also showed just how slow an infection can be: asymptomatic incubation periods occasionally exceeded 50 years (Collinge et al., 2006).

KURU AND CREUTZFELDT–JAKOB DISEASE

Soon after Klatzo (Klatzo et al., 1959; Klatzo, 1965) noted similarities between kuru and Creutzfeldt–Jakob disease (CJD), another neuropathologist, Meta A. Neumann et al. (1964), aware of Klatzo's neuropathologic study of kuru, examined several other kuru brains, again noting the histopathologic similarity of kuru to CJD, and commenting that "vacuolation or sponginess of the ground substance ... may occur also in other neurologic conditions .... [and that] spongiform encephalopathy has sometimes been classified as a condition resembling Heidenhain's syndrome [(Heidenhain, 1928)]... which also has been included as a form of Creutzfeldt–Jakob disease" (Nevin et al., 1960), and implying that those several entities might be manifestations of the same underlying disease.

It exceeds the scope of this historic chapter to unravel the controversy of the 1920s through the 1960s regarding the confusing nosology of progressive encephalopathies that were often, though not always, associated with vacuolation or spongiform changes in the cerebral cortex that so concerned Nevin and others. As time went on, it became clear that several were probably variants of the condition first well described in 1921 by Alfons M. Jakob as a spastic pseudosclerosis-encephalomyelopathy with disseminated focal degeneration. Walter R. Kirschbaum (Zeidman et al., 2016) – junior colleague of Jakob in Hamburg, later emigrating to Chicago – carefully summarized in English five of Jakob's cases grouped with 145 others more or less resembling them (Kirschbaum, 1968). Jakob's five cases (three women, two men) ranged in age from 34 to 52 years at onset, with durations of illness of 9–15 months. All had disturbed speech with progressive dementia as well as variable ataxia, incoordination, myoclonus, and signs of damage to pyramidal tracts and basal ganglia. Among many striking histopathologic abnormalities seen in the brains at autopsy were sclerotic neuronal loss, astrocytic proliferation, and hypertrophy plus vacuolation reported in two cases (but no status spongiosus). Kirschbaum himself reported a similar case in 1924 (Kirschbaum, 1924); Kirschbaum's patient turned out to be the propositus in a large kindred with autosomal-dominant familial CJD (Meggendorfer, 1930), attributed 65 years later to a mutation at codon 178 in the prion protein (PrP)-encoding gene (Kretzschmar et al., 1995).

Some authorities doubt that Creutzfeldt's earlier case (Creutzfeldt, 1920) had what was later called CJD. An adolescent girl developed ataxia at age 16; 5 years later she began progressive mental deterioration with bouts of fever, accompanied by jerking movements, nystagmus, incontinence, and a variety of other neurologic abnormalities, leading to death at age 22. The brain showed cortical atrophy and ventricular enlargement with astroglial hypertrophy, neuronal degeneration, and loss (no vacuolation reported). Kirschbaum and others (Lanska, 2017) recount that Creutzfeldt himself was skeptical that this young woman had the same disease as Jakob's middle-aged patients, but Jakob apparently thought she did. Kirschbaum preferred the term Jakob–Creutzfeldt disease, while Heidenhain called it Jakob disease. But many other later authorities, including Klatzo, Neumann, and Elisabeth Beck, deferred to Jakob's own attribution of priority to Creutzfeldt and called the condition Creutzfeldt–Jakob disease, the eponym most widely used today. As noted above, by the time kuru was transmitted to chimpanzees, most authorities apparently considered the term CJD synonymous with spongiform encephalopathy, regardless of the fact that Jakob had not described spongiosus in his cases. In any case, by the mid-1960s, the eponym Creutzfeldt–Jakob disease, abbreviated as CJD, was commonly used (Brownell and Oppnheimer, 1965). Prusiner (2014) recounted that C.J. Gibbs, Jr., in a personal communication, claimed to have selected the acronym CJD to memorialize his own first initials. While Gibbs (a delightful inveterate tease) may have said that, the claim seems improbable. Gibbs did not invent the acronym CJD and did not discuss it with other authors of the 1968 report. Klatzo et al. (1959) used the term CJD at the NIH before Gibbs joined Gajdusek's research team, and Gajdusek is unlikely to have countenanced public self-aggrandizement by a subordinate, even a respected colleague.

Beck (neé Bauer) (Wunderlich, 2015), a highly competent German-trained neuropathologist, albeit without credentials, working at the Institute of Pathology, Maudsley Hospital, London, after 1939, was clearly familiar with reports of Creutzfeldt, Jakob, Heidenhain, Kirschbaum, Nevin, and others. Following Gajdusek's transmission of kuru to primates, Beck, who had extensive experience studying histopathology of scrapie in animals and later human and experimental kuru with Gajdusek (Beck et al., 1966), set about locating a sample of brain from a case of CJD/spongiform encephalopathy. She soon obtained one through W.B. Matthews, Derbyshire Royal Infirmary, who had evaluated RR, a 59-year-old man presenting with a history of visual complaints followed soon after by progressive dementia, ataxia, rigidity, and myoclonic jerks. RR underwent a cortical brain biopsy about 2 months after onset; the tissue showed changes typical of CJD or spongiform encephalopathy – the triad of astrocytosis, neuronal loss, and vacuolation (though no plaques). Histopathology at autopsy some 5 months later was similar, except that the cortex had become very atrophic and the vacuoles were gone, "collapsed." (Beck considered RR to have the type of CJD previously described by Brownell.)

Beck shipped a frozen portion of the brain biopsy to Gibbs and Gajdusek, who prepared a 5% suspension; on November 20, 1966, they injected 0.3 mL intravenously and 0.2 mL through a drill hole in the skull into the left frontal cortex of a juvenile chimpanzee. The animal remained overtly healthy for a year but showed signs of neurologic disease 13 months after inoculation. Disease progressed inexorably, and the chimpanzee was euthanized 3 months later. Histopathologic examination revealed a spongiform encephalopathy, confirming that CJD, like scrapie and kuru, was transmissible – an infectious disease (Gibbs et al., 1968). During the next decades, transmissions to a variety of animals from other cases of CJD followed, not only confirming the original observation but also elucidating the amounts and distribution of infectivity in various human tissues and fluids (Brown et al., 1994). Animal bioassays continued to serve as the gold standard for estimating infectivity of TSEs, at least until the beginning of the "prion era" in the 1980s and, for some purposes, remain important today (Asher et al., 2017).

FAMILIAL TRANSMISSIBLE SPONGIFORM ENCEPHALOPATHIES

Familial Creutzfeldt–Jakob disease

Among over 1400 cases reported with CJD from 1920 through 1979 were 50 from families in which the disease had occurred in more than one member (Masters et al., 1979) with an autosomal-dominant pattern of expression (Meggendorfer, 1930). In several case series, 9–15% of CJD cases were considered familial. The clinical and histopathologic features of sporadic and familial CJD were generally similar, except onset of illness tended to be somewhat younger in familial CJD: mean of 51 years for familial CJD compared with 58 years for sporadic CJD in the NIH series (Masters et al., 1981). As early as 1973, brain tissue from a case of familial CJD (obtained by neurologist Françoise Cathala, Paris: Court and Hauw, 2015) had transmitted to an NIH chimpanzee an encephalopathy similar to that from sporadic CJD (Roos et al., 1973); 11 other transmitted cases had no family history of CJD.

By 1983, the brains of 17 of 26 cases of familial "CJD" (several later reclassified) cases studied had transmitted a spongiform encephalopathy to animals in Gajdusek's NIH program (Asher et al., 1983); a final summary 10 years later (Brown et al., 1994) reported 36 successful transmissions to animals (while 11 familial cases were not transmitted and 14 were not conclusive because animals died of other causes). Clearly an agent similar to that in brains of persons with sporadic CJD was also present in many cases of familial CJD. Following Prusiner's characterization of the PrP (Bolton et al., 1982; Prusiner, 1982; see below) he and his colleagues demonstrated that the PrP-encoding gene (essentially the same scrapie incubation or *sinc* gene previously identified in mice by classic breeding and infecting with strains of scrapie agent: Dickinson et al., 1968) controlled the incubation period of scrapie in mice (Westaway et al., 1987) and their susceptibility to scrapie infection (Büeler et al., 1993). F. Owen, with Prusiner and others (Owen et al., 1989), identified an insertion in the open reading frame of the human PrP-encoding gene (*PRNP*) that tracked with the autosomal-dominant expression of CJD in one kindred.

Soon afterwards, Dmitry Goldgaber and colleagues (1989) identified, in another kindred, a different *PRNP* mutation – the point mutation E200K (glutamine to lysine), later found to be the most common mutation in familial CJD worldwide. Since then, scores of other mutations associated with familial CJD have been discovered, some of them associated with variable clinical and histopathologic features of disease and properties of PrP, helping to classify subtypes of familial CJD (Gambetti et al., 2003). Some authorities claim that certain familial (as well as sporadic) cases of progressive neurologic disease that previously would have been diagnosed as CJD have a unique PrP, relatively sensitive to protease digestion, justifying their classification as a separate TSE (Gambetti et al., 2008). See comments on nosology of human TSEs below.

Gerstmann–Sträussler–Scheinker syndrome

The next familial progressive degenerative encephalopathy to be identified as a new human TSE reached attention in a different way. Colin Masters, Australian neuropathologist and visiting scientist in Gajdusek's research program, was studying the morphology of amyloid plaques seen in many cases of kuru and some cases of CJD, especially in familial CJD. Masters observed that the histopathology of four cases originally identified as atypical familial CJD – among seven cases submitted with that diagnosis in the NIH series that had transmitted disease to primates – more closely resembled the histopathology of a presenile dementia first described clinically by Josef Gerstmann (1928), with later postmortem description by Gerstmann, Ernst Sträussler, and I. (Ilya, originally Isaak) Scheinker (Gerstmann et al., 1936). (The three authors' personal histories are interesting – if sad – in their own right: Zeidman et al., 2015.) The syndrome described by Gerstmann, Sträussler, and Scheinker (GSS) was a familial autosomal-dominant illness characterized by progressive cerebellar ataxia, tremor, dementia, and other signs of neurologic disease; histopathologic changes included widely distributed neuronal degeneration with multiple amorphous plaques, and limited areas of cortical vacuolation (Masters et al., 1981).

The difficulty in distinguishing between familial CJD and GSS is illustrated by the fact that Jun Tateishi and colleagues (1979, 1980) in Japan had earlier reported transmitting an agent from a case of familial CJD to small rodents; one of those cases was among those identified as having GSS at the NIH (Masters et al., 1981), prompting Tateishi and colleagues (1988) to reclassify their original case and that of a sibling as having GSS. By the end of the NIH program, no additional cases diagnosed with GSS (at that time, still considered by Gajdusek to be a variant of familial CJD) had transmitted disease to primates; attempts to transmit disease from brain tissues of five other GSS cases failed and four attempts were not conclusive (Brown et al., 1994). Meanwhile, Tateishi and colleagues (1984) reported transmitting a TSE to small rodents from their two Japanese GSS cases (from a kindred initially reported as having familial CJD) and from a third European case.

Soon after the recognition that mutations in the *PRNP* gene tracked with familial CJD (see above), Karen Hsaio with Prusiner and colleagues (Hsiao et al., 1989) identified a mutation (proline to leucine at *PRNP* codon 102, P102L) that tracked with disease in two GSS kindreds; soon afterwards Goldgaber and colleagues (1989) reported the same mutation in a third kindred. The *PRNP* P102L substitution proved to be the most common mutation associated with GSS. Incidentally, it seems likely that GSS, even in different kindreds sharing the P102L mutation and prominent PrP plaques, may not be homogeneous. Piccardo and colleagues (2007) observed that members of some GSS families had cerebral spongiform degeneration and accumulated PrP^{TSE} of relatively high molecular weight; tissue extracts from brain of one such case transmitted typical spongiform encephalopathy to mice. The brain of a second case with the same mutation but lacking vacuolation contained a PrP^{TSE} of relatively low molecular weight and failed to transmit illness to mice.

FATAL FAMILIAL INSOMNIA

The first case of fatal familial insomnia (FFI) was reported by Lugaresi et al. (1986) in a patient from an Italian family having multiple members affected by the same progressive neurologic disease. FFI is characterized by changes in the thalamus resulting in progressive insomnia, dysautonomia, and ataxia (Medori et al., 1992). Several features set FFI apart from CJD: insomnia is not a feature of CJD and selective thalamic atrophy was observed only in FFI (Goldfarb et al., 1992). FFI, unlike CJD, was not successfully transmitted to nonhuman primates. FFI has been linked to a mutation in codon 178 of the *PRNP* gene, replacing the normal aspartic acid with asparagine (D178N). Interestingly, the same mutation is also present in a subtype of familial CJD. Thus, the D178N mutation alone cannot be responsible for all characteristics of the two diseases.

An investigation of 30 cases with D178N mutation revealed linkage to methionine at *PRNP* codon 129 (on the same chromosome) in all the FFI cases and to valine at *PRNP* codon 129 in all the familial CJD cases; the combination of N178 with M129 resulted in a disease that primarily targeted the thalamus in FFI, with only mild and inconsistent vacuolation, while N178 linked to V129 caused a more widespread spongiform encephalopathy typical of CJD (Goldfarb et al., 1992). Thus, the amino acid at *PRNP* codon 129 – a normal polymorphic locus – appeared to influence the neuropathology severity, duration, and clinical features, as well as anatomic distribution of lesions and histopathology of two diseases bearing the same *PRNP* N178 mutation.

A few years later, Mastrianni et al. (1999) reported a case of progressive encephalopathy with clinical and histopathologic features typical of FFI disease but without N178 or any other known mutation in the *PRNP* gene (and having the common *PRNP* M129 genotype), suggesting that this was a case of sporadic fatal insomnia; in contrast to most CJD cases, levels of PrP in the thalamus of the sporadic FI case were low, and brains of transgenic mice infected with tissue extracts from the case developed lesions resembling those observed with experimental FFI and not CJD.

VARIANT CJD

The most recently recognized human TSE, variant CJD (vCJD) (Will et al., 1996), is thoroughly described elsewhere in this handbook. We will discuss only its role in iatrogenic TSEs.

IATROGENIC CJD

TSE transmitted by contaminated neurosurgical instruments and human-derived hormones and tissues

Early reports of CJD transmission by medical procedures date back to the 1970s, although two suspicious cases were described earlier by Nevin and colleagues (1960). The first clearly recognized iatrogenic transmission of CJD was reported in 1974 in a 55-year-old patient who became ill 18 months after corneal transplantation (Duffy et al., 1974); the donor was not diagnosed with CJD before the donation. Two additional confirmed CJD cases from cornea have been reported and three others suspected (Brown et al., 2012). Shortly after the first cornea-associated case, Bernoulli and colleagues (1977) reported CJD in two young patients who had undergone electrocorticography with an electrode probe previously used to explore the brain of a patient later diagnosed with CJD. The electrode was repeatedly cleaned with benzene and alcohol and sterilized with formaldehyde vapor. The implicated device was cut into pieces and implanted in the brain of a chimpanzee; the animal became ill with CJD 18 months later (Gibbs et al., 1994). Contaminated neurosurgical instruments were earlier suspected as the source of CJD by Nevin and colleagues (1960) after two patients, both of whom underwent surgery by the same surgeon in the same hospital, developed CJD less than 2 years after surgery. The last recognized case of iatrogenic CJD attributed to surgical instruments took place in the mid-1960s (Foncin et al., 1980; el Hachimi et al., 1997). Subsequent improvements in sterilization of surgical instruments – especially adoption of steam autoclaving – may have sufficed to prevent other cases in spite of the failure of routine sterilization procedures to free surfaces of TSE agent infectivity in experimental studies (Belay et al., 2010; Rutala and Weber, 2010a, b).

The greatest number of iatrogenic cases have involved two medical products accidentally contaminated with CJD agent: cadaveric human pituitary growth hormone and human dura mater allografts. Thadani and colleagues (1988) reported CJD in a 28-year-old woman who had received a cadaveric dura mater allograft 18 months earlier. Since then, a total of 238 cases of iatrogenic CJD in recipients of dura mater allografts have become known to the US Centers for Disease Control and Prevention (CDC) (Bonda et al., 2016), more than half of them in Japan.

Contaminated human cadaveric pituitary hormones have been another relatively common source of iatrogenic CJD. Cases of CJD following earlier treatment with growth hormone were first reported in 1985 by Koch et al. and Gibbs et al. Many similar cases were soon recognized, and the total number of iatrogenic CJD cases attributed to treatment with pituitary-derived growth hormone worldwide has reached at least 238 (Bonda et al., 2016). Cadaveric pituitaries were also used to extract gonadotropin (follicle-stimulating hormone) to treat infertility. In 1990, Cochius and colleagues described a case of CJD in an Australian woman treated with pituitary-derived follicle-stimulating hormone 13 years earlier (Cochius et al., 1992); three other cases of CJD in pituitary follicle-stimulating hormone recipients – all in Australia – were reported later (Brown et al., 2000). In the United States, no case of growth hormone-associated CJD has yet been identified among recipients who initiated treatment after 1977, when a chromatographic purification step was introduced to the pituitary extraction procedure (Brown et al., 2012). After 1985, recombinant growth hormone replaced the pituitary-derived product in the United States, eliminating the iatrogenic CJD risk.

TSEs transmitted by blood components

Most attempts to detect infectivity in blood or serum of animals with TSEs failed until 1978, when Elias Manuelidis and colleagues demonstrated the transmissible agent in crude buffy coat preparations from blood of 13 guinea pigs injected with brain material of other guinea pigs with experimental CJD; infectivity was detected throughout most of the incubation period. The guinea pigs injected with blood had long incubation periods (some over a year), suggesting that amounts of infectivity in donor guinea pig blood were probably very small. In 1983, NIH investigators demonstrated that the blood buffy coats of mice infected with a TSE agent derived from a patient with GSS – originally considered to have familial CJD – also contained infectivity, detectable from the middle of the incubation period through terminal illness (Kuroda et al., 1983). The finding of small amounts of TSE infectivity in blood was later confirmed in a variety of other animals, including sheep with naturally acquired scrapie (Hunter et al., 2002), experimental bovine spongiform encephalopathy (BSE) (Houston et al., 2000), chimpanzees injected with brain material from a GSS patient (Williams et al., 2007), and macaques experimentally infected with BSE agent

(Lasmézas et al., 2001). Although much of the infectivity was associated with nucleated cells (Brown et al., 1999, 2001; Brown, 2000; Holada et al., 2002), plasma contained substantial amounts as well (Gregori et al., 2004).

In an ongoing look-back study, the UK Transfusion Medicine Epidemiology Review (TMER) (Health Protection Agency UK, 2007; Urwin et al., 2016) traced 67 recipients of blood transfusions from 18 donors who later developed vCJD. In addition, TMER identified 11 vCJD donors who contributed plasma to 25 pools fractionated into plasma derivatives before 1999. The first UK case of transfusion-transmitted vCJD was recognized in 2003 in a recipient of nonleukoreduced red blood cells (Llewelyn et al., 2004). The implicated donation had been transfused 6.5 years earlier. The donor died demented with vCJD 3 years and 4 months after the donation. The recipient was homozygous for methionine at codon 129 of the *PRNP* gene.

A second case was reported in 2004, when another blood donor in the TMER cohort died of vCJD 18 months after donation (Peden et al., 2004). A recipient of nonleukoreduced red blood cells from that donation died of an aortic aneurysm without evidence of neurologic illness 5 years after transfusion; however, an unusually thorough examination of lymphoid tissues revealed accumulations of abnormal PrP (PrP^{TSE}) typical of vCJD, suggesting that infection was present but had not yet spread to the brain. This was the first report of a vCJD infection in a person heterozygous for methionine and valine at *PRNP* codon 129 among all those tested. (Homozygosity for methionine or valine at *PRNP* codon 129 is overrepresented in persons with iatrogenic and sporadic forms of CJD: Deslys et al., 1994.) One possible case of vCJD (Kaski et al., 2009) and another confirmed case of vCJD (Mok et al., 2017) have since been reported in nontransfused persons heterozygous for methionine and valine at *PRNP* codon 129.

A third donor in the TMER cohort had donated three units of nonleukoreduced red cells 21, 17, and 4 months before becoming ill with vCJD. The first two donations were transfused into two recipients who developed vCJD 7.5 and 8.5 years after receiving the implicated units. Both individuals were homozygous for methionine at codon 129 of the *PRNP* gene (Wroe et al., 2006). The last unit was transfused into a recipient who remains alive at the time of this writing, more than 15 years later (Health Protection Agency UK, 2007).

In all, four instances of probable transfusion-transmitted vCJD infection have been identified by the UK TMER, including three clinically overt cases and a fourth with a putative subclinical or preclinical infection. As of December 2017, 14 recipients survive transfusions of blood components from vCJD donors. Those four infections through blood transfusion identified to date (all in recipients of nonleukoreduced red blood cell concentrates) developed in a cohort of only 32 recipients who survived for at least 5 years after transfusion (Chohan et al., 2010). The survival of so many recipients suggests that amounts of infectivity in blood of vCJD-infected donors are likely to be very small, even late in the asymptomatic incubation period (Gregori et al., 2011).

Neither the TMER study (Urwin et al., 2016) nor a collaborative look-back study by the American Red Cross and the US CDC identified CJD in any recipient of transfusion from donors later found to have sporadic CJD (Crowder et al., 2017). A recent report of sporadic CJD in two hemophilia patients treated with plasma-derived coagulation factors in the United Kingdom, while anecdotal, is less reassuring (Urwin et al., 2017).

Possible latent vCJD infection in an asymptomatic UK patient with hemophilia

Postmortem examination of a UK adult with hemophilia who, at the time of death, had no neurologic illness suggestive of vCJD showed accumulation of PrP^{TSE} in the spleen (Peden et al., 2010). The patient had been exposed to several potential sources of vCJD infection; a formal risk assessment (Bennett and Ball, 2009) concluded that the most likely exposure was through repeated injections of UK-sourced human plasma-derived factor VIII. (One lot of factor VIII was prepared from a pool of plasma to which a donor later diagnosed with vCJD had contributed, but, because of the very large numbers of donors contributing plasma for fraction, other donors might also have been incubating vCJD.) The patient was heterozygous for methionine and valine at *PRNP* codon 129.

PrP^{TSE} in appendices of otherwise healthy persons in the UK: possible implications for prevalence of latent vCJD infections

New cases of vCJD diagnosed each year peaked in the United Kingdom in 1999 and deaths peaked the next year; rates declined in the following years. The current total number of cases meeting the UK definition for confirmed or probable vCJD (as of December 2017) stood at 228 worldwide (not counting presumed preclinical infections), of which 175 were resident in the United Kingdom (not counting the three transfusion-transmitted vCJD cases) (www.cjd.ed.ac.uk/). The country with the second highest number of vCJD cases is France. A more detailed analysis of vCJD cases is offered elsewhere in this handbook. No new cases were reported in either country in 2016 or 2017. No case of vCJD has been detected in any person born in the United Kingdom after 1989, suggesting that dietary exposure to the BSE agent must have been greatly reduced, if not eliminated, after that time.

Shortly after the first clinical and histopathologic descriptions of vCJD (Will et al., 1996), lymphoid tissues (spleen, lymph nodes) of a person who died with vCJD were found to contain accumulations of PrP^{TSE} (Hill et al., 1997, 1999) – not seen in other forms of CJD, though infectivity has been detected in lymphoid and other nonneural tissues in sporadic CJD (Brown et al., 1994). It is worth noting that both tonsils and appendix of the second presumptive transfusion-transmitted vCJD case contained no detectable PrP^{TSE} (Peden et al., 2004), suggesting that its frequent occurrence in those tissues of other cases resulted from the more common oral–intestinal route of exposure to the BSE agent in food. The appendix removed from an otherwise healthy person who developed signs of vCJD 8 months later also contained PrP^{TSE} (Hilton et al., 1998), as did another appendix removed 2 years before onset, although a third appendix removed 10 years before onset was negative (Hilton et al., 2002); those fortuitous findings suggested that a survey of archived tonsils and appendices might provide a useful estimate of the minimum number of persons with preclinical vCJD in the UK population.

Three major surveys of archived paraffin-embedded appendix samples tested for PrP^{TSE} by immunohistochemistry have been reported to date: the first yielded three PrP^{TSE}-positive samples among 12,674 appendices for an estimated rate of 237/million (95% confidence interval, 49–692/million), suggesting that as many as one in 4000 people in the United Kingdom might be latently infected with the vCJD agent (Hilton et al., 2004). A second appendix survey tested 32,441 samples, of which 16 were positive, for an estimated prevalence of approximately one in 2000 people (Gill et al., 2013). A more recent survey (UK Appendix III Study) reported finding seven PrP^{TSE}-positive samples among 29,516 tested, for an estimated prevalence of approximately one in 4200 people (Public Health England, 2016) – consistent with estimated prevalence from the previous two studies. Those results were unexpected and controversial, because all seven appendices were removed either before the assumed beginning of the BSE outbreak or from subjects born after exposure was thought to have ended in 1996; they were interpreted as suggesting either that the PrP^{TSE} detected in appendices may not result from latent vCJD infection or that exposures to the BSE agent, causing asymptomatic vCJD infections, began earlier and continued later than previously assumed. This topic is reviewed in greater detail elsewhere in this handbook.

THE UNCONVENTIONAL NATURE OF TSE AGENTS: HISTORY

Conceptions of the nature of the TSE agents have their own interesting history. Cuillé and Chelle (1936, 1939) and others showed convincingly, in the 1930s and 1940s, that the scrapie agent was transmissible from affected to normal animals and self-replicating in the sense that injection of small amounts of infectivity resulted in accumulation of large amounts in the tissues of the recipient animal even before onset of overt illness. Furthermore, scrapie infectivity passed through the pores of filters that retained bacteria – an important criterion, at the time, for concluding that an infectious agent must be a virus (Wilson et al., 1950). However, William S. Gordon's experience, in the mid-1930s (Gordon, 1946), summarized later (Wilson et al., 1950; Asher, 1999), with a veterinary flavivirus vaccine prepared from formalin-treated sheep tissue first revealed that the scrapie agent had a property not then associated with other viruses (Offit, 2005): resistance to inactivation by 0.35% formaldehyde for more than 3 months. (It later became clear that significant fractions of "conventional" viruses also resisted inactivation by formalin under certain circumstances; tragic experience with early poliovirus vaccines illustrates that resistance (Offit, 2005).) (Pattison (1965) later reported that some scrapie infectivity survived even exposures to 20% formalin for 18 hours and to 12% formalin for 28 months.) A second property not shared with viruses soon became evident: some scrapie agent remained infectious after boiling at 100°C for 30 minutes (DR Wilson, 1954, unpublished observations, cited and confirmed by Stamp and colleagues (1959), who demonstrated some residual infectivity in diluted scrapie-infected brain suspensions heated at 99.5°C for exposure as long as 8 hours). Other efforts at about the same time, by Eklund and colleagues (1963) and Hunter (1965), failed to confirm the finding that a fraction of the scrapie agent survived boiling. Years later, Rohwer (1984a), scrupulously maintaining scrapie agent in suspension, found that boiling reduced its infectivity to undetectable levels in less than 5 minutes, though the agent resisted inactivation at lower temperatures. Spores of some bacteria were long known to resist boiling for as long as 5 hours, thanks to the pioneering work of polymath John Tyndall in the 1870s (cited by Stanier et al., 1970), so the finding of resistance to boiling alone could not rule out the existence of a nucleic acid genome in the scrapie agent.

Stamp et al. (1959) also found that scrapie agent survived exposure to acetylethyleneamine, a substance thought to destroy infectivity of all known viruses by disrupting nucleoproteins, concluding that "it is difficult to accept that … results [with the scrapie agent] … are simply due to a virus." Five years later Pattison and Sansom (1964) added to growing doubt regarding the viral nature of the scrapie agent when they reported that, in four of six attempts, scrapie agent had passed through the 2.4-μm average diameter pores of dialysis casing. (When

Pattison presented results of his dialysis experiments at a symposium in 1964, they were greeted with skepticism; critics preferred the explanation that the dialysis casings had leaked (NINDB Symposium, 1965). (Previous studies had failed to force the agent through filters with nominal average pore diameters of 27 μm (Stamp et al., 1959) and 20–35 μm (Eklund et al., 1963) – a size consistent with those of small or medium-sized viruses.)

In 1965, Pattison speculated that, based on the totality of "unusual findings, it is likely that if the transmissible agent of scrapie is a living virus, it is a virus of a kind as yet unrecognized." Two years later, impressed by similarities in properties of the scrapie agent to those of the protein that elicited allergic encephalomyelitis (not an infectious disease), Pattison and Jones (1967) "concluded that the scrapie transmissible agent may be, or may be associated with, a small basic protein." Pattison attributed to H.B. Parry precedence for first suggesting, in 1962, that the scrapie agent might not be a virus (Parry, 1962). Parry proposed that "[s]crapie is both an infective and genetic disease...the clinically affected genotype contains a potentially infective, self-replicating pathogenic particle, which does not spread naturally...but can be transmitted artificially by inoculation." Parry dubbed the hypothetical particle a "provirus" but he did not specifically suggest that it might be a protein. Rohwer later presented data suggesting that those properties of the scrapie agent were not completely inconsistent with those of some conventional agents (Rohwer, 1984a, b).

Increasing doubt about the viral nature of the scrapie agent followed the work of Tikva Alper and colleagues studying the resistance of scrapie agent to inactivation by ionizing radiation (Alper et al., 1966) and ultraviolet light (Alper et al., 1967). She concluded, in early 1967, that the unusually high resistance of scrapie agent to irradiation suggested that any nucleic acid present in the agent must be improbably small in size– too small to be a virus – but that the agent could be a protein. Rohwer (1984b), informed by later molecular virological studies, modified the sizes that Alper assumed for viruses and concluded that the scrapie agent might be larger than she had estimated. Later that year, Gibbons and Hunter (1967) summarized information showing that the scrapie agent was uniquely resistant to both chemical and physical inactivation, agreeing with Alper that the agent was less likely to be a virus than a protein; Griffith (1967), in an accompanying article, suggested three possible theoretical models for a self-replicating pathogenic protein, reassuring skeptics that "there is no reason to fear that the existence of a protein agent would cause the whole structure of molecular biology to tumble down." So was born the "all-protein" theory for the nature of scrapie agent – the theory prevailing today, albeit in a somewhat modified form. Peter K. Lewin, repeatedly reminded, over 18 years starting in 1972 (Lewin, 1972, 1981, 1982, 1990), that TSE agents were likely to be peptides or small proteins. (We are not aware that Lewin himself ever attempted to validate the all-protein theory of TSE agents. We also do not know whether Lewin's periodic reminders played any role in stimulating research on the nature of TSE agents, but he was remarkably persistent.) In any case, searches for the putative protein agent began.

In 1981 Patricia Merz and colleagues, studying extracts of scrapie-infected rodent brains by negative-stain transmission electron microscopy, described peculiar paired and twisted filaments resembling but not identical to those seen in Alzheimer disease; they called them "scrapie-associated fibrils" or SAF and soon identified the same fibrils in preparations of brain from CJD cases (Merz et al., 1983). (SAF proved useful for diagnosing TSEs postmortem, and the electron-microscopic technique for veterinary diagnosis remained in use in Europe well into the BSE epidemic.)

The following year, Prusiner, with David Bolton and Michael McKinley (Bolton et al., 1982; Prusiner, 1982), described a protein extracted from the brains of scrapie-infected hamsters (but not in normal control hamsters) that, unlike most other proteins found in brain, resisted complete digestion with the proteolytic enzyme proteinase K. Prusiner coined the term "prion" – for proteinaceous infectious agent – to describe the protein and postulated that it was at least a component, if not the entire agent, of scrapie and, by extension, the agents of other TSEs. The finding and subsequent characterization of the PrP, especially the development of mouse monoclonal antibodies to the PrP (which also reacted with SAF) led to the development of Western immunoblots, immunohistochemistry, and enzyme-linked immunosorbent assay-based tests that soon revolutionized the clinical diagnosis of human TSEs (Brown et al., 1986). Expression of PrP was found to be required to infect animals with TSE agents (Büeler et al., 1993; Prusiner et al., 1993), and sequencing of PrP ultimately identified mutations in the *PRNP* gene that explained the susceptibility of members of families with familial TSEs and other previously puzzling features of the diseases and their agents (see section on familial TSEs, above). Prusiner (1998) has described in great detail and from a personal point of view the rationale and history of his seminal work over more than 30 years (Prusiner, 2014).

Several research groups, including Prusiner's, have since attempted to prove the all-protein (prion) hypothesis. Their efforts seem to fall into two general types: (1) engineering mutant *PRNP* genes of mice never exposed to natural TSE agents to express infectious prions de novo; and (2) synthesizing infectious variants of PrP in vitro, some employing a variety of non-PrP cofactors and protein amplification techniques yielding filamentous PrP, such as those generated by protein misfolding cyclical amplification (PMCA) (Soto et al., 2002) or real-time quaking-induced conversion (RTQuIC) (Atarashi et al., 2007).

While it is beyond the scope of this chapter and the abilities of its authors to summarize these efforts, we note that results of several studies are difficult to interpret because some transgenic mice used to assay scrapie infectivity – in both types of experiment – overexpress PrP and develop spontaneous neurologic illnesses (Hsiao et al., 1990) accelerated by intracerebral injections of misfolded PrP (Nazor et al., 2005). Furthermore, few efforts have convincingly confirmed putative de novo synthesis of agents claimed to recapitulate the important properties of TSE agents – self-replication demonstrated by serial passage and faithful eliciting of progressive illness with TSE pathology in wild-type animals (not just accumulations of misfolded PrP in brains of transgenic animals). At the moment, strong proponents of the prion hypothesis consider the theory to have been proven beyond reasonable doubt (Supattapone, 2014). Devoted skeptics – a few remain – continue to suspect that true replication of infectious TSE agents and seeded misfolding of amyloid proteins are separable phenomena that have been confused by the proponents of the prion hypothesis and that small nucleic acids may lurk undetected as the actual infectious agents of TSEs (Botsios et al., 2015). The disagreement awaits future resolution.

No less confusing is a related corollary hypothesis regarding the origin of sporadic TSEs. In recent years, some authorities have concluded that cases of both sporadic CJD and "atypical" BSE (and atypical scrapie) arise by spontaneous misfolding of normal PrP to yield transmissible prions. We are not aware that any actual evidence, except lack of documented previous exposure to a TSE agent, supports the concept of spontaneous generation of TSE agents. The spontaneous-generation corollary, unlike the prion hypothesis, has serious implications for public health, in that it discourages continued search for infective TSE agents in the environment as a source of sporadic TSEs. History demonstrates that outbreaks of TSEs have been ended by preventing exposure to the agent: outbreaks of transmissible mink encephalopathy, BSE in cattle, and kuru and vCJD in humans were all controlled or even eliminated by reducing opportunities for exposure to TSE agent in food. It remains possible that sporadic cases of BSE and CJD are infections acquired by exposure to TSE agents in the environment, uncommon exposures or having low attack rates. It would be unfortunate to cease looking for potentially preventable sources of exposure to TSE agents because of the predictions of a theory – however persuasive and exciting.

NOSOLOGY OF HUMAN TSES: COMMENT

The medical geneticist Victor McKusick (1969) remarked that "Nosologists in all fields tend to be either 'lumpers' or 'splitters'." Inevitably, students of human TSEs fall into both categories. Early on, splitters proposed that CJD be divided into different syndromes depending on clinical presentation, distribution of histopathologic lesions in the brain, and morphology of amyloid plaques. After the discovery of PrP, differences in its molecular mass and relative sensitivity to proteinase K digestion in different cases were proposed as defining new TSEs, although they all resembled CJD as originally described. (Even GSS and familial CJD were not clearly differentiated until different mutations in the *PRNP* genes were recognized.) The splitting of human TSEs into different subtypes is defensible if the classification better predicts duration of illness (prognosis) of individual cases, and splitting seems, at worst, harmless. For those involved in public health, a more meaningful advantage of splitting CJD and similar diseases into subtypes lies in identifying those that are more easily transmitted; for example, vCJD has been transmitted by blood transfusion while transmission of sporadic CJD has not been observed in an even larger number of at-risk blood recipients (see above). Especially problematic is the tendency by some authorities to lump together as possible "prion diseases" a variety of neurologic diseases, like Alzheimer and Parkinson disease, in which misfolded normal proteins also accumulate in the brain; none of those diseases has been found transmissible, at least not under natural conditions. We consider it unfortunate, from the standpoint of public health, to group TSEs together with other diseases associated with misfolded proteins based on that general histopathologic similarity rather than on a common etiology, because the avenues for possible eventual prevention seem so different.

CONCLUSION

The history of TSEs is beyond remarkable. In just over 60 years, the study of an exotic condition of sheep, scrapie, led to recognition that kuru, an obscure human disease in an isolated population, was a food-borne infection and that several other progressive degenerative diseases of the human nervous system, worldwide in distribution and previously of unknown etiology, were associated with similar unconventional infectious agents. The TSE agents are unique pathogens, whatever their molecular structure – prion or something else – and their self-replicating mechanism turn out to be. It is reassuring that the attack rates for both iatrogenic and food-borne TSEs of human origin and for zoonotic infections of humans with BSE agent were relatively low and eventually controlled effectively by simple traditional measures long known to public health: preventing exposure to the pathogenic agents. Mysteries remain regarding TSEs, for example, the origin of sporadic cases of CJD, BSE, and scrapie, as well as the origin of chronic wasting disease, its host range, and strategies to control its rapid spread. We are confident that future generations of research investigators will address and eventually solve these problems.

DISCLAIMER

The authors' contributions to this chapter are informal communications representing our own views that do not bind or obligate the US FDA.

References

Alper T, Haig DA, Clarke MC (1966). The exceptionally small size of the scrapie agent. BBRC 22: 278–284.

Alper T, Cramp WA, Haig DA et al. (1967). Does the agent of scrapie replicate without nucleic acid? Nature 214: 764–766.

Alpers MP (2008). The epidemiology of kuru: monitoring the epidemic from its peak to its end. Philos Trans R Soc Lond Biol Sci 363: 3707–3713.

Asher DM (1999). The transmissible spongiform encephalopathy agents: concerns and responses of United States regulatory agencies in maintaining the safety of biologics. Dev Biol Stand 100: 103–118.

Asher DM (2008). Kuru: memories of the NIH years. Philos Trans R Soc Lond Biol Sci 363: 3618–3625.

Asher DM, Oldstone MBA (2013). D. Carleton Gajdusek 1923–2008. A biographical memoir, Biographical memoirs of the [US] National Academy of Sciences. Available online at: www.nasonline.org/.../biographical-memoirs/memoir-pdfs/gajdusek-d-carleton.pdf.

Asher DM, Masters CL, Gajdusek DC et al. (1983). Familial spongiform encephalopathies. Res Publ Assoc Res Nerv Ment Dis 60: 273–291.

Asher DM, Piccardo P, Gregori L (2017). Nonhuman primates in research on transmissible spongiform encephalopathies. In: PP Liberski (Ed.), Neuromethods 129. Prion diseases. Humana Press/Springer Protocols, New York, pp. 49–63.

Atarashi R, Moore RA, Sim VL et al. (2007). Ultrasensitive detection of scrapie prion protein using seeded conversion of recombinant prion protein. Nature Methods 4: 645–650.

Beck E, Daniel PM, Alpers M et al. (1966). Experimental "kuru" in chimpanzees. A pathological report. Lancet 2: 1056–1059.

Belay E, Schonberger L, Brown P et al. (2010). Disinfection and sterilization of prion-contaminated medical instruments. Infect Control Hosp Epidemiol 31: 1304–1306.

Bennett P, Ball J (2009). vCJD risk assessment calculations for a patient with multiple routes of exposure, UK Department of Health, London, pp. 1–15. Available online at: http://webarchive.nationalarchives.gov.uk/20130124050233/http://www.dh.gov.uk/prod_consum_dh/groups/dh_digitalassets/documents/digitalasset/dh_100337.pdf:.

Bernoulli C, Siegfried J, Baumgartner G et al. (1977). Danger of accidental person-to-person transmission of Creutzfeldt–Jakob disease by surgery. Lancet 1: 478–479.

Bolton DC, McKinley MP, Prusiner SB (1982). Identification of a protein that purifies with the scrapie prion. Science 218: 1309–1311.

Bonda DJ, Manjila S, Mehndiratta P et al. (2016). Human prion diseases: surgical lessons learned from iatrogenic prion transmission. Neurosurg Focus 41: E10.

Botsios S, Tittman S, Manuelidis L (2015). Rapid chemical decontamination of infectious CJD and scrapie particles parallels treatments known to disrupt microbes and biofilms. Virulence 6: 787–801.

Brown P (2000). The risk of blood-borne Creutzfeldt–Jakob disease. Dev Biol Stand 102: 53–59.

Brown P, Bradley R (1998). 1755 and all that: a historical primer of transmissible spongiform encephalopathy. BMJ 317: 1688–1692.

Brown P, Coker-Vann M, Pomeroy K et al. (1986). Diagnosis of Creutzfeldt–Jakob disease by Western blot identification of marker protein in human brain tissue. N Engl J Med 314: 547–551.

Brown P, Gibbs Jr CJ, Rodgers-Johnson P et al. (1994). Human spongiform encephalopathy: the National Institutes of Health series of 300 cases of experimentally transmitted disease. Ann Neurol 35: 513–529.

Brown P, Cervenakova L, McShane LM et al. (1999). Further studies of blood infectivity in an experimental model of transmissible spongiform encephalopathy, with an explanation of why blood components do not transmit Creutzfeldt–Jakob disease in humans. Transfusion 39: 1169–1178.

Brown P, Preece M, Brandel JP et al. (2000). Iatroenic Creutzfeldt–Jakob disease at the millennium. Neurology 55: 1075–1081.

Brown P, Cervenakova L, Diringer H (2001). Blood infectivity and the prospects for a diagnostic screening test in Creutzfeldt–Jakob disease. J Lab Clin Med 137: 5–13.

Brown P, Brandel JP, Sato T et al. (2012). Iatrogenic Creutzfeldt–Jakob disease, final assessment. Emerg Infect Dis 18: 901–907.

Brownell B, Oppenheimer D (1965). An ataxic form of subacute presenile polioencephalopathy (Creutzfeldt–Jakob disease). J Neurol Neurosurg Psychiatry 28: 350–361.

Büeler H, Aguzzi A, Sailer A et al. (1993). Mice devoid of PrP are resistant to scrapie. Cell 73: 1339–1347.

Chohan G, Llewelyn C, Mackenzie J et al. (2010). Variant Creutzfeldt–Jakob disease in a transfusion recipient: coincidence or cause? Transfusion 50: 1003–1006.

Cochius JI, Burns RJ, Blumbergs PC et al. (1990). Creutzfeldt–Jakob disease in a recipient of human pituitary-derived gonadotrophin. Aust N Z J Med 20: 592–593.

Cochius JI, Hyman N, Esiri MM (1992). Creutzfeldt–Jakob disease in a recipient of human pituitary-derived gonadotrophin – a second case. J Neurol, Neurosurg Psychr 55: 1094–1095.

Collinge J, Whitfield J, McKintosh E et al. (2006). Kuru in the 21st century – an acquired human prion disease with very long incubation periods. Lancet 367: 2068–2074.

Court L, Hauw JJ (2015). Doctor Francoise Cathala and history of prions diseases. Rev Neurol (Paris) 171: 805–811.

Creutzfeldt HG (1920). Ueber eine eigenartige herdfoermige Erkrankung des Zentralnervensystems. Z gesamte Neurol Psychiatr 57: 1–18.

Crowder LA, Schonberger LB, Dodd RY et al. (2017). Creutzfeldt–Jakob disease lookback study: 21 years of surveillance for transfusion transmission risk. Transfusion 57: 1875–1878.

Cuillé J, Chelle P-L (1936). La tremblante du mouton est elle inoculable? Comptes Rendus de l' Academie des Sciences, Paris 203: 1552–1554.

Cuillé J, Chelle P-L (1939). Transmission experimentale de la tremblante à la chèvre. Comptes Rendus de l' Academie des Sciences, Paris 208: 1058–1060.

Deslys JP, Marce D, Dormont D (1994). Similar genetic susceptibility in iatrogenic and sporadic Creutzfeldt–Jakob disease. J Gen Virol 75: 23–27.

Dickinson AG, Meikle VMH, Fraser H (1968). Identification of a gene which controls the incubation period of some strain of scrapie agent in mice. J Comp Pathol 78: 293–299.

Duffy P, Collins G, Devoe AG et al. (1974). Possible person-to-person transmission of Creutzfeldt–Jakob disease. N Engl J Med 290: 693.

Eklund CM, Hadlow WJ, Kennedy RC (1963). Some properties of the scrapie agent and its behavior in mice. Proc Natl Acad Sci USA 112: 974–979.

el Hachimi KH, Chaunu MP, Cervenakova L et al. (1997). Putative neurosurgical transmission of Creutzfeldt–Jakob disease with analysis of donor and recipient: agent strains. C R Acad Sci III 320: 319–328.

Foncin J, Gaches J, Cathala F et al. (1980). Transmission iatrogene interhumaine possible de maladie de Creutzfeldt–Jakob avec atteinte de grains du cervelet. Revue Neurologique (Paris) 136: 280.

Fowler M, Robertson EG (1959). Observations on kuru. III. Pathological features in five cases. Australasian Ann Med 8: 16–26.

Gajdusek DC (1965). Kuru in New Guina and the origin of the NINDB study of slow, latent and temperate virus infections of the nerous system of man. In: NINDB Monograph 2. DC Gajdusek, CJ Gibbs Jr, MP Alpers (Eds.), Slow, Latent and Temperate Virus Infections, 1. US Government Printing Office, Washington, DC, pp. 3–12.

Gajdusek DC (1977). Unconventional viruses and the origin and disappearance of kuru. Science 197: 943–960.

Gajdusek D, Zigas V (1957). Degenerative disease of the central nervous system in New Guinea: epidemic occurrence of "kuru" in the native population. N Engl J Med 257: 974–978.

Gajdusek DC, Gibbs Jr CJ, Alpers M (1966). Experimental transmission of a kuru-like syndrome to chimpanzees. Nature 209: 794–796.

Gajdusek DC, Gibbs Jr CJ, Asher DM et al. (1968). Transmission of experimental kuru to the spider monkey (*Ateles geoffreyi*). Science 162: 693–694.

Gambetti P, Kong Q, Zou W et al. (2003). Sporadic and familial CJD: classification and characterisation. Br Med Bull 66: 213–239.

Gambetti P, Dong Z, Yuan J et al. (2008). A novel human disease with abnormal prion protein sensitive to protease. Ann Neurol 63: 697–708.

Gerstmann J (1928). Über ein noch nicht beschiebenes Reflexphänomen bei einer Erkrankung des zerebellaren Systems. Wiener Med Wochenschr 78: 906–908.

Gerstmann J, Sträussler E, Scheinker I (1936). Über eine eigenartige hereditär-familiäre Erkrankung des Zentralnervensystems. Zeitschrift für Neurologie 154: 736–762.

Gibbons RA, Hunter GD (1967). Nature of the scrapie agent. Nature 215: 1041–1043.

Gibbs Jr CJ, Gajdusek DC, Asher DM et al. (1968). Creutzfeldt–Jakob disease (spongiform encephalopathy): transmission to the chimpanzee. Science 161: 388–389.

Gibbs Jr CJ, Joy A, Heffner R et al. (1985). Clinical and pathological features and laboratory confirmation of Creutzfeldt–Jakob disease in a recipient of pituitary-derived human growth hormone. N Engl J Med 313: 734–738.

Gibbs Jr CJ, Asher DM, Kobrine A et al. (1994). Transmission of Creutzfeldt–Jakob disease to a chimpanzee by electrodes contaminated during neurosurgery. J Neurol Neurosurg Psychiatr 57: 757–758.

Gill O, Spencer Y, Richard-Loendt A et al. (2013). Prevalent abnormal prion protein in human appendixes after bovine spongiform encephalopathy epizootic: large scale survey. BMJ 3457: f5675.

Goldfarb LG, Petersen RB, Tabaton M et al. (1992). Fatal familial insomnia and familial Creutzfeldt–Jakob disease: disease phenotype determined by a DNA polymorphism. Science 258: 806–808.

Goldgaber D, Goldfarb LG, Brown P et al. (1989). Mutations in familial Creutzfeldt–Jakob disease and Gerstmann–Sträussler–Scheinker's syndrome. Exp Neurol 106: 204–206.

Gordon WS (1946). Advances in veterinary research. Louping ill, tick-borne fever and scrapie. Vet Rec 58: 516–518.

Gregori L, McCombie N, Palmer D et al. (2004). Effectiveness of leucoreduction for removal of infectivity of transmissible spongiform encephalopathies from blood. Lancet 364: 529–531.

Gregori L, Yang H, Anderson S (2011). Estimation of variant Creutzfeldt–Jakob disease infectivity titers in human blood. Transfusion 51: 2596–2602.

Griffith JS (1967). Self-replication and scrapie. Nature 215: 1043–1044.

Hadlow WJ (1959). Scrapie and kuru. Lancet 2: 289–290.

Hadlow WJ (1992). The scrapie-kuru connection: recollections of how it came about. In: SB Prusiner, J Collinge, J Powell et al. (Eds.), Prion diseases of humans and animals, 2. Ellis Horwood, Chichester, pp. 40–46.

Health Protection Agency UK (2007). Fourth case of variant CJD associated with blood transfusion. In: Eurosurveillance 12: pii3117.

Heidenhain A (1928). Klinische und anatomusche Untersuchungen über eine eigenartige organische Erkrankung des Zentralnervensystems im Presenium. Z. f. d. ges. Neur. u. Psych. 118: 49–114.

Hill AF, Zeidler M, Ironside J et al. (1997). Diagnosis of new variant Creutzfeldt–Jakob disease by tonsil biopsy. Lancet 349 (9045): 99–100.

Hill AF, Butterworth RJ, Joiner S et al. (1999). Investigation of variant Creutzfeldt–Jakob disease and other human prion diseases with tonsil biopsy samples. Lancet 353: 183–189.

Hilton DA, Fathers E, Edwards P et al. (1998). Prion immunoreactivity in appendix before clinical onset of variant Creutzfeldt–Jakob disease. Lancet 352: 703–704.

Hilton DA, Ghani AC, Conyers L et al. (2002). Accumulation of prion protein in tonsil and appendix: review of tissue samples. BMJ 325: 633–634.

Hilton DA, Ghani AC, Conyers L et al. (2004). Prevalence of lymphoreticular prion protein accumulation in UK tissue samples. J Pathol 203: 733–739.

Holada K, Vostal JG, Theisen PW et al. (2002). Scrapie infectivity in hamster blood is not associated with platelets. J Virol 76: 4649–4650.

Houston F, Foster JD, Chong A et al. (2000). Transmission of BSE by blood transfusion in sheep. Lancet 356: 999–1000.

Hsiao K, Baker HF, Crow TJ et al. (1989). Linkage of a prion protein missense variant to Gerstmann-Sträussler syndrome. Nature 338: 342–345.

Hsiao KK, Scott M, Foster D et al. (1990). Spontaneous neurodegeneration in transgenic mice with mutant prion protein. Science 250: 1587–1590.

Hunter GD (1965). Progress toward the isolation and characterization of the scrapie agent. In: DC Gajdusek, CJ Gibbs Jr, MP Alpers (Eds.), NINDB Monograph 2. Slow, Latent, and Temperate Virus Infections. US Government Printing Office, Washington, DC, pp. 259–262.

Hunter N, Foster J, Chong A et al. (2002). Transmission of prion diseases by blood transfusion. J Gen Virol 83: 2897–2905.

Jakob A (1921). Über eigenartige Erkrankungen des Zentralnervensystems mit bewerkenswertem anatomische Befunde (Spastische Pseudosklerose-Encephalomyelopathie mit disseminierten Degenerationsherden). Deutsche Zeitschrift für Nervenheilkunde 70: 132–146.

Kaski D, Mead S, Hyare H et al. (2009). Variant CJD in an individual heterozygous for PRNP codon 129. Lancet 374: 2128.

Kirschbaum W (1924). Zwei eigenartige Erkrankungen des Zentralnervensystems nach Art der spastischen Pseudosklerose (Jakob). Zeitschr f d ges Neurol u Psychiatr 92: 175–220.

Kirschbaum WR (1968). Jakob-Creutzfeldt disease, American Elsevier, New York.

Klatzo I (1965). Neuropathological findings in kuru. In: NINDB Monograph 2. Slow, Latent, and Temperate Virus Infections DC Gajdusek, CJ Gibbs Jr, MP Alpers (Eds.), US Government Printing Office, Washington, DC, pp. 83–84.

Klatzo I, Gajdusek DC, Zigas V (1959). Pathology of kuru disease. Lab Invest 8: 799–847.

Koch TK, Berg BO, De Armond SJ et al. (1985). Creutzfeldt–Jakob disease in a young adult with idiopathic hypopituitarism. Possible relation to the administration of cadaveric human growth hormone. N Engl J Med 313: 731–733.

Kretzschmar HA, Neumann M, Stavrou D (1995). Codon 178 mutation of the human prion protein gene in a German family (Backer family): sequencing data from 72-year-old celloidin-embedded brain tissue. Acta Neuropathol 89: 96–98.

Kuroda Y, Gibbs Jr CJ, Amyx HL et al. (1983). Creutzfeldt–Jakob disease in mice: persistent viremia and preferential replication of virus in low-density lymphocytes. Infection and Immunity 41: 154–161.

Lanska DJ (2017). Etymologia: Creutzfeldt–Jakob disease. Emerg Infect Dis 23: 1760–1761.

Lasmézas CI, Fournier JG, Nouvel V et al. (2001). Adaptation of the bovine spongiform encephalopathy agent to primates and comparison with Creutzfeldt–Jakob disease: implications for human health. Proc Natl Acad Sci USA 98: 4142–4147.

Lewin P (1972). Scrapie: an infective peptide? Lancet i 748.

Lewin PK (1981). Infectious peptides in slow virus infections: a hypothesis. Can Med Assoc J 124: 1436.

Lewin PK (1982). Infectious peptides: postulated mechanisms of protovirus replication in scrapie. Can Med Assoc J 127: 471–472.

Lewin PK (1990). Scrapie and human neurodegenerative diseases. Can Med Assoc J 142: 928.

Llewelyn CA, Hewitt PE, Knight RS et al. (2004). Possible transmission of variant Creutzfeldt–Jakob disease by blood transfusion. Lancet 363: 417–421.

Lugaresi E, Medori R, Montagna P et al. (1986). Fatal familial insomnia and dysautonomia with selective degeneration of thalamic nuclei. N Engl J Med 315: 997–1003.

Manuelidis EE, Gorgacs EJ, Manuelidis L (1978). Viremia in experimental Creutzfeldt–Jakob disease. Science 200: 1069–1071.

Masters CL, Harris JO, Gajdusek DC et al. (1979). Creutzfeldt–Jakob disease: patterns of world wide occurrence and the significance of familial and sporadic clustering. Ann Neurol 5: 177–188.

Masters CL, Gajdusek DC, Gibbs Jr CJ (1981). Creutzfeldt–Jakob disease virus isolation from the Gerstmann-Sträussler syndrome, with an analysis of the various forms of amyloid deposition in the virus-induced spongiform encephalopathies. Brain 104: 559–588.

Mastrianni JA, Nixon R, Layzer R et al. (1999). Prion protein conformation in a patient with sporadic fatal insomnia. N Engl J Med 340: 1630–1638.

McKusick VA (1969). On lumpers and splitters, or the nosology of genetic disease. Perspect Biol Med 12: 298–312.

Medori R, Montagna P, Tritschler HJ et al. (1992). Fatal familial insomnia: a second kindred with mutation of prion protein gene at codon 178. Neurology 42: 669–670.

Meggendorfer F (1930). Klinische und genealogische Beobachtungen bei einem Fall von spastischer

Pseudosklerose Jakobs. Z f d ges Neur u Psychiatr 128: 337–341.

Merz PA, Somerville RA, Wisniewski HM et al. (1981). Abnormal fibrils from scrapie-infected brain. Acta Neuropathol 54: 63–74.

Merz PA, Somerville RA, Wisniewski HM et al. (1983). Scrapie-associated fibrils in Creutzfeldt–Jakob disease. Nature 306: 474–476.

Mok T, Jaunmuktane Z, Joiner S et al. (2017). Variant Creutzfeldt–Jakob dsease in a patient with heterozygosity at PRNP codon 129. N Engl J Med 376: 292–294.

Nazor KE, Kuhn F, Seward T et al. (2005). Immunodetection of disease-associated mutant PrP, which accelerates disease in GSS transgenic mice. EMBO J 24: 2472–2480.

Neumann MA, Gajdusek DC, Zigas V (1964). Neuropathologic findings in exotic neurological disorders among natives of the highlands of New Guinea. Journal of Neuropathology and Exper Neurol 23: 486–507.

Nevin S, McMenemy WH, Behrman D et al. (1960). Subacute spongiform encephalopathy: a subacute form of encephalopathy attributed to vascular dysfunction (spongiform cerebral atrophy). Brain 83: 519–564.

NINDB Monograph 2 (1965). In: DC Gajdusek, CJ Gibbs Jr, MP Alpers (Eds.), Slow, Latent, and Temperate Virus Infections. US Government Printing Office, Washington, DC, pp. 225–257.

Offit PA (2005). The Cutter incident. In: How America's first polio vaccine led to the growing vaccine crisis, Yale University Press, New Haven, CT.

Owen F, Poulter M, Lofthouse R et al. (1989). Insertion in prion protein gene in familial Creutzfeldt–Jakob disease. Lancet 1 (8628): 51–52.

Parry HB (1962). Scrapie: a transmissible and hereditary disease of sheep. Heredity 17: 75–105.

Pattison IH (1965). Resistance of the scrapie agent to formalin. J Comp Pathol 75: 159–164.

Pattison IH, Jones KM (1967). The possible nature of the transmissible agent of scrapie. Vet Rec 80 (1): 2–9.

Pattison IH, Sansom BF (1964). Dialysis of the scrapie agent. Res Vet Sci 5: 340–347.

Peden AH, Head MW, Ritchie DL et al. (2004). Preclinical vCJD after blood transfusion in a PRNP codon 129 heterozygous patient. Lancet 364: 527–529.

Peden A, McCardle L, Head MW et al. (2010). Variant CJD infection in the spleen of a neurologically asymptomatic UK adult patient with haemophilia. Haemophilia 16: 296–304.

Piccardo P, Manson JC, King D et al. (2007). Accumulation of prion protein in the brain that is not associated with transmissible disease. Proc Natl Acad Sci USA 104: 4712–4717.

Poser CM (2002). Notes on the history of the prion disease. Clin Neurol Neurosurg 104: 1–9.

Prusiner SB (1982). Novel proteinaceous infectious particles cause scrapie. Science 216: 136–144.

Prusiner SB (1998). Prions. Proc Natl Acad Sci USA 95: 13363–13383.

Prusiner SB (2014). Madness and memory, Yale University Press, New Haven, CT.

Prusiner SB, Hadlow WJ, Eklund CM et al. (1977). Sedimentation properties of the scrapie agent. Proc Natl Acad Sci USA 74: 4656–4660.

Prusiner SB, Groth D, Serban A et al. (1993). Ablation of the prion protein (PrP) gene in mice prevents scrapie and facilitates production of anti-PrP antibodies. Proc Natl Acad Sci USA 90: 10608–10612.

Public Health England (2016). Summary results of the third national survey of abnormal prion protein prevalence in archived appendix specimens. Health Protection Report (Weekly Report) 10: 1–2.

Rohwer RG (1984a). Scrapie infectious agent is virus-like in size and susceptibility to inactivation. Nature 308: 658–662.

Rohwer RG (1984b). Virus-like sensitivity of scrapie agent to heat inactivation. Science 223: 600–602.

Roos R, Gajdusek DC, Gibbs Jr CJ (1973). The clinical characteristics of transmissible Creutzfeldt–Jakob disease. Brain 96: 1–20.

Rutala W, Weber D (2010a). Guideline for disinfection and sterilization of prion-contaminated medical instruments. Infect Control Hosp Epidemiology 31: 107–117.

Rutala W, Weber D (2010b). Reply to Belay et al. Infect Control Hosp Epidemiol 31: 1306–1308.

Sigurdsson B (1954a). Observations on three slow infections of sheep. BMJ [Clinical Research Ed.] 110: 255–270. 307–322, 341–354.

Sigurdsson B (1954b). Observations on three slow infections of sheep. 2. Paratuberculosis (Johne's disease of sheeo in Iceland. Immunological studies and observations on its mode of spread. Br Vet J 110: 307–322.

Sigurdsson B (1954c). Observations on three slow infections of sheep. 3. Rida, a chronic encephalitis of sheep, with general remarks on infections which develop slowly and some of their special characteristics. Br Vet J 110: 341–354.

Sigurdsson B (1954d). Observations on three slow infections of sheep. 1. Maedi, a slow progressive pneumonia of sheep: an epizootological and a pathological study. Br Vet J 110: 255–270.

Soto C, Saborio GP, Anderes L (2002). Cyclic amplification of protein misfolding: application to prion-related disorders and beyond. Trends Neurosci 25: 390–394.

Stamp JT, Brotherston JG, Zlotnik I et al. (1959). Further studies on scrapie. J Comp Pathol 69: 268–280.

Stanier RY, Doudoroff M, Adelberg EA (1970). The microbial world, Prentice-Hall, Englewood Cliffs, NJ.

Supattapone S (2014). Synthesis of high titer infectious prions with cofactor molecules. J Biol Chem 289: 19850–19854.

Tateishi J, Ohta M, Koga M et al. (1979). Transmission of chronic spongiform encephalopathy with kuru plaques from humans to small rodents. Ann Neurol 5: 581–584.

Tateishi J, Koga M, Sato Y et al. (1980). Properties of the transmissible agent derived from chronic spongiform encephalopathy. Ann Neurol 7: 390–391.

Tateishi J, Sato Y, Nagara H et al. (1984). Experimental transmission of human subacute spongiform encephalopathy to small rodents. IV. Positive transmission from a typical case of Gerstmann-Straussler-Scheinker's disease. Acta Neuropathol 64: 85–88.

Tateishi J, Kitamoto T, Hashiguchi H et al. (1988). Gerstmann-Straussler-Scheinker disease: immunohistological and experimental studies. Ann Neurol 24: 35–40.

Thadani V, Penar PL, Partington J et al. (1988). Creutzfeldt–Jakob disease probably acquired from a cadaveric dura mater graft. Case report. J Neurosurg 69: 766–769.

Urwin PJ, Mackenzie JM, Llewelyn CA et al. (2016). Creutzfeldt–Jakob disease and blood transfusion: updated results of the UK Transfusion Medicine Epidemiology Review Study. Vox Sang 110: 310–316.

Urwin P, Thanigaikumar K, Ironside JW et al. (2017). Sporadic Creutzfeldt–Jakob disease in 2 plasma product recipients, United Kingdom. Emerg Infect Dis 23: 893–897.

Westaway D, Goodman PA, Mirenda CA et al. (1987). Distinct prion proteins in short and long scrapie incubation period mice. Cell 51: 651–662.

Will RG, Ironside JW, Zeidler M et al. (1996). A new variant of Creutzfeldt–Jakob disease in the UK. Lancet 347: 921–925.

Williams L, Brown P, Ironside J et al. (2007). Clinical, neuropathological and immunohistochemical features of sporadic and variant forms of Creutzfeldt–Jakob disease in the squirrel monkey (*Saimiri sciureus*). J Gen Virol 88: 688–695.

Wilson DR, Anderson RD, Smith W (1950). Studies in scrapie. J Comp Pathol 60: 67–282.

Wroe SJ, Pal S, Siddique D et al. (2006). Clinical presentation and pre-mortem diagnosis of variant Creutzfeldt–Jakob disease associated with blood transfusion: a case report. Lancet 368: 2061–2067.

Wunderlich V (2015). Die Hirnforscherin Elisabeth Beck (1907–2002). Aus Deutschland vertrieben – in England zur erfolgreichen Wissenschaftlerin gereift. Schriftenreihe der Deutschen Gesellschaft für Geschichte der Nervenkrankheiten 21: 265–296.

Zeidman LA, Ziller MG, Shevell M (2015). "With a smile through tears." The uprooted career of the man behind Gerstmann syndrome. J History Neurosciences 24: 148–172.

Zeidman LA, Von Villiez A, Stellmann J-P et al. (2016). "History had taken such a large piece out of my life." Neuroscientist refugees from Hamburg during National Socialism. J History Neurosciences 25: 275–298.

Zigas V (1979). Origin of investigations on slow virus infections in man. In: SB Prusiner, WJ Hadlow (Eds.), Slow transmissible diseases of the nervous system, 2. Academic Press, New York, pp. 3–6.

Zigas V (1990). Laughing death, Springer/Humana Press, Clifton NJ.

Zigas V, Gajdusek D (1957). Kuru: clinical study of a new syndrome resembling paralysis agitans in natives of the Eastern Highlands of Australian New Guinea. Med J Austral 44: 744–754.

Section I

Pathophysiology of prions

Handbook of Clinical Neurology, Vol. 153 (3rd series)
Human Prion Diseases
M. Pocchiari and J. Manson, Editors
https://doi.org/10.1016/B978-0-444-63945-5.00002-7

Chapter 2

The cellular and pathologic prion protein

ANDREW C. GILL[1,2]* AND ANDREW R. CASTLE[2]

[1]*School of Chemistry, Joseph Banks Laboratories, University of Lincoln, Lincoln, United Kingdom*

[2]*Division of Neurobiology, The Roslin Institute and Royal (Dick) School of Veterinary Sciences, University of Edinburgh, Edinburgh, United Kingdom*

Abstract

The cellular prion protein, PrP^C, is a small, cell surface glycoprotein with a function that is currently somewhat ill defined. It is also the key molecule involved in the family of neurodegenerative disorders called transmissible spongiform encephalopathies, which are also known as prion diseases. The misfolding of PrP^C to a conformationally altered isoform, designated PrP^{TSE}, is the main molecular process involved in pathogenesis and appears to precede many other pathologic and clinical manifestations of disease, including neuronal loss, astrogliosis, and cognitive loss. PrP^{TSE} is also believed to be the major component of the infectious "prion," the agent responsible for disease transmission, and preparations of this protein can cause prion disease when inoculated into a naïve host. Thus, understanding the biochemical and biophysical properties of both PrP^C and PrP^{TSE}, and ultimately the mechanisms of their interconversion, is critical if we are to understand prion disease biology. Although entire books could be devoted to research pertaining to the protein, herein we briefly review the state of knowledge of prion biochemistry, including consideration of prion protein structure, function, misfolding, and dysfunction.

BACKGROUND

The prion protein is a relatively small glycoprotein that is tethered to the outer leaflet of the plasma membrane, where it appears to interact with various molecular partners to carry out what is currently rather an obscure function. It has a region of globular structure and a partially disordered region that can bind copper ions. It is monomeric, detergent-soluble, and, in many senses, it is rather unremarkable. However, the prion protein is also the primary player in a devastating class of neurodegenerative disorders known as transmissible spongiform encephalopathies (TSEs) or prion diseases. During pathogenesis of a prion disease the normal form of the prion protein (called PrP^C – the cellular prion protein) misfolds into an insoluble form that aggregates into large assemblies, including amyloid fibrils and plaques. The misfolded protein is known as PrP^{TSE} (the TSE isoform) and this form accumulates during disease in the brain of affected individuals, leading inextricably to death (Prusiner, 1998). In many prion diseases, accumulations of misfolded protein can also be detected in the lymphoreticular system (Mabbott, 2017). Prion diseases are not the only neurodegenerative disease caused by misfolded protein – other examples include Alzheimer, Parkinson, and Huntington diseases, as well as amyotrophic lateral sclerosis. Each disease involves the misfolding of a different protein. Thus, whilst there are common generic mechanisms in the different protein misfolding diseases (PMDs), there are also disease-specific mechanisms governed, at least in part, by the biochemistry and cell biology of the protein involved. In this chapter we focus briefly on biochemical details of both the cellular and pathologic forms of the prion proteins.

PRP^C

PrP^C expression and regulation

The gene encoding PrP^C is designated *PRNP* and is located on chromosome 20 (in humans). Within mammals

*Correspondence to: Andrew C. Gill, School of Chemistry, Joseph Banks Laboratories, University of Lincoln, Green Lane, Lincoln, Lincolnshire LN6 7DL, United Kingdom. Tel: +44-1522-835-258, E-mail: angill@lincoln.ac.uk

the gene is remarkably conserved (Wopfner et al., 1999), whilst other vertebrates have homologs that vary somewhat from mammals, in terms of sequence identity, but which have similar structural motifs (Calzolai et al., 2005). The *PRNP* gene has several features common to housekeeping genes that allow constitutive expression (Puckett et al., 1991; Sakudo et al., 2010), but there are also putative binding sites for numerous transcription factors upstream of the transcription start site that presumably allow partial dynamic control of expression. Potential transcription factors regulating PrP^C expression include Sp1 (Basler et al., 1986), activator protein 1 and activator protein 2 (Mahal et al., 2001), and forkhead box protein O3 (Liu et al., 2013), but this list is not exhaustive. These factors, alongside others, enable PrP^C expression to be modulated by, for example, growth factor signaling (Kuwahara et al., 2000; Zawlik et al., 2006; Liu et al., 2013) or a variety of stressors, including endoplasmic reticulum (ER), oxidative and genotoxic stress (Dery et al., 2013; Cichon and Brown, 2014; Bravard et al., 2015). Two additional homologs of *PRNP* in mammals have been discovered over the last 15 years or so, named *PRND* and *SPRN*. These genes encode proteins known as doppel and shadoo respectively. Whilst it seems likely that their structures, biochemical properties, and functions are intertwined with those of PrP^C, we do not have space to consider these proteins herein and direct interested readers to an excellent recent comparison of the three proteins (Ciric and Rezaei, 2015).

The highest level of expression of PrP^C is in the central nervous system (CNS), but both transcript and protein can be detected at lower levels in a variety of other tissue/cell types (Castle and Gill, 2017). In the brain, PrP^C expression appears important during development with expression reducing from early life towards adulthood (Sales et al., 2002; Adle-Biassette et al., 2006). Expression of PrP^C has been detected in most neural cell types, including astrocytes (Lima et al., 2007; Hartmann et al., 2013), oligodendrocytes (Moser et al., 1995; Bribian et al., 2012), and microglia (Adle-Biassette et al., 2006), in addition to the classic view that PrP^C is highly expressed in neurons. Brain-derived PrP^C can also be detected in endothelial cells in blood vessel walls (Adle-Biassette et al., 2006) and, in the peripheral nervous system (PNS), PrP^C expression has been reported in the dorsal and ventral root ganglia of the spinal cord (Tremblay et al., 2007; Peralta et al., 2012; Ganley et al., 2015), sensory and motor axons (Manson et al., 1992), and Schwann cells (Follet et al., 2002). Outside the nervous system, PrP^C expression has been detected in immune cells, including T lymphocytes, natural killer cells, and mast cells (Durig et al., 2000; Haddon et al., 2009), and also in multiple organs, including the heart, pancreas, intestine, spleen, liver, and kidneys (Peralta and Eyestone, 2009).

PrP^C primary structure, sequence motifs, and processing

PrP^C is expressed initially as a polypeptide of approximately 250 amino acids (Fig. 2.1A) and incorporates both N- and C-terminal signal peptides. Since PrP^C is ultimately to be secreted from the cell, it is synthesized and co-translationally translocated into the ER under direction of the N-terminal signal peptide, which is subsequently removed. Although the vast majority of protein is faithfully trafficked into the ER, inefficient ER targeting (Rane et al., 2004) can result in some PrP^C becoming localized to the cytoplasm or becoming ectopically integrated into the ER membrane and these forms appear to elicit toxic signaling (see below).

Nevertheless, when PrP^C is correctly translocated this allows the C-terminal signal peptide to be removed and a glycophosphatidylinositol (GPI) membrane anchor is attached to the new C-terminus. Removal of both signal sequences results in a mature protein of 208 amino acids (residues 23–230 of the precursor protein), which is composed of two domains that are approximately equally sized. The N-terminal region may possess poly-L-proline II structure (Gill et al., 2000; Blanch et al., 2004; Taubner et al., 2010), facilitating interactions with multiple partners (Bakkebo et al., 2015), but this region is often viewed as intrinsically disordered. Within the N-terminal domain are octapeptide repeats, which are highly conserved (Wopfner et al., 1999), and hence may be of functional significance. Between N- and C-terminal domains exists a ~20-residue stretch of hydrophobic amino acids, whilst the C-terminal domain has a classic globular structure, consisting of three α-helices and two β-strands (Riek et al., 1996; Haire et al., 2004). Within the C-terminal domain there is a single disulfide bond and two consensus sites of potential N-linked glycosylation. Whilst most PrP^C appears di-glycosylated, this may not apply to all cell types or in all tissues (Williams et al., 2004). The amino acid sequence of human PrP^C is shown in Fig. 2.1A), whilst structural features of PrP^C are shown diagrammatically in Figure 2.1B and C.

During its life cycle, a PrP^C molecule can undergo up to three cleavage events, the functional and pathologic significance of which are still under investigation. The approximate sites of each of the three types of cleavage of PrP^C are shown in Figure 2.1B. The first cleavage event to be discovered takes place enzymatically within the hydrophobic domain (Chen et al., 1995;

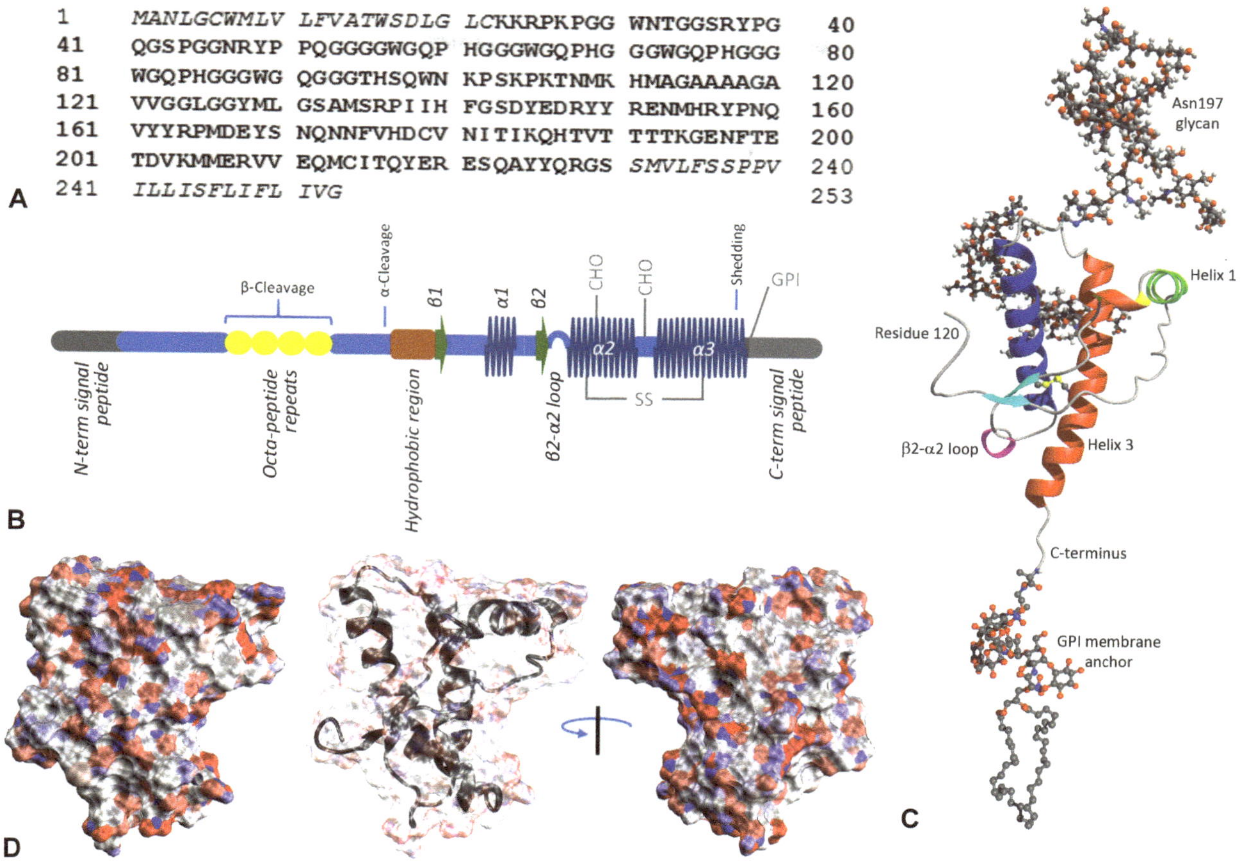

Fig. 2.1. (**A**) The amino acid sequence of human PrP^{C}, according to Uniprot entry P04156. The mature protein is in bold, whilst N- and C-terminal signal sequences are in italics. (**B**) Schematic of primary and secondary structural features of the mammalian prion protein. (**C**) Schematic of the tertiary structure of mammalian PrP^{C}, based on the ovine crystal structure solved by Haire et al. with Protein DataBank code 1UW3. Typical complex N-glycans were added to the two consensus sites and a typical GPI anchor structure to the C-terminus to illustrate these features, but their positions and conformations should not be taken literally. Note, the entire N-terminal region from residue 23 to 120 has been omitted from this model since its atomic-level structure has not been solved. (**D**) Molecular surfaces of the C-terminal, globular region of murine PrP, with the locations of positively (blue) and negatively (red) charged amino acids shown. The two surfaces show the molecule from the front and back to illustrate the compact core of the globular domain. A partially transparent surface with the backbone visible is included to allow the reader to orient the molecule correctly, in conjunction with (C). Images were prepared with MolMol or SwissPDB Viewer.

Watt et al., 2005; McDonald et al., 2014) and has been designated α-cleavage. There is some ambiguity as to the identity of the protease responsible for this cleavage (Beland et al., 2012; Wik et al., 2012), but disintegrin and metalloproteinase domain-containing protein (ADAM) family members are widely implicated (Vincent et al., 2001; Cisse et al., 2008; McDonald et al., 2014). The subcellular location in which α-cleavage takes place is also debated, with suggestions that it occurs in either an acidic endosomal compartment (Shyng et al., 1993) or within the Golgi apparatus (Walmsley et al., 2009). α-Cleavage produces the fragments N1 and C1 from the N- and C-termini respectively; N1 is released from the cell whilst C1 is trafficked to the cell membrane, similar to full-length PrP^{C} (Harris et al., 1993; Vincent et al., 2000; Laffont-Proust et al., 2006). Secondly, PrP^{C} can be cleaved within the octapeptide repeat region (β-cleavage), an event that seems to be driven by chemical, rather than enzymatic, mechanisms (McMahon et al., 2001; Mange et al., 2004; Watt et al., 2005; McDonald et al., 2014), but which does seem to occur physiologically. β-Cleavage results in fragments designated N2 and C2 and occurs at the cell surface, leading to C2 being retained on the cell membrane while N2 is released (Mange et al., 2004; Watt et al., 2005). Finally, PrP^{C} can also be shed from the cell surface through ADAM10-mediated cleavage close to the C-terminus, allowing the N-terminal protein fragment, sometimes known as N3, to be released into the extracellular matrix (Taylor et al., 2009; McDonald et al., 2014).

Variations and importance of posttranslational modifications in PrP^C

As indicated in the previous section and shown in Figure 2.1B and C, PrP^C undergoes posttranslational modifications (PTMs) during transit through the ER/ Golgi complex; a single disulfide bond is added, the C-terminal signal sequence is replaced by a GPI anchor and glycans are added to the two consensus sites for N-linked glycosylation. It was shown many years ago that these modifications are also present in PrP^{TSE} (Haraguchi et al., 1989; Stahl et al., 1992, 1993) and their impact on prion protein misfolding has been investigated extensively, the outcomes of which are described later.

However, somewhat less investigation has been performed on the impact of PTMs in the context of PrP^C cell biology and most studies that have been carried out are largely descriptive. It is generally accepted that removal of the single disulfide bond initiates misfolding (Jackson et al., 1999) and that PrP molecules lacking this bond are likely, therefore, to be targeted for degradation; we will not consider the disulfide bond further in this section but return to the question of whether the single disulfide bond is important in PrP^{TSE} later in the chapter.

Characterization of the GPI anchor attached to PrP^C (Stahl et al., 1992) was conducted in the 1990s, using mass spectrometric methods that were cutting edge at the time, but these studies warrant repeating at high definition. Nevertheless, from the early work it appears that PrP^C is slightly unusual in that its GPI anchor can be at least partially sialylated. There is recent evidence that the presence of sialic acid affects the localization and function of PrP^C (Bate et al., 2016a, c) and the level of sialylation seems to vary depending on context (Katorcha et al., 2016b). The GPI anchor of PrP^C has a heterogeneous sugar backbone common to other GPI-linked proteins (Stahl et al., 1992). Since in the early characterization work the lipid chains were cleaved from the PrP^C GPI anchor, nothing is known about the identity of these moieties, but it is reasonable to suspect that these are also heterogeneous, in line with other GPI-anchored proteins. Hence, it remains pertinent to ask what the spectrum of GPI anchors attached to PrP^C looks like and whether this spectrum differs in different situations (Katorcha et al., 2016b). However, even if the full range of GPI anchors present on PrP^C is completely defined using more modern mass spectrometric techniques, we still lack tools to allow targeted production of different forms by selective chemical and/or biochemical synthesis. Although this is an interesting area of prion biology, the importance of individual GPI anchors to a PrP^C molecule seems likely to remain unclear for some time to come.

A variety of studies have also been performed to assess the importance and structure of the N-linked glycans on PrP^C. In general, mature PrP^C that is attached to the cell surface is predominately di-glycosylated – both N-linked consensus sites are occupied – although various underglycosylated forms can be detected by analysis of total PrP^C levels in cells or tissues. It is likely that these underglycosylated forms are undergoing biosynthesis. An interesting facet of PrP^C glycosylation is that the glycan chains are highly heterogeneous in nature; over 60 sugar structures have been characterized that can occur at one or other site, or both (Rudd et al., 1999; Stimson et al., 1999; Ritchie et al., 2002). The glycans present at both sites are of the complex type that are matured in the Golgi complex and, like the GPI anchor, the glycan chains are multiply sialylated (Rudd et al., 1999; Stimson et al., 1999) and many carry core fucose residues. Because of the complexity of mass spectrometric analysis of carbohydrates, it is not clear whether there are cell-, tissue- or species-specific sugar structures present on PrP^C and the significance of the presence of such a wide variety of different chains is not known. Some of this is a little clearer for PrP^{TSE}, and will be discussed later. Little is known about the effect of individual sugar structures; however the generic effects of N-linked glycosylation on PrP^C have been investigated predominantly by genetic removal of one or other of the N-linked consensus sites or by molecular dynamic simulations. Removal of such N-linked consensus sites appears to affect trafficking of PrP^C and there is some evidence for delayed transit of aglycosyl PrP^C through the ER/Golgi complex and even retention of the protein in the ER/Golgi (Neuendorf et al., 2004), presumably because of the requirement for glycan-specific chaperone binding during trafficking. However, it is difficult to demonstrate that this is an effect of lack of glycosylation rather than the sequence variations made to remove the consensus sites. In concert with other glycoproteins, one putative role for the glycans is in maintaining protein stability on the cell surface. It remains to be determined whether the N-linked glycans effect the interaction of PrP^C with any functionally important interaction partners.

PrP^C secondary, tertiary, and quaternary structure

A key area of research over many years has been in defining the structures of all forms of the prion protein, whether these are the normal physiologic form, the pathogenic or toxic isoforms, or other isoforms produced by in vitro misfolding of recombinant protein under a variety of conditions. The reasonable rationale is that defining structures of all potential forms of PrP should allow us to determine more readily how or whether interconversion between each form takes place. As discussed later, defining structures of aberrantly folded isoforms has proved challenging, but it has been somewhat easier to solve the structure of PrP^C. Initial studies used nuclear magnetic resonance (NMR) analysis of recombinant prion protein (recPrP) expressed in *Escherichia coli* and refolded in vitro. The first studies focused on solving the structures of mouse, hamster, and human proteins (Riek et al., 1996; Donne et al., 1997; James et al., 1997), but there have since been a large range of studies of a wider range of different prion proteins (Wuthrich and Riek, 2001; Calzolai et al., 2005; Gossert et al., 2005; Lysek et al., 2005; Christen et al., 2008; Perez et al., 2010). The research has extended to X-ray crystallography for sheep (Eghiaian et al., 2004; Haire et al., 2004), human (Knaus et al., 2001; Antonyuk et al., 2009; Lee et al., 2010), and rabbit (Khan et al., 2010) proteins, amongst others and NMR studies of PrP^C purified from bovine brain have essentially confirmed that the results can be extended to endogenous, mammalian-expressed protein (Hornemann et al., 2004).

Overall, the structural studies have found that PrP^C is essentially a chimeric protein composed of an N-terminal domain that is highly flexible and a C-terminal domain that possesses a typical globular structure, as depicted in Figure 2.1C. The globular domain has three α-helices that fold around each other to produce a three-helix bundle. Helices 2 and 3 are linked together by the disulfide bond, which helps to constrain structural variability. Two short β-strands are present, which flank helix 1. The globular region is also framed by the two N-linked glycan chains. Overall, the globular domain spans residues ~125 to the mature C-terminus at residue ~230; this section is compact (Fig. 2.1D), with only short loops linking the secondary structural motifs, and the fold is highly conserved amongst those prion proteins that have been studied. Of interest in the context of disease is a loop that links the second β-strand with the second α-helix (β2–α2 loop), the flexibility of which depends on the exact amino acid sequence (Christen et al., 2013) and which may be modulated by distal parts of the globular domain (Christen et al., 2009).

Immediately N-terminal of the globular domain is a hydrophobic stretch of about 20 amino acids; prior to the first NMR analyses this hydrophobic region was postulated, from predictions of structure, to form an additional α-helix (Nguyen et al., 1995), but it is now well established that this region is rather flexible. Importantly, this region has also been modeled as a transmembrane region and is responsible for anchoring PrP^C in the ER membrane in forms that do not correctly translocate into the ER, as previously discussed (Hegde et al., 1998). The structure of this peptide is not known in these circumstances, but it may fold into helical conformations to facilitate membrane localization. On the N-terminal side of the hydrophobic region, PrP^C contains a section of approximately 80 amino acids that is traditionally viewed as intrinsically disordered. This region incorporates several imperfect, glycine/proline-rich octapeptide repeats that contribute to the flexibility of the N-terminal region. These regions have similarity to collagenous domains and there is some evidence for poly-L-proline II structure, similar to that found in collagen strands (Gill et al., 2000; Blanch et al., 2004; Taubner et al., 2010). The octapeptide repeats bind metal ions in vitro (Wong et al., 2000a) and possibly in vivo (Brown et al., 1997) producing more defined conformations (Brown et al., 2004; Younan et al., 2011). At the extreme N-terminal region there is a short section of highly basic amino acids, that appears important for PrP^C cell biology, and it has also been suggested that this region interacts with the globular domain of PrP^C either intra- or intermolecularly (Yao et al., 2003). These suggestions await robust confirmatory studies.

Finally, there have been some intriguing reports that PrP^C may exist, at least partially, as dimers (Priola et al., 1995; Meyer et al., 2000). The first crystal structure obtained for recPrP revealed a domain-swapped dimeric structure, but this may have been an artefact of the crystallization process (Knaus et al., 2001). Dimers of PrP^C is an attractive idea that would help to explain some facets of prion disease pathogenesis and more research in this area is needed to confirm that such interactions occur physiologically.

PrP^C function(s)

The function of PrP^C has been of long-standing interest, since disruption of this function may play a key role in prion disease pathogenesis (Leighton and Allison, 2016; Allison et al., 2017). However, targeted ablation of PrP^C expression in mice, by different techniques, produced animals that were viable, developmentally normal, and did not appear to suffer from major, deleterious phenotypes in the CNS or elsewhere (Bueler et al., 1992; Manson et al., 1994a). On detailed study of knockout mice, PrP^C-null goats, zebrafish models of PrP^C ablation, as well as PrP^C-expressing and nonexpressing cell lines, a range of phenotypes and potential functions for the protein emerged (for a recent review, see Castle and Gill, 2017); concomitantly, molecular studies produced a large and varied putative interactome of PrP^C (Rutishauser et al., 2009). Over time, the plethora of functions of this relatively small protein has grown, some

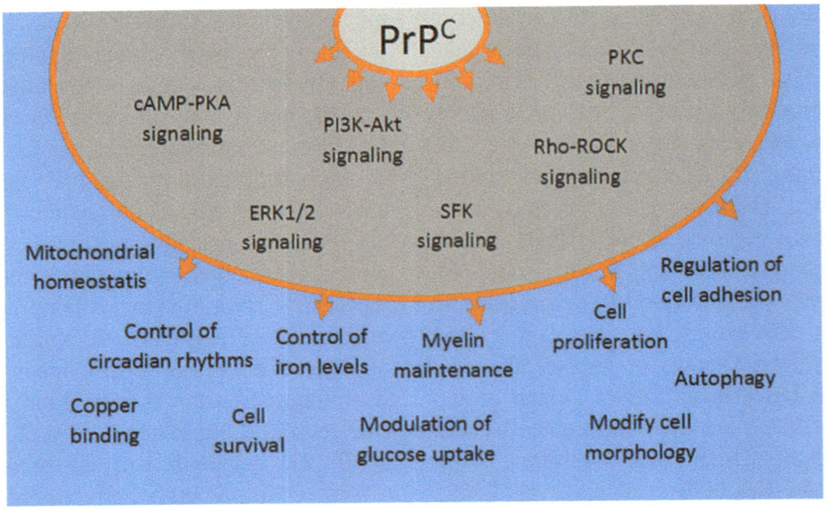

Fig. 2.2. Putative functions of the prion protein. PrP^C has been postulated to impact directly or indirectly a range of signaling pathways. Through these biochemical pathways, or others, PrP^C expression causes various downstream measurable effects, including, but not limited to, those shown on the figure. For a comprehensive recent review of PrP^C function, see Castle and Gill (2017).

of which are outlined in Figure 2.2, and we do not have space to cover all functions in detail. Below we briefly mention the most important areas, any of which (or none of which) may turn out to be an accurate reflection of the function of PrP^C. Further information can be found in the following comprehensive reviews of the subject (Bakkebo et al., 2015; Castle and Gill, 2017; Linden, 2017; Wulf et al., 2017).

The principal function that is frequently ascribed to PrP^C is that of (neuronal) protection against stress, a suggestion that has propagated partly because it fits neatly into the theory that loss of the protective effect of PrP^C during prion disease exacerbates any toxic effects of PrP^{TSE} on neurons. A range of studies has found that prion protein expression protects cells from the toxic effects of: serum withdrawal, through suppression of Bax-mediated apoptosis (Kim et al., 2004); staurosporin-induced cell death, through interaction with stress-induced phosphoprotein 1 (STI1) (Lopes et al., 2005); oxidative stress, including suppressing reactive oxygen species and oxidative DNA damage (Bertuchi et al., 2012; Bravard et al., 2015); and ER stress, upon which PrP^C expression may be upregulated through ER stress response elements in the promoter region of the *PRNP* gene (Dery et al., 2013). However, whilst the balance of literature is slightly in favor of a neuroprotective role for PrP^C, there are contradictory reports for many of the proposed stress response functions (Castle and Gill, 2017) and, overall, a direct function for PrP^C as a protein protecting against stress is unproven. It is also difficult to reconcile the cell surface expression of PrP^C with roles conferring protection for intracellular pathways directly. Far more likely is that PrP^C interacts with other cell surface molecules to transduce signals, one effect of which is to potentiate a cell's response to stressful events, in a context-specific manner (Linden, 2017).

In the light of the arguments presented, it is intriguing that PrP^C has been reported to interact with, and mediate the response of, several important cell surface receptor molecules. These include metabotropic glutamate, α7 nicotinic acetylcholine, kainate, α-amino-3-hydroxy-5-methyl-4-isoxazolepropionic acid (Kleene et al., 2007) and *N*-methyl-D-aspartate receptors (NMDARs) (Khosravani et al., 2008). PrP^C may inhibit the activity of NMDARs containing the GluN2D subunit, and since glutamate-related excitotoxicity may contribute to cell death during prion disease, as well as impacting various other physiologic processes, this raises the prospect that PrP^C functions to restrict glutamate-mediated excitotoxicity. In addition, PrP^C expression appears to restrict infarct volumes in ischemic stroke, during which excitotoxicity is a major cause of cell death (Weise et al., 2006). By contrast, the literature documenting the effect of PrP^C on kainate receptor activity is less consistent, with reports that PrP expression modulates (Carulla et al., 2011, 2015) responses to seizure-inducing treatments, but further suggestions that loss of genes flanking the *PRNP* locus, removed concomitantly with *PRNP* knockout, may be responsible (Striebel et al., 2013a, b).

Several studies report that PrP^C promotes neurite outgrowth through interactions with STI1 (Lopes et al., 2005), growth factor receptors (Llorens et al., 2013), or integrins (Loubet et al., 2012), amongst others, thereby activating or inhibiting downstream pathways, including the ROCK (Loubet et al., 2012) ERK1/2, PI3K-Akt, and protein kinase C signaling pathways (Lopes et al., 2005; Caetano et al., 2008; Beraldo et al., 2011;

Llorens et al., 2013). This may reflect a wider role of PrP^C in modulating cellular differentiation, since there is some evidence that PrP^C exerts influence on differentiation processes early during embryogenesis. PrP^C may regulate the epithelial-to-mesenchymal transition by indirectly modulating NCAM1 polysialylation (Mehrabian et al., 2015, 2016) and may promote guided differentiation of cultured human embryonic stem cells and neural precursors into neurons, astrocytes, and oligodendrocytes (Steele et al., 2006; Lee and Baskakov, 2014). A role in cell differentiation may explain findings that PrP^C knockdown or knockout results in altered expression of cytoskeletal proteins in cells (Provansal et al., 2010; Weiss et al., 2010; Mehrabian et al., 2014) and also in PrP^C-null liver tissues compared with wild-type controls (Arora et al., 2013). It may also explain findings that PrP^C has been shown to inhibit proliferation of oligodendrocyte precursors (Bribian et al., 2012), neuronal cells (Kim et al., 2005), and cells derived from the intestinal epithelium (Morel et al., 2008) since cellular differentiation impacts on cell cycle progression.

A relatively recently found phenotype of several lines of PrP^C knockout mice, apparently independent of how they were derived, is a widespread, adult-onset demyelination of the PNS (Bremer et al., 2010; Nuvolone et al., 2016), suggesting a role for PrP^C in myelin maintenance. Bremer et al. (2010) showed that neuron-specific PrP^C expression was sufficient to rescue demyelination and the interaction of the poly-basic N-terminal region (residues 23–33) and G-protein-coupled receptor 126 (GPR126) on the surface of Schwann cells (Kuffer et al., 2016) may be important for this activity. There is some evidence that α-cleavage of neuronal PrP^C is required to prevent PNS demyelination (Bremer et al., 2010), perhaps through binding of the released PrP^C N-terminus to promote receptor activation, thereby initiating signaling through the cyclic adenosine monophosphate–protein kinase A pathway (Kuffer et al., 2016). Despite reasonable levels of PNS demyelination, no myelin-related abnormalities were identified in the CNS of PrP^C knockout mice (Bremer et al., 2010), but this may be because CNS myelination is reported not to depend upon GPR126 activity (Monk et al., 2011).

Finally, as mentioned earlier, the octapeptide repeat region of the N-terminal domain has been reported to bind Cu^{2+} ions (Hornshaw et al., 1995a, b; Brown et al., 1997). Copper binding to PrP^C has been proposed to regulate NMDAR activity (Gasperini et al., 2015), astrocytic glutamate uptake (Brown and Mohn, 1999), protection against oxidative stress (Rachidi et al., 2003; Watt et al., 2007), and maintenance of Cu^{2+} homeostasis in the placenta (Alfaidy et al., 2013). Although the evidence for PrP^C binding to copper in vitro is overwhelming, it remains uncertain whether binding also occurs in vivo. PrP^C-dependent internalization of Cu^{2+} by cells requires Cu^{2+} concentrations above physiologically relevant levels (Rachidi et al., 2003). There is also evidence that PrP^C is involved in the physiologic uptake of iron by cells, possibly because of a regulatory role in ferritin and transferrin/transferrin receptor levels (Singh et al., 2009a, b). Furthermore, the liver, spleen, brain, and kidneys of Zurich I PrP^C-null mice have all been shown to have lower total levels of iron than wild-type controls (Singh et al., 2009a; Haldar et al., 2015).

The effect of sequence variations on PrP^C biochemistry

Sequence variations in the *PRNP* gene are discussed in detail elsewhere in this book, but we consider briefly here the effect that alterations to the amino acid sequence of PrP^C have on the biochemical properties of the protein. Amino acid differences can be categorized broadly as one of three different types: firstly, in humans there are amino acid changes that appear to lead inexorably to a prion disease – these mutations occur at various codons throughout the sequence of the prion protein and are covered in more detail later in this chapter. Secondly, in humans and a range of other species, there are polymorphisms in the *PRNP* gene that lead to coding changes, but which do not appear to cause disease. Instead, many of these changes impact the spatial/temporal pathogenesis of a prion disease, although some seem largely neutral. The archetypal species that expresses many allelic variants of the *PRNP* gene is sheep and a wide variety of amino acid substitutions are known to confer enhanced resistance or susceptibility to scrapie, but there are also polymorphisms in cervids, mice, and humans, amongst others. Notably, however, some species, such as cattle, appear to have little to no variation in *PRNP*.

Most investigations of the effect of amino acid changes in PrP^C have focused on whether the protein has differential potential to misfold, as discussed later, and relatively few studies have investigated the effect on the structure and function of PrP^C in its own right. In general, those amino acid substitutions associated with resistance to prion disease appear to decrease the stability of recombinant prion proteins in vitro (Thackray et al., 2004; Bujdoso et al., 2005; Paludi et al., 2007; Kirby et al., 2010). This may result in resistance-associated proteins having a shorter half-life in vivo, thereby reducing the levels of PrP^C available for misfolding during disease. By contrast, there are conflicting data on the ability of mutations associated with human familial disease to affect the structure of PrP^C (Inouye et al., 2000; Vanik and Surewicz, 2002; Apetri et al., 2004; Yin et al., 2007; Bae et al., 2009; van der Kamp and Daggett, 2010;

Rossetti et al., 2011) and interpreting these data mechanistically is not straightforward. It seems likely that the effect of individual amino acid changes depends on the specific substitution as well as the position within the sequence of PrP^C and it cannot be ruled out that amino acid alterations impact one of the putative functions of PrP^C.

Thirdly, although *PRNP* sequences between mammals have a high degree of homology, there tend to be several codons that differ between any two species and the resulting amino acid differences have been postulated to account for the barriers to prion infection across species. For instance, between mice and golden (Syrian) hamsters there are only 11 amino acid differences in their respective PrP^C sequence, and yet this is sufficient almost entirely to prevent cross-species prion infections. The molecular mechanisms behind the species barrier are not clear, but amino acids mismatches most probably impact negatively on the interaction between PrP^C and PrP^{TSE}. However, in the context of PrP^C biochemistry, there are two key areas of the protein where the structure of PrP^C appears most affected by the amino acid sequence of the protein: one is the β_2–α_2 loop region, highlighted in Figure 2.1C, which shows differential stability depending on the amino acids in and around the loop (Agarwal et al., 2015; Caldarulo et al., 2017); the second is the extreme C-terminal region which also appears differentially flexible depending on amino acid sequence, at least in vitro using non-GPI-anchored protein (Liu et al., 1999). The consequence of β2–α2 loop stability has been the subject of intense recent speculation (Christen et al., 2013; Kurt et al., 2014a; Agarwal et al., 2015; Caldarulo et al., 2017), but little is known about the how the flexibility of the C-terminus impacts PrP^C biology.

PRP^{TSE}

The abnormal isoform derived from conversion of PrP^C is designated PrP^{TSE} (The TSE deriving from the abbreviation of transmissible spongiform encephalopathy). PrP^{TSE} is a form that is intimately associated with prion diseases, since the ability to detect PrP^{TSE} is viewed as one of the diagnostic markers of a bona fide prion disease. It is also worth noting that animals that do not express PrP^C do not succumb to prion infections (Bueler et al., 1993; Manson et al., 1994b), underlining the key role of the PrP^C-to-PrP^{TSE} transition in disease. In contrast to PrP^C, PrP^{TSE} is partially insoluble in detergents, is resistant to proteases, readily forms aggregates and, as a result, is deposited as large aggregates in diseased tissues (Prusiner, 1998). These biophysical properties of PrP^{TSE} also give rise to alternative nomenclature for abnormal prion protein such as PrP^d ("d" stands for deposited or diseased) or PrP^{res} ("res" stands for resistant to proteases and in this context PrP^{sen} is a form of PrP that is sensitive to proteases) based on operational definitions. However, the term PrP^{TSE} is used herein as a "catch-all" of abnormally folded PrP molecules in vivo and this includes those forms that might have partial sensitivity to proteases but which are aberrantly folded (Sajnani and Requena, 2012). PrP^{TSE} is believed to form from PrP^C purely through a conformational/tertiary structural change, but this is not to say that the protein's primary structure and any modifications to this structure has no bearing, as outlined below. Crucially, it is widely believed that PrP^{TSE} is itself infectious and carries, within its conformation, all information necessary to initiate prion disease when it is administered to naïve individuals (Prusiner, 1998). Since PrP^{TSE} is most probably a collective of different forms of abnormal PrP, possibly with different conformations or morphologies, it is possible that only a subset of abnormally folded protein carries disease-specific information.

PrP^{TSE} primary structure and posttranslational modifications

Since PrP^{TSE} is derived posttranslationally from PrP^C, the basic amino acid sequences of the mature-length molecules are identical, because this sequence is encoded by the host's *PRNP* gene. Soon after the discovery of the prion protein, seminal research showed that both PrP^C and PrP^{TSE} carry similar PTMs; the single disulfide bond (Stahl et al., 1993), N-linked glycans (Haraguchi et al., 1989), and the GPI anchor (Stahl et al., 1992) are present in both forms of the protein. Since the studies that mapped the basic information, research has turned towards whether the detailed structures of the PTMs are different (in the case of the sugars and GPI) or whether specific variations to the PTMs in a small proportion of PrP^C molecules might initiate the misfolding cascade. The latter area is best exemplified by studies investigating the disulfide bond, where several lines of inquiry have explored whether disulfide removal plays a role in misfolding.

Whilst reduction of the disulfide bond in PrP^C has been suggested to be important for misfolding (Herrmann and Caughey, 1998; Welker et al., 2002; Lucassen et al., 2003; Hafner-Bratkovic et al., 2011) and loss of the disulfide from recPrP undoubtedly initiates misfolding in vitro, there is currently little convincing evidence to support a role for PrP^C disulfide reduction in vivo. However, since the disulfide bond is made posttranslationally in the ER, forms of the protein that do not correctly translocate into the ER (Rane et al., 2004) presumably lack this bond and these forms are reportedly highly toxic to cells. Trafficking abnormalities of PrP^C in which the two cysteines have been genetically mutated restrict the conclusions that can be drawn from studies in cells (Yanai et al., 1999) and this area of prion science warrants additional research. Conversely, N-linked glycosylation and the GPI anchor can be manipulated both in vitro and in vivo, allowing their role in PrP^{TSE} biology to be studied; a few molecular studies have also aimed to dissect the individual structures of glycans and GPI anchors on PrP^{TSE} to determine whether they are different to those associated with PrP^{C}.

Genetic removal of the C-terminal signal peptide prevents addition of the GPI anchor and results in secretion of PrP^{C} from the cell, instead of it being tethered to the cell membrane. Transgenic mice that express PrP^{C} without a GPI anchor (anchorless PrP^{C}) do not succumb to prion disease after scrapie inoculation and there is a lack of neurodegenerative phenotypes, but the mice do accumulate large amyloid plaques composed of anchorless PrP (Chesebro et al., 2005). These data suggest that the GPI anchor is not important for PrP misfolding per se, but that tethering of the protein to the cell surface plays an important role in neuronal toxicity (Caughey et al., 2009). However, preventing GPI anchor addition by removal of the C-terminal signal peptide also inhibits glycosylation of PrP^{C} and this may be a compounding factor in the lack of pathology and/or disease, as discussed below. Recent work using a cell-painting technique suggests that the structure and sialylation status of the GPI anchor may be important in dictating misfolding (Bate et al., 2016b, c), although this is currently an unresolved and complex area that warrants additional studies (Baskakov and Katorcha, 2016; Katorcha et al., 2016b; Srivastava et al., 2017).

There has been intense interest in the glycans attached to PrP^{TSE}, primarily because the two N-linked consensus sites are somewhat underoccupied in PrP^{TSE} compared to PrP^{C}. PrP^{C} tends to be almost completely di-glycosylated; that is, both potential N-linked sites have glycans attached. By contrast, the population of molecules that comprise PrP^{TSE} contains larger quantities of protein in which one or other site (or indeed both) is not occupied. Furthermore, different strains of prion disease, defined by different incubation periods, clinical signs, and targeting of neuropathology, also seem to produce PrP^{TSE} with subtly different levels of glycan site occupancy (Fig. 2.3). Thus, it has been hypothesized that either the level of N-glycan site occupancy or the specific sugars attached to either site might: (1) initiate prion protein misfolding or (2) encode strain-specific information to allow incubation periods and neural targeting to be faithfully replicated in naïve individuals. However, neither hypothesis seems to be accurate. Although initial studies suggested that expressing aglycosyl PrP^{C} in cells produced spontaneously misfolded protein (Lehmann and Harris, 1997), this may have been a consequence of overexpression. More recent work has failed to replicate this finding (Cancellotti et al., 2005), albeit some mutations used to remove the N-linked consensus sites produced PrP^{C} that was inefficiently trafficked through the cell, which essentially hampers interpretation of certain experiments (DeArmond et al., 1997; Capellari et al., 2000; Wong et al., 2000b; Cancellotti et al., 2005; Ikeda et al., 2008; Salamat et al., 2011). Transgenic mice that express appropriately trafficked aglycosyl PrP^{C} do not succumb to spontaneous disease, but are susceptible to several strains of prion disease (Neuendorf et al., 2004; Cancellotti et al., 2005). However, data from our laboratories suggest that mice in which glycosylation of PrP^{C} is removed from one or other site, or both, have shown differing susceptibility to certain prion strains (Tuzi et al., 2008). Furthermore, these studies also show that glycosylation on PrP^{C} is not required for strain targeting following intracranial injection but glycosylation of PrP^{C}/PrP^{TSE} may be important for either peripheral replication of PrP^{TSE} or for trafficking of the infection to the CNS (Cancellotti et al., 2010).

There have been several descriptive studies of the sugar structures attached to PrP^{TSE}, to attempt to

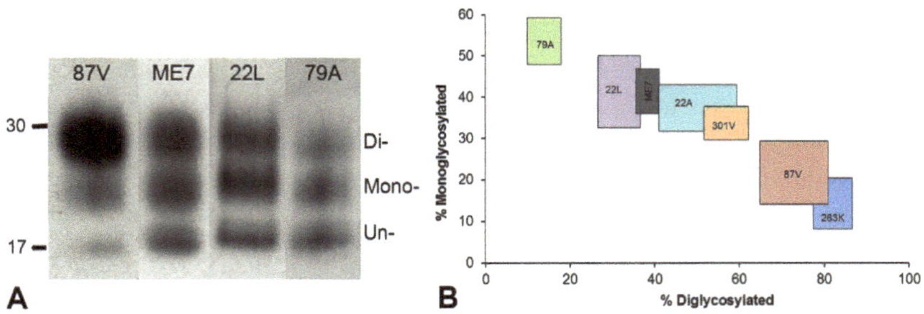

Fig. 2.3. (**A**) Composite Western blot analysis of PrP^{TSE} deposited in mouse brains during the pathogenesis of four different strains of mouse-passaged prion disease. In each case, three bands are seen that correspond to di-, mono-, and unglycosylated PrP^{C}, the different apparent molecular weights reflecting the mass shift caused by glycan addition. The PrP^{TSE} from each strain has subtly different levels of the three glycoforms. (**B**) Quantitation of the relative proportion of each of the three glycoforms of PrP^{TSE} from a range of prion strains. The relative proportion of monoglycosylated PrP^{TSE} is plotted against that of diglycosylated protein. PrP^{TSE} from each strain clusters in a discrete region of the graph.

determine whether the repertoire of structures expressed is different from PrP^{C} or whether PrP^{TSE} from different strains possesses different subsets of sugar chains. Some studies have used low-resolution techniques that report at a population-average level, and have found intriguing effects of glycan sialylation (Katorcha et al., 2014, 2015, 2016a). However, high-resolution work using mass spectrometric and/or high-performance liquid chromatography-based characterization has, thus far, not gone much beyond the initial stages of structure mapping of the different sugars present at each site (Rudd et al., 1999; Stimson et al., 1999; Ritchie et al., 2002), a direct result of the complexity and heterogeneity of the sugars themselves coupled with the comparative difficulty of glycoproteomic analyses. The studies have uncovered some evidence for PrP^{TSE} having a restricted set of glycan chains compared with PrP^{C}, but this subset are also all detected on PrP^{C}, suggesting a deficit in specific glycosyl transferases during prion infection rather than the presence of specific sugars that drive misfolding (Rudd et al., 1999). There are essentially no high-resolution data comparing glycan structures on PrP^{TSE} derived from animals infected with different prion strains.

PrP^{TSE} secondary, tertiary, and quaternary structure

After the conversion of PrP^{C} to PrP^{TSE}, the abnormal form possesses dramatically increased resistance to proteolytic digestion: when PrP^{TSE} is treated with the enzyme proteinase K, the N-terminal region is degraded to approximately residue 90, whilst the C-terminal region is largely preserved, indicating that it is this region that is primarily involved in the misfolding process (Prusiner, 1998). The reasons for the resistance to protease digestion are still not clear, but it presumably results from each protein molecule adopting a compact conformation that is resistant to degradation through steric factors or, more likely, from many protein molecules associating into a morphology that renders protease-susceptible sites inaccessible to proteases. Whilst this suggestion is consistent with antibody epitope exposure, our knowledge is lacking because there currently is no reliable, atomic-level structure(s) for PrP^{TSE}. This deficit results largely from the insolubility of PrP^{TSE}-containing aggregates and their heterogeneity. Techniques that have been used to solve structures of PrP^{C} – or most other proteins for that matter – rely on having high concentrations of soluble protein in a homogeneous conformation and such techniques, therefore, cannot reliably be used to study PrP^{TSE} without extensive, and potentially structurally detrimental, preliminary processing of samples.

By contrast, a range of low- to medium-resolution techniques have been used to probe PrP^{TSE} structure and this area has been the subject of an excellent recent review (Rodriguez et al., 2017). Early studies by Fourier transform infrared (FT-IR) spectroscopy analysis suggested that PrP^{TSE} possessed significantly more β-sheet structure than did PrP^{C}, but that around half of the α-helical content of PrP^{C} was retained during the misfolding to PrP^{TSE} (Caughey et al., 1991). Based on these studies and data from antibody-binding experiments, some model structures for PrP^{TSE} were produced in which the second and third α-helices of PrP^{C} were retained during the conversion process (Peretz et al., 1997; Guest et al., 2011).

Since these beginnings, various different models were produced, based on experimental investigations by electron crystallography (Wille et al., 2002) followed by threading the PrP protein sequence on to a left-handed β-helix (Govaerts et al., 2004) or based on molecular dynamics simulations (DeMarco and Daggett, 2004; Daggett, 2006), but all retained a significant level of helical structure. However, more recent data have cast doubt on whether α-helical sections are present in PrP^{TSE} (Smirnovas et al., 2011). Hydrogen/deuterium exchange rates in PrP^{TSE}, measured by mass spectrometry, are more consistent with β-sheet structure across the entire C-terminal domain (Smirnovas et al., 2009) and reinterpretation of FT-IR spectra agrees with these conclusions (Baron et al., 2011). Although this goes against what has been conventional wisdom of PrP^{TSE} secondary and tertiary structure for several decades, it has allowed novel structural models to be developed that includes a parallel, in register, β-sheet structure (Groveman et al., 2014) that seems to agree, in part, with empiric studies (Cobb et al., 2007, 2008). It is conceivable that there is heterogeneity amongst PrP^{TSE} molecules and that some retain helical sections whilst some do not and in the absence of atomic-level descriptions of the structure(s) of PrP^{TSE} such ambiguity cannot be solved (Rodriguez et al., 2017).

One of the facets of prion disease biology that is challenging to explain in molecular terms is how information is encoded for the multiple prion strains that exist (Bruce, 2003; Morales, 2017). As discussed above, various experiments have explored whether the intricacies of sugar structures might encode such information (Cancellotti et al., 2013), but it is more widely believed that the PrP^{TSE} associated with different prion strains possesses different secondary, tertiary, or quaternary structures (Morales, 2017; Morales et al., 2016). Since we do not have atomic-level detail of PrP^{TSE} structure, these assertions are impossible to verify with any conviction, but a range of indirect evidence supports this. By way of examples, it has been shown that PrP^{TSE} from different strains (1) is digested by proteases at subtly different places in the N-terminal region, suggesting that these regions have differential accessibility to proteases (Gielbert et al., 2009); (2) shows different stability against chaotrope-induced denaturation (Safar et al., 1998); and (3) has different levels of stability against thermal denaturation (Somerville and Gentles, 2011). Whilst "conformational differences" are frequently muted as a cause of these effects, it is equally possible that morphologic differences are driven by the inclusion of other molecules into the amyloid particles (see below) and we will only be clear on how strain properties are manifest at a molecular level when high-resolution structures for the various protein assemblies are available.

Sequence variations

As outlined earlier in this chapter, the human *PRNP* gene is subject to coding mutations that are causally related to development of familial forms of prion disease. Additionally, both humans and other mammals can express *PRNP* alleles that carry polymorphisms and encode amino acid substitutions that impact on susceptibility to an infecting prion disease. Although it is possible that these alterations in the primary structure of PrP^{C} cause instability in the fold (as outlined earlier), more research has been directed towards the hypothesis that amino acid changes promote one or other of the various misfolding pathways open to the protein. For instance, humans can express either methionine or valine at codon 129 and the amino acid present determines susceptibility to variant Creutzfeldt–Jakob disease as well as impacting pathogenesis of other human diseases. In vitro experiments show that human recPrP that incorporates valine at residue 129 fibrillizes significantly more rapidly than protein incorporating methionine (Baskakov et al., 2005), whilst the methionine-containing recPrP forms oligomers more readily (Tahiri-Alaoui et al., 2004). Whilst the mechanistic significance of these observations for disease is not clear, they provide evidence that amino acid changes can dictate the misfolding profile of the protein. Thus, when human PrP^{C} contains an amino acid substitution that causes a prion disease, it is believed that the mutation predisposes the protein to misfold to such an extent that the misfolding cascade is initiated in a carrier within the lifetime of the individual.

In vivo the evidence to support this hypothesis is somewhat contradictory, but the fact that certain transgenic mice expressing PrP-carrying disease-associated mutations succumb to spontaneous disease lends considerably more weight to the argument (Telling et al., 1996; Jackson et al., 2009). However, it must be cautioned that not all such mice accumulate abnormal PrP within their lifetime (Manson et al., 1999) and it is likely that expression levels of PrP^{C} impact on the extent of misfolding, with mice overexpressing wild-type PrP often succumbing to spontaneous neurologic disease driven, apparently, by prion protein misfolding.

Since we have no clear three-dimensional structure for PrP^{TSE}, we also do not know whether amino acid changes in PrP^{C} result in PrP^{TSE} that has different structures, although there is evidence that some human familial diseases produce PrP^{TSE} that possess rather different properties from classic PrP^{TSE} (Piccardo et al., 1998, 2001; Tagliavini et al., 2001). As with other aspects of prion disease pathogenesis, the mechanistic role that amino acid changes play in misfolding is likely to become apparent only when an atomic-level structure for PrP^{TSE} has been determined (Rodriguez et al., 2017).

The function of PrP^{TSE}: are protein aggregates toxic to cells?

Since PrP^{TSE} represents an isoform of the prion protein formed during disease pathogenesis, it is unlikely that it has a "function" in the traditional sense of the word. Presumably it has not evolved to catalyze chemical reactions like enzymes, to play an important role in signal transduction like kinases, nor to provide cellular structural integrity like cytoskeletal proteins. Nevertheless, an important question in prion diseases, and indeed in PMDs in general, is whether the misfolded proteins that are deposited during disease cause the loss of neurons directly. In other words, are these abnormal protein deposits neurotoxic? Does neurotoxicity represent a "gain of function" of PrP^{TSE} during a prion infection and, if so, what molecular mechanisms are involved (Winklhofer et al., 2008; Saa et al., 2016)?

One of the key problems in answering this question using in vivo experimentation is that assays for visualizing abnormal protein deposits are still not sufficiently sensitive. By the time we can detect overt PrP^{TSE} deposition then morphologic alterations to neurons have already taken place. In addition, there is significant morphologic heterogeneity associated with PrP^{TSE} and, as a result, many assays for proteo-toxicity have been undertaken in vitro where protein preparations can be more readily defined, at least to an extent. However, there now exists a variety of animal models of prion infection or PrP misfolding where the correlation between abnormal PrP deposition and prion pathology is less than perfect (Lasmezas et al., 1997; Chesebro et al., 2005; Barron et al., 2007, 2016; Piccardo et al., 2007, 2013; Jeffrey et al., 2012). Such models seem to suggest that classic PrP^{TSE} is neither necessary nor sufficient for prion disease-specific neurodegeneration and recent suspicion has fallen on the surrounding glial cells, the specific activity of which may represent a key switch between neuronal protection and neurodegeneration (Brown and Neher, 2010; Alibhai et al., 2016; Aguzzi and Zhu, 2017; Obst et al., 2017).

In vitro studies often use recPrP isoforms that have been misfolded in the laboratory, but there are many different methods for the preparation of protein aggregates, some or none of which may be physiologically relevant. Consequently, results must be interpreted with caution. Nevertheless, taken together, most molecular studies appear to support the view that prefibrillar, oligomeric protein species are toxic to cells (Bucciantini et al., 2002; Caughey and Lansbury, 2003; Simoneau et al., 2007; Zhang et al., 2010), whether this is oligomers of PrP (Simoneau et al., 2007; Sanghera et al., 2008; Huang et al., 2013) or of other proteins involved in neurodegenerative misfolding diseases (Dahlgren et al., 2002; Gunther and Strittmatter, 2010; Winner et al., 2011; Ugalde et al., 2016). Several studies have also found that fibrillar forms of PrP are toxic to neurons (Novitskaya et al., 2006; Kristiansen et al., 2007; Simoneau et al., 2007), but it is more widely believed that such isoforms are benign and that the formation of large fibrillar deposits is a protective mechanism to remove oligomeric protein (Douglas et al., 2008; Treusch et al., 2009; Marshall et al., 2014; Landreh et al., 2016). A plausible explanation for these apparently conflicting results is that if small, highly toxic oligomers can detach from the inert fibrils of certain morphologies, then the overall process may lead to cellular toxicity.

There is also little consensus on how different protein aggregates cause toxicity. Although there are reports of misfolded proteins – whether PrP or other misfolded proteins – causing cell death through apoptosis (Simoneau et al., 2007; Zhou et al., 2012; Saa et al., 2016), other reports suggest that excitotoxicity is important (Scallet and Ye, 1997; Molinuevo et al., 2005; Biasini et al., 2013; Esposito et al., 2013). Still more highlight ER stress (Doyle et al., 2011; Torres et al., 2015; Mays and Soto, 2016) or autophagy (Christensen et al., 2010; Liberski et al., 2011; Yao et al., 2013; Milisav et al., 2015; Cai et al., 2016; Martini-Stoica et al., 2016) as pathways that initiate the cell death cascade. Oligomeric proteins may physically disrupt membranes, thereby affecting calcium levels within the cell triggering apoptosis (Simoneau et al., 2007), but they may also insert into the phospholipid membrane and act as semiporous ion channels to disrupt the membrane potential (Quist et al., 2005). Since there is a wide variety of preparation methods of misfolded forms of PrP uniformity in approaches is desperately needed and the field generally needs to perform more extensive characterization upon any PrP isoforms prior to incubation with cells or inoculation into animals to reduce inconsistencies in the literature (Urbanc et al., 2002; Caughey and Lansbury, 2003).

Molecular mechanisms of conversion of PrP^C to PrP^{TSE}

Having considered structural and functional aspects of each of the two forms of the prion protein, we turn to how they interconvert. The early ideas of the molecular mechanisms involved in prion diseases were formulated in the "prion hypothesis," which suggested that PrP^{TSE} acts as a template upon which PrP^C misfolds, thereby propagating the structure of the PrP^{TSE} molecule (Prusiner, 1998). The basic premise is outlined in Figure 2.4. It was not until the mid-1990s, when seminal studies demonstrated that mixing immuno-isolated PrP^C with PrP^{TSE} that had been enriched biochemically from prion-infected animal brain in a suitable buffer system caused the PrP^C to take on characteristics of PrP^{TSE}, assayed for by resistance to protease digestion (Kocisko et al., 1994). The procedure was called the cell-free conversion assay and a series of experiments showed that this assay replicated some key details of prion diseases (Kirby et al., 2003), such as species barriers (Kocisko et al., 1995; Raymond et al., 2000), the effects of sequence variations (Bossers et al., 1997, 2000; Kirby et al., 2006), and the inhibitory effects of antiprion compounds (Kocisko et al., 2003).

These experiments provided compelling evidence for the central premise of the prion hypothesis, essentially proving that the presence of PrP^{TSE} (or something that co-purifies with it) instigates the misfolding of PrP^C. It is assumed that either direct or indirect physical interaction between the two protein isoforms is a prerequisite for conformational conversion and there is evidence to support this assumption (Horiuchi and Caughey, 1999; Baron et al., 2002; Solforosi et al., 2007; Taguchi and Schatzl, 2013). However, in some senses molecular models for how the process takes place have not advanced greatly beyond the hypothetic scenarios depicted in Figure 2.4, largely because the structure for PrP^{TSE} remains unknown. Nevertheless, it seems likely that PrP^C binds to a PrP^{TSE} aggregate, after which it is induced to misfold; a partial unfolding of PrP^C to an activated PrP* conformation in advance of its association with PrP^{TSE} may also take place (Gill et al., 2010). Fragmentation of aggregates, thereby generating new "seeds," is also believed to be an important part of the misfolding cascade (Knowles et al., 2009).

Given that PrP^C needs to unfold prior to refolding in a disease-associated conformation, various studies have sought to find factors that enhance PrP^C unfolding. Through combined in vivo, in vitro, and in silico approaches,

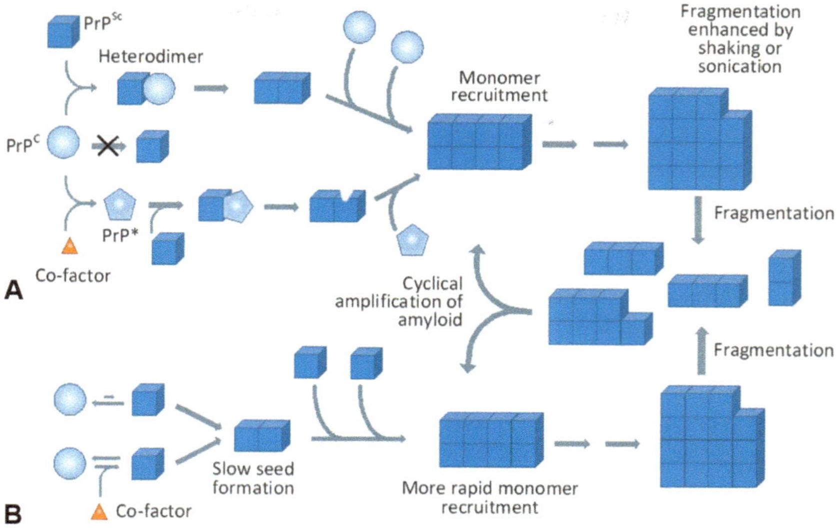

Fig. 2.4. Schematic of different proposed pathways of amyloidogenic protein misfolding (**A**). In this scheme, the interconversion between PrP^C and PrP^{TSE} is separated by a large energy barrier and cannot take place spontaneously. Instead, the interaction between a molecule of PrP^C and a molecule of PrP^{TSE} is required – the formation of this heterodimer catalyzes the conversion of the PrP^C to PrP^{TSE} and subsequent addition of PrP^C molecules creates a large fibril. Alternatively, a cofactor may partially unfold PrP^C to an activated PrP* conformation, which facilitates heterodimer formation. (**B**) An alternative postulated pathway involves PrP^C and PrP^{TSE} existing in an equilibrium that is heavily in favor of the PrP^C conformation. In the unlikely event of two or more PrP^{TSE} monomers coming into contact, they can form a seed, to which additional PrP^{TSE} monomers can add. Cofactors might help this process by shifting the equilibrium of monomers in favor of PrP^{TSE}. In both above pathways, large amyloids can become fragmented, resulting in additional PrP^{TSE} seeds, a process that is believed to be stimulated by shaking or sonication.

the stability of three spatially discrete, but structurally linked, motifs have emerged as candidates to underpin the earliest steps of the conformational conversion:

1. Structural studies have shown that helix 1 is held only loosely to the rest of the PrP^C structure and appears primed to unfold (Speare et al., 2003; Norstrom and Mastrianni, 2006; Tseng et al., 2009; Honda et al., 2014; Chamachi and Chakrabarty, 2017). Since this helix links the two β-strands, the result of this unfolding may be to extend the β-sheet dramatically and initiate the misfolding process.
2. The β2–α2 loop region also appears to be a key motif that can initiate unfolding of PrP^C and hence initiate the misfolding process (Sigurdson et al., 2011). Amino acid substitutions in this region can impact misfolding (Kurt et al., 2014a, b; Agarwal et al., 2015) and this loop forms part of an epitope that might bind molecular effectors of misfolding (Kaneko et al., 1997). The conformation of the loop is affected by the amino acid sequence of distal portions of the protein (Christen et al., 2009).
3. The compact structure of PrP^C is held together partly by a collection of amino acids with aromatic side chains that form the hydrophobic core of the protein (van der Kamp and Daggett, 2010). Molecular dynamics studies have suggested that disruption of this network is a key driver in unfolding of PrP^C prior to misfolding to PrP^{TSE} and the exposure of several hydrophobic amino acids as part of this process may aid intermolecular interactions (Cheng and Daggett, 2014).

These three possibilities are not necessarily mutually exclusive and may converge on a similar outcome (Cheng and Daggett, 2014) . A large body of work also suggests that other molecules help drive the conversion process by binding and destabilizing the native PrP^C fold (Fig. 2.4).

A role for cofactors in conversion

The cell-free conversion assay, described previously, is extremely inefficient and only small amounts of the input PrP^C are converted to a protease-resistant isoform (Kirby et al., 2003). Whilst low conversion rates may reflect what occurs in vivo and explain why prion disease incubation periods are so prolonged, increased efficiency of in vitro conversion can allow more rapid, robust scientific research. In the last decade or so, newer methods of converting PrP^C have been developed that generate significantly higher conversion rates and these methods fall into roughly two categories:

1. techniques that use a buffer system that includes chaotropes (to induce partial unfolding of the protein

substrate) and which also incorporate vigorous shaking, as a source of energy to greatly increase conversion efficiency (Colby et al., 2007; Breydo et al., 2008; Atarashi et al., 2011). These methods typically use natively folded recPrP as a substrate and result in the production of amyloid fibrils, but tend not to model important aspects of prion disease, such as species barriers (Makarava et al., 2007; Orru et al., 2015).

2. techniques that use high-powered sonication as a source of energy, and which use a more physiological buffer system (Saborio et al., 2001). Crucially, these latter methods also include tissue homogenate – typically brain homogenate – as a source of PrP^{C} substrate, but which also includes many other molecules that may assist the conformational transition of PrP^{C} to PrP^{TSE} (Fig. 2.4). These molecules are believed to act as cofactors that facilitate misfolding (Fig. 2.4) (Supattapone, 2014; Wang et al., 2017).

Over several years, the identity of potential cofactors has begun to become apparent and it seems likely that a polyanionic compound (such as glycosaminoglycans or nucleic acid) (Deleault et al., 2003, 2005) coupled with a lipidic environment (Wang et al., 2007; Deleault et al., 2012) promotes a misfolding pathway that is relevant to prion disease (Deleault et al., 2007). Cofactors appear to be an obligatory part of the environment that stimulates disease-specific misfolding, and recent evidence from in vitro misfolding experiments shows that molecules from different brain regions are differentially capable of stimulating PrP misfolding in line with in vivo prion strain-specific tropism, underlining the contribution from none-PrP^{C} molecular subsets in dictating misfolding pathways (Privat et al., 2017).

Indeed, in an appropriate biomolecular environment, recPrP can be induced to misfold, even in the absence of a seed of PrP^{TSE}, into a form that can initiate a prion-like disease after inoculation into naïve animals (Wang et al., 2010). This study, and others that use ex vivo-derived PrP^{TSE} as a template (Weber et al., 2007; Barria et al., 2009; Edgeworth et al., 2010), represent the closest that we have come to proving that misfolded PrP is the infectious agent in prion disease, but even if recPrP can be induced to form abnormal conformations in vitro in the presence of partially defined cofactors, the identities of the molecules playing this role in vivo are still elusive. Analysis of PrP^{TSE} preparations ex vivo, aimed at determining whether cofactors are integrated into the protein structures, has detected few molecules that might be potential cofactors; some proteins appear regularly to co-purify (Moore et al., 2010; Graham et al., 2011), but this may be because they have similar biochemical properties to PrP^{TSE}. In addition, an inert polysaccharide with structural similarity to glycogen has been suggested to be a constituent of PrP^{TSE} assemblies (Appel et al., 1999; Dumpitak et al., 2005) and trace amounts of two sphingolipids have been detected (Klein et al., 1998). Such molecules may represent the elusive cofactors, but still need complete characterization.

Do biochemical properties of PrP^{TSE} make prion diseases transmissible?

This chapter would be incomplete without considering briefly whether there are protein structural factors that might explain why prion diseases are transmissible in ways that other PMDs are not. A large body of work now exists to show that pathogenesis of other PMDs involves mechanisms that are highly similar to those involved in prion diseases (Lundmark et al., 2002; Meyer-Luehmann et al., 2006; Bolmont et al., 2007; Kordower et al., 2008; Li et al., 2008; Desplats et al., 2009; Eisele et al., 2009; Krammer et al., 2009; Sydow and Mandelkow, 2010; Grad et al., 2011; Guo and Lee, 2011; Munch et al., 2011), including template-associated misfolding of endogenous proteins, cell-to-cell spread of protein aggregates (Frost and Diamond, 2010), spatial targeting of neuronal loss and, in some cases, even the existence of distinct "strains" of pathologic proteins (Watts et al., 2014; Peelaerts et al., 2015). There are now a large number of reports of the initiation of the misfolding cascade of proteins (α-synuclein, Aβ, tau, etc.) in animals following the inoculation of preformed protein aggregates either intracranially or by peripheral administration. These results suggest that experimental "transmissibility" might be a generic property of protein aggregates, but thus far only prion diseases show natural transmission to wild-type animals and can justifiably be categorized as infectious diseases. Are there biochemical aspects of prion protein structure and/or function that explain why this is so? The simple answer is that it does not appear so.

Structurally, PrP^{C} is not particularly unusual – as outlined above, it has partially unstructured regions and a partially asparagine/glutamine-rich region, both of which do seem to lend themselves to misfolding, but such features are also common in other prion-like domains (Paul and Ross, 2015; Zambrano et al., 2015) and cannot reasonably account for the infectivity associated with PrP aggregates. Equally, what little we know of the structure of PrP^{TSE} suggests that it is rather typical of amyloid, with a cross-β core, which is common to fibrillar structures of other proteins (Chiti and Dobson, 2017). A potential key difference between the prion protein and other proteins involved in misfolding diseases relates to cellular expression profiles and cell biology of PrP^{C}, which is covered elsewhere in this book. It seems likely that the natural infectivity of prion diseases is governed by the ability of PrP^{TSE} to be secreted from individuals in biomaterials that are then capable of being taken up readily by naïve individuals. Potential examples of infected materials that are released by animals and that have been shown to harbor prion infectivity include saliva, urine, or blood (see, for example, Shaked et al., 2001; Haley et al., 2011; McCutcheon et al., 2011). There is currently little evidence for the presence of "infectious" assemblies of Aβ, α-synuclein, or SOD1 (for example) in such bodily secretions, even in individuals at terminal stages of disease.

After ingestion of infected tissues, prion infection also seems to be trafficked across the intestinal endothelium relatively readily (Da Costa Dias et al., 2011; Donaldson et al., 2015) where cells of the immune system, including follicular dendritic cells (Bruce et al., 2000; McCulloch et al., 2011), seem to be competent at amplifying PrP^{TSE}, thereby kick-starting the neuroinvasion cascade. It is not clear to what extent aggregates of other proteins can be translocated across the wall of the intestine and, if they are, whether the awaiting immune cells replicate these aggregates as opposed to destroying them. The field of prion-like mechanisms is still developing apace and it is reasonable to expect us to know why prions are infectious whilst other PMDs are not in the coming decade.

ACKNOWLEDGMENTS

ACG was funded, partly, through an Institute Strategic Programme Grant to the Roslin Institute from the Biotechnology and Biological Sciences Research Council (BBSRC), United Kingdom. ARC was funded by a doctoral training grant from BBSRC, United Kingdom. We thank Dr. Sandra McCutcheon for critical comments on the manuscript and Dr. James F. Graham for providing the Western blot images featured in Figure 2.3.

References

Adle-Biassette H, Verney C, Peoc'h K et al. (2006). Immunohistochemical expression of prion protein (PrPC) in the human forebrain during development. J Neuropathol Exp Neurol 65: 698–706.

Agarwal S, Doring K, Gierusz LA et al. (2015). Complex folding and misfolding effects of deer-specific amino acid substitutions in the beta2-alpha2 loop of murine prion protein. Sci Rep 5: 15528.

Aguzzi A, Zhu C (2017). Microglia in prion diseases. J Clin Invest 127: 3230–3239.

Alfaidy N, Chauvet S, Donadio-Andrei S et al. (2013). Prion protein expression and functional importance in developmental angiogenesis: role in oxidative stress and copper homeostasis. Antioxid Redox Signal 18: 400–411.

Alibhai J, Blanco RA, Barria MA et al. (2016). Distribution of misfolded prion protein seeding activity alone does not predict regions of neurodegeneration. PLoS Biol 14: e1002579.

Allison WT, DuVal MG, Nguyen-Phuoc K et al. (2017). Reduced abundance and subverted functions of proteins in prion-like diseases: gained functions fascinate but lost functions affect aetiology. Int J Mol Sci: 18.

Antonyuk SV, Trevitt CR, Strange RW et al. (2009). Crystal structure of human prion protein bound to a therapeutic antibody. Proc Natl Acad Sci U S A 106: 2554–2558.

Apetri AC, Surewicz K, Surewicz WK (2004). The effect of disease-associated mutations on the folding pathway of human prion protein. J Biol Chem 279: 18008–18014.

Appel TR, Dumpitak C, Matthiesen U et al. (1999). Prion rods contain an inert polysaccharide scaffold. Biol Chem 380: 1295–1306.

Arora AS, Zafar S, Schmitz M et al. (2013). Differential proteome analysis of cytoskeleton associated proteins in the liver of PrP knockout mice. Prion 7: 69.

Atarashi R, Sano K, Satoh K et al. (2011). Real-time quaking-induced conversion: a highly sensitive assay for prion detection. Prion 5: 150–153.

Bae SH, Legname G, Serban A et al. (2009). Prion proteins with pathogenic and protective mutations show similar structure and dynamics. Biochemistry 48: 8120–8128.

Bakkebo MK, Mouillet-Richard S, Espenes A et al. (2015). The cellular prion protein: a player in immunological quiescence. Front Immunol 6: 450.

Baron GS, Wehrly K, Dorward DW et al. (2002). Conversion of raft associated prion protein to the protease-resistant state requires insertion of PrP-res (PrP(Sc)) into contiguous membranes. EMBO J 21: 1031–1040.

Baron GS, Hughson AG, Raymond GJ et al. (2011). Effect of glycans and the glycophosphatidylinositol anchor on strain dependent conformations of scrapie prion protein: improved purifications and infrared spectra. Biochemistry 50: 4479–4490.

Barria MA, Mukherjee A, Gonzalez-Romero D et al. (2009). De novo generation of infectious prions in vitro produces a new disease phenotype. PLoS Pathog 5: e1000421.

Barron RM, Campbell SL, King D et al. (2007). High titers of transmissible spongiform encephalopathy infectivity associated with extremely low levels of PrPSc in vivo. J Biol Chem 282: 35878–35886.

Barron RM, King D, Jeffrey M et al. (2016). PrP aggregation can be seeded by pre-formed recombinant PrP amyloid fibrils without the replication of infectious prions. Acta Neuropathol 132: 611–624.

Baskakov IV, Katorcha E (2016). Multifaceted role of sialylation in prion diseases. Front Neurosci 10: 358.

Baskakov I, Disterer P, Breydo L et al. (2005). The presence of valine at residue 129 in human prion protein accelerates amyloid formation. FEBS Lett 579: 2589–2596.

Basler K, Oesch B, Scott M et al. (1986). Scrapie and cellular PRP isoforms are encoded by the same chromosomal gene. Cell 46: 417–428.

Bate C, Nolan W, McHale-Owen H et al. (2016a). Sialic acid within the glycosylphosphatidylinositol anchor targets the cellular prion protein to synapses. J Biol Chem 291: 17093–17101.

Bate C, Nolan W, Williams A (2016b). Does the tail wag the dog? How the structure of a glycosylphosphatidylinositol anchor affects prion formation. Prion 10: 127–130.

Bate C, Nolan W, Williams A (2016c). Sialic acid on the glycosylphosphatidylinositol anchor regulates PrP-mediated cell signaling and prion formation. J Biol Chem 291: 160–170.

Beland M, Motard J, Barbarin A et al. (2012). PrPC homodimerization stimulates the production of PrPC cleaved fragments PrPN1 and PrPC1. J Neurosci 32: 13255–13263.

Beraldo FH, Arantes CP, Santos TG et al. (2011). Metabotropic glutamate receptors transduce signals for neurite outgrowth after binding of the prion protein to laminin gamma 1 chain. FASEB J 25: 265–279.

Bertuchi FR, Bourgeon DM, Landemberger MC et al. (2012). PrPC displays an essential protective role from oxidative stress in an astrocyte cell line derived from PrPC knockout mice. Biochem Biophys Res Commun 418: 27–32.

Biasini E, Unterberger U, Solomon IH et al. (2013). A mutant prion protein sensitizes neurons to glutamate-induced excitotoxicity. J Neurosci 33: 2408–2418.

Blanch EW, Gill AC, Rhie AGO et al. (2004). Raman optical activity demonstrates poly(L-proline) II helix in the N-terminal region of the ovine prion protein: implications for function and misfunction. J Mol Biol 343: 467–476.

Bolmont T, Clavaguera F, Meyer-Luehmann M et al. (2007). Induction of tau pathology by intracerebral infusion of amyloid-beta-containing brain extract and by amyloid-beta deposition in APP x Tau transgenic mice. Am J Pathol 171: 2012–2020.

Bossers A, Belt P, Raymond GJ et al. (1997). Scrapie susceptibility-linked polymorphisms modulate the in vitro conversion of sheep prion protein to protease-resistant forms. Proc Natl Acad Sci U S A 94: 4931–4936.

Bossers A, de Vries R, Smits MA et al. (2000). Susceptibility of sheep for scrapie as assessed by in vitro conversion of nine naturally occurring variants of PrP. J Virol 74: 1407–1414.

Bravard A, Auvre F, Fantini D et al. (2015). The prion protein is critical for DNA repair and cell survival after genotoxic stress. Nucleic Acids Res 43: 904–916.

Bremer J, Baumann F, Tiberi C et al. (2010). Axonal prion protein is required for peripheral myelin maintenance. Nat Neurosci 13: 310–U319.

Breydo L, Makarava N, Baskakov IV (2008). Methods for conversion of prion protein into amyloid fibrils. Methods Mol Biol 459: 105–115.

Bribian A, Fontana X, Llorens F et al. (2012). Role of the cellular prion protein in oligodendrocyte precursor cell proliferation and differentiation in the developing and adult mouse CNS. PLoS One: 7.

Brown DR, Mohn CM (1999). Astrocytic glutamate uptake and prion protein expression. Glia 25: 282–292.

Brown GC, Neher JJ (2010). Inflammatory neurodegeneration and mechanisms of microglial killing of neurons. Mol Neurobiol 41: 242–247.

Brown DR, Qin K, Herms JW et al. (1997). The cellular prion protein binds copper in vivo. Nature 390: 684–687.

Brown DR, Guantieri V, Grasso G et al. (2004). Copper(II) complexes of peptide fragments of the prion protein. Conformation changes induced by copper(II) and the binding motif in C-terminal protein region. J Inorg Biochem 98: 133–143.

Bruce ME (2003). TSE strain variation. Br Med Bull 66: 99–108.

Bruce ME, Brown KL, Mabbott NA et al. (2000). Follicular dendritic cells in TSE pathogenesis. Immunol Today 21: 442–446.

Bucciantini M, Giannoni E, Chiti F et al. (2002). Inherent toxicity of aggregates implies a common mechanism for protein misfolding diseases. Nature 416: 507–511.

Bueler H, Fischer M, Lang Y et al. (1992). Normal development and behaviour of mice lacking the neuronal cell-surface PrP protein. Nature 356: 577–582.

Bueler H, Aguzzi A, Sailer A et al. (1993). Mice devoid of PrP are resistant to scrapie. Cell 73: 1339–1347.

Bujdoso R, Burke DF, Thackray AM (2005). Structural differences between allelic variants of the ovine prion protein revealed by molecular dynamics simulations. Proteins 61: 840–849.

Caetano FA, Lopes MH, Hajj GNM et al. (2008). Endocytosis of prion protein is required for ERK1/2 signaling induced by stress-inducible protein 1. J Neurosci 28: 6691–6702.

Cai Y, Arikkath J, Yang L et al. (2016). Interplay of endoplasmic reticulum stress and autophagy in neurodegenerative disorders. Autophagy 12: 225–244.

Caldarulo E, Barducci A, Wuthrich K et al. (2017). Prion protein beta2-alpha2 loop conformational landscape. Proc Natl Acad Sci U S A 114: 9617–9622.

Calzolai L, Lysek DA, Perez DR et al. (2005). Prion protein NMR structures of chickens, turtles, and frogs. Proc Natl Acad Sci U S A 102: 651–655.

Cancellotti E, Wiseman F, Tuzi NL et al. (2005). Altered glycosylated PrP proteins can have different neuronal trafficking in brain but do not acquire scrapie-like properties. J Biol Chem 280: 42909–42918.

Cancellotti E, Bradford BM, Tuzi NL et al. (2010). Glycosylation of PrPC determines timing of neuroinvasion and targeting in the brain following transmissible spongiform encephalopathy infection by a peripheral route. J Virol 84: 3464–3475.

Cancellotti E, Mahal SP, Somerville R et al. (2013). Post-translational changes to PrP alter transmissible spongiform encephalopathy strain properties. EMBO J 32: 756–769.

Capellari S, Zaidi SI, Long AC et al. (2000). The Thr183Ala mutation, not the loss of the first glycosylation site, alters the physical properties of the prion protein. J Alzheimers Dis 2: 27–35.

Carulla P, Bribian A, Rangel A et al. (2011). Neuroprotective role of PrPC against kainate-induced epileptic seizures and cell death depends on the modulation of JNK3 activation by GluR6/7-PSD-95 binding. Mol Biol Cell 22: 3041–3054.

Carulla P, Llorens F, Matamoros-Angles A et al. (2015). Involvement of PrP(C) in kainate-induced excitotoxicity in several mouse strains. Sci Rep 5: 11971.

Castle AR, Gill AC (2017). Physiological functions of the cellular prion protein. Front Mol Biosci 4: 19.

Caughey B, Lansbury PT (2003). Protofibrils, pores, fibrils, and neurodegeneration: separating the responsible protein aggregates from the innocent bystanders. Annu Rev Neurosci 26: 267–298.

Caughey BW, Dong A, Bhat KS et al. (1991). Secondary structure analysis of the scrapie-associated protein PrP 27-30 in water by infrared spectroscopy. Biochemistry 30: 7672–7680.

Caughey B, Baron GS, Chesebro B et al. (2009). Getting a grip on prions: oligomers, amyloids, and pathological membrane interactions. Annu Rev Biochem 78: 177–204.

Chamachi NG, Chakrabarty S (2017). Temperature-induced misfolding in prion protein: evidence of multiple partially disordered states stabilized by non-native hydrogen bonds. Biochemistry 56: 833–844.

Chen SG, Teplow DB, Parchi P et al. (1995). Truncated forms of the human prion protein in normal brain and in prion diseases. J Biol Chem 270: 19173–19180.

Cheng CJ, Daggett V (2014). Different misfolding mechanisms converge on common conformational changes: human prion protein pathogenic mutants Y218N and E196K. Prion 8: 125–135.

Chesebro B, Trifilo M, Race R et al. (2005). Anchorless prion protein results in infectious amyloid disease without clinical scrapie. Science 308: 1435–1439.

Chiti F, Dobson CM (2017). Protein misfolding, amyloid formation, and human disease: a summary of progress over the last decade. Annu Rev Biochem 86: 27–68.

Christen B, Perez DR, Hornemann S et al. (2008). NMR structure of the bank vole prion protein at 20 degrees C contains a structured loop of residues 165-171. J Mol Biol 383: 306–312.

Christen B, Hornemann S, Damberger FF et al. (2009). Prion protein NMR structure from tammar wallaby (*Macropus eugenii*) shows that the beta2-alpha2 loop is modulated by long-range sequence effects. J Mol Biol 389: 833–845.

Christen B, Damberger FF, Perez DR et al. (2013). Structural plasticity of the cellular prion protein and implications in health and disease. Proc Natl Acad Sci U S A 110: 8549–8554.

Christensen HM, Dikranian K, Li A et al. (2010). A highly toxic cellular prion protein induces a novel, nonapoptotic form of neuronal death. Am J Pathol 176: 2695–2706.

Cichon A-C, Brown DR (2014). Nrf-2 regulation of prion protein expression is independent of oxidative stress. Mol Cell Neurosci 63: 31–37.

Ciric D, Rezaei H (2015). Biochemical insight into the prion protein family. Front Cell Dev Biol 3: 5.

Cisse MA, Louis K, Braun U et al. (2008). Isoform-specific contribution of protein kinase C to prion processing. Mol Cell Neurosci 39: 400–410.

Cobb NJ, Sonnichsen FD, Mchaourab H et al. (2007). Molecular architecture of human prion protein amyloid: a parallel, in-register beta-structure. Proc Natl Acad Sci U S A 104: 18946–18951.

Cobb NJ, Apetri AC, Surewicz WK (2008). Prion protein amyloid formation under native-like conditions involves refolding of the C-terminal alpha-helical domain. J Biol Chem 283: 34704–34711.

Colby DW, Zhang Q, Wang S et al. (2007). Prion detection by an amyloid seeding assay. Proc Natl Acad Sci U S A 104: 20914–20919.

Da Costa Dias B, Jovanovic K, Weiss SF (2007). Alimentary prion infections: touchdown in the intestine. Prion 5: 6–9.

Daggett V (2006). Alpha-sheet: The toxic conformer in amyloid diseases? Acc Chem Res 39: 594–602.

Dahlgren KN, Manelli AM, Stine Jr WB et al. (2002). Oligomeric and fibrillar species of amyloid-beta peptides differentially affect neuronal viability. J Biol Chem 277: 32046–32053.

DeArmond SJ, Sanchez H, Yehiely F et al. (1997). Selective neuronal targeting in prion disease. Neuron 19: 1337–1348.

Deleault NR, Lucassen RW, Supattapone S (2003). RNA molecules stimulate prion protein conversion. Nature 425: 717–720.

Deleault NR, Geoghegan JC, Nishina K et al. (2005). Protease-resistant prion protein amplification reconstituted with partially purified substrates and synthetic polyanions. J Biol Chem 280: 26873–26879.

Deleault NR, Harris BT, Rees JR et al. (2007). Formation of native prions from minimal components in vitro. Proc Natl Acad Sci U S A 104: 9741–9746.

Deleault NR, Piro JR, Walsh DJ et al. (2012). Isolation of phosphatidylethanolamine as a solitary cofactor for prion formation in the absence of nucleic acids. Proc Natl Acad Sci U S A 109: 8546–8551.

DeMarco ML, Daggett V (2004). From conversion to aggregation: protofibril formation of the prion protein. Proc Natl Acad Sci U S A 101: 2293–2298.

Dery MA, Jodoin J, Ursini-Siegel J et al. (2013). Endoplasmic reticulum stress induces PRNP prion protein gene expression in breast cancer. Breast Cancer Res 15: R22.

Desplats P, Lee HJ, Bae EJ et al. (2009). Inclusion formation and neuronal cell death through neuron-to-neuron transmission of alpha-synuclein. Proc Natl Acad Sci U S A 106: 13010–13015.

Donaldson DS, Else KJ, Mabbott NA (2015). The gut-associated lymphoid tissues in the small intestine, not the large intestine, play a major role in oral prion disease pathogenesis. J Virol 89: 9532–9547.

Donne DG, Viles JH, Groth D et al. (1997). Structure of the recombinant full-length hamster prion protein PrP(29-231): the N terminus is highly flexible. Proc Natl Acad Sci U S A 94: 13452–13457.

Douglas PM, Treusch S, Ren HY et al. (2008). Chaperone-dependent amyloid assembly protects cells from prion toxicity. Proc Natl Acad Sci U S A 105: 7206–7211.

Doyle KM, Kennedy D, Gorman AM et al. (2011). Unfolded proteins and endoplasmic reticulum stress in neurodegenerative disorders. J Cell Mol Med 15: 2025–2039.

Dumpitak C, Beekes M, Weinmann N et al. (2005). The polysaccharide scaffold of PrP 27-30 is a common compound of natural prions and consists of alpha-linked polyglucose. Biol Chem 386: 1149–1155.

Durig J, Giese A, Schulz-Schaeffer W et al. (2000). Differential constitutive and activation-dependent expression of prion protein in human peripheral blood leucocytes. Br J Haematol 108: 488–496.

Edgeworth JA, Gros N, Alden J et al. (2010). Spontaneous generation of mammalian prions. Proc Natl Acad Sci U S A 107: 14402–14406.

Eghiaian F, Grosclaude J, Lesceu S et al. (2004). Insight into the PrPC–>PrPSc conversion from the structures of antibody-bound ovine prion scrapie-susceptibility variants. Proc Natl Acad Sci U S A 101: 10254–10259.

Eisele YS, Bolmont T, Heikenwalder M et al. (2009). Induction of cerebral beta-amyloidosis: intracerebral versus systemic Abeta inoculation. Proc Natl Acad Sci U S A 106: 12926–12931.

Esposito Z, Belli L, Toniolo S et al. (2013). Amyloid beta, glutamate, excitotoxicity in Alzheimer's disease: are we on the right track? CNS Neurosci Ther 19: 549–555.

Follet J, Lemaire-Vieille C, Blanquet-Grossard F et al. (2002). PrP expression and replication by Schwann cells: implications in prion spreading. J Virol 76: 2434–2439.

Frost B, Diamond MI (2010). Prion-like mechanisms in neurodegenerative diseases. Nat Rev Neurosci 11: 155–159.

Ganley RP, Iwagaki N, del Rio P et al. (2015). Inhibitory interneurons that express GFP in the PrP-GFP mouse spinal cord are morphologically heterogeneous, innervated by several classes of primary afferent and include lamina I projection neurons among their postsynaptic targets. J Neurosci 35: 7626–7642.

Gasperini L, Meneghetti E, Pastore B et al. (2015). Prion protein and copper cooperatively protect neurons by modulating NMDA receptor through S-nitrosylation. Antioxid Redox Signal 22: 772–784.

Gielbert A, Davis LA, Sayers AR et al. (2009). High-resolution differentiation of transmissible spongiform encephalopathy strains by quantitative N-terminal amino acid profiling (N-TAAP) of PK-digested abnormal prion protein. J Mass Spectrom 44: 384–396.

Gill AC, Ritchie MA, Hunt LG et al. (2000). Post-translational hydroxylation at the N-terminus of the prion protein reveals presence of PPII structure in vivo. EMBO J 19: 5324–5331.

Gill AC, Agarwal S, Pinheiro TJ et al. (2010). Structural requirements for efficient prion protein conversion: cofactors may promote a conversion-competent structure for PrP(C). Prion 4: 235–242.

Gossert AD, Bonjour S, Lysek DA et al. (2005). Prion protein NMR structures of elk and of mouse/elk hybrids. Proc Natl Acad Sci U S A 102: 646–650.

Govaerts C, Wille H, Prusiner SB et al. (2004). Evidence for assembly of prions with left-handed beta-helices into trimers. Proc Natl Acad Sci U S A 101: 8342–8347.

Grad LI, Guest WC, Yanai A et al. (2011). Intermolecular transmission of superoxide dismutase 1 misfolding in living cells. Proc Natl Acad Sci U S A 108: 16398–16403.

Graham JF, Kurian D, Agarwal S et al. (2011). Na+/K+-ATPase is present in scrapie-associated fibrils, modulates PrP misfolding in vitro and links PrP function and dysfunction. PLoS One 6: e26813.

Groveman BR, Dolan MA, Taubner LM et al. (2014). Parallel in-register intermolecular beta-sheet architectures for prion-seeded prion protein (PrP) amyloids. J Biol Chem 289: 24129–24142.

Guest WC, Plotkin SS, Cashman NR (2011). Toward a mechanism of prion misfolding and structural models of PrP(Sc): current knowledge and future directions. J Toxicol Environ Health A 74: 154–160.

Gunther EC, Strittmatter SM (2010). Beta-amyloid oligomers and cellular prion protein in Alzheimer's disease. J Mol Med (Berl) 88: 331–338.

Guo JL, Lee VM (2011). Seeding of normal tau by pathological tau conformers drives pathogenesis of Alzheimer-like tangles. J Biol Chem 286: 15317–15331.

Haddon DJ, Hughes MR, Antignano F et al. (2009). Prion protein expression and release by mast cells after activation. J Infect Dis 200: 827–831.

Hafner-Bratkovic I, Bester R, Pristovsek P et al. (2011). Globular domain of the prion protein needs to be unlocked by domain swapping to support prion protein conversion. J Biol Chem 286: 12149–12156.

Haire LF, Whyte SM, Vasisht N et al. (2004). The crystal structure of the globular domain of sheep prion protein. J Mol Biol 336: 1175–1183.

Haldar S, Tripathi A, Qian J et al. (2015). Prion protein promotes kidney iron uptake via its ferrireductase activity. J Biol Chem 290: 5512–5522.

Haley NJ, Mathiason CK, Carver S et al. (2011). Detection of chronic wasting disease prions in salivary, urinary, and intestinal tissues of deer: potential mechanisms of prion shedding and transmission. J Virol 85: 6309–6318.

Haraguchi T, Fisher S, Olofsson S et al. (1989). Asparagine-linked glycosylation of the scrapie and cellular prion proteins. Arch Biochem Biophys 274: 1–13.

Harris DA, Huber MT, Vandijken P et al. (1993). Processing of a cellular prion protein - identification of N-terminal and C-terminal cleavage sites. Biochemistry 32: 1009–1016.

Hartmann CA, Martins VR, Lima FRS (2013). High levels of cellular prion protein improve astrocyte development. FEBS Lett 587: 238–244.

Hegde RS, Mastrianni JA, Scott MR et al. (1998). A transmembrane form of the prion protein in neurodegenerative disease. Science 279: 827–834.

Herrmann LM, Caughey B (1998). The importance of the disulfide bond in prion protein conversion. Neuroreport 9: 2457–2461.

Honda RP, Yamaguchi K, Kuwata K (2014). Acid-induced molten globule state of a prion protein: crucial role of strand 1-helix 1-strand 2 segment. J Biol Chem 289: 30355–30363.

Horiuchi M, Caughey B (1999). Specific binding of normal prion protein to the scrapie form via a localized domain initiates its conversion to the protease-resistant state. EMBO J 18: 3193–3203.

Hornemann S, Schorn C, Wuthrich K (2004). NMR structure of the bovine prion protein isolated from healthy calf brains. EMBO Rep 5: 1159–1164.

Hornshaw MP, McDermott JR, Candy JM (1995a). Copper-binding to the N-terminal tandem repeat regions of mammalian and avian prion protein. Biochem Biophys Res Commun 207: 621–629.

Hornshaw MP, McDermott JR, Candy JM et al. (1995b). Copper-binding to the N-terminal tandem repeat region of mammalian and avian prion protein - structural studies using synthetic peptides. Biochem Biophys Res Commun 214: 993–999.

Huang P, Lian F, Wen Y et al. (2013). Prion protein oligomer and its neurotoxicity. Acta Biochim Biophys Sin Shanghai 45: 442–451.

Ikeda S, Kobayashi A, Kitamoto T (2008). Thr but Asn of the N-glycosylation sites of PrP is indispensable for its misfolding. Biochem Biophys Res Commun 369: 1195–1198.

Inouye H, Bond J, Baldwin MA et al. (2000). Structural changes in a hydrophobic domain of the prion protein induced by hydration and by ala–>Val and pro–>Leu substitutions. J Mol Biol 300: 1283–1296.

Jackson GS, Hill AF, Joseph C et al. (1999). Multiple folding pathways for heterologously expressed human prion protein. Biochim Biophys Acta 1431: 1–13.

Jackson WS, Borkowski AW, Faas H et al. (2009). Spontaneous generation of prion infectivity in fatal familial insomnia knockin mice. Neuron 63: 438–450.

James TL, Liu H, Ulyanov NB et al. (1997). Solution structure of a 142-residue recombinant prion protein corresponding to the infectious fragment of the scrapie isoform. Proc Natl Acad Sci U S A 94: 10086–10091.

Jeffrey M, McGovern G, Chambers EV et al. (2012). Mechanism of PrP-amyloid formation in mice without transmissible spongiform encephalopathy. Brain Pathol 22: 58–66.

Kaneko K, Zulianello L, Scott M et al. (1997). Evidence for protein X binding to a discontinuous epitope on the cellular prion protein during scrapie prion propagation. Proc Natl Acad Sci U S A 94: 10069–10074.

Katorcha E, Makarava N, Savtchenko R et al. (2014). Sialylation of prion protein controls the rate of prion amplification, the cross-species barrier, the ratio of PrPSc glycoform and prion infectivity. PLoS Pathog 10: e1004366.

Katorcha E, Makarava N, Savtchenko R et al. (2015). Sialylation of the prion protein glycans controls prion replication rate and glycoform ratio. Sci Rep 5: 16912.

Katorcha E, Daus ML, Gonzalez-Montalban N et al. (2016a). Reversible off and on switching of prion infectivity via removing and reinstalling prion sialylation. Sci Rep 6: 33119.

Katorcha E, Srivastava S, Klimova N et al. (2016b). Sialylation of glycosylphosphatidylinositol (GPI) anchors of mammalian prions is regulated in a host-, tissue-, and cell-specific manner. J Biol Chem 291: 17009–17019.

Khan MQ, Sweeting B, Mulligan VK et al. (2010). Prion disease susceptibility is affected by beta-structure folding propensity and local side-chain interactions in PrP. Proc Natl Acad Sci U S A 107: 19808–19813.

Khosravani H, Zhang YF, Tsutsui S et al. (2008). Prion protein attenuates excitotoxicity by inhibiting NMDA receptors. J Cell Biol 181: 551–565.

Kim BH, Lee HG, Choi JK et al. (2004). The cellular prion protein (PrPC) prevents apoptotic neuronal cell death and mitochondrial dysfunction induced by serum deprivation. Brain Res Mol Brain Res 124: 40–50.

Kim BH, Kim JI, Choi EK et al. (2005). A neuronal cell line that does not express either prion or Doppel proteins. Neuroreport 16: 425–429.

Kirby L, Birkett CR, Rudyk H et al. (2003). In vitro cell-free conversion of bacterial recombinant PrP to PrPres as a model for conversion. J Gen Virol 84: 1013–1020.

Kirby L, Goldmann W, Houston F et al. (2006). A novel, resistance-linked ovine PrP variant and its equivalent mouse variant modulate the in vitro cell-free conversion of rPrP to PrP(res). J Gen Virol 87: 3747–3751.

Kirby L, Agarwal S, Graham JF et al. (2010). Inverse correlation of thermal lability and conversion efficiency for five prion protein polymorphic variants. Biochemistry 49: 1448–1459.

Kleene R, Loers G, Langer J et al. (2007). Prion protein regulates glutamate-dependent lactate transport of Astrocytes. J Neurosci 27: 12331–12340.

Klein TR, Kirsch D, Kaufmann R et al. (1998). Prion rods contain small amounts of two host sphingolipids as revealed by thin-layer chromatography and mass spectrometry. Biol Chem 379: 655–666.

Knaus KJ, Morillas M, Swietnicki W et al. (2001). Crystal structure of the human prion protein reveals a mechanism for oligomerization. Nat Struct Biol 8: 770–774.

Knowles TP, Waudby CA, Devlin GL et al. (2009). An analytical solution to the kinetics of breakable filament assembly. Science 326: 1533–1537.

Kocisko DA, Come JH, Priola SA et al. (1994). Cell-free formation of protease-resistant prion protein. Nature 370: 471–474.

Kocisko DA, Priola SA, Raymond GJ et al. (1995). Species specificity in the cell-free conversion of prion protein to protease-resistant forms: a model for the scrapie species barrier. Proc Natl Acad Sci U S A 92: 3923–3927.

Kocisko DA, Baron GS, Rubenstein R et al. (2003). New inhibitors of scrapie-associated prion protein formation in a library of 2000 drugs and natural products. J Virol 77: 10288–10294.

Kordower JH, Chu Y, Hauser RA et al. (2008). Lewy body-like pathology in long-term embryonic nigral transplants in Parkinson's disease. Nat Med 14: 504–506.

Krammer C, Schatzl HM, Vorberg I (2009). Prion-like propagation of cytosolic protein aggregates: insights from cell culture models. Prion 3: 206–212.

Kristiansen M, Deriziotis P, Dimcheff DE et al. (2007). Disease-associated prion protein oligomers inhibit the 26S proteasome. Mol Cell 26: 175–188.

Kuffer A, Lakkaraju AK, Mogha A et al. (2016). The prion protein is an agonistic ligand of the G protein-coupled receptor Adgrg6. Nature 536: 464–468.

Kurt TD, Bett C, Fernandez-Borges N et al. (2014a). Prion transmission prevented by modifying the beta2-alpha2 loop structure of host PrPC. J Neurosci 34: 1022–1027.

Kurt TD, Jiang L, Bett C et al. (2014b). A proposed mechanism for the promotion of prion conversion involving a strictly conserved tyrosine residue in the beta2-alpha2 loop of PrPC. J Biol Chem 289: 10660–10667.

Kuwahara C, Kubosaki A, Nishimura T et al. (2000). Enhanced expression of cellular prion protein gene by insulin or nerve growth factor in immortalized mouse neuronal precursor cell lines. Biochem Biophys Res Commun 268: 763–766.

Laffont-Proust I, Hassig R, Haik S et al. (2006). Truncated PrPc in mammalian brain: interspecies variation and location in membrane rafts. Biol Chem 387: 297–300.

Landreh M, Sawaya MR, Hipp MS et al. (2016). The formation, function and regulation of amyloids: insights from structural biology. J Intern Med 280: 164–176.

Lasmezas CI, Deslys JP, Robain O et al. (1997). Transmission of the BSE agent to mice in the absence of detectable abnormal prion protein. Science 275: 402–405.

Lee YJ, Baskakov IV (2014). The cellular form of the prion protein guides the differentiation of human embryonic stem cells into neuron-, oligodendrocyte-, and astrocyte-committed lineages. Prion 8: 266–275.

Lee S, Antony L, Hartmann R et al. (2010). Conformational diversity in prion protein variants influences intermolecular beta-sheet formation. EMBO J 29: 251–262.

Lehmann S, Harris DA (1997). Blockade of glycosylation promotes acquisition of scrapie-like properties by the prion protein in cultured cells. J Biol Chem 272: 21479–21487.

Leighton PL, Allison WT (2016). Protein misfolding in prion and prion-like diseases: reconsidering a required role for protein loss-of-function. J Alzheimers Dis 54: 3–29.

Li JY, Englund E, Holton JL et al. (2008). Lewy bodies in grafted neurons in subjects with Parkinson's disease suggest host-to-graft disease propagation. Nat Med 14: 501–503.

Liberski PP, Sikorska B, Gibson P et al. (2011). Autophagy contributes to widespread neuronal degeneration in hamsters infected with the Echigo-1 strain of Creutzfeldt-Jakob disease and mice infected with the Fujisaki strain of Gerstmann-Straussler-Scheinker (GSS) syndrome. Ultrastruct Pathol 35: 31–36.

Lima FRS, Arantes CP, Muras AG et al. (2007). Cellular prion protein expression in astrocytes modulates neuronal survival and differentiation. J Neurochem 103: 2164–2176.

Linden R (2017). The biological function of the prion protein: a cell surface scaffold of signaling modules. Front Mol Neurosci 10: 77.

Liu H, Farr-Jones S, Ulyanov NB et al. (1999). Solution structure of Syrian hamster prion protein rPrP(90-231). Biochemistry 38: 5362–5377.

Liu T, Yi WJ, Feng BY et al. (2013). IGF-1-induced enhancement of PRNP expression depends on the negative regulation of transcription factor FOXO3a. PLoS One: 8.

Llorens F, Carulla P, Villa A et al. (2013). PrPC regulates epidermal growth factor receptor function and cell shape dynamics in Neuro2a cells. J Neurochem 127: 124–138.

Lopes MH, Hajj GN, Muras AG et al. (2005). Interaction of cellular prion and stress-inducible protein 1 promotes neuritogenesis and neuroprotection by distinct signaling pathways. J Neurosci 25: 11330–11339.

Loubet D, Dakowski C, Pietri M et al. (2012). Neuritogenesis: the prion protein controls beta 1 integrin signaling activity. FASEB J 26: 678–690.

Lucassen R, Nishina K, Supattapone S (2003). In vitro amplification of protease-resistant prion protein requires free sulfhydryl groups. Biochemistry 42: 4127–4135.

Lundmark K, Westermark GT, Nystrom S et al. (2002). Transmissibility of systemic amyloidosis by a prion-like mechanism. Proc Natl Acad Sci U S A 99: 6979–6984.

Lysek DA, Schorn C, Nivon LG et al. (2005). Prion protein NMR structures of cats, dogs, pigs, and sheep. Proc Natl Acad Sci U S A 102: 640–645.

Mabbott NA (2017). Immunology of prion protein and prions. Prog Mol Biol Transl Sci 150: 203–240.

Mahal SP, Asante EA, Antoniou M et al. (2001). Isolation and functional characterisation of the promoter region of the human prion protein gene. Gene 268: 105–114.

Makarava N, Lee CI, Ostapchenko VG et al. (2007). Highly promiscuous nature of prion polymerization. J Biol Chem 282: 36704–36713.

Mange A, Beranger F, Poec'h K et al. (2004). Alpha- and beta-cleavages of the amino-terminus of the cellular prion protein. Biol Cell 96: 125–132.

Manson J, West JD, Thomson V et al. (1992). The prion protein gene - a role in mouse embryogenesis. Development 115: 117–122.

Manson JC, Clarke AR, Hooper ML et al. (1994a). 129/Ola mice carrying a null mutation in PrP that abolishes mRNA production are developmentally normal. Mol Neurobiol 8: 121–127.

Manson JC, Clarke AR, McBride PA et al. (1994b). PrP gene dosage determines the timing but not the final intensity or distribution of lesions in scrapie pathology. Neurodegeneration 3: 331–340.

Manson JC, Jamieson E, Baybutt H et al. (1999). A single amino acid alteration (101L) introduced into murine PrP dramatically alters incubation time of transmissible spongiform encephalopathy. EMBO J 18: 6855–6864.

Marshall KE, Marchante R, Xue WF et al. (2014). The relationship between amyloid structure and cytotoxicity. Prion: 8.

Martini-Stoica H, Xu Y, Ballabio A et al. (2016). The autophagy-lysosomal pathway in neurodegeneration: a TFEB perspective. Trends Neurosci 39: 221–234.

Mays CE, Soto C (2016). The stress of prion disease. Brain Res 1648: 553–560.

McCulloch L, Brown KL, Bradford BM et al. (2011). Follicular dendritic cell-specific prion protein (PrP) expression alone is sufficient to sustain prion infection in the spleen. PLoS Pathog 7: e1002402.

McCutcheon S, Alejo Blanco AR, Houston EF et al. (2011). All clinically-relevant blood components transmit prion disease following a single blood transfusion: a sheep model of vCJD. PLoS One 6: e23169.

McDonald AJ, Dibble JP, Evans EGB et al. (2014). A new paradigm for enzymatic control of alpha-cleavage and beta-cleavage of the prion protein. J Biol Chem 289: 803–813.

McMahon HEM, Mange A, Nishida N et al. (2001). Cleavage of the amino terminus of the prion protein by reactive oxygen species. J Biol Chem 276: 2286–2291.

Mehrabian M, Brethour D, MacIsaac S et al. (2014). CRISPR-Cas9-based knockout of the prion protein and its effect on the proteome. PLoS One: 9.

Mehrabian M, Brethour D, Wang H et al. (2015). The prion protein controls polysialylation of neural cell adhesion molecule 1 during cellular morphogenesis. PLoS One: 10.

Mehrabian M, Brethour D, Williams D et al. (2016). Prion protein deficiency causes diverse proteome shifts in cell models that escape detection in brain tissue. PLoS One: 11.

Meyer RK, Lustig A, Oesch B et al. (2000). A monomer-dimer equilibrium of a cellular prion protein (PrPC) not observed with recombinant PrP. J Biol Chem 275: 38081–38087.

Meyer-Luehmann M, Coomaraswamy J, Bolmont T et al. (2006). Exogenous induction of cerebral beta-amyloidogenesis is governed by agent and host. Science 313: 1781–1784.

Milisav I, Suput D, Ribaric S (2015). Unfolded protein response and macroautophagy in Alzheimer's, Parkinson's and prion diseases. Molecules 20: 22718–22756.

Molinuevo JL, Llado A, Rami L (2005). Memantine: targeting glutamate excitotoxicity in Alzheimer's disease and other dementias. Am J Alzheimers Dis Other Demen 20: 77–85.

Monk KR, Oshima K, Jors S et al. (2011). Gpr126 is essential for peripheral nerve development and myelination in mammals. Development 138: 2673–2680.

Moore RA, Timmes A, Wilmarth PA et al. (2010). Comparative profiling of highly enriched 22L and Chandler mouse scrapie prion protein preparations. Proteomics 10: 2858–2869.

Morales R (2017). Prion strains in mammals: different conformations leading to disease. PLoS Pathog 13: e1006323.

Morales R, Hu PP, Duran-Aniotz C et al. (2016). Strain-dependent profile of misfolded prion protein aggregates. Sci Rep 6: 20526.

Morel E, Fouquet S, Strup-Perrot C et al. (2008). The cellular prion protein PrPc is involved in the proliferation of epithelial cells and in the distribution of junction-associated proteins. PLoS One: 3.

Moser M, Colello RJ, Pott U et al. (1995). Developmental expression of the prion protein gene in glial-cells. Neuron 14: 509–517.

Munch C, O'Brien J, Bertolotti A (2011). Prion-like propagation of mutant superoxide dismutase-1 misfolding in neuronal cells. Proc Natl Acad Sci U S A 108: 3548–3553.

Neuendorf E, Weber A, Saalmueller A et al. (2004). Glycosylation deficiency at either one of the two glycan attachment sites of cellular prion protein preserves susceptibility to bovine spongiform encephalopathy and scrapie infections. J Biol Chem 279: 53306–53316.

Nguyen J, Baldwin MA, Cohen FE et al. (1995). Prion protein peptides induce alpha-helix to beta-sheet conformational transitions. Biochemistry 34: 4186–4192.

Norstrom EM, Mastrianni JA (2006). The charge structure of helix 1 in the prion protein regulates conversion to pathogenic PrPSc. J Virol 80: 8521–8529.

Novitskaya V, Bocharova OV, Bronstein I et al. (2006). Amyloid fibrils of mammalian prion protein are highly toxic to cultured cells and primary neurons. J Biol Chem 281: 13828–13836.

Nuvolone M, Hermann M, Sorce S et al. (2016). Strictly co-isogenic C57BL/6J-Prnp(-/-) mice: a rigorous resource for prion science. J Exp Med 213: 313–327.

Obst J, Simon E, Mancuso R et al. (2017). The role of microglia in prion diseases: a paradigm of functional diversity. Front Aging Neurosci 9: 207.

Orru CD, Groveman BR, Raymond LD et al. (2015). Bank vole prion protein as an apparently universal substrate for RT-QuIC-based detection and discrimination of prion strains. PLoS Pathog 11: e1004983.

Paludi D, Thellung S, Chiovitti K et al. (2007). Different structural stability and toxicity of PrP(ARR) and PrP(ARQ) sheep prion protein variants. J Neurochem 103: 2291–2300.

Paul KR, Ross ED (2015). Controlling the prion propensity of glutamine/asparagine-rich proteins. Prion 9: 347–354.

Peelaerts W, Bousset L, Van der Perren A et al. (2015). Alpha-synuclein strains cause distinct synucleinopathies after local and systemic administration. Nature 522: 340–344.

Peralta OA, Eyestone WH (2009). Quantitative and qualitative analysis of cellular prion protein (PrPC) expression in bovine somatic tissues. Prion 3: 161–170.

Peralta OA, Huckle WR, Eyestone WH (2012). Developmental expression of the cellular prion protein (PrPC) in bovine embryos. Mol Reprod Dev 79: 488–498.

Peretz D, Williamson RA, Matsunaga Y et al. (1997). A conformational transition at the N terminus of the prion protein features in formation of the scrapie isoform. J Mol Biol 273: 614–622.

Perez DR, Damberger FF, Wuthrich K (2010). Horse prion protein NMR structure and comparisons with related variants of the mouse prion protein. J Mol Biol 400: 121–128.

Piccardo P, Dlouhy SR, Lievens PM et al. (1998). Phenotypic variability of Gerstmann-Straussler-Scheinker disease is associated with prion protein heterogeneity. J Neuropathol Exp Neurol 57: 979–988.

Piccardo P, Liepnieks JJ, William A et al. (2001). Prion proteins with different conformations accumulate in Gerstmann-Straussler-Scheinker disease caused by A117V and F198S mutations. Am J Pathol 158: 2201–2207.

Piccardo P, Manson JC, King D et al. (2007). Accumulation of prion protein in the brain that is not associated with transmissible disease. Proc Natl Acad Sci U S A 104: 4712–4717.

Piccardo P, King D, Telling G et al. (2013). Dissociation of prion protein amyloid seeding from transmission of a spongiform encephalopathy. J Virol 87: 12349–12356.

Priola SA, Caughey B, Wehrly K et al. (1995). A 60-kDa prion protein (PrP) with properties of both the normal and scrapie-associated forms of PrP. J Biol Chem 270: 3299–3305.

Privat N, Levavasseur E, Yildirim S et al. (2017). Region-specific protein misfolding cyclic amplification reproduces brain tropism of prion strains. J Biol Chem 292: 16688–16696.

Provansal M, Roche S, Pastore M et al. (2010). Proteomic consequences of expression and pathological conversion of the prion protein in inducible neuroblastoma N2a cells. Prion 4: 292–301.

Prusiner SB (1998). Prions. Proc Natl Acad Sci U S A 95: 13363–13383.

Puckett C, Concannon P, Casey C et al. (1991). Genomic structure of the human prion protein gene. Am J Hum Genet 49: 320–329.

Quist A, Doudevski I, Lin H et al. (2005). Amyloid ion channels: a common structural link for protein-misfolding disease. Proc Natl Acad Sci U S A 102: 10427–10432.

Rachidi W, Vilette D, Guiraud P et al. (2003). Expression of prion protein increases cellular copper binding and antioxidant enzyme activities but not copper delivery. J Biol Chem 278: 9064–9072.

Rane NS, Yonkovich JL, Hegde RS (2004). Protection from cytosolic prion protein toxicity by modulation of protein translocation. EMBO J 23: 4550–4559.

Raymond GJ, Bossers A, Raymond LD et al. (2000). Evidence of a molecular barrier limiting susceptibility of humans, cattle and sheep to chronic wasting disease. EMBO J 19: 4425–4430.

Riek R, Hornemann S, Wider G et al. (1996). NMR structure of the mouse prion protein domain PrP(121-231). Nature 382: 180–182.

Ritchie MA, Gill AC, Deery MJ et al. (2002). Precursor ion scanning for detection and structural characterization of heterogeneous glycopeptide mixtures. J Am Soc Mass Spectrom 13: 1065–1077.

Rodriguez JA, Jiang L, Eisenberg DS (2017). Toward the atomic structure of PrPSc. Cold Spring Harb Perspect Biol: 9.

Rossetti G, Cong X, Caliandro R et al. (2011). Common structural traits across pathogenic mutants of the human prion protein and their implications for familial prion diseases. J Mol Biol 411: 700–712.

Rudd PM, Endo T, Colominas C et al. (1999). Glycosylation differences between the normal and pathogenic prion protein isoforms. Proc Natl Acad Sci U S A 96: 13044–13049.

Rutishauser D, Mertz KD, Moos R et al. (2009). The comprehensive native interactome of a fully functional tagged prion protein. PLoS One 4: e4446.

Saa P, Harris DA, Cervenakova L (2016). Mechanisms of prion-induced neurodegeneration. Expert Rev Mol Med 18: e5.

Saborio GP, Permanne B, Soto C (2001). Sensitive detection of pathological prion protein by cyclic amplification of protein misfolding. Nature 411: 810–813.

Safar J, Wille H, Itri V et al. (1998). Eight prion strains have PrP(Sc) molecules with different conformations. Nat Med 4: 1157–1165.

Sajnani G, Requena JR (2012). Prions, proteinase K and infectivity. Prion 6: 430–432.

Sakudo A, Xue GA, Kawashita N et al. (2010). Structure of the prion protein and its gene: an analysis using bioinformatics and computer simulation. Curr Protein Pept Sci 11: 166–179.

Salamat MK, Dron M, Chapuis J et al. (2011). Prion propagation in cells expressing PrP glycosylation mutants. J Virol 85: 3077–3085.

Sales N, Hassig R, Rodolfo K et al. (2002). Developmental expression of the cellular prion protein in elongating axons. Eur J Neurosci 15: 1163–1177.

Sanghera N, Wall M, Venien-Bryan C et al. (2008). Globular and pre-fibrillar prion aggregates are toxic to neuronal cells and perturb their electrophysiology. Biochim Biophys Acta 1784: 873–881.

Scallet AC, Ye X (1997). Excitotoxic mechanisms of neurodegeneration in transmissible spongiform encephalopathies. Ann N Y Acad Sci 825: 194–205.

Shaked GM, Shaked Y, Kariv-Inbal Z et al. (2001). A protease-resistant prion protein isoform is present in urine of animals and humans affected with prion diseases. J Biol Chem 276: 31479–31482.

Shyng SL, Huber MT, Harris DA (1993). A prion protein cycles between the cell-surface and an endocytic compartment in cultured neuroblastoma-cells. J Biol Chem 268: 15922–15928.

Sigurdson CJ, Joshi-Barr S, Bett C et al. (2011). Spongiform encephalopathy in transgenic mice expressing a point mutation in the beta2-alpha2 loop of the prion protein. J Neurosci 31: 13840–13847.

Simoneau S, Rezaei H, Sales N et al. (2007). In vitro and in vivo neurotoxicity of prion protein oligomers. PLoS Pathog 3: e125.

Singh A, Kong QZ, Luo X et al. (2009a). Prion protein (PrP) knock-out mice show altered iron metabolism: a functional role for PrP in iron uptake and transport. PLoS One: 4.

Singh A, Mohan ML, Isaac AO et al. (2009b). Prion protein modulates cellular iron uptake: a novel function with implications for prion disease pathogenesis. PLoS One: 4.

Smirnovas V, Kim JI, Lu X et al. (2009). Distinct structures of scrapie prion protein (PrPSc)-seeded versus spontaneous recombinant prion protein fibrils revealed by hydrogen/deuterium exchange. J Biol Chem 284: 24233–24241.

Smirnovas V, Baron GS, Offerdahl DK et al. (2011). Structural organization of brain-derived mammalian prions examined by hydrogen-deuterium exchange. Nat Struct Mol Biol 18: 504–506.

Solforosi L, Bellon A, Schaller M et al. (2007). Toward molecular dissection of PrPC-PrPSc interactions. J Biol Chem 282: 7465–7471.

Somerville RA, Gentles N (2011). Characterization of the effect of heat on agent strains of the transmissible spongiform encephalopathies. J Gen Virol 92: 1738–1748.

Speare JO, Rush 3rd TS, Bloom ME et al. (2003). The role of helix 1 aspartates and salt bridges in the stability and conversion of prion protein. J Biol Chem 278: 12522–12529.

Srivastava S, Katorcha E, Daus ML et al. (2017). Sialylation controls prion fate in vivo. J Biol Chem 292: 2359–2368.

Stahl N, Baldwin MA, Hecker R et al. (1992). Glycosylinositol phospholipid anchors of the scrapie and cellular prion proteins contain sialic acid. Biochemistry 31: 5043–5053.

Stahl N, Baldwin MA, Teplow DB et al. (1993). Structural studies of the scrapie prion protein using mass spectrometry and amino acid sequencing. Biochemistry 32: 1991–2002.

Steele AD, Emsley JG, Ozdinler PH et al. (2006). Prion protein (PrPc) positively regulates neural precursor proliferation during developmental and adult mammalian neurogenesis. Proc Natl Acad Sci U S A 103: 3416–3421.

Stimson E, Hope J, Chong A et al. (1999). Site-specific characterization of the N-linked glycans of murine prion protein by high-performance liquid chromatography/electrospray mass spectrometry and exoglycosidase digestions. Biochemistry 38: 4885–4895.

Striebel JF, Race B, Chesebro B (2013a). Prion protein and susceptibility to kainate-induced seizures: genetic pitfalls in the use of PrP knockout mice. Prion 7: 280–285.

Striebel JF, Race B, Pathmajeyan M et al. (2013b). Lack of influence of prion protein gene expression on kainate-induced seizures in mice: studies using congenic, coisogenic and transgenic strains. Neuroscience 238: 11–18.

Supattapone S (2014). Elucidating the role of cofactors in mammalian prion propagation. Prion 8: 100–105.

Sydow A, Mandelkow EM (2010). 'Prion-like' propagation of mouse and human tau aggregates in an inducible mouse model of tauopathy. Neurodegener Dis 7: 28–31.

Tagliavini F, Lievens PM, Tranchant C et al. (2001). A 7-kDa prion protein (PrP) fragment, an integral component of the PrP region required for infectivity, is the major amyloid protein in Gerstmann-Straussler-Scheinker disease A117V. J Biol Chem 276: 6009–6015.

Taguchi Y, Schatzl HM (2013). Identifying critical sites of PrP(c)-PrP(Sc) interaction in prion-infected cells by dominant-negative inhibition. Prion 7: 452–456.

Tahiri-Alaoui A, Gill AC, Disterer P et al. (2004). Methionine 129 variant of human prion protein oligomerizes more rapidly than the valine 129 variant: implications for disease susceptibility to Creutzfeldt-Jakob disease. J Biol Chem 279: 31390–31397.

Taubner LM, Bienkiewicz EA, Copie V et al. (2010). Structure of the flexible amino-terminal domain of prion protein bound to a sulfated glycan. J Mol Biol 395: 475–490.

Taylor DR, Parkin ET, Cocklin SL et al. (2009). Role of ADAMs in the ectodomain shedding and conformational conversion of the prion protein. J Biol Chem 284: 22590–22600.

Telling GC, Haga T, Torchia M et al. (1996). Interactions between wild-type and mutant prion proteins modulate neurodegeneration in transgenic mice. Genes Dev 10: 1736–1750.

Thackray AM, Yang S, Wong E et al. (2004). Conformational variation between allelic variants of cell-surface ovine prion protein. Biochem J 381: 221–229.

Torres M, Matamala JM, Duran-Aniotz C et al. (2015). ER stress signaling and neurodegeneration: at the intersection between Alzheimer's disease and prion-related disorders. Virus Res 207: 69–75.

Tremblay P, Bouzamondo-Bernstein E, Heinrich C et al. (2007). Developmental expression of PrP in the post-implantation embryo. Brain Res 1139: 60–67.

Treusch S, Cyr DM, Lindquist S (2009). Amyloid deposits: protection against toxic protein species? Cell Cycle 8: 1668–1674.

Tseng CY, Yu CP, Lee HC (2009). Integrity of H1 helix in prion protein revealed by molecular dynamic simulations to be especially vulnerable to changes in the relative orientation of H1 and its S1 flank. Eur Biophys J 38: 601–611.

Tuzi NL, Cancellotti E, Baybutt H et al. (2008). Host PrP glycosylation: a major factor determining the outcome of prion infection. PLoS Biol 6: e100.

Ugalde CL, Finkelstein DI, Lawson VA et al. (2016). Pathogenic mechanisms of prion protein, amyloid-beta and alpha-synuclein misfolding: the prion concept and neurotoxicity of protein oligomers. J Neurochem 139: 162–180.

Urbanc B, Cruz L, Le R et al. (2002). Neurotoxic effects of thioflavin S-positive amyloid deposits in transgenic mice and Alzheimer's disease. Proc Natl Acad Sci U S A 99: 13990–13995.

van der Kamp MW, Daggett V (2010). Pathogenic mutations in the hydrophobic core of the human prion protein can promote structural instability and misfolding. J Mol Biol 404: 732–748.

Vanik DL, Surewicz WK (2002). Disease-associated F198S mutation increases the propensity of the recombinant prion protein for conformational conversion to scrapie-like form. J Biol Chem 277: 49065–49070.

Vincent B, Paitel E, Frobert Y et al. (2000). Phorbol ester-regulated cleavage of normal prion protein in HEK293 human cells and murine neurons. J Biol Chem 275: 35612–35616.

Vincent B, Paitel E, Saftig P et al. (2001). The disintegrins ADAM10 and TACE contribute to the constitutive and phorbol ester-regulated normal cleavage of the cellular prion protein. J Biol Chem 276: 37743–37746.

Walmsley AR, Watt NT, Taylor DR et al. (2009). Alpha-cleavage of the prion protein occurs in a late compartment of the secretory pathway and is independent of lipid rafts. Mol Cell Neurosci 40: 242–248.

Wang F, Yang F, Hu Y et al. (2007). Lipid interaction converts prion protein to a PrPSc-like proteinase K-resistant conformation under physiological conditions. Biochemistry 46: 7045–7053.

Wang F, Wang X, Yuan CG et al. (2010). Generating a prion with bacterially expressed recombinant prion protein. Science 327: 1132–1135.

Wang F, Wang X, Orru CD et al. (2017). Self-propagating, protease-resistant, recombinant prion protein conformers with or without in vivo pathogenicity. PLoS Pathog 13: e1006491.

Watt NT, Taylor DR, Gillott A et al. (2005). Reactive oxygen species-mediated beta-cleavage of the prion protein in the cellular response to oxidative stress. J Biol Chem 280: 35914–35921.

Watt NT, Routledge MN, Wild CP et al. (2007). Cellular prion protein protects against reactive-oxygen-species-induced DNA damage. Free Radic Biol Med 43: 959–967.

Watts JC, Condello C, Stohr J et al. (2014). Serial propagation of distinct strains of Abeta prions from Alzheimer's disease patients. Proc Natl Acad Sci U S A 111: 10323–10328.

Weber P, Giese A, Piening N et al. (2007). Generation of genuine prion infectivity by serial PMCA. Vet Microbiol 123: 346–357.

Weise J, Sandau R, Schwarting S et al. (2006). Deletion of cellular prion protein results in reduced Akt activation, enhanced postischemic caspase-3 activation, and exacerbation of ischemic brain injury. Stroke 37: 1296–1300.

Weiss E, Ramljak S, Asif AR et al. (2010). Cellular prion protein overexpression disturbs cellular homeostasis in SH-sy5y neuroblastoma cells but does not alter p53 expression: a proteomic study. Neuroscience 169: 1640–1650.

Welker E, Raymond LD, Scheraga HA et al. (2002). Intramolecular versus intermolecular disulfide bonds in prion proteins. J Biol Chem 277: 33477–33481.

Wik L, Klingeborn M, Willander H et al. (2012). Separate mechanisms act concurrently to shed and release the prion protein from the cell. Prion: 6.

Wille H, Michelitsch MD, Guenebaut V et al. (2002). Structural studies of the scrapie prion protein by electron crystallography. Proc Natl Acad Sci U S A 99: 3563–3568.

Williams WM, Stadtman ER, Moskovitz J (2004). Ageing and exposure to oxidative stress in vivo differentially affect cellular levels of PrPc in mouse cerebral microvessels and brain parenchyma. Neuropathol Appl Neurobiol 30: 161–168.

Winklhofer KF, Tatzelt J, Haass C (2008). The two faces of protein misfolding: gain- and loss-of-function in neurodegenerative diseases. EMBO J 27: 336–349.

Winner B, Jappelli R, Maji SK et al. (2011). In vivo demonstration that alpha-synuclein oligomers are toxic. Proc Natl Acad Sci U S A 108: 4194–4199.

Wong BS, Venien-Bryan C, Williamson RA et al. (2000a). Copper refolding of prion protein. Biochem Biophys Res Commun 276: 1217–1224.

Wong NK, Renouf DV, Lehmann S et al. (2000b). Glycosylation of prions and its effects on protein conformation relevant to amino acid mutations. J Mol Graph Model 18: 126–134. 163–125.

Wopfner F, Weidenhofer G, Schneider R et al. (1999). Analysis of 27 mammalian and 9 avian PrPs reveals high conservation of flexible regions of the prion protein. J Mol Biol 289: 1163–1178.

Wulf MA, Senatore A, Aguzzi A (2017). The biological function of the cellular prion protein: an update. BMC Biol 15: 34.

Wuthrich K, Riek R (2001). Three-dimensional structures of prion proteins. Adv Protein Chem 57: 55–82.

Yanai A, Meiner Z, Gahali I et al. (1999). Subcellular trafficking abnormalities of a prion protein with a disrupted disulfide loop. FEBS Lett 460: 11–16.

Yao Y, Ren J, Jones IM (2003). Amino terminal interaction in the prion protein identified using fusion to green fluorescent protein. J Neurochem 87: 1057–1065.

Yao H, Zhao D, Khan SH et al. (2013). Role of autophagy in prion protein-induced neurodegenerative diseases. Acta Biochim Biophys Sin Shanghai 45: 494–502.

Yin S, Pham N, Yu S et al. (2007). Human prion proteins with pathogenic mutations share common conformational changes resulting in enhanced binding to glycosaminoglycans. Proc Natl Acad Sci U S A 104: 7546–7551.

Younan ND, Klewpatinond M, Davies P et al. (2011). Copper(II)-induced secondary structure changes and reduced folding stability of the prion protein. J Mol Biol 410: 369–382.

Zambrano R, Conchillo-Sole O, Iglesias V et al. (2015). PrionW: a server to identify proteins containing glutamine/asparagine rich prion-like domains and their amyloid cores. Nucleic Acids Res 43: W331–337.

Zawlik I, Witusik M, Hulas-Bigoszewska K et al. (2006). Regulation of PrPc expression: Nerve growth factor (NGF) activates the prion gene promoter through the MEK1 pathway in PC12 cells. Neurosci Lett 400: 58–62.

Zhang C, Jackson AP, Zhang ZR et al. (2010). Amyloid-like aggregates of the yeast prion protein ure2 enter vertebrate cells by specific endocytotic pathways and induce apoptosis. PLoS One 5: e12529.

Zhou M, Ottenberg G, Sferrazza GF et al. (2012). Highly neurotoxic monomeric alpha-helical prion protein. Proc Natl Acad Sci U S A 109: 3113–3118.

Handbook of Clinical Neurology, Vol. 153 (3rd series)
Human Prion Diseases
M. Pocchiari and J. Manson, Editors
https://doi.org/10.1016/B978-0-444-63945-5.00003-9
2018 Published by Elsevier B.V.

Chapter 3

Cell biology of prion infection

SUZETTE A. PRIOLA*
Laboratory of Persistent Viral Diseases, National Institute of Allergy and Infectious Diseases, Hamilton, MT, United States

Abstract

The development of multiple cell culture models of prion infection over the last two decades has led to a significant increase in our understanding of how prions infect cells. In particular, new techniques to distinguish exogenous from endogenous prions have allowed us for the first time to look in depth at the earliest stages of prion infection through to the establishment of persistent infection. These studies have shown that prions can infect multiple cell types, both neuronal and nonneuronal. Once in contact with the cell, they are rapidly taken up via multiple endocytic pathways. After uptake, the initial replication of prions occurs almost immediately on the plasma membrane and within multiple endocytic compartments. Following this acute stage of prion replication, persistent prion infection may or may not be established. Establishment of a persistent prion infection in cells appears to depend upon the achievement of a delicate balance between the rate of prion replication and degradation, the rate of cell division, and the efficiency of prion spread from cell to cell. Overall, cell culture models have shown that prion infection of the cell is a complex and variable process which can involve multiple cellular pathways and compartments even within a single cell.

INTRODUCTION

The establishment of in vitro cell culture models of infection can be a daunting task but, once established, they are much more easily manipulated and controlled than in vivo models of infection. As such, they are critical tools for understanding the myriad of processes which underlie how infectious agents infect, and sometimes kill, cells. Data from studies using cell culture models can be used to design and implement studies in animals where the in vitro results can often – although by no means always – be recapitulated. Indeed, in vitro cell-based systems are an important component of translational research and continue to be used as model systems to identify compounds that can be used for prophylactic or therapeutic treatments of a wide variety of infections as well as for the development and propagation of vaccines to prevent infection.

The development of cell culture models of prion infection has, in many ways, been more difficult than that of viruses and bacteria. This is due in part to the unusual nature of the infectious agent and the mechanism by which it replicates. The causative agents of these diseases are known as prions and are distinguished from more conventional viruses and bacteria by the composition of the infectious particle. Prions are composed largely, if not entirely, of an abnormally refolded, insoluble, and protease-resistant form (PrP^{TSE}) of the mammalian prion protein (PrP). PrP^{TSE} itself is a conformationally distinct form of the soluble and protease-sensitive cellular prion protein (PrP^{C}) which is expressed in almost every cell type in the body. As described in greater detail elsewhere in this volume, PrP^{TSE}, and thus prions, replicate via a conversion process called seeded polymerization. In seeded polymerization, aggregates of PrP^{TSE} interact with PrP^{C} in the host cell and, through a poorly

*Correspondence to: Suzette A. Priola, National Institute of Allergy and Infectious Diseases, Laboratory of Persistent Viral Diseases, TSE/Prion Molecular Biology Section, Rocky Mountain Laboratories, Hamilton MT 59840, United States. Tel: +1-406-363-9319, Fax: +1-406-363-9286, E-mail: spriola@nih.gov

understood process, refold the host PrP^C into the PrP^{TSE} conformer, thus incorporating it into the PrP^{TSE} aggregate. This process is repeated until PrP^{TSE} accumulates to levels that eventually lead to disease.

Prion replication is thus dependent upon the host's PrP^C molecule. One consequence of this is that, once a prion infects a cell, the process of prion replication inevitably leads to the host PrP^C molecule being incorporated into the incoming PrP^{TSE} prion. Furthermore, if persistent infection is established, all PrP^{TSE} in the cell will eventually be derived solely from its host PrP^C precursor. Studying prion replication in a cell therefore requires being able to distinguish three types of PrP molecules: the exogenous PrP^{TSE} that comprises the infectious prion, the PrP^C molecule of the host cell, and the newly made PrP^{TSE} that is derived from the host's own PrP^C. Distinguishing these different types of PrP molecules has proven to be very difficult in live cells since the differences are not necessarily dependent upon differences in the amino acid sequence of the PrP molecule but rather on differences in how the protein is folded (i.e., its conformation). Most studies of prion-infected cells have therefore used either fixed cells and denaturing treatments to distinguish PrP^{TSE} from PrP^C microscopically or infected cell lysates treated with proteases to distinguish PrP^C from PrP^{TSE} biochemically. This has in many ways limited our ability to fully understand the process of prion infection using cell-based models.

Nevertheless, over the last two decades there has been a large increase in the number of cell culture models of prion infection, including the development of established cell lines that do not express PrP^C and the identification of highly susceptible cell lines. New techniques have been developed to distinguish host cell PrP from exogenous PrP^{TSE} that have allowed us to look at the earliest stages of prion infection. These approaches have greatly enhanced our understanding of the process of prion infection from the initial contact of prions with the cell to the establishment of persistent infection.

GENERAL CELL MODELS OF PRION INFECTION

Brain cell culture

The earliest cell models of prion infection were developed in the 1960s and 1970s, decades prior to the identification of the prion protein. At that time, prion diseases were known as TSEs and the infectious agent was believed to be a slow virus. In 1965, Gustafson and Kanitz isolated transmissible spongiform encephalopathy (TSE)-infected cells by taking portions of scrapie-infected sheep or mouse brain, dissociating the cells using trypsin, and adding the resulting suspension to cell growth media. After 23 serial passages, media from adherent cell cultures which grew out of the scrapie-positive sheep brain transmitted disease to mice. Similarly, media removed from scrapie-positive mouse brain cell culture after 38 days in culture also transmitted disease to mice. Experiments using cells that grew out of either human Creutzfeldt–Jakob disease (CJD) brain explants or brain cells from chimpanzees infected with CJD or kuru demonstrated that human TSE infectivity could also be maintained in cell culture for months (Gajdusek et al., 1972). Although it was not possible in either of these experiments to discount the possibility that transmission of infectivity was due to residual infectivity from the brain as opposed to newly made infectious particles (Gajdusek et al., 1972), these experiments nonetheless suggested that the scrapie agent could be maintained in culture.

Using similar techniques, Clarke and Haig (1970a) isolated spontaneously immortalized cell lines from the brains of mice infected with a mouse-adapted strain of sheep scrapie called Chandler (also known as RML). Consistent with the cells being persistently infected with the Chandler scrapie agent, titratable and stable infectivity could be detected in these scrapie mouse brain (SMB) cells up to at least 150 passages (Clarke and Haig, 1970a; Clarke, 1979). Early studies with these cells were the first to look at the replication kinetics of scrapie infection and suggested that each round of agent replication doubled the amount of Chandler scrapie, with multiplication of Chandler closely linked to multiplication of the cells (Clarke and Haig, 1970b). Thus, studies in SMB cells were the first to demonstrate definitively that the scrapie agent could replicate and be maintained in cultured cells. SMB cells have also been utilized to study strain-specific aspects of prion infection. Once cured of prion infection, they can be reinfected de novo with multiple strains of mouse prions (Birkett et al., 2001).

Attempts to establish cell lines from prion-infected hamster brains were less successful and resulted in a cell line, known as HaB, that contained PrP^C but not PrP^{TSE} (Taraboulos et al., 1990). Dependent upon the temperature at which they were cultured, HaB cells could be infected with hamster prions (Taraboulos et al., 1990) but ultimately were unable to stably support persistent prion infection (Taraboulos et al., 1992). Brain tissue has not been the only source of prion-infected cell cultures based on tissue explant. More recently, stromal cells derived from the bone marrow of rats infected with rat-adapted sporadic CJD (sCJD), mice infected with mouse-adapted bovine spongiform encephalopathy (BSE) or CJD, and a human sCJD patient have been shown to persistently accumulate PrP^{TSE} in vitro (Takakura et al., 2008). Thus, cells of multiple lineages explanted from prion-infected hosts can support persistent prion infection in vitro. In the case of SMB cells, these cells have become an established cell line used to study persistent prion infection.

Established cell lines

The most successful in vitro models of prion infection have resulted from the exposure of immortalized and easily attainable cell lines to brain homogenates from prion-infected animals. Since PrP^C is absolutely required for prion infection (Bueler et al., 1993) and is expressed in almost all cell types, it could be assumed that any cell expressing PrP^C would be able to support prion infection. However, it has proven surprisingly difficult to persistently infect cells with prions. Expression of PrP^C does not correlate with susceptibility to prion infection and only a subset of prion strains has been successfully transmitted to cells (Table 3.1). Thus, the susceptibility of a cell to prion infection must be determined empirically by testing different cell type and prion strain combinations, a task which can be quite daunting to undertake. For example, one recent study tested the susceptibility of 33 different PrP^C-expressing cell lines to infection with five different prion agents. Only two cell lines were found that could support persistent prion infection: murine neuroblastoma cells (N2a) infected with RML mouse prions and the bovine kidney cell line PES infected with sheep scrapie (Oelschlegel et al., 2015). Fortunately, while many cell lines are resistant to prion infection, extensive testing over the last 30 years has led to the identification of over 20 cell lines of various lineages that can support persistent prion infection (Table 3.1).

Since prion agents replicate to high titers in tissues of the central nervous system (CNS), cells from these tissues were among the first tested for susceptibility to prion infection and there are now several CNS-derived cell lines that have been shown to be susceptible to prion infection (Table 3.1). The first such cell lines identified were mouse neuroblastoma cells which were found to be susceptible to multiple strains of mouse prions including RML (Race et al., 1987; Butler et al., 1988; Bosque and Prusiner, 2000), 139A (Nishida et al., 2000), 22L (Nishida et al., 2000; Klohn et al., 2003), as well as mouse-adapted strains of human Gerstmann–Straussler–Scheinker (GSS), hamster 263K, and BSE prions (Arjona et al., 2004; Manuelidis et al., 2009). Prion-infected murine neuroblastoma cells were used in most of the early studies of prion infection and remain the cells most commonly used to study the process of prion infection and PrP^{TSE} formation. In fact, one murine neuroblastoma cell subclone, N2aPK1, is highly susceptible to infection with multiple strains of mouse prions and is the basis of the first widely accepted in vitro prion titration assay (Mahal et al., 2007).

Other neuronal cell lines that have proven susceptible to multiple mouse-adapted prion agents include GT1 cells, which are murine CNS-derived gonadotropin-releasing hormone neurons (Schatzl et al., 1997; Nishida et al., 2000; Arjona et al., 2004; Manuelidis et al., 2009), the septal neuron cell line SN56 (Baron et al., 2006), and the mixed microglial/neuronal mouse cerebellar cell line CRBL (Mays et al., 2008). At least three neural cell lines that can be differentiated into neurons can also be persistently infected with prions. Differentiated murine CAD5 cells can be infected with multiple strains of mouse prions as well as mouse-adapted BSE (Mahal et al., 2007), while differentiated rat PC12 cells (Rubenstein et al., 1984, 1992) and mouse 1C11 cells (Mouillet-Richard et al., 2008) are susceptible to mouse prions and are useful for studying how different neuronal subtypes respond to prion infection (Rubenstein et al., 1992; Mouillet-Richard et al., 2008). Finally, nonneuronal cells of the CNS and peripheral nervous system can also be infected with prions. Schwann cells from the peripheral nervous system of mice (Follet et al., 2002) and sheep (Archer et al., 2004) are susceptible to mouse and sheep prions, respectively, as are immortalized, CNS-derived microglial cells from mice (Iwamaru et al., 2007) and sheep (Munoz-Gutierrez et al., 2015).

Somewhat surprisingly, given that prion disease is primarily associated with the nervous system of the host, fibroblast and epithelial cells are among the cell lines most susceptible to prion infection (Table 3.1) (Vorberg et al., 2004b). NIH 3T3 fibroblast cells can be infected with the 22L strain of mouse prions (Vorberg et al., 2004b) while mouse L929 fibroblast cells are susceptible to 22L, ME7, and RML mouse prions (Vorberg et al., 2004b). One of the cell lines most susceptible to prion infection is derived from a species that is actually highly resistant to natural prion infection. Rabbit kidney epithelial cells (RK13) do not express rabbit PrP^C (Vilette et al., 2001), the presence of which can significantly inhibit PrP^{TSE} formation (Vorberg et al., 2003). However, stable expression in RK13 cells of PrP^C from other species, including sheep (Vilette et al., 2001; Courageot et al., 2008), mouse (Courageot et al., 2008; Lawson et al., 2008), bank vole (Courageot et al., 2008), and elk (Bian et al., 2010), renders RK13 cells susceptible to infection with prions of the corresponding species. Clearly, tissue origin does not predispose a cell to support prion infection, a point amply illustrated by the recent findings that Madin-Darby bovine kidney cell clones are susceptible to BSE (Tark et al., 2015) and sheep scrapie (Oelschlegel et al., 2015); mouse bone marrow-derived mesenchymal-like stem cells and spleen-derived stromal cells can be infected with mouse-adapted CJD (Akimov et al., 2008, 2009; Cervenakova et al., 2011); and rat bone marrow stromal cells are susceptible to rat-adapted human GSS (Takakura et al., 2008).

Table 3.1

Prion-susceptible cell lines

Cell line	Cell type	Susceptible to:	Resistant to:	Notes	Reference
N2a	Neuroblastoma	RML, Fu-1	M1000, BSE, scrapie, ME7		Race et al. (1987); Butler et al. (1988); Bosque and Prusiner (2000); Lewis et al. (2009); Oelschlegel et al. (2015)
		Fu-1, RML, 22L, 139A	87V, 22A	N2a58 subclone	Nishida et al. (2000); Arjona et al. (2004)
		RML, 22L	ME7, 22A, 301C, mo-263K	N2aPK1 subclone	Klohn et al. (2003)
		RML		C1300 subclone	Butler et al. (1988)
RK13	Epithelial	Scrapie		Rov cells	Vilette et al. (2001)
		Fu-1, RML, 22L	ME7	Mov cells	Courageot et al. (2008)
		M1000		moRK13 cells	Vella et al. (2007)
		M1000	CJD	huRK13 cells	Lawson et al. (2008)
		BSE, scrapie		voRK13 cells	Courageot et al. (2008)
		CWD		Elk RK13 cells	Bian et al. (2010)
GT1	Hypothalamic neurons	RML		GT1-trk cells	Schatzl et al. (1997)
		Fu-1		GT1-1 subclone	Arjona et al. (2004)
		RML, 139A, 22L, Fu-1, M1000, SY-CJD, mo-vCJD, mo-263K, Obihiro	87V, 22A	GT1-7 subclone	Nishida et al. (2000); Vella et al. (2007); Manuelidis et al. (2009); Elhelaly et al. (2013a)
SMB	Mesodermal	Chandler[a], 139A, 79A, 22F		Spontaneously immortalized Chandler-infected mouse brain cells	Clarke and Haig (1970a, b); Birkett et al. (2001)
SN56	Septal neurons	ME7, RML, 22L	263K		Magalhaes et al. (2005); Baron et al. (2006)
L929	Fibroblast	ME7, 22L, RML	301C		Clarke and Millson (1976); Vorberg et al. (2004b); Mahal et al. (2007); Piccardo et al. (2011)
NIH 3T3	Fibroblast	22L	M1000		Vorberg et al. (2004b); Lewis et al. (2009); Piccardo et al. (2011)
MG20	Immature microglia	RML, ME7, Obihiro, mo-BSE		Overexpress moPrP^C	Iwamaru et al. (2007)
MDBK	Bovine kidney	BSE		Overexpress boPrP^C	Tark et al. (2015)
		Sheep scrapie	BSE	PES subclone	Oelschlegel et al. (2015)
hTERT	Ovine microglia	Sheep scrapie			Munoz-Gutierrez et al. (2015)
MDB	Mule deer fibroblast	CWD		Immortalized brain cell	Raymond et al. (2006)
MOV	Schwann cell-like	Sheep scrapie		Overexpress shPrP^C	Archer et al. (2004)
MSC 80	Schwann cell	RML			Follet et al. (2002)
PC12	Rat pheochromocytoma	139A, ME7	263K, 139R		Rubenstein et al. (1984, 1992)

C2C12	Differentiated myotube	RML, ME7, 22L	Hyper		Dlakic et al. (2007); Herbst et al. (2013)
CRBL	Mixed neuron, glial	139A (SMB cell lysate)	RML (BH)		Mays et al. (2008)
NS-1	Lymphoblast	139A		Not stable	Elleman (1984)
CAD5	Cath-a-differentiated	RML, 22L, 79A, ME7, 301C			Mahal et al. (2007)
TR6Bc1	Neural cell	RML, Obihiro			Elhelaly et al. (2013a)
SH-SY5Y		CJD			Ladogana et al. (1995)
Min 6	Pancreatic B cell	RML			Rouvinski et al. (2014)
1C11	Neuroectodermal progenitor	RML, 22L, Fu-1	ME7, 22A		Mouillet-Richard et al. (2008)
HpL 3-4	Hippocampal neural precursor	22L		PrP^{KO} cells + $moPrP^C$	Maas et al. (2007)
NpL2	Hippocampal cells	22L, RML		PrP^{KO} cells + $moPrP^C$	Marshall et al. (2017)
CF10	Neural progenitor cells	22L		PrP^{KO} cells + $moPrP^C$	McNally et al. (2009)

[a]Chandler is an alternative designation for the mouse prion strain RML. The two terms are interchangeable.

$boPrP^C$, bovine PrP^C; BSE, bovine spongiform encephalopathy; CJD, Creutzfeldt–Jakob disease; CWD, chronic wasting disease; Fu, Fukuoka mouse-adapted; GSS, Gerstmann–Straussler–Scheinker; mo, mouse adapted; $moPrP^C$, mouse PrP^C; BH, brain homogenate; PrP^{KO} cells, cells derived from brain of embryonic mice in which the *PRNP* gene has been ablated; $shPrP^C$, sheep PrP^C.

Primary cell culture

The literature on the susceptibility of primary cells to scrapie infection is much more limited than that of established cells. Primary neuronal cells cannot be passaged and are difficult to maintain in culture for more than a few weeks. Therefore, differentiating exogenous PrP^{TSE} in the infectious inoculum from PrP^{TSE} generated by the cells requires diluting out the initial inoculum by routine replacement of the cell media over several weeks and looking for an increase in PrP^{TSE} levels over time (Cronier et al., 2004). The first successful infection of primary neurons utilized cerebellar granular neurons isolated from transgenic mice overexpressing sheep or mouse PrP^{C}. These cells were susceptible to sheep prions and mouse prions respectively, as demonstrated by a steady increase in PrP^{TSE} and prion infectivity levels over 3–4 weeks (Cronier et al., 2004). Primary cerebellar granular neurons derived from transgenic mice overexpressing hamster and human PrP^{C} were also found to be susceptible to infection with prions, with the latter cells being one of the only instances in the literature of successful infection of cells with human CJD (Cronier et al., 2007). Interestingly, while primary neurons derived from wild-type mice are also susceptible to infection with multiple mouse prion strains (Hannaoui et al., 2013; Tanaka et al., 2016; Victoria et al., 2016), there are strain-specific differences in susceptibility depending upon whether the neurons are cerebellar granular neurons, cortical or striatal (Hannaoui et al., 2013). Finally, primary astrocytes alone (Cronier et al., 2004; Victoria et al., 2016) as well as mixed cultures of primary neurons and astrocytes (Cronier et al., 2012; Victoria et al., 2016) are susceptible to prion infection. Unlike most prion-infected cell lines, prion-infected primary neuronal cultures (Cronier et al., 2004) as well as mixed neuronal–astrocyte cultures (Cronier et al., 2012) exhibit signs of apoptosis, suggesting that they could be useful for studying prion-associated cell death.

Multicellular three-dimensional cell culture

The development of more complex, multicellular in vitro systems of prion infection also shows some promise as models of prion-associated neurodegeneration. Complex clusters of nestin-positive neural stem cells (neurospheres) derived from wild-type mice or transgenic mice overexpressing mouse PrP^{C} are susceptible to multiple mouse prion strains (Herva et al., 2010; Iwamaru et al., 2013) as well as mouse-adapted BSE (Iwamaru et al., 2013) and GSS (Collins and Haigh, 2017). Neurospheres are only susceptible to infection following differentiation (Herva et al., 2010; Iwamaru et al., 2013) when they develop into complex cellular clusters with externally located quiescent, immature cells underneath which is a layer of astrocytes, neuronal precursors, and mature neurons (Collins and Haigh, 2017). Prion infection of neurospheres leads to focal degeneration reminiscent of prion pathology (Iwamaru et al., 2013) as well as apoptosis-associated astrocyte cell death (Iwamaru et al., 2013; Collins and Haigh, 2017). Thus, they may be useful models for prion infection-associated cell loss.

Organotypic slice cultures represent one of the most promising in vitro systems to study prion-associated pathogenesis. Thick cerebellar tissue slices, isolated from mice that are several days old and maintained in culture for several weeks, are susceptible to persistent prion infection with a variety of mouse and mouse prion-adapted strains (Falsig et al., 2008; Wolf et al., 2015b). While prion-infected cerebellar slices remain viable, they nonetheless exhibit multiple prion strain-specific morphologic changes, including diffuse and plaque-like deposition of PrP^{TSE}, selective neuronal loss, vacuolation, astrogliosis, and loss of dendritic spines (Falsig et al., 2008; Campeau et al., 2013; Wolf et al., 2015b). As such, they can be used as an in vitro model system of prion-associated neurodegeneration and have been used to demonstrate a role for microglia in degradation of PrP^{TSE} (Falsig et al., 2008) and calpains in neurotoxicity (Falsig et al., 2012).

DETERMINANTS OF CELLULAR SUSCEPTIBILITY TO PRION INFECTION

Expression of PrP^{C}

Deletion of the prion protein gene (*PRNP*) in mice renders those mice resistant to prion infection (Bueler et al., 1993) and restoration of the *PRNP* gene locus restores susceptibility to prion infection (Manson et al., 1994; Weissmann et al., 1994; Sakaguchi et al., 1995; Fischer et al., 1996; Raeber et al., 1997), results which have been recapitulated using cell culture models. There are now several established cell lines where the *PRNP* gene locus has been ablated (Table 3.1), all of which were derived from mouse brain (Kuwahara et al., 1999; Greil et al., 2008; Nishimura et al., 2008). PrP^{C} knockout cells are also resistant to prion infection unless mouse PrP^{C} expression is restored, after which they are susceptible to infection with mouse prions (Maas et al., 2007; McNally et al., 2009; Marshall et al., 2017). Expression of endogenous host PrP^{C} is therefore an absolute requirement for a productive prion infection in vivo and in cell-based models of prion infection in vitro.

However, expression of PrP^{C} is not sufficient for a cell to be susceptible to prion infection. There are cell lines which express PrP^{C} but remain refractory to prion infection (e.g., Piccardo et al., 2011; Oelschlegel et al., 2015), cell lines that can be infected with one strain of prion but not another (Table 3.1), and even instances of prion-resistant subclones being derived from susceptible cell lines (Bosque and Prusiner, 2000; Klohn et al., 2003). A threshold level of PrP^C expression could explain this lack of correlation but multiple studies have shown that PrP^C expression level does not in fact predict whether or not a cell can be infected with prions. Cell lines with relatively low levels of PrP^C can be infected with prions just as well as cell lines with relatively high levels of PrP^C (Vorberg et al., 2004b; Chasseigneaux et al., 2008; Piccardo et al., 2011; Oelschlegel et al., 2015). While the quantity of PrP^C may not be a driving factor in a cell's susceptibility to prion infection, the quality of PrP^C can influence susceptibility. Cell lines where a proteolytically cleaved PrP^C product known as C1 is present at a higher proportion to full-length PrP^C were less susceptible to persistent prion infection, likely because the C1 fragment is much less efficiently converted to PrP^{TSE} (Lewis et al., 2009). Thus, the relative proportions of different PrP^C species may influence PrP^{TSE} replication (Yadavalli et al., 2004) and the susceptibility of a cell to prion infection (Lewis et al., 2009).

Cell-based determinants of susceptibility to prion infection

There are only a handful of studies which have looked for genes that are either uniquely expressed or whose expression level is altered in cells susceptible to prion infection. Doh-ura et al. (1995) utilized subtractive DNA hybridization to analyze cDNAs from five RML mouse scrapie-infected neuroblastoma cell lines and five noninfected mouse neuroblastoma cell lines. They found no genes that were uniquely expressed in the scrapie-infected cells. However, they did identify almost 100 genes whose expression was altered in the scrapie-positive cells when compared to scrapie-negative cells, including heat shock protein 70 and chromogranin B. However, expression of these genes was also quite variable in some, but not necessarily all, of the noninfected cell clones (Doh-ura et al., 1995). Chasseigneaux et al. (2008) did a similar study comparing both karyotype and gene expression of six 22L mouse scrapie-infected neuroblastoma cell lines and two noninfected mouse neuroblastoma cell lines. They also identified a set of genes that were differentially expressed between infected and noninfected cells lines but again were unable to identify a gene profile that was specific to cell lines susceptible to prion infection.

These studies strongly suggested that susceptible cells do not express a specific cellular receptor that is required for prion infection. One implication of these early data was that susceptibility to infection might involve alterations to one or more cellular pathways. If these cellular alterations varied subtly between different cell/prion strain combinations, they could be difficult to distinguish without a deeper genomic or proteomic analysis.

Two more recent studies suggest that this may indeed be the case. One used mRNA microarray and quantitative polymerase chain reaction (qPCR) analysis to determine the relative gene expression level in several RML-infected mouse N2a cell clones. By comparing prion replication rates in susceptible versus less susceptible cell clones, a group of genes associated both directly and indirectly with homeostasis of the extracellular matrix (ECM) was identified (Marbiah et al., 2014). Upregulation of these genes, which included fibronectin-1, integrin α8, and 3'-phospho-adenosine-5'-phosphosulphate synthase 2 (PAPS), was closely associated with decreased rates of prion replication and decreased susceptibility to infection. When these genes were experimentally silenced in less susceptible cells using RNA knockdown technology, the rate of prion replication subsequently increased, suggesting an increase in susceptibility to prion infection (Marbiah et al., 2014). Importantly, several of the genes identified also had altered expression levels in both 22L prion-infected N2a cells and CAD5 cells infected with RML prions (Marbiah et al., 2014), suggesting that between cell types there were some commonalities in the pathways involved.

A second study used RNA-seq analysis and reverse transcription qPCR to compare relative gene expression levels in sheep scrapie-susceptible and resistant cell clones derived from the hTERT sheep microglial cell line (Munoz-Gutierrez et al., 2016). Once again, using prion replication rates to define relative susceptibility to prion infection, cells that were less permissive to prion infection had increased expression levels of fibronectin-1 and other genes involved in proteolysis and remodeling of the ECM (Munoz-Gutierrez et al., 2016).

These studies link rate of prion replication to susceptibility to prion infection and provide a possible mechanism based on the genes identified. For example, the enzyme PAPS was overexpressed in N2a cells more resistant to prion replication (Marbiah et al., 2014). PAPS is required for the sulfation of ECM proteins (Wang et al., 2012) and loss of functional PAPS leads to undersulfation of the ECM proteoglycan heparin and increased susceptibility to prion infection (Marbiah et al., 2014). This was inconsistent with an earlier study demonstrating that inhibition of glycosaminoglycan (GAG) sulfation reduced the level of PrP^{TSE} in persistently infected N2a cells (Gabizon et al., 1993). The level of activation of specific metalloproteases regulated by fibronectin 1 can also affect the composition of ECM proteins and alter the level of PrP^C in the ECM that is available for conversion to PrP^{TSE} (Marbiah et al., 2014; Munoz-Gutierrez et al., 2016). Overall, the implication from these studies is that processes associated with ECM homeostasis, including posttranslational modifications and protein degradation, help to determine susceptibility to prion infection most likely by limiting the location and amount of PrP^C and thus the rate of prion replication.

ACUTE PRION INFECTION

For the purposes of this chapter, the process by which prions infect cells in vitro has been broadly divided into three stages. The first, acute stage of infection encompasses the earliest events which must occur for a cell to become infected. These include the initial interaction of PrP^{TSE} with the cell, PrP^{TSE} uptake and trafficking, and the initial conversion of the host PrP^C molecule to PrP^{TSE}, i.e., prion replication. In vitro, the acute phase of infection for established cell lines is generally defined as the time period, ranging anywhere from 0 to 96 hours, from the first exposure of cells to infectious prions up to the first passage of the cells (Vorberg et al., 2004a). The second phase of infection is initiated after the first cell passage. It involves the transition from acute to persistent infection, a period which might encompass several cell passages and one where protein degradation, prion replication rate, and prion spread are all critical issues. The final stage is a persistent infection that can be stably maintained over many months and many, many cell passages.

Cellular binding and uptake of PrP^{TSE}

To study the process by which PrP^{TSE} interacts with and is taken up by cells, cells in culture are exposed to exogenous PrP^{TSE} that may or may not be purified from prion-infected brain homogenate and the cellular association, uptake, and trafficking of PrP^{TSE} are assayed over time. In experiments such as these, it is critical to be able to distinguish exogenous PrP^{TSE} from both the host cell's PrP^C as well as any PrP^{TSE} that has been derived from the host PrP^C molecule once prion replication begins. Several different approaches have been used to accomplish this, including the use of established cell lines which express either extremely low levels of PrP^C (Hijazi et al., 2005; Paquet et al., 2007) or cell lines in which PrP^C expression has been ablated (Greil et al., 2008). Differences in antibody reactivity between the exogenous PrP^{TSE} molecules and the host PrP^C molecules (Goold et al., 2011; Greil et al., 2008; Horonchik et al., 2005; Taraboulos et al., 1990) have also been utilized (Fig. 3.1A). Finally, purified PrP^{TSE} that has been cross-linked with fluorescently labeled dyes has been used to study the uptake and trafficking of PrP^{TSE} in both live and fixed cells (Magalhaes et al., 2005; Gousset et al., 2009; Jen et al., 2010; Yamasaki et al., 2014).

Several studies have analyzed whether or not molecules known to bind PrP^{TSE} such as PrP^C, GAGs, the laminin receptor protein (LRP 37/67 kDa), and the low-density lipoprotein receptor-related protein (LRP1) act as receptors for PrP^{TSE} binding and uptake. As discussed earlier, PrP^C expression level does not necessarily correlate with susceptibility to prion infection (Vorberg et al., 2004b; Chasseigneaux et al., 2008; Piccardo et al., 2011; Oelschlegel et al., 2015), suggesting that it does not act as a cellular receptor for PrP^{TSE}. An early study looking at the uptake of hamster PrP^{TSE} by Chinese hamster ovary (CHO) cells, which do not express detectable levels of PrP^C, found that they bound hamster PrP^{TSE} as efficiently as CHO cells which had been transfected to express hamster PrP^C (Hijazi et al., 2005).

A similar result was seen using RK13 cells, another cell line which does not express detectable levels of PrP^C (Paquet et al., 2007). In that study, PrP^{TSE} uptake in wild-type RK13 cells was compared to RK13 cells which express sheep PrP^C under the control of a doxycycline inducible promoter (Rov cells). Induction of sheep PrP^C expression did not alter the uptake of sheep PrP^{TSE}. Similarly, stimulation of PrP^C expression in murine macrophage and microglial cells lines also did not affect mouse PrP^{TSE} uptake (Gilch et al., 2007).

A later study looked at the uptake of epitope-tagged PrP^{TSE} from three different strains of mouse prions by neural cells derived from PrP^C knockout mice (CF10 cells) versus CF10 cells overexpressing PrP^C or fibroblast cells expressing wild-type levels of endogenous PrP^C (Greil et al., 2008). The kinetics of PrP^{TSE} uptake were similar for all three cell types, again suggesting that PrP^C expression was not required for PrP^{TSE} uptake and that PrP^C expression level did not influence the rate of uptake.

Overall, a majority of studies agree that PrP^C is not acting as a receptor for PrP^{TSE} (Hijazi et al., 2005; Magalhaes et al., 2005; Paquet et al., 2007; Greil et al., 2008; Langevin et al., 2010). However, there is some evidence that PrP^C, while not essential, may still influence the efficiency of PrP^{TSE} uptake. In the aforementioned Rov cell study, PrP^{TSE} derived from BSE-infected transgenic mice expressing sheep PrP^C was taken up less efficiently than sheep PrP^{TSE} (Paquet et al., 2007). In murine SN56 cells, the uptake and trafficking of hamster PrP^{TSE} were less efficient than that of PrP^{TSE} from two different mouse prion strains (Magalhaes et al., 2005). Thus, while not essential for PrP^{TSE} uptake, in some cell types PrP^C may modulate PrP^{TSE} uptake in a prion strain and species-dependent manner.

Many different viruses use cellular GAGs as receptors to infect a cell (Liu and Thorp, 2002). GAGs are also obvious candidates for cellular PrP^{TSE} receptors. They are known to bind PrP (Gabizon et al., 1993; Imamura et al., 2016) and can act either as cofactors in the conversion of PrP^C to PrP^{TSE} (Wong et al., 2001;

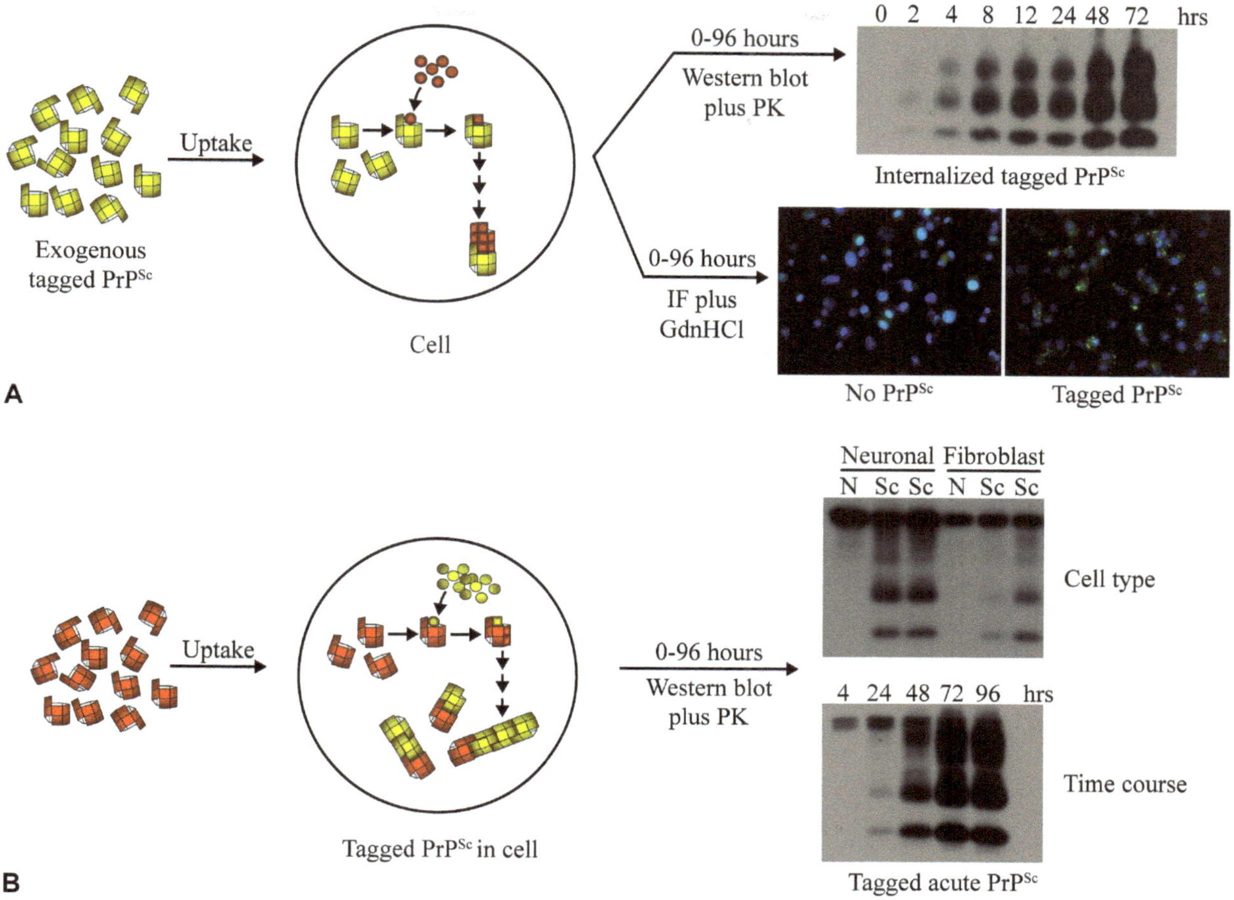

Fig. 3.1. Modeling acute prion infection in vitro. (**A**) Modeling PrP^{TSE} uptake. Exogenous PrP^{TSE} which has been uniquely tagged with a fluorescent dye or antibody epitope (PrP^{Sc}, yellow squares) is added to cells expressing PrP^{C} which is not tagged (red circles). Exogenous PrP^{TSE} binds PrP^{C} to form new PrP^{TSE} molecules (red squares) which are not tagged. The amount of exogenous PrP^{TSE} associated with the cell over several days can then be analyzed either by Western blot following proteinase K (PK) digestion of the cell lysate or immunofluorescence (IF) following treatment of the cells with guanidine hydrochloride (GdnHCl). Using antibodies specific to the tagged PrP^{TSE} molecules, only exogenous PrP^{TSE} will be detected. (**B**) Modeling acute PrP^{TSE} formation. Exogenous PrP^{TSE} (red squares) is added to different cell types, in this example neuronal or fibroblast cells, expressing a PrP^{C} molecule tagged with a unique antibody epitope. Exogenous PrP^{TSE} binds tagged PrP^{C} to form new, tagged PrP^{TSE} molecules (yellow squares). The amount of newly formed PrP^{TSE} can then be analyzed over several days using antibodies specific to the tagged PrP^{TSE} molecules by Western blot following PK digestion of the cell lysate. Under these conditions, only acutely formed PrP^{TSE} will be detected. hrs, hours; N, cells not exposed to exogenous PrP^{TSE}; Sc, cells exposed to exogenous PrP^{TSE}.

Imamura et al., 2016) or as inhibitors of the conversion process (Priola and Caughey, 1994). In CHO cells, PrP^{TSE} binding was significantly decreased in the presence of heparin and there was very little binding of PrP^{TSE} to CHO cells lacking either GAGs or the specific GAG heparin sulfate (Hijazi et al., 2005). In N2a cells exposed to purified hamster PrP^{TSE}, PrP^{TSE} uptake was decreased in the presence of heparin sulfate and by treatment with heparinase III (Horonchik et al., 2005). Similarly, binding of purified mouse PrP^{TSE} to GT1 cells was also reduced in the presence of heparinase III (Horonchik et al., 2005) and treatment of the cells with sodium chlorate, which inhibits sulfation of GAGs, reduced PrP^{TSE} binding. Thus, these studies suggested that a heparinase III-sensitive, sulfated heparin sulfate proteoglycan was crucial for the binding and uptake of PrP^{TSE} by several cell types (Horonchik et al., 2005).

However, in CHO cells exposed to hamster PrP^{TSE} there was also clearly a GAG-independent mechanism for PrP^{TSE} uptake. PrP^{TSE} binding was not completely abolished even in GAG-negative cells and at higher PrP^{TSE} concentrations GAGs were not even required for PrP^{TSE} to interact with the cells (Hijazi et al., 2005). Moreover, Wolf et al. (2015a) demonstrated that in N2a cells and L929 fibroblast cells exposed to PrP^{TSE} from RML and 22L-infected mouse brain homogenates, treatment with either dextran sulfate or sodium chlorate did not reduce PrP^{TSE} uptake. Additionally, there was no difference in the uptake of 22L and RML mouse PrP^{TSE} when wild-type CHO cells were compared to GAG-deficient CHO cells (Wolf et al., 2015a). While the data support a role for GAGs in the uptake of at least some strains of prions, clearly PrP^{TSE} uptake can occur via GAG-independent mechanisms.

Cell surface LRP 37 kDa/67 kDA (LRP) may also play a role in PrP^{TSE} uptake. LRP binds PrP^{C} and, with heparin sulfate proteoglycan as a cofactor, internalizes it via clathrin-coated pits or caveolae (Gauczynski et al., 2001; Hundt et al., 2001) (Fig. 3.2). Antisense or siRNA inhibition of LRP RNA in RML scrapie-infected GT1

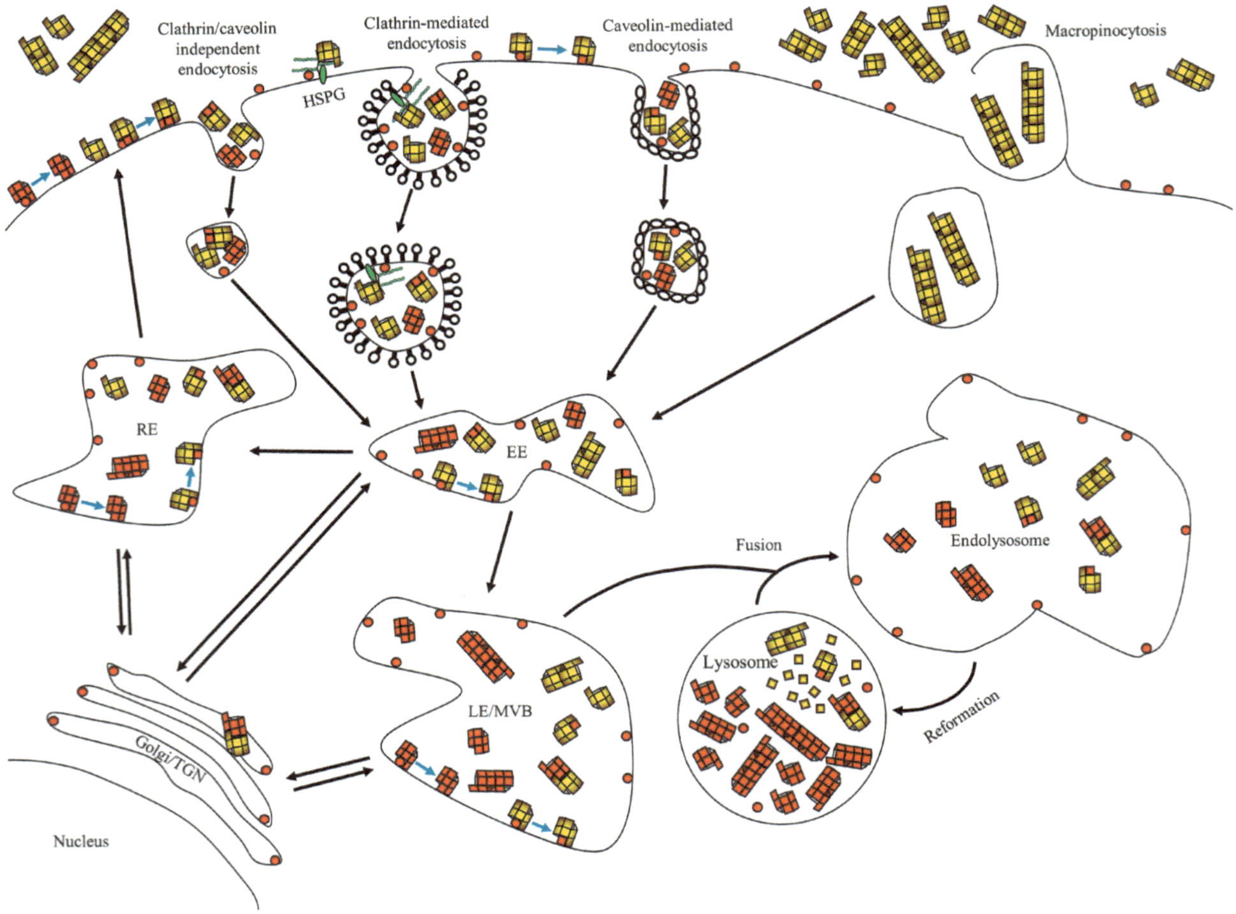

Fig. 3.2. Cell biology of prion infection. Prion infection of a cell from the initial exposure of the cell to infectious prions to the establishment of persistent prion infection is shown. Exogenous PrP^{TSE} (yellow square aggregates), composed of a heterogeneous mix of aggregates is taken up by the cell via clathrin and caveolin-dependent and -independent mechanisms as well as macropinocytosis. The pathway used may depend upon the size of the PrP^{TSE} aggregate. In some instances, PrP^{TSE} may also bind to low-density lipoprotein receptor-related protein (LRP1, not shown) or heparin sulfate proteoglycans (HSPG: small chain of blue circles) on the cell surface, possibly in association with the laminin receptor protein (LRP, green oval). Following binding, it is then taken up by clathrin or caveolin-mediated endocytosis. Once in the cell, exogenous PrP^{TSE} enters both the endolysosomal and endocytic recycling pathway and is found in early endosomes (EE), endolysosomes, late endosomes/multivesicular bodies (LE/MVB), and lysosomes where a significant percentage of it is degraded. Exogenous PrP^{TSE} is also trafficked to the recycling endosomes (RE) where it can be recycled back to the plasma membrane. Once exogenous PrP^{TSE} comes into contact with the cell, it binds to cellular PrP^{C} (red circles) leading to the formation of acute PrP^{TSE} (mixed yellow and red square aggregates). Acute PrP^{TSE} can be formed on the cell surface, following either the initial contact of exogenous PrP^{TSE} with the cell or recycling of exogenous PrP^{TSE} to the plasma membrane, as well as within EE, LE/MVB, and RE. Acutely formed PrP^{TSE} can be recycled to the cell surface likely via the endocytic recycling/trans-Golgi network (TGN) pathway where it can trigger PrP^{TSE} formation and then eventually accumulate in the lysosome. Over time as the cells are passaged, PrP^{TSE} in the cell is derived solely from the cell's own PrP^{C} molecules and a persistent infection is established (red square aggregates). As with exogenous PrP^{TSE}, persistent PrP^{TSE} is endocytosed via clathrin and caveolin-dependent and -independent mechanisms and eventually accumulates in the lysosome where it has a longer half-life (>24 hours) than nonhost-derived PrP^{TSE}. Similarly to acute PrP^{TSE}, persistent PrP^{TSE} is also made on the plasma membrane, REs, and possibly LE/MVB, but does not appear to be made in EE.

cells reduced both PrP^{C} and PrP^{TSE}, suggesting that LRP could play a role in the propagation of PrP^{TSE}, possibly by affecting PrP^{C} trafficking (Leucht et al., 2003). LRP could also be directly interacting with PrP^{TSE}, a possibility supported by the observation that uptake of PrP^{TSE} by the human enterocyte-like cell line Caco-2/TC7 could be inhibited by an antibody against LRP (Morel et al., 2005).

Baby hamster kidney cells (BHK) transfected with mouse LRP exhibited dose-dependent binding of mouse PrP^{TSE} that was blocked by GAG inhibitors (Gauczynski et al., 2006). However, this inhibition was independent of LRP expression, suggesting that PrP^{TSE} (Gauczynski et al., 2006) was interacting with GAGs on the cell surface, including the heparin sulfate proteoglycan associated with LRP (Gauczynski et al., 2006).

Finally, there is one study suggesting that the low-density lipoprotein receptor-related protein (LRP1) can also act as a receptor for PrP^{TSE}. In both primary neuron cultures and hippocampal organ cultures, the uptake of fluorescently labeled PrP^{TSE} derived from the ME7 strain of mouse scrapie was blocked by inhibiting LRP1 with the receptor-associated protein RAP (Jen et al., 2010).

Overall, there is no consensus on the cellular component most likely to bind PrP^{TSE} upon its initial interaction with the cell. This could be the result of the variety of different cellular systems used to study PrP^{TSE} uptake. However, it is more likely that, at least in part as a consequence of its highly aggregated and heterogeneous nature, PrP^{TSE} can interact with multiple molecules on the cell surface. When one of those molecules is unavailable, another is used. Thus, PrP^{TSE} likely enters the cell in a variety of ways that can be both dependent and independent of GAGs, LRP, LRP1 or other as yet unidentified PrP^{TSE}-binding partners.

PrP^{TSE} uptake

Multiple studies have shown that PrP^{TSE} uptake is temperature-sensitive, indicating a general, active cellular process such as endocytosis (Magalhaes et al., 2005; Greil et al., 2008). Since PrP^{TSE} does not appear to have a preferred cellular binding partner, its uptake could occur via any of a variety of endocytic processes, including clathrin-mediated endocytosis, clathrin-independent endocytosis, phagocytosis, and macropinocytosis (Fig. 3.2). In nonphagocytic cells, particle size can determine which of these endocytic pathways is utilized as well as the efficiency and rate of uptake and the downstream fate of the endocytosed particle (Rejman et al., 2004). For example, internalization of microspheres by clathrin-mediated endocytosis is very rapid and occurs almost immediately for microspheres between 50 and 100 nm in size, but is slower for 200-nm particles. By contrast, particles >200 nm in size are internalized very slowly over the course of hours via caveolae-mediated endocytosis and possibly micropinocytosis (Rejman et al., 2004). Once internalized, the 50–200-nm particles are then trafficked to late endosomes/lysosomes (Rejman et al., 2004).

The restriction of internalization of microspheres by size suggests that, since PrP^{TSE} is a heterogeneous mix of different-sized aggregates, PrP^{TSE} aggregate size would have a significant influence on its mode and rate of uptake. Studies using either fluorescently labeled or epitope-tagged PrP^{TSE} have clearly shown that this is the case. When primary mouse neurons or SN56 cells were exposed to fluorophore cross-linked PrP^{TSE} aggregates from several species, uptake of the fluorescent aggregates occurred very slowly over the course of several days (Magalhaes et al., 2005; Baron et al., 2006). This process did not appear to be receptor or lipid raft-mediated but was more consistent with macropinocytosis (Magalhaes et al., 2005).

By contrast, when murine fibroblast or neural cells were exposed to murine PrP^{TSE} prion strains that contained the epitope to the hamster-specific anti-PrP antibody (PrP-3F4^{Sc}), PrP-3F4^{Sc} uptake was easily detectable after 2 hours with most PrP^{TSE} internalized by 24 hours (Greil et al., 2008). Conjugating PrP-3F4^{Sc} to a fluorophore led to a significant increase in PrP-3F4^{Sc} aggregate size and poor internalization, suggesting that the different rates of PrP^{TSE} uptake were related to artificial aggregation of PrP^{TSE} during conjugation of PrP^{TSE} to the fluorophore (Greil et al., 2008). Indeed, when fluorescently labeled PrP^{TSE} was sonicated and the larger aggregates removed, its uptake was much more rapid, easily detectable after 2 hours (Magalhaes et al., 2005; Baron et al., 2006; Yamasaki et al., 2014), and occurred via clathrin-mediated endocytosis (Yamasaki et al., 2014). Overall, the majority of studies are consistent with PrP^{TSE} internalization being a rapid process consistent with endocytosis (Taraboulos et al., 1990; Mohan et al., 2005; Rybner-Barnier et al., 2006; Greil et al., 2008; Langevin et al., 2010; Elhelaly et al., 2013b; Choi et al., 2014), suggesting that most sources of PrP^{TSE} contain abundant particles of under 200 nm in size.

Consistent with size being a critical factor for PrP^{TSE} uptake, one study has shown that the pool of PrP^{TSE} internalized by the cells is limited by aggregate size (Choi and Priola, 2013). Approximately 80% of PrP^{TSE} sedimented from prion-infected brain homogenates using discontinuous sucrose gradient fractionation is found in the bottom three fractions of the gradient, indicating that the majority of PrP^{TSE} aggregates are quite large. However, when cells were exposed to those same brain homogenates, analysis of cell-associated PrP^{TSE} 2 hours postexposure showed that the majority of PrP^{TSE} internalized by the cell sedimented in a single fraction of the gradient (Choi and Priola, 2013). This fraction was not representative of the largest PrP^{TSE} aggregates in the starting brain homogenate (Choi and Priola, 2013). Thus, the cells selectively internalized only PrP^{TSE} aggregates within a certain size range, indicating a particle size-based restriction of PrP^{TSE} uptake.

The influence of PrP^{TSE} aggregate size on uptake may also explain why some studies indicate that macropinocytosis is the mechanism of PrP^{TSE} uptake (Magalhaes et al., 2005; Wadia et al., 2008; Rouvinski et al., 2014) while others do not (Paquet et al., 2007) and why there are conflicting results regarding whether or not PrP^{TSE} uptake is prion strain or species-dependent (Magalhaes et al., 2005; Paquet et al., 2007; Greil et al., 2008). While differences in the cell culture systems used between studies could contribute to these discrepancies, the fact that when PrP^{TSE} aggregate size is similar between samples the kinetics of PrP^{TSE} uptake appear to be similar and independent of prion strain and cell type (Greil et al., 2008; Choi and Priola, 2013; Yamasaki et al., 2014; Wolf et al., 2015a) makes this less likely. Overall, the data strongly support a role for PrP^{TSE} aggregate size significantly influencing both the kinetics and endocytic mechanism of prion uptake by the cell.

One other factor that influences the kinetics of PrP^{TSE} uptake and efficiency of infection is related to how PrP^{TSE} is presented to the cells. Purified PrP^{TSE} is less efficiently internalized than PrP^{TSE} present in brain homogenate (Greil et al., 2008) or PrP^{TSE} -containing brain microsomes (Baron et al., 2006). Exposure of cells to prion-infected brain homogenate leads to the most efficient uptake of PrP^{TSE} (Greil et al., 2008). These data suggest that there may be a cofactor or specific PrP^{TSE} microenvironment, such as cholesterol-rich lipid (Baron et al., 2006), that may facilitate prion uptake which is lost when PrP^{TSE} is purified.

PrP^{TSE} trafficking

Depending upon the cell type, anywhere from 10% to 20% (Greil et al., 2008; Choi and Priola, 2013; Choi et al., 2014) to 80% (Paquet et al., 2007) of the input PrP^{TSE} is internalized. The reason for this variation is unclear but could be due to multiple factors such as PrP^{TSE} aggregate size and the endocytic/phagocytic activity of the cell. The percentage of cells in a culture which initially take up PrP^{TSE} also varies between different cell culture systems (Magalhaes et al., 2005; Greil et al., 2008; Wolf et al., 2015a). Variation in the susceptibility of an individual cell within a culture to prion infection may at least partially explain why PrP^{TSE} is not internalized by all cells in the culture. Early studies in N2a cells demonstrated that only a subpopulation of cells in the culture were susceptible to prion infection (Butler et al., 1988; Race et al., 1988; Bosque and Prusiner, 2000) and subcloning is routinely used to isolate cells from cell lines that are either stably infected (Butler et al., 1988; Race et al., 1988) or highly susceptible to initial prion infection (Bosque and Prusiner, 2000; Nishida et al., 2000; Mahal et al., 2007). However, cells that are resistant to prion infection can also internalize PrP^{TSE} (Horonchik et al., 2005; Greil et al., 2008) so susceptibility to infection is unlikely to be the only explanation for cell-to-cell variability in taking up PrP^{TSE}.

There is much better agreement between cell models as to how PrP^{TSE} is trafficked once it has been internalized by the cell. A study by Yamasaki et al. (2014) shows that, at 2 hours postexposure, fluorescently labeled PrP^{TSE} added to N2a cells can be found in multiple Rab-positive compartments, including early endosomes, recycling endosomes, and late endosomes (Fig. 3.2). This indicates that the input PrP^{TSE} is being trafficked very rapidly through multiple endocytic compartments (Yamasaki et al., 2014). For several hours postexposure, PrP^{TSE} co-localizes with the transferrin receptor indicating the involvement of clathrin-mediated endocytosis and trafficking of PrP^{TSE} to early endosomes followed by recycling to the plasma membrane where, shortly after inoculation, ~20% of the input PrP^{TSE} is found (Yamasaki et al., 2014).

In addition to the transferrin receptor, fluorescently labeled PrP^{TSE} also co-localizes with low-density lipoprotein (LDL) after its initial uptake. However, at 30 hours postexposure almost all of the PrP^{TSE} co-localizes with LDL and not transferrin, suggesting that at later timepoints PrP^{TSE} has been trafficked to lysosomes and late endosomes (Yamasaki et al., 2014) where LDL is known to be degraded (Ikonen, 2008). Fluorescently labeled, exogenous mouse PrP^{TSE} is also trafficked after several days to late endosomes/lysosomes in SN56 cells and primary neurons (Magalhaes et al., 2005; Jen et al., 2010). In addition, in both human tonsil-derived follicular dendritic type cells (HK cells) and the human astrocyte cell line SVG, PrP^{TSE} is found almost exclusively in lysosomal compartments 24 hours postexposure (Choi et al., 2014; Krejciova et al., 2014). Murine PrP^{TSE} taken up by mouse macrophages similarly localizes to lysosomes by 24 hours postexposure (Mayer-Sonnenfeld et al., 2008; Sassa et al., 2010). Thus, the data suggest that, during acute infection, exogenous PrP^{TSE} is trafficked at early timepoints through recycling and endolysosomal endocytic pathways to both the cell surface and endolysosomes, but that at later timepoints almost all of the exogenous PrP^{TSE} has entered the endolysosomal pathway and is localized to late endosomes/lysosomes (Yamasaki et al., 2014).

PrP^{TSE} degradation

The localization of exogenous PrP^{TSE} to late endosomal and lysosomal compartments several hours after uptake suggests that it has been targeted for degradation. Surprisingly, given the extremely high protease resistance of PrP^{TSE}, a large percentage of internalized PrP^{TSE} is in fact degraded by the cell. Phagocytic murine bone marrow-derived dendritic cells, plasmacytoid dendritic cells, and macrophages all degrade exogenous PrP^{TSE} from various species within 2–4 days (Luhr et al., 2002; Mohan et al., 2005; Rybner-Barnier et al., 2006; Gilch et al., 2007; Gousset et al., 2009; Langevin et al., 2010; Elhelaly et al., 2013b), as do the macrophage cell lines J774 and Raw (Gilch et al., 2007; Sassa et al., 2010; Elhelaly et al., 2013b) and the murine microglial cell line BV2 (Gilch et al., 2007).

PrP^{TSE} degradation in phagocytic cells may depend upon the maturity of the cells, as mouse XS106 cells, which have a mature Langerhans cell phenotype, can degrade the ME7 strain of mouse PrP^{TSE}, while the immature Langerhans cell line XS52 cannot (Mohan et al., 2005). Somewhat surprisingly, cells that are not professional phagocytic cells can also degrade PrP^{TSE}, including hamster CHO cells (Mayer-Sonnenfeld et al., 2008), human embryonic stem cells (Krejciova et al., 2011), human SVG astrocyte cells (Choi et al., 2014), murine neuroblastoma cells (Elhelaly et al., 2013b; Yamasaki et al., 2014), and murine neural (Choi and Priola, 2013; Elhelaly et al., 2013b), intestinal (Elhelaly et al., 2013b), and fibroblast cells (Elhelaly et al., 2013b).

In macrophages, degradation of PrP^{TSE} is inhibited at low temperature and dependent upon cholesterol (Elhelaly et al., 2013b) but occurs independently of PrP^{C} expression (Rybner-Barnier et al., 2006; Mayer-Sonnenfeld et al., 2008), suggesting that it involves PrP^{C}-independent trafficking to an intracellular compartment. The most likely compartment is the lysosome. Lysosomal inhibitors leupeptin (Luhr et al., 2004; Sassa et al., 2010) and E64-d (Sassa et al., 2010) inhibit PrP^{TSE} degradation consistent with it being degraded by lysosomal cathepsin proteases. Degradation of PrP^{TSE} in lysosomes is also supported by the observation that, in CHO cells, tilorone-induced accumulation of sulfated GAGs in the lysosome blocks clearance of PrP^{TSE} (Mayer-Sonnenfeld et al., 2008). Some PrP^{TSE} may also be degraded via the proteosomal pathway as proteasome activity is decreased at low temperature (Elhelaly et al., 2013b) and the proteosomal inhibitors MG132 and ALLN reduced PrP^{TSE} degradation in mouse macrophages (Sassa et al., 2010). Thus, trafficking of exogenous PrP^{TSE} via the endolysosomal pathway to the lysosome is likely the primary mechanism for its degradation and clearance, although degradation via proteasomes may also have an impact.

The mechanism by which lysosomes can degrade exogenous PrP^{TSE} is unclear. In CF10 cells with or without PrP^{C}, PrP^{TSE} particles are disaggregated over time even as the amount of PrP^{TSE} taken up by the cell continues to increase (Choi and Priola, 2013). The rate of disaggregation does not appear to be dependent on the relative stability of the PrP^{TSE} aggregate since more stable PrP^{TSE} aggregates can be disaggregated more rapidly than less stable PrP^{TSE} aggregates (Choi and Priola, 2013). Moreover, the relative protease resistance of the PrP^{TSE} particle did not appear to correlate with its rate of degradation (Choi et al., 2014), suggesting that factors other than protease-sensitivity may be influencing how rapidly PrP^{TSE} is degraded. This somewhat paradoxical result could be explained if the acidic pH of the lysosome leads to the loss of conformational determinants that contribute to the protease resistance of PrP^{TSE}. Alternatively, since disaggregation of PrP^{TSE} appears to precede its degradation (Choi and Priola, 2013), protein or nonprotein cofactors which stabilize PrP^{TSE} may be degraded/removed by lysosomal enzymes, leading to destabilization and increased sensitivity of the PrP^{TSE} particle to proteolysis. While no specific protein cofactors have been associated with PrP^{TSE} (Moore et al., 2010), GAGs interact with and stabilize PrP^{TSE} (Caspi et al., 1998; Beringue et al., 2000; Mayer-Sonnenfeld et al., 2008) and accumulation of sulfated GAGs in lysosomes reduces the clearance of PrP^{TSE} (Mayer-Sonnenfeld et al., 2008). Thus, clearance of PrP^{TSE} by the lysosome may first involve the removal of stabilizing molecules such as GAGs leading to disaggregation and increased protease-sensitivity of PrP^{TSE} allowing its degradation by lysosomal proteases.

Acute PrP^{TSE} formation

The final step in the process of prion infection of a cell is the initiation of prion replication. Even though prion diseases take months or years to develop in vivo, in cells in vitro the initiation of prion replication via the formation of new PrP^{TSE} is a surprisingly rapid process. Exposure of fibroblast or N2a cells expressing a uniquely epitope-tagged murine PrP^{C} molecule (PrP^{C}-3F4) to brain homogenates containing wild-type PrP^{TSE} (e.g., Fig. 3.1B) resulted in the acute formation of epitope-tagged PrP^{TSE} -3F4 (Vorberg et al., 2004a). Consistent with the rapid cellular uptake of PrP^{TSE}, acute PrP^{TSE} formation could be detected by immunoblot 4 hours post-exposure (Vorberg et al., 2004a), suggesting that new

PrP^{TSE} formation was initiated almost immediately upon exposure of the cells to PrP^{TSE}. Indeed, two other immunofluorescent microscopy-based studies have suggested that acute PrP^{TSE} is formed in cells either 2 hours (Yamasaki et al., 2014) or 1 minute (Goold et al., 2011) after exposure to PrP^{TSE}. In all studies, acute PrP^{TSE} formation appeared to be independent of cell type (Fig. 3.1B) and prion strain (Vorberg et al., 2004a; Goold et al., 2011; Elhelaly et al., 2013a; Yamasaki et al., 2014).

Acute PrP^{TSE} formation must take place in cellular locations where PrP^{C} is trafficked since PrP^{C} and PrP^{TSE} must directly interact for new PrP^{TSE} to be made (Fig. 3.2). Synthesis and trafficking of PrP^{C} to the cell surface involves the secretory pathway while its removal from the cell surface utilizes clathrin-dependent and independent endocytosis as well as endocytosis via caveolae. It then enters either the endolysosomal pathway to be degraded or the recycling endosomal pathway, where it may be trafficked back to the cell surface (for review, see Prado et al., 2004). Thus, acute PrP^{TSE} could theoretically be generated at any point along these multiple pathways.

In highly susceptible N2aPK1 cells exposed to the RML strain of prions the plasma membrane is the primary site of acute PrP^{TSE} formation which requires GPI-anchored, cell surface PrP^{C} and most likely occurs in a lipid raft environment (Goold et al., 2011). In this model, which uses PrP^{C} tagged with the MYC epitope, acute PrP^{TSE} formation occurs within 1 minute and reaches maximum levels by 2 hours (Goold et al., 2011). By contrast, another study using neuroblastoma N2a cells exposed to the 22L and Obihiro strains of mouse prions suggests that early, late, and recycling endosomes, but not the plasma membrane, are the primary site of acute PrP^{TSE} formation (Yamasaki et al., 2014) and that acute PrP^{TSE} levels continue to increase over the first 72 hours of infection (Vorberg et al., 2004a; Yamasaki et al., 2014) (Fig. 3.1B). As further evidence against the plasma membrane being the primary site of acute PrP^{TSE} formation, PrP^{C} without the GPI anchor can also form PrP^{TSE} during acute infection, albeit at a lower efficiency (McNally et al., 2009). The reason for these contradictory results is unclear, but it could be due to differences in the cells and prion strains used as well as the techniques utilized to distinguish acute, epitope-tagged PrP^{TSE} from epitope-tagged PrP^{C}.

Despite the contradictory data on the initial location and rate of formation of acute PrP^{TSE}, there is relatively good agreement as to how it is trafficked after its formation (Fig. 3.2). Acute PrP^{TSE} on the plasma membrane is endocytosed via a pathway involving GM1-enriched membranes (Goold et al., 2013) and enters both the endolysosomal and endocytic recycling pathways (Goold et al., 2013; Yamasaki et al., 2014). Over time, the amount of acute PrP^{TSE} found in early and recycling endosomes increases (Goold et al., 2013; Yamasaki et al., 2014) with some transferring from endosomes to the trans-Golgi and Golgi (but not the endoplasmic reticulum), indicating retrograde trafficking (Goold et al., 2013). There is also evidence that acute PrP^{TSE} can be formed in late endosomes and/or be recycled back to the cell surface where it can trigger more PrP^{TSE} formation (Goold et al., 2013; Yamasaki et al., 2014). In addition, acute PrP^{TSE} can be targeted to the lysosome via either the endolysosomal pathway (Yamasaki et al., 2014) or a recycling/retrograde pathway involving endosomes and the trans-Golgi network (Goold et al., 2013). Thus, as with exogenously added PrP^{TSE}, acutely formed PrP^{TSE} can also be degraded over time (Vorberg et al., 2004a; Goold et al., 2013; Yamasaki et al., 2014).

ESTABLISHMENT OF PERSISTENT INFECTION

Adaptation

Intriguingly, formation of acute PrP^{TSE} does not always lead to persistent PrP^{TSE} formation and chronic infection of a cell (Vorberg et al., 2004a). This suggests that there may be prion strain-specific or cell-specific factors that can control the switch from acute prion infection to persistent prion infection. In N2a cells that are resistant to infection with 22L mouse prions, acute PrP^{TSE} is detectable at 24 hours but then decreases in amount over the next 72 hours. This suggests that prion replication is either inefficient or unable to keep pace with PrP^{TSE} degradation. By contrast, in fibroblast cells that are susceptible to 22L prion infection, PrP^{TSE} is detectable by 24 hours and increases steadily over the next 72 hours. This increase is not accompanied by an increase in the number of infected cells, suggesting that it represents increasingly efficient formation of PrP^{TSE} (Vorberg et al., 2004a). In addition to the quantitative change in PrP^{TSE} levels in susceptible cells, there is a qualitative change. PrP^{TSE} derived from distinct prion strains has a reproducible glycosylation profile, i.e., the relative ratio of the diglycosylated and monoglyosylated forms of PrP^{TSE} (Collinge et al., 1996; Somerville et al., 1997; Kuczius et al., 1998). During the first 96 hours of PrP^{TSE} formation in 22L susceptible fibroblasts this ratio is highly variable but, following passage, the glycosylation profile appears to stabilize (Vorberg et al., 2004a). Since the glycosylation profile of PrP^{C} can dictate the glycosylation profile of PrP^{TSE} (Tuzi et al., 2008), one interpretation of these data is that acute PrP^{TSE} formation may be occurring in multiple cellular compartments with different pools of PrP^{C} (Vorberg et al., 2004a). The fact that acute PrP^{TSE} formation occurs in early, late, and recycling endosomes (Goold et al., 2011; Yamasaki et al., 2014) as well as on the plasma membrane (Goold et al., 2011) (Fig. 3.2) is consistent with this interpretation. The quantitative and qualitative differences observed in acute PrP^{TSE} formation between resistant and susceptible cells suggest that, in susceptible cells, PrP^{TSE} is "adapting" to the cell by finding a cellular environment that allows for efficient prion replication and thus the establishment of persistent infection.

Role of PrP^{C}

Prion strain-specific cofactors could dictate whether or not a given prion strain can establish a persistent infection in vitro and thus might control the switch from acute to persistent prion infection. However, no strain-specific protein cofactors have been found in close association with PrP^{TSE} (Moore et al., 2010) and there is no evidence of nonprotein molecules interacting with PrP^{TSE} in a prion strain-specific manner. By contrast, there is some evidence that GPI anchoring of PrP^{C} to the plasma membrane is necessary for the transition from acute to persistent prion infection in vitro. Changing the GPI anchor of PrP^{C} to a transmembrane anchor inhibits its conversion to PrP^{TSE} (Taraboulos et al., 1995; Kaneko et al., 1997; Marshall et al., 2017), suggesting that the localization of PrP^{C} to lipid rafts via its GPI anchor is necessary for PrP^{TSE} formation. By contrast, during the acute phase of prion infection PrP^{C} without the GPI anchor can be converted to PrP^{TSE}, albeit with a lower efficiency, suggesting that membrane anchoring is not required for acute PrP^{TSE} formation (McNally et al., 2009). However, cells expressing PrP^{C} without the GPI anchor cannot support either persistent replication of GPI anchorless PrP^{TSE} or persistent prion infection unless wild-type GPI-anchored PrP^{C} is present (McNally et al., 2009). Thus, while the GPI anchor is not essential for formation of PrP^{TSE} in vitro, the presence of GPI-anchored PrP^{TSE} appears to be required in the transition from acute to persistent prion infection.

Cell-specific factors

Currently, no specific cell factors have been identified that enable the transition from acute to persistent prion infection. GAGs have been identified as cofactors in PrP^{TSE} formation (Caughey and Raymond, 1993; Priola and Caughey, 1994; Wong et al., 2001) and may influence PrP^{TSE} metabolism (Wolf et al., 2015a). As discussed earlier, inhibition of GAG sulfation reduces the level of PrP^{TSE} in persistently infected N2a cells (Gabizon et al., 1993), suggesting that the level of GAG sulfation influences prion replication in vitro. Sulfation of GAGs may also be important in the establishment of prion infection. Treatment of fibroblast cells with inhibitors of GAG sulfation prior to infection with mouse prions had no effect on PrP^{TSE} uptake (Paquet et al., 2007; Wolf et al., 2015a) but did decrease the amount of PrP^{TSE} made after two passages (Wolf et al., 2015a). These results suggest that the inhibitors target events after PrP^{TSE} uptake and that undersulfation of GAGs may impair the establishment of persistent prion infection (Wolf et al., 2015a).

Once a persistent prion infection is established, efficient replication of prions is obviously critical to maintaining that infection, especially since only a small percentage of PrP^{C} is converted to PrP^{TSE} (Caughey and Raymond, 1991; Caughey et al., 1991; Borchelt et al., 1992). A balance between the rate of PrP^{TSE} conversion, cell division, PrP^{TSE} degradation, and cell-to-cell spread is likely required for a prion infection to persist in cells in vitro (Ghaemmaghami et al., 2007). Thus, if the rate of conversion is less than the rate of cell division or PrP^{TSE} degradation, the cells will be unable to maintain a persistent infection. For example, in N2a cells persistently infected with 22L prions, acute PrP^{TSE} levels increase over the first 96 hours, suggesting that the rate of new PrP^{TSE} formation and/or cell-to-cell spread are outpacing PrP^{TSE} clearance (Vorberg et al., 2004a). By contrast, in N2a cells exposed to mouse 22L prions that did not become persistently infected, the degradation of newly made PrP^{TSE} over 96 hours suggests that the rate of PrP^{TSE} clearance was faster than the rate of new PrP^{TSE} formation or spread, thus preventing the establishment of persistent infection (Vorberg et al., 2004a). Overall, the data suggest that a complex interplay between multiple cellular pathways may be critical for the establishment of persistent prion infection in vitro, although the cellular factors enabling the switch from acute to chronic prion infection remain poorly understood.

PERSISTENT PRION INFECTION

Cellular location of PrP^{TSE} formation

Not surprisingly, the cellular compartments where prion replication can occur in chronically infected cells are almost identical to those implicated in acute PrP^{TSE} formation (Fig. 3.2). Early studies in RML prion-infected N2a cells demonstrated that PrP^{TSE} formation was temperature-dependent and was inhibited if the cells were treated with proteases or phosphatidylinositol phospholipase C, which cleaves GPI membrane-anchored proteins at the cell surface (Borchelt et al., 1990, 1992; Caughey and Raymond, 1991; Taraboulos et al., 1992). More recent live cell imaging studies in mouse prion-infected SMB and GT1 cells have demonstrated PrP^{TSE} on the cell surface co-localizing with caveolin-1 (Rouvinski et al., 2014). Pulse chase studies using biotinylated or ^{35}S-radiolabeled prion-infected cells showed that PrP^{TSE} present on the cell surface was internalized (Borchelt et al., 1990, 1992; Caughey and Raymond, 1991; Caughey et al., 1991; Taraboulos et al., 1992) via either clathrin-dependent (Kaneko et al., 1997) or independent (Naslavsky et al., 1997) endocytic pathways. Following internalization, PrP^{TSE} accumulates in a lysosomal compartment (Caughey and Raymond, 1991; Caughey et al., 1991; McKinley et al., 1991; Borchelt et al., 1992). Thus, analogous with acute PrP^{TSE} formation, these early studies suggested that persistent PrP^{TSE} formation occurs at the cell surface and/or along the endocytic pathway.

However, it is important to distinguish which cellular compartments on the plasma membrane or along the endocytic pathway support PrP^{TSE} formation and which compartments are simply accumulating PrP^{TSE}. One clue comes from the fact that, unlike PrP^{TSE} isolated from brain, all PrP^{TSE} made in persistently infected cells is truncated at the N-terminus (Caughey and Raymond, 1991; Caughey et al., 1991; Taraboulos et al., 1992). This truncation can be blocked by inhibitors of lysosomal proteases (Caughey et al., 1991; Taraboulos et al., 1992) or calpain proteases (Yadavalli et al., 2004), indicating that PrP^{C} has acquired protease resistance at a point along the endocytic pathway prior to reaching the lysosome. Thus, lysosomes appear to be a site for accumulation of PrP^{TSE} rather than a cellular compartment where PrP^{TSE} is formed.

Inhibition of cholesterol and sphingolipid metabolism (Vey et al., 1996), imaging of cells using immunofluorescent and electron microscopy (McKinley et al., 1991; Veith et al., 2009), as well as cell biologic studies comparing the effect of transmembrane and GPI-anchored PrP^{C} on persistent PrP^{TSE} formation (Taraboulos et al., 1995; Kaneko et al., 1997; Marshall et al., 2017) all indicate that membrane domains rich in cholesterol are sites of PrP^{TSE} formation. Cholesterol-rich domains are present in plasma membrane lipid rafts, caveolae and caveolae-like domains, clathrin-coated pits, and late endosomes and recycling endosomes. PrP^{TSE} has been identified in all of these compartments (McKinley et al., 1991; Arnold et al., 1995; Veith et al., 2009) and any one of them could theoretically support PrP^{TSE} formation.

Antibody binding to cell surface PrP^{C} at the N-terminus (Kim et al., 2004) or C-terminus (Enari et al., 2001; Peretz et al., 2001) decreases PrP^{TSE} formation. Since conversion occurs almost immediately after PrP^{C} and PrP^{TSE} interact on the cell surface (Vorberg et al., 2004a; Goold et al., 2011; Yamasaki et al., 2014), this suggests that at least some PrP^{TSE} is made within lipid rafts at the plasma membrane. This would be consistent with the identification of the cell surface, lipid raft membrane-anchored heparin sulfate proteoglycan glypican-1 as a cofactor in PrP^{TSE} formation (Taylor et al., 2009). It is also consistent with the co-localization of full-length PrP^{TSE} with caveolin-1 on the cell surface (Rouvinski et al., 2014).

Impairment of recycling of PrP to the plasma membrane and stimulation of retrograde transport to the endoplasmic reticulum and Golgi increases PrP^{TSE} levels (Beranger et al., 2002). Since PrP^{TSE} is generally not localized to either the endoplasmic reticulum or Golgi in persistently infected cells (McKinley et al., 1991; Taraboulos et al., 1992; Marijanovic et al., 2009), this suggests that cellular compartments involved in retrograde transport prior to the endoplasmic reticulum and trans-Golgi network are sites of PrP^{TSE} formation (Beranger et al., 2002). Indeed, in RML-infected GT1-1 cells and 139A-infected CAD5 cells, loss of PrP^{TSE} is associated with inhibition of trafficking from the early endosome to the endosomal recycling compartment. This suggests that PrP^{TSE} is not made in early endosomes but rather recycling endosomes (Godsave et al., 2008; Marijanovic et al., 2009) with no requirement for being recycled back to the cell surface (Marijanovic et al., 2009). Localization of PrP^{TSE} to flotillin-1-positive, LAMP1-negative vesicles in RML-infected GT1 cells is also consistent with PrP^{TSE} formation occurring in recycling endosomes (Pimpinelli et al., 2005), as is the presence of N-terminally truncated PrP^{TSE} on the cell surface (Rouvinski et al., 2014). Recycling endosomes fit the requirement for a cellular site of PrP^{TSE} formation as they retain GPI-anchored proteins such as PrP^{C} and are cholesterol- and sphingolipid-rich (Mayor et al., 1998; Chatterjee et al., 2001).

However, sites of PrP^{TSE} formation may differ somewhat between cell types and/or prion strains. For example, in 22L-infected N2a cells, recycling endosomes do not appear to be an important site of persistent PrP^{TSE} formation (Marijanovic et al., 2009; Yim et al., 2015) and PrP^{TSE} is not present in flotillin-1-positive, LAMP1-negative vesicles in RML-infected N2a cells (Pimpinelli et al., 2005). Inhibition of multivesicular body (MVB) maturation leads to a nondegradative loss of PrP^{TSE} in 22L-infected SMB and N2a cells, suggesting that the late endosome/MVB may be a site of conversion of PrP^{C} into PrP^{TSE} (Yim et al., 2015). In prion-infected N2a cells and GT1 cells, PrP^{TSE} may be recycled back to the plasma membrane to convert cell surface PrP^{C} to PrP^{TSE} (Goold et al., 2013; Rouvinski et al., 2014) while in growth-inhibited prion-infected GT1 cells PrP^{TSE} is almost exclusively localized to the cell surface (Rouvinski et al., 2014). Thus, there may be many different cellular compartments where PrP^{TSE} formation can occur and which ones predominate may depend upon multiple factors, including prion strain, cell type, and the metabolic activity of the cell.

PrP^{TSE} degradation

In persistently infected cells, radiolabel pulse-chase studies have shown that PrP^{TSE} has a half-life of >24 hours, much longer than that of PrP^{C} which has a half-life of 4–6 hours (Borchelt et al., 1990; Caughey and Raymond, 1991). Thus, degradation of PrP^{TSE} is slow, with little or no detectable turnover within a 24-hour period (Caughey and Raymond, 1991). This is in stark contrast to exogenous PrP^{TSE} added during the acute infection of cells where, as described earlier in this chapter, a significant percentage of PrP^{TSE} is degraded within the first 24–48 hours. The reasons for this are unclear, but it may be due to differences in cofactors available to stabilize PrP^{TSE} aggregates (e.g., GAGs). Established cells in culture are derived from a single cell type while brain-derived PrP^{TSE} can potentially be made in multiple cell types. Heterogeneity in the population of PrP^{TSE} may therefore be a contributing factor and PrP^{TSE} in cells in vitro may simply be more homogeneous and thus more stable. Regardless of the explanation, there is clearly a difference in the cell's ability to degrade endogenous PrP^{TSE} versus exogenous PrP^{TSE}.

There are two protein degradation pathways in a cell: the ubiquitin/proteasome system and the autophagosome/lysosome system. No matter where it is formed, PrP^{TSE} is eventually trafficked to the lysosome (Caughey et al., 1991; McKinley et al., 1991; Borchelt et al., 1992; Taraboulos et al., 1992; Veith et al., 2009), suggesting that PrP^{TSE} degradation occurs via the autophagosome/lysosome pathway. Several lines of evidence are consistent with this. Increased numbers of autophagic vesicles are present in RML-infected GT1 cells when compared to uninfected cells (Schatzl et al., 1997). Treatment of prion-infected cells with compounds that induce autophagy such as imatinib (Ertmer et al., 2004), trehalose (Aguib et al., 2009), rapamycin (Aguib et al., 2009), or lithium (Heiseke et al., 2009) decreases PrP^{TSE} levels and can reduce the half-life of PrP^{TSE} in the cell from > 24 hours to < 9 hours (Ertmer et al., 2004). Mechanistically, the data support either mTOR-dependent or independent autophagy in PrP^{TSE} clearance (Aguib et al., 2009; Heiseke et al., 2009; Ishibashi et al., 2015; Xu et al., 2016). The mTOR-dependent pathway likely involves PI3K/MEK signaling (Ishibashi et al., 2015) as well as p62 (sequestosome 1), a cytosolic protein involved in the formation of aggresomes that has been linked to mTOR-dependent autophagy (Bjorkoy et al., 2005). In prion-infected N2a and MG20 cells, p62 is increased in abundance and associated with PrP^{TSE}-containing aggresomes and acceleration of PrP^{TSE} clearance (Homma et al., 2014).

Complicating matters somewhat is the fact that prion strain or cell variation may influence the pathway by which PrP^{TSE} is degraded. For example, PrP^{TSE} in N2a cells persistently infected with the mouse-adapted human GSS prion strain Fukuoka-1 (Fu-1) is degraded by mTOR-dependent autophagy but PrP^{TSE} in N2a cells infected with RML or 22L mouse prions is not (Ishibashi et al., 2015). However, other studies using RML-infected N2a cells indicate that PrP^{TSE} is cleared via autophagy in these cells (Aguib et al., 2009; Heiseke et al., 2009). Thus, prion strain and/or variation between different N2a cell lines may influence how PrP^{TSE} is degraded. As another example, tamoxifen treatment of RML-infected GT1 cells led to a significant decrease in PrP^{TSE} levels with no concomitant increase of PrP^{TSE} in autolysosomes (Marzo et al., 2013). Since tamoxifen treatment of prion-infected cells does not affect autophagy but does inhibit the release of cholesterol from lysosomes and increase the level of PrP^{TSE} in lysosomes, this suggests an autophagy-independent mechanism whereby PrP^{TSE} reaches the lysosome for clearance (Marzo et al., 2013).

The evidence of a role for proteasomes in PrP^{TSE} degradation is both limited and mixed. PrP^{TSE} inhibits proteasome function due to its highly aggregated state (Kristiansen et al., 2007; Deriziotis et al., 2011) and chemical inhibitors of proteasomes such as MG132 have no effect on PrP^{TSE} levels in N2a cells infected with RML or 22L mouse prions (Ishibashi et al., 2015). On the other hand, in N2aPK1 cells infected with RML, proteasome inhibition does lead to increased levels of PrP^{TSE}, suggesting that proteasomes contribute to PrP^{TSE} clearance in these cells (Goold et al., 2013). Overall, while current data suggest that the autophagosome/lysosome system is mostly responsible for PrP^{TSE} degradation in cells persistently infected with prions, other pathways may also come into play depending upon the prion strain and cell line.

Prion spread in cell culture

The efficient spread of prion infectivity from cell to cell is critical to maintaining persistent prion infection in established cell lines. In vitro, cellular spread of prions could occur horizontally via either cell-to-cell contact or release of prions into the media. Alternatively, prions could spread vertically from mother to daughter cell during cell division. Consistent with these mechanisms of spread, cell-free studies of PrP^{TSE} formation suggest that, during initial infection of a cell, PrP^{TSE} may need to interact with a host cell membrane either via direct cell-to-cell contact or via uptake of membrane particles containing PrP^{TSE} (Baron et al., 2002). However, as with other aspects of the cell biology of prion infection discussed earlier in this chapter, cellular spread of prions appears to be a complex process that may involve more than one mechanism of spread.

For example, when green fluorescent protein-expressing N2a cells were mixed for up to 5 weeks with nonfluorescently labeled N2a cells infected with RML mouse prions, PrP^{TSE} was detected almost exclusively in nonfluorescent cells (Ghaemmaghami et al., 2007). This suggested that the primary means of prion spread in N2a cells was from mother to daughter cell, with the rate of cell division much faster than the rate of any potential horizontal cell-to-cell spread (Ghaemmaghami et al., 2007). Another study showed that PrP^{TSE} present in membrane-derived microvesicles shed into the supernatant from the plasma membrane of RML-infected N2a cells could infect naïve N2a cells (Mattei et al., 2009) while a third study showed that exosomes shed from 22L prion-infected N2a cells could transmit infection to naïve cells (Alais et al., 2008). Thus, the data in N2a cells suggest that the primary means of prion spread is vertical but that, independent of prion strain, horizontal transmission via small membrane vesicles can also occur.

There is a significant body of work demonstrating that prions can be released into the cellular supernatant to spread infectivity horizontally and without the requirement of cell-to-cell contact. This type of spread was first demonstrated in RML-infected GT1 cells (Schatzl et al., 1997) and has since been identified as a mode of prion spread in RK13 cells (Fevrier et al., 2004), HpL3-4 cells (Maas et al., 2007), primary and established microglial cells (Stanton et al., 2008), primary neurons and astrocytes (Victoria et al., 2016), SN56 cells (Baron et al., 2006), N2a cells (Alais et al., 2008), and CAD5 cells (Victoria et al., 2016). Studies in sheep prion-infected Rov and Mov cells (Fevrier et al., 2004) and GT1 cells infected with Fu-1 (Vella et al., 2007; Arellano-Anaya et al., 2015) demonstrated that prion infectivity in the supernatant was associated with PrP^{TSE}-positive exosomes. Moreover, studies using highly purified exosomal fractions from prion-infected cells provide compelling evidence that exosomes are the primary vesicles for transporting prion infectivity between cells (Coleman et al., 2012).

Exosomes are lipid raft-rich microvesicles of endocytic origin which are produced during maturation of endosomes when invaginations into the endosomal lumen lead to the formation of MVBs. MVBs can fuse with lysosomes but exosomes are the intraluminal vesicles released when MVBs fuse with the plasma membrane (Thery et al., 2002; Gruenberg and Stenmark, 2004; Raposo and Stoorvogel, 2013). The presence of PrP^{TSE} in exosomes is therefore not very surprising as it is associated with lipid raft membrane domains and can be found in all the cellular compartments involved in the exosome life cycle. Exosomal vesicles are heterogeneous (Colombo et al., 2013) but there is some evidence to suggest that exosomes containing PrP^{TSE}, while also heterogeneous, are a distinct exosomal subpopulation (Coleman et al., 2012). The amount of PrP^{TSE} released in exosomes has been estimated at $<3\%$ of the total PrP^{TSE} in the cell (Fevrier et al., 2004; Arellano-Anaya et al., 2015), although the level of exosomal PrP^{TSE} can be increased if the cells are co-infected with a retrovirus (Leblanc et al., 2006; Alais et al., 2008; Stanton et al., 2008). Given the low level of PrP^{TSE}, spread of prion infectivity by exosomes is generally not as efficient as spread by direct contact between cells and often requires prolonged exposure or passage of recipient cells to detect transmission (Fevrier et al., 2004; Baron et al., 2006).

Indeed, in GT1 cells infected with Fu-1 (Nishida et al., 2005; Miyazawa et al., 2011), mouse-adapted hamster 263K (Miyazawa et al., 2011), or 22L prions (Nishida et al., 2005), PrP^{TSE} in the media contributes only minimally to prion transmission and transmission by mother to daughter cell division predominates (Nishida et al., 2005; Miyazawa et al., 2011). In experiments studying the spread of prions secreted into the medium of infected CAD5 cells or primary astrocytes, cell-to-cell contact was more efficient in transmitting prions from CAD5 cells to primary astrocytes while cell-to-cell contact and exposure to conditioned media from prion-infected primary astrocytes were equally efficient at transmitting prions to CAD5 cells (Victoria et al., 2016). Thus, cell type may help determine how efficiently secreted and/or exosome-associated PrP^{TSE} can spread prion infection to other cells.

Mechanistically, exosomal secretion of prions involves the endososomal sorting complex required for transport (ESCRT) system, a cellular pathway involved in MVB generation (Raiborg and Stenmark, 2009; Schmidt and Teis, 2012). In several different prion-infected cell lines, knocking down expression of HRS, a subunit of ESCRT-0, decreases PrP^{TSE} levels significantly (Vilette et al., 2015; Yim et al., 2015), as does silencing of the ESCRT-1 subunit tumor susceptibility gene 101 (Tsg101) (Vilette et al., 2015). HRS depletion also leads to a reduction in the ABCA1 transporter protein which is involved in cholesterol homeostasis and is known to affect prion replication (Kumar et al., 2008; Cui et al., 2014). A lipid raft-based mechanism involving ceramide (Trajkovic et al., 2008), but not ESCRT, may also contribute to the formation of PrP^{TSE}-containing exosomes. Inhibiting neutral sphingomyelinase, an enzyme involved in ceramide metabolism, decreased PrP^{TSE}-containing exosomes in the cellular supernatant (Vilette et al., 2015; Guo et al., 2016) and intercellular transmission of prion infectivity (Guo et al., 2016) without affecting prion replication (Vilette et al., 2015). Thus, both ESCRT-dependent and independent mechanisms appear to be involved in the generation of PrP^{TSE}-containing exosomes and intercellular transmission of prion infectivity.

Cell-to-cell contact independent of cellular division (Kanu et al., 2002) is another potential mechanism of prion spread in vitro. Direct contact between cellular membranes (Kanu et al., 2002) and cellular projections known as tunneling nanotubes has been identified as mechanisms of prion spread between cells (Gousset et al., 2009; Langevin et al., 2010; Zhu et al., 2015). Tunneling nanotubes (TNT) are long, thin, intercellular projections containing actin that transport vesicles, organelles, and even viruses between cells (Davis and Sowinski, 2008). When CAD5 cells infected with the mouse prion strain 139A were mixed with naïve CAD cells expressing a fluorescent protein, there was little evidence of PrP^{TSE} being transferred via exosomes or direct cellular contact. Rather, PrP^{TSE} was found in TNT that connected the infected cell with the indicator cell, suggesting that PrP^{TSE} was being transferred cell to cell via TNT (Gousset et al., 2009). Preventing TNT formation by inhibition of actin polymerization blocked the transfer of PrP^{TSE} between cells, supporting the idea that the PrP^{TSE}-positive projections were TNT (Gousset et al., 2009). Similar results were seen when bone marrow-derived dendritic cells were exposed to fluorescently labeled PrP^{TSE} and mixed with uninfected CAD5 cells (Gousset et al., 2009) or primary neurons (Langevin et al., 2010). Consistent with the cellular compartments where PrP^{TSE} can be found, PrP^{TSE} in TNT is largely associated with either recycling endosomes or lysosomes, with a smaller percentage found in early endosomes (Zhu et al., 2015). TNTs thus provide one mechanism, dependent upon cellular contact but independent of cellular division, by which prions can spread cell to cell in vitro.

ACKNOWLEDGMENTS

The author would like to thank Anita Mora for technical assistance in preparation of the figures. This work was supported by the National Institutes of Health intramural research program.

REFERENCES

Aguib Y, Heiseke A, Gilch S et al. (2009). Autophagy induction by trehalose counteracts cellular prion infection. Autophagy 5: 361–369.

Akimov S, Yakovleva O, Vasilyeva I et al. (2008). Persistent propagation of variant Creutzfeldt-Jakob disease agent in murine spleen stromal cell culture with features of mesenchymal stem cells. J Virol 82: 10959–10962.

Akimov S, Vasilyeva I, Yakovleva O et al. (2009). Murine bone marrow stromal cell culture with features of mesenchymal stem cells susceptible to mouse-adapted human TSE agent, Fukuoka-1. Folia Neuropathol 47: 205–214.

Alais S, Simoes S, Baas D et al. (2008). Mouse neuroblastoma cells release prion infectivity associated with exosomal vesicles. Biol Cell 100: 603–615.

Archer F, Bachelin C, Andreoletti O et al. (2004). Cultured peripheral neuroglial cells are highly permissive to sheep prion infection. J Virol 78: 482–490.

Arellano-Anaya ZE, Huor A, Leblanc P et al. (2015). Prion strains are differentially released through the exosomal pathway. Cell Mol Life Sci 72: 1185–1196.

Arjona A, Simarro L, Islinger F et al. (2004). Two Creutzfeldt-Jakob disease agents reproduce prion protein-independent identities in cell cultures. Proc Natl Acad Sci U S A 101: 8768–8773.

Arnold JE, Tipler C, Laszlo L et al. (1995). The abnormal isoform of the prion protein accumulates in late-endosome-like organelles in scrapie-infected mouse brain. J Pathol 176: 403–411.

Baron GS, Wehrly K, Dorward DW et al. (2002). Conversion of raft associated prion protein to the protease-resistant state requires insertion of PrP-res (PrP(Sc)) into contiguous membranes. EMBO J 21: 1031–1040.

Baron GS, Magalhaes AC, Prado MA et al. (2006). Mouse-adapted scrapie infection of SN56 cells: greater efficiency with microsome-associated versus purified PrP-res. J Virol 80: 2106–2117.

Beranger F, Mange A, Goud B et al. (2002). Stimulation of PrP(C) retrograde transport toward the endoplasmic reticulum increases accumulation of PrP(Sc) in prion-infected cells. J Biol Chem 277: 38972–38977.

Beringue V, Adjou KT, Lamoury F et al. (2000). Opposite effects of dextran sulfate 500, the polyene antibiotic MS-8209, and Congo red on accumulation of the protease-resistant isoform of PrP in the spleens of mice inoculated intraperitoneally with the scrapie agent. J Virol 74: 5432–5440.

Bian J, Napier D, Khaychuck V et al. (2010). Cell-based quantification of chronic wasting disease prions. J Virol 84: 8322–8326.

Birkett CR, Hennion RM, Bembridge DA et al. (2001). Scrapie strains maintain biological phenotypes on propagation in a cell line in culture. EMBO J 20: 3351–3358.

Bjorkoy G, Lamark T, Brech A et al. (2005). p62/SQSTM1 forms protein aggregates degraded by autophagy and has a protective effect on huntingtin-induced cell death. J Cell Biol 171: 603–614.

Borchelt DR, Scott M, Taraboulos A et al. (1990). Scrapie and cellular prion proteins differ in their kinetics of synthesis and topology in cultured cells. J Cell Biol 110: 743–752.

Borchelt DR, Taraboulos A, Prusiner SB (1992). Evidence for synthesis of scrapie prion proteins in the endocytic pathway. J Biol Chem 267: 16188–16199.

Bosque PJ, Prusiner SB (2000). Cultured cell sublines highly susceptible to prion infection. J Virol 74: 4377–4386.

Bueler H, Aguzzi A, Sailer A et al. (1993). Mice devoid of PrP are resistant to scrapie. Cell 73: 1339–1347.

Butler DA, Scott MR, Bockman JM et al. (1988). Scrapie-infected murine neuroblastoma cells produce protease-resistant prion proteins. J Virol 62: 1558–1564.

Campeau JL, Wu G, Bell JR et al. (2013). Early increase and late decrease of Purkinje cell dendritic spine density in prion-infected organotypic mouse cerebellar cultures. PLoS One 8: e81776.

Caspi S, Halimi M, Yanai A et al. (1998). The anti-prion activity of Congo red. Putative mechanism. J Biol Chem 273: 3484–3489.

Caughey B, Raymond GJ (1991). The scrapie-associated form of PrP is made from a cell surface precursor that is both protease- and phospholipase-sensitive. J Biol Chem 266: 18217–18223.

Caughey B, Raymond GJ (1993). Sulfated polyanion inhibition of scrapie-associated PrP accumulation in cultured cells. J Virol 67: 643–650.

Caughey B, Raymond GJ, Ernst D et al. (1991). N-terminal truncation of the scrapie-associated form of PrP by lysosomal protease(s): implications regarding the site of conversion of PrP to the protease-resistant state. J Virol 65: 6597–6603.

Cervenakova L, Akimov S, Vasilyeva I et al. (2011). Fukuoka-1 strain of transmissible spongiform encephalopathy agent infects murine bone marrow-derived cells with features of mesenchymal stem cells. Transfusion 51: 1755–1768.

Chasseigneaux S, Pastore M, Britton-Davidian J et al. (2008). Genetic heterogeneity versus molecular analysis of prion susceptibility in neuroblasma N2a sublines. Arch Virol 153: 1693–1702.

Chatterjee S, Smith ER, Hanada K et al. (2001). GPI anchoring leads to sphingolipid-dependent retention of endocytosed proteins in the recycling endosomal compartment. EMBO J 20: 1583–1592.

Choi YP, Priola SA (2013). A specific population of abnormal prion protein aggregates is preferentially taken up by cells and disaggregated in a strain-dependent manner. J Virol 87: 11552–11561.

Choi YP, Head MW, Ironside JW et al. (2014). Uptake and degradation of protease-sensitive and -resistant forms of abnormal human prion protein aggregates by human astrocytes. Am J Pathol 184: 3299–3307.

Clarke MC (1979). Infection of cell cultures with scrapie agent. In: SB Prusiner, WJ Hadlow (Eds.), Slow transmissible diseases of the central nervous system, Academic Press, New York, pp. 225–233.

Clarke MC, Haig DA (1970a). Evidence for the multiplication of scrapie agent in cell culture. Nature 225: 100–101.

Clarke MC, Haig DA (1970b). Multiplication of scrapie agent in cell culture. Res Vet Sci 11: 500–501.

Clarke MC, Millson GC (1976). Infection of a cell line of mouse L fibroblasts with scrapie agent. Nature 261: 144–145.

Coleman BM, Hanssen E, Lawson VA et al. (2012). Prion-infected cells regulate the release of exosomes with distinct ultrastructural features. FASEB J 26: 4160–4173.

Collinge J, Sidle KC, Meads J et al. (1996). Molecular analysis of prion strain variation and the aetiology of 'new variant' CJD. Nature 383: 685–690.

Collins SJ, Haigh CL (2017). Simplified murine 3D neuronal cultures for investigating neuronal activity and neurodegeneration. Cell Biochem Biophys 75: 3–13.

Colombo M, Moita C, van Niel G et al. (2013). Analysis of ESCRT functions in exosome biogenesis, composition and secretion highlights the heterogeneity of extracellular vesicles. J Cell Sci 126: 5553–5565.

Courageot MP, Daude N, Nonno R et al. (2008). A cell line infectible by prion strains from different species. J Gen Virol 89: 341–347.

Cronier S, Laude H, Peyrin JM (2004). Prions can infect primary cultured neurons and astrocytes and promote neuronal cell death. Proc Natl Acad Sci U S A 101: 12271–12276.

Cronier S, Beringue V, Bellon A et al. (2007). Prion strain- and species-dependent effects of antiprion molecules in primary neuronal cultures. J Virol 81: 13794–13800.

Cronier S, Carimalo J, Schaeffer B et al. (2012). Endogenous prion protein conversion is required for prion-induced neuritic alterations and neuronal death. FASEB J 26: 3854–3861.

Cui HL, Guo B, Scicluna B et al. (2014). Prion infection impairs cholesterol metabolism in neuronal cells. J Biol Chem 289: 789–802.

Davis DM, Sowinski S (2008). Membrane nanotubes: dynamic long-distance connections between animal cells. Nat Rev Mol Cell Biol 9: 431–436.

Deriziotis P, Andre R, Smith DM et al. (2011). Misfolded PrP impairs the UPS by interaction with the 20S proteasome and inhibition of substrate entry. EMBO J 30: 3065–3077.

Dlakic WM, Grigg E, Bessen RA (2007). Prion infection of muscle cells in vitro. J Virol 81: 4615–4624.

Doh-ura K, Perryman S, Race R et al. (1995). Identification of differentially expressed genes in scrapie-infected mouse neuroblastoma cells. Microb Pathog 18: 1–9.

Elhelaly AE, Inoshima Y, Ishiguro N (2013a). Alteration of cell responses to PrP(Sc) in prolonged cell culture and its effect on transmission of PrP(Sc) to neural cells. Arch Virol 158: 651–658.

Elhelaly AE, Inoshima Y, Ishiguro N (2013b). Characterization of early transient accumulation of PrP(Sc) in immune cells. Biochem Biophys Res Commun 439: 340–345.

Elleman CJ (1984). Attempts to establish the scrapie agent in cell lines. Vet Res Commun 8: 309–316.

Enari M, Flechsig E, Weissmann C (2001). Scrapie prion protein accumulation by scrapie-infected neuroblastoma cells abrogated by exposure to a prion protein antibody. Proc Natl Acad Sci U S A 98: 9295–9299.

Ertmer A, Gilch S, Yun SW et al. (2004). The tyrosine kinase inhibitor STI571 induces cellular clearance of PrPSc in prion-infected cells. J Biol Chem 279: 41918–41927.

Falsig J, Julius C, Margalith I et al. (2008). A versatile prion replication assay in organotypic brain slices. Nat Neurosci 11: 109–117.

Falsig J, Sonati T, Herrmann US et al. (2012). Prion pathogenesis is faithfully reproduced in cerebellar organotypic slice cultures. PLoS Pathog 8: e1002985.

Fevrier B, Vilette D, Archer F et al. (2004). Cells release prions in association with exosomes. Proc Natl Acad Sci U S A 101: 9683–9688.

Fischer M, Rulicke T, Raeber A et al. (1996). Prion protein (PrP) with amino-proximal deletions restoring susceptibility of PrP knockout mice to scrapie. EMBO J 15: 1255–1264.

Follet J, Lemaire-Vieille C, Blanquet-Grossard F et al. (2002). PrP expression and replication by Schwann cells: implications in prion spreading. J Virol 76: 2434–2439.

Gabizon R, Meiner Z, Halimi M et al. (1993). Heparin-like molecules bind differentially to prion-proteins and change their intracellular metabolic fate. J Cell Physiol 157: 319–325.

Gajdusek DC, Gibbs Jr CJ, Rogers NG et al. (1972). Persistence of viruses of kuru and Creutzfeldt-Jakob disease in tissue cultures of brain cells. Nature 235: 104–105.

Gauczynski S, Peyrin JM, Haik S et al. (2001). The 37-kDa/67-kDa laminin receptor acts as the cell-surface receptor for the cellular prion protein. EMBO J 20: 5863–5875.

Gauczynski S, Nikles D, El-Gogo S et al. (2006). The 37-kDa/67-kDa laminin receptor acts as a receptor for infectious prions and is inhibited by polysulfated glycanes. J Infect Dis 194: 702–709.

Ghaemmaghami S, Phuan PW, Perkins B et al. (2007). Cell division modulates prion accumulation in cultured cells. Proc Natl Acad Sci U S A 104: 17971–17976.

Gilch S, Schmitz F, Aguib Y et al. (2007). CpG and LPS can interfere negatively with prion clearance in macrophage and microglial cells. FEBS J 274: 5834–5844.

Godsave SF, Wille H, Kujala P et al. (2008). Cryo-immunogold electron microscopy for prions: toward identification of a conversion site. J Neurosci 28: 12489–12499.

Goold R, Rabbanian S, Sutton L et al. (2011). Rapid cell-surface prion protein conversion revealed using a novel cell system. Nat Commun 2: 281.

Goold R, McKinnon C, Rabbanian S et al. (2013). Alternative fates of newly formed PrPSc upon prion conversion on the plasma membrane. J Cell Sci 126: 3552–3562.

Gousset K, Schiff E, Langevin C et al. (2009). Prions hijack tunnelling nanotubes for intercellular spread. Nat Cell Biol 11: 328–336.

Greil CS, Vorberg IM, Ward AE et al. (2008). Acute cellular uptake of abnormal prion protein is cell type and scrapie-strain independent. Virology 379: 284–293.

Gruenberg J, Stenmark H (2004). The biogenesis of multivesicular endosomes. Nat Rev Mol Cell Biol 5: 317–323.

Guo BB, Bellingham SA, Hill AF (2016). Stimulating the release of exosomes increases the intercellular transfer of prions. J Biol Chem 291: 5128–5137.

Gustafson DP, Kanitz CL (1965). Evidence of the presence of scrapie in cell cultures of brain. In: DC Gajdusek, CJ Gibbs, M Alpers (Eds.), Slow, latent, and temperate virus infections, US Department of Health, Education, and Welfare, Washington, DC, pp. 221–236.

Hannaoui S, Maatouk L, Privat N et al. (2013). Prion propagation and toxicity occur in vitro with two-phase kinetics specific to strain and neuronal type. J Virol 87: 2535–2548.

Heiseke A, Aguib Y, Riemer C et al. (2009). Lithium induces clearance of protease resistant prion protein in prion-infected cells by induction of autophagy. J Neurochem 109: 25–34.

Herbst A, Banser P, Velasquez CD et al. (2013). Infectious prions accumulate to high levels in non proliferative C2C12 myotubes. PLoS Pathog 9: e1003755.

Herva ME, Relano-Gines A, Villa A et al. (2010). Prion infection of differentiated neurospheres. J Neurosci Methods 188: 270–275.

Hijazi N, Kariv-Inbal Z, Gasset M et al. (2005). PrPSc incorporation to cells requires endogenous glycosaminoglycan expression. J Biol Chem 280: 17057–17061.

Homma T, Ishibashi D, Nakagaki T et al. (2014). Increased expression of p62/SQSTM1 in prion diseases and its association with pathogenic prion protein. Sci Rep 4: 4504.

Horonchik L, Tzaban S, Ben-Zaken O et al. (2005). Heparan sulfate is a cellular receptor for purified infectious prions. J Biol Chem 280: 17062–17067.

Hundt C, Peyrin JM, Haik S et al. (2001). Identification of interaction domains of the prion protein with its 37-kDa/67-kDa laminin receptor. EMBO J 20: 5876–5886.

Ikonen E (2008). Cellular cholesterol trafficking and compartmentalization. Nat Rev Mol Cell Biol 9: 125–138.

Imamura M, Tabeta N, Kato N et al. (2016). Heparan sulfate and heparin promote faithful prion replication in vitro by binding to normal and abnormal prion proteins in protein misfolding cyclic amplification. J Biol Chem 291: 26478–26486.

Ishibashi D, Homma T, Nakagaki T et al. (2015). Strain-dependent effect of macroautophagy on abnormally folded prion protein degradation in infected neuronal cells. PLoS One 10: e0137958.

Iwamaru Y, Takenouchi T, Ogihara K et al. (2007). Microglial cell line established from prion protein-overexpressing mice is susceptible to various murine prion strains. J Virol 81: 1524–1527.

Iwamaru Y, Takenouchi T, Imamura M et al. (2013). Prion replication elicits cytopathic changes in differentiated neurosphere cultures. J Virol 87: 8745–8755.

Jen A, Parkyn CJ, Mootoosamy RC et al. (2010). Neuronal low-density lipoprotein receptor-related protein 1 binds and endocytoses prion fibrils via receptor cluster 4. J Cell Sci 123: 246–255.

Kaneko K, Vey M, Scott M et al. (1997). COOH-terminal sequence of the cellular prion protein directs subcellular trafficking and controls conversion into the scrapie isoform. Proc Natl Acad Sci U S A 94: 2333–2338.

Kanu N, Imokawa Y, Drechsel DN et al. (2002). Transfer of scrapie prion infectivity by cell contact in culture. Curr Biol 12: 523–530.

Kim CL, Karino A, Ishiguro N et al. (2004). Cell-surface retention of PrPC by anti-PrP antibody prevents protease-resistant PrP formation. J Gen Virol 85: 3473–3482.

Klohn PC, Stoltze L, Flechsig E et al. (2003). A quantitative, highly sensitive cell-based infectivity assay for mouse scrapie prions. Proc Natl Acad Sci U S A 100: 11666–11671.

Krejciova Z, Pells S, Cancellotti E et al. (2011). Human embryonic stem cells rapidly take up and then clear exogenous human and animal prions in vitro. J Pathol 223: 635–645.

Krejciova Z, De Sousa P, Manson J et al. (2014). Human tonsil-derived follicular dendritic-like cells are refractory to human prion infection in vitro and traffic disease-associated prion protein to lysosomes. Am J Pathol 184: 64–70.

Kristiansen M, Deriziotis P, Dimcheff DE et al. (2007). Disease-associated prion protein oligomers inhibit the 26S proteasome. Mol Cell 26: 175–188.

Kuczius T, Haist I, Groschup MH (1998). Molecular analysis of bovine spongiform encephalopathy and scrapie strain variation. J Infect Dis 178: 693–699.

Kumar R, McClain D, Young R et al. (2008). Cholesterol transporter ATP-binding cassette A1 (ABCA1) is elevated in prion disease and affects PrPC and PrPSc concentrations in cultured cells. J Gen Virol 89: 1525–1532.

Kuwahara C, Takeuchi AM, Nishimura T et al. (1999). Prions prevent neuronal cell-line death. Nature 400: 225–226.

Ladogana A, Liu Q, Xi YG et al. (1995). Proteinase-resistant protein in human neuroblastoma cells infected with brain material from Creutzfeldt-Jakob patient. Lancet 345: 594–595.

Langevin C, Gousset K, Costanzo M et al. (2010). Characterization of the role of dendritic cells in prion transfer to primary neurons. Biochem J 431: 189–198.

Lawson VA, Vella LJ, Stewart JD et al. (2008). Mouse-adapted sporadic human Creutzfeldt-Jakob disease prions propagate in cell culture. Int J Biochem Cell Biol 40: 2793–2801.

Leblanc P, Alais S, Porto-Carreiro I et al. (2006). Retrovirus infection strongly enhances scrapie infectivity release in cell culture. EMBO J 25: 2674–2685.

Leucht C, Simoneau S, Rey C et al. (2003). The 37 kDa/67 kDa laminin receptor is required for PrP(Sc) propagation in scrapie-infected neuronal cells. EMBO Rep 4: 290–295.

Lewis V, Hill AF, Haigh CL et al. (2009). Increased proportions of C1 truncated prion protein protect against cellular M1000 prion infection. J Neuropathol Exp Neurol 68: 1125–1135.

Liu J, Thorp SC (2002). Cell surface heparan sulfate and its roles in assisting viral infections. Med Res Rev 22: 1–25.

Luhr KM, Wallin RP, Ljunggren HG et al. (2002). Processing and degradation of exogenous prion protein by CD11c(+) myeloid dendritic cells in vitro. J Virol 76: 12259–12264.

Luhr KM, Nordstrom EK, Low P et al. (2004). Scrapie protein degradation by cysteine proteases in CD11c+ dendritic cells and GT1-1 neuronal cells. J Virol 78: 4776–4782.

Maas E, Geissen M, Groschup MH et al. (2007). Scrapie infection of prion protein-deficient cell line upon ectopic expression of mutant prion proteins. J Biol Chem 282: 18702–18710.

Magalhaes AC, Baron GS, Lee KS et al. (2005). Uptake and neuritic transport of scrapie prion protein coincident with infection of neuronal cells. J Neurosci 25: 5207–5216.

Mahal SP, Baker CA, Demczyk CA et al. (2007). Prion strain discrimination in cell culture: the cell panel assay. Proc Natl Acad Sci U S A 104: 20908–20913.

Manson JC, Clarke AR, McBride PA et al. (1994). PrP gene dosage determines the timing but not the final intensity or distribution of lesions in scrapie pathology. Neurodegeneration 3: 331–340.

Manuelidis L, Liu Y, Mullins B (2009). Strain-specific viral properties of variant Creutzfeldt-Jakob disease (vCJD) are encoded by the agent and not by host prion protein. J Cell Biochem 106: 220–231.

Marbiah MM, Harvey A, West BT et al. (2014). Identification of a gene regulatory network associated with prion replication. EMBO J 33: 1527–1547.

Marijanovic Z, Caputo A, Campana V et al. (2009). Identification of an intracellular site of prion conversion. PLoS Pathog 5: e1000426.

Marshall KE, Hughson A, Vascellari S et al. (2017). PrP knockout cells expressing transmembrane PrP resist prion infection. J Virol 91: 301686–301716.

Marzo L, Marijanovic Z, Browman D et al. (2013). 4-hydroxytamoxifen leads to PrPSc clearance by conveying both PrPC and PrPSc to lysosomes independently of autophagy. J Cell Sci 126: 1345–1354.

Mattei V, Barenco MG, Tasciotti V et al. (2009). Paracrine diffusion of PrP(C) and propagation of prion infectivity by plasma membrane-derived microvesicles. PLoS One 4: e5057.

Mayer-Sonnenfeld T, Avrahami D, Friedman-Levi Y et al. (2008). Chemically induced accumulation of GAGs delays PrP(Sc) clearance but prolongs prion disease incubation time. Cell Mol Neurobiol 28: 1005–1015.

Mayor S, Sabharanjak S, Maxfield FR (1998). Cholesterol-dependent retention of GPI-anchored proteins in endosomes. EMBO J 17: 4626–4638.

Mays CE, Kang HE, Kim Y et al. (2008). CRBL cells: establishment, characterization and susceptibility to prion infection. Brain Res 1208: 170–180.

McKinley MP, Taraboulos A, Kenaga L et al. (1991). Ultrastructural localization of scrapie prion proteins in cytoplasmic vesicles of infected cultured cells. Lab Invest 65: 622–630.

McNally KL, Ward AE, Priola SA (2009). Cells expressing anchorless prion protein are resistant to scrapie infection. J Virol 83: 4469–4475.

Miyazawa K, Emmerling K, Manuelidis L (2011). Replication and spread of CJD, kuru and scrapie agents in vivo and in cell culture. Virulence 2: 188–199.

Mohan J, Hopkins J, Mabbott NA (2005). Skin-derived dendritic cells acquire and degrade the scrapie agent following in vitro exposure. Immunology 116: 122–133.

Moore RA, Timmes A, Wilmarth PA et al. (2010). Comparative profiling of highly enriched 22L and Chandler mouse scrapie prion protein preparations. Proteomics 10: 2858–2869.

Morel E, Andrieu T, Casagrande F et al. (2005). Bovine prion is endocytosed by human enterocytes via the 37 kDa/67 kDa laminin receptor. Am J Pathol 167: 1033–1042.

Mouillet-Richard S, Nishida N, Pradines E et al. (2008). Prions impair bioaminergic functions through serotonin- or catecholamine-derived neurotoxins in neuronal cells. J Biol Chem 283: 23782–23790.

Munoz-Gutierrez JF, Schneider DA, Baszler TV et al. (2015). hTERT-immortalized ovine microglia propagate natural scrapie isolates. Virus Res 198: 35–43.

Munoz-Gutierrez JF, Pierle SA, Schneider DA et al. (2016). Transcriptomic determinants of scrapie prion propagation in cultured ovine microglia. PLoS One 11: e0147727.

Naslavsky N, Stein R, Yanai A et al. (1997). Characterization of detergent-insoluble complexes containing the cellular prion protein and its scrapie isoform. J Biol Chem 272: 6324–6331.

Nishida N, Harris DA, Vilette D et al. (2000). Successful transmission of three mouse-adapted scrapie strains to murine neuroblastoma cell lines overexpressing wild-type mouse prion protein. J Virol 74: 320–325.

Nishida N, Katamine S, Manuelidis L (2005). Reciprocal interference between specific CJD and scrapie agents in neural cell cultures. Science 310: 493–496.

Nishimura T, Sakudo A, Xue G et al. (2008). Establishment of a new glial cell line from hippocampus of prion protein gene-deficient mice. Biochem Biophys Res Commun 377: 1047–1050.

Oelschlegel AM, Geissen M, Lenk M et al. (2015). A bovine cell line that can be infected by natural sheep scrapie prions. PLoS One 10: e0117154.

Paquet S, Daude N, Courageot MP et al. (2007). PrPc does not mediate internalization of PrPSc but is required at an early stage for de novo prion infection of Rov cells. J Virol 81: 10786–10791.

Peretz D, Williamson RA, Kaneko K et al. (2001). Antibodies inhibit prion propagation and clear cell cultures of prion infectivity. Nature 412: 739–743.

Piccardo P, Cervenakova L, Vasilyeva I et al. (2011). Candidate cell substrates, vaccine production, and transmissible spongiform encephalopathies. Emerg Infect Dis 17: 2262–2269.

Pimpinelli F, Lehmann S, Maridonneau-Parini I (2005). The scrapie prion protein is present in flotillin-1-positive vesicles in central- but not peripheral-derived neuronal cell lines. Eur J Neurosci 21: 2063–2072.

Prado MA, Alves-Silva J, Magalhaes AC et al. (2004). PrPc on the road: trafficking of the cellular prion protein. J Neurochem 88: 769–781.

Priola SA, Caughey B (1994). Inhibition of scrapie-associated PrP accumulation. Probing the role of glycosaminoglycans in amyloidogenesis. Mol Neurobiol 8: 113–120.

Race RE, Fadness LH, Chesebro B (1987). Characterization of scrapie infection in mouse neuroblastoma cells. J Gen Virol 68: 1391–1399.

Race RE, Caughey B, Graham K et al. (1988). Analyses of frequency of infection, specific infectivity, and prion protein biosynthesis in scrapie-infected neuroblastoma cell clones. J Virol 62: 2845–2849.

Raeber AJ, Race RE, Brandner S et al. (1997). Astrocyte-specific expression of hamster prion protein (PrP) renders PrP knockout mice susceptible to hamster scrapie. EMBO J 16: 6057–6065.

Raiborg C, Stenmark H (2009). The ESCRT machinery in endosomal sorting of ubiquitylated membrane proteins. Nature 458: 445–452.

Raposo G, Stoorvogel W (2013). Extracellular vesicles: exosomes, microvesicles, and friends. J Cell Biol 200: 373–383.

Raymond GJ, Olsen EA, Lee KS et al. (2006). Inhibition of protease-resistant prion protein formation in a transformed deer cell line infected with chronic wasting disease. J Virol 80: 596–604.

Rejman J, Oberle V, Zuhorn IS et al. (2004). Size-dependent internalization of particles via the pathways of clathrin- and caveolae-mediated endocytosis. Biochem J 377: 159–169.

Rouvinski A, Karniely S, Kounin M et al. (2014). Live imaging of prions reveals nascent PrPSc in cell-surface, raft-associated amyloid strings and webs. J Cell Biol 204: 423–441.

Rubenstein R, Carp RI, Callahan SM (1984). In vitro replication of scrapie agent in a neuronal model: infection of PC12 cells. J Gen Virol 65: 2191–2198.

Rubenstein R, Deng H, Race RE et al. (1992). Demonstration of scrapie strain diversity in infected PC12 cells. J Gen Virol 73: 3027–3031.

Rybner-Barnier C, Jacquemot C, Cuche C et al. (2006). Processing of the bovine spongiform encephalopathy-specific prion protein by dendritic cells. J Virol 80: 4656–4663.

Sakaguchi S, Katamine S, Shigematsu K et al. (1995). Accumulation of proteinase K-resistant prion protein (PrP) is restricted by the expression level of normal PrP in mice inoculated with a mouse-adapted strain of the Creutzfeldt-Jakob disease agent. J Virol 69: 7586–7592.

Sassa Y, Yamasaki T, Horiuchi M et al. (2010). The effects of lysosomal and proteasomal inhibitors on abnormal forms of prion protein degradation in murine macrophages. Microbiol Immunol 54: 763–768.

Schatzl HM, Laszlo L, Holtzman DM et al. (1997). A hypothalamic neuronal cell line persistently infected with scrapie prions exhibits apoptosis. J Virol 71: 8821–8831.

Schmidt O, Teis D (2012). The ESCRT machinery. Curr Biol 22: R116–R120.

Somerville RA, Chong A, Mulqueen OU et al. (1997). Biochemical typing of scrapie strains. Nature 386: 564.

Stanton JB, Knowles DP, O'Rourke KI et al. (2008). Small-ruminant lentivirus enhances PrPSc accumulation in cultured sheep microglial cells. J Virol 82: 9839–9847.

Takakura Y, Yamaguchi N, Nakagaki T et al. (2008). Bone marrow stroma cells are susceptible to prion infection. Biochem Biophys Res Commun 377: 957–961.

Tanaka M, Fujiwara A, Suzuki A et al. (2016). Comparison of abnormal isoform of prion protein in prion-infected cell lines and primary-cultured neurons by PrPSc-specific immunostaining. J Gen Virol 97: 2030–2042.

Taraboulos A, Serban D, Prusiner SB (1990). Scrapie prion proteins accumulate in the cytoplasm of persistently infected cultured cells. J Cell Biol 110: 2117–2132.

Taraboulos A, Raeber AJ, Borchelt DR et al. (1992). Synthesis and trafficking of prion proteins in cultured cells. Mol Biol Cell 3: 851–863.

Taraboulos A, Scott M, Semenov A et al. (1995). Cholesterol depletion and modification of COOH-terminal targeting sequence of the prion protein inhibit formation of the scrapie isoform. J Cell Biol 129: 121–132.

Tark D, Kim H, Neale MH et al. (2015). Generation of a persistently infected MDBK cell line with natural bovine spongiform encephalopathy (BSE). PLoS One 10: e0115939.

Taylor DR, Whitehouse IJ, Hooper NM (2009). Glypican-1 mediates both prion protein lipid raft association and disease isoform formation. PLoS Pathog 5: e1000666.

Thery C, Zitvogel L, Amigorena S (2002). Exosomes: composition, biogenesis and function. Nat Rev Immunol 2: 569–579.

Trajkovic K, Hsu C, Chiantia S et al. (2008). Ceramide triggers budding of exosome vesicles into multivesicular endosomes. Science 319: 1244–1247.

Tuzi NL, Cancellotti E, Baybutt H et al. (2008). Host PrP glycosylation: a major factor determining the outcome of prion infection. PLoS Biol 6: e100.

Veith NM, Plattner H, Stuermer CA et al. (2009). Immunolocalisation of PrPSc in scrapie-infected N2a mouse neuroblastoma cells by light and electron microscopy. Eur J Cell Biol 88: 45–63.

Vella LJ, Sharples RA, Lawson VA et al. (2007). Packaging of prions into exosomes is associated with a novel pathway of PrP processing. J Pathol 211: 582–590.

Vey M, Pilkuhn S, Wille H et al. (1996). Subcellular colocalization of the cellular and scrapie prion proteins in caveolae-like membranous domains. Proc Natl Acad Sci U S A 93: 14945–14949.

Victoria GS, Arkhipenko A, Zhu S et al. (2016). Astrocyte-to-neuron intercellular prion transfer is mediated by cell-cell contact. Sci Rep 6: 20762.

Vilette D, Andreoletti O, Archer F et al. (2001). Ex vivo propagation of infectious sheep scrapie agent in heterologous epithelial cells expressing ovine prion protein. Proc Natl Acad Sci U S A 98: 4055–4059.

Vilette D, Laulagnier K, Huor A et al. (2015). Efficient inhibition of infectious prions multiplication and release by targeting the exosomal pathway. Cell Mol Life Sci 72: 4409–4427.

Vorberg I, Groschup MH, Pfaff E et al. (2003). Multiple amino acid residues within the rabbit prion protein inhibit formation of its abnormal isoform. J Virol 77: 2003–2009.

Vorberg I, Raines A, Priola SA (2004a). Acute formation of protease-resistant prion protein does not always lead to persistent scrapie infection in vitro. J Biol Chem 279: 29218–29225.

Vorberg I, Raines A, Story B et al. (2004b). Susceptibility of common fibroblast cell lines to transmissible spongiform encephalopathy agents. J Infect Dis 189: 431–439.

Wadia JS, Schaller M, Williamson RA et al. (2008). Pathologic prion protein infects cells by lipid-raft dependent macropinocytosis. PLoS One 3: e3314.

Wang W, Li F, Wang K et al. (2012). PAPSS2 promotes alkaline phosphates activity and mineralization of osteoblastic MC3T3-E1 cells by crosstalk and Smads signal pathways. PLoS One 7: e43475.

Weissmann C, Bueler H, Fischer M et al. (1994). Susceptibility to scrapie in mice is dependent on PrPC. Philos Trans R Soc Lond B Biol Sci 343: 431–433.

Wolf H, Grassmann A, Bester R et al. (2015a). Modulation of glycosaminoglycans affects PrPSc metabolism but does not block PrPSc uptake. J Virol 89: 9853–9864.

Wolf H, Hossinger A, Fehlinger A et al. (2015b). Deposition pattern and subcellular distribution of disease-associated prion protein in cerebellar organotypic slice cultures infected with scrapie. Front Neurosci 9: 410.

Wong C, Xiong LW, Horiuchi M et al. (2001). Sulfated glycans and elevated temperature stimulate PrP(Sc)-dependent cell-free formation of protease-resistant prion protein. EMBO J 20: 377–386.

Xu Y, Tian C, Sun J et al. (2016). FBXW7-induced MTOR degradation forces autophagy to counteract persistent prion infection. Mol Neurobiol 53: 706–719.

Yadavalli R, Guttmann RP, Seward T et al. (2004). Calpain-dependent endoproteolytic cleavage of PrPSc modulates scrapie prion propagation. J Biol Chem 279: 21948–21956.

Yamasaki T, Baron GS, Suzuki A et al. (2014). Characterization of intracellular dynamics of inoculated PrP-res and newly generated PrP(Sc) during early stage prion infection in Neuro2a cells. Virology 450–451: 324–335.

Yim YI, Park BC, Yadavalli R et al. (2015). The multivesicular body is the major internal site of prion conversion. J Cell Sci 128: 1434–1443.

Zhu S, Victoria GS, Marzo L et al. (2015). Prion aggregates transfer through tunneling nanotubes in endocytic vesicles. Prion 9: 125–135.

Handbook of Clinical Neurology, Vol. 153 (3rd series)
Human Prion Diseases
M. Pocchiari and J. Manson, Editors
https://doi.org/10.1016/B978-0-444-63945-5.00004-0

Chapter 4

Experimental models of human prion diseases and prion strains

ABIGAIL B. DIACK[1]* AND JASON C. BARTZ[2]

[1]*Infection and Immunity, The Roslin Institute, University of Edinburgh, Easter Bush, United Kingdom*

[2]*Department of Medical Microbiology and Immunology, School of Medicine, Creighton University, Omaha, NE, United States*

Abstract

Prion strains occur in natural prion diseases, including prion diseases of humans. Prion strains can correspond with differences in the clinical signs and symptoms of disease and the distribution of prion infectivity in the host and are hypothesized to be encoded by strain-specific differences in the conformation of the disease-specific isoform of the host-encoded prion protein, PrP^{TSE}. Prion strains can differ in biochemical properties of PrP^{TSE} that can include the relative sensitivity to digestion with proteinase K and conformational stability in denaturants. These strain-specific biochemical properties of field isolates are maintained upon transmission to experimental animal models of prion disease. Experimental human models of prion disease include traditional and gene-targeted mice that express endogenous PrP^{C}. Transgenic mice that express different polymorphs of human PrP^{C} or mutations in human PrP^{C} that correspond with familial forms of human prion disease have been generated that can recapitulate the clinical, pathologic, and biochemical features of disease. These models aid in understanding disease pathogenesis, evaluating zoonotic potential of animal prion diseases, and assessing human-to-human transmission of disease. Models of sporadic or familial forms of disease offer an opportunity to define mechanisms of disease, identify key neurodegenerative pathways, and assess therapeutic interventions.

Prion diseases are a group of fatal neurodegenerative diseases caused by the misfolding of the endogenous prion protein, PrP^{C} to PrP^{TSE}. They exist as a number of prion strains. Variation in prion strains was first described by Pattison and Millson (1961a, b) when they observed different disease phenotypes in goats and sheep inoculated with scrapie. This phenomenon has been most extensively characterized and studied in rodent-adapted prion disease (reviewed by Bruce, 1993). Prion strain variation is now recognized to play a major role in disease pathogenesis and transmission.

PRION STRAIN BIOLOGY

Prion strains are defined as a heritable phenotype of disease under a controlled set of agent and host parameters. Not all disease phenotypes are characteristic for a strain; for example, distinct strains can have similar incubation periods and/or clinical signs of disease (Ayers et al., 2011). The relative intensity and distribution of spongiform degeneration in select areas of the central nervous system (CNS) are the most accepted criteria to distinguish prion strains and are the basis of the lesion profile (Fraser and Dickinson, 1967, 1968). Lesion profile analysis is a robust and highly reproducible technique that has been successfully used for nearly 50 years. A disadvantage of this operational definition of prion strains is that the degree to which the disease phenotype has to vary to be considered a unique strain is subjective.

Distinct conformations of PrP^{TSE} may encipher prion strain diversity. Studies of prions in rodents were the first to suggest that unique biochemical properties of PrP^{TSE} correspond with different prion strains (Kascsak et al., 1987). Studies of the hyper (HY) and drowsy (DY) strains of hamster-adapted Transmissible Mink Encephalopathy (TME) were the first to reveal strain-specific

*Correspondence to: Abigail B. Diack, Infection and Immunity, The Roslin Institute and R(D)SVS, University of Edinburgh, Easter Bush, Midlothian EH25 9RG, United Kingdom. Tel: +44-131-651-9100, E-mail: abigail.diack@roslin.ed.ac.uk

differences in the proteinase K (PK) digestion site, relative PK resistance, and detergent solubility of PrP^{TSE} (Bessen and Marsh, 1992a, b, 1994). In human prion disease, strain-specific differences in the migration of PrP^{TSE} of human prion isolates were preserved upon transmission to transgenic mice expressing chimeric mouse-human PrP^{C}, further suggesting that the conformation of PrP^{TSE} differed between prion strains (Telling et al., 1996b). Structural studies of PrP^{TSE} have identified strain-specific differences in PrP^{TSE} secondary structure, fibril morphology, and aggravation state (Caughey et al., 1998; Sim and Caughey, 2009; Tixador et al., 2010; Moore et al., 2011; Laferrière et al., 2013). The conformation-dependent immunoassay has identified strain-specific differences in PrP^{TSE} conformation from several rodent-adapted prion strains (Safar et al., 1998). Additionally, strain-specific differences in PrP^{TSE} conformational stability, from a wide range of natural and synthetic prion strains, are observed (Peretz et al., 2001; Thackray et al., 2007; Colby et al., 2009; Ayers et al., 2011; Gonzalez-Montalban et al., 2011; Ghaemmaghami et al., 2013). Binding of luminescent conjugated polythiophenes (LCPs) to PrP^{TSE} from different prion strains can result in strain-specific LCP emission wavelength spectra, suggesting strain-specific differences in tertiary or quaternary structure of PrP^{TSE} (Sigurdson et al., 2007). While these assays are all consistent with the hypothesis that strain-specific differences in PrP^{TSE} encode strain diversity, the relationship between the strain-specific conformation of PrP^{TSE} and the phenotype of disease is not understood.

Strain-specific cofactors may contribute to prion strain diversity. This hypothesis predicts that the strain-specific conformation of PrP^{TSE} requires a unique cellular cofactor, or combination of cofactors, to stably maintain strain properties. Current work indicates that cellular cofactors can alter the rate of PrP^{TSE} formation (Deleault et al., 2010; Saa et al., 2012; Gonzalez-Montalban et al., 2013). The rate of murine PrP^{TSE} formation in vitro is increased in the presence of phosphatidylethanolamine (PE) (Deleault et al., 2012a). There is increasing evidence suggesting that cellular cofactors can contribute to prion strain diversity. Propagation of three prion strains using protein misfolding cyclic amplification (PMCA) that contained PE as the cofactor resulted in the convergence to a single indistinguishable strain (Deleault et al., 2012b). The properties of this strain, when passaged in animals, differed compared to the input strains and indicate that cofactors can modify strain properties in vitro that are maintained in vivo (Deleault et al., 2012b). What remains to be determined is if these cellular cofactors are involved in natural disease and if the distribution of cofactors in the host influences cellular tropism of prions.

Strain-specific rates of PrP^{TSE} formation can occur. The rate of prion accumulation in tissues from animals infected with different natural and experimental prion strains have been observed; however, the relative contribution of prion formation and clearance to the overall change in prion abundance is unknown (Hadlow et al., 1987, van Keulen et al., 2000). To overcome this limitation, the efficiency of PrP^{TSE} formation can be determined using PMCA, which only measures prion formation and not clearance (Shikiya et al., 2014). Short-incubation-period prion strains have a correspondingly higher efficiency of PrP^{TSE} formation in PMCA compared to strains with long incubation periods (Makarava et al., 2010; Shikiya et al., 2010; Ayers et al., 2011; Gonzalez-Montalban et al., 2011). The structural features of PrP^{TSE} that contribute to these observations are unknown. Interestingly, sialation of PrP N-linked glycosylation can influence the rate of PrP^{TSE} formation in vitro and it is hypothesized that strain-specific differences in PrP sialation may influence the rate of PrP^{TSE} formation in vivo (Katorcha et al., 2014). Strain-specific differences in the effect of RNA in the formation of PrP^{TSE} have been identified, further suggesting that cellular cofactors can influence the rate of prion formation (Deleault et al., 2010; Piro and Supattapone, 2011; Saa et al., 2012; Gonzalez-Montalban et al., 2013). Fragmentation of PrP^{TSE} is hypothesized to be a requirement of PrP^{TSE} propagation. Studies of yeast prions indicated that the rate of [PSI+] strain propagation inversely corresponded to low conformational stability, suggesting that prions with low stabilities fragment more easily and can recruit monomeric protein into the growing fibril more rapidly (Tanaka et al., 2004).

Consistent with the results of yeast prions, murine prion strains with shorter incubation periods have PrP^{TSE} with a lower conformational stability compared to PrP^{TSE} from long-incubation-period murine strains, suggesting that low conformational stability PrP^{TSE} can fragment more readily, facilitating the rapid formation of PrP^{TSE} compared to PrP^{TSE} from long-incubation-period strains (Colby et al., 2009; Colby and Prusiner, 2011; Ghaemmaghami et al., 2011). Subsequent work examining hamster-adapted and human prion strains found that short-incubation-period strains have high PrP^{TSE} conformational stabilities compared to long-incubation-period strains (Peretz et al., 2001; Ayers et al., 2011; Cescatti et al., 2016).

These apparently contradictory findings from murine, hamster, and human strains have several possible interpretations. First, relatively high or low PrP^{TSE} conformational stabilities could enhance fragmentation, resulting in higher rates of PrP^{TSE} formation and shorter incubation periods. Second, these studies correlate PrP^{TSE} conformational stability with incubation period; however, the role of PrP^{TSE} conformational stability in prion clearance may also contribute to the observed differences

(Ayers et al., 2011; Choi et al., 2014). Finally, the PrP^{TSE} conformational stability assay may be measuring a property of PrP^{TSE} unrelated to fragmentation.

PRION STRAIN TROPISM

Differences in the regional deposition of PrP^{TSE} within the CNS are strain-specific. Lesion profile analysis is a defining characteristic of prion strains; however, it does not always reflect strain-specific differences in prion neuronal tropism since neurons can contain high levels of PrP^{TSE} at terminal disease, yet fail to develop spongiform degeneration (van Keulen et al., 1995). Histoblot analysis can identify strain-specific regional differences in the distribution of PrP^{TSE} in the CNS (Hecker et al., 1992; DeArmond et al., 1993). High-resolution anatomic localization and cellular distribution of PrP^{TSE} are provided by PrP^{TSE} immunohistochemistry and have revealed strain-specific differences in the patterns of PrP^{TSE} immunoreactivity (Jeffrey et al., 2001, 2003; Siso et al., 2010). Additional detail is provided by using a panel of anti-PrP antibodies that span from the N- to the C-terminus of PrP that can reveal strain-specific forms of truncated PrP^{TSE} within neurons and glia (Jeffrey et al., 2006; Jeffrey and Gonzalez, 2007; Ayers et al., 2011).

The extraneural tropism of prions is a determinate of prion strains. Sheep naturally infected with classic or atypical scrapie have differences in the distribution of PrP^{TSE} in spleen and lymph nodes (Benestad et al., 2003; Klingeborn et al., 2006; Andreoletti et al., 2011). In experimentally infected animals, the distribution of infectivity and PrP^{TSE} in HY TME-infected hamsters is detected in brain, lymphoreticular system, skeletal muscle, nasal secretions, and blood (Bessen and Marsh, 1992a; Marsh and Bessen, 1994; Mulcahy et al., 2004; Bessen et al., 2010; Elder et al., 2013, 2015). In striking contrast, in DY TME-infected hamsters, infectivity and PrP^{TSE} are restricted to the CNS (Bartz et al., 2003, 2004; Bessen et al., 2009).

The mechanism of PrP^{TSE} tropism is not understood. One possibility is that strain-specific routes of prion spread result in the strain-specific differences in the distribution of PrP^{TSE} at terminal disease. In the CNS, the temporal and spatial spread of PrP^{TSE} and spongiform degeneration are consistent with spread along neuroanatomic tracks independent of the initial site of inoculation (Fraser and Dickinson, 1985; Scott and Fraser, 1989; Beekes et al., 1998; Andréoletti et al., 2000; Beekes and McBride, 2000; van Keulen et al., 2000; Bartz et al., 2003; Kincaid and Bartz, 2007). Inoculation of the sciatic nerve with either the HY or DY TME strains indicated that both of these strains were specifically transported along the same four descending motor pathways; however, at terminal disease, strain-specific differences in PrP^{TSE} distribution in the CNS occurred (Ayers et al., 2009). This result suggested that strain-specific differences in susceptibility of neurons to infection contributed to the difference in PrP^{TSE} distribution at terminal disease. Further experiments indicated that populations of neurons that did not contain detectable PrP^{TSE} following sciatic nerve inoculation could support PrP^{TSE} infection following intracerebral inoculation (Ayers et al., 2009). These data suggest that strain-specific differences in axonal transport or the ability of neurons to support PrP^{TSE} formation do not contribute to the pattern of PrP^{TSE} deposition at terminal disease.

These data are consistent with the clinical target area hypothesis, where strain-specific differences in neurodegeneration determine the length of incubation period and the clinical phenotype of disease. In this scenario, during the incubation period of disease, PrP^{TSE} is transported along neuroanatomic pathways, and the final distribution of PrP^{TSE} at terminal disease is determined by the extent of PrP^{TSE} spread when the clinical target areas are infected and destroyed (Kimberlin et al., 1987a; Kimberlin and Walker, 1988; Mirabile et al., 2015). At this time, it is unclear what role strain-specific cofactors contribute to the final distribution of PrP^{TSE} in neurons and glia (Deleault et al., 2012b; Miller et al., 2013; Supattapone, 2014). Less is known about the mechanism underlying tropism in cells other than neurons and glia. It is possible that strain-specific receptors, cell-specific PrP^{TSE} conversion cofactors, or inhibitors control PrP^{TSE} formation. Alternatively, strain-specific differences in the relative rates of PrP^{TSE} formation and clearance may influence tropism (Choi and Priola, 2013).

PRION STRAINS IN NATURAL PRION DISEASES OF LIVESTOCK AND CERVIDS

Prion strain variation was initially observed in ruminants. The sheep scrapie brain pool 1 (SSBP/1) is a mixture of brain homogenate from three individual sheep that was serially passaged in sheep without measurable changes in the phenotype of disease (Dickinson, 1976). Transmission of SSBP/1 to goats produced two distinct disease phenotypes, labeled drowsy and scratching (Pattison and Millson, 1961b). Serial transmission of the scratching and drowsy isolates in goats maintained the clinical phenotype of disease, providing convincing evidence for strains in natural prion disease. Experimental transmission of SSBP/1 to mice produces several distinct strains, suggesting that more than one strain of sheep scrapie is present in the inoculum (Thackray et al., 2011, 2012). Passage of sheep scrapie to transgenic mice expressing ovine PrP^{C} preserves distinctive strain properties of the inoculum, providing further evidence for strain diversity in scrapie (Thackray et al., 2011, 2012). Atypical sheep scrapie, also known as Nor98, has a different clinical presentation of disease and histopathologic features, and has PrP^{TSE} that is more sensitive to PK digestion compared to classic forms of scrapie (Benestad et al., 2003; Klingeborn et al., 2006).

Several strains of bovine spongiform encephalopathy (BSE) are recognized. Classic BSE was first identified in 1986 and is naturally transmissible to several species, including humans, in the form of variant Creutzfeldt–Jakob disease (vCJD) (Wells et al., 1987; Bruce et al., 1997; Hill et al., 1997; Scott et al., 1999). Surveillance efforts in cattle resulted in the identification of two additional forms of BSE. Bovine amyloidotic spongiform encephalopathy (BASE), also known as L-type BSE, has PrP^{TSE} that migrates faster (i.e., lower) compared to PrP^{TSE} from classic BSE (Casalone et al., 2004; Buschmann et al., 2006). The distribution of PrP^{TSE} in the CNS from BASE differs from classic BSE and is characterized by the presence of amyloid plaques (Casalone et al., 2004). The third form of BSE, H-type, has PrP^{TSE} that migrates slower (i.e., higher) compared to PrP^{TSE} from classic BSE (Biacabe et al., 2004). Transmission of H- or L-type BSE field isolates to transgenic mice expressing bovine PrP^{C} preserves the strain-specific migration of PrP^{TSE}, indicating that these are distinct BSE strains (Buschmann et al., 2006). The atypical forms of BSE largely occur in older cattle, leading to the hypothesis that they have a sporadic etiology, especially in light of the low pathogenicity of atypical BSE to cattle via the oral route (Brown et al., 2006; Biacabe et al., 2008; Okada et al., 2017). Interestingly, experimental transmission studies suggest that BASE may be the origin of TME, classic BSE, and some forms of sporadic CJD; however, more work is required to firmly establish a causal link (Baron et al., 2007; Béringue et al., 2007; Capobianco et al., 2007; Mestre-Francés et al., 2012).

Strains of CWD have been identified following experimental passage in animals. Initial transmission studies of CWD to transgenic mice expressing cervid PrP^{C} hinted at the existence of CWD strain diversity (Browning et al., 2004; LaFauci et al., 2006; Tamguney et al., 2006). A subsequent study that passaged a large cohort of CWD isolates to transgenic mice expressing cervid PrP provided the first evidence for two strains of CWD (Angers et al., 2010). While these CWD strains have different neuropathologic features, the biochemical properties of PrP^{TSE} are similar between the two strains, making identification of these strains in the natural host difficult.

Recent work suggests that the occupancy of amino acid 95 can influence the emergence of a novel CWD strain (Duque Velásquez et al., 2015). Interestingly, this strain has an increased pathogenicity for animals that contain serine at amino acid 96, a genotype thought to be relatively resistant to CWD infection (Meade-White et al., 2007; Race et al., 2011). It is unclear if this novel strain of CWD represents a strain that was newly formed based on the amino acid differences between the inoculum PrP^{TSE} and host PrP^{C} or if this strain pre-existed in the original field isolate. Regardless, these data indicate that the cervid PrP genotype can select for strains similar to what has been observed in sheep and mice (Dickinson and Meikle, 1971; Goldmann et al., 1994; Hunter et al., 1996).

PRION STRAINS IN HUMANS

Six subgroups of sporadic CJD (sCJD) are recognized in humans. Two major forms of PK-resistant PrP^{TSE} are found in CJD. The unglycosylated PrP^{TSE} polypeptide of type 1 PrP^{TSE} migrates at 21 kDa while the same PrP^{TSE} polypeptide from type 2 migrates at 19 kDa (Parchi et al., 1996). These differences in PrP^{TSE} migration are due to corresponding differences in the PK cleavage of PrP^{TSE} at amino acid 82 in type 1 and 97 in type 2 (Parchi et al., 2000). These two subtypes are further classified based on the *PRNP* codon 129 methionine (M)/ valine (V) polymorphism into six subtypes that correspond with specific clinical and pathologic features (Parchi et al., 1996, 1999). Experimental transmission of these subtypes largely maintains the biochemical properties of PrP^{TSE}, suggesting that the observed PrP^{TSE} differences in the field isolates represent distinct CJD strains (Telling et al., 1996b; Nonno et al., 2006; Kobayashi et al., 2010; Parchi et al., 2010; Moda et al., 2012).

Transmission of the six subgroups of sCJD to transgenic mice representing the diversity of codon 129 variability originally identified four distinct strains (Bishop et al., 2010), with an additional subgroup and strain later identified (Moda et al., 2012). The in vivo findings from Bishop et al. are consistent with previous work suggesting the biochemical properties of PrP^{TSE} from sCJD cases clustered into four subtypes (Uro-Coste et al., 2008; Bishop et al., 2010). However, recent work using novel experimental approaches have identified biochemical features that may expand this grouping (Cescatti et al., 2016; Cracco et al., 2017).

EXPERIMENTAL MODELS OF HUMAN PRION DISEASE

The "human" mouse

The most commonly used in vivo model of prion disease is the mouse. Unlike mouse models of other neurodegenerative diseases, such as Alzheimer's or Parkinson's disease, which only partially recapitulate the pathology of the human disease, the prion mouse model undergoes a bona fide prion infection. Prion-infected mice recapitulate the clinical, neuropathologic (TSE vacuolation, PrP deposition, gliosis), biochemical, and infectious features of a prion disease in a higher species such as humans. One of the advantages of the prion mouse model is that it can use the infectious nature of the disease via inoculation of the isolate of interest to start the disease process. Initially transmission studies were carried out in wild-type mice to assess strain and infectivity potential; however, this approach provides limited data on the effects of host genotype, zoonotic potential, and transmissibility between individuals. The development of transgenic mice expressing human PrP or human PrP with specific familial mutations has overcome these limitations.

The first transgenic mouse model for use in prion research overexpressed hamster PrP introduced by random integration into the mouse genome on the endogenous murine PrP background. When inoculated with hamster scrapie, these mice had significantly shorter incubation times than control mice (Scott et al., 1989). This was the first evidence that the species barrier could be overcome and demonstrated that sequence identity between host and donor PrP is important in determining species barriers and transmission potential. These seminal studies led the way for the use of transgenic mouse models in prion research. The production of PrP null mouse lines in which endogenous murine PrP was removed further allowed the development of transgenic mouse lines whist avoiding the problems associated with endogenous murine PrP interactions and illustrated the requirement of PrP^{C} for prion conversion (Bueler et al., 1992; Manson et al., 1994). A number of different transgenic models expressing human PrP or associated genetic mutations have now been produced. Each model has its own merits and can be divided into two broad categories: gene-targeted and conventional transgenic mice.

Gene-targeted models

The gene-targeted or knock-in mouse models are produced via homologous recombination into a specific locus in the target genome (reviewed in Capecchi, 2005). Expression of the mutant gene is at physiologic levels and is under control of the elements that normally regulate the expression of the PrP gene. Alterations in prion disease susceptibility or pathogenesis can therefore be attributed to the mutant gene, allowing for direct comparison of different genotypes of the mutant protein. A disadvantage of this system is long incubation periods that can be beyond the natural lifespan of the mouse.

Conventional transgenic mice

Conventional transgenic mouse models use random integration in which the transgene is integrated randomly into the genome. These models can have varying levels of expression and PrP expression may not follow normal CNS expression patterns. Although increased expression of PrP is associated with shortened incubation periods which can prove useful, overexpression of PrP can also cause spontaneous disease and can impact on strain characteristics (Le Dur et al., 2017). The variation in expression levels and patterns makes comparison between models difficult.

Common polymorphisms and mutations of human PrP

There are a large number of polymorphisms and mutations in the human *PRNP* gene (reviewed in Kobayashi et al., 2015). Some are nonpathogenic, such as the polymorphisms at codon 129; methionine or valine or codon 219; glutamic acid and lysine. These polymorphisms are now recognized as being important in disease susceptibility and phenotypes of acquired and sporadic prion diseases. Other mutations can lead to genetic forms of diseases such as Gerstmann–Sträussler–Scheinker (GSS) and fatal familial insomnia (FFI). These diseases can be modeled in mice using a transgenic approach or via inducing disease through inoculation of the agent.

Understanding and overcoming the species barrier in acquired diseases

Although prion diseases tend to transmit more efficiently within a species, some strains are able to transmit between species, albeit with large variation in efficiency. The inefficient transmission of a prion agent to a new species is often described as the species barrier and is associated with low attack rates and long incubation periods (Pattison, 1966; Kimberlin and Walker, 1979; Kimberlin et al., 1987b). Upon subsequent passage, attack rates increase and incubation periods can decrease. What determines the extent of the species barrier is still unknown but sequence identity between the PrP of the host and agent, glycosylation status, and specific mutations can all play a role. The transmission of BSE to zoo animals and humans most likely through contaminated food products highlights the risk of animal prion diseases crossing the species barrier, with the transmission of BSE to humans the only recognized instance of a zoonotic prion disease to date (Bruce et al., 1994, 1997).

In order to assess the zoonotic potential of animal prion diseases, a number of transgenic mouse models in which human PrP is expressed have been produced. There is a large number of both conventional and gene-targeted models expressing one of the *PRNP* codon 129 genotypes. The polymorphism at codon 129 is of particular interest in humans as certain genotypes are associated with phenotypes of sCJD or FFI or are over-represented in cases of vCJD. Although the normal frequencies of codon 129 polymorphism are 42% MM, 47% MV, and 11% VV in the UK population (Nurmi et al., 2003), all definite/probable clinical cases of vCJD, with the exception of one, have been methionine homozygote, suggesting a link between genotype and susceptibility.

Transmission studies of BSE have utilized both gene-targeted and overexpression models of human PrP. Whereas gene-targeted models expressing human PrP codon 129 MM, MV, or VV, referred to as HuM, HuMV, and HuV mice respectively, did not show any evidence of BSE transmission (Table 4.1) (Bishop et al., 2006), mice overexpressing 129VV and 129VVTg-152 exhibited low transmission rates (38%) and longer incubation periods than wild-type (FVB) mice – 602 versus 371 days respectively (Hill et al., 1997). These studies indicate that a significant species barrier exists between human PrP and cattle BSE consistent with the limited numbers of identified cases of probable/definite vCJD (178 cases in the United Kingdom as of April 2018; National CJD Research and Surveillance Unit, 2018) compared to the large numbers of cattle BSE. In comparison, the transmission of BSE after it has been passed through an intermediate species such as sheep is more efficient. In human PrP^{C} overexpressing mice, sheep BSE transmits with reduced incubation periods and increased susceptibility when compared to cattle BSE (Padilla et al., 2011). Similarly, in gene-targeted mice, 16/23 HuM mice showed evidence of disease compared with 0/18 mice inoculated with cattle BSE (Table 4.1) (Plinston et al., 2011). These results suggest that if BSE transmits through an intermediate species, the zoonotic potential could be greater than cattle BSE.

Although scrapie appears to have been endemic in the sheep population since 1732, transmission to humans has not been identified (reviewed in Liberski, 2012). However, experimental evidence arising from studies of overexpression models has provided conflicting results. When challenged with scrapie, mice which overexpress human PrP by four- (TgMet/Val129) or six- (Tg650 Met) fold showed evidence of disease transmission and, upon serial passage, increased susceptibility was observed (Cassard et al., 2014). This may be a consequence of the levels of PrP expression affecting the species barrier, i.e., higher levels may lead to a lowering of the barrier. However, it means that the risk of scrapie to human health cannot be absolutely dismissed. In contrast, transmission studies of natural and atypical scrapie in gene-targeted models found no evidence of disease transmission (Table 4.1) (Plinston et al., 2011; Wilson et al., 2012).

Chronic wasting disease (CWD) has become increasingly common in North America and has now been identified in Europe, raising concerns over zoonotic transmission both through consumption of contaminated meat and/or exposure to contaminated materials and the environment by hunters and agricultural workers (Benestad et al., 2016; Ricci et al., 2017). Although no specific bans are in place, there are a number of

Table 4.1

Transmission of animal transmissible spongiform encephalopathy (TSE) isolates to gene-targeted mice expressing human PrP

	Gene-targeted mouse line						
	HuM		HuMV		HuV		
Strain of agent	IP	TSE pathology[a]	IP	TSE pathology[a]	IP	TSE pathology[a]	Reference
BSE	>765	0/18	>749	0/23	>793	0/22	Bishop et al. (2006)
Sheep BSE	>750	16/23	>708	0/24	>650	0/23	Plinston et al. (2011)
BASE	>687	0/24	>672	0/24	>763	0/24	Wilson et al. (2012)
BSE-H	>722	0/24	>708	0/24	>722	0/24	Wilson et al. (2012)
Natural scrapie (VRQ/VRQ)	>730	0/24	>682	0/24	>710	0/24	Plinston et al. (2011)
Atypical scrapie (ARR/ARR)	>651	0/23	>724	0/21	>829	0/24	Wilson et al. (2012)
CWD	>680	0/24	>730	0/24	>722	0/24	Wilson et al. (2012)

[a]TSE pathology confirmed by either immunohistochemistry or TSE vacuolation.

BASE, bovine amyloidotic spongiform encephalopathy; BSE, bovine spongiform encephalopathy; CWD, chronic wasting disease; IP, incubation period.

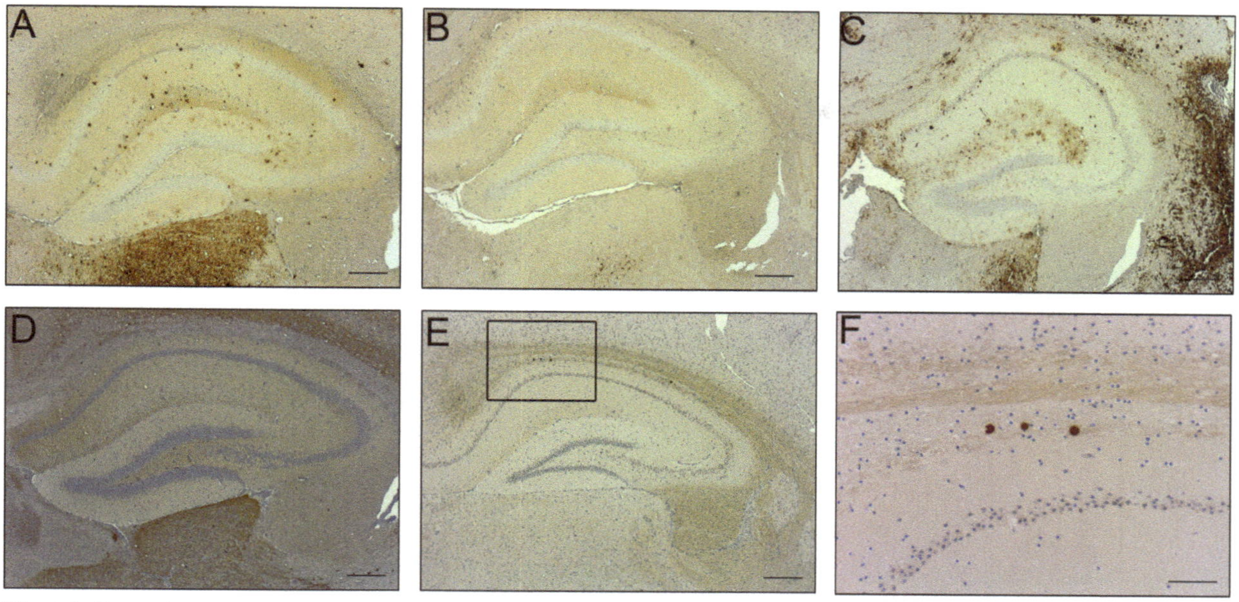

Fig. 4.1. Examples of abnormal PrP deposition in transgenic mice expressing the human *PRNP* codon 129 genotypes challenged with human prion diseases. (**A**) HuM mouse challenged with variant Creutzfeldt–Jakob disease (vCJD). (**B**) HuMV mouse challenged with vCJD. (**C**) HuV mouse challenged with vCJD. (**D**) HuV mouse challenged with sporadic Creuttzfeldt–Jakob disease VV2. (**E** and **F**) HuV mouse challenged with UK case of variably protease-sensitive prionopathy; (**F**) is magnification of area indicated in box. Immunohistochemistry was performed with (**A–C**) 6H4 anti-PrP antibody or (**D–F**) 3F4 anti-PrP antibody. Representative sections are shown through the hippocampus/thalamus. Scale bars: (**A–E**) 200 μm; (**F**) 50 μm.

recommendations regarding testing of carcasses and subsequent consumption. No recognized cases of CWD transmission to humans have occurred, but as the disease spreads to new cervid species the zoonotic potential may rise. Although no positive transmission of CWD to gene-targeted mice expressing human PrP has been demonstrated (Table 4.1), there have been early reports of disease transmission to mice overexpressing 129MM or 129VV PrP (Kong et al., 2016). In comparison, in vitro model systems have provided evidence that CWD has zoonotic potential. Although less efficient than classic BSE, CWD was able to convert human PrP from human brain, human cell homogenates, and transgenic mouse brain expressing human PrP in the PMCA assay. The resulting PMCA reaction product resembled that of type 1 PrP^{res} similar to that of sCJD (Barria et al., 2014). These results not only appear to suggest that CWD does have zoonotic potential but also demonstrate the difficulties in interpreting data from both in vivo and in vitro studies and assessing risks of transmission.

Modeling intraspecies transmission in humans

The generation of transgenic mice expressing human PrP allows us to model transmission between individuals and the impact of codon 129 on transmission potential. Variant CJD transmits both to mice overexpressing human PrP and to gene-targeted models, demonstrating that susceptibility to disease varies according to host genotype (Fig. 4.1, A–C). Bishop et al. (2006) used gene-targeted mice to show that susceptibility decreased in the order HuM > HuMV > HuV and provided evidence that the 129MV and 129VV genotypes may exhibit longer incubations and that individuals of all genotypes may remain asymptomatic during life (Table 4.2). Retrospective studies of fixed appendix and lymphoreticular tissues have now given estimates that up to 1 in 2000 individuals have evidence of abnormal PrP in their appendices (Hilton et al., 2004; Gill et al., 2013). The most recent study has indicated that these individuals are from a range of birth cohorts and genotypes (Gill et al., 2013).

There have been four probable cases of vCJD transmission associated with the transfusion of infected red blood cells and one likely case through infected factor VIII products, indicating that individuals are infective during the presymptomatic phase of disease. Gene-targeted mice which were challenged with material from an individual who developed vCJD as a result of suspected blood transfusion indicated that transmission through a 129MM individual had not resulted in an adaptation to the host since the numbers of mice with vacuolation were similar between a primary case of vCJD and a transfusion recipient: 6/16 HuM, 1/15 HuMV, and 1/15 HuV mice and 8/15 HuM, 0/17 HuMV, and 0/17 HuV respectively (Bishop et al., 2006, 2008). Serial passage

Table 4.2

Transmission of vCJD, sCJD, or VPSPr to gene-targeted mice expressing human PrP

			Gene-targeted mouse line						
			HuM		HuMV		HuV		
Name	Features of disease	Inocula (*PRNP* genotype/ PrP^{res} type)	IP	TSE pathology[a]	IP	TSE pathology[a]	IP	TSE pathology[a]	Reference
vCJD	Early, persistent psychiatric symptoms Severe spongiform change in the caudate nucleus and putamen Multiple florid plaques	vCJD 2B	>401	11/17	>600	11/16	–	1/16	Bishop et al. (2006)
Classic CJD	Rapidly progressive dementia Synaptic-type PrP staining	sCJD MM1 sCJD MV1	446±3 446±5	13/13 16/16	457±11 475±10	14/14 17/18	588±21 603±34	14/16 15/18	Bishop et al. (2010)
Ataxic variant	Ataxia at onset with late dementia Plaque-like focal deposits of PrP and perineuronal staining	sCJD VV2	582±8	15/17	450	5/15	274 ± 4	16/16	Bishop et al. (2010)
Kuru plaques variant	Ataxia and progressive dementia Consistent plaque-like focal deposits of PrP with the presence of amyloid kuru plaques	sCJD MV2	563±2	10/11	575±37	15/17	288±3	16/16	Bishop et al. (2010)
Thalamic variant	Insomnia, ataxia, cognitive impairment Atrophy of the thalamus, absent or focal spongiosis and lower amounts of PrP than other variants	sCJD MM2	535±32	13/14	ND	ND	ND	ND	Moda et al. (2012)
Cortical variant	Progressive dementia Large confluent vacuoles, perivacuolar PrP deposition	sCJD MM2	–	0/15 0//16	–	2/18 ND	–	3/17 ND	Bishop et al. (2010); Moda et al. (2012)
Rare	Progressive dementia Pathology in the cerebral cortex, faint synaptic PrP deposition	sCJD VV1	–	2/16	557±11	9/14	568±0	7/14	Bishop et al. (2010)
VPSPr	Atypical dementia-like. Accumulation of microplaques. "Ladder-like" profile on Western blot and ~8-kDa fragment	VPSPr VV VPSPr MV	– –	1/15 0/15	– –	2/14 0/14	– –	5/14 0/14	Diack et al. (2014)

[a]Transmissible spongiform encephalopathy (TSE) pathology confirmed by either immunohistochemistry or TSE vacuolation.
– indicates no clinical signs; CJD, Creutzfeldt–Jakob disease; IP, incubation period; ND, not done; sCJD, sporadic Creutzfeldt–Jakob disease; vCJD, variant Creutzfeldt–Jakob disease; VPSPr, variably protease-sensitive prionopathy.

of vCJD through gene-targeted mice has also shown a lack of adaptation to the presence of human PrP (Diack, unpublished observations).

The recent identification of vCJD in a codon 129 heterozygous individual has raised concerns of a second wave of vCJD. The age at onset of disease was 36 years, which is older than the average age in 129MM individuals, suggestive of a longer incubation period (Mok et al., 2017). An earlier case of asymptomatic vCJD in a heterozygous individual in which abnormal PrP was only observed in the spleen and a lymph node showed that the abnormal PrP in the spleen was capable of transmitting infectivity to HuM mice, albeit at lower rates than spleen material from 129MM individuals (Peden et al., 2004; Bishop et al., 2013). Assessing both the transmissibility of the recent MV case and understanding the significance of other peripheral accumulations of abnormal PrP in the appendix studies is now of great importance in assessing the risks of vCJD infectivity to the population and the impact this may have on public health.

Sporadic diseases

At present the only method of studying or modeling human sporadic prion diseases is through inoculation of the appropriate mouse model. Diseases such as sCJD are rare, with sCJD appearing at a rate of 1.5 cases per million per annum (Ladogana et al., 2005), and it is hypothesized that they occur as a result of a random conversion event of the normal PrP protein to the abnormal form. Early transmission studies of sCJD to wild-type mice demonstrated low attack rates at primary passage (Bruce et al., 1997), whereas transmission to bank voles proved more successful, with MM1 and MV1 behaving as a single strain, but limited or no transmission occurred with MV2 and VV2 (Nonno et al., 2006).

Using a combination of gene-targeted mice and the traditional strain-typing approach, Bishop et al. (2010) and Moda et al. (2012) established that the sCJD subtypes could be transmitted to at least one genotype of mouse and classified into different strains of disease (Table 4.2 and Fig. 4.1D). Five strains of sCJD appear to occur: $M1^{CJD}$; MM1 and MV1, $V2^{CJD}$; MV2 and VV2, $M2^{CJD}$; MM2, $V1^{CJD}$; VV1 (Bishop et al., 2010) and MM1 thalamic (Moda et al., 2012). These studies not only highlighted the need for awareness of iatrogenic transmission of sCJD but also provided a standard dataset which other atypical or sporadic forms of prion disease could be compared against.

In 2008, a novel prion disease, variably protease-sensitive prionopathy (VPSPr), was described in the United States (Gambetti et al., 2008) and later identified in Europe (Head et al., 2009). The most distinctive features of VPSPr PrP^{TSE} are the electrophoretic profile and resistance to PK digestion. Western blot analysis of PrP^{TSE} VPSPr results in a distinctive ladder-like profile with the presence of a low-molecular-weight fragment at approximately 8 kDa, similar to GSS. Unlike GSS, mutations in the PrP gene have not been identified in patients with VPSPr. VPSPr can occur in all codon 129 genotypes, with the highest number of cases in the 129VV genotype. Different codon 129 genotype occupancy appears to give slightly different clinical symptoms, disease duration, relative resistance of PrP^{TSE} to PK digestion, and histopathologic features (Zou et al., 2010).

As a novel prion disease, assessing the transmissibility of the agent is important for public health. Two transmission studies have been completed using either conventional transgenic mice or gene-targeted mice. Although neither study found evidence of pathologically confirmed clinical disease, TSE vacuolation and abnormal PrP deposition were identified in the conventional transgenic mice (Notari et al., 2014), whereas only abnormal PrP deposition was identified in the gene-targeted mouse lines (Table 4.2 and Fig. 4.1, E and F) (Diack et al., 2014). In both studies, material from individuals of the 129VV genotype appeared to favor the same genotypes. Both studies concluded that VPSPr is a transmissible prion disease but is relatively inefficient and that it held unique strain properties. These studies emphasize the need for continuing surveillance for novel prion diseases.

Modeling inherited/genetic forms of prion disease

Genetic forms of prion disease are associated with mutations in the *PRNP* gene and account for 10–15% of all cases. There are a number of commonly recognized genetic forms of disease, including familial CJD (fCJD), GSS, and FFI. The three forms can be distinguished by clinical symptoms, neuropathologic changes, and the biochemical properties of PrP^{TSE}. Although some diseases can be transmitted to nontransgenic mice, the production of transgenic mice expressing specific genetic mutations has been a slow process and some models can only recapitulate certain aspects of the human disease or fail to develop clinical or pathologic disease (Hsiao et al., 1990; Dossena et al., 2008; Asante et al., 2009; Bouybayoune et al., 2015).

Familial CJD

The E200K-129M haplotype is the most common genetic mutation that can cluster in ethnic populations or geographic locations (Hsiao et al., 1991). The generation of a transgenic mouse line in which the E to K mutation was inserted at codon 199 (equivalent to the E200K mutation) in a chimeric human/mouse model has led to a model which shares certain phenotypic characteristics of the human disease. The TgMMHu2-ME199K lines show a progressive neurodegenerative disease from 5 to 6 months old which further deteriorates to a terminal state at approximately 11–14 months old (Friedman-Levi et al., 2011). Neuropathologic analysis revealed gliosis, intraneuronal deposition of abnormal PrP (similar to human cases), neuronal and synaptic loss, and biochemical analysis provides evidence of truncated PrP^{res} (Friedman-Levi et al., 2011; Fainstein et al., 2016). In addition brain material proved infectious when inoculated into wild-type mice, further confirming the presence of a typical prion disease. As this model appears to recapitulate the phenotype of the human disease, it has been used to assess therapeutic treatments for genetic CJD and has given some insight into potential targets (Mizrahi et al., 2014).

A more recent model uses transgenic mice expressing bank vole prion protein containing the E200K mutation. Bank vole PrP is susceptible to conversion to PrP^{TSE} by prions from a large number of species (Nonno et al., 2006; Di Bari et al., 2008, 2013; Watts et al., 2014). The Tg(BvPrPI109,E200K) mouse model develops a spontaneous neurologic disease at between ~120 and 560 days, dependent upon the specific mouse line used, with small rounded aggregates of PrP^{TSE} accompanied by spongiform vacuolation. PrP^{res} could also be detected in clinically ill mice (Watts et al., 2016). This unique approach to producing transgenic models of genetic prion diseases could prove useful in testing therapeutics.

A less frequent familial form of CJD is caused by a valine-to-isoleucine substitution (V210I) at codon 210 of *PRNP* (Pocchiari et al., 1993; Ripoll et al., 1993). Inoculation of V210I brain material into transgenic mice expressing a chimeric human–mouse transgene (Tg(MHu2M)Prnp0/0) produced a clinical disease with pathology unlike that of E200K or FFI but more akin to sCJD. The data from this transmission study suggest that different pathogenic mutations could lead to different PrP^{TSE} conformations and result in different prion strains (Mastrianni et al., 2001).

Gerstmann–Sträussler–Scheinker disease

GSS disease is associated with a number of point mutations (>16) in the *PRNP* gene. The most common mutation is the P102L mutation, which was the first to be identified in 1989 (Hsiao et al., 1989) and has been extensively studied in transgenic mice. The corresponding mouse mutation P101L has been modeled in conventional mice that develop a spontaneous disease with misfolded PrP but little or no PrP^{TSE} in the brains (Hsiao et al., 1990; Telling et al., 1996a). This suggested that the 101L mutation may result in an unstable PrP protein conformation. Gene-targeted models (101LL) show no evidence of spontaneous disease but are susceptible to inoculation with GSS. Clinical disease occurs at ~290 days with spongiform vacuolation, variable amounts of abnormal PrP deposition, and low levels of PrP^{res} present (Manson et al., 1999). Inoculation with GSS from individuals in which no spongiform degeneration is apparent and only an 8-kDa PrP^{res} fragment is observed results in a nonclinical phenotype without spongiform degeneration but PrP-amyloid plaques can be observed (Piccardo et al., 2007). These results have questioned the relationship between PrP accumulation and infectivity.

Asante et al. (2009) produced conventional transgenic mice expressing human PrP 102LL on a mouse background (102LL Tg27 mice) which again did not produce a spontaneous disease. Inoculation with GSS gives rise to a clinical disease with incubation periods of 185–191 days. Although PrP deposition was observed, it was reminiscent of the multicentric plaques commonly observed in GSS cases (Asante et al., 2009). Although not fully recapitulating all the phenotypes of the human disease, these mouse models have proved useful in understanding the role of PrP confirmation and strains of agent in GSS.

Fatal familial insomnia

FFI is clinically characterized by alterations in the sleep–wake cycle causing progressive insomnia and dementia. It is associated with the D178N mutation in combination with methionine at codon 129. If the D178N mutation occurs in combination with valine at codon 129 then an fCJD phenotype manifests. The first mouse models of FFI used gene targeting to replace the mouse open reading frame with a mutant D177N allele (the mouse equivalent of D178N) and also included the L108M, V111M human mutation which gave an epitope for the human-specific 3F4 antibody (Jackson et al., 2009). These mice, ki-3F4-FFI, exhibited age-related changes in behavior which were more prominent at night, including alterations in sleep which started as early as 5 months of age and disruption in body temperature control, reminiscent of the abnormalities observed in human FFI cases.

Neuropathologic analysis revealed neuronal loss in the thalamus and reactive astrogliosis in the thalamus and cerebellum, again similar to human FFI cases. However, immunohistochemistry and biochemical analysis failed to detect the presence of abnormal PrP deposition or PrP^{res}. Tga20 mice are susceptible to infection, confirming the presence of an infectious agent (Jackson et al., 2009). Transgenic mice expressing mouse PrP at one and two times normal expression (FFI-26 mice) also develop a neurologic phenotype with thalamic and cerebellar degeneration and PrP deposition could be observed (Bouybayoune et al., 2015).

More recently, transgenic mice expressing bank vole prion protein and the D178N mutation, similar to the E200K model discussed above, were produced. As with the E200K model, this model appears to recapitulate the FFI phenotype, gliosis, PrP deposition, and vacuolation. A 8-kDa PrP^{res} fragment was observed upon Western blot analysis, which appears to be a feature of the bank vole model rather than the disease phenotype, i.e., FFI cases normally exhibit PrP^{res} at 27–30 kDa (Watts et al., 2016). Although no mouse model to date appears to fully recapitulate a genetic prion disease in particular, the presence of PrP^{res}, the examples discussed here, and the many other models that exist provide a means of understanding and dissecting the mechanisms behind spontaneous prion formation and may be useful in assessing therapeutic approaches or identifying targets.

Identification and assessment of therapeutic targets

Transgenic mice can be used to model human prion diseases and provide an opportunity to define mechanisms of disease, identify therapeutic targets, and test the efficacy of antiprion compounds. The use of mice in which tissue- and/or temporal-specific knockdown of the *Prnp* gene occurs during the course of disease has demonstrated that disease can be halted. Using the Cre-lox system to deplete neuronal PrP in mice which had been inoculated with Rocky Mountain Laboratory prion strain, Mallucci et al. (2003, 2007) observed that behavioral and neuropathologic effects were reversed and disease appeared to be halted. These elegant studies suggest that there is scope for therapeutic intervention even after the appearance of pathology. Later studies have exploited specific pathways such as the unfolded protein response that mediate PrP neurotoxicity and demonstrate that targeting key mediators of this pathway can extend survival rates (Moreno et al., 2012, 2013).

Although a number of compounds have appeared to be effective as prion therapeutics in wild-type mouse models with scrapie strains, they have not always been as effective when assessed in wild-type or chimeric mice challenged with human strains such as sCJD, suggesting that treatments may be highly strain-specific (Berry et al., 2013; Lu et al., 2013; Giles et al., 2016). Using transgenic models expressing human PrP and challenged with human isolates may overcome these issues.

CONCLUSION

Prion strains are operationally defined as a heritable phenotype of disease under controlled transmission conditions. Several biochemical features of the infectious agent, PrP^{TSE}, correspond with distinct prion strains, consistent with the hypothesis that prion strain diversity is encoded in the conformation of PrP^{TSE}. Work on prion strain diversity and many other aspects of prion biology would not be possible without the development and advancement of powerful transgenic animal models of prion disease. Transgenic mice expressing exogenous PrP^C have allowed for a wide range of investigative studies into the impact of human polymorphisms and/or mutations on disease transmission and pathogenesis. These models allow us to define disease processes with the aim of identifying therapeutic targets and ultimately disease interventions. It is only with a combination of an increased understanding of prion strain diversity, basic prion biology, and use of transgenic models that we will become closer to a cure for these devastating diseases.

References

Andréoletti O, Berthon P, Marc D et al. (2000). Early accumulation of PrPSc in gut-associated lymphoid and nervous tissues of susceptible sheep from a Romanov flock with natural scrapie. J Gen Virol 81: 3115–3126.

Andreoletti O, Orge L, Benestad SL et al. (2011). Atypical/Nor98 scrapie infectivity in sheep peripheral tissues. PLoS Pathog 7: e1001285.

Angers RC, Kang HE, Napier D et al. (2010). Prion strain mutation determined by prion protein conformational compatibility and primary structure. Science 328: 1154–1158.

Asante EA, Gowland I, Grimshaw A et al. (2009). Absence of spontaneous disease and comparative prion susceptibility of transgenic mice expressing mutant human prion proteins. J Gen Virol 90: 546–558.

Ayers JI, Kincaid AE, Bartz JC (2009). Prion strain targeting independent of strain-specific neuronal tropism. J Virol 83: 81–87.

Ayers JI, Schutt CR, Shikiya RA et al. (2011). The strain-encoded relationship between PrPSc replication, stability and processing in neurons is predictive of the incubation period of disease. PLoS Pathog 7: e1001317.

Baron T, Bencsik A, Biacabe A-G et al. (2007). Phenotypic similarity of transmissible mink encephalopathy in cattle and L-type bovine spongiform encephalopathy in a mouse model. Emerg Infect Dis 13: 1887–1894.

Barria MA, Balachandran A, Morita M et al. (2014). Molecular barriers to zoonotic transmission of prions. Emerg Infect Dis 20: 88–97.

Bartz JC, Kincaid AE, Bessen RA (2003). Rapid prion neuroinvasion following tongue infection. J Virol 77: 583–591.

Bartz JC, Aiken JM, Bessen RA (2004). Delay in onset of prion disease for the HY strain of transmissible mink encephalopathy as a result of prior peripheral inoculation with the replication-deficient DY strain. J Gen Virol 85: 265–273.

Beekes M, McBride PA (2000). Early accumulation of pathological PrP in the enteric nervous system and gut-associated lymphoid tissue of hamsters orally infected with scrapie. Neurosci Lett 278: 181–184.

Beekes M, Mcbride PA, Baldauf E (1998). Cerebral targeting indicates vagal spread of infection in hamsters fed with scrapie. J Gen Virol 79: 601–607.

Benestad SL, Sarradin P, Thu B et al. (2003). Cases of scrapie with unusual features in Norway and designation of a new type, Nor98. Vet Rec: 153.

Benestad SL, Mitchell G, Simmons M et al. (2016). First case of chronic wasting disease in Europe in a Norwegian free-ranging reindeer. Vet Res 47: 1–7.

Béringue V, Andréoletti O, Le Dur A et al. (2007). A bovine prion acquires an epidemic bovine spongiform encephalopathy strain-like phenotype on interspecies transmission. J Neurosci 27: 6965–6971.

Berry DB, Lu D, Geva M et al. (2013). Drug resistance confounding prion therapeutics. Proc Natl Acad Sci U S A 110: E4160–E4169.

Bessen RA, Marsh RF (1992a). Biochemical and physical properties of the prion protein from two strains of the transmissible mink encephalopathy agent. J Virol 66: 2096–2101.

Bessen RA, Marsh RF (1992b). Identification of two biologically distinct strains of transmissible mink encephalopathy in hamsters. J Gen Virol 73: 329–334.

Bessen RA, Marsh RF (1994). Distinct PrP properties suggest the molecular-basis of strain variation in transmissible mink encephalopathy. J Virol 68: 7859–7868.

Bessen RA, Martinka S, Kelly J et al. (2009). Role of the lymphoreticular system in prion neuroinvasion from the oral and nasal mucosa. J Virol 83: 6435–6445.

Bessen RA, Shearin H, Martinka S et al. (2010). Prion shedding from olfactory neurons into nasal secretions. PLoS Pathog 6: e1000837.

Biacabe A-G, Laplanche J-L, Ryder S et al. (2004). Distinct molecular phenotypes in bovine prion diseases. EMBO Rep 5: 110–115.

Biacabe A-G, Morignat E, Vulin J et al. (2008). Atypical bovine spongiform encephalopathies, France, 2001–2007. Emerg Infect Dis 14: 298–300.

Bishop MT, Hart P, Aitchison L et al. (2006). Predicting susceptibility and incubation time of human-to-human transmission of vCJD. Lancet Neurol 5: 393–398.

Bishop MT, Ritchie DL, Will RG et al. (2008). No major change in vCJD agent strain after secondary transmission via blood transfusion. PLoS ONE 3: e2878.

Bishop MT, Will RG, Manson JC (2010). Defining sporadic Creutzfeldt-Jakob disease strains and their transmission properties. Proc Natl Acad Sci U S A 107: 12005–12010.

Bishop MT, Diack AB, Ritchie DL et al. (2013). Prion infectivity in the spleen of a PRNP heterozygous individual with subclinical variant Creutzfeldt-Jakob disease. Brain 136: 1139–1145.

Bouybayoune I, Mantovani S, Del Gallo F et al. (2015). Transgenic fatal familial insomnia mice indicate prion infectivity-independent mechanisms of pathogenesis and phenotypic expression of disease. PLoS Pathog 11: e1004796.

Brown P, Mcshane LM, Zanusso G et al. (2006). On the question of sporadic or atypical bovine spongiform encephalopathy and Creutzfeldt-Jakob disease. Emerg Infect Dis 12: 1816–1821.

Browning SR, Mason GL, Seward T et al. (2004). Transmission of prions from mule deer and elk with chronic wasting disease to transgenic mice expressing cervid PrP. J Virol 78: 13345–13350.

Bruce ME (1993). Scrapie strain variation and mutation. Br Med Bull 49: 822–838.

Bruce M, Chree A, McConnell I et al. (1994). Transmission of bovine spongiform encephalopathy and scrapie to mice: strain variation and the species barrier. Philos Trans R Soc Lond Ser B Biol Sci 343: 405–411.

Bruce ME, Will RG, Ironside JW et al. (1997). Transmissions to mice indicate that 'new variant' CJD is caused by the BSE agent. Nature 389: 498–501.

Bueler H, Fischer M, Lang Y et al. (1992). Normal development and behaviour of mice lacking the neuronal cell-surface PrP protein. Nature 356: 577–582.

Buschmann A, Gretzschel A, Biacabe AG et al. (2006). Atypical BSE in Germany – proof of transmissibility and biochemical characterization. Vet Microbiol 117: 103–116.

Capecchi MR (2005). Gene targeting in mice: functional analysis of the mammalian genome for the twenty-first century. Nat Rev Genet 6: 507–512.

Capobianco R, Casalone C, Suardi S et al. (2007). Conversion of the BASE prion strain into the BSE strain: the origin of BSE? PLoS Pathog 3: e31.

Casalone C, Zanusso G, Acutis P et al. (2004). Identification of a second bovine amyloidotic spongiform encephalopathy: molecular similarities with sporadic Creutzfeldt-Jakob disease. Proc Natl Acad Sci U S A 101: 3065–3070.

Cassard H, Torres J-M, Lacroux C et al. (2014). Evidence for zoonotic potential of ovine scrapie prions. Nat Commun: 5.

Caughey B, Raymond GJ, Bessen RA (1998). Strain-dependent differences in β-sheet conformations of abnormal prion protein. J Biol Chem 273: 32230–32235.

Cescatti M, Saverioni D, Capellari S et al. (2016). Analysis of conformational stability of abnormal prion protein aggregates across the spectrum of Creutzfeldt-Jakob disease prions. J Virol 90: 6244–6254.

Choi YP, Priola SA (2013). A specific population of abnormal prion protein aggregates is preferentially taken up by cells and disaggregated in a strain-dependent manner. J Virol 87: 11552–11561.

Choi YP, Head MW, Ironside JW et al. (2014). Uptake and degradation of protease-sensitive and -resistant forms of abnormal human prion protein aggregates by human astrocytes. Am J Pathol 184: 3299–3307.

Colby DW, Prusiner SB (2011). De novo generation of prion strains. Nat Rev Microbiol 9: 771–777.

Colby DW, Giles K, Legname G et al. (2009). Design and construction of diverse mammalian prion strains. Proc Natl Acad Sci U S A 106: 20417–20422.

Cracco L, Notari S, Cali I et al. (2017). Novel strain properties distinguishing sporadic prion diseases sharing prion protein genotype and prion type. Sci Rep 7: 38280.

DeArmond SJ, Yang SL, Lee A et al. (1993). Three scrapie prion isolates exhibit different accumulation patterns of the prion protein scrapie isoform. Proc Natl Acad Sci U S A 90: 6449–6453.

Deleault NR, Kascsak R, Geoghegan JC et al. (2010). Species-dependent differences in cofactor utilization for formation of the protease-resistant prion protein in vitro. Biochemistry 49: 3928–3934.

Deleault NR, Piro JR, Walsh DJ et al. (2012a). Isolation of phosphatidylethanolamine as a solitary cofactor for prion formation in the absence of nucleic acids. Proc Natl Acad Sci U S A 109: 8546–8551.

Deleault NR, Walsh DJ, Piro JR et al. (2012b). Cofactor molecules maintain infectious conformation and restrict strain properties in purified prions. Proc Natl Acad Sci U S A 109: E1938–E1946.

Diack AB, Ritchie DL, Peden AH et al. (2014). Variably protease-sensitive prionopathy, a unique prion variant with inefficient transmission properties. Emerg Infect Dis 20: 1969–1979.

Di Bari MA, Chianini F, Vaccari G et al. (2008). The bank vole (*Myodes glareolus*) as a sensitive bioassay for sheep scrapie. J Gen Virol 89: 2975–2985.

Di Bari MA, Nonno R, Castilla J et al. (2013). Chronic wasting disease in bank voles: characterisation of the shortest incubation time model for prion diseases. PLoS Pathog 9: e1003219.

Dickinson AG (1976). Scrapie in sheep and goats. Front Biol 44: 209–241.

Dickinson AG, Meikle VM (1971). Host-genotype and agent effects in scrapie incubation: change in allelic interaction with different strains of agent. Mol Gen Genet 112: 73–79.

Dossena S, Imeri L, Mangieri M et al. (2008). Mutant prion protein expression causes motor and memory deficits and abnormal sleep patterns in a transgenic mouse model. Neuron 60: 598–609.

Duque Velásquez C, Kim C, Herbst A et al. (2015). Deer prion proteins modulate the emergence and adaptation of chronic wasting disease strains. J Virol 89: 12362–12373.

Elder AM, Henderson DM, Nalls AV et al. (2013). In vitro detection of prionemia in TSE-infected cervids and hamsters. PLoS One 8: e80203.

Elder AM, Henderson DM, Nalls AV et al. (2015). Immediate and ongoing detection of prions in the blood of hamsters and deer following oral, nasal, or blood inoculations. J Virol 89: 7421–7424.

Fainstein N, Dori D, Frid K et al. (2016). Chronic progressive neurodegeneration in a transgenic mouse model of prion disease. Front Neurosci: 10.

Fraser H, Dickinson AG (1967). Distribution of experimentally induced scrapie lesions in the brain. Nature 216: 1310–1311.

Fraser H, Dickinson AG (1968). The sequential development of the brain lesion of scrapie in three strains of mice. J Comp Pathol 78: 301–311.

Fraser H, Dickinson AG (1985). Targeting of scrapie lesions and spread of agent via the retino-tectal projection. Brain Res 346: 32–41.

Friedman-Levi Y, Meiner Z, Canello T et al. (2011). Fatal prion disease in a mouse model of genetic E200K Creutzfeldt-Jakob disease. PLoS Pathog 7: e1002350.

Gambetti P, Dong Z, Yuan J et al. (2008). A novel human disease with abnormal prion protein sensitive to protease. Ann Neurol 63: 697–708.

Ghaemmaghami S, Watts JC, Nguyen H-O et al. (2011). Conformational transformation and selection of synthetic prion strains. J Mol Biol 413: 527–542.

Ghaemmaghami S, Colby DW, Nguyen H-OB et al. (2013). Convergent replication of mouse synthetic prion strains. Am J Pathol 182: 866–874.

Giles K, Berry DB, Condello C et al. (2016). Optimization of aryl amides that extend survival in prion-infected mice. J Pharmacol Exp Ther 358: 537–547.

Gill ON, Spencer Y, Richard-Loendt A et al. (2013). Prevalent abnormal prion protein in human appendixes after bovine spongiform encephalopathy epizootic: large scale survey. BMJ: 347.

Goldmann W, Hunter N, Smith G et al. (1994). PrP genotype and agent effects in scrapie: change in allelic interaction with different isolates of agent in sheep, a natural host of scrapie. J Gen Virol 75: 989–995.

Gonzalez-Montalban N, Makarava N et al. (2011). Relationship between conformational stability and amplification efficiency of prions. Biochemistry 50: 7933–7940.

Gonzalez-Montalban N, Lee YJ, Makarava N et al. (2013). Changes in prion replication environment cause prion strain mutation. FASEB J 27: 3702–3710.

Hadlow WJ, Race RE, Kennedy RC (1987). Temporal distribution of transmissible mink encephalopathy virus in mink inoculated subcutaneously. J Virol 61: 3235–3240.

Head MW, Knight R, Zeidler M et al. (2009). A case of protease sensitive prionopathy in a patient in the UK. Neuropathol Appl Neurobiol 35: 628–632.

Hecker R, Taraboulos A, Scott M et al. (1992). Replication of distinct scrapie prion isolates is region specific in brains of transgenic mice and hamsters. Genes Dev 6: 1213–1228.

Hill AF, Desbruslais M, Joiner S et al. (1997). The same prion strain causes vCJD and BSE. Nature 448–450 (526): 389.

Hilton DA, Ghani AC, Conyers L et al. (2004). Prevalence of lymphoreticular prion protein accumulation in UK tissue samples. J Pathol 203: 733–739.

Hsiao K, Baker HF, Crow TJ et al. (1989). Linkage of a prion protein missense variant to Gerstmann-Straussler syndrome. Nature 338: 342–345.

Hsiao K, Scott M, Foster D et al. (1990). Spontaneous neurodegeneration in transgenic mice with mutant prion protein. Science 250: 1587–1590.

Hsiao K, Hsiao K, Meiner Z (1991). Mutation of the prion protein in Libyan Jews with Creutzfeldt–Jakob disease. N Engl J Med 324: 1091–1097.

Hunter N, Foster JD, Goldmann W et al. (1996). Natural scrapie in a closed flock of Cheviot sheep occurs only in specific PrP genotypes. Arch Virol 141: 809–824.

Jackson WS, Borkowski AW, Faas H et al. (2009). Spontaneous generation of prion infectivity in fatal familial insomnia knockin mice. Neuron 63: 438–450.

Jeffrey M, Gonzalez L (2007). Classical sheep transmissible spongiform encephalopathies: pathogenesis, pathological phenotypes and clinical disease. Neuropathol Appl Neurobiol 33: 373–394.

Jeffrey M, Martin S, Gonzalez L et al. (2001). Differential diagnosis of infections with the bovine spongiform encephalopathy (BSE) and scrapie agents in sheep. J Comp Pathol 125: 271–284.

Jeffrey M, Martin S, Gonzalez L (2003). Cell-associated variants of disease-specific prion protein immunolabelling are found in different sources of sheep transmissible spongiform encephalopathy. J Gen Virol 84: 1033–1045.

Jeffrey M, Martin S, Gonzalez L et al. (2006). Immunohistochemical features of PrP(d) accumulation in natural and experimental goat transmissible spongiform encephalopathies. J Comp Pathol 134: 171–181.

Kascsak RJ, Rubenstein R, Merz PA et al. (1987). Mouse polyclonal and monoclonal antibody to scrapie-associated fibril proteins. J Virol 61: 3688–3693.

Katorcha E, Makarava N, Savtchenko R et al. (2014). Sialylation of prion protein controls the rate of prion amplification, the cross-species barrier, the ratio of PrPSc glycoform and prion infectivity. PLoS Pathog 10: e1004366.

Kimberlin RH, Walker CA (1979). Pathogenesis of scrapie: agent multiplication in brain at the first and second passage of hamster scrapie in mice. J Gen Virol 42: 107–117.

Kimberlin RH, Walker CA (1988). Incubation periods in six models of intraperitoneally injected scrapie depend mainly on the dynamics of agent replication within the nervous system and not the lymphoreticular system. J Gen Virol 69: 2953–2960.

Kimberlin RH, Cole S, Walker CA (1987a). Pathogenesis of scrapie is faster when infection is intraspinal instead of intracerebral. Microb Pathog 2: 405–415.

Kimberlin RH, Cole S, Walker CA (1987b). Temporary and permanent modifications to a single strain of mouse scrapie on transmission to rats and hamsters. J Gen Virol 68: 1875–1881.

Kincaid AE, Bartz JC (2007). The nasal cavity is a route for prion infection in hamsters. J Virol 81: 4482–4491.

Klingeborn M, Wik L, Simonsson M et al. (2006). Characterization of proteinase K-resistant N- and C-terminally truncated PrP in Nor98 atypical scrapie. J Gen Virol 87: 1751–1760.

Kobayashi A, Sakuma N, Matsuura Y et al. (2010). Experimental verification of a traceback phenomenon in prion infection. J Virol 84: 3230–3238.

Kobayashi A, Teruya K, Matsuura Y et al. (2015). The influence of PRNP polymorphisms on human prion disease susceptibility: an update. Acta Neuropathol 130: 159–170.

Kong Q, Cali I, Qing L et al. (2016). Zoonotic potential of CWD prions: an update. Prion 2016 Conference Tokyo.

Ladogana A, Puopolo M, Croes EA et al. (2005). Mortality from Creutzfeldt-Jakob disease and related disorders in Europe, Australia, and Canada. Neurology 64: 1586–1591.

LaFauci G, Carp RI, Meeker HC et al. (2006). Passage of chronic wasting disease prion into transgenic mice expressing Rocky Mountain elk (*Cervus elaphus nelsoni*) PrPC. J Gen Virol 87: 3773–3780.

Laferrière F, Tixador P, Moudjou M et al. (2013). Quaternary structure of pathological prion protein as a determining factor of strain-specific prion replication dynamics. PLoS Pathog 9: e1003702.

Le Dur A, Lai TL, Stinnakre MG et al. (2017). Divergent prion strain evolution driven by PrPC expression level in transgenic mice. Nat Commun 8: 14170.

Liberski PP (2012). Historical overview of prion diseases: a view from afar. Folia Neuropathol 50: 1–12.

Lu D, Giles K, Li Z et al. (2013). Biaryl amides and hydrazones as therapeutics for prion disease in transgenic mice. J Pharmacol Exp Ther 347: 325–338.

Makarava N, Kovacs GG, Bocharova O et al. (2010). Recombinant prion protein induces a new transmissible prion disease in wild-type animals. Acta Neuropathol 119: 177–187.

Mallucci G, Dickinson A, Linehan J et al. (2003). Depleting neuronal PrP in prion infection prevents disease and reverses spongiosis. Science 302: 871–874.

Mallucci GR, White MD, Farmer M et al. (2007). Targeting cellular prion protein reverses early cognitive deficits and neurophysiological dysfunction in prion-infected mice. Neuron 53: 325–335.

Manson JC, Clarke AR, Hooper ML et al. (1994). 129/Ola mice carrying a null mutation in PrP that abolishes mRNA production are developmentally normal. Mol Neurobiol 8: 121–127.

Manson JC, Jamieson E, Baybutt H et al. (1999). A single amino acid alteration (101L) introduced into murine PrP dramatically alters incubation time of transmissible spongiform encephalopathy. EMBO J 18: 6855–6864.

Marsh RF, Bessen RA (1994). Physicochemical and biological characterizations of distinct strains of the transmissible mink encephalopathy agent. Philos Trans R Soc Lond Ser B Biol Sci 343: 413–414.

Mastrianni JA, Capellari S, Telling GC et al. (2001). Inherited prion disease caused by the V210I mutation: Transmission to transgenic mice. Neurology 57: 2198–2205.

Meade-White K, Race B, Trifilo M et al. (2007). Resistance to chronic wasting disease in transgenic mice expressing a naturally occurring allelic variant of deer prion protein. J Virol 81: 4533–4539.

Mestre-Francés N, Nicot S, Rouland S et al. (2012). Oral transmission of L-type bovine spongiform encephalopathy in primate model. Emerg Infect Dis 18: 142–145.

Miller MB, Wang, Wang DW et al. (2013). Cofactor molecules induce structural transformation during infectious prion formation. Structure 21: 2061–2068.

Mirabile I, Jat PS, Brandner S et al. (2015). Identification of clinical target areas in the brainstem of prion-infected mice. Neuropathol Appl Neurobiol 41: 613–630.

Mizrahi M, Friedman-Levi Y, Larush L et al. (2014). Pomegranate seed oil nanoemulsions for the prevention and treatment of neurodegenerative diseases: the case of genetic CJD. Nanomedicine: Nanotechnology. Biology and Medicine 10: 1353–1363.

Moda F, Suardi S, Di Fede G et al. (2012). MM2-thalamic Creutzfeldt-Jakob disease: neuropathological, biochemical and transmission studies identify a distinctive prion strain. Brain Pathol 22: 662–669.

Mok T, Jaunmuktane Z, Joiner S et al. (2017). Variant Creutzfeldt–Jakob disease in a patient with heterozygosity at PRNP codon 129. N Engl J Med 376: 292–294.

Moore RA, Timmes AG, Wilmarth PA et al. (2011). Identification and removal of proteins that co-purify with infectious prion protein improves the analysis of its secondary structure. Proteomics 11: 3853–3865.

Moreno JA, Radford H, Peretti D et al. (2012). Sustained translational repression by eIF2alpha-P mediates prion neurodegeneration. Nature 485: 507–511.

Moreno JA, Halliday M, Molloy C et al. (2013). Oral treatment targeting the unfolded protein response prevents neurodegeneration and clinical disease in prion-infected mice. Sci Transl Med 5: 206ra138.

Mulcahy ER, Bartz JC, Kincaid AE et al. (2004). Prion infection of skeletal muscle cells and papillae in the tongue. J Virol 78: 6792–6798.

CJD Research and Surveillance Unit National (2018). Creutzfeldt-Jakob disease in the UK (http://www.cjd.ed.ac.uk), Available online at http://www.cjd.ed.ac.uk/sites/default/files/figs_4.pdf (accessed 16/04/2018).

Nonno R, Di Bari MA, Cardone F et al. (2006). Efficient transmission and characterization of Creutzfeldt-Jakob disease strains in bank voles. PLoS Pathog 2: e12.

Notari S, Xiao X, Espinosa JC et al. (2014). Transmission characteristics of variably protease-sensitive prionopathy. Emerg Infect Dis 20: 2006–2014.

Nurmi MH, Bishop M, Strain L et al. (2003). The normal population distribution of PRNP codon 129 polymorphism. Acta Neurol Scand 108: 374–378.

Okada H, Iwamaru Y, Imamura M et al. (2017). Oral transmission of L-type bovine spongiform encephalopathy agent among cattle. Emerg Infect Dis 23: 284–287.

Padilla D, Beringue V, Espinosa JC et al. (2011). Sheep and goat BSE propagate more efficiently than cattle BSE in human PrP transgenic mice. PLoS Pathog 7: e1001319.

Parchi P, Castellani R, Capellari S et al. (1996). Molecular basis of phenotypic variability in sporadic Creutzfeldt-Jakob disease. Ann Neurol 39: 767–778.

Parchi P, Giese A, Capellari S et al. (1999). Classification of sporadic Creutzfeldt-Jakob disease based on molecular and phenotypic analysis of 300 subjects. Ann Neurol 46: 224–233.

Parchi P, Zou W, Wang W et al. (2000). Genetic influence on the structural variations of the abnormal prion protein. Proc Natl Acad Sci U S A 97: 10168–10172.

Parchi P, Cescatti M, Notari S et al. (2010). Agent strain variation in human prion disease: insights from a molecular and pathological review of the National Institutes of Health series of experimentally transmitted disease. Brain 133: 3030–3042.

Pattison IH (1966). The relative susceptibility of sheep, goats and mice to two types of the goat scrapie agent. Res Vet Sci 7: 207–212.

Pattison IH, Millson GC (1961a). Further experimental observations on scrapie. J Comp Pathol 71: 350–359.

Pattison IH, Millson GC (1961b). Scrapie produced experimentally in goats with special reference to the clinical syndrome. J Comp Pathol 71: 101–109.

Peden AH, Head MW, Ritchie DL et al. (2004). Preclinical vCJD after blood transfusion in a PRNP codon 129 heterozygous patient. Lancet 364: 527–529.

Peretz D, Scott MR, Groth D et al. (2001). Strain-specified relative conformational stability of the scrapie prion protein. Protein Sci 10: 854–863.

Piccardo P, Manson JC, King D et al. (2007). Accumulation of prion protein in the brain that is not associated with transmissible disease. Proc Natl Acad Sci U S A 104: 4712–4717.

Piro JR, Supattapone S (2011). Photodegradation illuminates the role of polyanions in prion infectivity. Prion 5: 49–51.

Plinston C, Hart P, Chong A et al. (2011). Increased susceptibility of human-PrP transgenic mice to bovine spongiform encephalopathy infection following passage in sheep. J Virol 85: 1174–1181.

Pocchiari M, Salvatore M, Cutruzzola F et al. (1993). A new point mutation of the prion protein gene in Creutzfeldt-Jakob disease. Ann Neurol 34: 802–807.

Race B, Meade-White K, Miller MW et al. (2011). In vivo comparison of chronic wasting disease infectivity from deer with variation at prion protein residue 96. J Virol 85: 9235–9238.

Ricci A, Allende A, Bolton D et al. (2017). Chronic wasting disease (CWD) in cervids. EFSA Journal, 15: e04667-n/a.

Ripoll L, Laplanche J-L, Salzmann M et al. (1993). A new point mutation in the prion protein gene at codon 210 in Creutzfeldt-Jakob disease. Neurology 43: 1934.

Saa P, Sferrazza GF, Ottenberg G et al. (2012). Strain-specific role of RNAs in prion replication. J Virol 86: 10494–10504.

Safar J, Wille H, Itri V et al. (1998). Eight prion strains have PrP(Sc) molecules with different conformations. Nat Med 4: 1157–1165.

Scott JR, Fraser H (1989). Transport and targeting of scrapie infectivity and pathology in the optic nerve projections following intraocular infection. Prog Clin Biol Res 317: 645–652.

Scott M, Foster D, Mirenda C et al. (1989). Transgenic mice expressing hamster prion protein produce species-specific scrapie infectivity and amyloid plaques. Cell 59: 847–857.

Scott MR, Will R, Ironside J et al. (1999). Compelling transgenic evidence for transmission of bovine spongiform encephalopathy prions to humans. Proc Natl Acad Sci U S A 96: 15137–15142.

Shikiya RA, Ayers JI, Schutt CR et al. (2010). Coinfecting prion strains compete for a limiting cellular resource. J Virol 84: 5706–5714.

Shikiya RA, Eckland TE, Young AJ et al. (2014). Prion formation, but not clearance, is supported by protein misfolding cyclic amplification. Prion 8: 415–420.

Sigurdson CJ, Nilsson KPR, Hornemann S et al. (2007). Prion strain discrimination using luminescent conjugated polymers. Nat Methods 4: 1023–1030.

Sim VL, Caughey B (2009). Ultrastructures and strain comparison of under-glycosylated scrapie prion fibrils. Neurobiol Aging 30: 2031–2042.

Siso S, Jeffrey M, Martin S et al. (2010). Characterization of strains of ovine transmissible spongiform encephalopathy with a short PrPd profiling method. J Comp Pathol 142: 300–310.

Supattapone S (2014). Synthesis of high titer infectious prions with cofactor molecules. J Biol Chem 289: 19850–19854.

Tamguney G, Giles K, Bouzamondo-Bernstein E et al. (2006). Transmission of elk and deer prions to transgenic mice. J Virol 80: 9104–9114.

Tanaka M, Chien P, Naber N et al. (2004). Conformational variations in an infectious protein determine prion strain differences. Nature 428: 323–328.

Telling GC, Haga T, Torchia M et al. (1996a). Interactions between wild-type and mutant prion proteins modulate neurodegeneration in transgenic mice. Genes Dev 10: 1736–1750.

Telling GC, Parchi P, Dearmond SJ et al. (1996b). Evidence for the conformation of the pathologic isoform of the prion protein enciphering and propagating prion diversity. Science 274: 2079–2082.

Thackray AM, Hopkins L, Klein MA et al. (2007). Mouse-adapted ovine scrapie prion strains are characterized by different conformers of PrPSc. J Virol 81: 12119–12127.

Thackray AM, Hopkins L, Lockey R et al. (2011). Emergence of multiple prion strains from single isolates of ovine scrapie. J Gen Virol 92: 1482–1491.

Thackray AM, Lockey R, Beck KE et al. (2012). Evidence for co-infection of ovine prion strains in classical scrapie isolates. J Comp Pathol 147: 316–329.

Tixador P, Herzog L, Reine F et al. (2010). The physical relationship between infectivity and prion protein aggregates is strain-dependent. PLoS Pathog 6: e1000859.

Uro-Coste E, Cassard H, Simon S et al. (2008). Beyond PrP res type 1/type 2 dichotomy in Creutzfeldt-Jakob disease. PLoS Pathog 4: e1000029.

Van Keulen LJM, Schreuder BEC, Meloen RH et al. (1995). Immumohistochemical detection and localization of prion protein in brain tissue of sheep with natural scrapie. Veterinary Pathology Online 32: 299–308.

Van Keulen LJM, Schreuder BEC, Vromans MEW et al. (2000). Pathogenesis of natural scrapie in sheep. In: MH Groschup, HA Kretzschmar (Eds.), Prion diseases: diagnosis and pathogenesis. Springer Vienna, Vienna.

Watts JC, Giles K, Patel S et al. (2014). Evidence that bank vole PrP is a universal acceptor for prions. PLoS Pathog 10: e1003990.

Watts JC, Giles K, Bourkas MEC et al. (2016). Towards authentic transgenic mouse models of heritable PrP prion diseases. Acta Neuropathol 132: 593–610.

Wells GA, Scott AC, Johnson CT et al. (1987). A novel progressive spongiform encephalopathy in cattle. Vet Rec 121: 419–420.

Wilson R, Plinston C, Hunter N et al. (2012). Chronic wasting disease and atypical forms of bovine spongiform encephalopathy and scrapie are not transmissible to mice expressing wild-type levels of human prion protein. J Gen Virol 93: 1624–1629.

Zou WQ, Puoti G, Xiao X et al. (2010). Variably protease-sensitive prionopathy: a new sporadic disease of the prion protein. Ann Neurol 68: 162–172.

Handbook of Clinical Neurology, Vol. 153 (3rd series)
Human Prion Diseases
M. Pocchiari and J. Manson, Editors
https://doi.org/10.1016/B978-0-444-63945-5.00005-2

Chapter 5

The role of the immune system in prion infection

NEIL A. MABBOTT[1]*, JAMES D. ALIBHAI[2], AND JEAN MANSON[3]
[1]*The Roslin Institute and Royal (Dick) School of Veterinary Sciences, University of Edinburgh, Easter Bush, United Kingdom*
[2]*The National CJD Research and Surveillance Unit, Centre for Clinical Brain Sciences, University of Edinburgh, Edinburgh, United Kingdom*
[3]*Centre for Clinical Brain Sciences, University of Edinburgh, Edinburgh, United Kingdom*

Abstract

Prion diseases are a unique group of chronic neurodegenerative diseases that affect humans and certain domestic and free-ranging animal species. Many natural prion diseases are acquired peripherally, such as by ingestion of contaminated food or pasture. Although the pathology during prion disease appears to be restricted to the central nervous system, where it causes extensive neurodegeneration, some prion diseases accumulate to high levels within the secondary lymphoid tissues of the host's immune system as they make their journey from the site of infection to the brain. The replication of prions within these tissues is essential for the efficient spread of disease to the brain. Moreover, the immune system has a profound influence on the development of disease within the central nervous system. This chapter describes the interactions between prions and the host's immune system. Particular emphasis is given to studies which have helped to identify the key tissues, cells, and molecules which the prions exploit to facilitate their propagation from peripheral sites of exposure (such as the intestine) to the brain. This chapter also describes how prion disease pathogenesis and susceptibility may be influenced by inflammation, co-infection with other pathogens, and aging. A thorough understanding of the factors which influence prion disease susceptibility is important as it may help to identify important targets for therapeutic intervention and to help determine the risk of susceptibility to novel peripherally acquired prion diseases.

PRIONS AND THE PRION PROTEIN

Prion diseases, or transmissible spongiform encephalopathies, are infectious chronic neurodegenerative diseases that affect humans and several domestic and free-ranging animal species (Table 5.1). During prion disease aggregations of PrP^{TSE}, abnormally folded isoforms of the host cellular prion protein (PrP^{C}), accumulate in affected tissues and appear to constitute the major component of the infectious agent (Bolton et al., 1982; Legname et al., 2004). The cellular PrP^{C} glycoprotein is encoded by the *PRNP* gene, and host cells must express PrP^{C} in order to replicate prions (Prusiner et al., 1993; Manson et al., 1994b). The secondary structure of PrP^{C} is rich in α-helical content with relatively little β-pleated sheet (Pan et al., 1993; Riek et al., 1997).

During prion disease changes occur in the secondary, tertiary, and quaternary structures of the PrP molecule, increasing the amount of β-pleated sheet (Caughey et al., 1991; Pan et al., 1993). These changes dramatically affect the physicochemical and biologic characteristics of the PrP molecule. As a consequence, disease-specific PrP^{TSE} is relatively resistant to proteinase digestion, accumulates in affected tissues in insoluble aggregates, and is neurotoxic. In this chapter, several terms are used to describe the presence of prions. PrP^{TSE} is used where evidence of proteinase resistance was demonstrated.

*Correspondence to: Neil A. Mabbott, The Roslin Institute and Royal (Dick) School of Veterinary Sciences, University of Edinburgh, Easter Bush, Midlothian EH25 9RG, United Kingdom. Tel: +44-131-651-9100, Fax: +44-131-651-9105, E-mail: neil.mabbott@roslin.ed.ac.uk

Table 5.1

Prion diseases of humans and animals

Prion disease	Affected species	Route of transmission
Iatrogenic Creutzfeldt–Jakob disease	Human	Accidental medical exposure to CJD-contaminated tissues or tissue products
Sporadic Creutzfeldt–Jakob disease	Human	Unknown. Theories include somatic mutation or spontaneous conversion of PrP^{c} to PrP^{TSE}
Variant Creutzfeldt–Jakob disease	Human	Ingestion of BSE-contaminated food or transfusion of blood or blood products from CJD-infected blood donor
Familial Creutzfeldt–Jakob disease	Human	Germline mutations of the *PRNP* gene
Gerstmann–Sträussler–Scheinker syndrome	Human	Germline mutations of the *PRNP* gene
Kuru	Human	Ritualistic cannibalism
Fatal familial insomnia	Human	Germline mutations of the *PRNP* gene
Bovine spongiform encephalopathy	Cattle	Ingestion of contaminated food
Scrapie	Sheep, goats, mouflon	Acquired. Ingestion, horizontal transmission, vertical transmission unclear
Chronic wasting disease	Elk, deer, moose	Acquired. Ingestion, horizontal transmission, vertical transmission unclear
Transmissible mink encephalopathy	Mink	Acquired (ingestion) source unknown
Feline spongiform encephalopathy	Domestic and zoologic cats	Ingestion of BSE-contaminated food
Exotic ungulate encephalopathy	Nyala, kudu	Ingestion of BSE-contaminated food

BSE, bovine spongiform encephalopathy; CJD, Creutzfeldt–Jakob disease; *PRNP*, the gene that encodes the cellular prion protein PrP^{C}.

Disease-specific PrP, or PrP^{d}, is used where it was not possible to confirm the proteinase resistance of the PrP accumulations. The term "infectious prions" is only used when disease transmission was demonstrated.

Within the immune system PrP^{C} is expressed on lymphocytes, leukocytes, granulocytes, and stromal cells, where it may play a role in cell activation (Cashman et al., 1990; Mabbott et al., 1997; Martínez del Hoyo et al., 2006), T-cell differentiation (Jouvin-Marche et al., 2006), intercellular interactions (Ballerini et al., 2006), and phagocytosis (de Almeida et al., 2005; Nakato et al., 2012). Despite these potential roles, PrP^{C}-deficient mice display no obvious immune deficit in vivo (McCulloch et al., 2013). Within the central nervous system (CNS) PrP^{C} plays an important role in promoting myelin homeostasis via the G-protein-coupled receptor Gpr126 (Adgrg6) in Schwann cells (Küffer et al., 2016). Although many other roles for PrP^{C} in the CNS have also been reported, PrP-deficient mice develop normally, suggesting that PrP^{C} is not an essential protein or that its loss can be compensated for by other proteins (Prusiner et al., 1993, 1998; Manson et al., 1994a; Lasmezas, 2003) (the physiologic function/s of PrP^{C} and its role in prion diseases are discussed in Chapters 3 and 2, respectively).

The ubiquitous cellular expression of PrP^{C} has important immunologic consequences. The PrP protein is tolerated by the host's immune system preventing the development of specific immune responses against PrP^{C} and, importantly, prion disease-specific PrP^{TSE}. As a consequence, no specific immunity to prions has been reported in affected animals despite the persistence of high levels of prions within some of their secondary lymphoid organs (SLO) throughout the disease (Clarke and Haig, 1966; Tsukamoto et al., 1985). However, it is possible that anti-PrP antibodies are generated in some prion disease-affected animals during the clinical (terminal) phase (Sassa et al., 2010).

Many prion strains accumulate in SLO before neuroinvasion

Many natural prion diseases such as natural sheep scrapie and chronic wasting disease (CWD) in cervids are acquired, for example after oral exposure, or via lesions to skin or mucous membranes (see Sections II and III of this publication for detailed accounts on the different prion diseases). The oral consumption of feed contaminated with bovine spongiform encephalopathy (BSE) prions was most likely involved in the spread of this devastating disease amongst cattle (Wilesmith et al., 1991). This disease also has zoonotic potential, demonstrated by the emergence of variant Creutzfeldt–Jakob disease (vCJD) in the UK human population (Bruce et al., 1997; Hill et al., 1997a) (the zoonotic potential of prion diseases is discussed in Chapter 25).

After infection by a peripheral route, many prion diseases first replicate within the SLO before infecting the CNS (a process termed neuroinvasion). For example, studies using experimental mice show that after oral exposure (ingestion), scrapie prions first accumulate in the gut-associated lymphoid tissues (GALT) such as the Peyer's patches in the small intestine (Mabbott et al., 2003; Prinz et al., 2003b; Glaysher and Mabbott, 2007) (Fig. 5.1A). Similarly, PrP^{TSE} is first detected in the GALT following experimental oral infection of mule deer fawns (*Odocoileus hemionus*) with CWD (Sigurdson et al., 1999) or sheep with some strains of natural scrapie (van Keulen et al., 1999; Andreoletti et al., 2000; Heggebø et al., 2000). In humans, the accumulation of vCJD prions in the GALT before the onset of clinical signs has also been described (Hilton et al., 1998).

Studies in the 1970s demonstrated that prion disease survival times after intraperitoneal injection were extended in mice which lacked the spleen (Fraser and Dickinson, 1970, 1978). An absence of Peyer's patches similarly impairs the neuroinvasion of orally acquired scrapie prions from the gut lumen (Prinz et al., 2003b; Glaysher and Mabbott, 2007; Donaldson et al., 2015, 2016). These studies revealed that prion accumulation within SLO was important for the efficient transmission of disease to the CNS after peripheral exposure. Indeed, studies suggest that prions exploit certain cells within the SLO in order to achieve efficient host infection. The sections below describe the key components of the SLO which are considered to play an essential role in the transmission of peripherally acquired prions to the CNS. As the splenectomy studies first indicated, treatments which block prion accumulation in the SLO can impede the neuroinvasion of prions. Therefore, a thorough understanding of the key components of SLO which aid the transmission of peripherally acquired prions to the CNS, may identify novel targets for intervention in these currently untreatable diseases. This information will also enhance our understanding of transmission risks and aid the design of preclinical diagnostics.

Identifying the key cellular and molecular components required for prion accumulation within, and neuroinvasion from, the SLO

B and T cells

Mice which lack mature B and T cells, such as severe combined immunodeficient (SCID) mice, Rag-$1^{-/-}$, Rag-$2^{-/-}$, and $Agr^{-/-}$ mice (Kitamoto et al., 1991; Fraser and Brown, 1994; Fraser et al., 1996; Klein et al., 1997; Mohan et al., 2004), are refractory to peripheral infection with prions. However, prion disease pathogenesis is unaffected in mice deficient in T cells alone (McFarlin et al., 1971; Fraser and Dickinson, 1978; Klein et al., 1997, 1998). T cells appear to lack the necessary cellular requirements to sustain prion infection. Even the ectopic expression of high levels of PrP^C specifically in T cells (20 × copies of the *Prnp* gene) is insufficient to enable prion replication within them (Raeber et al., 1999).

In the SLO of some prion-infected hosts heavy accumulations of disease-specific PrP are detectable within the B-cell follicles (Kitamoto et al., 1991; McBride et al., 1992; Hilton et al., 1998; Sigurdson et al., 1999; Andreoletti et al., 2000). In the specific absence of B cells the accumulation of prions in the spleen and subsequent neuroinvasion are significantly impeded (Klein et al., 1997). However, B cells also do not replicate prions as transgenic mice which express high levels of PrP^C only on B cells are similarly unable to support prion replication (Montrasio et al., 2001). This implied that the role of B cells in prion disease pathogenesis was most likely indirect, perhaps through their provision of homeostatic support to other cell populations within the SLO.

Follicular dendritic cells

The SLO of SCID mice (and other B-cell-deficient mouse strains) are also indirectly deficient in follicular dendritic cells (FDC) as they require constitutive stimulation from B cells to maintain their differentiated state (Kapasi et al., 1993; Chaplin and Fu, 1998; Mackay and Browning, 1998; Tumanov et al., 2002). The reconstitution of SCID mice with wild-type (immunocompetent) bone marrow restores the B and T cells in these mice, and by doing so, indirectly induces the maturation of FDC in their SLO (Kapasi et al., 1993). The reconstitution of SCID mice with wild-type bone marrow also renders them susceptible to peripheral prion infections (Fraser et al., 1996; Klein et al., 1998; Brown et al., 1999; Mohan et al., 2004).

FDC are important stromal cells that reside within the B-cell follicles and germinal centers of SLO. FDC differentiate from ubiquitous perivascular precursor cells (pericytes) and are a distinct lineage from bone marrow-derived conventional dendritic cells (DC)(Shortman and Liu, 2002; Mabbott et al., 2011; Krautler et al., 2012). Prions accumulate upon PrP^C-expressing FDC in the SLO of experimentally infected mice (Fig. 5.1A), some sheep with natural scrapie, cervids with CWD, and patients with vCJD (Kitamoto et al., 1991; McBride et al., 1992; Hilton et al., 1998; Sigurdson et al., 1999; Andreoletti et al., 2000).

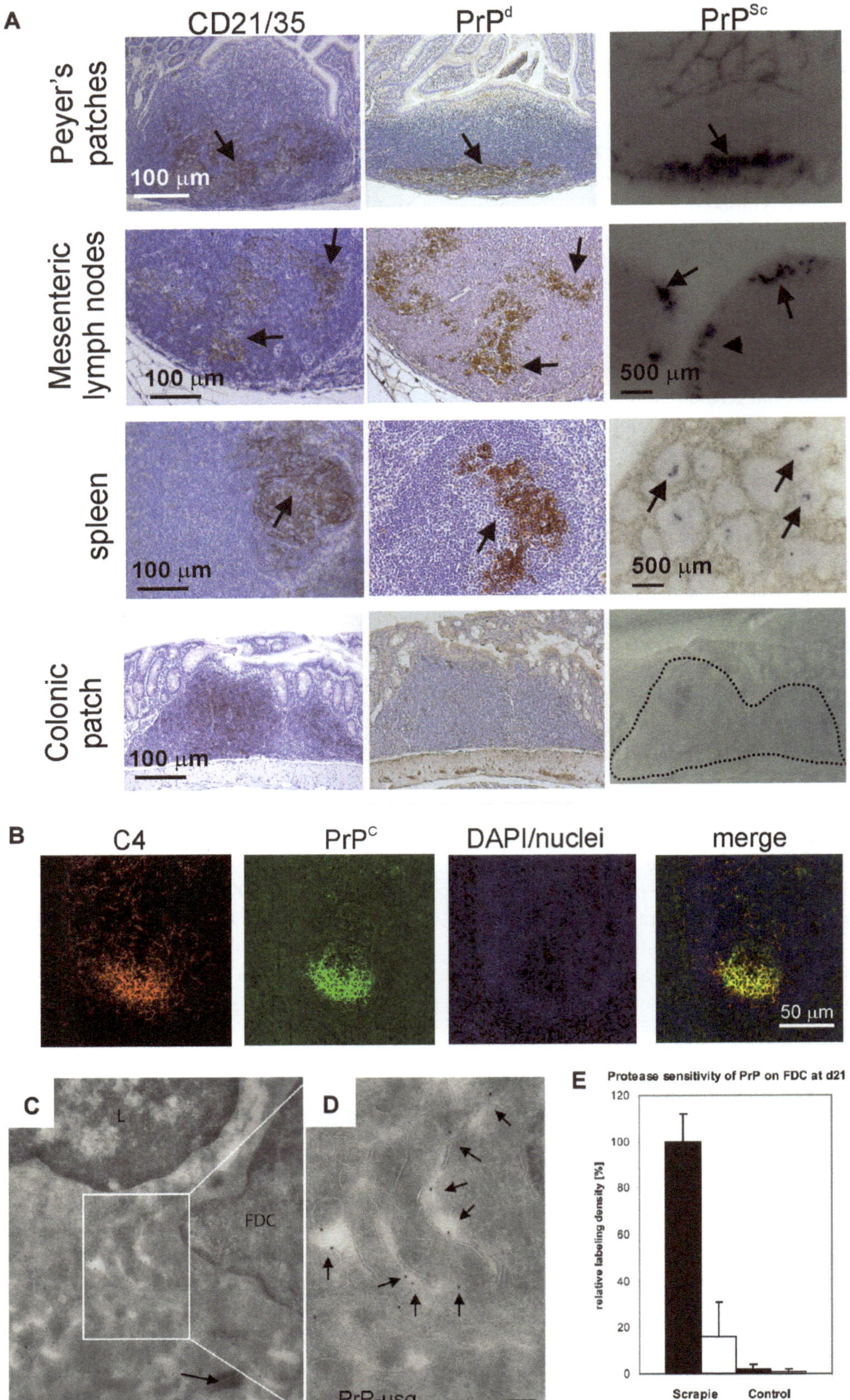

Fig. 5.1. PrP^{TSE} accumulates on the surface of follicular dendritic cells (FDC) in the secondary lymphoid organs of prion-infected mice. (**A**) Mice were orally exposed to ME7 scrapie prions and Peyer's patches, mesenteric lymph nodes, spleens,

B cells produce tumor necrosis factor-α (TNF-α) and lymphotoxins (LT) which are the essential stimuli which maintain FDC in their differentiated state (Mackay and Browning, 1998). In the absence of stimulation from these cytokines the FDC rapidly de-differentiate (Mackay and Browning, 1998). Prion accumulation in SLO and neuroinvasion are significantly impeded in mice deficient in TNF-α or LT stimulation, suggesting an important role for FDC in the establishment of prion infections (Mabbott et al., 2000b; Prinz et al., 2002; Glaysher and Mabbott, 2007). Prion accumulation in SLO and disease susceptibility are also reduced when FDC are temporarily de-differentiated by treatments which block LT- or TNF-α-mediated signaling between B cells and FDC (Mabbott et al., 2000a, 2002, 2003; Montrasio et al., 2000; Prinz et al., 2003a; Mohan et al., 2005).

FDC characteristically trap and retain native antigens on their surfaces for long periods which they display to B cells within the germinal center. The long-term retention of antigens by FDC helps to promote immunoglobulin (antibody) isotype class switching, affinity maturation of naïve B cells, and the maintenance of immunologic memory (Heesters et al., 2014). The ability of FDC to retain native antigens for long periods raised the possibility that they might also simply trap and retain prions which had been produced by other infected cell populations, such as neurones.

A series of independent studies exploited the nonhematopoietic origin of FDC to help address this issue. Mismatches were created in *Prnp* expression between the FDC-containing stromal and lymphocyte/leukocyte-containing compartments of SLO by grafting hematopoietic cells from PrP^C-deficient mice into PrP^C-expressing (wild-type) mice, and vice versa (Klein et al., 1998; Brown et al., 1999; Mohan et al., 2004). In these studies the FDC were recipient-derived, whereas all the hematopoietic cell lineages were derived from the donor bone marrow. Prion accumulation upon FDC was only detected in the spleens of mice which had a PrP^C-expressing stromal compartment, providing further evidence that FDC are important sites of prion accumulation. In a subsequent study, transgenic mice were created in which PrP^C expression was "switched on" or "switched off" only in FDC (McCulloch et al., 2011). The expression of PrP^C only on FDC was sufficient to sustain high levels of prion replication in the spleen. Conversely, prion replication in the spleen was blocked when PrP^C expression was specifically ablated only on the FDC. Together, these studies demonstrate that FDC were the essential sites of prion replication in SLO.

The role of FDC in prion disease pathogenesis appears to be to amplify the prions above the threshold required for neuroinvasion. After their replication upon FDC, the prions subsequently infect both the sympathetic and parasympathetic nervous systems and spread within them to the CNS where they ultimately cause neurodegeneration (Beekes and McBride, 2000; Glatzel et al., 2001; McBride et al., 2001; Kujala et al., 2011). How the prions subsequently infect the peripheral nervous system is uncertain as there are few, if any, physical contacts between FDC and nerves (see Neuroinvasion, below).

and colonic patches collected at 15 weeks after infection. High levels of PrP^d (brown) were detected in association with F'DC (CD21/35-positive cells; brown) in the Peyer's patches, mesenteric lymph nodes and spleen at this time after prion infection (arrows). Analysis of adjacent sections by paraffin-embedded tissue immunoblot analysis confirmed the presence of protease K-resistant PrP^{TSE} (blue/black). In contrast, no PrP^d or PrP^{TSE} was detected in the large intestinal gut-associated lymphoid tissues such as the colonic patches at this time after oral exposure. Sections were counterstained with hematoxylin to detect cell nuclei (blue). (**B**) FDC (complement C4-retaining cells, red) express high levels of the cellular form of the prion protein (PrPC, green) in the secondary lymphoid organs of uninfected control mice. Sections counterstained with 4',6-diamidino-2-phenylindole (DAPI) to detect cell nuclei (blue). (**C–E**) Analysis of Peyer's patches by cryo-electron microscopy. Peyer's patches collected at 21 days post oral infection with ME7 scrapie prions. Increased PrP labeling was observed on the cell surface of FDC. Arrow in panel **C** indicates a desmosome. Panel **D** shows an inset in **C** at higher magnification. Arrows in panel **D** show silver-enhanced PrP-specific monoclonal antibody 6H4-conjugated to UltraSmall gold PrP label (PrP-usg). (**E**) Peyer's patches were collected at 21 days post oral infection with prions and the FDC plasma membrane-bound PrP-specific gold was counted in untreated and trypsin-treated cryosections. Treatment with trypsin enabled discrimination of prion disease-specific, relatively proteinase-resistant, PrP^{TSE}: the remaining PrP after trypsin treatment is indicative for protease-resistant disease-related PrP^{TSE}. After trypsin treatment (white bar; scrapie +T) some PrP-specific label was evident on the plasma membranes of FDC from prion-infected mice when compared to untreated sections (black bar; scrapie –T; 100%). Untreated (black bar, control –T) and trypsin-treated (gray bar, control +T) sections from uninfected control mice show little PrP-specific label. Ten mature FDC cells were randomly selected and 50 μm of plasma membrane was analyzed/cell. Data presented as relative labeling density/membrane length ± SED. Scale bars: **C**, 500 nm; **D**, 200 nm. Data in (**A**) were reproduced from (Donaldson et al. (2015) under the terms of the Creative Commons Attribution 3.0 Unported (CC BY 3.0) Licence. Data in (**B**) were reproduced with permission from McCulloch et al. (2013). Data in panels (**C–E**) were reproduced from (Kujala et al. (2011) under the terms of the Creative Commons Attribution Licence.

FDC acquire prions as complement-opsonized complexes

FDC express high levels of PrP^C (Klein et al., 1998; Brown et al., 1999, 2012; McCulloch et al., 2011) (Fig. 5.1B), but many other cell lineages also express PrP^C highly and do not play an essential role in prion disease pathogenesis. Clearly other FDC characteristics were important to enable them to sustain prion replication. FDC have many slender and long dendritic processes which can extend throughout the B-cell follicle. These dendrites enable FDC to trap and retain large amounts of native antigens upon their surfaces in the form of immune complexes, consisting of antigen–antibody and/or opsonizing complement components (Fig. 5.1B). Complement component C1q can bind to PrP^{TSE} (Mitchell et al., 2007; Sim et al., 2007), and the specific absence of opsonizing complement components (C1q, C2, C3, and C4) or complement receptor (CR2/1) expression on FDC impedes prion accumulation in the spleen and delays neuroinvasion (Klein et al., 2001; Mabbott et al., 2001; Zabel et al., 2007; Michel et al., 2012a, 2013). This suggests that soon after the prions infect the host they are bound by opsonizing complement components and subsequently acquired by FDC in a CR-dependent manner (Klein et al., 2001; Mabbott et al., 2001; Zabel et al., 2007; Michel et al., 2012a).

After being acquired by FDC, immune complexes are initially internalized before undergoing cyclic rounds of display on the cell surface (Heesters et al., 2013). This cyclic mode of immune complex expression may help to protect the native antigens from degradation, enabling their long-term retention (Heesters et al., 2014). However, high-resolution immunohistochemical analyses indicate that prion replication occurs upon the FDC surface, as PrP^{TSE} has not been detected within them (Jeffrey et al., 2000b; McGovern et al., 2004, 2009; Kujala et al., 2011) (Fig. 5.1C). This appears to contrast with prion infection nerves, where PrP^{TSE} conversion can occur intracellularly within endosomal recycling compartments (Marijanovic et al., 2009).

FDC-independent prion accumulation and neuroinvasion

Although many prion isolates in different host species appear to replicate first upon FDC in the SLO before neuroinvasion, there are examples where this can occur independently of FDC. The factors which determine the requirement for FDC in prion disease pathogenesis are uncertain but this may be influenced by prion agent strain, host species, *PRNP* genotype, and exposure route. High doses of prions can also bypass the requirement for amplification within SLO prior to neuroinvasion (Fraser et al., 1996; Prinz et al., 2002). The infecting prion strain and the *PRNP* genotype of the host can each influence disease pathogenesis in sheep (Andreoletti et al., 2000; Heggebø et al., 2002). Some prion diseases, such as sporadic CJD in humans, do not appear to be associated with early prion accumulation in the periphery (Glatzel et al., 2003), and susceptibility of mice to the FU strain of CJD prions was unaffected by deficiency in B cells and FDC (Schlomchik et al., 2001).

BSE prions were also considered to have little involvement in SLO during the preclinical phase (Somerville et al., 1997), although PrP^{TSE} and/or infectious prions have been detected in the small intestines of most cattle after experimental (oral) infection and some naturally infected cattle (Wells et al., 1994; Terry et al., 2003; Hoffmann et al., 2011). However, when BSE prions are transmitted to other species such as humans (in the form of vCJD), sheep, and mice, their accumulation in SLO is a characteristic feature (Hill et al., 1997b; Foster et al., 2001; Brown and Mabbott, 2014). Under certain circumstances mouse passaged Rocky Mountain Laboratory (RML) prions can also accumulate in association with high endothelial venules in lymph nodes (Prinz et al., 2002; O'Connor et al., 2012). Inflammatory stromal cells have also been shown to have the potential to replicate prions under certain circumstances (Heikenwalder et al., 2008). Despite the presence of FDC within the nasal-associated lymphoid tissues, prion neuroinvasion after exposure via the tongue or nasal cavity appears to occur independently of SLO, implying direct infection of the nervous system (Bessen et al., 2009; Haybaeck et al., 2011).

The propagation of prions to and within SLO

For prions to establish infection upon FDC after peripheral exposure, they must first be propagated to the local SLO, such as the Peyer's patches in the small intestine after oral exposure. Many studies have attempted to identify the mechanisms involved, and although important knowledge gaps exist, some common themes have emerged. Of course, the contribution of certain cell populations to this process may vary depending on the host species, prion agent strain, and exposure route.

Establishing infection within Peyer's patches after oral exposure

In order for prions to establish infection upon the FDC within the GALT after oral exposure they must first cross the gut epithelium. The follicle-associated epithelium which covers the GALT contains a unique population of highly phagocytic epithelial cells, termed M cells. These cells are specialized for the transcytosis of particulate antigens and microorganisms from the gut lumen into the GALT (Mabbott et al., 2013) and are important for the initiation of efficient mucosal immune responses against certain pathogenic bacteria (Hase et al., 2009) and the commensal microflora (Rios et al., 2016). However, some pathogens appear to exploit M cells to enter host tissues (Westphal et al., 2008; Nakato et al., 2012; Tahoun et al., 2012; Gonzalez-Hernandez et al., 2014; Kolawole et al., 2015). Data show that prions also exploit M cells to establish host infection (Heppner et al., 2001; Miyazawa et al., 2010; Takakura et al., 2011; Donaldson et al., 2012, 2016). Furthermore, the accumulation of ME7 scrapie prions in the GALT and disease susceptibility after oral exposure were both reduced in mice that lacked M cells, or mice in which they were transiently depleted before exposure (Donaldson et al., 2012, 2016). Independent in vivo and in vitro studies using mouse-passaged RML scrapie prions (Heppner et al., 2001), Fukuoka-1 Gerstmann–Sträussler–Scheinker (GSS) prions (Takakura et al., 2011), BSE prions (Miyazawa et al., 2010), and 263K hamster prions (Beekes and McBride, 2000) also suggest a role for M cells in the initial transfer of other prion agent across the gut epithelium.

Certain pathogenic bacteria (Tahoun et al., 2012; Bennet et al., 2016) or inflammatory stimuli such as cholera toxin (Terahara et al., 2008) can increase M-cell density in the gut epithelium. M-cell differentiation is dependent on stimulation from underlying stromal cells via their production of the cytokine RANKL (Knoop et al., 2009; Rios et al., 2016). When mice were treated with RANKL to increase the abundance of M cells throughout the intestine, the uptake of prions from the gut lumen was enhanced and disease susceptibility was increased by approximately 10-fold (Donaldson et al., 2016). This suggests that factors that increase M-cell density in the gut epithelium, such as concurrent pathogen infection (see below) or inflammation, may dramatically enhance susceptibility to orally acquired prion infections. The binding of CWD prions to certain types of soil particles in the environment can also increase the uptake of prions from the gut lumen (Wyckoff et al., 2016). Whether the binding of prions to soil particles enhanced their transfer across the gut epithelium by M cells remains to be determined.

Data on the role of M cells in the initial uptake of prions from the gut lumen have occasionally been conflicting. Whereas some immunohistologic tracing studies have suggested that M cells are the initial sites of prion uptake in the gut epithelium (Foster and Macpherson, 2010; Takakura et al., 2011), other studies in lambs (Jeffrey et al., 2006) and mice (Kujala et al., 2011) have suggested M-cell-independent mechanisms may also play a role. The reasons for these discrepancies are uncertain. In vitro studies have shown that undifferentiated gut epithelial cell lines (Caco-2 cells) act as a barrier to prion uptake (Heppner et al., 2001), but transcytosis of PrP^{TSE} was evident when it was complexed with ferritin (Mishra et al., 2004). However, if prions predominantly exploit enterocytes or other M-cell-independent routes to establish host infection, one would not expect oral prion disease susceptibility to be blocked in the specific absence of M cells (Donaldson et al., 2012, 2016).

Antigen-sampling M cells have also been described in the epithelia covering the nasal-associated lymphoid tissue (Mutoh et al., 2016; Nair et al., 2016). After intranasal exposure of hamsters to 263K scrapie prions, transient prion uptake by M cells in the epithelium covering the nasal-associated lymphoid tissue was observed. However, a greater abundance of paracellular transport was evident (Kincaid et al., 2012), indicating that the requirement for M-cell-mediated prion uptake may vary depending on the route of exposure.

Studies using extremely sensitive PrP^{TSE}-based detection assays (see Chapter 22) have detected low/trace levels of prions in the blood stream within minutes of oral exposure (Elder et al., 2015; Urayama et al., 2016). The mechanism by which the prions initially contaminated the blood stream was not determined, but the authors proposed that the amount of PrP^{TSE} that was initially present was sufficient to establish infection in the CNS (Urayama et al., 2016). However, this conclusion contrasts with data, described above, which show that prion amplification within the GALT is essential to establish host infection and achieve neuroinvasion (Mabbott et al., 2003; Prinz et al., 2003b; Horiuchi et al., 2006; Glaysher and Mabbott, 2007; Raymond et al., 2007; Donaldson et al., 2015). Thus, although highly sensitive assays may detect PrP^{TSE} in the blood stream shortly after oral exposure (Elder et al., 2015; Urayama et al., 2016), the levels that are first detected within it are insufficient to directly establish host infection and achieve neuroinvasion.

M cells express a range of receptors on their apical surfaces which can specifically bind certain pathogenic microorganisms (Mabbott et al., 2013). Whether prion uptake by M cells is also receptor-mediated is uncertain. M cells express PrP^C highly (Nakato et al., 2009, 2012), but PrP^C deficiency within the gut epithelium does not affect PrP^{TSE} uptake from the intestine (Kujala et al., 2011; Takakura et al., 2011).

The demonstration that M cells play an important role in the initial uptake of prions from the gut lumen in order to establish host infection suggests they may represent an important prophylactic target against orally acquired prion infections.

Conventional dendritic cells propagate prions towards FDC in SLO

Antigens that have been transported across the gut epithelium by M cells are released into the basolateral pocket beneath them and sampled by the mononuclear phagocytes within it (Sakhon et al., 2015). Mononuclear phagocytes differentiate from bone marrow precursor cells and comprise a heterogeneous population of monocytes, conventional DC, and tissue macrophages. Conventional DC are a distinct lineage from the stromal-derived FDC (Shortman and Liu, 2002; Mabbott et al., 2011; Krautler et al., 2012), and are strategically positioned to sample their local environment for pathogens and their antigens. After antigen uptake, these cells undergo maturation and migrate towards the local SLO tissue to initiate an immune response. Conventional DC are also involved in the transport of antigens both within Peyer's patches and on towards the mesenteric lymph nodes (Liu and MacPherson, 1993; Banchereau et al., 2000; Cerovic et al., 2015). These migratory characteristics are exploited by some pathogens to facilitate their delivery to SLO (Wu et al., 2000; Ho et al., 2001, 2011; Steinman et al., 2003).

The ability of conventional DC to capture and retain unprocessed antigens (Wykes et al., 1998; Macpherson and Uhr, 2004) and migrate into B-cell follicles (Berney et al., 1999; Saeki et al., 2000; Leon et al., 2012) suggested that they may also propagate prions to and within SLO. This hypothesis was supported by the observation some DC migrating in the lymphatic fluid draining from the intestine had acquired PrP^{TSE} after its injection into the gut lumen (Huang et al., 2002). Subsequent studies showed that the early replication of prions upon FDC in the local SLO was impeded when conventional DC were transiently depleted at the time of exposure (Raymond et al., 2007; Sethi et al., 2007; Cordier-Dirikoc and Chabry, 2008; Wathne et al., 2012). This suggested that prions may also exploit conventional DC to establish host infection after peripheral exposure, perhaps using them as "Trojan horses."

Chemokines help to attract lymphocytes and conventional DC to SLO and control their positioning within them. The chemokine CXCL13 is expressed by FDC and other stromal cells in the B-cell follicles of SLO and recruits CXCR5-expressing cells towards them (Gunn et al., 1998; Ansel et al., 2000). The migration of certain populations of conventional DC towards the FDC-containing B-cell follicles is also mediated by CXCL13-CXCR5 signaling (Saeki et al., 2000; Yu et al., 2002; Leon et al., 2012). In the specific absence of CXCR5-expressing conventional DC the early accumulation of prions upon FDC in Peyer's patches was impaired, and disease susceptibility reduced (Bradford et al., 2017). This suggests that once the prions have been transferred across the gut epithelium by M cells they are subsequently acquired by conventional DC (Raymond et al., 2007; Kujala et al., 2011) and propagated by them towards FDC in Peyer's patches (Bradford et al., 2017). Once the prions have been propagated towards the B-cell follicles by conventional DC it is uncertain how they are subsequently transferred to FDC. Conventional DC can retain PrP^{TSE} both intracellularly and on the cell surface (Michel et al., 2012b). The higher expression level of CR on FDC may enable them to strip complement-opsonized prions from the surfaces of conventional DC.

The positioning of conventional DC within the interfollicular T-cell regions of Peyer's patches, and their steady-state migration from Peyer's patches to the mesenteric lymph nodes, are both dependent upon CCR7-CCL19/CCL21 signaling (Jang et al., 2006). Consistent with the demonstrations that T cells do not influence prion disease pathogenesis (Klein et al., 1997), prion neuroinvasion from the intestine is unaffected in the absence of CCR7-CCL19/CCL21 signaling (Levavasseur et al., 2007).

Whether specific conventional DC subsets propagate prions to and within SLO is uncertain. However, CD8+ conventional DC are unlikely to play a role as they are rarely encountered within the subepithelial dome region immediately beneath the M-cell-containing follicle-associated epithelium (Iwasaki and Kelsalla, 2000), and their specific depletion does not influence oral prion disease pathogenesis (Sethi et al., 2007). Similarly, although prion pathogenesis following infection via skin lesions was impaired in the specific absence of $CD11c^{+}langerin^{-}$ dermal DC, the absence of epidermal Langerhans cells or $langerin^{+}$ dermal DC had no effect (Wathne et al., 2012). High levels of infectious prions have also been detected within splenic plasmacytoid DC (Castro-Seoane et al., 2012), but these cells are unlikely to contribute to prion propagation as they do not migrate in the lymphatics (Yrlid et al., 2006).

Mononuclear phagocytes express cellular PrP^{C} (Burthem et al., 2001; Miyazawa et al., 2007; Cordier-Dirikoc et al., 2008), but the propagation of prions to FDC is not affected by the lack of PrP^{C} expression in hematopoietic cells (Klein et al., 1998; Brown et al., 1999; Mohan et al., 2004; Loeuillet et al., 2010; McCulloch et al., 2011; Michel et al., 2012b). This demonstrates that prions are acquired by conventional DC in a PrP^{C}-independent manner, and also that they are not important sites of prion replication. Conventional DC can acquire prions after their opsonization by complement components such as C1q and C3 (Flores-Lagnarica et al., 2009; Michel et al., 2012b). Depending on their location, phenotype, and activation status, conventional DC can express a variety of complement-binding receptors, including CR1 (CD35), CR2 (CD21), CR4 (CD11c/CD18), calreticulin, CD93, and SIGN-R1 (CD209b). Whether some of these receptors mediate the uptake of prions by conventional DC is uncertain (Flores-Lagnarica et al., 2009; Michel et al., 2012b), but SIGN-R1 does not appear to be involved (Bradford et al., 2016). Conventional DC might simply acquire prions non-specifically by fluid-phase micropinocytosis as they constitutively sample their microenvironment.

Phagocytosis and destruction of prions by macrophages

While some mononuclear phagocytes such as conventional DC can propagate infectious prions to FDC within SLO, other populations appear to phagocytose and destroy them (Carp and Callahan, 1981, 1982). The tingible body macrophages within germinal centers are characteristically loaded with the remnants of phagocytosed apoptotic lymphocytes (tingible bodies), and during prion disease also contain heavy PrP^{TSE} accumulations within their endosomal compartments (McGovern et al., 2009; Kujala et al., 2011; McCulloch et al., 2011). The depletion of macrophages before peripheral prion enhances the accumulation of PrP^{TSE} within SLO (Beringue et al., 2000; Maignien et al., 2005), suggesting that macrophages typically scavenge and degrade prions in an attempt to protect the host from infection.

The accumulation of infectious prions within the SLO rapidly reaches a plateau level within a few weeks of exposure, and persists for the duration of the infection (Brown et al., 1999; Mabbott et al., 2000b). How this plateau is maintained is uncertain. It is plausible that a competitive state is reached whereby the rate of prion amplification upon FDC matches the rate of degradation by macrophages (Carp and Callahan, 1982; Maignien et al., 2005).

Cell-free

Although the data above suggest that prions are propagated to and within SLO by cell-associated mechanisms, the possibility that a proportion of the prions also reach these tissues in a cell-free manner cannot also be excluded (Gossner et al., 2005; Kincaid et al., 2012; Michel et al., 2012b; Wathne et al., 2012).

Orally acquired prions accumulate first in the GALT of the upper gastrointestinal tract before spreading most other SLO

Mouse transmissions show that FDC within Peyer's patches are the essential early sites of prion replication and neuroinvasion, as oral disease susceptibility is blocked in their absence (Prinz et al., 2003b; Horiuchi et al., 2006; Glaysher and Mabbott, 2007; Donaldson et al., 2015, 2016). Many natural prion diseases also accumulate upon FDC in the large intestinal GALT after oral exposure, such as within the rectoanal mucosa-associated lymphoid tissues (RAMALT) of scrapie-affected sheep and goats, and CWD-affected deer and elk (Espenes et al., 2006; Gonzalez et al., 2006, 2009; Spraker et al., 2006; Wolfe et al., 2007; Thomsen et al., 2012; Monello et al., 2013). The detection of PrP^{TSE} within the GALT has helped to identify prion-infected animals during the preclinical phase (Hilton et al., 1998; Espenes et al., 2006; Gonzalez et al., 2006; Spraker et al., 2006; Wolfe et al., 2007; Dennis et al., 2009), and has been used in the United Kingdom to estimate the prevalence of vCJD in the human population (Hilton et al., 2002, 2004; Gill et al., 2013). However, the large intestinal GALT are not early sites of prion accumulation or neuroinvasion from the intestine (Donaldson et al., 2015) (Fig. 5.1A). In sheep with natural scrapie, prions are first detected in the GALT of the upper gastrointestinal tract before spreading to the local lymph nodes and onwards to other SLO such as the spleen. Large intestinal GALT, such as the cecal patches, were not early sites of prion accumulation in these studies (van Keulen et al., 2000, 2002, 2008a; Tabouret et al., 2010).

A similar temporal distribution was observed after oral exposure of sheep to BSE (Van Keulen et al., 2008b). Similar analyses of RAMALT biopsies from scrapie-infected goats (Gonzalez et al., 2009) and CWD-infected white-tailed deer (Keane et al., 2009; Thomsen et al., 2012) show lower incidences of prion accumulation at the earlier stages of disease. A study of CWD prevalence in elk showed PrP^{TSE} was not reliably detected in the RAMALT until it was also detectable in the CNS (Monello et al., 2013), consistent with the conclusion that the large intestinal GALT become infected with prions much later in the disease process (Spraker et al., 2006, 2009a). The possibility therefore cannot be excluded that the analysis of large intestinal GALT biopsy specimens may miss infected individuals if sampled during the early stages after oral prion exposure and underestimate the disease prevalence.

Antigens acquired from the intestinal lumen may be delivered directly to the mesenteric lymph nodes (Huang et al., 2000; Houston et al., 2016). Prions are similarly detected upon FDC in the mesenteric lymph nodes and spleen soon after oral exposure. The absence of the mesenteric lymph nodes does not affect prion neuroinvasion or disease susceptibility (Glaysher and Mabbott, 2007; Donaldson et al., 2015, 2016), indicating that the levels of prions initially delivered to them immediately after oral exposure are insufficient to establish infection upon the FDC within them. Absence of the spleen also does not influence oral prion disease pathogenesis or susceptibility in mice (Kimberlin and

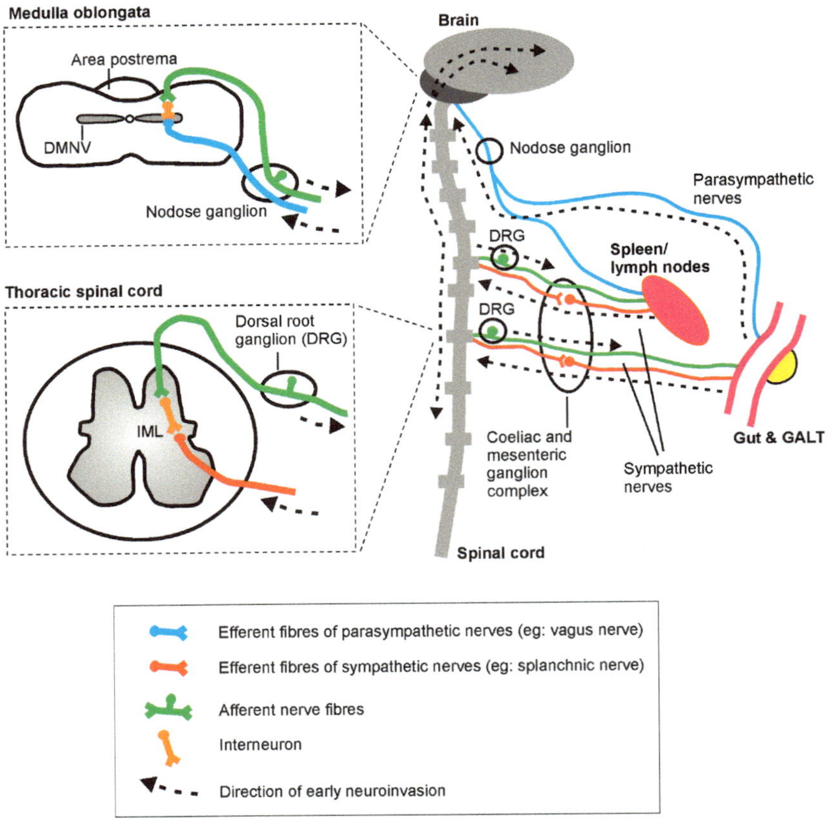

Fig. 5.2. Initial pathways of prion neuroinvasion from the intestine. After oral exposure the prions accumulate within the gut-associated lymphoid tissues (GALT) in the small intestine such as the Peyer's patches, and subsequently spread from these to infect other secondary lymphoid organs, including the mesenteric lymph nodes and spleen. After establishing infection and replication upon the follicular dendritic cells within the GALT, the prions then infect the peripheral nervous system and spread from the intestine to the central nervous system (CNS) via two distinct neuroanotomic pathways. In each case, the initial spread occurs in a retrograde direction along efferent (motor) pathways in a stepwise manner between synaptically linked sets of nerves. One route to the CNS occurs along sympathetic fibers of the splanchnic nerve to the intermediolateral cell column (IML) of the mid thoracic spinal cord. Subsequently the agent spreads to the brain in a caudal to cranial direction along the spinal cord. Neuroinvasion from the intestine can also occur independently of the spinal cord. In this case, the agent spreads along parasympathetic fibers of the vagus nerve to the dorsal motor nucleus of the vagus nerve (DMNV) within the medulla oblongata of the brain. (Adapted with permission from Mabbott NA, MacPherson GG (2006) Prions and their lethal journey to the brain. Nat Rev Microbiol 4: 201–211.)

Walker, 1989; Bradford et al., 2017), consistent with the conclusion that the GALT of the upper gastrointestinal tract are the essential sites of prion accumulation and neuroinvasion (Fig. 5.2).

After residing in Peyer's patches, B cells migrate to the mesenteric lymph nodes and then return to the circulation (Schmidt et al., 2013). B cells can recirculate between SLO for several weeks (Turner et al., 1997) and often acquire antigens from FDC as they travel through the germinal centers within them (Suzuki et al., 2009). When the migration of B cells between SLO was specifically blocked, the dissemination of prions from the draining SLO was also blocked (Mok et al., 2012). Thus, recirculating B cells appear to mediate the initial propagation of prions from the draining lymphoid tissue to other SLO. Prions have also been detected in association with lymphocytes (Andreoletti et al., 2012; Douet et al., 2016) and B cells in the blood of sheep with scrapie (Edwards et al., 2010) and deer with CWD (Mathiason et al., 2010).

Neuroinvasion

Circumventricular organs are important sites of molecular exchange between the blood stream and the CNS. The detection of prion disease-specific PrP within the circumventricular organs of the brain has been described in some scrapie-affected sheep (Sisó et al., 2006). However, monocytic infiltration into the circumventricular organs is not observed in prion disease-affected hosts, and an absence of recruitment of circulating monocytes does not influence CNS prion disease (Gomez-Nicola et al., 2014). This argues against the direct cell-associated hematogenous spread of prions into the CNS. In vCJD patients the spatial distribution of the PrP^{TSE} deposits in the brain in relation to the blood vessels also does not suggest a major role (Armstrong et al., 2003). The hematogenous spread of prions directly into the CNS cannot be entirely excluded, however, as low/trace levels of PrP^{TSE} may be initially detected in the brain soon after exposure using highly sensitive assays (Urayama et al., 2016). The SLO, including the GALT, are highly innervated (Felten and Felten, 1991). Detailed immunohistochemical tracing studies show that, after replication upon FDC in the GALT, orally acquired prions establish infection in the CNS via the enteric nervous system by spreading along efferent fibers of both the sympathetic (e.g., splanchnic) and parasympathetic (e.g., vagus) nervous systems (Beekes et al., 1996, 1998; Baldauf et al., 1997; McBride and Beekes, 1999; Beekes and McBride, 2000; Kujala et al., 2011; McBride et al., 2001) (Fig. 5.2). Furthermore, the specific depletion of sympathetic nerves impairs prion neuroinvasion from SLO (Glatzel et al., 2001). Conversely, prion disease pathogenesis is exacerbated in mice in which sympathetic nerve density in SLO is increased (Glatzel et al., 2001), or in which the distance between FDC and sympathetic nerves is reduced (Prinz et al., 2003a).

How prion infection initially spreads from the FDC to peripheral nerves in vivo is uncertain, but a role for conventional DC or other mononuclear phagocytes has been proposed (Aucouturier et al., 2001; Gousset et al., 2009; Langevin et al., 2010; Tanaka et al., 2012). Tunneling nanotubes (TNT) are thin membrane-bound cylinders of cytoplasm which can connect cells to enable cell-to-cell communication and the intercellular transfer of plasma membrane or cytoplasmic components. TNT are exploited by human immunodeficiency virus type 1 (HIV-1) to aid intercellular transfer between T cells (Sowinski et al., 2008), and to shuttle virus-encoded immunosuppressive factors from infected macrophages to B cells (Xu et al., 2009). In vitro studies show infectious prions can be transferred between conventional DC and neurones via endolysosomal vesicles within TNT (Gousset et al., 2009; Langevin et al., 2010; Tanaka et al., 2012; Zhu et al., 2015). Whether TNT mediate the intercellular transfer of prions in vivo remains to be determined. Infectious prions can also be released from infected cells in association with small endosomal-derived vesicles, termed exosomes (Fevrier et al., 2004), which have the potential to infect neighboring cells (Castro-Seoane et al., 2012). However, the relative contribution of exosomes to this process in vivo is uncertain and may be prion strain-dependent (Arellano-Anaya et al., 2015).

Effects of inflammation and pathogen co-infection on prion disease pathogenesis

Many studies have described the role of the immune system in prion disease pathogenesis during steady-state conditions, but inflammation can significantly impact on the pathogenesis. For example, pathology to the gut mucosa such as bacterial colitis (Sigurdson et al., 2009), enhanced M-cell density (Donaldson et al., 2016), and lesions to the mucosal surfaces of the oral (Denkers et al., 2011) or nasal cavities (Crowell et al., 2015) can enhance disease susceptibility by increasing prion uptake. Mitogen stimulation or repetitive immunization (against antigens other than PrP) can also enhance prion disease susceptibility (Dickinson et al., 1978; Bremer et al., 2009). Chronic inflammation can also expand the distribution of prions within the infected host by inducing the formation of additional sites of prion replication (FDC-containing ectopic tertiary lymphoid tissues) (Heikenwalder et al., 2005; Ligios et al., 2005; Seeger et al., 2005; Glaysher and Mabbott, 2007; Donaldson et al., 2015).

Enteritis may also influence oral prion disease susceptibility. For example, concurrent infection with the enteroinvasive bacterium *Salmonella enterica* serovar Typhimurium (*S.* Typhimurium) increased oral prion disease susceptibility (Sigurdson et al., 2009). Although this was originally attributed to the colitis induced by the pathogen in the large intestine, a similar effect on prion disease pathogenesis was not observed in an independent study using the large intestine-restricted helminth pathogen *Trichuris muris* (Donaldson et al., 2015). Data show that *S.* Typhimurium can rapidly transform gut epithelial cells into M cells to facilitate host infection (Tahoun et al., 2012). Since an increased abundance of M cells in the small intestine can enhance oral prion disease pathogenesis and susceptibility (Donaldson et al., 2016), the effects of *S.* Typhimurium on the M-cell-mediated uptake of prions cannot be excluded in the above study (Sigurdson et al., 2009).

The effects of inflammation or pathogen co-infection on prion disease pathogenesis may have other important consequences. Although prions may be secreted into the milk of some prion-infected hosts (Konold et al., 2008, 2013, 2016), this is enhanced in scrapie-infected sheep with mastitis (Ligios et al., 2005) and can transmit disease to suckling lambs (Ligios et al., 2011). Chronic inflammation in the kidney may lead to enhanced environmental contamination due to excretion of prions in urine, and aid the horizontal transmission of disease (Seeger et al., 2005).

Effects of host age on prion disease pathogenesis and susceptibility

Clinical vCJD cases have almost exclusively occurred in young adults (median age at disease onset = 26 years). However, this age-related incidence of vCJD is not simply due to the exposure of young adults to greater levels of BSE prions through dietary preference (Boelle et al., 2004). Aging is accompanied by a decline in immune function, termed immunosenescence (Mabbott et al., 2015). As a consequence, the elderly respond less effectively to vaccination, and have increased susceptibility to viral and bacterial infections and increased incidence of cancer and autoimmune diseases. Immunosenescence can also influence the pathogenesis of peripherally acquired prion infections, by impeding prion accumulation and replication in SLO and reducing disease susceptibility (Brown et al., 2009, 2012; Avrahami and Gabizon, 2011; Brown and Mabbott, 2014). Data from the analysis of sheep, cattle, cervids, and humans also show an association between GALT development and susceptibility to peripheral exposure to natural prion infections (St. Rose et al., 2006). For example, in Cheviot sheep a reduction in ileal Peyer's patch size and lymphoid follicle density is apparent from the onset of puberty (St. Rose et al., 2007).

In aged mice (≥600 days old) the functional status of key immune cell populations which aid prion neuroinvasion is adversely affected. The expression of PrP^{C} by aged FDC is reduced (Brown et al., 2009), and due to disturbances to the microarchitecture of the spleen, the delivery of immune complexes to FDC is adversely affected in aged mice (Brown et al., 2012; Brown and Mabbott, 2014; Turner and Mabbott, 2017). The functional maturation of M cells in aged Peyer's patches is also impaired, substantially reducing the uptake of particulate antigens from the gut lumen (Kobayashi et al., 2013). These aging-related impairments to M cells and FDC coincide with the dramatically reduced accumulation of infectious prions in the SLO of aged mice and their significantly reduced susceptibility to peripheral prion infections (Brown et al., 2009, 2012; Brown and Mabbott, 2014).

The effects of immunosenescence may also affect the ability to reliably detect prion-infected animals during the preclinical phase. Although PrP^{TSE} was detected in the brains of many peripherally infected aged mice despite the absence of clinical signs, PrP^{TSE} was undetectable in many of their spleens (Brown et al., 2009). This has important implications for the reliability of preclinical diagnostic tests based on the detection of PrP^{TSE} in the SLO, as these may be much less sensitive when used on elderly individuals. For example, low numbers of lymphoid follicles were detected in RAMALT specimens from older CWD-affected elk (*Cervus elaphus nelson*; >8.5 years old) (Spraker et al., 2009b) and mule deer (*Odocoileus hemionus*; ≥ 3 years old) (Geremia et al., 2015), reducing the reliability of the histopathologic detection of PrP^{TSE}.

At the other end of the aging spectrum (pre-weaning), the developmental status of the GALT or intestine can also influence oral prion disease susceptibility. As a consequence of the underdeveloped status of their FDC, prion accumulation in the SLO of neonatal mice is reduced and neuroinvasion is delayed (Outram et al., 1973; Ierna et al., 2006). The GALT tissues are more developed in neonatal sheep when compared to mice. Furthermore, the incidence of clinical prion disease is greater in lambs orally exposed to BSE prions during the pre-weaning stage, when compared to those exposed post-weaning (Hunter et al., 2012). Multiple factors are likely to contribute to this age-related difference in susceptibility, but mouse studies show that the presence of maternal immunoglobulin during the weaning period can enhance PrP^{TSE} transfer across the gut epithelium (Ano et al., 2010).

Involvement of the immune system in CNS prion pathogenesis

In the CNS, prion aggregates accumulate to high levels and are considered to eventually overwhelm the nerves within it, leading to neurodegeneration and death. Although differences between prion agent strains may exist, the neurodegeneration process is slow and progressive. Synapses appear to be most vulnerable to degeneration early in disease, occurring before signs of axonal retraction, cell body atrophy, and neuronal loss (Jeffrey et al., 2000a; Jamieson et al., 2001; Cunningham et al., 2003; Šišková et al., 2013). The mechanisms of neurodegeneration are uncertain and many neuronal cell processes appear to be compromised and/or activated. For example, one study showed that PrP^{TSE} accumulation in the CNS causes persistent translational repression of global protein synthesis via the eukaryotic translation initiation factor, eIF2 (Moreno et al., 2012).

One of the earliest pathologic signs during CNS prion disease is the activation of the glial cells, microglia, and astrocytes (Betmouni et al., 1996). Furthermore, neurodegeneration was observed to occur only in the brains of prion-infected mice when PrP^{TSE} accumulation was associated with an upregulated innate immune response by the microglia within the same region (Alibhai et al., 2016) (Fig. 5.3). Microglia are the resident mononuclear phagocytes of the CNS and play important roles in the maintenance of neuronal homeostasis, synaptic remodeling, and the removal of dead and dying cells and also provide a first line of defense against pathogens (Kranich

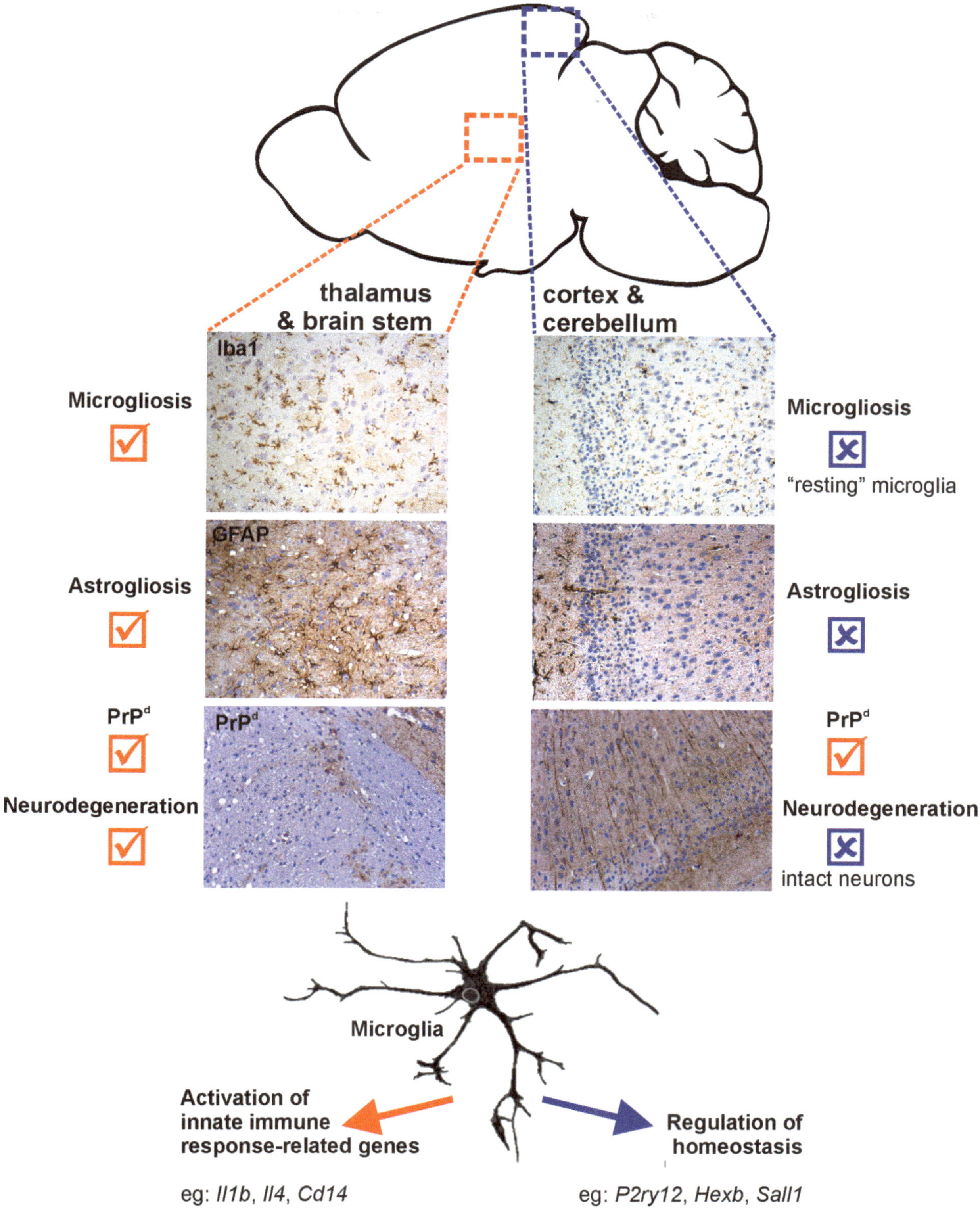

Fig. 5.3. During prion disease, neurodegeneration and morphologic glial cell responses are restricted to specific brain regions. A specific mouse model of prion disease (Gerstmann–Sträussler–Scheinker (Georgsson et al., 1993) disease in mice with a proline to leucine alteration at codon 101 of murine PrP) was used to study the impact of disease-specific PrP (PrP^d) accumulations and glia cell responses (astrogliosis and microgliosis) on neurodegeneration in the central nervous system (Alibhai et al., 2016). In this model accumulations of PrP^d were detected in all brain regions from an early stage of the disease. However, neurodegeneration

(Continued)

et al., 2010; Prinz and Priller, 2014; Zhan et al., 2014; De Lucia et al., 2016). Resting microglia typically display a ramified appearance, whereas upon activation they display shortened processes and hypertrophied cell bodies (Boche et al., 2013).

A change in microglial status from resting to activated is one of the earliest neuropathologic features of prion disease and precedes the onset of neuropathology (Vincenti et al., 2016). The activated microglia in the prion-affected CNS express elevated levels of a wide range of activation and signaling receptors, including Trem2, SiglecF, CD200R, and Fcγ receptors (Lunnon et al., 2011). The microglial characteristics during CNS prion disease are typical of the anti-inflammatory profile exhibited by macrophages following their engulfment of apoptotic cells (Fadok et al., 1998) and appear to be mediated by the transforming growth factor-β and prostaglandin E_2-dominated cytokine milieu which is induced in the brain during infection (Minghetti et al., 2000; Walsh et al., 2000; Boche et al., 2003; Cunningham et al., 2003). Furthermore, prion disease pathogenesis is exacerbated in mice deficient in the anti-inflammatory cytokines interleukin (IL)-4, IL-10, IL-13 (Thackray et al., 2004; Tamguney et al., 2008).

It is important to note, however, that a proinflammatory response is not completely absent. Whereas deficiency in characteristic proinflammatory mediators such as TNF-α or its receptor TNFR1 (Klein et al., 1997; Mabbott et al., 2000b), complement components (Klein et al., 2001; Mabbott et al., 2001; Mabbott and Bruce, 2004; Michel et al., 2012a, 2013), the chemokine receptors CCR2 and CCR5 (Tamguney et al., 2008), IL-6 (Mabbott et al., 2000b), IL-12p35 and IL-12p40 (Tribouillard-Tanvier et al., 2012), the negative regulator of IL-1, IL1-Ra (Carroll et al., 2015), the inflammasome (Nuvolone et al., 2015), treatment with anti-interferon antibody (Gresser et al., 1983), and an absence of canonic NF-κB signaling in the neurons, astrocytes, and oligodendrocytes (Julius et al., 2008) do not influence CNS prion disease pathogenesis, survival times are extended in mice deficient in IL-1R type 1 (Tamguney et al., 2008) or the chemokine receptor CXCR3 (Reimer et al., 2008).

Transcriptional analyses of stimulated macrophages show that their activation states present as a spectrum which extends beyond the M1 (classically activated; proinflammatory) versus M2 (alternatively activated; anti-inflammatory/tissue repair and remodeling) model (Xue et al., 2014). The available evidence indicates that a unique prion disease-specific microglial response is induced in the CNS with both anti-inflammatory and proinflammatory components (Alibhai et al., 2016; Vincenti et al., 2016). Whether these contrasting responses are displayed by the same or distinct populations of microglia within the same brain regions is uncertain; co-expression of pro- and anti-inflammatory genes by individual mononuclear phagocyte populations is evident at the transcriptional level (Mabbott et al., 2010; Xue et al., 2014).

The absence of significant evidence of circulating monocytes into the CNS during prion disease indicates that CNS-resident cells are the major/sole immune regulators (Gomez-Nicola et al., 2014). Microglia are not the only CNS-resident cell type which can engage in an immune response during neurodegenerative diseases. Mice deficient in the chemokine receptor CCR2 have deficits in perivascular macrophage recruitment, but the pathologic manifestation of CNS prion disease in these mice is not affected (Gomez-Nicola et al., 2014), suggesting that perivascular macrophages do not play a role. Astrocytes may also contribute to the innate immune response in the prion-affected CNS. For example, co-culture of prion-exposed astrocytes and primary neurons could induce the migration of N11 microglial cells (Marella and Chabry, 2004). This suggests that astrocyte and/or neuronal signaling might aid the recruitment and activation of microglia to sites of prion infection. Other studies showed that the prion disease-associated astrogliosis was attenuated in IL-1R type 1-deficient mice (Schultz et al., 2004). Whether astrocytes play an important role in stimulating microglial activation during CNS prion disease, or whether microglial activation stimulates astrogliosis, remains to be determined.

As mentioned earlier, in the absence of macrophages the accumulation of PrP^{TSE} within SLO is enhanced (Beringue et al., 2000; Maignien et al., 2005). Similarly, in mice deficient in astrocyte-derived MFGE-8, the inability of microglia to sequester apoptotic cell remnants in the CNS leads to accelerated prion pathogenesis (Kranich et al., 2010). Furthermore, the depletion of

Fig. 5.3—cont'd specifically occurred only in areas such as the thalamus and brainstem. Other parts of the brain, such as the cortex or cerebellum, remained unaffected despite the presence of PrP^d. Transcriptional analyses of the cellular responses in each brain region indicated that the major cellular response originated from the microglia. However, the microglial response was complex and comprised at least two separate signatures. One signature suggested the activation of the innate immune response-related genes, and was specifically restricted to brain regions undergoing neurodegeneration and exhibiting morphologic glial cell responses. The alternate signature suggested the upregulation of many genes involved in regulating homeostasis.

microglia in cerebellar organotypic cultured slices enhances prion accumulation (Falsig et al., 2008) and CNS prion disease pathogenesis is exacerbated in vivo in the absence of microglia (Zhu et al., 2016). Conversely, selective inhibition of CSF1R-signaling enhances the expression of certain anti-inflammatory microglial markers during CNS prion disease, delaying the onset of clinical signs and extending survival times (Gomez-Nicola et al., 2013). The growing body of evidence indicates that during CNS prion disease a predominantly anti-inflammatory cytokine milieu is induced in the brain to stimulate the microglia within it to provide a protective role by scavenging and clearing prions and prion-affected cells, and maintain homeostasis. However, in regions of neurodegeneration, transcriptional analyses indicate that the microglia enter into a cycle of innate immune activation (Alibhai et al., 2016) (Fig. 5.3). These data also suggest that manipulation of the microglial response during CNS prion disease could be a credible target for therapeutic intervention.

Exciting data show that the composition of the commensal bacterial microbiota in the intestine can influence the status of microglia in the brain (Erny et al., 2015). It is currently uncertain whether similar changes to the composition of the commensal bacterial microbiota can influence CNS prion disease (Donaldson and Mabbott, 2016). However, systemic inflammation such as that induced by bacterial lipopolysaccharide can induce the expression of proinflammatory cytokines and cytotoxic mediators in the CNS during prion disease. These have the effect of switching the neuroprotective phenotype of the microglia within the prion-affected CNS to a more proinflammatory phenotype, leading to exacerbated neuropathology (Combrinck et al., 2002; Cunningham et al., 2005).

CONCLUDING REMARKS

Substantial advances have been made during the past 40 or more years in our understanding of the role of the immune system in prion diseases. Major aims have been to identify the key tissues, cells, and molecules which play an essential role in the propagation of prions from the site of exposure to the CNS where they ultimately cause disease. Data from such studies have several important practical implications. The identification of sites of prion accumulation and replication in non-CNS tissues helps in the assessment of the potential risk of disease transmission. For example, the identification that B cells and SLO played an important role in prion disease pathogenesis (Klein et al., 1997), and that vCJD prions also accumulated in human SLO during disease (Hill et al., 1997b), correctly raised concern that blood or blood components from vCJD-affected individuals might have the potential to transmit disease via blood transfusion (Peden et al., 2004; Llewelyn et al., 2004; Wroe et al., 2006). Experimental evidence shows that treatments that block prion accumulation in SLO can reduce disease susceptibility or extend survival times (Montrasio et al., 2000; Mabbott et al., 2000a, 2002, 2003; Mohan et al., 2005; Raymond et al., 2007; Cordier-Dirikoc and Chabry, 2008; Donaldson et al., 2012; Wathne et al., 2012). Unfortunately, many of these treatments cause transient periods of immunosuppression which may increase susceptibility to other pathogens and, importantly, are only effective when used during the interval between exposure and neuroinvasion.

However, the identification of a neuroprotective role for the microglia during CNS prion disease indicates that therapeutic strategies which enhance this activity may represent a novel strategy to prevent or intervene in these currently untreatable diseases. Both passive (White et al., 2003) and active immunization against PrP (Sigurdsson et al., 2002) can impede experimental prion disease pathogenesis in mice, suggesting that immunization is a realistic approach. However, important issues remain to be resolved in the development of effective antiprion vaccines, especially overcoming T-cell tolerance towards host PrP^C (Mabbott, 2015) (Chapter 7 provides an indepth discussion on immunization against prions.)

Despite all the progress that has been made in our understanding of prion disease pathogenesis, significant knowledge gaps exist (for detailed discussion, see Requena et al., 2016). Subsequent outbreaks of novel and emerging prion diseases in the future are likely to be orally acquired. It is therefore essential to insure that during these outbreaks we fully understand the factors that influence susceptibility to peripherally acquired prion infections and those which influence the risk of disease transmission to other host species.

REFERENCES

Alibhai J, Blanco RA, Barria MA et al. (2016). Distribution of misfolded prion protein seeding activity alone does not predict regions of neurodegeneration. PLoS Biol 14: e1002579.

Andreoletti O, Berthon P, Marc D et al. (2000). Early accumulation of PrPSc in gut-associated lymphoid and nervous tissues of susceptible sheep from a Romanov flock with natural scrapie. J Gen Virol 81: 3115–3126.

Andreoletti O, Litaise C, Simmons H et al. (2012). Highly efficient prion transmission by blood transfusion. PLoS Pathog 8: e1002782.

Ano Y, Sakudo A, Uraki R et al. (2010). Enhanced enteric invasion of scrapie agents into the villous columnar epithelium via maternal immunoglobulin. Int J Mol Med 26: 845–851.

Ansel KM, Ngo VN, Hyman PL et al. (2000). A chemokine-driven feedback loop organizes lymphoid follicles. Nature 406: 309–314.

Arellano-Anaya ZE, Huor A, Leblanc P et al. (2015). Prion strains are differentially released through the exosomal pathway. Cell Mol Life Sci 72: 1185–1196.

Armstrong RA, Cairns NJ, Ironside JW et al. (2003). Does the neuropathology of human patients with variant Creutzfeldt–Jakob disease reflect haematogenous spread of the disease. Neurosci Lett 348: 37–40.

Aucouturier P, Geissmann F, Damotte D et al. (2001). Infected splenic dendritic cells are sufficient for prion transmission to the CNS in mouse scrapie. J Clin Investig 108: 703–708.

Avrahami D, Gabizon R (2011). Age-related alterations affect the susceptibility of mice to prion infection. Neurobiol Aging 32: 2006–2015.

Baldauf E, Beekes M, Diringer H (1997). Evidence for an alternative direct route of access for the scrapie agent to the brain bypassing the spinal cord. J Gen Virol 78: 1187–1197.

Ballerini C, Gourdain P, Bachy V et al. (2006). Functional implication of cellular prion protein in antigen-driven interactions between T cells and dendritic cells. J Immunol 176: 7254–7262.

Banchereau J, Briere F, Caux C et al. (2000). Immunobiology of dendritic cells. Annu Rev Immunol 18: 767–811.

Beekes M, McBride PA (2000). Early accumulation of pathological PrP in the enteric nervous system and gut-associated lymphoid tissue of hamsters orally infected with scrapie. Neurosci Lett 278: 181–184.

Beekes M, Baldauf E, Diringer H (1996). Sequential appearance and accumulation of pathognomonic markers in the central nervous system of hamsters orally infected with scrapie. J Gen Virol 77: 1925–1934.

Beekes M, McBride PA, Baldauf E (1998). Cerebral targeting indicates vagal spread of infection in hamsters fed with scrapie. J Gen Virol 79: 601–607.

Bennet KM, Parnell EA, Sanscartier C et al. (2016). Induction of colonic M cells during intestinal inflammation. Am J Pathol 186: 166–179.

Beringue V, Demoy M, Lasmezas CI et al. (2000). Role of spleen macrophages in the clearance of scrapie agent early in pathogenesis. J Pathol 190: 495–502.

Berney C, Herren S, Power CA et al. (1999). A member of the dendritic cell family that enters B cell follicles and stimulates primary antibody responses identified by a mannose receptor fusion protein. J Exp Med 190: 851–860.

Bessen RA, Martinka S, Kelly J et al. (2009). Role of the lymphoreticular system in prion neuroinvasion from the oral and nasal mucosa. J Virol 83: 6435–6445.

Betmouni S, Perry VH, Gordon JL (1996). Evidence for an early inflammatory response in the central- nervous-system of mice with scrapie. Neuroscience 74: 1–5.

Boche D, Cunningham C, Gauldie J et al. (2003). Transforming growth factor-beta 1-mediated neuroprotection against excitotoxic injury in vivo. J Cereb Blood Flow Metab 23: 1174–1182.

Boche D, Perry VH, Nicoll JA (2013). Review: activation patterns of microglia and their identification in the human brain. Neuropathol Appl Neurobiol 39: 3–18.

Boelle P-Y, Cesbron J-Y, Valleron A-J (2004). Epidemiological evidence of higher susceptibility to vCJD in the young. BMC Infect Dis 4: 7.

Bolton DC, McKinley MP, Prusiner SB (1982). Identification of a protein that purifies with the scrapie prion. Science 218: 1309–1311.

Bradford BM, Brown KL, Mabbott NA (2016). Prion pathogenesis is unaltered following down-regulation of SIGN-R1. Virology 497: 337–345.

Bradford BM, Reizis B, Mabbott NA (2017). Oral prion disease pathogenesis is impeded in the specific absence of CXCR5-expressing dendritic cells. J Virol 91: e001224-17.

Bremer J, Heikenwalder M, Haybaeck J et al. (2009). Repetitive immunization enhances the susceptibility of mice to peripherally administered prions. PLoS One 4: e7160.

Brown KL, Mabbott NA (2014). Evidence of subclinical prion disease in aged mice following exposure to bovine spongiform encephalopathy. J Gen Virol 95: 231–243.

Brown KL, Stewart K, Ritchie D et al. (1999). Scrapie replication in lymphoid tissues depends on PrP-expressing follicular dendritic cells. Nat Med 5: 1308–1312.

Brown KL, Wathne GJ, Sales J et al. (2009). The effects of host age on follicular dendritic cell status dramatically impair scrapie agent neuroinvasion in aged mice. J Immunol 183: 5199–5207.

Brown KL, Gossner A, Mok S et al. (2012). The effects of host age on the transport of complement-bound complexes to the spleen and the pathogenesis of intravenous scrapie infection. J Virol 86: 1228–1237.

Bruce ME, Will RG, Ironside JW et al. (1997). Transmissions to mice indicate that 'new variant' CJD is caused by the BSE agent. Nature 389: 498–501.

Burthem J, Urban B, Pain A et al. (2001). The normal cellular prion protein is strongly expressed by myeloid dendritic cells. Blood 98: 3733–3738.

Carp RI, Callahan SM (1981). In vitro interaction of scrapie agent and mouse peritoneal macrophages. Intervirology 16: 8–13.

Carp RI, Callahan SM (1982). Effect of mouse peritoneal macrophages on scrapie infectivity during extended in vitro incubation. Intervirology 17: 201–207.

Carroll JA, Striebel JF, Race B et al. (2015). Prion infection of mouse brain reveals multiple new upregulated genes involved in neuroinflammation or signal transduction. J Virol 89: 2388–2404.

Cashman NR, Loertscher R, Nalbantoglu J et al. (1990). Cellular isoform of the scrapie agent protein participates in lymphocyte activation. Cell 61: 185–192.

Castro-Seoane R, Hummerich H, Sweeting T et al. (2012). Plasmacytoid dendritic cells sequester high prion titres at early stages of prion infection. PLoS Pathog 8: e1002538.

Caughey BW, Dong A, Bhat KS et al. (1991). Secondary structure analysis of the scrapie-associated protein PrP

27–30 in water by infrared spectroscopy. Biochemistry 30: 7672–7680.
Cerovic V, Houston SA, Westlund J et al. (2015). Lymph-borne CD8+ dendritic cells are uniquely able to cross-prime CD8+ T cells with antigen acquired from intestinal epithelial cells. Mucosal Immunol 8: 38–48.
Chaplin DD, Fu Y-X (1998). Cytokine regulation of secondary lymphoid organ development. Curr Opin Immunol 10: 289–297.
Clarke MC, Haig DA (1966). Attempts to demonstrate neutralising antibodies in the sera of scrapie-infected animals. Vet Rec (19): 647–649.
Combrinck MI, Perry VH, Cunningham C (2002). Peripheral infection evokes exaggerated sickness behaviour in preclinical murine prion disease. Neuroscience 112: 7–11.
Cordier-Dirikoc S, Chabry J (2008). Temporary depletion of CD11c+ dendritic cells delays lymphoinvasion after intraperitoneal scrapie infection. J Virol 82: 8933–8936.
Cordier-Dirikoc S, Zsürger N, Cazareth J et al. (2008). Expression profiles of prion and doppel proteins and of their receptors in mouse splenocytes. Eur J Immunol 38: 1–11.
Crowell J, Wiley JA, Bessen RA (2015). Lesion of the olfactory epithelium accelerates prion neuroinvasion and disease onset when prion replication is restricted to neurons. PLoS One 10: e0119863.
Cunningham C, Deacon R, Wells H et al. (2003). Synaptic changes characterize early behavioural signs of the ME7 model of muring prion disease. Eur J Neurosci 17: 2147–2155.
Cunningham C, Wilcockson DC, Campion S et al. (2005). Central and systemic endotoxin challenges exacerbate the local inflammatory response and increase neuronal death during chronic neurodegeneration. J Neurosci 25: 9275–9284.
de Almeida CJG, Chiarini LB, da Silva JP et al. (2005). The cellular prion protein modulates phagocytosis and inflammatory response. J Leukoc Biol 77: 238–246.
De Lucia C, Rinchon A, Olmos-Alsonso A et al. (2016). Microglia regulate hippocampal neurogenesis during chronic neurodegeneration. Brain Behav Immun 55: 179–190.
Denkers ND, Telling GC, Hoover EA (2011). Minor oral lesions facilitate transmission of chronic wasting disease. J Virol 85: 1396–1399.
Dennis MM, Thomsen BV, Marshall KL et al. (2009). Evaluation of immunohistochemical detection of prion protein in rectoanal mucosa-associated lymphoid tissue for diagnosis of scrapie in sheep. Am J Vet Res 70: 63–72.
Dickinson AG, Fraser H, McConnell I et al. (1978). Mitogenic stimulation of the host enhances susceptibility to scrapie. Nature 272: 54–55.
Donaldson DS, Mabbott NA (2016). The influence of the commensal and pathogenic gut microbiota on prion disease pathogenesis. J Gen Virol 97: 1725–1738.
Donaldson DS, Kobayashi A, Ohno H et al. (2012). M cell depletion blocks oral prion disease pathogenesis. Mucosal Immunol 5: 216–225.
Donaldson DS, Else KJ, Mabbott NA (2015). The gut-associated lymphoid tissues in the small intestine, not the large intestine, play a major role in oral prion disease pathogenesis. J Virol 15: 9532–9547.
Donaldson DS, Sehgal A, Rios D et al. (2016). Increased abundance of M cells in the gut epithelium dramatically enhances oral prion disease susceptibility. PLoS Pathog 12: e1006075.
Douet JY, Lacroux C, Litaise C et al. (2016). Mononucleated blood cell populations display different abilities to transmit prion disease by the transfusion route. J Virol 90: 3439–3445.
Edwards JC, Moore SJ, Hawthorne JA et al. (2010). PrP(Sc) is associated with B cells in the blood of scrapie-infected sheep. Virology 405: 110–119.
Elder AM, Henderson DM, Nalls AV et al. (2015). Immediate and ongoing detection of prions in the blood of hamsters and deer following oral, nasal and blood inoculations. J Virol 89: 7421–7424.
Erny D, Hrabe de Angelis AL, Jaitin D et al. (2015). Host microbiota constantly control maturation and function of microglia in the CNS. Nat Neurosci 18: 965–977.
Espenes A, McL.Press, Landsverk et al. (2006). Detection of PrPSc in rectal biopsy and necroscopy samples from sheep with experimental scrapie. J Comp Pathol 134: 115–125.
Fadok VA, Bratton DL, Konowal A et al. (1998). Macrophages that have ingested apoptotic cells in vitro inhibit proinflammatory cytokine production through autocrine/paracrine mechanisms involving TGF-beta, PGE2, and PAF. J Clin Investig 101: 890–898.
Falsig J, Julius C, Margalith I et al. (2008). A versatile prion replication assay in organotypic brain slices. Nat Neurosci 11: 109–117.
Felten SY, Felten DL (1991). Innervation of lymphoid tissue. In: Psychoneuroimmunology, 2nd edn. Academic Press, London, UK.
Fevrier B, Vilette D, Archer F et al. (2004). Cells release prions in association with exosomes. Proc Natl Acad Sci, USA 101: 9683–9688.
Flores-Lagnarica A, Sebti Y, Mitchell DA et al. (2009). Scrapie pathogenesis: the role of complement C1q in scrapie agent uptake by conventional dendritic cells. J Immunol 182: 1305–1313.
Foster N, Macpherson GG (2010). Murine cecal patch M cells transport infectious prions in vivo. J Infect Dis 202: 1916–1919.
Foster JD, Parnham DW, Hunter N et al. (2001). Distribution of the prion protein in sheep terminally affected with BSE following experimental oral transmission. J Gen Virol 82: 2319–2326.
Fraser H, Brown K (1994). Peripheral pathogenesis of scrapie in normal and immunocompromised mice. Animal Technology 45: 21–22.
Fraser H, Dickinson AG (1970). Pathogenesis of scrapie in the mouse: the role of the spleen. Nature 226: 462–463.
Fraser H, Dickinson AG (1978). Studies on the lymphoreticular system in the pathogenesis of scrapie: the role of spleen and thymus. J Comp Pathol 88: 563–573.

Fraser H, Brown KL, Stewart K et al. (1996). Replication of scrapie in spleens of SCID mice follows reconstitution with wild-type mouse bone marrow. J Gen Virol 77: 1935–1940.

Georgsson G, Gisladóttir E, Árnadóttir S (1993). Quantitative assessment of the astrocytic response in natural scrapie of sheep. J Comp Pathol 108: 229–240.

Geremia C, Hoeting JA, Wolfe LL et al. (2015). Age and repeated biopsy influence antemortem PrPCWD testing in mule deer (*Odocoileus hemionus*) in Colorado, USA. J Wildl Dis 51: 801–810.

Gill ON, Spencer Y, Richard-Loendt A et al. (2013). Prevelent abnormal prion protein in human appendixes after bovine spongiform encephalopathy epizootic: large scale survey. Br Med J f5675: 347.

Glatzel M, Heppner FL, Albers KM et al. (2001). Sympathetic innervation of lymphoreticular organs is rate limiting for prion neuroinvasion. Neuron 31: 25–34.

Glatzel M, Abela E, Maissen M et al. (2003). Extraneural pathological prion protein in sporadic Creutzfeldt–Jakob disease. N Engl J Med 349: 1812–1820.

Glaysher BR, Mabbott NA (2007). Role of the GALT in scrapie agent neuroinvasion from the intestine. J Immunol 178: 3757–3766.

Gomez-Nicola D, Fransen NL, Suzzi S et al. (2013). Regulation of microglial proliferation during chronic neurodegeneration. J Neurosci 33: 2481–2493.

Gomez-Nicola D, Schetters STT, Perry VH (2014). Differential role of CCR2 in the dynamics of microglia and perivascular macrophages during prion disease. GLIA 62: 1041–1052.

Gonzalez L, Dagleish MP, Bellworthy SJ et al. (2006). Postmortem diagnosis of preclinical and clinical scrapie in sheep by the detection of disease-associated PrP in their rectal mucosa. Vet Rec 158: 325–331.

Gonzalez L, Martin S, Siso S et al. (2009). High prevalence of scrapie in a dairy goat herd: tissue distribution of disease-associated PrP and effect of PRNP genotype and age. Vet Res 40: 65.

Gonzalez-Hernandez MB, Liu T, Payne HC et al. (2014). Efficient norovirus and reovirus replication in the mouse intestine requires microfold (M) cells. J Virol 88: 6934–6943.

Gossner A, Hunter N, Hopkins J (2005). Role of lymph-borne cells in the early stages of scrapie agent dissemination from the skin. Vet Immunol Immunopathol 109: 267–278.

Gousset K, Schiff E, Langevin C et al. (2009). Prions hijack tunnelling nanotubes for intercellular spread. Nat Cell Biol 11: 328–336.

Gresser I, Maury C, Chandler RL (1983). Failure to modify scrapie in mice by administration of interferon or anti-interferon globulin. J Gen Virol 64: 1387–1389.

Gunn MD, Ngo VN, Ansel KM et al. (1998). A B-cell-homing chemokine made in lymphoid follicles activates Burkitt's lymphoma receptor-1. Nature 391: 799–803.

Hase K, Kawano K, Nochi T et al. (2009). Uptake through glycoprotein 2 of FimH+ bacteria by M cells initiates mucosal immune responses. Nature 462: 226–231.

Haybaeck J, Heikenwalder M, Klevenz B et al. (2011). Aerosols transmit prions to immunocompetent and immunodeficient mice. PLoS Pathog 7: e1001257.

Heesters BA, Chatterjee P, Kim YA et al. (2013). Endocytosis and recycling of immune complexes by follicular dendritic cells enhances B cell antigen binding and activation. Immunity 38: 1164–1175.

Heesters BA, Myers RC, Carroll MC (2014). Follicular dendritic cells: dynamic antigen libraries. Nat Rev Immunol 14: 495–504.

Heggebø R, Press CM, Gunnes G et al. (2000). Distribution of prion protein in the ileal Peyer's patch of scrapie-free lambs and lambs naturally and experimentally exposed to the scrapie agent. J Gen Virol 81: 2327–2337.

Heggebø R, Press CM, Gunnes G et al. (2002). Distribution and accumulation of PrP in gut-associated and peripheral lymphoid tissue of scrapie-affected Suffolk sheep. J Gen Virol 83: 479–489.

Heikenwalder M, Zeller N, Seeger H et al. (2005). Chronic lymphocytic inflammation specifies the organ tropism of prions. Science 307: 1107–1110.

Heikenwalder M, Kurrer MO, Margalith I et al. (2008). Lymphotoxin-dependent prion replication in inflammatory stromal cells of granulomas. Immunity 29: 998–1008.

Heppner FL, Christ AD, Klein MA et al. (2001). Transepithelial prion transport by M cells. Nat Med 7: 976–977.

Hill AF, Desbruslais M, Joiner S et al. (1997a). The same prion strain causes vCJD and BSE. Nature 389: 448–450.

Hill AF, Zeidler M, Ironside J et al. (1997b). Diagnosis of new variant Creutzfeldt–Jakob disease by tonsil biopsy. Lancet 349: 99–100.

Hilton D, Fathers E, Edwards P et al. (1998). Prion immunoreactivity in appendix before clinical onset of variant Creutzfeldt–Jakob disease. Lancet 352: 703–704.

Hilton DA, Ghani AC, Conyers L et al. (2002). Accumulation of prion protein in tonsil and appendix: review of tissue samples. Br Med J 325: 633–634.

Hilton DA, Ghani AC, Conyers L et al. (2004). Prevalence of lymphoreticular prion protein accumulation in UK tissue samples. J Pathol 203: 733–739.

Ho L-J, Wang J-J, Shaio M-F et al. (2001). Infection of human dendritic cells by dengue virus causes cell maturation and cytokine production. J Immunol 166: 1499–1506.

Ho AW, Prabhu N, Betts RJ et al. (2011). Lung CD103+ dendritic cells efficiently transport infuenza virus to the lymph node and load viral antigen onto MHC class I for presentation to CD8 T cells. J Immunol 187: 6011–6021.

Hoffmann C, Eiden M, Kaatz M et al. (2011). BSE infectivity in jejunum, ileum and ileocaecal junction of incubating cattle. Vet Res 42: 21.

Horiuchi M, Furuoka H, Kitamura N et al. (2006). Alymphoplasia mice are resistant to prion infection via oral route. Jpn J Vet Res 53: 149–157.

Houston SA, Cerovic V, Thomson C et al. (2016). The lymph nodes draining the small intestine and colon are anatomically separate and immunologically distinct. Mucosal Immunol 9: 468–478.

Huang F-P, Platt N, Wykes M et al. (2000). A discrete subpopulation of dendritic cells transports apoptotic intestinal epithelial cells to T cell areas of mesenteric lymph nodes. J Exp Med 191: 435–443.

Huang F-P, Farquhar CF, Mabbott NA et al. (2002). Migrating intestinal dendritic cells transport PrPSc from the gut. J Gen Virol 83: 267–271.

Hunter N, Houston F, Foster J et al. (2012). Susceptibility of young sheep to oral infection with bovine spongiform encephalopathy decreases significantly after weaning. J Virol 86: 11856–11862.

Ierna MI, Farquhar CF, Outram GW et al. (2006). Resistance of neonatal mice to scrapie is associated with inefficient infection of the immature spleen. J Virol 80: 474–482.

Iwasaki A, Kelsalla BA (2000). Localization of distinct Peyer's patch dendritic cell subsets and their recruitment by chemokines macrophage inflammatory protein (MIP)-3, MIP-3ß, and secondary lymphoid organ chemokine. J Exp Med 191: 1381–1394.

Jamieson E, Jeffrey M, Ironside JW et al. (2001). Apoptosis and dendritic dysfunction precede prion protein accumulation in 87V scrapie. Neuroreport 12: 2147–2153.

Jang MH, Sougawa N, Tanaka T et al. (2006). CCR7 is critically important for migration of dendritic cells in intestinal lamina propria to mesenteric lymph nodes. J Immunol 176: 803–810.

Jeffrey M, Halliday WG, Bell J et al. (2000a). Synapse loss associated with abnormal PrP precedes neuronal degeneration in the scrapie-infected hippocampus. Neuropathol Appl Neurobiol 26: 41–54.

Jeffrey M, McGovern G, Goodsir CM et al. (2000b). Sites of prion protein accumulation in scrapie-infected mouse spleen revealed by immuno-electron microscopy. J Pathol 191: 323–332.

Jeffrey M, González L, Espenes A et al. (2006). Transportation of prion protein across the intestinal mucosa of scrapie-susceptible and scrapie-resistant sheep. J Pathol 209: 4–14.

Jouvin-Marche E, Attuli-Audenis V, Aude-Garcia C et al. (2006). Overexpression of cellular prion protein induces and antioxidant environment altering T cell development in the thymus. J Immunol 176: 3490–3497.

Julius C, Heikenwalder M, Schwarz P et al. (2008). Prion propagation in mice lacking central nervous system NF-kappaB signalling. J Gen Virol 89: 1545–1550.

Kapasi ZF, Burton GF, Schultz LD et al. (1993). Induction of functional follicular dendritic cell development in severe combined immunodeficiency mice. J Immunol 150: 2648–2658.

Keane D, Barr D, Osborn R et al. (2009). Validation of use of rectoanal mucosa-associated lymphoid tissue for immunohistochemical diagnosis of chronic wasting disease in white-tailed deer (*Odocoileus virginianus*). J Clin Microbiol 47: 1412–1417.

Kimberlin RH, Walker CA (1989). Pathogenesis of scrapie in mice after intragastric infection. Virus Res 12: 213–220.

Kincaid AE, Hudson KF, Richey MW et al. (2012). Rapid transepithelial transport of prions following inhalation. J Virol 86: 12731–12740.

Kitamoto T, Muramoto T, Mohri S et al. (1991). Abnormal isoform of prion protein accumulates in follicular dendritic cells in mice with Creutzfeldt–Jakob disease. J Virol 65: 6292–6295.

Klein MA, Frigg R, Flechsig E et al. (1997). A crucial role for B cells in neuroinvasive scrapie. Nature 390: 687–691.

Klein MA, Frigg R, Raeber AJ et al. (1998). PrP expression in B lymphocytes is not required for prion neuroinvasion. Nat Med 4: 1429–1433.

Klein MA, Kaeser PS, Schwarz P et al. (2001). Complement facilitates early prion pathogenesis. Nat Med 7: 488–492.

Knoop KA, Kumar N, Butler BR et al. (2009). RANKL is necessary and sufficient to initiate development of antigen-sampling M cells in the intestinal epithelium. J Immunol 183: 5738–5747.

Kobayashi A, Donaldson DS, Erridge C et al. (2013). The functional maturation of M cells is dramatically reduced in the Peyer's patches of aged mice. Mucosal Immunol 6: 1027–1037.

Kolawole AO, Gonzalez-Hernandez MB, Turula H et al. (2015). Oral norovirus infection is blocked in mice lacking Peyer's patches and mature M cells. J Virol 90: 1499–1506.

Konold T, Moore SJ, Bellworthy SJ et al. (2008). Evidence of scrapie transmission via milk. BMC Vet Res 4: 14.

Konold T, Moore SJ, Bellworthy SJ et al. (2013). Evidence of effective scrapie transmission via colostrum and milk in sheep. BMC Vet Res 9: 99.

Konold T, Thorne L, Simmons HA et al. (2016). Evidence of scrapie transmission to sheep via goat milk. BMC Vet Res 208: 208.

Kranich J, Krautler NJ, Falsig J et al. (2010). Engulfment of cerebral apoptotic bodies controls the course of prion disease in a mouse strain-dependent manner. J Exp Med 207: 2271–2281.

Krautler NJ, Kana V, Kranich J et al. (2012). Follicular dendritic cells emerge from ubiquitous perivascular precursors. Cell 150: 194–206.

Küffer A, Lakkraju AK, Mogha A et al. (2016). The prion protein is an agonistic ligand of the G protein-coupled receptor Adgrg6. Nature 536: 464–468.

Kujala P, Raymond C, Romeijn M et al. (2011). Prion uptake in the gut: identification of the first uptake and replication sites. PLoS Pathog 7: e1002449.

Langevin C, Gousset K, Costanzo M et al. (2010). Characterization of the role of dendritic cells in prion transfer to primary neurons. Biochem J 431: 189–198.

Lasmezas CI (2003). Putative functions of PrPC. Br Med Bull 66: 61–70.

Legname G, Baskakov IV, Nguyen H-OB et al. (2004). Synthetic mammalian prions. Science 305: 673–676.

Leon B, Ballesteros-Tato A, Browning JL et al. (2012). Regulation of T(H)2 development by CXCR5+ dendritic cells and lymphotoxin-expressing B cells. Nat Immunol 13: 681–690.

Levavasseur E, Matharom P, Dorban G et al. (2007). Experimental scrapie in 'plt' mice: an assessment of the role of dendritic-cell migration in the pathogenesis of prion diseases. J Gen Virol 88: 2353–2360.

Ligios C, Sigurdson C, Santucciu C et al. (2005). PrPSc in mammary glands of sheep affected by scrapie and mastitis. Nat Med 11: 1137–1138.

Ligios C, Cancedda MG, Carta A et al. (2011). Sheep with scrapie and mastitis transmit infectious prions through the milk. J Virol 85: 1136–1139.

Liu M, MacPherson GG (1993). Antigen acquisition by dendritic cells: intestinal dendritic cells acquire antigen administered orally and can prime naive T cells in vivo. J Exp Med 177: 1299–1307.

Llewelyn CA, Hewitt PE, Knight RSG et al. (2004). Possible transmission of variant Creutzfeldt–Jakob disease by blood transfusion. Lancet 363: 417–421.

Loeuillet C, Lemaire-Vielle C, Naquet P et al. (2010). Prion replication in the hematopoietic compartment is not required for neuroinvasion in scrapie mouse model. PLoS One 5: e13166.

Lunnon K, Teeling JL, Tutt AL et al. (2011). Systemic inflammation modulates Fc receptor expression on microglia during chronic neurodegeneration. J Immunol 186: 7215–7224.

Mabbott NA (2015). Prospects for safe and effective vaccines against prion diseases. Expert Rev Vaccines 14: 1–4.

Mabbott NA, Bruce ME (2004). Complement component C5 is not involved in scrapie pathogenesis. Immunobiology 209: 545–549.

Mabbott NA, MacPherson GG (2006). Prions and their lethal journey to the brain. Nat Rev Microbiol 4: 201–211.

Mabbott NA, Brown KL, Manson J et al. (1997). T lymphocyte activation and the cellular form of the prion protein. Immunology 92: 161–165.

Mabbott NA, Mackay F, Minns F et al. (2000a). Temporary inactivation of follicular dendritic cells delays neuroinvasion of scrapie. Nat Med 6: 719–720.

Mabbott NA, Williams A, Farquhar CF et al. (2000b). Tumor necrosis factor-alpha-deficient, but not interleukin-6-deficient, mice resist peripheral infection with scrapie. J Virol 74: 3338–3344.

Mabbott NA, Bruce ME, Botto M et al. (2001). Temporary depletion of complement component C3 or genetic deficiency of C1q significantly delays onset of scrapie. Nat Med 7: 485–487.

Mabbott NA, McGovern G, Jeffrey M et al. (2002). Temporary blockade of the tumour necrosis factor signaling pathway impedes the spread of scrapie to the brain. J Virol 76: 5131–5139.

Mabbott NA, Young J, McConnell I et al. (2003). Follicular dendritic cell dedifferentiation by treatment with an inhibitor of the lymphotoxin pathway dramatically reduces scrapie susceptibility. J Virol 77: 6845–6854.

Mabbott NA, Baillie JC, Hume DA et al. (2010). Meta-analysis of co-expressed gene signatures in mouse leukocyte populations. Immunobiology 215: 724–736.

Mabbott NA, Bailie JK, Kobayashi A et al. (2011). Expression of mesenchyme-specific gene signatures by follicular dendritic cells: insights from the meta-analysis of microarray data from multiple mouse cell populations. Immunology 133: 482–498.

Mabbott NA, Donaldson DS, Ohno H et al. (2013). Microfold (M) cells: important immunosurveillance posts in the intestinal epithelium. Mucosal Immunol 6: 666–677.

Mabbott NA, Kobayashi A, Sehgal A et al. (2015). Aging and the mucosal immune system in the intestine. Biogerontology 16: 133–145.

Mackay F, Browning JL (1998). Turning off follicular dendritic cells. Nature 395: 26–27.

Macpherson AJ, Uhr T (2004). Induction of protective IgA by intestinal dendritic cells carrying commensal bacteria. Science 303: 1662–1665.

Maignien T, Shakweh M, Calvo P et al. (2005). Role of gut macrophages in mice orally contaminated with scrapie or BSE. Int J Pharm 298: 293–304.

Manson JC, Clarke AR, Hooper ML et al. (1994a). 129/Ola mice carrying a null mutation in PrP that abolishes mRNA production are developmentally normal. Mol Neurobiol 8: 121–127.

Manson JC, Clarke AR, McBride PA et al. (1994b). PrP gene dosage determines the timing but not the final intensity or distribution of lesions in scrapie pathology. Neurodegeneration 3: 331–340.

Marella M, Chabry J (2004). Neurons and astrocytes respond to prion infection by inducing microglia recruitment. J Neurosci 243: 620–627.

Marijanovic Z, Caputo A, Campana V et al. (2009). Identification of an intracellular site of prion conversion. PLoS Pathog 5: e1000426.

Martínez del Hoyo G, López-Bravo M, Metharom P et al. (2006). Prion protein expression by mouse dendritic cells is restricted to the nonplasmacytoid subsets and correlates with the maturation state. J Immunol 177: 6137–6142.

Mathiason CK, Hayes-Klug J, Hays SA et al. (2010). B cells and platelets harbour prion infectivity in the blood of deer infected with chronic wasting disease. J Virol 84: 5097–5107.

McBride PA, Beekes M (1999). Pathological PrP is abundant in sympathetic and sensory ganglia of hamsters fed with scrapie. Neurosci Lett 265: 135–138.

McBride P, Eikelenboom P, Kraal G et al. (1992). PrP protein is associated with follicular dendritic cells of spleens and lymph nodes in uninfected and scrapie-infected mice. J Pathol 168: 413–418.

McBride PA, Schulz-Shaeffer WJ, Donaldson M et al. (2001). Early spread of scrapie from the gastrointestinal tract to the central nervous system involves autonomic fibers of the splanchnic and vagus nerves. J Virol 75: 9320–9327.

McCulloch L, Brown KL, Bradford BM et al. (2011). Follicular dendritic cell-specific prion protein (PrPC) expression alone is sufficient to sustain prion infection in the spleen. PLoS Pathog 7: e1002402.

McCulloch L, Brown KL, Mabbott NA (2013). Ablation of the cellular prion protein, PrPC, specifcally on follicular dendritic cells has no effect on their maturation or function. Immunology 138: 246–257.

McFarlin DE, Raff MC, Simpson E et al. (1971). Scrapie in immunologically deficient mice. Nature 233: 336.

McGovern G, Brown KL, Bruce ME et al. (2004). Murine scrapie infection causes an abnormal germinal centre reaction in the spleen. J Comp Pathol 130: 181–194.

McGovern G, Mabbott NA, Jeffrey M (2009). Scrapie affects the maturation cycle and immune complex trapping by follicular dendritic cells in mice. PLoS One 4: e8186.

Michel B, Ferguson A, Johnson T et al. (2012a). Genetic depletion of complement receptors CD21/35 prevents terminal prion disease in a mouse model of chronic wasting disease. J Immunol 189: 4520–4527.

Michel B, Meyerett-Reid C, Johnson T et al. (2012b). Incunabular immunological events in prion trafficking. Sci Rep 2: 440.

Michel B, Ferguson A, Johnson T et al. (2013). Complement protein C3 exacerbates prion disease in a mouse model of chronic wasting disease. Int Immunol 25: 697–702.

Minghetti L, Greco A, Cardone F et al. (2000). Increased brain synthesis of prostaglandin E2 and F2-isoprostane in human and experimental transmissible spongiform encephalopathies. J Neuropathol Exp Neurol 59: 866–871.

Mishra RS, Basu S, Gu Y et al. (2004). Protease-resistant human prion protein and ferritin are cotransported across Caco-2 epithelial cells: Implications for species barrier in prion uptake from the intestine. J Neurosci 24: 11280–11290.

Mitchell DA, Kirby L, Paulin SM et al. (2007). Prion protein activates and fixes complement directly via the classical pathway: Implications for the mechanism of scrapie agent propagation in lymphoid tissue. Mol Immunol 44: 2997–3004.

Miyazawa K, Kanaya T, Tanaka S et al. (2007). Immunohistochemical characterization of cell types expressing the cellular prion protein in the small intestine of cattle and mice. Histocem Cell Biol 127: 291–301.

Miyazawa K, Kanaya T, Takakura I et al. (2010). Transcytosis of murine-adapted bovine spongiform encephalopathy agents in an in vitro bovine M cell model. J Virol 84: 12285–12291.

Mohan J, Brown KL, Farquhar CF et al. (2004). Scrapie transmission following exposure through the skin is dependent on follicular dendritic cells in lymphoid tissues. J Dermatol Sci 35: 101–111.

Mohan J, Bruce ME, Mabbott NA (2005). Follicular dendritic cell dedifferentiation reduces scrapie susceptibility following inoculation via the skin. Immunology 114: 225–234.

Mok SW, Proia RL, Brinkmann V et al. (2012). B cell-specific S1PR1 deficiency blocks prion dissemination between secondary lymphoid organs. J Immunol 188: 5032–5040.

Monello RJ, Powers JG, Hobbs NT et al. (2013). Efficacy of antemortem rectal biopsies to diagnose and estimate prevalence of chronic wasting disease in free-ranging cow elk (*Cervus elaphus nelsoni*). J Wildl Dis 49: 270–278.

Montrasio F, Frigg R, Glatzel M et al. (2000). Impaired prion replication in spleens of mice lacking functional follicular dendritic cells. Science 288: 1257–1259.

Montrasio F, Cozzio A, Flechsig E et al. (2001). B-lymphocyte-restricted expression of the prion protein does not enable prion replication in PrP knockout mice. Proc Natl Acad Sci, USA 98: 4034–4037.

Moreno JA, Radford H, Peretti D et al. (2012). Sustained translational repression by eIF2-P mediates prion neurodegeneration. Nature 485: 507–511.

Mutoh M, Kimura S, Takashi-Iwanaga H et al. (2016). RANKL regulates differentiation of microfold cells in mouse nasopharynx-associated lymphoid tissue (NALT). Cell Tissue Res 364: 175–184.

Nair VR, Franco LH, Zacharia VM et al. (2016). Microfold cells actively translocate Mycobacterium tuberculosis to initiate infection. Cell Rep 16: 1253–1258.

Nakato G, Fukuda S, Hase K et al. (2009). New approach for M-cell-specific molecules by screening comprehensive transcriptome analysis. DNA Res 16: 227–235.

Nakato G, Hase K, Suzuki M et al. (2012). Cutting edge: *Brucella abortus* exploits a cellular prion protein on intestinal M cells as an invasive receptor. J Immunol 189: 1540–1544.

Nuvolone M, Sorce S, Schwarz P et al. (2015). Prion pathogenesis in the absence of NLRP3/ASC inflammasomes. PLoS One 10: e0117208.

O'Connor T, Frei N, Sponarova J et al. (2012). Lymphotxin, but not TNF, is required for prion invasion of lymph nodes. PLoS Pathog 8: e1002867.

Outram GW, Dickinson AG, Fraser H (1973). Developmental maturation of susceptibility to scrapie in mice. Nature 241: 536–537.

Pan K-M, Baldwin M, Nguyen J et al. (1993). Conversion of alpha-helices into beta-sheets features in the formation of the scrapie prion protein. Proc Natl Acad Sci, USA 90: 10962–10966.

Peden AH, Head MW, Ritchie DL et al. (2004). Preclinical vCJD after blood transfusion in a PRNP codon 129 heterozygous patient. Lancet 354: 527–529.

Prinz M, Priller J (2014). Microglia and brain macrophages in the molecular age: from origin to neuropsychiatric disease. Nat Rev Neurosci 15: 300–312.

Prinz M, Montrasio F, Klein MA et al. (2002). Lymph nodal prion replication and neuroinvasion in mice devoid of follicular dendritic cells. Proc Natl Acad Sci, USA 99: 919–924.

Prinz M, Heikenwalder M, Junt T et al. (2003a). Positioning of follicular dendritic cells within the spleen controls prion neuroinvasion. Nature 425: 957–962.

Prinz M, Huber G, Macpherson AJS et al. (2003b). Oral prion infection requires normal numbers of Peyer's patches but not of enteric lymphocytes. Am J Pathol 162: 1103–1111.

Prusiner SB, Groth D, Serban A et al. (1993). Ablation of the prion protein (PrP) gene in mice prevents scrapie and facilitates production of anti-PrP antibodies. Proceedings of the National Academy of Sciences USA 90: 10608–10612.

Prusiner SB, Scott MR, DeArmond SJ et al. (1998). Prion protein biology. Cell 93: 337–348.

Raeber AJ, Sailer A, Hegyi I et al. (1999). Ectopic expression of prion protein (PrP) in T lymphocytes or hepatocytes of PrP knockout mice is insufficient to sustain prion replication. Proceedings of the National Academy of Sciences. USA 96: 3987–3992.

Raymond CR, Aucouturier P, Mabbott NA (2007). In vivo depletion of CD11c+ cells impairs scrapie agent neuroinvasion from the intestine. J Immunol 179: 7758–7766.

Reimer C, Schultz J, Burwinkel M et al. (2008). Accelerated prion replication in, but prolonged survival times of, prion-infected CXCR3-/- mice. J Virol 82: 12464–12471.

Requena JR, Kristensson K, Korth C et al. (2016). The priority position paper: protecting Europe's food chain from prions. Prion 10: 165–181.

Riek R, Hornemann S, Wider G et al. (1997). NMR characterization of the full-length recombinant murine prion protein, mPrP. FEBS Lett 413: 282–288.

Rios D, Wood MB, Li J et al. (2016). Antigen sampling by intestinal M cells is the principal pathway initiating mucosal IgA production to commensal enteric bacteria. Mucosal Immunol 9: 907–916.

Saeki H, Wu M, Olasz E et al. (2000). A migratory population of skin-derived dendritic cells expresses CXCR5, responds to B lymphocyte chemoattractant in vitro, and co-localizes to B cell zones in lymph nodes in vivo. Eur J Immunol 30: 2808–2814.

Sakhon OS, Ross B, Gusti V et al. (2015). M cell-derived vesicles suggest a unique pathway for trans-epithelial antigen delivery. Tissue Barriers 3: e1004975.

Sassa Y, Kataoka N, Inoshima Y et al. (2010). Anti-PrP antibodies detected at terminal stage of prion-affected mouse. Cell Immunol 263: 212–218.

Schlomchik MJ, Radebold K, Duclos N et al. (2001). Neuroinvasion by a Creutzfeldt–Jakob disease agent in the absence of B cells and follicular dendritic cells. Proc Natl Acad Sci, USA 98: 9289–9294.

Schmidt TH, Bannard O, Gray EE et al. (2013). CXCR4 promotes B cell egress from Peyer's patches. J Exp Med 210: 1099–1107.

Schultz J, Schwarz A, Neidhold S et al. (2004). Role of interleukin-1 in prion disease-associated astrocyte activation. Am J Pathol 165: 671–678.

Seeger H, Heikenwalder M, Zeller N et al. (2005). Coincident scrapie infection and nephritis lead to urinary prion excretion. Science 310: 324–326.

Sethi S, Kerksiek KM, Brocker T et al. (2007). Role of the CD8+ dendritic cell subset in transmission of prions. J Virol 81: 4877–4880.

Shortman K, Liu Y-J (2002). Mouse and human dendritic cell subtypes. Nat Rev Immunol 2: 151–161.

Sigurdson CJ, Williams ES, Miller MW et al. (1999). Oral transmission and early lymphoid tropism of chronic wasting disease PrPres in mule deer fawns (*Odocoileus hemionus*). J Gen Virol 80: 2757–2764.

Sigurdson CJ, Heikenwalder M, Manco G et al. (2009). Bacterial colitis increases susceptibility to oral prion pathogenesis. J Infect Dis 199: 243–252.

Sigurdsson EM, Brown DR, Daniels M et al. (2002). Immunization delays the onset of prion disease in mice. Am J Pathol 161: 13–17.

Sim RB, Kishore U, Villiers CL et al. (2007). C1q binding and complement activation by prions and amyloid. Immunobiology 212: 355–362.

Šišková Z, Reynolds RA, O'Connor V et al. (2013). Brain region specific pre-synaptic and post-synaptic degeneration are early components of neuropathology in prion disease. PLoS One 8: e55004.

Sisó S, González L, Jeffrey M et al. (2006). Prion protein in kidneys of scrapie-infected sheep. Vet Rec 159: 327–328.

Somerville RA, Birkett CR, Farquhar CF et al. (1997). Immunodetection of PrPSc in spleens of some scrapie-infected sheep but not BSE-infected cows. J Gen Virol 78: 2389–2396.

Sowinski S, Jolly C, Berninghausen O et al. (2008). Membrane nanotubes physically connect T cells over long distances presenting a novel route for HIV-1 transmission. Nat Cell Biol 10: 211–219.

Spraker TR, Gidlewski TL, Balachandran A et al. (2006). Detection of PrPCWD in postmortem rectal lymphoid tissues in Rocky Mountain elk (*Cervus elaphus nelsoni*) infected with chronic wasting disease. J Vet Diagn Investig 18: 553–557.

Spraker TR, VerCauteren KC, Gidlewski T et al. (2009a). Antermortem detection of PrPCWD in preclinical, ranch-raised Rocky Mountain elk (*Cervus elaphus nelsoni*) by biopsy of the rectal mucosa. J Vet Diagnost Invest 21: 15–24.

Spraker TR, VerCauteren KC, Gidlewski TL et al. (2009b). Impact of age and sex of Rocky Mountain elk (*Cervus elaphus nelsoni*) on follicle counts from rectal mucosal biopsies for preclinical detection of chronic wasting disease. J Vet Diagnost Invest 21: 868–870.

St. Rose S, Hunter N, Matthews D et al. (2006). Comparative evidence for a link between Peyer's patch development and susceptibility to transmissible spongiform encephalopathies. BMC Infect Dis 6: 5.

St. Rose SG, Hunter N, Foster JD et al. (2007). Quantification of Peyer's patches in Cheviot sheep for future scrapie pathogenesis studies. Vet Immunol Immunopathol 116: 163–171.

Steinman RM, Granelli-Piperno A, Pope M et al. (2003). The interaction of immunodeficiency viruses with dendritic cells. Curr Top Microbiol Immunol 276: 1–30.

Suzuki K, Grigorova I, Phan TG et al. (2009). Visualizing B cell capture of cognate antigen from follicular dendritic cells. J Exp Med 206: 1485–1493.

Tabouret G, Lacroux C, Lugan S et al. (2010). Relevance of oral experimental challenge with classical scrapie in sheep. J Gen Virol 91: 2139–2144.

Tahoun A, Mahajan S, Paxton E et al. (2012). Salmonella transforms follicle-associated epithelial cells into M cells to promote intestinal invasion. Cell Host Microbe 12: 645–666.

Takakura I, Miyazawa K, Kanaya T et al. (2011). Orally administered prion protein is incorporated by M cells and spreads to lymphoid tissues with macrophages in prion protein knockout mice. Am J Pathol 179: 1301–1309.

Tamguney G, Giles K, Glidden DV et al. (2008). Genes contributing to prion pathogenesis. J Gen Virol 98: 1777–1788.

Tanaka Y, Sadaike T, Inoshima Y et al. (2012). Characterisation of PrPSc transmission from immune cells to neuronal cells. Cell Immunol 279: 145–150.

Terahara K, Yoshida M, Igarashi O et al. (2008). Comprehensive gene expression profiling of Peyer's patch M cells, villous M-like cells, and intestinal epithelial cells. J Immunol 180: 7840–7846.

Terry LA, Marsh S, Ryder SJ et al. (2003). Detection of disease-specific PrP in the distal ileum of cattle exposed orally to the agent of bovine spongiform encephalopathy. Vet Rec 152: 387–392.

Thackray AM, McKenzie AN, Klein MA et al. (2004). Accelerated prion disease pathogenesis in the absence of interleukin-10. J Virol 78: 13697–13707.

Thomsen BV, Schneider DA, O'Rourke KI et al. (2012). Diagnostic accuracy of rectal mucosa biopsy testing for chronic wasting disease within white-tailed deer (*Odocoileus virginianus*) herds in North America: effects of age, sex, polymorphism at PRNP codon 96, and disease progression. J Vet Diagnost Invest 24: 878–887.

Tribouillard-Tanvier D, Race B, Striebel JF et al. (2012). Early cytokine elevation, PrPres deposition, and gliosis in mouse scrapie: no effect on disease by deletion of cytokine genes IL-12p40 and IL-12p35. J Virol 86: 10377–10383.

Tsukamoto T, Diringer H, Ludwig H (1985). Absence of autoantibodies against neurofilament proteins in the sera of scarpie infected mice. Tohoku J Exp Med (4): 483–484.

Tumanov AV, Kuprash DV, Lagarkova MA et al. (2002). Distinct role of surface lymphotoxin epxressed by B cells in the organization of secondary lymphoid tissues. Immunity 239: 239–250.

Turner VM, Mabbott NA (2017). Ageing adversely affects the migration and function of marginal zone B cells. Immunology 151: 349–362.

Turner M, Gulbranson-Judge A, Quinn ME et al. (1997). Syk tyrosine kinase is required for the positive selection of immature B cells into the recirculating B cell pool. J Exp Med 186: 2013–2021.

Urayama A, Concha-Marambio L, Khan U et al. (2016). Prions efficiently cross the intestinal barrier after oral administration: Study of the bioavailability, and cellular tissue distribution in vivo. Sci Rep 6: 32338.

van Keulen LJM, Schreuder BEG, Vromans MEW et al. (1999). Scrapie-associated prion protein in the gastro-intestinal tract of sheep with scrapie. J Comp Pathol 121: 55–63.

van Keulen LJ, Schreuder BE, Vromans ME et al. (2000). Pathogenesis of natural scrapie in sheep. Arch Virol Supplementum 16: 57–71.

Van Keulen LJM, Vromans MEW, van Zijderveld FG (2002). Ealry and late pathogenesis of natural scrapie infection in sheep. APMIS 110: 23–32.

Van Keulen LJM, Bossers A, Van Zijderveld FG (2008a). TSE pathogenesis in cattle and sheep. Vet Res 39: 24.

Van Keulen LJM, Vromans MEW, Dolstra CH et al. (2008b). Pathogenesis of bovine spongiform encephalopathy in sheep. Arch Virol 153: 445–453.

Vincenti JE, Murphy L, Grabert K et al. (2016). Defining the microglial response during the time course of chronic neurodegeneration. J Virol 90: 3003–3017.

Walsh DT, Perry VH, Minghetti L (2000). Cyclooxygenase-2 is highly expressed in microglia-like cells in a murine model of prion disease. GLIA 29: 392–396.

Wathne GJ, Kissenpfennig A, Malissen B et al. (2012). Determining the role of mononuclear phagocytes in prion neuroinvasion from the skin. J Leukoc Biol 91: 817–828.

Wells GAH, Dawson M, Hawkins SAC et al. (1994). Infectivity in the ileum of cattle challenged orally with bovine spongiform encephalopathy. Vet Rec 135: 40–41.

Westphal S, Lugering A, von Wedel J et al. (2008). Resistance of chemokine receptor 6-deficient mice to *Yersinia enterocolitica* infection. Evidence of defective M-cell formation in vivo. Am J Path 172: 671–680.

White AR, Enever P, Tayebi M et al. (2003). Monoclonal antibodies inhibit prion replication and delay the development of prion disease. Nature 422: 80–83.

Wilesmith JW, Ryan JB, Atkinson MJ (1991). Bovine spongiform encephalopathy: epidemiological studies of the origin. Vet Rec 218: 199–203.

Wolfe LL, Spraker TR, González L et al. (2007). PrPCWD in rectal lymphoid tissue of deer (*Odocoileus* spp.). J Gen Virol 88: 2078–2082.

Wroe SJ, Pal S, Siddique D et al. (2006). Clinical presentation and pre-mortem diagnosis of variant Creutzfeldt–Jakob disease associated with blood transfusion: a case report. Lancet 368: 2061–2067.

Wu S-JL, Grouard-Vogel G, Sun W et al. (2000). Human skin Langerhans cells are targets of dengue virus infection. Nat Med 6: 816–820.

Wyckoff AC, Kane S, Lockwood K et al. (2016). Clay components in soil dictate environmental stability and bioavailability of cervid prions in mice. Front Microbiol 7: 1885.

Wykes M, Pombo A, Jenkins C et al. (1998). Dendritic cells interact directly with Naive B lymphocytes to transfer antigen and initiate class switching in a primary T-dependent response. J Immunol 161: 1313–1319.

Xu W, Santini PA, Sullivan JS et al. (2009). HIV-1 evades virus-specific IgG2 and IgA responses by targeting systemic conduits and intestinal B cells via long-range intercellular conduits. Nat Immunol 10: 1008–1017.

Xue J, Schmidt SV, Sander J et al. (2014). Transcriptome-based network analysis reveals a spectrum model of human macrophage activation. Immunity 40: 274–288.

Yrlid U, Cerovic V, Milling S et al. (2006). Plasmacytoid dendritic cells do not migrate in intestinal or hepatic lymph. J Immunol 177: 6115–6121.

Yu P, Wang Y, Chin RK et al. (2002). B cells control the migration of a subset of dendritic cells into B cell follicles via CXC chemokine ligand 13 in a lymphotoxin-dependent fashion. J Immunol 168: 5117–5123.

Zabel MD, Heikenwalder M, Prinz M et al. (2007). Stromal complement receptor CD21/35 facilitates lymphoid prion colonization and pathogenesis. J Immunol 179: 6144–6152.

Zhan Y, Paolocelli RC, Sfronazzini F et al. (2014). Deficient neuron-microglia signaling results in impaired functional brain connectivity and social behaviour. Nat Neurosci 17.

Zhu S, Victoria GS, Marzo L et al. (2015). Prion aggregates transfer through tunneling nanotubes in endocytic vesicles. Prion 9: 125–135.

Zhu C, Hermann US, Falsig J et al. (2016). A neuroprotective role for microglia during prion diseaes. J Exp Med 213: 1047–1059.

Section II

Animal prion diseases (clinical, epidemiology, neuropathological, biochemical, biomarker, and genotypes)

Handbook of Clinical Neurology, Vol. 153 (3rd series)
Human Prion Diseases
M. Pocchiari and J. Manson, Editors
https://doi.org/10.1016/B978-0-444-63945-5.00006-4

Chapter 6

Classic and atypical scrapie – a genetic perspective

WILFRED GOLDMANN*

Neurobiology Division, The Roslin Institute and Royal (Dick) School of Veterinary Studies, University of Edinburgh, Easter Bush, United Kingdom

Abstract

Scrapie was the first prion disease to be recognised and the study of this disease in sheep and goats has provided a wealth of information not only for scrapie but also for the other prion diseases. All prion diseases are under strong genetic control of the prion gene *PRNP*, independent of whether they are typical or atypical scrapie and which of the different prion strains is causing infection. Decades of studies using experimental disease challenges and field surveys have established disease association models, in which species-specific amino acid variations in the prion or PrP protein, encoded by the *PRNP* gene, can predict disease susceptibility or resistance. *PRNP* genetics represents an important and successful basis for implementing scrapie eradication strategies in sheep and goats.

In general terms these studies have revealed that there appear to be many more amino acid changes in PrP leading to increased resistance than to higher susceptibility. Most changes are in the globular part of PrP protein and three regions appear to have major influence. This knowledge can be transferred into prion diseases of other species to facilitate genetic control strategies. However, an obstacle remains with the lack of fully understanding the underlying molecular mechanism, impeding our ability to deal with the difference in the genetic control between typical and atypical forms of scrapie or to predict association in newly infected species. This chapter will discuss the advances in both typical and atypical scrapie from a genetic perspective.

INTRODUCTION

Scrapie in sheep was the first prion disease to be recognized, as early as 1732 (Leopoldt, 1750), and was identified in goats by 1942 (Chelle, 1942). Two forms of scrapie are now recognized, known as classic and atypical scrapie, which both occur throughout Europe (EFSA Panel on Biological Hazards (BIOHAZ), 2014) and almost worldwide. Scrapie was proven to be a transmissible agent in 1936 by Cuille and Chelle (1938a, b). In 1967 a protein was proposed as the infectious agent (Pattison and Jones, 1967) and the protein-only hypothesis was put forward (Griffith, 1967), followed by the virino hypothesis (Dickinson and Outram, 1979). The importance of the prion protein (PrP) in controlling susceptibility and resistance to scrapie was recognized in a series of important experiments. Prusiner (1982) introduced the term prion and Oesch et al. (1985) identified the cellular gene encoding the PrP. The PrP gene was then demonstrated to be the major factor controlling incubation time of disease (Dickinson et al., 1968; Carlson et al., 1986; Hunter et al., 1987; Westaway et al., 1987; Moore et al., 1998).

Classic scrapie usually affects sheep around 3–5 years of age. Sheep infected with scrapie can scratch excessively and show patches of wool loss and lesions on the skin, which led to the name scrapie. Progressive neurodegeneration and chronic systemic disease follow, leading to death. Histologic analysis of the central nervous system post mortem shows accumulation of the PrP and abnormal forms of the protein accumulation are detected biochemically in both the central nervous system (CNS) and peripheral tissues. The pattern of CNS pathology is both host gene- (the PrP gene, *PRNP*) and scrapie agent-specific (Begara-McGorum et al., 2002;

*Correspondence to: Wilfred Goldmann, Neurobiology Division, The Roslin Institute, University of Edinburgh, Easter Bush, Midlothian EH25 9RG, United Kingdom. E-mail: wilfred.goldmann@roslin.ed.ac.uk

Ligios et al., 2002). The genetics and control of scrapie in goats are current areas of focus in Europe (Ricci et al., 2017).

A number of strains of classic scrapie have been identified through mouse transmission studies (Bruce, 2003) and, although there is no epidemiologic evidence that scrapie affects humans, a report on transmission of scrapie to transgenic mice expressing the human prion gene (Cassard et al., 2014) suggests that there may not be an absolute barrier to transmission of ovine scrapie to humans, although whether such transmission would occur naturally is not known. The mechanism of transmission between animals has been studied extensively, with evidence for both vertical and horizontal transmission. Environmental contamination is a key source of sheep-to-sheep transmission (van Keulen et al., 2002; Gough and Maddison, 2010; Maddison et al., 2010), along with other routes of transmission, including maternal transmission (Hoinville et al., 2010; Foster et al., 2013; Spiropoulos et al., 2014).

Extensive European surveillance has led to the identification of a different form of scrapie in sheep, known as Nor98 (Benestad et al., 2003) or atypical scrapie, which tends to occur in older animals and animals considered to be resistant to classic scrapie based on *PRNP* genotype (Saunders et al., 2006; Benestad et al., 2008). Retrospective studies demonstrated that this was not a new disease but had already existed as early as 1972 (Chong et al., 2015). Atypical scrapie can be distinguished from classic scrapie both clinically and pathologically. In atypical scrapie cases, the PrP^{TSE} deposition appears as fine punctate to coarse granular deposits in both gray and white matter when examined by immunohistochemistry. Intraneuronal staining has never been reported and the brainstem at the level of the obex has been described as totally negative, contrasting with most of the classic scrapie isolates. The biochemical properties of the disease-associated PrP also differ between classic and atypical scrapie, with the disease-associated PrP showing less resistance to protease K and characteristic low-molecular-weight bands (7–12 kDa) on Western blots, which are not found in classic scrapie (Le Dur et al., 2005).

Differences in the PrP gene have not only led to a greater understanding of the prion diseases in general and the importance of the prion gene in the control of disease, but have also led to specific breeding programs in the United Kingdom and continental Europe with the aim of eradicating scrapie from sheep flocks and populations. This chapter will focus on genetic studies.

GENETIC STUDIES OF SCRAPIE SUSCEPTIBILITY

For the development of scrapie disease and agent replication, PrP has to be expressed (Bueler et al., 1993). The genetics of the *PRNP* gene, which encodes this protein and regulates its expression in various tissues, is therefore crucial for pathogenesis and propagation of the scrapie agent. Consequently, other genes that control the *PRNP* gene or the posttranslational processing of cellular PrP (PrP^C) will also contribute to disease phenotypes and need to be considered in disease.

Disease onset for sheep and goats falls within the reproductive period of the animals and genetic selection may have played a significant role in the distribution of *PRNP* alleles found around the world. Additionally, the *PRNP* gene has normal physiologic functions (Westergard et al., 2007; Bakkebø et al., 2015; Castle and Gill, 2017), which, although largely unknown in detail, may also influence the degree of tolerated allelic variation. Breeding for genetic resistance to scrapie in sheep will ultimately shift allelic frequencies away from their natural balance and gene variants may eventually be lost.

Breeding for typical scrapie resistance in sheep has been applied in Europe for over a decade and, based on the decreasing number of scrapie cases, this method appears very successful (Dawson et al., 2008; Hagenaars et al., 2010). Application of similar selection regimes in goats is currently under consideration (Ricci et al., 2017). All these programs have focused on the natural variation of the *PRNP* gene and evidence from experimental and natural scrapie studies for the association with disease resistance. Whether the progress of genome-editing methods, particularly in livestock species, will become a useful addition to the strategies of scrapie eradication remains to be seen, but this will depend on fully understanding and appreciating the complexity of genetic control of scrapie and PrP^C biology.

The ovine/caprine *PRNP* gene open reading frame consists of 256 amino acid codons. After co- and posttranslational modifications are completed, mature PrP^C protein comprises 210 amino acids. Two N-linked carbohydrate structures and a C-terminal glycolipid membrane anchor result in an apparent molecular weight of 33–35 kDa. Further proteolytic modifications lead to several different secreted and membrane-attached fragments of PrP^C, of which only the full-length protein is able to act as substrate for the pathogenic conversion found in prion diseases (reviewed in Goldmann, 1993; Liang and Kong, 2012).

Three types of polymorphism have been found in ruminant PrP. Single-nucleotide polymorphisms in the DNA lead to amino acid substitution (missense) or translational stop (nonsense), and precise in-frame insertions or deletions of octapeptide repeats of the type PHGGGWGQ in the N-terminal domain.

Compared to other genes, an unusually high number of complete ovine (*Ovis aries*) and caprine (*Capra hircus*) *PRNP* open reading frame sequences have been determined in the past decades, upwards of 30,000 worldwide (Figs 6.1–6.3). These studies revealed a total of 118 polymorphisms, of which 14 are shared between the two species. The current account includes two mutations leading to premature termination of translation in goats (Papasavva-Stylianou et al., 2011; Benestad et al., 2012), three octapeptide repeat number variants (Goldmann et al., 1998; Saunders et al., 2006; Papasavva-Stylianou et al., 2011), and 113 amino acid substitutions (reviewed up to 2008/2009 in Goldmann, 2008; Vaccari et al., 2009b; since then, Serrano et al., 2009; Andrade et al., 2011; Guan et al., 2011; Frootan et al., 2012; Hautaniemi et al., 2012; Piestrzynska-Kajtoch et al., 2012; Taore et al., 2012; Zhao et al., 2012; Acin et al., 2013; Meydan et al., 2013, 2017; Kipanyula et al., 2014; Lan et al., 2014; Maestrale et al., 2015). These amino acid substitutions have been found in 78 out of 256 codons (30%), but the distribution of the polymorphisms is not equal throughout the protein sequence.

High variability is apparent in the highly structured, globular C-terminal domain, with 65 substitutions between codons 126 and 175 and very low variability in the flexible N-terminal domain, with only five

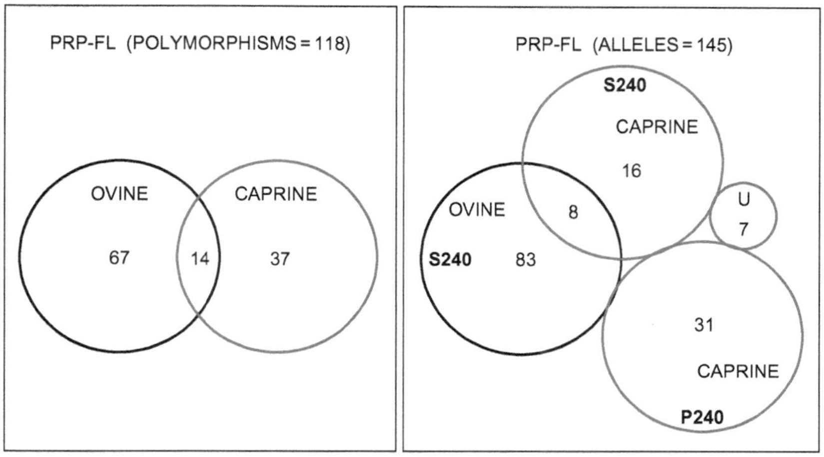

Fig. 6.1. Prion protein (PrP) amino acid variation in sheep and goats. Studies of full-length PrP (PrP-FL) with a length of 256 amino acids have so far revealed 118 polymorphisms and 145 alleles (haplotypes). Alleles in goats are separated into S240 and P240 encoding sequences. U represents caprine sequences undefined at codon 240.

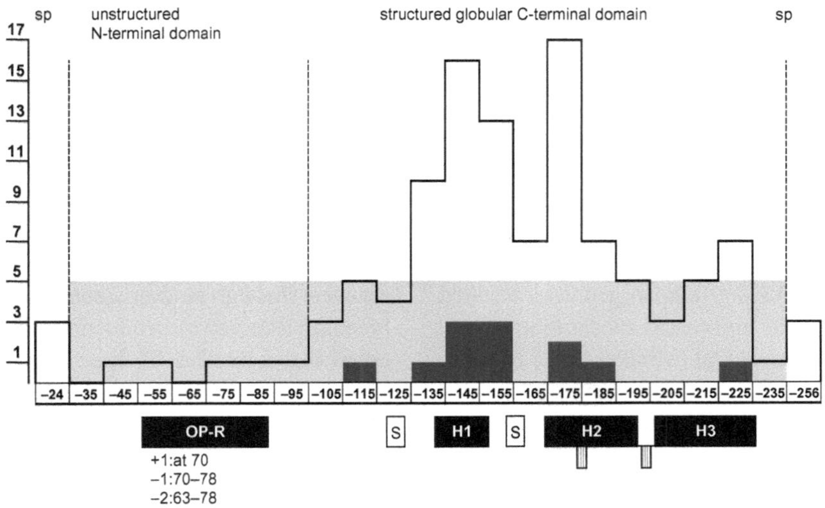

Fig. 6.2. Histogram showing the distribution of amino acid polymorphisms in sheep and goats over the length of the prion protein sequence. The sequence is shown in 10 amino acid steps, with the exception of the N- and C-terminal signal peptides (sp). The structural elements of the protein are depicted at the bottom with three helices (H1, H2, and H3) and two strands (S). The N-terminal domain contains octapeptide repeats (OP-R) which vary in number as indicated. The light-gray shaded area indicates a theoretic equal distribution over the entire sequence of all polymorphisms. The dark-gray shaded area represents amino acids proven to be associated with scrapie susceptibility.

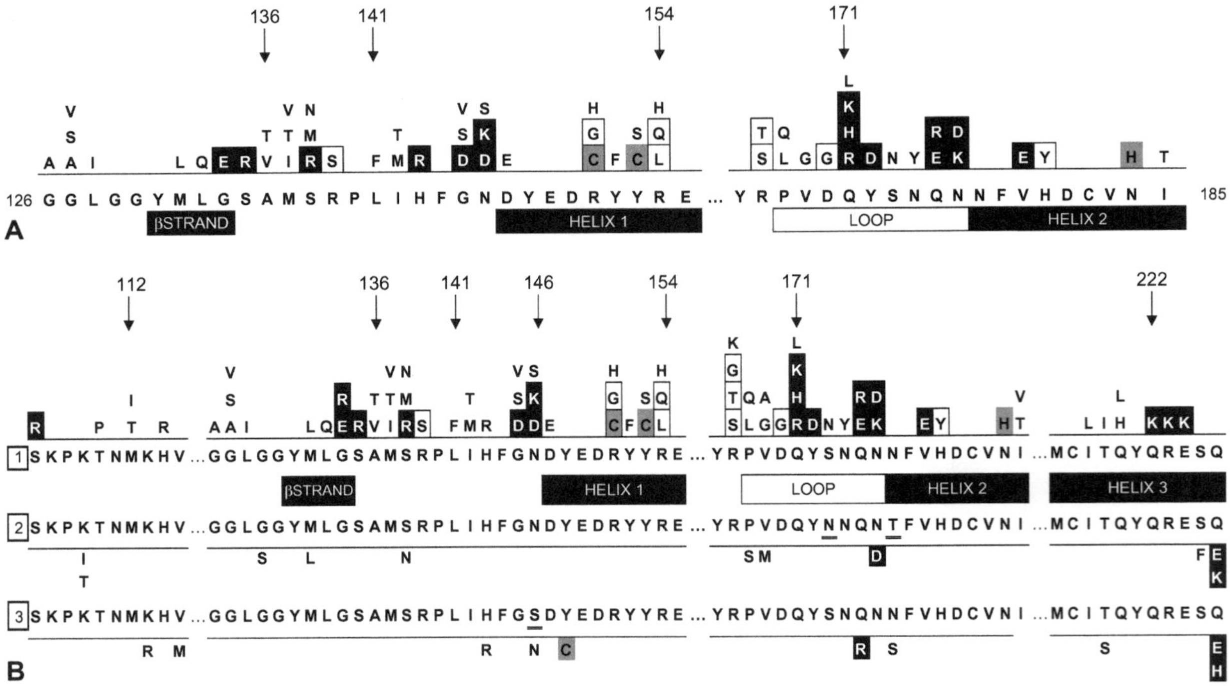

Fig. 6.3. Amino acid changes in prion protein (PrP) core region between codons 126 to 155 and 166 to 185 in sheep and goats. (**A**) The baseline shows the wild-type sheep/goat sequence. White on black background: polymorphisms that introduce or change charged amino acids. Boxed: polymorphisms that remove charged amino acids. Gray shading: new amino acids create or remove posttranslational modification sites. (**B**) (1) is the same as in (**A**) but added for comparison are the equivalent regions of cervine (2) and bovine (3) PrP sequence and known polymorphisms.

substitutions between codons 25 and 94. Altogether 145 different alleles have been found in both species combined, when the entire open reading frame for PrP is considered. However, some of the polymorphisms reside within the N-terminal and C-terminal signal peptides, which are cleaved off during protein maturation. It follows that the mature PrP exists in at least 125 unique variants in these two domesticated ruminants. Whether this sequence variability is exceptional or present in other proteins is currently difficult to say, as few, if any, mammalian proteins have been sequenced to that extent. *PRNP* in other ruminants, such as bovine or cervine species, appears much less variable (Clawson et al., 2006; Robinson et al., 2012). However, analysis of 600,000 human genomes resulted in 180 PrP variants, with amino acid substitutions found in 109 out of 153 codons (43%) (Minikel et al., 2014).

The N-terminus of PrP normally contains three copies of the octapeptide PHGGGWGQ enclosed by two nonapeptides P(Q/H)GGGGWGQ (9-8-8-8-9). Within this configuration the number of octapeptide repeats is polymorphic. While variation in the number of total repeats between four and six is not exceptional amongst species, only one ovine allele with six repeats has been found (Saunders et al., 2006). In goats, two alleles are known with either three or four repeats (Goldmann et al., 1998; Papasavva-Stylianou et al., 2011). An association of scrapie susceptibility and variation in repeat number between three and six remains unproven but possible, whereas variation above eight repeats has been associated in humans with increased risk of developing Creutzfeldt–Jakob disease (Lloyd et al., 2011).

The published record shows ~30% more ovine PrP variants than for caprine PrP, but this is more likely a reflection of the number of surveyed animals for each species than a true variability difference of the sequences. Of course, not all alleles have equal frequencies and a large number appear to be rare, often found in only one or two animals within the surveyed population. However, rare polymorphisms may be maintained rather than lost through random genetic drift because livestock breeding is driven by production values. It should also be noted that a number of these polymorphisms have not been validated by observing the polymorphism in additional samples unrelated to the original set of chromosomes surveyed to define the polymorphism. The resulting ascertainment bias may be considerable for rare *PRNP* alleles.

By common agreement, *PRNP* gene haplotypes are mostly referred to as alleles, particularly in sheep, where they are referred to by amino acids in codons 136, 154, and 171, e.g., ARQ (Hunter, 2003). Additional polymorphisms are sometimes included, for example, L141 or

K176 containing alleles will be described as $AL_{141}RQ$ or $ARQK_{176}$, respectively. While this type of terminology is less commonly used for the caprine *PRNP* gene, references can be found to the wild-type allele as IRRQS (codons 142, 154, 211, 222, 240) or similar (Corbière et al., 2013).

Association of *PRNP* amino acid polymorphisms with scrapie susceptibility/resistance

Genetically modified PrP knockout mouse lines, which do not produce any PrP, do not develop prion disease (Bueler et al., 1993). It is therefore reasonable to assume that sheep and goats without PrP^C expression will be resistant to any prion disease. This benefical effect of a PrP knockout mutation regarding scrapie resistance may however be small compared to potential health defects that *PRNP* null animals may exhibit under normal living conditions. *PRNP* knockout cattle have been produced for research (Richt et al., 2007), but this approach has not yet been used to eradicate scrapie from small ruminant livestock.

Nonsense polymorphisms have been found in a goat on Cyprus (Q163stop) (Papasavva-Stylianou et al., 2011) and in Norwegian white dairy goats (G32stop) (Benestad et al., 2012; Kipanyala et al., 2014). There is so far no evidence from genotyping surveys of European goats that these nonsense mutations occur in any other breeds. Whereas the 163stop mutation was only found in one animal in a heterozgous genotype, the identical mutation found in human early-onset dementia cases suggests that a truncated PrP^C protein is produced from this haplotype with detrimental effects to health. In contrast, the G32stop mutation carriers fail to produce any PrP^C protein, as has been shown for homozygotes. Their susceptibility to scrapie and general health status are currently under investigation, but it would be rather surprising if disease resistance as found in mice would not be the result in these goats.

There are specific *PRNP* genotypes that associate with scrapie susceptibility and incubation period length, but the underlying mechanisms are not fully understood. Major studies in the 1990s, particularly in the United Kingdom, the Netherlands, and France, demonstrated association of scrapie susceptibility with common natural PrP variants in codons 136, 154, and 171 (Goldmann et al., 1991, 1994; Laplanche et al., 1993; Belt et al., 1995). Based on the five alleles found in these sheep populations (ARQ, AHQ, ARR, ARH, VRQ), 15 genotypes were defined i.e., ARR/ARR, VRQ/ARQ, ARH/AHQ, etc. The association of these genotypes with scrapie was established first in experimental scrapie models, but it was soon shown that they are effectively transferred to natural disease (Baylis and Goldmann, 2004). Later, a risk classification system was developed (R1–R5) for sheep (Dawson et al., 2008), which was applied in breeding and scrapie eradication programs in several countries and ultimately led to European Union regulations on *PRNP* genotyping for the control of scrapie and potentially bovine spongiform encephalopathy (BSE) in sheep (Regulation (EC) No 999/2001, 2001).

PRNP genotyping efforts in many countries worldwide uncovered a wide range of novel PrP variants in a large number of breeds and there is as yet no adjustment of the risk group assignment to these new *PRNP* genotypes. For example, it is now known that the number of alleles based on codons 136, 154, and 171 is not five but at least 13 (TRQ (sheep, goat) or ARK, ALQ, AQQ, ARL, VRR, TRR, AHR (sheep)) (Goldmann, 2008; Guan et al., 2011; Zhao et al., 2012). None of these additional variants can be associated unambiguously with disease susceptibility, highlighting our lack of understanding of the underlying molecular mechanisms leading to resistance and the molecular interactions with various scrapie strains.

It was also established in the past decade that on average almost 25% of ovine/caprine ARQ alleles have additional polymorphisms, with fewer variants recognized for the ARR, VRQ, and AHQ alleles (Goldmann, 2008; Vaccari et al., 2009b). Although some of the alleles are low in frequency and consequently the frequency of certain genotype combinations will be very low, it is worth mentioning that at the level of individual flocks/herds their allele frequencies could become significant through founder effects, such as the introduction of a specific ram/buck.

All *PRNP* alleles fall into three fundamental categories: (1) an allele that will enhance susceptibility and/or decrease the incubation period length; (2) an allele that will reduce susceptibility and/or lengthen the incubation period duration, ultimately leading to resistance; and (3) an allele that is neutral with regard to these scrapie disease phenotypes. Of course, there are also alleles for which there are as yet no data to assign them to these categories. The categories are based on relative values and therefore need a reference point, which is normally the wild-type ARQ allele. A further important aspect is the genotype–phenotype relationship due to dominant or recessive alleles.

Category 1: highly susceptible

Rather surprisingly, there are only three alleles known to increase scrapie susceptibility significantly. The first one is the ovine VRQ allele, associated with high susceptibility to many typical scrapie strains. VRQ is dominant over the ARQ allele and codominant with AHQ and ARR, which results in VRQ/ARR and VRQ/AHQ sheep developing disease with longer incubation periods than VRQ/ARQ in experimental scrapie; they also show older age at onset and lower attack rates than VRQ/ARQ in natural scrapie (Baylis and Goldmann, 2004). The VRQ allele defines the highest-risk group in sheep (R5), which are animals that are at greatest risk of developing scrapie themselves and will pass on high susceptibility to their offspring (Dawson et al., 1998). It is however important to note that VRQ/VRQ sheep can survive for a normal lifespan when kept in a scrapie-free environment (Hunter et al., 1997; Hunter and Cairns, 1998).

The other two alleles are $AL_{141}RQ$ and AHQ (ovine and caprine), which enhance the susceptibility to atypical scrapie; both alleles appear dominant over ARQ (Moum et al., 2005).

Category 2: reduced susceptibility or resistance

This category contains several alleles in both species, with a wide range of phenotypes, from delayed clinical disease presentation to lengthened incubation periods to lowered attack rates to almost complete resistance.

Very high resistance is associated with the ovine ARR and caprine ARQ-K_{222} alleles. Both are found exceedingly rarely in natural typical scrapie cases. Only four ARR/ARR animals with natural typical scrapie have ever been confirmed worldwide, covering several thousand scrapie cases collected over a period of almost 30 years (Ikeda et al., 1995; Groschup et al., 2007; Andrade et al., 2015). ARQ-K_{222}/ARQ-K_{222} goats with natural typical scrapie have not yet been found, but heterozygous ARR/ARQ sheep and ARQ-K_{222}/ARQ goats are occasionally observed and are therefore only partially resistant (Baylis and Goldmann, 2004; Corbière et al., 2013). Both alleles have also been associated with complete survival or low attack rates and very long incubation periods after experimental challenges (Acutis et al., 2012; Lacroux et al., 2014, 2017; Aguilar-Calvo et al., 2015). R1 sheep (only ARR/ARR genotype) are the most resistant and when bred randomly their offspring will remain partially resistant (risk groups R1–R4) (Dawson et al., 1998).

It was recently shown that ARR/ARR sheep (Aguilar-Calvo et al., 2015) and ARQ-K_{222}/ARQ-K_{222} goats (Lacroux et al., 2014) can become infected when experimentally challenged by intracerebral inoculation with typical scrapie, but with low attack rates of 5/15 in sheep and 1/5 in goats, and incubation periods of 6–8 years for both species. The significance of this resistance becomes clear when compared to wild-type animals, which have 100% attack rates and incubation times of about a year following an identical inoculation regime.

Strong resistance is also associated with the caprine $AS_{146}RQ$ and $AD_{146}RQ$ alleles, found at high frequencies in Cyprus (Papasavva-Stylianou et al., 2011; Ortiz-Pelaez et al., 2014) and in the Boer goat breed in other European countries (Goldmann et al., 2011). Homozygous $AS_{146}RQ/AS_{146}RQ$ or $AD_{146}RQ/AD_{146}RQ$ goats with natural scrapie have never been confirmed and heterozygotes have extended incubation periods after experimental challenge (White et al., 2012; Papasavva-Stylianou et al., 2017). A few codon 146 heterozygote goats have been found with scrapie and all codon 146 genotypes are susceptible after intracerebral challenge (Papasavva-Stylianou et al., 2017). The $AS_{146}RQ$ allele has also been reported in sheep and is likely to produce a resistance-associated phenotype in sheep too.

Longer incubation periods and lower attack rates of typical scrapie compared to wild type have also been reported for other ovine/caprine alleles, amongst them $T_{112}ARQ$, $AT_{137}RQ$, $AM_{142}RQ$, $AD_{145}RQ$, $AC_{151}RQ$, $ARP_{168}Q$, $ARQK_{176}$ (Goldmann et al., 1996, 2006; Thorgeirsdottir et al., 1999; Saunders et al., 2009; Vaccari et al., 2009a; Maestrale et al., 2015). Interestingly, increased resistance to typical scrapie and ovine BSE is associated with alleles AHQ and $AF_{141}RQ$ (Hunter et al., 2012; Tan et al., 2012), a reversal of their association with atypical scrapie (Colussi et al., 2008). Similarly, it appears that the VRQ allele may have a slight protective effect against atypical scrapie (Moum et al., 2005; Saunders et al., 2006). Lower protection appears to be associated with $S_{127}ARQ$ (Dassanayake et al., 2015), $G_{102}ARQ$ (3 repeats) (Goldmann et al., 1998), and $AR_{143}RQ$ (Billinis et al., 2002).

Category 3: neutral

The assignment as presented above leaves approximately 100 alleles without clear disease association. Whether there are truly disease-neutral substitutions remains to be established. Candidates for neutrality may be substitutions between codons 25 and 85, while studies of chronic wasting disease in deer confirmed that substitutions at N-terminal positions 95/96 are important in disease susceptibility (Robinson et al., 2012). With so many unclassified alleles, it is unlikely that all of them or even the majority can be tested directly for their association with scrapie resistance. Alternatively, theoretic considerations, such as the position of a change relative to established disease-associated substitutions or species comparisons, may lead to clues for their classifications. They will however represent low confidence predictions as the overall PrP sequence in each species is different and single substitutions may only work in a particular sequence context. Ultimately, only investigations of the underlying molecular mechanisms will enhance our predictive ability.

Other factors and genes

The *PRNP* gene in sheep and goats is composed of three exons and has been mapped to chromosome 13. A recently established high-resolution transcriptome atlas for sheep (Clark et al., 2017) has revealed substantial amounts of *PRNP* transcript outside the brain, which may be crucially important for the peripheral pathogenesis of scrapie in sheep and by inference in goats. The amount of PrP, PrP tissue distribution, and temporal availability are all genetically controlled by the gene promoter and enhance/silencer elements. For example, protein DNA-binding studies revealed that two ovine promoter polymorphisms significantly change the binding characteristics of transcription factors and mRNA levels in cell culture (Burgess et al., 2009), but there is as yet no confirmation of an association with transcript levels in vivo or that these polymorphisms are associated with sheep scrapie. An association between *PRNP* transcription level, PrP^C amount, and disease was however found for BSE in cattle (Sander et al., 2005; Juling et al., 2006) and for scrapie in *PRN-P*$^{+/-}$ hemizygous mouse models (Bueler et al., 1994; Tuzi et al., 2004).

Because the availability of full-length PrP^C for disease is essential, any fragmentation of PrP^C is likely to have consequences for scrapie susceptibility or at least for the pathogenesis and thus for incubation period length. Evidence supporting this assumption comes from a study of the resistant ARR/ARR genotype. These sheep exhibited a significantly higher percentage of truncated PrP^C fragment C1 linked to a lower percentage of fragment C2 than wild-type ARQ/ARQ sheep (Campbell et al., 2013). These findings would be in line with our understanding that C1 fragment does not contribute to the prion conversion, whereas C2 may represent a precursor of disease-related PrP^{Sc}.

Shedding of PrP^C from the membrane is another post-translational mechanism that is likely to interfere with the conversion of PrP^{Sc} (Altmeppen et al., 2015). Only a few of the genes responsible for PrP^C processing are known (e.g., *ADAM10*) (Altmeppen et al., 2011); others remain to be discovered, but it is reasonable to speculate that genetic variation in these genes will lead to new genetic associations with disease. Decrease of PrP^C protein during pathogenesis has been shown to occur in parallel to a decrease of the shadoo protein (Mays et al., 2014), encoded by the *SPRN* gene. Sequence variation of shadoo in sheep (Stewart et al., 2009) and goats is known and has already been shown to be associated with resistance in goats (Peletto et al., 2012) and humans (Beck et al., 2008). Further studies of these and similar genes surely will reveal new genetic influences on scrapie in ruminants, most likely in the peripheral replication, pathogenesis, and transport of infection. Of course, studies of experimental scrapie have given the impression that the contribution of PrP^C to disease development is so overwhelming that other genes may have little additional effect. Future investigations of natural TSEs may prove this a false conclusion. Novel genes may lead to finally resolving the genetic control and modulation of atypical and sporadic prion diseases.

CONCLUSIONS

Investigating the general and species-specific mechanisms that link susceptibility of classic and atypical forms of TSEs to genetic variation of the *PRNP* gene encoding the prion or PrP protein has been carried out to predict host disease response and to improve risk assessments and breeding strategies. While scrapie eradication through *PRNP* breeding has been successfully applied to sheep populations throughout the world, other livestock and free-ranging species with TSE disease outbreaks have not yet benefitted from similar genetic selection programs. However, the vast knowledge and experience gained from understanding the genetic control of scrapie provide a platform for the potential control of other prion diseases. Options of genetic control in goat scrapie and chronic wasting disease in American deer are currently under investigation. Genetics studies are being used to understand and predict the spread of chronic wasting disease in deer populations in both North America and in Europe. Moreover, since chronic wasting disease is present in wild deer populations the potential susceptibility of scavengers and carnivores to prion agents is also under investigation through genetic studies.

References

Acin C, Martin-Burriel I, Monleon E et al. (2013). Prion protein gene variability in Spanish goats. Inference through susceptibility to classical scrapie strains and pathogenic distribution of peripheral PrPsc. PLoS One 8: e1118.

Acutis PL, Martucci F, D'Angelo A et al. (2012). Resistance to classical scrapie in experimentally challenged goats carrying mutation K222 of the prion protein gene. Vet Res 43: 8.

Aguilar-Calvo P, Fast C, Tauscher K et al. (2015). Effect of Q211 and K222 PRNP polymorphic variants in the susceptibility of goats to oral infection with goat bovine spongiform encephalopathy. J Infect Dis 212: 664–672.

Altmeppen H, Prox J, Puig B et al. (2011). Lack of a-disintegrin- and -metalloproteinase ADAM10 leads to intracellular accumulation and loss of shedding of the cellular prion protein in vivo. Mol Neurodegener 6: 36.

Altmeppen HD, Prox J, Krasemann S et al. (2015). The sheddase ADAM10 is a potent modulator of prion disease. elife 4: E04260.

Andrade de CP, Almeida LL, Castro LA et al. (2011). Single nucleotide polymorphisms at 15 codons of the prion protein gene from a scrapie-affected herd of Suffolk sheep in Brazil. Pesqui Vet Bras 31: 893–898.

Andrade de CP, de Oliveira EC, Leal JS et al. (2015). Report of outbreaks of classical scrapie in Dorper sheep and associated prion protein gene polymorphisms in affected flocks. Trop Anim Health Prod 47: 1203–1212.

Bakkebø MK, Mouillet-Richard S, Espenes A et al. (2015). The prion protein: a player in immunological quiescence? Front Immunol 6: 450.

Baylis M, Goldmann W (2004). The genetics of scrapie in sheep and goats. Curr Mol Med 4: 385–39625.

Beck JA, Campbell TA, Adamson G et al. (2008). Association of a null allele of SPRN with variant Creutzfeldt-Jakob disease. J Med Genet 45: 813–817.

Begara-McGorum I, Gonzalez L, Simmons M et al. (2002). Vacular lesion profile in sheep scrapie: factors influencing its variation and relationship to disease specific PrP accumulation. J Comp Pathol 127: 59–68.

Belt PBGM, Muileman IH, Schreuder BEC et al. (1995). Identification of five allelic variants of the sheep PrP gene and their association with natural scrapie. J Gen Virol 76: 509–517.

Benestad SL, Sarradin P, Thu B et al. (2003). Cases of scrapie with unusual features in Norway and designation of a new type, Nor98. Vet Rec 153: 202–208.

Benestad SL, Arsca JN, Goldmann W et al. (2008). Atypical/Nor98 scrapie properties of the agent, genetics and epidemiology. Vet Res 39: 19.

Benestad SL, Austbo L, Tranulis MA et al. (2012). Healthy goats naturally devoid of prion protein. Vet Res 43: 87.

Billinis C, Panagiotidis CH, Psychas V et al. (2002). Prion protein gene polymorphisms in natural goat scrapie. J Gen Virol 83: 713–721.

Bruce ME (2003). TSE strain variation. Br Med Bull 66: 99–108.

Bueler H, Aguzzi A, Sailer A et al. (1993). Mice devoid of PrP are resistant to scrapie. Cell 73: 1339–1347.

Bueler H, Raeber A, Sailer A et al. (1994). High prion and PrPSc levels but delayed onset of disease in scrapie-inoculated mice heterozygous for a disrupted PrP gene. Mol Med 1: 19–30.

Burgess S, Shen C, Ferguson LA et al. (2009). Identification of adjacent binding sites for the YY1 and E4BP4 transcription factors in the ovine prp (prion) gene promoter. J Biol Chem 284: 6716–6724.

Campbell L, Gill AC, McGovern G et al. (2013). The PrPC C1 fragment derived from the ovine A136R171 PRNP allele is highly abundant in sheep brain and inhibits fibrillisation of full-length PrPC protein in vitro. Biochimica et Biophysica Acta. Molecular Basis of Disease (BBAdis) 1832: 826–836.

Carlson G, Kingsbury DT, Goodman PA et al. (1986). Linkage of prion protein and scrapie incubation time genes. Cell 46: 503–511.

Cassard H, Torres JM, Lacroux C et al. (2014). Evidence for zoonotic potential of ovine scrapie prions. Nat Commun 5: 5821.

Castle AR, Gill AC (2017). Physiological functions of the cellular prion protein. Front Mol Biosci 4: 19.

Chelle PL (1942). Un cas de tremblante chez la chèvre. Bull Acad Vet Fr 15: 294–295.

Chong A, Kennedy I, Goldmann W et al. (2015). Atypical scrapie found in a mixed infection of a sheep in 1972. J Gen Virol 96: 3165–3178.

Clark EL, Bush SJ, McCulloch MEB et al. (2017). A high resolution atlas of gene expression in the domestic sheep (*Ovis aries*). PLoS Genet 13: e1006997.

Clawson ML, Heaton MP, Keele JW et al. (2006). Prion gene haplotypes of US cattle. BMC Genet 7: 51.

Colussi S, Vaccari G, Maurella C et al. (2008). Histidine at codon 154 of the prion protein gene is a risk factor for Nor98 scrapie in goats. J Gen Virol 89: 3173–3176.

Corbière F, Perrin-Chauvineau C, Lacroux C et al. (2013). PrP-associated resistance to scrapie in five highly infected goat herds. J Gen Virol 94: 241–245.

Cuille J, Chelle PL (1938a). La tremblante du mouton est-elle déterminé par un virus filterable? CR Acad Sci 206: 1687–1688.

Cuille J, Chelle PL (1938b). Le tremblante du mouton est bien inculable. CR Acad Sci 206: 78–79.

Dassanayake RP, White SN, Madsen-Bouterse SA et al. (2015). Role of the PRNP S127 allele in experimental infection of goats with classical caprine scrapie. Anim Genet 46: 341.

Dawson M, Hoinville L, Hosie BD et al. (1998). Guidance on the use of PrP genotyping as an aid to the control of clinical scrapie. Scrapie Information Group. Vet Rec 142: 623–625.

Dawson M, Moore RC, Bishop SC (2008). Progress and limits of PrP gene selection policy. Vet Res 39: 1–12.

Dickinson AG, Outram GW (1979). The scrapie replication site hypothesis and its implication for pathogenesis. In: SB Prusiner, WJ Hadlow (Eds.), Slow transmissible disease of the nervous system: pathogenesis, immunology, virology and molecular biology of spongiform encephalopathies. vol 2. Academic Press, New York.

Dickinson AG, Meikle VM, Fraser H (1968). Identification of a gene which controls the incubation time of scrapie in mice. J Comp Pathol 78: 293–299.

EFSA Panel on Biological Hazards (BIOHAZ), (2014). Scientific opinion on the scrapie situation in the EU after 10 years of monitoring and control in sheep and goats. EFSA Journal 12 (7): 3781–3935.

Foster J, Goldmann W, Hunter N (2013). Evidence for prenatal transmission of SSBP/1 scrapie to lambs from infected ewes. PLoS One 8: e79433.

Frootan F, Nikbakhat G, Özgentürk NÖ et al. (2012). Prion protein coding gene (PRNP) variability in sheep from Turkey and Iran. Biochem Genet 50: 277–284.

Goldmann W (1993). PrP gene and its association with spongiform encephalopathies. Br Med Bull 49: 839–859.

Goldmann W (2008). PrP genetics in ruminant transmissible spongiform encephalopathies. Vet Res 39: 30.

Goldmann W, Hunter N, Benson G et al. (1991). Different scrapie-associated fibril proteins (PrP) are encoded by lines of sheep selected for different alleles of the Sip gene. J Gen Virol 72: 2411–2417.

Goldmann W, Hunter N, Smith G et al. (1994). PrP genotype and agent effects in scrapie: change in allelic interaction with different isolates of agent in sheep, a natural host of scrapie. J Gen Virol 75: 989–995.

Goldmann W, Martin T, Foster J et al. (1996). Novel polymorphisms in the caprine PrP gene: a codon 142 mutation associated with scrapie incubation period. J Gen Virol 77: 2885–2891.

Goldmann W, Chong A, Foster J et al. (1998). The shortest known prion protein gene allele occurs in goats has only three octapeptide repeats and is non-pathogenic. J Gen Virol 79: 3173–3176.

Goldmann W, Houston F, Stewart P et al. (2006). The ovine prion (PrP) protein variant A136R154L168Q171 increases resistance to experimental challenge with bovine spongiform encephalopathy (BSE) agent. J Gen Virol 87: 3741–3745.

Goldmann W, Ryan K, Stewart P et al. (2011). Caprine prion gene polymorphisms are associated with decreased incidence of classical scrapie in goat herds in the United Kingdom. Vet Res 42: 110.

Gough KC, Maddison BC (2010). Prion transmission and occurrence in the environment. Prion 4: 275–282.

Griffith JS (1967). Self-replication and scrapie. Nature 215: 1043–1044.

Groschup MH, Lacroux C, Buschmann A et al. (2007). Classic scrapie in sheep with the ARR/ARR prion genotype in Germany and France. Emerg Infect Dis 13: 1201–1207.

Guan F, Pan L, Li J et al. (2011). Polymorphisms of the prion protein gene and their effects on litter size and risk evaluation for scrapie in Chinese Hu sheep. Virus Genes 43: 147–152.

Hagenaars TJ, Melchior MB, Bossers A et al. (2010). Scrapie prevalence in sheep of susceptible genotype is declining in a population subject to breeding for resistance. BMC Vet Res 6: 25.

Hautaniemi M, Tapiovaara H, Korpenfelt SL et al. (2012). Genotyping and surveillance for scrapie in Finnish sheep. BMC Vet Res 8: 12.

Hoinville LJ, Tongue SC, Wilesmith JW (2010). Evidence for maternal transmission of scrapie in naturally affected flocks. Prev Vet Med 93: 121–128.

Hunter N (2003). Scrapie and experimental BSE. Br Med Bull 66: 171–183.

Hunter N, Cairns D (1998). Scrapie-free Merino and Poll Dorset sheep from Australia and New Zealand have normal frequencies of scrapie-susceptible PrP genotypes. J Gen Virol 79: 2079–2082.

Hunter N, Hope J, McConnell I et al. (1987). Linkage of the scrapie associated fibril protein (PrP) gene and Sine using congenic mice and restriction fragment length polymorphism analysis. J Gen Virol 68: 2711–2716.

Hunter N, Cairns D, Foster J et al. (1997). Is scrapie solely a genetic disease? Nature 386: 137.

Hunter N, Houston F, Foster J et al. (2012). Susceptibility of young sheep to oral infection with bovine spongiform encephalopathy decreases significantly after weaning. J Virol 86: 11856–11862.

Ikeda T, Horiuchi M, Ishiguro N, et al. (1995). Amino acid polymorphisms of PrP with reference to onset of scrapie in Suffolk and Corriedale sheep in Japan. J Gen Virol 76: 2577–2581.

Juling K, Schwarzenbacher H, Williams JL et al. (2006). A major genetic component of BSE susceptibility. BMC Biol 4: 33.

Kipanyula MJ, Chuma IS, Brundtland E et al. (2014). Prion protein (PrP) gene polymorphisms in small East African and Norwegian white goats. Small Rumin Res 121: 200–206.

Lacroux C, Perrin-Chauvineau C, Corbière F et al. (2014). Genetic resistance to scrapie infection in experimentally challenged goats. J Virol 88: 2406–2413.

Lacroux C, Cassard H, Simmons H et al. (2017). Classical scrapie transmission in ARR/ARR genotype sheep. J Gen Virol 98: 2200–2204.

Lan Z, Li J, Sun C et al. (2014). Allelic variants of PRNP in 16 Chinese local sheep breeds. Arch Virol 159: 2141–2144.

Laplanche JL, Chatelain J, Westaway D et al. (1993). PrP polymorphisms associated with natural scrapie discovered by denaturing gradient gel electrophoresis. Genomics 15: 30–37.

Le Dur, Beringue V, Andreoltti O et al. (2005). A newly identified type of scrapie can naturally infect sheep with resistant PrP genotypes. Proc Natl Acad Sci U S A 102: 16031–16036.

Leopoldt JG (1750). Nutzliche und auf die Erfahrung gegrundete Einleitung zu der Land-Wirthschafft, vol. 5. Johann Gottlieb Rothen, Sorau.

Liang J, Kong Q (2012). α-Cleavage of cellular prion protein. Prion 6: 453–460.

Ligios C, Jeffrey M, Ryder SJ et al. (2002). Distinction of scrapie phenotypes by lesion profiling. J Com Pathol 127: 45–57.

Lloyd S, Mead S, Collinge J (2011). Genetics of prion disease. Top Curr Chem 305: 1–22.

Maddison BC, Baker CA, Terry LA et al. (2010). Environmental sources of scrapie prions. J Virol 84: 11560–11562.

Maestrale C, Cancedda MG, Pintus D et al. (2015). Genetic and pathological follow-up study of goats experimentally and naturally exposed to a sheep scrapie isolate. J Virol 89: 10044–10052.

Mays CE, Kim C, Haldimann T et al. (2014). Prion disease tempo determined by host-dependent substrate reduction. J Clin Investig 124: 847–858.

Meydan H, Özkan MM, Yildiz MA et al. (2013). Novel polymorphism in ovine prion protein gene. Anim Genet 44: 588–591.

Meydan H, Pehlivan E, Özkan MM et al. (2017). Prion protein gene polymorphisms in Turkish native goat breeds. J Genet 96: 299–305.

Minikel EV, Zerr I, Collins SJ et al. (2014). Ascertainment bias causes false signal of anticipation in genetic prion disease. Am J Hum Genet 95: 371–382.

Moore RC, Hope J, McBride PA et al. (1998). Mice with gene targetted prion protein alterations show that Prnp, Sinc and Prni are congruent. Nat Genet 18: 118–125.

Moum T, Olsaker I, Hopp P et al. (2005). Polymorphisms at codons 141 and 154 in the ovine prion protein gene are associated with scrapie Nor98 cases. J Gen Virol 86: 231–235.

Oesch B, Westaway D, Wuchli M et al. (1985). A cellular gene encodes scrapie PrP 27-30. Protein Cell 40: 735–746.

Ortiz-Pelaez A, Georgiadou S, Simmons MM et al. (2014). Allelic variants at codon 146 in the PRNP gene show significant differences in the risk for natural scrapie in Cypriot goats. Epidemiol Infect 143: 1304–1310.

Papasavva-Stylianou P, Windl O, Saunders G et al. (2011). PrP gene polymorphisms in Cyprus goats and their association with resistance or susceptibility to natural scrapie. Vet J 187: 245–250.

Papasavva-Stylianou P, Simmons MM, Ortiz-Palaez A et al. (2017). Effect of polymorphisms at codon 146 of the goat PRNP gene on susceptibility to challenge with classical scrapie by different routes. J Virol 91: 22. 12e01142-17.

Peletto S, Bertolini S, Maniaci MG et al. (2012). Association of an indel polymorphism in the 3'UTR of the caprine SPRN gene with scrapie positivity in the central nervous system. J Gen Virol 93: 1620–1623.

Pattison IH, Jones KM (1967). The possible nature of the transmissible agent of scrapie. Vet Rec 80 (1): 2–9.

Piestrzynska-Kajtoch A, Gurgul A, Polak MP et al. (2012). Characterization of PRNP and SPRN coding regions from atypical scrapie cases diagnosed in Poland. Mol Biol Rep 39: 2575–2583.

Prusiner SB (1982). Novel proteinaceous infectious particles cause scrapie. Science 216: 136–144.

Regulation (EC) No 999/2001 (2001) Regulation (EC) No 999/2001 of the European Parliament and of the Council of 22 May 2001 laying down rules for the prevention, control and eradication of certain transmissible spongiform encephalopathies. Official Journal of the European Union L147, 1–40. Retrieved on 21 November 2017 from http://eur-lex.europa.eu/legal-content/EN/ALL/?uri=CELEX:32001R0999.

Ricci A, Allende A, Bolton D et al. (2017). Genetic resistance to transmissible spongiform encephalopathies (TSE) in goats. EFSA J 15: 4962.

Richt JA, Kasinathan P, Hamir AN et al. (2007). Production of cattle lacking prion protein. Nat Biotechnol 25: 132–138.

Robinson SJ, Samuel MD, O'Rourke KI et al. (2012). The role of genetics in chronic wasting disease of North American cervids. Prion 6: 1–10.

Sander P, Hamann H, Drögemüller C et al. (2005). Bovine prion protein gene (PRNP) promoter polymorphisms modulate PRNP expression and may be responsible for differences in bovine spongiform encephalopathy susceptibility. J Biol Chem 280: 37408–37414.

Saunders GC, Cawthraw S, Mountjoy SJ et al. (2006). PrP genotypes of atypical scrapie cases in Great Britain Journal of General Virology 87: 3141–3149.

Saunders GC, Lantier I, Cawthraw S et al. (2009). Protective effect of the T112 PrP variant in sheep challenged with bovine spongiform encephalopathy. J Gen Virol 90: 2569–2574.

Serrano C, Hammouchi M, Benomar A et al. (2009). PRNP haplotype distribution in Moroccan goats. Anim Genet 40: 565–568.

Spiropoulos J, Hawkins SAC, Simmons MM et al. (2014). Evidence of in utero transmission of classical scrapie in sheep. J Virol 88: 4591–4594.

Stewart P, Shen C, Zhao D et al. (2009). Genetic analysis of the SPRN gene in ruminants reveals polymorphisms in the alanine-rich segment of shadoo protein. J Gen Virol 90: 2575–2580.

Tan BC, Alejo-Blanco AR, Houston EF et al. (2012). Codon 141 in the ovine PRNP gene modulates incubation time in sheep orally infected with BSE. J Gen Virol 93: 2749–2756.

Taore A, Royo LJ, Kabore A et al. (2012). Prion protein gene polymorphism in four West African sheep populations. Trop Anim Health Prod 44: 1469–1472.

Thorgeirsdottir S, Sigurdarson S, Thorisson HM et al. (1999). PrP gene polymorphism and natural scrapie in Icelandic sheep. J Gen Virol 80: 2527–2534.

Tuzi NL, Clarke AR, Bradford B et al. (2004). Cre-loxP mediated control of PrP to study transmissible spongiform encephalopathy diseases. Genesis 40: 1–6.

Vaccari G, Scavia G, Sala M et al. (2009a). Protective effect of the AT137RQ and ARQK176 PrP allele against classical scrapie in Sarda breed sheep. Vet Res 40 (3): 19–29.

Vaccari G, Panagiotidis CH, Acin C et al. (2009b). State-of-the-art review of goat TSEs in the European Union, with special emphasis on PrP genetics. Vet Res 40: 48.

Van Keulen LJM, Vromans MEW, van Zijderveld (2002). Early and late pathogenesis of natural scrapie infection in sheep. Eur J Immunol 110: 23–32.

Westaway D, Goodman PA, Mirenda CA et al. (1987). Distinct prion proteins in short and long scrapie incubation period mice. Cell 51 (4): 651–662.

Westergard L, Christensen HM, Harris DA (2007). The cellular prion protein (PrPC): its physiological function and role in disease. Biochim Biophys Acta 1772: 629–644.

White SN, Reynolds JO, Waldron DF et al. (2012). Extended scrapie incubation time in goats singly heterozygous for PRNP S146 or K222. Gene 501: 49–51.

Zhao CL, Wu R, Liu L et al. (2012). Ovine prion protein genotype frequencies in north-western China. Genet Mol Res 11: 1671–1681.

Handbook of Clinical Neurology, Vol. 153 (3rd series)
Human Prion Diseases
M. Pocchiari and J. Manson, Editors
https://doi.org/10.1016/B978-0-444-63945-5.00007-6

Chapter 7

Atypical and classic bovine spongiform encephalopathy

CRISTINA CASALONE[1]* AND JAMES HOPE[2]*
[1]*Istituto Zooprofilattico del Piemonte, Liguria e Valle d'Aosta, Turin, Italy*
[2]*One Health, Norwich, Norfolk, United Kingdom*

Abstract

This chapter describes the prion diseases of cattle, or bovine transmissible spongiform encephalopathies (BoTSEs). "Classic" bovine spongiform encephalopathy (C-BSE), the major prion protein disorder of Bovidae, was first described in 1986. We also describe the spatiotemporal correlation of C-BSE to a novel form of human prion disease, variant Creutzfeldt–Jakob disease (vCJD), which led to the classification of BSE as a zoonotic disease (and the "cause" of vCJD) in 1996. From isolated cases first identified retrospectively in May 1985, a major bovine spongiform encephalopathy (BSE) epidemic peaked within the British Isles in 1991, and has so far led to over 195,000 confirmed cases in cattle, and several thousand more cases within Europe and a few elsewhere. By 2017, the disease had been essentially eradicated below the level of surveillance detection in Europe, although sporadic cases are still predicted to show up for several years to come. By 2004, other forms of BSE, H-type and L-type, had been recognized and, in the absence of information to the contrary, are also included in the classification of BSE as a zoonotic prion disease of bovine origin. This chapter aims to cover the clinical, epidemiologic, neuropathologic, biochemical, biomarker, and pathogenetic aspects of the bovine prion disease and gives a brief, but important, description of the surveillance of BSE and other animal TSEs in Europe.

INTRODUCTION

Bovine spongiform encephalopathy (BSE) has ravaged the UK cattle industry for more than 30 years. From isolated cases first reported in 1986, and some retrospectively identified in May 1985, a major epidemic was under way by 1988 which has so far led to over 195,000 confirmed cases in cattle within the British Isles, and several thousand more cases within Europe; a true estimate of the number of infected animals over this period, and the number entering the human food chain, is difficult to calculate but it is likely to be several million cattle at various stages of a protracted, asymptomatic incubation period (Donnelly et al., 2002; Adkin et al., 2016).[1] The disease produces a progressive degeneration of the central nervous system (CNS) and was named because of the sponge-like appearance of BSE brain tissue when seen under the light microscope (Wells et al., 1987) before its confirmation as a prion disease by transmission to laboratory mice (Fraser et al., 1988) and high-resolution, biochemical studies on aggregates of the abnormal bovine prion protein (BoPrP) (Hope et al., 1988). This chapter aims to cover the clinical, epidemiologic, neuropathologic, biochemical, biomarker,

[1]A mathematical model (C-TSEMM) has been developed to estimate, for the European Union, the number of BSE-infected cattle slaughtered in a given year by birth cohort and the number of BSE-infected animals entering undetected into the food and feed chains. Current surveillance sensitivity in key EU member states exceeds detection of 1 BSE case in 100,000 animals, the OIE "A" type surveillance criterion [1].

*Correspondence to: Cristina Casalone, DVM, Via Bologna 148, Turin 10143, Italy. Tel: +39-0112686341, E-mail: Cristina.Casalone@izsto.it and James Hope, c/o Jane Witz, Animal and Plant Health Agency, Pentland Science Park, Midlothian, UK, EH26 0PZ. E-mail: jameshope8@outlook.com

and pathogenetic aspects of the bovine prion disease and gives a brief, but important, description of the surveillance of BSE and other animal TSEs in Europe and the challenges it faces.

BSE surveillance testing of cattle for abnormal PrP in Europe has allowed the identification of two further, distinct types of cattle TSE, termed H- and L- (or bovine amyloidotic spongiform encephalopathy (BASE)) type BSE (Biacabe et al., 2004; Casalone et al., 2004; Jacobs et al., 2007; Ducrot et al., 2008; Polak et al., 2008; Sala et al., 2012). Similar cases were also detected outside Europe (in Japan and the United States) (Hagiwara et al., 2007; Clawson et al., 2008). About 104 atypical BSE cases have been described worldwide.

CLINICAL SIGNS OF BSE

Observations by stockmen, farmers, or local veterinarians (passive surveillance) have historically played a key role in the early detection and management of BSE. Warning signs of the illness include changes in the behavior, sensation, and locomotion of the cattle. The affected animal becomes increasingly apprehensive and has problems of movement and posture, especially of its hind limbs. The cow (or bull) has increased sensitivity to touch and sound, loss of weight and, as the disease takes hold of its nervous system, paralysis sets in. This clinical phase of BSE may last from a fortnight to over 6 months (Konold et al., 2004). In various investigations to strengthen the clinical diagnosis of BSE, Konold and colleagues (2010) scored 60 clinical signs and behavior combinations in over 500 experimentally exposed cattle and compared outcomes to the confirmation or not of disease at postmortem; they found the intensity of vacuolar pathology and abnormal PrP immunohistochemistry in the brain – the laboratory diagnostic criteria – progressed in tandem with signs indicative of BSE suspects, particularly overreactivity to external stimuli and ataxia. Intriguingly, BSE-like signs or sign combinations occurred in some inoculated animals that could not be confirmed by statutory lab testing; such discordance has been observed to a limited extent in other cattle exposure studies and remains to be fully explained (Czub et al., personal communication).

To maintain awareness of the disease across Europe, the EU TSE [transmissible spongioform encephalopathy] Reference Laboratory curates a section of video clips available for download on various aspects of clinical, classic BSE in cattle on its website (https://science.vla.gov.uk/tse-lab-net/training.html) and these have recently been supplemented by examples of experimental atypical H- and L-type BSE. In cattle transmission experiments, H- and L-type BSE clinically affected cattle with a shorter survival time displayed a "nervous" form, whereas cattle with a longer survival time displayed a "dull" form of disease. Intriguingly, Konold and his colleagues (2014) found in a second passage of "nervous" or "dull" forms of disease by intracerebral injection that while biochemical and histopathologic features were maintained irrespective of BSE type, these clinical distinctions were not maintained. This again emphasizes a general feature of TSEs, noted 30 years ago in the context of "clinical target areas," that no simple relationship exists between clinical disease and pathology (Kimberlin and Walker, 1988).

EPIDEMIOLOGY OF BSE

Classic BSE

From the perspective of 25 years, it is now apparent that, although the majority of animals affected with BSE have been dairy cows, this neurologic disease can occur in either sex with a modal age of onset of 4–4.5 years (range 1.8–18 years). Most early cases of BSE occurred in cattle between the ages of 3 and 5 years in Great Britain, but as the epidemic has waned and level of exposure declined, the average age of cattle with confirmed signs of disease has increased gradually to over 12 years (EFSA, 2009). BSE has occurred in different European countries at different times and reflects the staggered nature of the BSE epidemics that have spread throughout Europe from the United Kingdom. For most of its development time the disease gives no telltale sign of its presence (Wilesmith et al., 1988) and the inability to detect the asymptomatic carrier of BSE has limited, and continues to limit, refinement of the measures which can be taken to prevent infected bovine tissues from use in feed and pharmaceutical products.

Epidemiologic analyses of BSE-affected herds identified a protein feed supplement as the most likely source of infection (Kimberlin and Wilesmith, 1994). During the late 1970s changes in the rendering process which salvages compounds of nutritional and commercial value from abattoir waste are thought to have led to a less efficient system for inactivating prion-infected offal and, in turn, to a contaminated protein supplement, meat and bone meal (MBM). Subsequent recycling of BSE-infected cattle waste in this process may have contributed to the persistence of the disease. Although MBM can be seen retrospectively to have been the major vector for the spread of BSE in the United Kingdom and to the rest of the world, it was recognized very early on that prions in an infected bovine subject to the rendering process would be scattered throughout many of the primary byproducts derived from that process. Tallow, a fat fraction important in the food and animal feed industries, is an example of a bovine byproduct initially classified as "negligible" risk in epidemiologic terms but which, as an allowed additive in calf milk replacer, emerged in the tailing edge of the epidemic as a likely source of infection in BSE cases in Denmark (Willeberg et al., 2011).

Ruminant feed legislation aimed at removing the source of infection from cattle born after 1988 was introduced in 1989–1990 in the United Kingdom, and reinforced throughout Europe in October 2000. At its peak, over 1000 cases were reported each week in Great Britain in 1993 and this has now dwindled to below the detection level of the current EU surveillance systems, with no confirmed cases of BSE in Great Britain in 2016. Although the feed bans have had a dramatic effect on the epidemic curve, cases of BSE continued to be confirmed in cattle born after the reinforced bans of 2000 and illegal or unknowing feeding of contaminated protein to calves is suspected as the reason for most of these "born after the real ban" (BARB) cases. Their biologic and biochemical characteristics of BARBs appear similar to those seen earlier in the epidemic and differ from those of atypical BSE cases that have been recognized recently (see below).

From the United Kingdom, classic BSE (C-BSE) spread to at least 28 other countries, mostly in Europe, with occasional cases also confirmed in Asia (Japan), the Middle East (Israel), and North America. To date, more than 115 million animals have been examined in Europe, and more than 185,000 cases of BSE have been confirmed in the United Kingdom, 7891 in Europe, and 60 cases in the rest of the world (Brazil, Canada, Israel, and Japan). The World Organisation for Animal Health (OIE) reported only 7 cases of BSE worldwide in 2015, 5 in 2016, and 4 in 2017 (for an updated number of BSE cases, see the OIE website at http://www.oie.int/en/animal-health-in-the-world/bse-specific-data/).

Atypical forms of BSE

The origins of atypical BSEs remain obscure, and it has therefore been postulated that they represent a spontaneous TSE in cattle, comparable to most sporadic CJD cases in humans. They are mainly detected in cattle that are 8 years of age or older. Data on atypical BSE cases reported in the EU BSE databases since 2001 show that a total of 60 cases of L-type and 44 of H-type BSE have been identified in Europe. The prevalence of atypical BSE cases in the rest of the world is unknown because there are no official surveillance requirements or systematic reports from different countries, but atypical cases have been reported in the United States, Canada, Brazil, and Japan.

In France, a retrospective study of all the TSE-positive cattle identified through the compulsory EU surveillance program between 2001 and 2007 has been published (Biacabe et al., 2008), and updated with a focus on H- and L-type BSE epidemiology (Sala et al., 2012). The 2008 study indicated that all BSE H and L cases detected by rapid tests were observed in animals over 8 years old (Casalone et al. 2004) in either the "at-risk" or "healthy slaughtered" surveillance target group. In this study, the reported frequency of H- and L-type BSE was respectively 1.9 and 1.7 cases per million of tested animals over 8 years old. In the later study (Sala et al., 2012), "the median age at detection for L-BSE and H-BSE cases was 12.4 (range 8.4–18.7) and 12.5 (8.3–18.2) years respectively, with no significant difference between the two distributions. However, this median age differed significantly from that of classical BSE 7.0 (range 3.5–15.4) years," and while the risk of L-type BSE increased with age, no age-related effect on the incidence of H-type BSE was evident.

The distribution of H- and L-type cases in France by year of birth differs markedly from that for C-BSE and could be interpreted to indicate that both forms of atypical BSE are sporadic diseases which arise spontaneously. These speculations extend to the origins of C-BSE too, and they are fueled by the apparent sporadic occurrence of C-BSE (as well as atypical BSE) as numbers of cases decline exponentially in Europe (Arnold et al., 2017) and at least one "mutant" bovine PrP allele encoding K211 (equivalent to the sporadic CJD human K200 allotype) has been linked to clinical disease in the United States (Nicholson et al., 2008; Ferguson-Smith and Richt, 2009.

Atypical BSE cases are uncommon but found worldwide and evidence from laboratory studies has been interpreted to support the idea that the European epidemic of what we now call C-BSE may have been initiated by a "spontaneous" case of L-type BSE (Casalone et al., 2004). Cases of H- and L- (or BASE) type BSE have been transmitted by intracerebral challenge to inbred mice and transgenic (Tg) mice expressing bovine and ovine PrP. L-type BSE has also been transmitted to Tg mice expressing alleles of the human PrP (Fig. 7.1) (Beringue et al., 2006, 2007; Bushmann et al., 2006; Kong et al., 2008). Transmission and serial passage in inbred mice and Tg VRQ mice have been interpreted to indicate that, after interspecies passage, L-type BSE could generate C-BSE (Beringue et al., 2007; Capobianco et al., 2007). However, it should be noted that L-BSE–C-BSE phenotypic convergence has not been observed in other Tg mice, including mice expressing the ARQ allele of sheep PrP (Bushmann et al., 2006; Beringue et al., 2007). This phenomenon needs to be confirmed in an independent set of experiments but does raise the issue of a possible C-BSE re-emergence originating from atypical BSE cases.

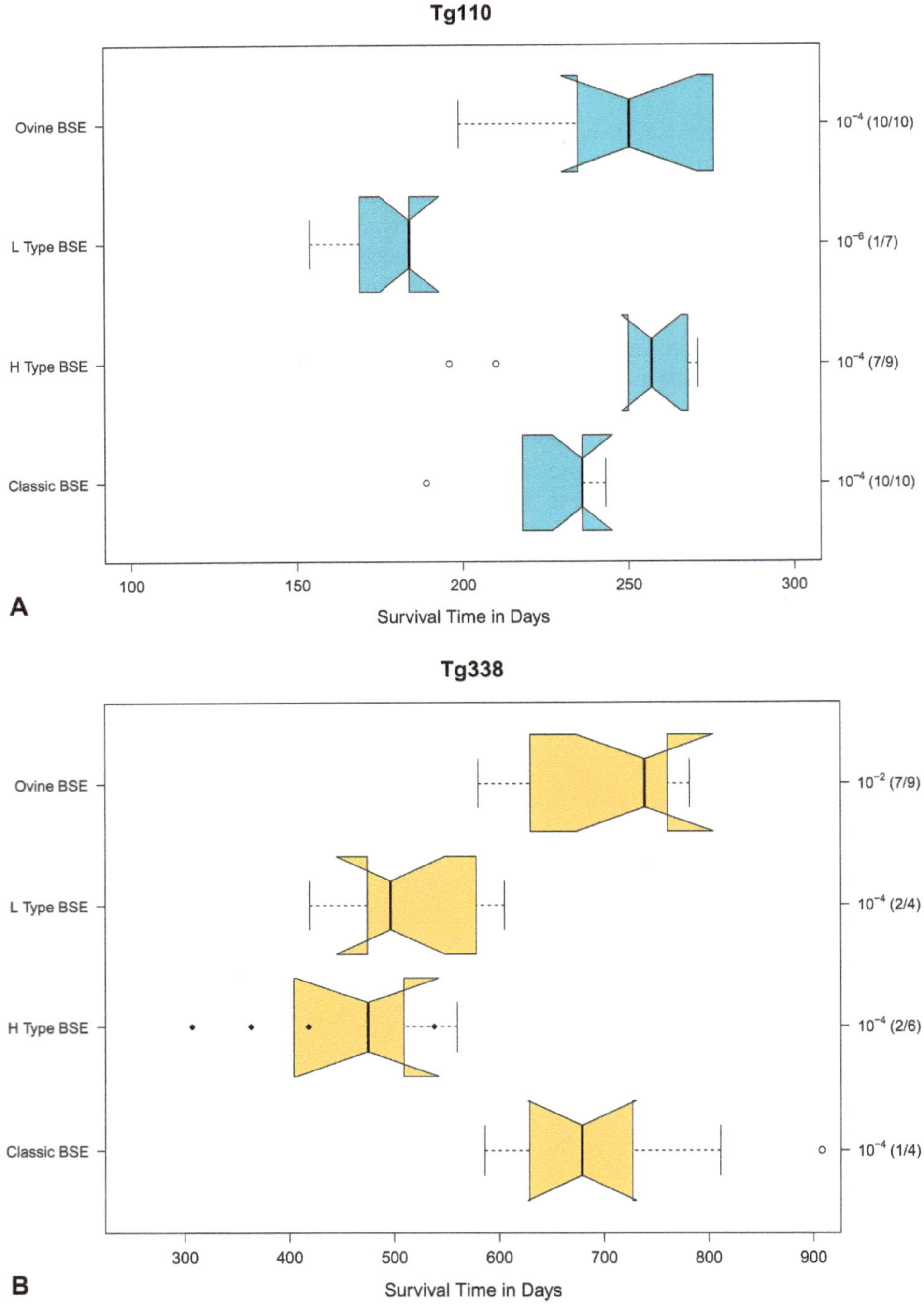

Fig. 7.1. Survival times and attack rates of ovine bovine spongiform encephalopathy (BSE), C-, L-, and H-type BSE prions in transgenic mice overexpressing bovine (Tg110: **A**) or the VRQ allele of ovine prion protein (Tg338: **B**). Each transgenic mouse line is allocated its own figure (**A**: Tg110; and **B**: Tg338), with their survival times in days for each of the four BSE inocula at the 10^{-1} dilution represented as a box plot; box plots show the interquartile range (IQR), and the notch displays the confidence interval around the median (line). Where the confidence interval (median $\pm$ 1.57 $\times$ IQR) extends beyond the 25th and 75th percentiles, the notch is displayed "inside out." Whisker marks show greatest and least values up to 1.5 $\times$ IQR with outliers displayed as open circles. Culled mice negative for all laboratory tests are shown as black diamonds. The attack rates of the highest dilution to produce clinical disease are shown on the right-hand side of the figures and give a crude approximation of prion titer for that particular mouse line/type of prion model. (Reproduced from Hope J, Witz J, Griffiths P, et al. (2017) Creating a panel of animal prion inocula to characterise and compare transgenic mouse lines. Prion 2017, Edinburgh (available at www.elsevier.org/xyz).

PATHOGENESIS AND GENOME

Pathogenesis

C-BSE is a neurologic disease but its main route of transmission is via the oral route and, although the tissue tropism of the BSE prion can be largely reproduced by the more convenient, intracerebral route of infection, much time and expense have been applied to measuring the titer of bovine brain prion extracts and defining spread of disease following feeding of this infected material to cattle.

Experimental oral dosing of cattle with BSE-affected cattle brain homogenates has confirmed that as little as 1 mg of brain (with $\sim$ 10–100 mouse intracerebral ID_{50} units) can induce disease after extended incubation periods of 8–10 years (Arnold et al., 2009; Konold et al., 2012). Larger doses (up to 100 grams) have been used to study oral pathogenesis of BSE in cattle in the United Kingdom (Wells et al., 2007), Japan (Okada et al, 2011a, b), and Germany (Hoffmann et al., 2007; Kaatz et al., 2012). These studies have confirmed by PrP immunohistochemistry and bioassay that there is limited early distribution of prions to parts of the lower alimentary tract (distil ileum, jejunum) and spread via the autonomic nervous system from the gastrointestinal tract to the CNS via either the celiac and mesenteric ganglion complex, splanchnic nerves and the lumbal/caudal thoracic spinal cord or via the vagal nerve. This experimental tissue distribution of infectivity has been used to refine the list of specified risk materials from various age cohorts of cattle banned for human consumption and has underpinned several assessments of human and animal exposure risk that have defined UK and European policy for control and management of BSE over the years (Fig. 7.2) (European Commission, 2017). Similar mappings of H- and L-type prions in orally infected cattle have been used to support risk assessment of atypical BSE exposures and the European Food Safety Authority has published a protocol detailing the scale and scope of further investigations into the pathogenesis of atypical BSE in cattle required to improve our understanding of these variants (EFSA, 2014).

Genome

Pioneering work by Dickinson and Fraser (1969) identified a murine gene locus, *Sinc*, with two alleles, s7 and p7, controlling incubation period of TSEs induced by serially passaged sheep sources of prions and the co-genicity of *Sinc* and the *Prn-i/Prnp* locus followed the discovery of the PrP in the 1980s (Westaway et al., 1987; Dickinson and Outram, 1988; Hope and Hunter, 1988). Goldmann and colleagues (1990, 1991) showed a similar co-relation between the natural and experimental survival times of sheep exposed to field and laboratory strains of scrapie prions and different allotypes/alleles of the ovine PrP/gene, notably the relative resistance to disease of ARR/ARR

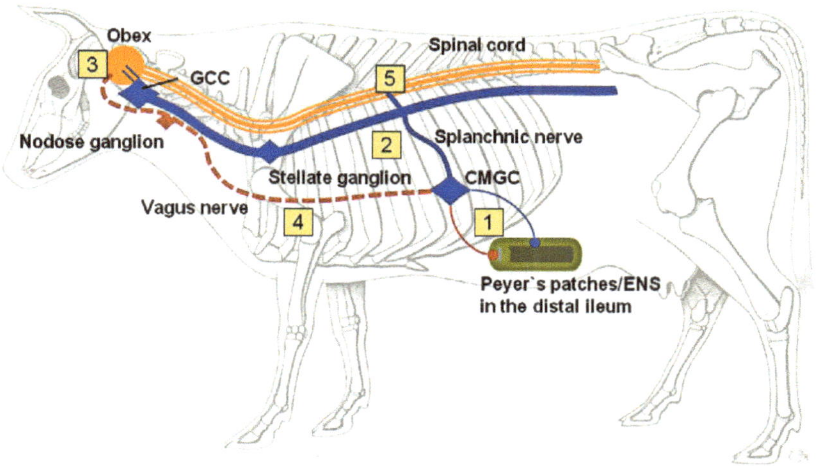

Fig. 7.2. Spread of classic bovine spongiform encephalopathy (BSE) prions in cattle after oral exposure. Prions in the bovine alimentary tract (green; ENS—enteric nervous system) cross the intestinal mucosa and spread via sympathetic (blue) and parasympathetic (red) nerve projections to the celiac mesenteric ganglion complex (CMGC), and thence into the central nervous system (CNS) (orange) directly via the splanchic nerve or the cranial cervical ganglia (GCC), at the level of the obex, to the dorsal motor nucleus of the vagus (DMNV). Alternatively, prions may spread directly to the CNS from the gut via the vagus nerve. The DMNV is the area pathologists target when confirming diagnosis of BSE, and it is often compromised by autolysis in fallen stock, leading to an "inconclusive" diagnosis. Understanding of BSE pathogenesis and its timing underpins current EU strategies for the removal of specified risk material to minimize the exposure of humans to material from infected but undetected cases of BSE. (Reproduced from Kaatz M, Fast C, Ziegler U, et al. (2012) Spread of classic BSE prions from the gut via the peripheral nervous system to the brain. Am J Pathol 181: 515–524.)

homozygous sheep. Therefore, it was prudent to look for a genetic determinant of BSE susceptibility within the bovine PrP open reading frame (ORF) at the outbreak of BSE in the mid-1980s.

Early investigation of a relationship between cattle PrP gene polymorphisms and BSE prion susceptibility found a restricted genetic diversity of the PrP locus in commercial cattle breeds within the United Kingdom (Goldmann et al., 1991; Hunter et al., 1994), although deletion alleles of a 23-basepair insertion/deletion (indel) polymorphism in the bovine *PRNP* promoter region and of a 12-basepair indel within intron 1 were later associated with incidence of C-BSE (Sander et al., 2005; Juling et al., 2006). These polymorphisms lie within *PRNP* but outside the PrP ORF and may exert their effects on disease pathogenesis by modulating levels of bovine PrP in different cell types within the animal; these indels are highly conserved in many cattle populations (Murdoch et al., 2010).

Bovine PrP ORF and indel sequencing of UK BARB case DNA have not identified a germline mutation in these cases, as proposed by the mutational hypothesis for the origin of the BSE epidemic (BSE Inquiry, 2001; Ferguson-Smith, 2003; Saunders et al., 2007).

The pathogenicity of the K222 mutation described in an Alabama cow in 2009 (Ferguson-Smith and Richt, 2009) is still under investigation by the US Department of Agriculture in a carrier daughter cow (Richt, personal communication). Interestingly, the Alabama cow was a cross of *Bos taurus* and *B. indicus* species and the species origin of the K222 allele has not been published to date. Since 2009, the whole-genome sequences of *B. taurus* and *B. indicus*, and subspecies, have been published (Elsik et al., 2009; Tellam et al., 2009) and some ~1.3% of each of the nucleotide sequence of bovine ORFs sequences was found to be polymorphic. Whole-genome sequencing of a proportion of bovine samples from confirmed cases and control animals might then identify the putative mutations suggested in the PrP ORF or noncoding regions (such as the K222 PrP Alabama bovine mutation) or elsewhere. However, interpretation of such mutations as causative and possible origin of disease would require further verification; recent sequencing studies and analysis of human PrP ORFs have shown such "prion disease" mutations may be far more common in the human genome than the incidence of human TSE disease (Minikel et al., 2014, 2016).

LABORATORY METHODS FOR BSE DIAGNOSIS

Historically, BSE diagnosis has relied on histopathologic confirmation of vacuolation in diverse anatomic regions of formalin-fixed brain samples (Wells et al., 1989). The discovery of PrP aggregates (scrapie-associated fibrils) and the production of antibody against PrPs and peptides in the early 1980s led to improved methods for testing for TSEs (Merz et al., 1981; Bode et al., 1985); however, PrP-antibody-based techniques (Western blotting (WB), enzyme-linked immunoassay, and immunohistochemistry) began to replace histology in routine diagnosis only after BSE was confirmed as a PrP-related disease (Wells et al., 1989) and a European-wide initiative to harmonize surveillance methodologies in 2001 was implemented (EU Regulation (EC) no. 999/2001).

Sampling and rapid tests

The preferred sampling site for testing is the brainstem at the level of the obex (the more aboral portion of the brainstem) because PrP^{TSE} accumulation in the CNS begins in these nuclei. Sampling is not recommended if the obex is absent, since samples from other brainstem portions will not show the early accumulation of PrP^{TSE}, thus precluding the certainty of a negative result. The obex can be accessed through the foramen magnum using a proprietary sampling spoon. The brainstem sample is divided longitudinally along its midline: one-half is fixed in 10% buffered formaldehyde solution for histologic and immunohistochemistry analysis, and the other half is used for rapid testing and then frozen at –20°C for WB analysis.

Under EC Regulation no. 999/2001, each Member State must have an annual TSE monitoring program in place that includes a rapid test screening procedure. Rapid tests are approved by the EU Commission after they have been evaluated by the European Reference Laboratory according to the scientific protocol validated by the European Food Safety Authority. These tests have high sensitivity and can be completed within 24 hours, making them suitable for high-throughput testing.

Confirmatory tests

Confirmatory tests are performed by a recognized national reference laboratory or central reference laboratory. The tests have high specificity and serve to confirm clinical suspicion of disease or positive or inconclusive rapid test results. Histologic and immunohistochemistry analysis, scrapie-associated fibril detection, and WB analysis OIE manual and subsequently updates are the recommended confirmatory test methods.

Histologic examination is performed on formalin-fixed, paraffin-embedded brain sections that are stained with hematoxylin and eosin. Optical microscopy reveals the histologic C-BSE changes in the CNS: vacuolation of gray-matter neuropil (spongiform change) and/or neuron vacuolation, with a predilection for certain neuroanatomic locations (Wells et al., 1989; Wells and Wilesmith, 1995), astrocytosis, and neuronal degeneration (Simmons et al., 1996). The target areas at the level of the obex are the

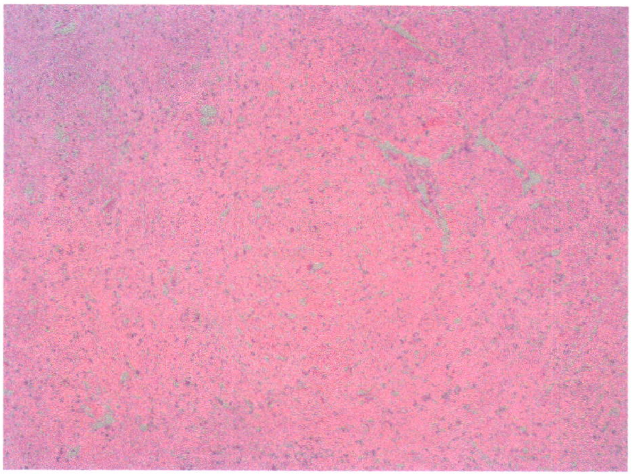

Fig. 7.3. Hematoxylin and eosin: presence of spongiosis in the neuropil of classic bovine spongiform encephalopathy. Nucleus of the solitary tract, brainstem (10 ×).

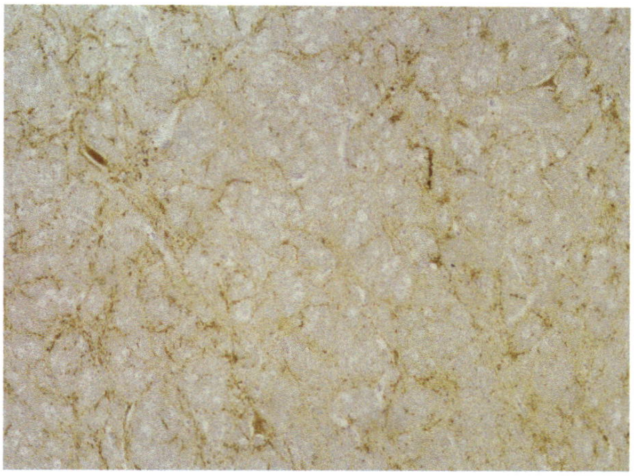

Fig. 7.4. Immunohistochemistry: patterns of PrP^{TSE} of classic bovine spongiform encephalopathy, characterized by granular, intraneuronal deposits, and linear tracts. Reticular formation, brainstem. Immunodetection performed by monoclonal antibody F99/97.6.1 (VMRD, United States) (10 ×).

solitary tract nucleus and the spinal tract nucleus of the trigeminal nerve (Fig. 7.3). Vacuolation may be observed also in the central gray matter of the midbrain and mild spongiform changes of the neuropil at the level of the thalamus in some cases.

In natural cases of L-type BSE, spongiosis is not consistently found in the brainstem, the obex, or the more rostral areas. The frontal, parietal, and occipital cortices are apparently spared, and vacuolation is absent in the olfactory bulb, piriform cortex, and hippocampus (Casalone et al., 2004). In experimental L-type BSE cases, the central gray matter (periaqueductal gray) and rostral colliculus are more severely involved but not the vestibular nuclear complex. Prominent changes may be noted in the olfactory areas, amygdalae, hippocampi, and dorsal horns of spinal cords, but not in the ventral and dorsal roots (Lombardi et al., 2008). In experimental H-type BSE, vacuolar changes are generally observed in all areas of the brain: major vacuolation in the thalamic nuclei and neuropil of the central gray matter of the midbrain, and mild vacuolation in the caudal cerebral and cerebellar cortices. In the vestibular and pontine nuclei, spongy changes are not as prominent as in the other brainstem nuclei (Okada et al., 2011a).

Immunohistochemical analysis on paraffin-embedded brain tissues reveals the presence of PrP^{TSE} accumulation. Various immunohistochemical types of PrP^{TSE} deposition can be observed in the brain of cattle affected by C-BSE (Casalone et al., 2006) (Fig. 7.4):

- glial type labeling with PrP^{TSE} deposits branching out from the nucleus of glial cells along their processes confers them a stellate appearance
- granular type, characterized by granular PrP^{TSE} accumulations in the neuropil
- intraneuronal type with PrP^{TSE} immunoreactivity throughout the neuronal cytoplasm
- perineuronal type, characterized by PrP^{TSE} deposits around single neuronal perikarya and neuritis
- linear tract, characterized by PrP^{TSE} deposits along neuronal processes
- coalescing type, arising from the merging of granular PrP^{TSE} deposits that form amorphous or mesh-like masses
- intraglial type, with fine punctate PrP^{TSE} adjacent to glial nuclei.

A distinctive feature of natural L-type BSE cases is the prevalent deposition of PrP^{TSE} in the more rostral portions of the brain than that seen in C-BSE. The punctate and granular types are the prevalent PrP^{TSE} deposition patterns at the level of the brainstem (Porcario et al., 2011). Glial, intraneuronal, perineuronal, and linear tracts are also frequently observed in several areas of the brain. The hallmark characteristic of L-type BSE is the presence of PrP-positive amyloid plaques, which appear as dense, unicentric or, less frequently, multicentric rounded structures up to 25 μm in diameter, with a pale core and a dark radial periphery. They are predominantly found in the thalamus, subcortical white matter, deeper layers of cerebral cortices, and olfactory bulb (Casalone et al., 2004). In experimental L-type BSE cattle, abundant amyloid PrP plaques are observed in the subcortical white matter and deep gray nuclei, as observed in natural L-type BSE, but are absent in the olfactory glomeruli, cerebellum, and spinal cord (Fig. 7.5) (Lombardi et al., 2008).

Natural H-type BSE is characterized by granular, intraneuronal, linear, intraglial, and punctate PrP^{TSE} deposits in the brainstem (Porcario et al., 2011) (Fig. 7.6). Differently, large amounts of PrP^{TSE} are diffusely deposited in the cerebral cortex, basal ganglia, thalamus, hypothalamus,

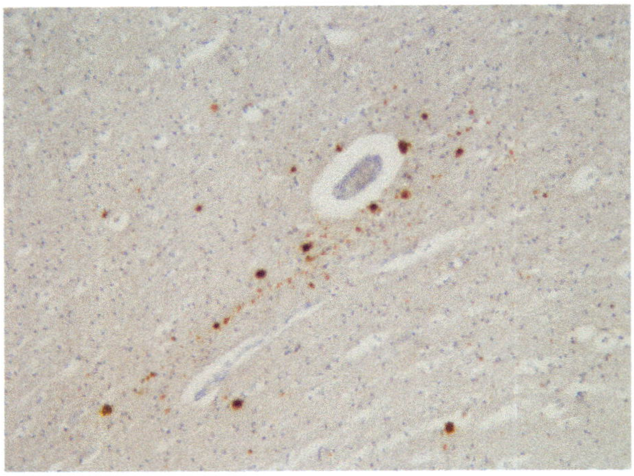

Fig. 7.5. Immunohistochemistry: patterns of PrP^{TSE} of L-type bovine spongiform encephalopathy, characterized by amyloid plaques. Basal ganglia. Immunodetection performed by monoclonal antibody F99/97.6.1 (VMRD, United States) (20 ×).

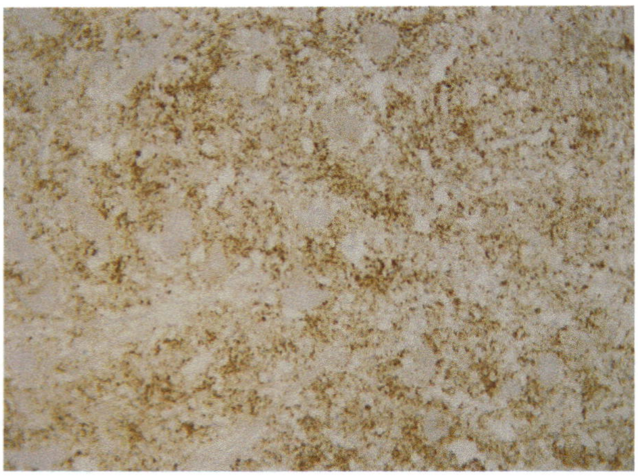

Fig. 7.6. Immunohistochemistry: pattern of PrP^{TSE} of H-type bovine spongiform encephalopathy, characterized by granular and intraglial prion deposition. Reticular formation, brainstem. Immunodetection performed by monoclonal antibody F99/97.6.1 (VMRD, United States) (20 ×).

brainstem, and spinal cord in experimental H-type BSE, in which the most conspicuous type of PrP^{TSE} depositions are fine or coarse particulate type, linear, perineuronal, intraneuronal, glial type and intraglial type. PrP^{TSE}-positive plaques may also be seen in some cases (Okada et al., 2011a).

Negative-contrast electron microscopy, because of its low sensitivity, is seldom used for the detection of purified scrapie-associated fibrils, although it can be an alternative method for examining autolyzed samples or when only formalin tissue is available.

In WB analysis, antibody specific for PrP is used for the detection of PrP^{TSE} in homogenates of unfixed CNS tissue, whereby PrP^{c} and PrP^{TSE} are distinguished through an enzyme digestion step that removes PrP^{c}. Based on electrophoresis, WB can measure the molecular weight of PrP^{TSE} and display its glycosylation pattern. In positive cases, confirmatory WB shows an electrophoretic pattern consisting of three bands that correspond to the di-, mono-, and nonglycosylated forms of PrP^{TSE} that migrate at approximately 30, 25, and 19 kDa, respectively. (Hayashi et al., 2004). Immunoblotting methods are useful for evaluating the molecular features of PrP^{TSE} and to discriminate between classic and atypical BSE isolates. The H-type is characterized by the significantly higher molecular size of the nonglycosylated PrP^{TSE} form and a conventional glycopattern, whereas the L-type has a slightly lower molecular size of the nonglycosylated and a predominance of the monoglycosylated moiety (Biacabe et al., 2004; Casalone et al., 2004) (Fig. 7.7).

New amplification techniques

In prion-affected animals, PrP^{TSE} can be detected in a variety of peripheral tissues and body fluids, including blood, urine, saliva, cerebrospinal fluid, and nasal fluids; however, a validated diagnostic test for antemortem diagnosis of animal prion diseases is not yet available. Because biochemical and immunocytochemical assays have low sensitivity and may yield inconclusive results, they are not reliable in a clinical or preclinical setting of prion-infected hosts. In contrast, in vitro amplification techniques can be used to determine whether a tissue contains any prion seeding activity. Two highly efficient procedures to amplify prions in a test tube are protein misfolding cyclic amplification (PMCA) and real-time quaking-induced conversion (RT-QuIC) (described in detail in Chapter 19).

These methods allow the detection of minute amounts of PrP^{TSE} in biologic tissues or fluid samples, including blood, urine, and cerebrospinal fluid from many prion-

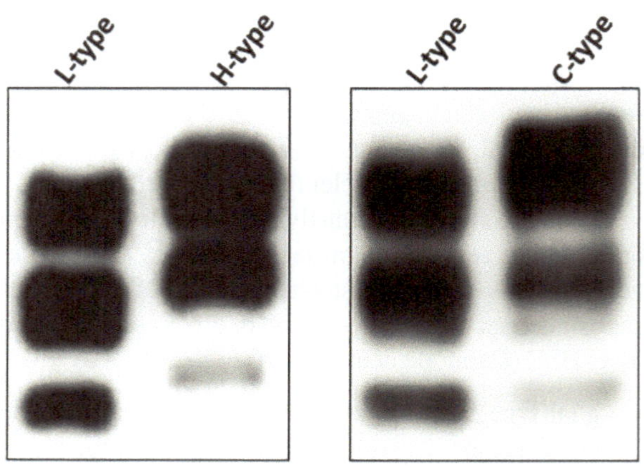

Fig. 7.7. Western Blotting analysis of PrP^{TSE} from classic (C-type), low (L-type), and high (H-type) bovine spongiform encephalopathy. Immunodetection performed by monoclonal antibody 6H4 (Prionics, Switzerland).

infected species. PMCA has sufficient sensitivity for PrP^{TSE} detection in blood in the asymptomatic stages of BSE (Lacroux et al., 2014). Furthermore, recent studies have adapted RT-QuIC assays to the sensitive detection and discrimination of C-BSE, L-BSE, and H-BSE (Orru et al., 2015; Masujin et al., 2016). In brain tissues from cattle affected by these strains tested by the RT-QuIC assay, it was found that all these forms can be detected and distinguished using particular rPrP substrates.

Future areas of focus for the antemortem diagnosis of TSE in animals of farm interest are:

- identification of the most noninvasive and economic biologic peripheral matrix for prion testing in living subjects
- recognition of classic and atypical forms of PrP^{TSE} with the use of a common protocol to have a single diagnostic assay for TSE diseases
- collection of preclinical and clinical data from subjects testing PrP^{TSE}-positive in peripheral matrices to better define the distribution of peripheral TSE infectivity.

INACTIVATION OF BSE PRIONS AND RISK ASSESSMENT

The physical heterogeneity of prions has been one of the major drawbacks preventing their molecular characterization but it is generally accepted that transmission of disease depends on the propagation of abnormal aggregates of the PrP. During fractionation of tissue homogenates of infected brain by centrifugation, infectivity ranges in size from 40S to > 500S, and this behavior is probably due to its association with the PrP. The range in size observed may be due to the interaction of this protein with various membrane fragments and cell debris. The use of filters, ultracentrifugation, gel filtration, and other sizing techniques to define the minimum size of the pathogen has been hindered by this problem.

Physical and chemical treatments of infectious fractions can alter the pathogenesis of infection in the animals used in the quantal titration of infectivity, and these complex effects are often neglected when fractionation/titer data are analyzed. For example, boiling reduces the titer of inocula as measured by an intracerebral route but not by peripheral inoculation (Dickinson and Fraser, 1969), and removal of water or lipid prior to or during heating can radically affect the extent and rate of thermal inactivation (Gale, 2006; Fernie et al., 2007). The cellular and molecular basis of these effects on titer are poorly understood and hence much of our knowledge on inactivation is anecdotal and difficult to interpret in terms of molecular structure. Critically, the stability of prions in one species may change on transmission to another and, ideally, prion inactivation procedures should be validated by bioassay using the most relevant strain/host model (Giles et al., 2008); of course, this is impractical for strains of BSE and experimentation using tissues from natural cases of these diseases and bioassay in transgenic mice expressing bovine PrP transgenes has been used to infer stability in these cases.

Current public health guidelines in the United Kingdom recommend steam autoclaving at 136–138°C for 18 minutes for the sterilization of possible CJD-exposed instruments and materials, and Table 7.1 summarizes the heat stability of BSE agents during standard laboratory autoclaving conditions (133°C for 20 minutes at 3 bar pressure), showing these conditions are effective in inactivating H- and L-type BSE prions as well as destroying the prions causing classic BSE: the impact of autoclaving on titer was: (log10 reduction in infectivity: C-BSE, 7.03; L-type BSE, > 9.65 (lower 95% confidence interval (CI)); H-type BSE, > 3.94 (lower 95% CI)). For comparison, parallel studies investigating the thermal stability of sheep scrapie prions found the impact of these autoclaving conditions on titer to be: (log10 reduction in infectivity: classic scrapie, 6.39; DAW scrapie, 6.33; and atypical scrapie, 7.22). This has given confidence to European risk managers concerned about the persistence of infectivity in animal byproducts after heat treatment (Spiropoulos et al., 2016).

EUROPEAN SURVEILLANCE FOR ANIMAL PRION DISEASES

Current statutory surveillance for TSEs, including BSE

EU TSE surveillance follows EU Regulation (EC) 999/2001,[2] laying down the rules for prevention, control, and eradication of certain TSEs.

The case definition of a TSE has broadened qualitatively over the past 25 years from a description of an animal with neurologic signs and vacuolation of the brainstem to include healthy slaughter animals with minimal histologic change (vacuolation) in brain but where detection of deposits of abnormal bovine PrP provides a definitive diagnosis. In the research laboratory, the TSE spectrum has been expanded further to include disease produced by overexpression of wild-type PrP or normal levels of expression of mutant forms where clinical disease is associated with little or no protease-resistant PrP (where abnormality is defined operationally in terms of protease resistance). Currently, the case definition of a

[2]As amended by Regulation EC 727/2007 (June 26, 2007).

Table 7.1

Heat stability of bovine spongiform encephalopathy (BSE) agents during standard laboratory autoclaving conditions

	Dilution factor (95% CI)	
Inoculum	Using attack rate data only	Using attack rate and incubation period data
Classic BSE	−7.31 (−11.59, −4.91)	−7.03 (−8.38, −5.87)
L-type BSE	−8.97 (lower 95% CI)	−9.65 (lower 95% CI)
H-type BSE	−4.21 (lower 95% CI)	−3.94 (lower 95% CI)
Classic scrapie	−6.39 (−8.58, −5.44)	−6.39 (−7.56, −5.72)
Atypical scrapie	–	−7.22[a]
DAW scrapie	−5.26[a]	−6.33[a]

(Reproduced from Spiropoulos J, Witz J, Arnold M, et al. (2016) Inactivation of atypical and classical BSE prions by laboratory-scale autoclaving. Prion 2016, Tokyo (available at www.elsevier.org/xyz).)

[a]Confidence interval (CI) unable to be evaluated due to insufficient data.

The approach developed in Arnold et al. (2009) was used to estimate the incubation period and probability of infection versus dose from the titration data. The Arnold et al. approach was then used to estimate the titer of the autoclaved samples (and hence the effect of autoclaving on the titer). This method uses both the incubation period and proportion infected to estimate the titer and so has greater statistical power than using either mortality data or incubation period assay alone. Inconclusive samples or samples where no tissue was available were excluded from the analysis. For L- and H-type BSE, the autoclaved samples had no positives for any dilution, and so the titer of the inoculum in these cases was not possible. Instead, the upper 95% CI of the titer was calculated, i.e., the lower 95% CI of the effect of autoclaving.

BSE/TSE disease does not include all of the characteristics encountered in these experimental models but it is legitimate to continue to speculate on the power of any surveillance system's ability to detect such novel forms of TSE if they were to exist in domestic farm animals, particularly in view of their zoonotic potential and their extensive animal health and economic impact.

Types of surveillance and the detection of emerging forms of prion disease

Surveillance schemes are conceptually divided into those that monitor incidence or distribution of known forms of a disease and those that seek to identify new diseases or novel presentations of existing diseases. The first of these is generally known as targeted surveillance. Targeted surveillance requires the availability of accurate tests of known sensitivity that can be applied to epidemiologically and numerically significant, and relevant, risk groups. The second type is scanning surveillance and this is necessary for the detection of TSE disease forms or emerging strains which lie outside the currently recognized spectrum of clinical, biochemical, and pathologic characteristics of disease. Over the years, surveillance for C-BSE has evolved from purely passive surveillance through to targeted, active surveillance of cohorts defined by birth year. The sheer numbers of cases in the early decades precluded any sophisticated categorization of suspect animals based on differing phenotype, and atypical forms of BSE were only detected late in the European epidemic; they were named H-type or L-type (or BASE) to reflect their biochemical and histologic characteristics.

Targeted surveillance

Targeted surveillance and statutory diagnostic methods for TSE/prion diseases are based on measuring abnormal PrP that may, by extrapolation from experimental models, differ qualitatively and/or quantitatively from PrP forms found in normal brains. Such measurements are potentially ineffective for monitoring the emergence of new prion diseases or perhaps novel strains of currently recognized prion diseases. By definition, novel TSEs with physicochemical forms of PrP that are substantially different from those forms currently tested for may evade existing rapid tests. At least one type of cattle disease outside the classification of C-, H-, and L-type BSE remains under investigation as a novel prion disease and two cases, in aged cattle (15 and 8 years of age), were originally identified in Switzerland (Boujon et al., 2016).

Scanning surveillance

Scanning surveillance of novel TSEs starts with field clinical recognition of unusual neurologic disease and is backed up by formal morphologic pathology. At present few adult cattle (or goat and deer) brains arising from neurologic sick individuals undergo postmortem examination. While significantly more examinations of brains of neurologically sick adult sheep are undertaken: (1) it is a matter of uncertainty whether or not they are examined in sufficient numbers to detect (an undefined) low-frequency disease such as the BSE prion in sheep; and (2) (without having a priori a case definition) it is not possible to know what rigor of investigation would be required to diagnose a neurologically sick sheep of undetermined cause as a new TSE disease. Natural BSE prions have not been confirmed in sheep in the EU, although two cases of BSE in goats have been reported (Eloit et al., 2005; Gonzalez et al., 2009), and small ruminant (or experimental) cervid BSE will not be considered here.

The mechanisms in place for targeted disease surveillance within the EU appear to be effective in monitoring alteration in numeric frequency and geographic range of known strains and sources of prion diseases of ruminants, including BSE. However, again by definition, the impacts of missed diagnosis of novel diseases are unquantifiable, and so estimating suitable levels of sampling and supporting logistics for scanning surveillance is inevitably a difficult judgment exercise. These considerations are critical to any discussion of how to effectively combat the re-emergence of BSE or a derivative form of the disease in the European cattle population.

Laboratory testing for BSE

C-BSE of cattle cases is confidently recognized by the presence of distinctive brainstem vacuolation and accumulation of abnormal PrP by WB. Using currently available methodologies, abnormal forms of PrP can usually be detected in prion disease brains and some viscera. Normal host PrP (PrP^c) obtained from nonprion-infected brains by detergent centrifugation is completely digested by proteinase K and is operationally defined as PrPsen (PrP sensitive to proteases). In contrast, PrP aggregates extracted in the same way from classic TSE/prion-affected brains are incompletely degraded by protease enzymes under the same conditions (e.g., times, proteinase concentrations, temperatures, salt concentration, pH) used to digest PrPsen. The operational term used to denote this form of PrP is protease-resistant PrP (PrPres). However, no simple relationship exists between infectivity or clinical disease and PrPres, and this can easily be demonstrated by the wide range of responses for BSE and other farm animal prions following experimental transmission to lines of laboratory mice. Figure 7.1 (Hope et al., 2017) shows the range of attack rates and survival times elicited by the same mass of different forms of BSE prion in two types of transgenic mice overexpressing the bovine PrP (tg110, Fig. 7.1A) or the VRQ allele of ovine PrP (tg338, Fig. 7.1B). This diversity of response complicates the efforts to quantify the effective levels of prion exposure, human and animal, which underpins the "proportionate" management approach to BSE promulgated by the EU.

Methods for statutory testing biochemically for PrPres in classic prion diseases are defined in several publications, manuals, and websites, including that of the EU TSE Reference Laboratory at Animal and Plant Health Agency (APHA) Weybridge in the United Kingdom (see APHA website). Immunohistochemistry may also be used to detect abnormal forms of PrP. However, more recently, natural and experimental studies have broadened the spectrum of biochemical and pathologic features of these PrP-related diseases (for example, idiopathic brainstem neurone chromatolysis of cattle (Jeffrey et al., 2015).

CONCLUSION

The spread of C-BSE has been confirmed as a common source epidemic linked to feed. To date the numbers of C-BSE have declined rapidly in Europe, and this could be related to the strict controls on ruminant protein and its use in animal feed.

The lack of an in vivo test is still a big gap in the diagnostic system, which hopefully will be filled by new ongoing research, to increase the efficacy of surveillance plans and simultaneously reduce their costs.

Atypical BSE cases have been also identified: two different molecular PrP^{TSE} patterns have been described, the L-BSE and H-BSE, but there is limited information about the clinical signs and pathology of these cases. Data are instead more detailed in studies of C-BSE.

Laboratory transmission experiments indicate that the L-BSE agent has a significant zoonotic potential, which appears even higher than that of the C-BSE agent. There are insufficient epidemiologic data with which to undertake any effective risk assessment.

It is important to further investigate the real significance of atypical BSEs and its potential role in causing a new "BSE crisis." Many fundamental questions remain unanswered; in particular, it is speculated that the origin of these atypical cases is sporadic and the possibility of the spread of disease is still unclear.

ACKNOWLEDGMENTS

Our sincere thanks to Jane Witz, APHA Lasswade, UK for her expertise and perseverance in composing Figure 7.1.

References

Adkin A, Simons R, Arnold M (2016). Assessing the sensitivity of European surveillance for detecting BSE in cattle according to international standards. Prev Vet Med 135: 113–122.

Arnold ME, Hawkins SAC, Green R et al. (2009). Pathogenesis of experimental bovine spongiform encephalopathy (BSE): estimation of tissue infectivity according to incubation period. Vet Res 40: 8.

Arnold ME, Simons RRL, Hope J et al. (2017). Is there a decline in bovine spongiform encephalopathy cases born after reinforced feed bans? A modelling study in EU member states. Epidemiol Infect 145: 2280–2286.

Beringue V, Bencsik A, Le Dur A et al. (2006). Isolation from cattle of a prion strain distinct from that causing bovine spongiform encephalopathy. PLoS Pathog 2: e112.

Beringue V, Andreoletti O, Le Dur A et al. (2007). A bovine prion acquires an epidemic bovine spongiform encephalopathy strain-like phenotype on interspecies transmission. J Neurosci 27: 6965–6971.

Biacabe A-G, Laplanche J-L, Ryder S et al. (2004). Distinct molecular phenotypes in bovine prion diseases. EMBO Rep 5: 110–115.

Biacabe A-G, Morignat E, Vulin J et al. (2008). Atypical bovine spongiform encephalopathies, France, 2001-2007. Emerg Infect Dis 14: 298–300.

Bode L, Pocchiari M, Gelderblom H et al. (1985). Characterization of antisera against scrapie-associated fibrils (SAF) from affected hamster and cross-reactivity with SAF from scrapie-affected mice and from patients with Creutzfeldt–Jakob disease. J Gen Virol 66: 2471–2478.

Boujon C, Serra F, Seuberlich T (2016). Atypical variants of bovine spongiform encephalopathy: rare diseases with consequences for BSE surveillance and control. Schweiz Arch Tierheilkd 158: 171–177.

BSE Inquiry (2001). webarchive.nationalarchives.gov.uk. Accessed: 19 April 2018.

Buschmann A, Gretzschel A, Biacabe AG et al. (2006). Atypical BSE in Germany–proof of transmissibility and biochemical characterization. Vet Microbiol 117 (2–4): 103–116.

Capobianco R, Casalone C, Suardi S et al. (2007). Conversion of the BASE prion strain into the BSE strain: the origin of BSE? PLoS Pathog 3: e31.

Casalone C, Zanusso G, Acutis P et al. (2004). Identification of a second bovine amyloidotic spongiform encephalopathy: molecular similarities with sporadic Creutzfeldt–Jakob disease. Proc Natl Acad Sci U S A 101: 3065–3070.

Casalone C, Caramelli M, Crescio MI et al. (2006). BSE immunohistochemical patterns in the brainstem: a comparison between UK and Italian cases. Acta Neuropathol 111: 444–449.

Clawson ML, Richt JA, Baron T et al. (2008). Association of a bovine prion gene haplotype with atypical BSE. PLoS One 3: e1830.

Dickinson AG, Fraser H (1969). Modification of the pathogenesis of scrapie in mice by treatment of the agent. Nature 222: 892–893.

Dickinson AG, Outram GW (1988). Genetic aspects of unconventional virus infections: the basis of the virino hypothesis. Ciba Found Symp 135: 63–83.

Donnelly CA, Ferguson NA, Ghani AC et al. (2002). Implications of the BSE infection screening data for the scale of the British BSE epidemic and current European infection levels. Proc Biol Sci R Soc: 2179–2190.

Ducrot C, Arnold M, de Koeijer A et al. (2008). Review on the epidemiology and dynamics of BSE epidemics. Vet Res 39: 15.

EFSA (2009). Scientific opinion of the panel on biological hazards on a request from the EC on the updated risk for human and animal health related to the revision of the BSE monitoring regime in some member states. The EFSA Journal 1059: 1–40.

EFSA (2014). Protocol for further laboratory investigations into the distribution of infectivity of Atypical BSE. EFSA Journal 12 (7): 3798, pp. 55. https://doi.org/10.2903/j.efsa.2014.3789.

Eloit M, Adjou K, Coulpier M et al. (2005). BSE agent signatures in a goat. Vet Rec 156: 523–524.

Elsik CG, Tellam RL, Worley KC et al. (2009). The genome sequence of taurine cattle: a window to ruminant biology and evolution. Science 324: 522–528.

European Commission (2017). https://ec.europa.eu/food/ Control of TSEs (including BSE and scrapie).

Ferguson-Smith MA (2003). Continuing anxiety about BSE. Vet Rec 153: 723.

Ferguson-Smith MA, Richt JA (2009). Rare BSE mutation raises concerns over risks to public health. Nature 457: 1079.

Fernie K, Steele PJ, Taylor DM et al. (2007). Comparative studies on the thermostability of five strains of transmissible-spongiform-encephalopathy agent. Biotechnol Appl Biochem 47: 175–183.

Fraser H, McConnell I, Wells GA et al. (1988). Transmission of bovine spongiform encephalopathy to mice. Vet Rec 123: 472.

Gale P (2006). The infectivity of transmissible spongiform encephalopathy agent at low doses: the importance of phospholipid. J Appl Microbiol 101: 261–274.

Giles K, Glidden DV, Beckwith R et al. (2008). Resistance of bovine spongiform encephalopathy (BSE) prions to inactivation. PLoS Pathog 4: e1000206.

Goldmann W, Hunter N, Foster JD et al. (1990). Two alleles of a neural protein gene linked to scrapie in sheep. Proc Natl Acad Sci U S A 87: 2476–2480.

Goldmann W, Hunter N, Benson G et al. (1991). Different scrapie-associated fibril proteins (PrP) are encoded by lines of sheep selected for different alleles of the Sip gene. J Gen Virol 72: 2411–2417.

Gonzalez L, Martin S, Siso S et al. (2009). High prevalence of scrapie in a dairy goat herd: tissue distribution of disease-associated PrP and effect of PRNP genotype and age. Vet Res 40: 65.

Hagiwara K, Yamakawa Y, Sato Y et al. (2007). Accumulation of mono-glycosylated form-rich, plaque-forming PrPSc in the second atypical bovine spongiform encephalopathy case in Japan. Jpn. J Infect Dis 60: 305–308.

Hayashi H, Takata M, Iwamaru Y et al. (2004). Effect of tissue deterioration on postmortem BSE diagnosis by immunobiochemical detection of an abnormal isoform of prion protein. J Vet Med Sci 66: 515–520.

Hoffmann C, Ziegler U, Buschmann A et al. (2007). Prions spread via the autonomic nervous system from the gut to the central nervous system in cattle incubating bovine spongiform encephalopathy. J Gen Virol 88: 1048–1055.

Hope J, Hunter N (1988). Scrapie-associated fibrils. PrP protein and the Sinc gene Ciba Found Symp 135: 146–163.

Hope J, Reekie LJ, Hunter N et al. (1988). Fibrils from brains of cows with new cattle disease contain scrapie-associated protein. Nature 336: 390–392.

Hope J., Witz J., Griffiths P., et al. (2017) Creating a panel of animal prion inocula to characterise and compare transgenic mouse lines. Prion 2017, Edinburgh (available at www.elsevier.org/xyz).

Hunter N, Goldmann W, Smith G et al. (1994). Frequencies of PrP gene variants in healthy cattle and cattle with BSE in Scotland. Vet Rec 135: 400–403.

Jacobs JG, Langeveld JPM, Biacabe A-G et al. (2007). Molecular discrimination of atypical bovine spongiform encephalopathy strains from a geographical region spanning a wide area in Europe. J Clin Microbiol 45: 1821–1829.

Jeffrey M, Piccardo P, Ritchie DL et al. (2015). A naturally occurring bovine tauopathy is geographically widespread in the UK. PLoS One 10: e0129499.

Juling K, Schwarzenbacher H, Williams JL et al. (2006). A major genetic component of BSE susceptibility. BMC Biol 4: 33.

Kaatz M, Fast C, Ziegler U et al. (2012). Spread of classic BSE prions from the gut via the peripheral nervous system to the brain. Am J Pathol 181: 515–524.

Kimberlin RH, Walker CA (1988). Pathogenesis of experimental scrapie. Ciba Found Symp 135: 37–62.

Kimberlin RH, Wilesmith JW (1994). Bovine spongiform encephalopathy. Epidemiology, low dose exposure and risks Ann N Y Acad Sci 724: 210–220.

Kong Q, Zheng M, Casalone C et al. (2008). Evaluation of the human transmission risk of an atypical bovine spongiform encephalopathy prion strain. J Virol 82: 3697–3701.

Konold T, Bone G, Ryder S et al. (2004). Clinical findings in 78 suspected cases of bovine spongiform encephalopathy in Great Britain. Vet Rec 155: 659–666.

Konold T, Sayers AR, Sach A et al. (2010). Relationship between clinical signs and postmortem test status in cattle experimentally infected with the bovine spongiform encephalopathy agent. BMC Vet Res 6: 53.

Konold T, Arnold ME, Austin AR et al. (2012). Bovine spongiform encephalopathy: the effect of oral exposure dose on attack rate and incubation period in cattle - an update. BMC Res Notes 5: 674.

Konold T, Phelan LJ, Clifford D et al. (2014). The pathological and molecular but not clinical phenotypes are maintained after second passage of experimental atypical bovine spongiform encephalopathy in cattle. BMC Vet Res 10: 243.

Lacroux C, Comoy E, Moudjou M et al. (2014). Preclinical detection of variant CJD and BSE prions in blood. PLoS Pathog 10: e1004202.

Lombardi G, Casalone C, D'Angelo A et al. (2008). Intraspecies transmission of BASE induces clinical dullness and amyotrophic changes. PLoS Pathog 4: e1000075.

Masujin K, Orru CD, Miyazawa K et al. (2016). Detection of atypical H-type bovine spongiform encephalopathy and discrimination of bovine prion strains by real-time quaking-induced conversion. J Clin Microbiol 54: 1407.

Merz PA, Somerville RA, Wisniewski HM et al. (1981). Abnormal fibrils from scrapie-infected brain. Acta Neuropathol 54: 63–74.

Minikel EV, Zerr I, Collins SJ et al. (2014). Ascertainment bias causes false signal of anticipation in genetic prion disease. Am J Hum Genet 95: 371–382.

Minikel Vallabh SM, Lek M et al. (2016). Quantifying prion disease penetrance using large population control cohorts. Sci Transl Med 8: 322ra9.

Murdoch BM, Clawson ML, Yue S et al. (2010). PRNP haplotype associated with classical BSE incidence in European Holstein cattle. PLoS One 5.

Nicholson EM, Brunelle BW, Richt JA et al. (2008). Identification of a heritable polymorphism in bovine PRNP associated with genetic transmissible spongiform encephalopathy: evidence of heritable BSE. PLoS One 3: e2912.

Okada H, Iwamaru Y, Imamura M et al. (2011a). Experimental H-type bovine spongiform encephalopathy characterized by plaques and glial- and stellate-type prion protein deposits. Vet Res 42: 79.

Okada H, Iwamaru Y, Imamura M et al. (2011b). Neuroanatomical distribution of disease-associated prion protein in cases of bovine spongiform encephalopathy detected by fallen stock surveillance in Japan. J Vet Med Sci 73: 1465–1471.

Orru CD, Favole A, Corona C et al. (2015). Detection and discrimination of classical and atypical L-type bovine spongiform encephalopathy by real-time quaking-induced conversion. J Clin Microbiol 53: 1115–1120.

Polak MP, Zmudzinski JF, Jacobs JG et al. (2008). Atypical status of bovine spongiform encephalopathy in Poland: a molecular typing study. Arch Virol 153: 69–79.

Porcario C, Hall SM, Martucci F et al. (2011). Evaluation of two sets of immunohistochemical and Western blot confirmatory methods in the detection of typical and atypical BSE cases. BMC Res Notes 4: 376.

Sala C, Morignat E, Oussaid N et al. (2012). Individual factors associated with L- and H-type bovine spongiform encephalopathy in France. BMC Vet Res 8: 74.

Sander P, Hamann H, Drogemuller C et al. (2005). Bovine prion protein gene (PRNP) promoter polymorphisms modulate PRNP expression and may be responsible for differences in bovine spongiform encephalopathy susceptibility. J Biol Chem 280: 37408–37414.

Saunders GC, Griffiths PC, Cawthraw S et al. (2007). Polymorphisms of the prion protein gene coding region in born-after-the-reinforced-ban (BARB) bovine spongiform encephalopathy cattle in Great Britain. J Gen Virol 88: 1374–1378.

Simmons MM, Harris P, Jeffrey M et al. (1996). BSE in Great Britain: consistency of the neurohistopathological findings in two random annual samples of clinically suspect cases. Vet Rec 138: 175–177.

Spiropoulos J, Witz J, Arnold M et al. (2016). Inactivation of atypical and classical BSE prions by laboratory-scale autoclaving, Prion 2016, Tokyo (available at www.elsevier.org/xyz).

Tellam RL, Lemay DG, Van Tassell CP et al. (2009). Unlocking the bovine genome. BMC Genomics 10: 193.

Wells GA, Wilesmith JW (1995). The neuropathology and epidemiology of bovine spongiform encephalopathy. Brain Pathol 5: 91–103.

Wells GA, Scott AC, Johnson CT et al. (1987). A novel progressive spongiform encephalopathy in cattle. Vet Rec 121: 419–420.

Wells GA, Hancock RD, Cooley WA et al. (1989). Bovine spongiform encephalopathy: diagnostic significance of vacuolar changes in selected nuclei of the medulla oblongata. Vet Rec 125: 521–524.

Wells GAH, Konold T, Arnold ME et al. (2007). Bovine spongiform encephalopathy: the effect of oral exposure dose on attack rate and incubation period in cattle. J Gen Virol 88: 1363–1373.

Westaway D, Goodman PA, Mirenda CA et al. (1987). Distinct prion proteins in short and long scrapie incubation period mice. Cell 51: 651–662.

Wilesmith JW, Wells GA, Cranwell MP et al. (1988). Bovine spongiform encephalopathy: epidemiological studies. Vet Rec 123: 638–644.

Willeberg P, Paisley LG, Lind P (2011). Epidemiological models to support animal disease surveillance activities. Rev Sci Tech 30: 603–614.

Handbook of Clinical Neurology, Vol. 153 (3rd series)
Human Prion Diseases
M. Pocchiari and J. Manson, Editors
https://doi.org/10.1016/B978-0-444-63945-5.00008-8

Chapter 8

Chronic wasting disease: an evolving prion disease of cervids

SYLVIE L. BENESTAD[1] AND GLENN C. TELLING[2]*
[1]*Norwegian Veterinary Institute, Oslo, Norway*
[2]*Prion Research Center (PRC) and the Department of Microbiology, Immunology, and Pathology, Colorado State University, Fort Collins, CO, United States*

Abstract

Chronic wasting disease (CWD) is a relatively new and burgeoning prion epidemic of deer, elk, reindeer, and moose, which are members of the cervid family. While the disease was first described in captive deer, its subsequent discovery in various species of free-ranging animals makes it the only currently recognized prion disorder of both wild and farmed animals. In addition to its expanding range of host species, CWD continues to spread from North America to new geographic areas, including South Korea, and most recently Norway, marking the first time this disease was detected in Europe. Its unparalleled efficiency of contagious transmission, combined with high densities of deer in certain areas, complicates strategies for controlling CWD, raising concerns about its potential for spread to new species. Because there is a high prevalence of CWD in deer and elk, which are commonly hunted and consumed by humans, and since prions from cattle with bovine spongiform encephalopathy have been transmitted to humans causing variant Creutzfeldt–Jakob disease, the possibility of zoonotic transmission of CWD is particularly concerning. Here we review the clinical and pathologic features of CWD and its disturbing epidemiology, and discuss features that affect its transmission, including genetic susceptibility, pathogenesis, and agent strain variability. Finally, we discuss evidence that speaks to the potential for zoonotic transmission of this emerging disease.

CLINICAL SIGNS OF CHRONIC WASTING DISEASE

Diseased, free-ranging cervids are actually rarely observed, and the clinical signs that have been described for chronic wasting disease (CWD) have primarily been defined in captive elk and mule deer from North America. Animals manifesting clinical signs of CWD are usually older than 16 months. The incubation period is thought to vary from 2 to 4 years, and the duration of clinical disease can vary from a few days or months to, in some cases, 1 year. However, in most cases death occurs within 4 months of the onset of clinical disease. Diagnosis cannot be made solely on the basis of clinical signs because they are not specific, and are only suggestive of CWD. Behavioral changes, while they may be subtle, can be the first noticeable clinical signs. These include loss of fear of humans, generalized depression, and occasionally mild aggressive behavior towards other animals (Williams, 2003). The next clinical feature is progressive weight loss by loss of fat, and later muscle mass (hence the term "wasting disease"), which occurs typically over several weeks to months.

Necropsy observation of the rumens of diseased animals suggests that they continue to eat until death occurs. Weight loss is progressive throughout the course of disease, but it is important to recognize that CWD may be present in cervids that are not emaciated. On the other hand, wild cervids unaffected by CWD may manifest with poor condition, for example as a result of harsh seasonal weather conditions. Late in the disease, affected animals exhibit excessive thirst (polydipsia), urinate

*Correspondence to: Glenn Telling, BA, MA (Oxon.), PhD, 1619 Campus Delivery, Microbiology, Immunology and Pathology, Colorado State University, Fort Collins CO 80523, United States. Tel: +1-859-333-8076, E-mail: glenn.telling@colostate.edu

frequently (polyuria), and have saliva dripping from their mouths (sialorrhea or excessive drooling). Features such as low head carriage, drooped ears, fixed staring gaze, and grinding of the teeth are also commonly observed. Affected animals may show persistent aimless walking and may have periods of standing somnolence.

In CWD, as in other prion diseases, clinical signs result from pathologic processes in the central nervous system (CNS) causing neurologic disturbances (Williams, 2005). Animals show variable locomotor signs such as generalized incoordination (especially posterior ataxia) and head tremors, probably due to degeneration of the cerebellum and weakness (emaciation) of the skeletal muscles. Sick animals can be found lying down and unable to rise. Nevertheless, brainworm (*Elaphostrongylus rangiferi* in reindeer) or *Listeria monocytogenes* infections may also cause signs consistent with CNS dysfunction, including ataxia and hind-limb paresis, which may be confused with the signs of CWD. Death has been reported after routine chasing and chemical immobilization, even in animals in the early clinical stages of CWD. Aspiration pneumonia may be the only presenting clinical sign and is often the cause of death. Therefore, in cervids with aspiration pneumonia, CWD should be suspected (Williams, 2005). While pruritus and bilateral wool loss are sometimes the dominant signs of classic scrapie in sheep, this does not seem to be a feature of CWD. Although poor body condition associated with a rough and dry coat, and shedding of winter hair coat may be observed in cervids in the terminal stage of CWD, numerous other chronic conditions, including copper deficiency, can also cause abnormal shedding, especially in elk.

HISTOPATHOLOGY OF CWD

The histologic lesions in cervids with CWD are similar to those observed in other transmissible spongiform encephalopathies of animals and humans, characterized by vacuolation in the gray matter of the CNS. The earliest lesions can be found in the dorsal motor nucleus of the vagus nerve and with a mild hypertrophy and proliferation of astrocytes followed by spongiform degeneration of the neuropil and neurons (Williams and Young, 1993). Subsequently affected areas include the hypothalamic nuclei, followed by adjacent nuclei of the brainstem, thalamus, and olfactory cortex. The basal ganglia, cerebrum, and spinal cord are affected next, while lesions in the hippocampus are minimal. The cerebellum is the last region of the brain to be affected. Amyloid plaques, with pale eosinophilic fibrillar foci within the neuropil, can be seen within brain and spinal cord tissue sections. These plaques can be surrounded by vacuoles on hematoxylin and eosin-stained slides.

PATHOGENESIS OF CWD

After uptake from the gastrointestinal tract, the infectious agent, comprised of abnormal prion protein (PrP^{TSE}), is thought to cross the alimentary epithelium and migrate relatively quickly by two neuroanatomic pathways. The first is along the vagus nerve to the dorsal motor nucleus of the vagus nerve in the brain, and the second pathway is along the splanchnic nerve to the intermediolateral cell column of the midthoracic (McBride et al., 2001; Sigurdson et al., 2002). Ultimately, prions spread throughout the lymphoid tissues and CNS.

As in all prion diseases, histopathologic changes are only observed in the CNS. While brain lesions occur relatively late in disease, PrP^{TSE} can be detected earlier than histopathologic vacuolation, and before the animal displays signs of disease, and is therefore a better diagnostic tool. In the brain, PrP^{TSE} is predominantly found in the gray matter, especially perineuronal and perivascular, in the medulla oblongata, diencephalon, and olfactory cortex. In the medulla oblongata, several neuronal nuclei are affected, but most prominently the dorsal motor nucleus of the vagus nerve. The cerebral cortex and the hippocampus are less heavily affected. Large PrP^{TSE} aggregates in the form of amyloid plaques are particularly prominent in white-tailed deer (Guiroy et al., 1991).

Pathology and PrP^{TSE} distribution in CWD appear to be very similar to that observed in sheep affected with classic scrapie, with involvement of the lymphoreticular system preceding that of the CNS (Williams and Young, 1993; Sigurdson et al., 1999, 2002; Fox et al., 2006). However, CWD pathogenesis seems to vary between deer and elk, with less PrP^{TSE} deposition in the lymphoid tissues of elk compared with deer (Race et al., 2007). In lymphoid tissues, PrP^{TSE} is detected in lymph nodes, rectoanal mucosa-associated lymphoid tissue, tonsils, and spleen, particularly in germinal centers, with increased accumulation and over the course of disease. Using a range of conventional methods (immunohistochemistry, Western blot, enzyme-linked immunosorbent assay, or bioassay) or newer methods like protein misfolding cyclic amplification (PMCA) or real-time quaking-induced conversion (RT-QuIC), PrP^{TSE} is detected in a large number of other peripheral organs, such as the pancreas, adrenal glands, thyroid gland, heart, skeletal muscles, tongue, liver, retina, lungs, kidneys, antler velvet, bladder, and gastrointestinal tract (Sigurdson et al., 2001; Angers et al., 2006, 2009; Fox et al., 2006; Jewell et al., 2006; Daus et al., 2011; Mitchell et al., 2012). In addition, PrP^{TSE} and/or infectivity has been demonstrated in blood, saliva, fecal material, and urine (Mathiason et al., 2006; Haley et al., 2009a, b; Tamguney et al., 2009; Haley and Hoover, 2015; Plummer et al., 2017), suggesting their important role in the dissemination of the disease.

NATURAL TRANSMISSION

CWD was first identified in the late 1960s as a fatal wasting syndrome of captive mule deer (*Odocoileus hemionus*) and black-tailed deer (*O. hemionus columbianus*) in several wild-life facilities in northern Colorado. Microscopic evaluation of the CNS of diseased animals revealed the aforementioned neuropathologic features typical of prion diseases (Williams and Young, 1980). A subsequent retrospective study also revealed CWD infection of mule deer and black-tailed deer that resided at the Toronto Zoo between 1973 and 2003 (Dube et al., 2006). After its detection in wild-life facilities in northern Colorado, the disease was also identified in mule deer in a research facility in Wyoming and in Rocky Mountain elk (*Cervus elaphus nelsoni*) in both the Colorado and Wyoming wild-life facilities, and thereafter in free-ranging mule deer and elk in southeastern Wyoming and northeastern Colorado (Williams and Young, 1980, 1982, 1992), and in white-tailed deer (*O. virginianus*) in Nebraska and South Dakota in 2001 (Williams, 2005). Surveillance and modeling studies have indicated that CWD occurred endemically among free-ranging deer and elk in a contiguous area encompassing northeastern Colorado, southeastern Wyoming, and western Nebraska, and that CWD was most likely present in free-ranging cervids in this "endemic region" several decades prior to its detection (Miller et al., 2000).

Long thought to be limited to this endemic region, a new area of CWD infection was identified in 1996 in Saskatchewan, Canada, in a captive elk that was imported from the United States (Williams and Miller, 2002), while in 2002 CWD was detected for the first time in free-ranging populations of white-tailed deer east of the Mississippi, in southern Wisconsin (Joly et al., 2003). In September 2005, CWD was identified for the first time in a wild, hunter-killed Shira's moose (*Alces alces shirasi*) in Colorado, and in two additional free-ranging moose in October 2006 (Baeten et al., 2007). In February 2013, CWD was identified for the first time in a road-killed moose in Alberta, Canada (http://aep.alberta.ca/fish-wildlife/wildlife-diseases/chronic-wasting-disease/cwd-updates/documents/CWDinMooseAlberta-InfoSheet-Feb2013B.pdf).

The current spread of CWD in North America appears to be irreversible. At the time of writing, the geographic range of disease in both wild and farm-raised cervids includes 24 North American states and two Canadian provinces and is considered likely to continue to grow (https://www.cdc.gov/prions/cwd/occurrence.html). Additional foci of disease in free-ranging animals, distant from the endemic region, have been identified, including Wisconsin, New Mexico, New York, West Virginia, Missouri, Minnesota, and Arkansas. This discontinuous, patchy spread of the disease, with apparently unaffected regions between two geographically distant endemic regions, can be attributed to human translocation of infected captive deer and elk. While spread of this contagious disease by natural migration and, in particular, human transportation of infected cervids to other locations almost certainly plays a role in the emergence of CWD in new areas, the ultimate origins of CWD remain a mystery in North America. This is not the case, however, for CWD in the Republic of Korea. Here, importation of subclinically infected elk and deer from Canada was the means by which outbreaks of disease occurred (Sohn et al., 2002; Kim et al., 2005). In 2010, additional Korean CWD cases were observed in red deer (*Cervus elaphus*), sika deer (*C. nippon*), and crossbred sika and red deer (Lee et al., 2013).

In 2016, CWD was unexpectedly identified in a free-ranging Norwegian reindeer (*Rangifer tarandus tarandus*), marking the first time this disease was detected in Europe (Benestad et al., 2016). In the following months, two additional cases were detected in European moose (*A. alces alces*), as well as three additional cases in free-ranging reindeer. Like CWD in North America, the origin of European CWD remains a mystery. It is noteworthy that CWD prevalence worldwide is not well defined, and is probably underestimated at present since the disease is at a low incidence and the amount of sampling may not be adequate to detect it.

In the wild, the highly efficient transmission of CWD appears unparalleled among prion diseases (Williams and Young, 1980; Miller et al., 2000; Miller and Williams, 2003). The remarkably contagious nature of CWD has been documented in a captive mule deer population wherein 90% of the mule deer present for more than 2 years ultimately developed disease (Williams and Young, 1980). While the maximum incubation period of CWD in naturally infected animals is unknown, most cases occur in animals between 3 and 7 years of age, with the majority of animals probably developing the disease within 3 years of infection (Miller et al., 1998). CWD prevalence can be as high as 30% in some areas of Colorado (Williams, 2005), and wild-life management efforts to contain or eradicate CWD in the state have proven unsuccessful (Conner et al., 2007). Based on hunter-harvested animal surveillance, the prevalence of CWD in the endemic area from 1996 through 1999 was estimated at approximately 5% in mule deer, 2% in white-tailed deer, and <1% in elk (Spraker et al., 1997). Several studies have attempted to address the impact of CWD on cervid populations. Experimental studies show that CWD lowers deer survival, and can depress population growth rates when prevalence becomes sufficiently high (Miller et al., 2008; Dulberger et al., 2010).

Modeling approaches provide conflicting predictions based on the consequences of CWD to infected populations (Wasserberg et al., 2009; Almberg et al., 2011; Geremia et al., 2015).

Although the natural route of transmission is not precisely known, lateral transmission (Williams and Miller, 2002) by ingestion of forage or water contaminated by secretions, excretions, or other sources, for example CWD-infected carcasses (Miller et al., 2004), has long been thought the most plausible natural route. PrP^{TSE} in CWD-affected animals is readily detected in various lymphoid tissues, including those of the digestive tract (tonsils, Peyer's patches, and mesenteric lymph nodes). This distribution pattern suggests that CWD prions may be shed during incubation of the agent through the alimentary tract, and points to excreta as possible mediators of transmission. The presence of CWD prions in saliva, blood, urine, and feces (Mathiason et al., 2006; Haley et al., 2009a, b, 2011; Tamguney et al., 2009; Plummer et al., 2017) is consistent with this mechanism of contagious lateral transmission. Maternal transmission may occur (Nalls et al., 2013), but appears to be relatively rare. The detection of CWD prions in elk antler velvet, and the annual shedding of this material, raises the possibility that it may also play a role in CWD transmission (Angers et al., 2009). Recently developed, highly sensitive methods for CWD detection based on a standardized RT-QuIC assay, are likely to greatly facilitate epidemiologic studies (Haley et al., 2014; Henderson et al., 2015a).

Pertinent to the issue of disease transmission is the seemingly indefinite persistence of CWD in the environment (Miller et al., 2004; Seidel et al., 2007), a feature that is linked to the unusual and extreme resistance of prions to degradation. Residual infectivity in contaminated environments is therefore likely to be crucial in sustaining epidemics (Miller et al., 2004; Mathiason et al., 2006; Saunders et al., 2008). Coupled with this, prions bind avidly to soil particles, particularly montmorillonite clay and quartz (Smith et al., 2011), and remain infectious after oral consumption (Johnson et al., 2006b, 2007; Saunders et al., 2012). Of note, there appears to be a close correlation between these soil types and CWD prevalence (Saunders et al., 2012). Binding requires the flexible amino-terminus of PrP^{TSE} and cleavage with proteinase K effectively releases prions from soil particles (Saunders et al., 2011). Environmental shedding by CWD-infected animals brings into question the role of plant contamination in transmission. To address this, Pritzkow and colleagues (2015) analyzed the binding and retention of PrP^{TSE} to plants. This study found that even small quantities of prions in diluted brain homogenate or in urine and feces bind to wheat grass roots and leaves for several weeks, and that animals were efficiently infected by ingestion of prion-contaminated plants. These features apply to prions from diverse origins, including CWD. Moreover, root uptake of prions from contaminated soil is followed by transport to the stem and leaves.

EXPERIMENTAL TRANSMISSION

Transmission to natural hosts

While CWD has been shown to be experimentally transmissible after intracerebral inoculation of mule deer with incubation periods up to 2 years (Williams and Young, 1992), limited transmission studies have indicated that CWD developed ~25% more rapidly in orally challenged elk than deer (16 months for mule deer and 12 months for elk) (Williams, 2003). Levels of PrP^{TSE} were found to be higher in the tonsil and retropharyngeal lymph nodes of CWD-infected deer than elk (Race et al., 2007). Since this finding correlates with the natural prevalence of CWD in these species, the authors of this study speculated that CWD-infected deer may be more likely than elk to transmit the disease. While three captive Shira's moose (*A. alces shirasi*) orally inoculated with CWD from diseased mule deer died of causes unrelated to CWD, the presence of spongiform degeneration, and lymphoid and CNS PrP^{TSE} accumulation, was consistent with CWD replication (Kreeger et al., 2006).

Other cervid species have been shown to be sus ceptible to CWD following experimental challenge, including European red deer (*Cervus elaphus elaphus*) (Martin et al., 2009), muntjac deer (*Muntiacus reevesi*) (Nalls et al., 2013), and reindeer (Mitchell et al., 2012). Naïve reindeer exposed to reindeer infected with CWD from white-tailed deer, mule deer, or elk were susceptible regardless of source species, with horizontal transmission occurring through direct contact or indirectly through the environment (Moore et al., 2016). Brain material from CWD-infected white-tailed deer and elk produced disease in only 4 of 13 intracerebrally inoculated fallow deer (*Dama dama*) (Hamir et al., 2008), and the same species appeared resistant when co-housed in paddocks with CWD-affected mule deer (Rhyan et al., 2011), suggesting relative resistance of this cervid species to CWD. Subsequent full reports of transmission to this species, however, indicated that despite the fact that fallow deer might be less susceptible and clinical signs not as pronounced as in other deer species, intracerebrally inoculated fallow deer not only amplify CWD prions, but also develop lesions of spongiform encephalopathy (Hamir et al., 2011). Claims of CWD resistance in this species should therefore be interpreted with caution.

Transmission to noncervid species

Experimental transmission to other (noncervid) species has yielded mixed results. Studies by the late Dr. Richard Marsh in the mid-1980s at the University of Wisconsin, and later investigators at Colorado State University, demonstrated that the CWD agent was transmitted to Syrian golden hamsters, ferrets, mink, and squirrel monkeys (Bartz et al., 1998; Marsh et al., 2005; Sigurdson et al., 2008). Other susceptible species include several species of voles, white-footed mice, deer mice, cats, raccoons, squirrel monkeys, and pigs (Hamir et al., 2003, 2007; Race et al., 2009b, 2014; Heisey et al., 2010; Di Bari et al., 2013; Mathiason et al., 2013; Moore et al., 2017). While mice have been reported to be resistant to CWD infection (Browning et al., 2004), limited infection of the VM/Dk inbred strain of mice by elk CWD has been reported (Lee et al., 2013).

Whether the natural host range of CWD extends beyond the family Cervidae is currently unclear. However, the remarkably high rate of CWD prion transmission brings into question the risk posed to livestock from developing a novel CWD-related prion disease via shared grazing of CWD-contaminated rangeland. This issue has been addressed by transmitting CWD to cattle (Hamir et al., 2001, 2005, 2006c, 2007) and sheep (Hamir et al., 2006b). In the case of cattle, PrP^{TSE} was detected in ~40% of intracerebrally inoculated animals. Low rates of disease also occurred in intracerebrally inoculated sheep, and host genotype appeared to affect transmission. Transgenic (Tg) mice expressing ovine or bovine PrP were also challenged with CWD, with negative outcomes (Tamguney et al., 2006). Davenport and coworkers (2015) employed the RT-QuIC assay to compare the conversion properties of CWD and bovine spongiform encephalopathy (BSE), as well as feline-adapted versions of these prions. CWD, BSE, and feline-adapted CWD most effectively seeded cervid, bovine, and feline bacterially expressed recombinant PrP (rPrP) respectively, while feline spongiform encephalopathy (FSE) prions more efficiently converted bovine than feline rPrP. To model the potential of these prions to convert human PrP, human rPrP was used as a substrate in RT-QuIC. Remarkably, CWD, feline-adapted CWD, BSE, and FSE all converted human rPrP, although not as efficiently as sporadic Creutzfeldt–Jakob disease (CJD) prions.

Transgenic mouse models of CWD

The expense of housing cervids under prion-free conditions for long periods and the highly communicable nature of CWD present significant challenges for using deer as experimental hosts. Since expression of foreign PrP in Tg mice was known to be an extremely efficient means of abrogating prion species barriers, Tg mice expressing deer PrP were created to eliminate the known barrier to CWD prion transmission. Prototype Tg mice, referred to as Tg(CerPrP)1536 mice, developed signs of neurologic dysfunction ~230 days following intracerebral inoculation with four CWD isolates from either deer or elk (Browning et al., 2004). The brains of sick Tg(CerPrP)1536 mice recapitulated the cardinal neuropathologic features of CWD. Following this seminal report, several other groups reported similar results using comparable Tg mouse models (Kong et al., 2005; LaFauci et al., 2006; Tamguney et al., 2006; Meade-White et al., 2007). For the first time, the availability of CWD-susceptible Tg mouse models has also provided a means of quantifying CWD infectivity by endpoint titration (Angers et al., 2009). The availability of CWD-susceptible Tg mice greatly facilitated detection of CWD prions in tissues and bodily fluids of infected deer and elk, including deer skeletal muscle (Angers et al., 2006), elk antler velvet (Angers et al., 2009), urine and saliva (Haley et al., 2009b; Tamguney et al., 2012), feces (Tamguney et al., 2009), and fat (Race et al., 2009a). CWD has also been transmitted, albeit with less efficiency, to Tg mice overexpressing mouse (Sigurdson et al., 2006) or Syrian hamster PrP (Raymond et al., 2007).

In vitro amplification of CWD prions

Following the development of Tg(CerPrP)1536 mice, studies were initiated to evaluate the feasibility of expediting studies of CWD prion transmission by combining the resources of PMCA (Saborio et al., 2001) with Tg mouse models of prion disease. During PMCA, the normal form of PrP, PrP^{C}, is converted into protease-resistant PrP using small amounts of infectious PrP^{TSE}. Continued recruitment and conversion of PrP^{C} by PrP^{TSE} are accomplished by sonication in a process analogous to amplification of DNA by the polymerase chain reaction. In seminal studies, deer PrP^{C} expressed in the brains of Tg mice was used for amplification of CWD prions by PMCA. Using Tg(CerPrP) mice to characterize this in vitro-generated infectivity, PMCA was shown to enable high-fidelity amplification of CWD prions with apparently unaltered strain properties (Green et al., 2008b). These studies extended previous reports using Tg(CerPrP)1536 (Kurt et al., 2007) by showing that PMCA-derived CWD prions induce disease and the production of $CerPrP^{TSE}$ in Tg(CerPrP) mice as efficiently as prions isolated from the CNS of deer with CWD. Adaptation of the process whereby successive rounds of PMCA are performed using fresh brain homogenate substrate (serial PMCA), with ultimate evaluation by Western blotting added additional sensitivity to CWD detection (Angers et al., 2009; Haley et al., 2011).

In vitro amplification enhanced the sensitivity of CWD prion detection by several orders of magnitude greater than Western blotting, and has been used to confirm the presence of CWD prions in muscle (Daus et al., 2011), and feces (Pulford et al., 2012). Inclusion of Teflon beads in the PMCA reaction (PMCAb) increased the sensitivity of CWD detection without compromising assay specificity. PMCAb was demonstrated to be five orders of magnitude more sensitive than bioassay in Tg mice (Johnson et al., 2012). Using this approach, CWD prions were detected in the cerebrospinal fluid of CWD-exposed deer (Haley et al., 2013), and the urine and feces of elk, mule, and white-tailed deer by 6 months post inoculation (Plummer et al., 2017). Baculovirus-expressed PrP has also been successfully used as a source of substrate for PMCA conversion of CWD prions (Faburay et al., 2014).

As an alternative to whole-brain homogenates expressing PrP^C, and as part of a larger attempt to address the minimal components required for prion propagation, bacterially expressed rPrP has been used as a substrate for amplification, and CWD prion detection. In RT-QuIC (Atarashi et al., 2008), prion seeds are thought to induce rPrP to adopt a β-sheet structure. Thioflavin T, added to the reaction, is incorporated into the growing amyloid, causing an altered spectrofluorimetric emission pattern, which is monitored over time. RT-QuIC has been extensively applied to detection of CWD prions in tissues, body fluids, and excreta, including lymphoid tissue (Haley et al., 2014), cerebrospinal fluid (Haley et al., 2013), blood (Elder et al., 2013), saliva (Henderson et al., 2013), and urine and feces from preclinical animals (John et al., 2013; Cheng et al., 2016). Using these methods, Henderson and colleagues (2015a, b) estimated that urine and saliva from CWD-infected deer both contained 1–5 LD_{50} per 10 mL, suggesting substantial environmental contamination during the several-year course of an infection. Analysis of rectoanal mucosa-associated lymphoid tissue biopsy specimens and, to a lesser extent, nasal brushings, indicated that, like immunohistochemical analysis, RT-QuIC is a relatively sensitive assay for detection of CWD prions in rectoanal mucosa-associated lymphoid tissue biopsy specimens with potential for large-scale and rapid automated testing of antemortem samples for CWD (Haley et al., 2016).

THE ROLE OF HOST GENETICS IN CWD

To date, the sequence of the open reading frame of the gene encoding PrP, referred to as *PRNP*, has been studied in several cervid species currently infected by CWD, as well as those for which susceptibility is currently unknown. While the *PRNP* coding sequence (cds) is remarkably conserved among cervids, several key polymorphisms have been identified that are associated with lower rates and/or slower progression of CWD infection. Early work on the impact of cervid *PRNP* genetics occurred at the height of the BSE epidemic, prior to which CWD was merely a veterinary curiosity. In initial genetic analyses, Schatzl and coworkers (1997) reported that the PrP gene of North American elk (*Cervus elaphus canadensis*), otherwise referred to as wapiti, encodes leucine (L) at residue 132, while methionine (M) was found at this position in sika deer (*C. nippon dybowskii*). This finding was of interest in light of the fact that codon 132 is equivalent to codon 129 in the human *PRNP* cds, which can encode either M or valine (V) (Owen et al., 1990). This dimorphism has significant effects on human prion disease presentation (Collinge et al., 1991; Palmer et al., 1991).

Shortly thereafter, analysis of the *PRNP* cds of mule deer and Rocky Mountain elk by Cervenáková and colleagues (1997) revealed that the predicted amino acid sequence of PrP of these two species was identical, with the exception of a single difference at codon 226, encoding glutamine (Q) and glutamic acid (E) respectively. The occurrence of the L or M dimorphism at codon 132 in Rocky Mountain elk was confirmed by O'Rourke and colleagues (1998), and the same group showed that homozygosity of codon 132 encoding M was over-represented in both free-ranging and farm-raised CWD-affected elk when compared to unaffected control groups, suggesting relative protection against CWD in animals expressing L at this position (O'Rourke et al., 1999). The relatively protective effects of the L132 allele against CWD were confirmed in subsequent oral transmission experiments in this species (Hamir et al., 2006a; O'Rourke et al., 2007). However, arguing against safeguard from CWD by the 132L allele, in a survey of free-ranging elk in Colorado each codon genotype was represented in CWD-positive animals in proportion to their frequency in the population (Perucchini et al., 2008).

Subsequent large-scale genetic analyses of *PRNP* from mule deer (Brayton et al., 2004) revealed the presence of polymorphisms at codons 20 (encoding either aspartate (D) or glycine (G)), and at codon 225 (encoding serine (S) or phenylalanine (F)). Determination of *PRNP* alleles from 47 CWD-positive deer showed the predominant allele encoded D and S at codons 20 and 225 respectively at a frequency of 0.85. However, this study also showed that genetic analysis of CWD susceptibility alleles in this species was complicated by the nearly universal presence of a processed, but unexpressed, pseudogene, referred to as *PRNPψ*, which also contained a dimorphism (either asparagine (N) or S) at codon 138 (Brayton et al., 2004).

In Colorado and Wyoming, deer homozygous for the 225S allele developed CWD at a rate 30 times greater than heterozygous 225S/225F deer; the frequency of 225SF and 225FF genotypes in CWD-negative deer was 9.3%, but only 0.3% in CWD-positive deer (Jewell et al., 2005). In experimental transmissions, Fox and colleagues (2006) showed that, while PrP^{TSE} accumulation and distribution were similar in 225S/225S and 225S/225F deer, CNS PrP^{TSE} deposition was markedly delayed in heterozygotes, and while 225S/225S deer developed spongiform lesions after ~19 months, 225S/225F deer remained asymptomatic and free of neuropathologic lesions for up to 25 months. Studies comparing CWD susceptibility in 225S/225S and 225F/225F mule deer showed differences in clinical disease presentation, as well as more subtle, atypical traits in CWD-affected 225F/225F deer (Wolfe et al., 2014).

The presence of the *PRNPψ* pseudogene was confirmed in captive white-tailed deer (O'Rourke et al., 2004). In this study, two *PRNPψ* alleles encoding five or six copies of the octapeptide repeat were identified. In addition, this study identified four *PRNP* alleles, with substitutions at codons 95 (encoding either Q or histidine (H)); 96 (encoding either G or S) and 116 (encoding either alanine (A) or G). The pseudogene was not correlated with CWD status. The description of *PRNP* polymorphisms by O'Rourke and colleagues was consistent with earlier reports of *PRNP* status in smaller deer cohorts (Raymond et al., 2000; Heaton et al., 2003; Johnson et al., 2003), although in those studies functional genotypes could not be determined since primers were used that failed to discriminate *PRNP* from *PRNPψ*. Genetic analyses of free-ranging, Wisconsin white-tailed deer revealed a further polymorphism encoding lysine (K) at residue 226 (Johnson et al., 2006a). By comparing allelic frequencies in Wisconsin CWD-affected and unaffected deer, this study also suggested that occupancy of S and H at residues 96 and 95 was associated with reduced susceptibility to CWD.

Notwithstanding the fact that brains of CWD-affected deer that were heterozygous for the 96S/96G dimorphism contained lower amounts of PrP^{TSE} than CWD-affected 96G/96G deer, identification of a CWD-positive deer homozygous for the 96S allele indicated that this substitution did not provide complete resistance. Additional epidemiologic and genetic studies consistently reported lower CWD prevalence associated with the 96S compared with the 96G allele (Keane et al., 2008; Robinson et al., 2012), and experimental challenges revealed a longer CWD incubation period in deer expressing not only the 96S, but also the 95H alleles (Johnson et al., 2011). While the 95H and 116G alleles occur at relatively low frequencies, lower rates of CWD infection in populations expressing these alleles also suggested relative protection from these expressed variants against disease (O'Rourke et al., 2004; Johnson et al., 2006a; Kelly et al., 2008; Wilson et al., 2009).

Interestingly, while the residue 138 polymorphism encoding either N or S was originally thought to be unique to the *PRNPψ* pseudogene, the same polymorphism was subsequently detected in *PRNP* of reindeer and fallow deer but not in white-tailed or mule deer, which only carry the allele encoding S (Rhyan et al., 2011; Mitchell et al., 2012). Since fallow deer and mule deer/white-tailed deer differ only at position 138, this suggests that N at this position may confer relative resistance to CWD. In accordance with genetic protection from 138N, experimentally inoculated reindeer with at least one 138N allele were also relatively protected against developing CWD (Mitchell et al., 2012). Of possible relevance to disease management in threatened Canadian caribou populations, a significantly higher frequency of the 138N allele was detected in one of nine Albertan populations of woodland caribou (Cheng et al., 2017).

Modeling the effects of host genetic variability in transgenic mice

Tg mouse modeling provided an experimental means of assessing the role of these cervid PrP gene polymorphisms on CWD pathogenesis. In work combining studies in Tg mice, the natural host, cell-free prion amplification and molecular modeling approaches, the effects of deer PrP polymorphisms on CWD propagation and susceptibility to prions from different species were assessed (Angers et al., 2014). Reflecting the general authenticity of the Tg modeling approach, the properties of CWD prions were faithfully maintained in deer following their passage through Tg mice expressing cognate PrP. Moreover, the protective influences of naturally occurring deer PrP polymorphisms at codons 95, 96, and 225 on CWD susceptibility were accurately reproduced in Tg mice or during cell-free amplification. The resistance of Tg mice expressing deer PrP S96 to CWD in this study, referred to as Tg(DeerPrP-S96)7511 mice, was consistent with previously generated tg60 mice expressing serine at residue 96 (Meade-White et al., 2007). Interestingly, in the studies of Angers and colleagues (2014), whereas substitutions at residues 95 and 96 inhibited CWD propagation, they did not affect replication of sheep SSBP/1 prions in Tg mice. The residue 96 polymorphism also had no effect on the susceptibility of deer to SSBP/1 (Angers et al., 2014).

To more fully address the influence of the elk 132M/L polymorphism on CWD pathogenesis, transmissibility of CWD prions was assessed in Tg mice expressing cervid PrP^C encoding L or M at residue 132 (Green et al., 2008a). Paralleling the results of studies of the residue 95 and 96 dimorphisms reported by Angers and colleagues (2014), while Tg mice expressing CerPrP-L132 afforded partial resistance to CWD, SSBP/1 sheep scrapie prions transmitted efficiently to Tg mice expressing CerPrP-L132, suggesting that the elk 132M/L polymorphism also controls prion susceptibility at the level of prion strain selection. The contrasting ability of CWD and SSBP/1 prions to overcome the inhibitory effects of the CerPrPL132 allele is reminiscent of studies describing the effects of the human codon 129 methionine M/V polymorphism on variant CJD/BSE prion propagation in Tg mice expressing human PrP, which concluded that human PrP V129 severely restricts propagation of the BSE prion strain (Wadsworth et al., 2004). It therefore collectively appears that amino acid substitutions in the unstructured region of PrP, including at residues 95 and 96 in deer, and 132 and 129 in elk and humans respectively, affect PrP^C-to-PrP^{TSE} conversion in a strain-specific manner.

The susceptibility of Tg(DeerPrP-S96)7511 mice to CWD prions (Angers et al., 2014), albeit with incomplete attack rates and long incubation times, is at odds with previous work showing complete resistance of tg60 mice (Meade-White et al., 2007; Race et al., 2011). This apparent discrepancy is most likely related to the low transgene expression in tg60 mice, reported to be 70% the levels found in deer. As previously mentioned, CWD occurs naturally in deer homozygous for the PrP-S96 allele (Keane et al., 2008), which is clearly inconsistent with a completely protective effect of this substitution, suggesting that Tg(DeerPrP-S96)7511 mice represent an accurate Tg model in which to assess the effects of the S96 substitution.

In accordance with a role for the unstructured PrP region in strain selection, in subsequent studies, Tg mice expressing wild-type deer PrP (tg33) or tg60 were challenged with CWD prions from experimentally infected deer with varying polymorphisms at residues 95 and 96 (Duque Velasquez et al., 2015). Passage of deer CWD prions into tg33 mice expressing wild-type deer PrP resulted in 100% attack rates, with CWD prions from deer expressing H95 or S96 having significantly longer incubation periods. Remarkably, otherwise resistant tg60 mice (Meade-White et al., 2007; Race et al., 2011) developed disease only when inoculated with prions from deer expressing H95/Q95 and H95/S96 PrP genotypes.

The findings of Angers and coworkers (2014) also showed that residues 225 and 226 play a critical role in PrP^C-to-PrP^{TSE} conversion and strain propagation, but that the mechanism controlling their effects is distinct from that governing the effects of H95Q, G95S, and M132L polymorphisms in the unstructured PrP region. Structural analyses show that residues 225 and 226 are located in the distal region of α-helix 3. This region, referred to as the β2–α2 loop, participates with the loop region linking the second beta-sheet (β2) with the alpha2-helix (α2), to form a solvent-accessible contiguous epitope (Perez et al., 2010). High-resolution structural studies also revealed the β2–α2 loop of cervid PrP to be extremely well defined compared to most other species, raising the possibility that this structural characteristic correlates with the unusually facile contagious transmission of CWD (Gossert et al., 2005).

To address this notion, Tg mice were produced that expressed mouse PrP in which the β2–α2 loop was replaced by the corresponding region from cervid species. These mice spontaneously developed prion disease (Sigurdson et al., 2009). Additional studies have consistently pointed to the importance of the β2–α2 loop in regulating transmission barriers, including that of humans to CWD (Kurt et al., 2009, 2014, 2015; Sigurdson et al., 2010). However, subsequent work suggested a more complex mechanism involving participation of the β2–α2 loop with the distal region of α-helix 3 to form a solvent-accessible contiguous epitope (Perez et al., 2010). These and later studies (Christen et al., 2009) ascribed greater importance to the plasticity of this discontinuous epitope. For example, substitution of D found in horse, which contains a similarly structured loop region, by S at residue 170 of mouse (elk PrP numbering) loop, increased not only the structural order of the loop, but also the long-range interaction with Y228 in α-helix 3. Underscoring the importance of long-range β2–α2 loop/α-helix 3 interactions, similar structural connections occur between this residue, which is alanine (A) in Tammar wallaby PrP, and residue 169, which is isoleucine (I) in this species (19). Stabilizing long-range interactions between the β2–α2 loop and α-helix 3 also occur in rabbit PrP, a species generally regarded as resistant to prion infection. X-ray crystallographic analyses showed the rabbit β2–α2 loop to be clearly ordered and indicated that hydrophobic interactions between the side chains of

V169 and, in this case Y221 (elk PrP numbering) of α-helix 3, contributed to the stability of the β2–α2 loop/α helix 3 epitope (Khan et al., 2010).

Consistent with a role for this epitope in PrP conversion, Angers and colleagues (2014) showed that these polymorphisms severely impact replication of both SSBP/1 and, to variable degrees, CWD. In the case of Tg mice expressing deerPrP-F225, referred to as Tg(DeerPrP-F225), SSBP/1 incubation times were prolonged threefold, whereas inoculation with CWD produced incomplete attack rates or prolonged and variable incubation times in small numbers of mice. In those Tg(DeerPrP-F225) mice that did succumb to CWD, PrP^{TSE} distribution patterns were altered compared with Tg(DeerPrP) mice.

To address the effects of substitution of E for Q at residue 226, Angers and colleagues in separate studies also assessed whether Tg mice expressing wild-type elk or deer PrP, which differ only at this residue, diverged in their responses to CWD. These studies showed that this difference at residue 226 also affected CWD replication, but to a lesser degree than the residue 225 polymorphism. In this study disease onset was prolonged by 20–46% in CWD-inoculated Tg(DeerPrP) compared with Tg(ElkPrP) mice, and PrP^{TSE} distribution and neuropathology was different in each case (Angers et al., 2009). In contrast to Tg(DeerPrP) mice which are susceptible to SSBP/1 (Green et al., 2008a), Tg(ElkPrP) were completely resistant (Angers et al., 2009), although the resistance of elk PrP^C to propagation of SSBP/1 was overcome following adaptation in deer or Tg(DeerPrP) mice. Passage in Tg mice expressing E226 or Q226 profoundly affected the ability of SSBP/1 to reinfect Tg mice expressing sheep PrP^C. These studies paralleled aspects of previously published studies, indicating that amino acid differences at residue 226 controlled the manifestation of CWD quasi-species or closely related strains (Angers et al., 2010).

Collectively, these findings therefore point to an important role for residues 225 and 226 in PrP^C-to-PrP^{TSE} conversion, and in the manifestation of prion strain properties. They also substantiate the interpretation of structural analyses, which suggested that long-range interactions between the β2–α2 loop and α-helix 3 provide protection against prion infection. Finally, they suggest a likely mechanism to account for the protective effects of the F225 polymorphism. Molecular dynamics analyses (Angers et al., 2014) showed that the S225F and E226Q substitutions in deer alter the orientations of D170 in the β2–α2 loop and Y228 in α-helix 3. This structural change allows hydrogen bonding between the side chains of these residues, which results in reduced plasticity of the β2–α2 loop/α-helix 3 epitope compared with deer or elk PrP structures. This suggests that the increased stability of this tertiary structural epitope precludes PrP^C-to-PrP^{TSE} conversion of deerPrP-F225.

CWD STRAINS

Increasingly, Tg mice are used for typing strains in human and animal prion isolates (Telling, 2010). As mentioned previously, several Tg mouse lines expressing either elk or deer PrP have been developed in which the species barrier to CWD has been eliminated, enabling assessment of CWD strain prevalence. Although original transmission studies of CWD into Tg mice (Browning et al., 2004) and subsequent work (LaFauci et al., 2006) raised the possibility of CWD strain variation, the limited number of isolates and the lack of detailed strain analyses in those studies meant that this hypothesis remained speculative.

Subsequent studies supported the feasibility of using Tg(CerPrP)1536 mice for characterizing naturally occurring CWD strains, CWD prions generated by PMCA, and novel cervid prions (Green et al., 2008b). The prevalence of CWD prion strains in a large collection of captive and wild cervids from different species and geographic North American locations was assessed by bioassay in Tg mice (Angers et al., 2010). The findings provided substantial evidence for two prevalent CWD prion strains, referred to as CWD1 and CWD2, with distinct clinical and neuropathologic profiles. Remarkably, primary transmissions of CWD prions from elk produced either CWD1 or CWD2 profiles, while transmission of deer inocula favored the production of mixed, intra-study incubation times and CWD1 and CWD2 neuropathologies. These findings indicated that elk may be infected with either CWD1 or CWD2, while deer brains tend to harbor CWD1/CWD2 strain mixtures. Interestingly, previous limited CWD transmission studies in Tg mice also suggested that cervid brain inocula might be composed of strain mixtures (Tamguney et al., 2006).

Although certain strains are associated with distinct conformers and/or glycoform profiles of PrP^{TSE}, not all strains that can be biologically distinguished are composed of PrP^{TSE} with recognizably different biochemical properties. Despite consistent differences in incubation time and neuropathologic profiles, the electrophoretic migration patterns of PrP^{TSE} from the brains of mice infected by either CWD1 or CWD2 were indiscernible. PrP^{TSE} associated with CWD1 and CWD2 was composed of equivalent proportions of di-, mono-, and α-glycosyl forms, and had similar unfolding characteristics after treatment with guanidinium hydrochloride. When CWD1 or CWD2 elk isolates were transmitted to Tg mice expressing elk PrP, stabilities of the resulting PrP^{TSE} remained indistinguishable, but were distinct from PrP^{TSE} in Tg(CerPrP)1536 mice expressing deer PrP.

Duque Velasquez and coworkers (2015) evaluated the transmission properties of CWD prions derived experimentally from deer of four *PRNP* genotypes (variations at codons 95 and 96) in Tg mice expressing wild-type deer PrP, or PrP containing the S96 polymorphism. Disease signs and neuropathologic and PrP^{TSE} profiles in infected Tg mice expressing wild-type PrP were similar between groups, indicating that a prion strain (Wisc-1) common to all CWD inocula was amplified. In contrast, tg60 mice developed prion disease only when inoculated with CWD prions from animals with the H95/wt and H95/S96 genotypes. Serial passage in tg60 mice resulted in propagation of a novel CWD strain, referred to as H95(+), while transmission to tg33 mice, expressing wild-type PrP, produced two disease phenotypes consistent with propagation of two strains.

Additional studies also support the existence of multiple CWD strains. Infection of ferrets with two ferret-adapted CWD isolates indicated the existence of distinct strains with different clinical properties, distribution of PrP^{TSE} in the CNS and periphery, and proteinase K sensitivity of PrP^{TSE} (Perrott et al., 2012). CWD has also been transmitted, albeit with varying efficiency, to Tg mice overexpressing mouse PrP, referred to as Tga20 mice (Sigurdson et al., 2006; Tamguney et al., 2006). In the former study, a single mule deer isolate produced disease in all inoculated Tga20 mice. On successive passages, incubation times dropped to ~160 days. In the second study, an elk isolate from a total of 8 deer and elk CWD isolates induced disease in 75% of inoculated Tg mice overexpressing mouse PrP, referred to as Tg(MoPrP) 4053 mice. It is worth noting that the distribution of lesions in both studies appeared to resemble the CWD1 pattern.

Low-efficiency CWD prion transmission was also recorded in hamsters and Tg mice expressing Syrian hamster PrP (Raymond et al., 2007). In that study, during serial passage of mule deer CWD, fast and slow incubation time strains with different patterns of brain pathology and PrP^{TSE} deposition were also isolated. In yet other studies, serial passages of CWD from white-tailed deer into Tg mice expressing hamster PrP, and then Syrian golden hamsters produced a strain, referred to as "wasting" (WST), characterized by a prominent preclinical wasting disease, similar to cachexia, which the authors propose is due to a prion-induced endocrinopathy (Bessen et al., 2011). These same investigators identified a second strain, defined as "cheeky" (CKY), derived from infection of Tg mice that express hamster PrP (Crowell et al., 2015). The CKY strain had a shorter incubation period than WST, but after transmission to hamsters, the incubation period of CKY became 150 days longer than WST. In this case, proteinase K digestion revealed strain-specific PrP^{TSE} signatures that were maintained in both hosts, but the solubility and conformational stability of PrP^{TSE} differed for the CWD strains in a host-dependent manner. In addition to supporting the view that there are multiple CWD strains, these findings suggest the importance of host-specific pathways, independent of PrP, that participate in the selection and propagation of distinct strains.

Studies in cell culture support the existence of CWD strains. Quinacrine was found to alter the transmission properties of CWD prions, as well as the biochemical characteristics of the constitutive PrP^{TSE} (Bian et al., 2014). Despite accumulating significantly higher prion titers, quinacrine-treated (Q-CWD) prions from $Elk21^+$ cells produced prolonged incubation times, and altered neuropathologic profiles in Tg(DeerPrP) and Tg(ElkPrP) mice compared to CWD prions from untreated cells. This outcome is consistent with quinacrine affecting the intrinsic strain properties of CWD prions. Previous studies showed that strain properties are enciphered within the conformation of PrP^{TSE} (Telling et al., 1996; Green et al., 2008b), and that cervid prion incubation times positively correlate with PrP^{TSE} conformational stability (Green et al., 2008b). It is therefore significant that the longer incubation times of Q-CWD prions and altered patterns of PrP^{TSE} deposition in both Tg models were associated with an increase in the relative stability of PrP^{TSE} conformers constituting Q-CWD prions. The properties of Q-CWD prions provided convincing evidence for conformational mutation that were suggested, but could not be observed, in previous studies of mouse-adapted scrapie prions in cell cultures treated with swainsonine, an inhibitor of Golgi α-mannosidase II (Li et al., 2010).

In accordance with Western blotting-based analyses showing higher conformational stabilities of PrP^{TSE} produced in the brains of CWD-infected Tg(DeerPrP) mice compared with Tg(ElkPrP) mice (Angers et al., 2010), cell-based conformational stability assays confirmed that the conformation of deer PrP^{TSE} in RK13 cells expressing deer PrP (RKD^+) was more stable than elk PrP^{TSE} produced during infection of $Elk21^+$. Because $Elk21^+$ and RKD^+ propagated CWD prions from the same source, these differences in conformational stability result from the effects of residue 226, the sole primary structural difference between elk and deer PrP.

Novel cervid prion strains have been experimentally generated by adaptation of prions from other species by several means. Tg mice expressing deer, but not elk, PrP are sensitive to infection with SSBP/1 (Green et al., 2008a; Angers et al., 2014). Transmission of SSBP/1 to deer was also facile, with all inoculated animals developing within 19–20 months (Angers et al., 2014), which is in accordance with susceptibility of deer to a US scrapie isolate with a similar time to disease onset (Greenlee et al., 2011). Adaptation of mouse Rocky Mountain Lab (RML) prions, which required two passages in Tg(CerPrP) mice, was also accomplished by in vitro amplification of deer PrP^C by PMCA (Green et al., 2008b). In both cases the biologic and conformational strain properties of deer-adapted SSBP/1 and RML were distinct from those of CWD. Using PMCA, Zabel and coworkers spontaneously generated a novel strain of cervid prions which, upon inoculation into Tg(CerPrP) mice, displayed biochemical characteristics distinct from other cervid prion strains (Meyerett-Reid et al., 2017). These findings suggest that de novo prions resulted from the spontaneous misfolding of cervid PrP^C during PMCA.

ZOONOTIC POTENTIAL OF CWD

The identification and characterization of distinct CWD strains, and the influence of PrP primary structure on their stabilities, are of importance when considering the potential for interspecies transmission. The appearance of variant CJD following human exposure to BSE (Bruce et al., 1997; Hill et al., 1997) places the human species barrier to other animal prion diseases, particularly CWD, at the forefront of public health concerns. Since North American hunters harvest thousands of deer and elk each year, and it is not currently mandatory to have these animals tested, the demonstration of CWD prions in skeletal muscle and fat of deer (Angers et al., 2006; Race et al., 2009a) makes it likely that humans consume CWD prions. The substantial market for elk antler velvet in traditional Asian medicine also warrants concern (Angers et al., 2009).

Several strategies have been employed to assess the zoonotic potential of CWD, and estimates of how likely CWD prions might transmit to humans are currently mixed. While epidemiologic studies do not currently support a link between CWD and development of CJD, given the likelihood of a long incubation period, should transmission occur, current results cannot be taken as conclusive. Several case studies investigated unusual CJD cases in young adults, and cases with a history of hunting and/or venison consumption in areas where CWD is known to be present, but in all cases causes were determined to be genetic or sporadic (Belay et al., 2001; Anderson et al., 2007). In a 6-year follow-up of 81 individuals exposed to a CWD-infected deer in an upstate New York community, no CJD was documented (Olszowy et al., 2014). Using Colorado death certificate data from 1979 through 2001 to evaluate rates of death from CJD, Mawhinney and colleagues (2006) found no increase in the relative risk of CJD for residents of CWD-endemic county residents, and the rate of CJD did not increase over time.

In vitro conversion studies offer an indirect assessment of the transmissibility of CWD prions to humans. While initial cell-free conversion studies suggested that the ability of CWD prions to transform human PrP^C into protease-resistant PrP was low or failed to occur (Raymond et al., 2000; Luers et al., 2013), subsequent results showed that cervid PrP^{TSE} induced the conversion of human PrP^C by PMCA, following CWD prion strain stabilization by successive passages in vitro or in vivo (Barria et al., 2011). These results have implications for the human species barrier to CWD, and underscore the role of strain adaptation on interspecies transmission barriers. Consistent with these studies, Davenport and coworkers (2015) used RT-QuIC to model the transmission barrier of CWD to human rPrP. Their findings suggest that, at the level of protein–protein interactions, CWD adapts to a new species more readily than does BSE, and that the barrier preventing transmission of CWD to humans may be less robust than estimates from other approaches.

In vivo transmission approaches to model the species barrier to CWD prions have employed either nonhuman primate models (squirrel monkeys or *Cynomolgus* macaques) or Tg mice expressing human PrP. In two studies, squirrel monkeys challenged with CWD by intracerebral inoculation and oral exposure developed prion disease (Marsh et al., 2005; Race et al., 2009b). In contrast, macaques challenged by intracerebral, oral, and intradermal routes showed no indication of prion disease for periods ranging from 1.5 to more than 10 years (Race et al., 2009b, 2014). Additional studies using Tg mice expressing human PrP^C showed that CWD failed to induce disease following intracerebral CWD infection (Kong et al., 2005; Tamguney et al., 2006; Sandberg et al., 2010). However, the work of Kurt and colleagues (2015), which evaluated the effects of amino acid residues in the $\beta2$–$\alpha2$ loop sequence segment of human PrP, found that two specific amino acids had a significant impact on the efficiency of conversion by CWD.

CONCLUDING REMARKS

While CWD is, in many respects, the most enigmatic of all prion diseases, recent years have witnessed the development of specific research tools, including Tg mouse models and in vitro-based systems, for studying CWD prions and understanding the biology of this disease. Nonetheless, many significant questions and challenges remain. The origins of CWD in North America and Europe remain mysterious. Related to this, in the immediate future it will be important to determine whether the properties of prions causing disease in Norwegian reindeer and moose are distinct from those of prions causing CWD in US, Canadian, and South Korean deer and elk. Since the spread of CWD in wild North American cervids has been difficult, if not impossible, to check, the likelihood of similar CWD epidemics in Europe with unpredictable ecologic and public health consequences cannot be underestimated. CWD appears to have an unusually facile ability to affect a wide range of species. While currently confined to members of the cervid family, it will be of substantial importance to continue to monitor susceptibility of species that come into close contact with affected wild cervids. Current estimates of the zoonotic potential of CWD are mixed, but given the wide distribution of prions in diseased animals, and the fact that cervids are hunted, farmed, and consumed by humans, the likelihood of exposure, especially in select communities with close associations with such animals, remains high.

References

Almberg ES, Cross PC, Johnson CJ et al. (2011). Modeling routes of chronic wasting disease transmission: environmental prion persistence promotes deer population decline and extinction. PLoS One 6: e19896.

Anderson CA, Bosque P, Filley CM et al. (2007). Colorado surveillance program for chronic wasting disease transmission to humans: lessons from 2 highly suspicious but negative cases. Arch Neurol 64: 439–441.

Angers RC, Browning SR, Seward TS et al. (2006). Prions in skeletal muscles of deer with chronic wasting disease. Science 311: 1117.

Angers RC, Seward TS, Napier D et al. (2009). Chronic wasting disease prions in elk antler velvet. Emerg Infect Dis 15: 696–703.

Angers RC, Kang HE, Napier D et al. (2010). Prion strain mutation determined by prion protein conformational compatibility and primary structure. Science 328: 1154–1158.

Angers R, Christiansen J, Nalls AV et al. (2014). Structural effects of PrP polymorphisms on intra- and interspecies prion transmission. Proc Natl Acad Sci U S A 111: 11169–11174.

Atarashi R, Wilham JM, Christensen L et al. (2008). Simplified ultrasensitive prion detection by recombinant PrP conversion with shaking. Nat Methods 5: 211–212.

Baeten LA, Powers BE, Jewell JE et al. (2007). A natural case of chronic wasting disease in a free-ranging moose (*Alces alces shirasi*). J Wildl Dis 43: 309–314.

Barria MA, Telling GC, Gambetti P et al. (2011). Generation of a new form of human PrP(Sc) in vitro by interspecies transmission from cervid prions. J Biol Chem 286: 7490–7495.

Bartz JC, Marsh RF, McKenzie DI et al. (1998). The host range of chronic wasting disease is altered on passage in ferrets. Virology 251: 297–301.

Belay ED, Gambetti P, Schonberger LB et al. (2001). Creutzfeldt-Jakob disease in unusually young patients who consumed venison. Arch Neurol 58: 1673–1678.

Benestad SL, Mitchell G, Simmons M et al. (2016). First case of chronic wasting disease in Europe in a Norwegian free-ranging reindeer. Vet Res 47: 88.

Bessen RA, Robinson CJ, Seelig DM et al. (2011). Transmission of chronic wasting disease identifies a prion strain causing cachexia and heart infection in hamsters. PLoS One 6: e28026.

Bian J, Kang HE, Telling GC (2014). Quinacrine promotes replication and conformational mutation of chronic wasting disease prions. Proc Natl Acad Sci U S A 111: 6028–6033.

Brayton KA, O'Rourke KI, Lyda AK et al. (2004). A processed pseudogene contributes to apparent mule deer prion gene heterogeneity. Gene 326: 167–173.

Browning SR, Mason GL, Seward T et al. (2004). Transmission of prions from mule deer and elk with chronic wasting disease to transgenic mice expressing cervid PrP. J Virol 78: 13345–13350.

Bruce ME, Will RG, Ironside JW et al. (1997). Transmissions to mice indicate that 'new variant' CJD is caused by the BSE agent. Nature 389: 498–501.

Cervenáková L, Rohwer R, Williams S et al. (1997). High sequence homology of the PrP gene in mule deer and Rocky Mountain elk. Lancet 350: 219–220.

Cheng YC, Hannaoui S, John TR et al. (2016). Early and non-invasive detection of chronic wasting disease prions in elk feces by real-time quaking induced conversion. PLoS One 11: e0166187.

Cheng YC, Musiani M, Cavedon M et al. (2017). High prevalence of prion protein genotype associated with resistance to chronic wasting disease in one Alberta woodland caribou population. Prion 11: 136–142.

Christen B, Hornemann S, Damberger FF et al. (2009). Prion protein NMR structure from tammar wallaby (*Macropus eugenii*) shows that the beta2-alpha2 loop is modulated by long-range sequence effects. J Mol Biol 389: 833–845.

Collinge J, Palmer MS, Dryden AJ (1991). Genetic predisposition to iatrogenic Creutzfeldt-Jakob disease. Lancet 337: 1441–1442.

Conner MM, Miller MW, Ebinger MR et al. (2007). A meta-BACI approach for evaluating management intervention on chronic wasting disease in mule deer. Ecol Appl 17: 140–153.

Crowell J, Hughson A, Caughey B et al. (2015). Host determinants of prion strain diversity independent of prion protein genotype. J Virol 89: 10427–10441.

Daus ML, Breyer J, Wagenfuehr K et al. (2011). Presence and seeding activity of pathological prion protein (PrP(TSE)) in skeletal muscles of white-tailed deer infected with chronic wasting disease. PLoS One 6: e18345.

Davenport KA, Henderson DM, Bian J et al. (2015). Insights into chronic wasting disease and bovine spongiform encephalopathy species barriers by use of real-time conversion. J Virol 89: 9524–9531.

Di Bari MA, Nonno R, Castilla J et al. (2013). Chronic wasting disease in bank voles: characterisation of the shortest incubation time model for prion diseases. PLoS Pathog 9: e1003219.

Dube C, Mehren KG, Barker IK et al. (2006). Retrospective investigation of chronic wasting disease of cervids at the Toronto Zoo, 1973-2003. Can Vet J 47: 1185–1193.

Dulberger J, Hobbs NT, Swanson HM et al. (2010). Estimating chronic wasting disease effects on mule deer recruitment and population growth. J Wildl Dis 46: 1086–1095.

Duque Velasquez C, Kim C, Herbst A et al. (2015). Deer prion proteins modulate the emergence and adaptation of chronic wasting disease strains. J Virol 89: 12362–12373.

Elder AM, Henderson DM, Nalls AV et al. (2013). In vitro detection of prionemia in TSE-infected cervids and hamsters. PLoS One 8: e80203.

Faburay B, Tark D, Kanthasamy AG et al. (2014). In vitro amplification of scrapie and chronic wasting disease PrP(res) using baculovirus-expressed recombinant PrP as substrate. Prion 8: 393–403.

Fox KA, Jewell JE, Williams ES et al. (2006). Patterns of PrPCWD accumulation during the course of chronic wasting disease infection in orally inoculated mule deer (*Odocoileus hemionus*). J Gen Virol 87: 3451–3461.

Geremia C, Miller MW, Hoeting JA et al. (2015). Bayesian modeling of prion disease dynamics in mule deer using population monitoring and capture-recapture data. PLoS One 10: e0140687.

Gossert AD, Bonjour S, Lysek DA et al. (2005). Prion protein NMR structures of elk and of mouse/elk hybrids. Proc Natl Acad Sci U S A 102: 646–650.

Green KM, Browning SR, Seward TS et al. (2008a). The elk PRNP codon 132 polymorphism controls cervid and scrapie prion propagation. J Gen Virol 89: 598–608.

Green KM, Castilla J, Seward TS et al. (2008b). Accelerated high fidelity prion amplification within and across prion species barriers. PLoS Pathog 4: e1000139.

Greenlee JJ, Smith JD, Kunkle RA (2011). White-tailed deer are susceptible to the agent of sheep scrapie by intracerebral inoculation. Vet Res 42: 107.

Guiroy DC, Williams ES, Yanagihara R et al. (1991). Topographic distribution of scrapie amyloid-immunoreactive plaques in chronic wasting disease in captive mule deer (*Odocoileus hemionus hemionus*). Acta Neuropathol (Berl) 81: 475–478.

Haley NJ, Hoover EA (2015). Chronic wasting disease of cervids: current knowledge and future perspectives. Annu Rev Anim Biosci 3: 305–325.

Haley NJ, Mathiason CK, Zabel MD et al. (2009a). Detection of sub-clinical CWD infection in conventional test-negative deer long after oral exposure to urine and feces from CWD+ deer. PLoS One 4: e7990.

Haley NJ, Seelig DM, Zabel MD et al. (2009b). Detection of CWD prions in urine and saliva of deer by transgenic mouse bioassay. PLoS One 4: e4848.

Haley NJ, Mathiason CK, Carver S et al. (2011). Detection of CWD prions in salivary, urinary, and intestinal tissues of deer: potential mechanisms of prion shedding and transmission. J Virol 85: 6309–6318.

Haley NJ, Van de Motter A, Carver S et al. (2013). Prion-seeding activity in cerebrospinal fluid of deer with chronic wasting disease. PLoS One 8: e81488.

Haley NJ, Carver S, Hoon-Hanks LL et al. (2014). Detection of chronic wasting disease in the lymph nodes of free-ranging cervids by real-time quaking-induced conversion. J Clin Microbiol 52: 3237–3243.

Haley NJ, Siepker C, Hoon-Hanks LL et al. (2016). Seeded amplification of chronic wasting disease prions in nasal brushings and recto-anal mucosa-associated lymphoid tissues from elk by real-time quaking-induced conversion. J Clin Microbiol 54: 1117–1126.

Hamir AN, Cutlip RC, Miller JM et al. (2001). Preliminary findings on the experimental transmission of chronic wasting disease agent of mule deer to cattle. J Vet Diagn Investig 13: 91–96.

Hamir AN, Miller JM, Cutlip RC et al. (2003). Experimental inoculation of scrapie and chronic wasting disease agents in raccoons (*Procyon lotor*). Vet Rec 153: 121–123.

Hamir AN, Kunkle RA, Cutlip RC et al. (2005). Experimental transmission of chronic wasting disease agent from mule deer to cattle by the intracerebral route. J Vet Diagn Investig 17: 276–281.

Hamir AN, Gidlewski T, Spraker TR et al. (2006a). Preliminary observations of genetic susceptibility of elk (*Cervus elaphus nelsoni*) to chronic wasting disease by experimental oral inoculation. J Vet Diagn Investig 18: 110–114.

Hamir AN, Kunkle RA, Cutlip RC et al. (2006b). Transmission of chronic wasting disease of mule deer to Suffolk sheep following intracerebral inoculation. J Vet Diagn Investig 18: 558–565.

Hamir AN, Kunkle RA, Miller JM et al. (2006c). Experimental second passage of chronic wasting disease (CWD(mule deer)) agent to cattle. J Comp Pathol 134: 63–69.

Hamir AN, Miller JM, Kunkle RA et al. (2007). Susceptibility of cattle to first-passage intracerebral inoculation with chronic wasting disease agent from white-tailed deer. Vet Pathol 44: 487–493.

Hamir AN, Kunkle RA, Nicholson EM et al. (2008). Preliminary observations on the experimental transmission of chronic wasting disease (CWD) from elk and white-tailed deer to fallow deer. J Comp Pathol 138: 121–130.

Hamir AN, Greenlee JJ, Nicholson EM et al. (2011). Experimental transmission of chronic wasting disease (CWD) from elk and white-tailed deer to fallow deer by intracerebral route: final report. Can J Vet Res 75: 152–156.

Heaton MP, Leymaster KA, Freking BA et al. (2003). Prion gene sequence variation within diverse groups of U.S. sheep, beef cattle, and deer. Mamm Genome 14: 765–777.

Heisey DM, Mickelsen NA, Schneider JR et al. (2010). Chronic wasting disease (CWD) susceptibility of several North American rodents that are sympatric with cervid CWD epidemics. J Virol 84: 210–215.

Henderson DM, Manca M, Haley NJ et al. (2013). Rapid antemortem detection of CWD prions in deer saliva. PLoS One 8: e74377.

Henderson DM, Davenport KA, Haley NJ et al. (2015a). Quantitative assessment of prion infectivity in tissues and body fluids by real-time quaking-induced conversion. J Gen Virol 96: 210–219.

Henderson DM, Denkers ND, Hoover CE et al. (2015b). Longitudinal detection of prion shedding in saliva and urine by chronic wasting disease-infected deer by real-time quaking-induced conversion. J Virol 89: 9338–9347.

Hill AF, Desbruslais M, Joiner S et al. (1997). The same prion strain causes vCJD and BSE. Nature 389: 448–450.

Jewell JE, Conner MM, Wolfe LL et al. (2005). Low frequency of PrP genotype 225SF among free-ranging mule deer (*Odocoileus hemionus*) with chronic wasting disease. J Gen Virol 86: 2127–2134.

Jewell JE, Brown J, Kreeger T et al. (2006). Prion protein in cardiac muscle of elk (*Cervus elaphus nelsoni*) and white-tailed deer (*Odocoileus virginianus*) infected with chronic wasting disease. J Gen Virol 87: 3443–3450.

John TR, Schatzl HM, Gilch S (2013). Early detection of chronic wasting disease prions in urine of pre-symptomatic deer by real-time quaking-induced conversion assay. Prion 7: 253–258.

Johnson C, Johnson J, Clayton M et al. (2003). Prion protein gene heterogeneity in free-ranging white-tailed deer within the chronic wasting disease affected region of Wisconsin. J Wildl Dis 39: 576–581.

Johnson C, Johnson J, Vanderloo JP et al. (2006a). Prion protein polymorphisms in white-tailed deer influence susceptibility to chronic wasting disease. J Gen Virol 87: 2109–2114.

Johnson CJ, Phillips KE, Schramm PT et al. (2006b). Prions adhere to soil minerals and remain infectious. PLoS Pathog 2: e32.

Johnson CJ, Pedersen JA, Chappell RJ et al. (2007). Oral transmissibility of prion disease is enhanced by binding to soil particles. PLoS Pathog 3: e93.

Johnson CJ, Herbst A, Duque-Velasquez C et al. (2011). Prion protein polymorphisms affect chronic wasting disease progression. PLoS One 6: e17450.

Johnson CJ, Aiken JM, McKenzie D et al. (2012). Highly efficient amplification of chronic wasting disease agent by protein misfolding cyclic amplification with beads (PMCAb). PLoS One 7: e35383.

Joly DO, Ribic CA, Langenberg JA et al. (2003). Chronic wasting disease in free-ranging Wisconsin white-tailed deer. Emerg Infect Dis 9: 599–601.

Keane DP, Barr DJ, Bochsler PN et al. (2008). Chronic wasting disease in a Wisconsin white-tailed deer farm. J Vet Diagn Investig 20: 698–703.

Kelly AC, Mateus-Pinilla NE, Diffendorfer J et al. (2008). Prion sequence polymorphisms and chronic wasting disease resistance in Illinois white-tailed deer (*Odocoileus virginianus*). Prion 2: 28–36.

Khan MQ, Sweeting B, Mulligan VK et al. (2010). Prion disease susceptibility is affected by beta-structure folding propensity and local side-chain interactions in PrP. Proc Natl Acad Sci U S A 107: 19808–19813.

Kim TY, Shon HJ, Joo YS et al. (2005). Additional cases of chronic wasting disease in imported deer in Korea. J Vet Med Sci 67: 753–759.

Kong Q, Huang S, Zou W et al. (2005). Chronic wasting disease of elk: transmissibility to humans examined by transgenic mouse models. J Neurosci 25: 7944–7949.

Kreeger TJ, Montgomery DL, Jewell JE et al. (2006). Oral transmission of chronic wasting disease in captive Shira's moose. J Wildl Dis 42: 640–645.

Kurt TD, Perrott MR, Wilusz CJ et al. (2007). Efficient in vitro amplification of chronic wasting disease PrPRES. J Virol 81: 9605–9608.

Kurt TD, Telling GC, Zabel MD et al. (2009). Trans-species amplification of PrP(CWD) and correlation with rigid loop 170N. Virology 387: 235–243.

Kurt TD, Bett C, Fernandez-Borges N et al. (2014). Prion transmission prevented by modifying the beta2-alpha2 loop structure of host PrPC. J Neurosci 34: 1022–1027.

Kurt TD, Jiang L, Fernandez-Borges N et al. (2015). Human prion protein sequence elements impede cross-species chronic wasting disease transmission. J Clin Invest 125: 1485–1496.

LaFauci G, Carp RI, Meeker HC et al. (2006). Passage of chronic wasting disease prion into transgenic mice expressing Rocky Mountain elk (*Cervus elaphus nelsoni*) PrPC. J Gen Virol 87: 3773–3780.

Lee YH, Sohn HJ, Kim MJ et al. (2013). Experimental chronic wasting disease in wild type VM mice. J Vet Med Sci 75: 1107–1110.

Li J, Browning S, Mahal SP et al. (2010). Darwinian evolution of prions in cell culture. Science 327: 869–872.

Luers L, Bannach O, Stohr J et al. (2013). Seeded fibrillation as molecular basis of the species barrier in human prion diseases. PLoS One 8: e72623.

Marsh RF, Kincaid AE, Bessen RA et al. (2005). Interspecies transmission of chronic wasting disease prions to squirrel monkeys (*Saimiri sciureus*). J Virol 79: 13794–13796.

Martin S, Jeffrey M, Gonzalez L et al. (2009). Immunohistochemical and biochemical characteristics of BSE and CWD in experimentally infected European red deer (*Cervus elaphus elaphus*). BMC Vet Res 5: 26.

Mathiason CK, Powers JG, Dahmes SJ et al. (2006). Infectious prions in the saliva and blood of deer with chronic wasting disease. Science 314: 133–136.

Mathiason CK, Nalls AV, Seelig DM et al. (2013). Susceptibility of domestic cats to chronic wasting disease. J Virol 87: 1947–1956.

Mawhinney S, Pape WJ, Forster JE et al. (2006). Human prion disease and relative risk associated with chronic wasting disease. Emerg Infect Dis 12: 1527–1535.

McBride PA, Schulz-Schaeffer WJ, Donaldson M et al. (2001). Early spread of scrapie from the gastrointestinal tract to the central nervous system involves autonomic fibers of the splanchnic and vagus nerves. J Virol 75: 9320–9327.

Meade-White K, Race B, Trifilo M et al. (2007). Resistance to chronic wasting disease in transgenic mice expressing a naturally occurring allelic variant of deer prion protein. J Virol 81: 4533–4539.

Meyerett-Reid C, Wyckoff AC, Spraker T et al. (2017). De novo generation of a unique cervid prion strain using protein misfolding cyclic amplification. mSphere 2.

Miller MW, Williams ES (2003). Prion disease: horizontal prion transmission in mule deer. Nature 425: 35–36.

Miller MW, Wild MA, Williams ES (1998). Epidemiology of chronic wasting disease in captive Rocky Mountain elk. J Wildl Dis 34: 532–538.

Miller MW, Williams ES, McCarty CW et al. (2000). Epizootiology of chronic wasting disease in free-ranging cervids in Colorado and Wyoming. J Wildl Dis 36: 676–690.

Miller M, Williams E, Hobbs N et al. (2004). Environmental sources of prion transmission in mule deer. Emerging Infectious Diseases [serial on the Internet]: 10.

Miller MW, Swanson HM, Wolfe LL et al. (2008). Lions and prions and deer demise. PLoS One 3: e4019.

Mitchell GB, Sigurdson CJ, O'Rourke KI et al. (2012). Experimental oral transmission of chronic wasting disease to reindeer (*Rangifer tarandus tarandus*). PLoS One 7: e39055.

Moore SJ, Kunkle R, Greenlee MH et al. (2016). Horizontal transmission of chronic wasting disease in reindeer. Emerg Infect Dis 22: 2142–2145.

Moore SJ, West Greenlee MH, Kondru N et al. (2017). Experimental transmission of the chronic wasting disease agent to swine after oral or intracranial inoculation. J Virol 91: pii. e00926-17.

Nalls AV, McNulty E, Powers J et al. (2013). Mother to offspring transmission of chronic wasting disease in Reeves' muntjac deer. PLoS One 8: e71844.

O'Rourke KI, Baszler TV, Miller JM et al. (1998). Monoclonal antibody F89/160.1.5 defines a conserved epitope on the ruminant prion protein. J Clin Microbiol 36: 1750–1755.

O'Rourke KI, Besser TE, Miller MW et al. (1999). PrP genotypes of captive and free-ranging Rocky Mountain elk (*Cervus elaphus nelsoni*) with chronic wasting disease. J Gen Virol 80 (Pt 10): 2765–2769.

O'Rourke KI, Spraker TR, Hamburg LK et al. (2004). Polymorphisms in the prion precursor functional gene but not the pseudogene are associated with susceptibility to chronic wasting disease in white-tailed deer. J Gen Virol 85: 1339–1346.

O'Rourke KI, Spraker TR, Zhuang D et al. (2007). Elk with a long incubation prion disease phenotype have a unique PrPd profile. Neuroreport 18: 1935–1938.

Olszowy KM, Lavelle J, Rachfal K et al. (2014). Six-year follow-up of a point-source exposure to CWD contaminated venison in an Upstate New York community: risk behaviours and health outcomes 2005-2011. Public Health 128: 860–868.

Owen F, Poulter M, Collinge J et al. (1990). Codon 129 changes in the prion protein gene in Caucasians. Am J Hum Genet 46: 1215–1216.

Palmer MS, Dryden AJ, Hughes JT et al. (1991). Homozygous prion protein genotype predisposes to sporadic Creutzfeldt-Jakob disease. Nature 352: 340–342.

Perez DR, Damberger FF, Wuthrich K (2010). Horse prion protein NMR structure and comparisons with related variants of the mouse prion protein. J Mol Biol 400: 121–128.

Perrott MR, Sigurdson CJ, Mason GL et al. (2012). Evidence for distinct chronic wasting disease (CWD) strains in experimental CWD in ferrets. J Gen Virol 93: 212–221.

Perucchini M, Griffin K, Miller MW et al. (2008). PrP genotypes of free-ranging wapiti (*Cervus elaphus nelsoni*) with chronic wasting disease. J Gen Virol 89: 1324–1328.

Plummer IH, Wright SD, Johnson CJ et al. (2017). Temporal patterns of chronic wasting disease prion excretion in three cervid species. J Gen Virol 98: 1932–1942.

Pritzkow S, Morales R, Moda F et al. (2015). Grass plants bind, retain, uptake, and transport infectious prions. Cell Rep 11: 1168–1175.

Pulford B, Spraker TR, Wyckoff AC et al. (2012). Detection of PrPCWD in feces from naturally exposed Rocky Mountain elk (*Cervus elaphus nelsoni*) using protein misfolding cyclic amplification. J Wildl Dis 48: 425–434.

Race BL, Meade-White KD, Ward A et al. (2007). Levels of abnormal prion protein in deer and elk with chronic wasting disease. Emerg Infect Dis 13: 824–830.

Race B, Meade-White K, Race R et al. (2009a). Prion infectivity in fat of deer with chronic wasting disease. J Virol 83: 9608–9610.

Race B, Meade-White KD, Miller MW et al. (2009b). Susceptibilities of nonhuman primates to chronic wasting disease. Emerg Infect Dis 15: 1366–1376.

Race B, Meade-White K, Miller MW et al. (2011). In vivo comparison of chronic wasting disease infectivity from deer with variation at prion protein residue 96. J Virol 85: 9235–9238.

Race B, Meade-White KD, Phillips K et al. (2014). Chronic wasting disease agents in nonhuman primates. Emerg Infect Dis 20: 833–837.

Raymond GJ, Bossers A, Raymond LD et al. (2000). Evidence of a molecular barrier limiting susceptibility of humans, cattle and sheep to chronic wasting disease. EMBO J 19: 4425–4430.

Raymond GJ, Raymond LD, Meade-White KD et al. (2007). Transmission and adaptation of chronic wasting disease to hamsters and transgenic mice: evidence for strains. J Virol 81: 4305–4314.

Rhyan JC, Miller MW, Spraker TR et al. (2011). Failure of fallow deer (*Dama dama*) to develop chronic wasting disease when exposed to a contaminated environment and infected mule deer (*Odocoileus hemionus*). J Wildl Dis 47: 739–744.

Robinson SJ, Samuel MD, Johnson CJ et al. (2012). Emerging prion disease drives host selection in a wildlife population. Ecol Appl 22: 1050–1059.

Saborio GP, Permanne B, Soto C (2001). Sensitive detection of pathological prion protein by cyclic amplification of protein misfolding. Nature 411: 810–813.

Sandberg M, Al-Doujaily H, Sigurdson C et al. (2010). Chronic wasting disease prions are not transmissible to transgenic mice over-expressing human prion protein. J Gen Virol 91: 2651–2657.

Saunders SE, Bartz JC, Telling GC et al. (2008). Environmentally-relevant forms of the prion protein. Environ Sci Technol 42: 6573–6579.

Saunders SE, Bartz JC, Vercauteren KC et al. (2011). An enzymatic treatment of soil-bound prions effectively inhibits replication. Appl Environ Microbiol 77: 4313–4317.

Saunders SE, Bartelt-Hunt SL, Bartz JC (2012). Occurrence, transmission, and zoonotic potential of chronic wasting disease. Emerg Infect Dis 18: 369–376.

Schatzl HM, Wopfner F, Gilch S et al. (1997). Is codon 129 of prion protein polymorphic in human beings but not in animals? Lancet 349: 1603–1604.

Seidel B, Thomzig A, Buschmann A et al. (2007). Scrapie agent (strain 263K) can transmit disease via the oral route after persistence in soil over years. PLoS One 2: e435.

Sigurdson CJ, Williams ES, Miller MW et al. (1999). Oral transmission and early lymphoid tropism of chronic wasting disease PrPres in mule deer fawns (*Odocoileus hemionus*). J Gen Virol 80: 2757–2764.

Sigurdson CJ, Spraker TR, Miller MW et al. (2001). PrP (CWD) in the myenteric plexus, vagosympathetic trunk and endocrine glands of deer with chronic wasting disease. J Gen Virol 82: 2327–2334.

Sigurdson CJ, Barillas-Mury C, Miller MW et al. (2002). PrP (CWD) lymphoid cell targets in early and advanced chronic wasting disease of mule deer. J Gen Virol 83: 2617–2628.

Sigurdson CJ, Manco G, Schwarz P et al. (2006). Strain fidelity of chronic wasting disease upon murine adaptation. J Virol 80: 12303–12311.

Sigurdson CJ, Mathiason CK, Perrott MR et al. (2008). Experimental chronic wasting disease (CWD) in the ferret. J Comp Pathol 138: 189–196.

Sigurdson CJ, Nilsson KP, Hornemann S et al. (2009). De novo generation of a transmissible spongiform encephalopathy by mouse transgenesis. Proc Natl Acad Sci U S A 106: 304–309.

Sigurdson CJ, Nilsson KP, Hornemann S et al. (2010). A molecular switch controls interspecies prion disease transmission in mice. J Clin Invest 120: 2590–2599.

Smith CB, Booth CJ, Pedersen JA (2011). Fate of prions in soil: a review. J Environ Qual 40: 449–461.

Sohn HJ, Kim JH, Choi KS et al. (2002). A case of chronic wasting disease in an elk imported to Korea from Canada. J Vet Med Sci 64: 855–858.

Spraker TR, Miller MW, Williams ES et al. (1997). Spongiform encephalopathy in free-ranging mule deer (*Odocoileus hemionus*), white-tailed deer (*Odocoileus virginianus*), and Rocky Mountain elk (*Cervus elaphus nelsoni*) in northcentral Colorado. J Wildl Dis 33: 1–6.

Tamguney G, Giles K, Bouzamondo-Bernstein E et al. (2006). Transmission of elk and deer prions to transgenic mice. J Virol 80: 9104–9114.

Tamguney G, Miller MW, Wolfe LL et al. (2009). Asymptomatic deer excrete infectious prions in faeces. Nature 461: 529–532.

Tamguney G, Richt JA, Hamir AN et al. (2012). Salivary prions in sheep and deer. Prion 6: 52–61.

Telling GC (2010). Nucleic acid-free mutation of prion strains. Prion 4: 252–255.

Telling GC, Parchi P, DeArmond SJ et al. (1996). Evidence for the conformation of the pathologic isoform of the prion protein enciphering and propagating prion diversity. Science 274: 2079–2082.

Wadsworth JD, Asante EA, Desbruslais M et al. (2004). Human prion protein with valine 129 prevents expression of variant CJD phenotype. Science 306: 1793–1796.

Wasserberg G, Osnas EE, Rolley RE et al. (2009). Host culling as an adaptive management tool for chronic wasting disease in white-tailed deer: a modelling study. J Appl Ecol 46: 457–466.

Williams ES (2003). Scrapie and chronic wasting disease. Clin Lab Med 23: 139–159.

Williams ES (2005). Chronic wasting disease. Vet Pathol 42: 530–549.

Williams ES, Miller MW (2002). Chronic wasting disease in deer and elk in North America. Rev Sci Tech 21: 305–316.

Williams ES, Young S (1980). Chronic wasting disease of captive mule deer: a spongiform encephalopathy. J Wildl Dis 16: 89–98.

Williams ES, Young S (1982). Spongiform encephalopathy of Rocky Mountain elk. J Wildl Dis 18: 465–471.

Williams ES, Young S (1992). Spongiform encephalopathies in Cervidae. Rev Sci Tech Off Int Epiz 11: 551–567.

Williams ES, Young S (1993). Neuropathology of chronic wasting disease of mule deer (*Odocoileus hemionus*) and elk (*Cervus elaphus nelsoni*). Vet Pathol 30: 36–45.

Wilson GA, Nakada SM, Bollinger TK et al. (2009). Polymorphisms at the PRNP gene influence susceptibility to chronic wasting disease in two species of deer (*Odocoileus* spp.) in western Canada. J Toxicol Environ Health A 72: 1025–1029.

Wolfe LL, Fox KA, Miller MW (2014). "Atypical" chronic wasting disease in PRNP genotype 225FF mule deer. J Wildl Dis 50: 660–665.

Section III

Human prion diseases (clinical, epidemiology, neuropathological, biochemical, biomarker, and genotypes)

Handbook of Clinical Neurology, Vol. 153 (3rd series)
Human Prion Diseases
M. Pocchiari and J. Manson, Editors
https://doi.org/10.1016/B978-0-444-63945-5.00009-X

Chapter 9

Sporadic Creutzfeldt–Jakob disease

INGA ZERR[1]* AND PIERO PARCHI[2]

[1]*Department of Neurology, University Hospital, Georg-August-University, Goettingen, Germany*

[2]*Department of Experimental, Diagnostic and Specialty Medicine, University of Bologna and IRCCS Institute of Neurological Sciences, Bologna, Italy*

Abstract

Sporadic Creutzfeldt–Jakob disease (CJD), the most common human prion disease, is generally regarded as a spontaneous neurodegenerative illness, arising either from a spontaneous *PRNP* somatic mutation or a stochastic PrP structural change. Alternatively, the possibility of an infection from animals or other source remains to be completely ruled out. Sporadic CJD is clinically characterized by rapidly progressive dementia with ataxia, myoclonus, or other neurologic signs and, neuropathologically, by the presence of aggregates of abnormal prion protein, spongiform change, neuronal loss, and gliosis. Despite these common features the disease shows a wide phenotypic variability which was recognized since its early descriptions. In the late 1990s the identification of key molecular determinants of phenotypic expression and the availability of a large series of neuropathologically verified cases led to the characterization of definite clinicopathologic and molecular disease subtypes and to an internationally recognized disease classification. By showing that these disease subtypes correspond to specific agent strain–host genotype combinations, recent transmission studies have confirmed the biologic basis of this classification. The introduction of brain magnetic resonance imaging techniques such as fluid-attenuated inversion recovery and diffusion-weighted imaging sequences and cerebrospinal fluid biomarker assays for the detection of brain-derived proteins as well as real-time quaking-induced conversion assay, allowing the specific detection of prions in accessible biologic fluids and tissues, has significantly contributed to the improved accuracy of the clinical diagnosis of sporadic CJD in recent years.

INTRODUCTION

Creutzfeldt–Jakob disease (CJD) is a rare, fatal, rapidly progressive neurodegenerative human disorder occurring in sporadic, genetic, and acquired forms. Sporadic CJD (sCJD), by far the most common form, is typically characterized by a rapidly progressive clinical course and widespread brain deposition of abnormal prion protein (PrP^{TSE}) aggregates leading to spongiform change, gliosis, and neuronal loss. Despite these common features, however, the disease shows a wide phenotypic variability. The application of molecular techniques, the collection of large case series, and the completion of experimental disease transmissions provided the identification and characterization of definite clinicopathologic sCJD subtypes, novel insight into their molecular basis, and the formulation of a systematic disease classification. Significant advances have also been made in the clinical diagnosis of the disease. Indeed, while the full characterization of the disease histotype and PrP^{TSE} type still requires postmortem tissue analysis, the clinical diagnosis can nowadays be substantiated with high accuracy in the majority of cases by a variety of tests such as magnetic resonance imaging (MRI) and cerebrospinal fluid (CSF) analyses.

*Correspondence to: Inga Zerr, Department of Neurology, University Hospital, Georg-August-University, Robert-Koch-Straße 40, 37075 Goettingen, Germany. Tel: +49-551-39-66636, E-mail: epicjd@med.uni-goettingen.de

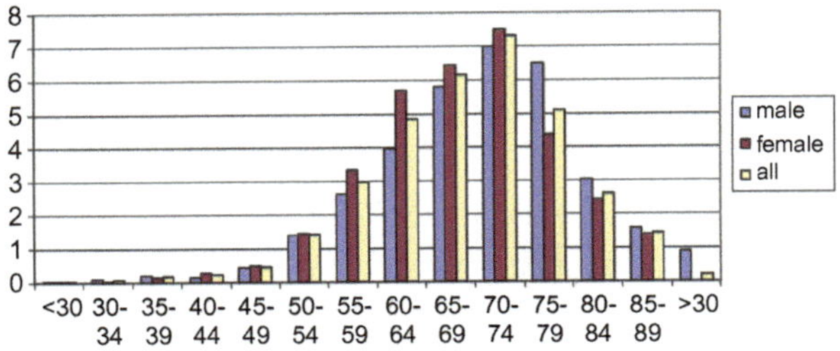

Fig. 9.1. Distribution of the age- and gender-specific mortality rate in sporadic Creutzfeldt–Jakob disease.

EPIDEMIOLOGY

sCJD is a rare disease, having an annual incidence of about two cases per million worldwide (Minikel et al., 2016). The disease is rare in young people (Will et al., 1998; Boesenberg et al., 2005; Ladogana et al., 2005; Heinemann et al., 2007).

The distribution of the yearly age- and gender-specific mortality rates revealed peak mortality in the 60–79-year age group (Ladogana et al., 2005) (Fig. 9.1). The analysis of pooled data for three time periods (1993–1995, 1996–1998, and 1999–2002) in a large multinational study showed mortality rates from sCJD increasing with time in all age groups. However, this effect was most prominent in the age group of 70 years and older (Ladogana et al., 2005). Improved clinical diagnosis, increased awareness, and establishment of surveillance programs may have contributed to this phenomenon (Will et al., 1996; Cousens et al., 1997; Brandel et al., 2000; Collins et al., 2002).

sCJD is slightly more frequent in women than in men (1.4:1). The difference remains even when gender-specific mortality rates are calculated. The median disease duration is 6 months, but cases with dramatic short disease duration as well as prolonged courses are also relatively frequent. Predicting factors of survival have been studied in a large, multicenter study: a longer survival was associated with female gender, younger age at onset of illness, and methionine-valine heterozygosity at codon 129 of the *PRNP* (Pocchiari et al., 2004). Given the significant difference in disease duration, age at onset, and, possibly, gender prevalence among sCJD subtypes segregating with distinct codon 129 genotypes (Parchi et al., 1999b, 2009) (see paragraph on molecular sCJD subtypes, below), the above-mentioned associations likely reflect this fundamental biologic heterogeneity of the disease.

GENETIC ASPECTS

The human prion protein (PrP) is encoded by a gene located on the short arm of chromosome 20. It consists of two exons and one intron of 13 kbp in length. The entire protein-coding part of the gene (open reading frame) is located in exon 2.

In addition to pathogenic mutation associated with genetic CJD, silent or influential *PRNP* polymorphisms are numerous (Capellari et al., 2011). The most important with respect to susceptibility and phenotypic expression is the methionine (M) or valine (V) polymorphism at codon 129 (Palmer et al., 1991). Among Caucasians approximately 51% of individuals are heterozygotes, 38% M homozygotes, and the remaining 11% V homozygotes. In contrast, the MM genotype (methionine homozygosity) is the most frequently occurring genotype in sCJD (Alpérovitch et al., 1999; Ladogana et al., 2005). The frequency of the M allele varies among populations, ranging from 0.55 in Africans to more than 0.9 in Asians (Capellari et al., 2011).

Table 9.1

Clinical findings in sporadic Creutzfeldt–Jakob disease at onset and during course[a]

	Onset (%)	Course (%)
Dementia	72	91
Ataxia	72	83
Pyramidal signs	40	77
Myoclonus	40	84
Visual/oculomotor	38	58
Extrapyramidal signs	36	75
Akinetic mutism	9	45
Paresthesia	13	16
Epileptic fits	3	12

[a]Onset = first 2 months of the disease; course = symptoms developed later than 2 months after disease onset.

CLINICAL FEATURES

Given its biologic heterogeneity, sCJD encompasses a wide phenotypic spectrum regarding age of onset, presenting features, rate of progression, and appearance of other clinical manifestations.

At disease onset, symptoms and signs are various and often not specific; however, during the disease course most patients develop dementia, ataxia and/or visual signs, myoclonus, and muscle tone abnormalities (Table 9.1) (Brown et al., 1994; de Silva, 1996; Parchi et al., 1999a; Zerr and Poser, 2002; Knight et al., 2004; Boesenberg et al., 2005).

The onset of definite neurologic signs is, sometimes, preceded by a prodromal phase characterized by unspecific behavioral changes, unspecified fear, adynamia, as well as headaches or dizziness. Many patients also complain about sleep disturbances or relatives might notice eating abnormalities and weight loss. These signs together with altered social behavior and depressive mood changes might point toward an organic depression at this phase.

Early stage

Impairment of higher cognitive functions is the most common neurologic presentation and may involve all domains. Due to the major involvement of the occipital lobe in the most common sCJD subtype, the presentation with central visual symptoms and signs (up to cortical anopia) is relatively frequent. This clinical phenotype was known earlier as Heidenhain variant of sCJD (Heidenhain, 1929; Kropp et al., 1999; Parchi et al., 1999b; Tsuji et al., 2004; Baiardi et al., 2016). In another frequent clinical phenotype, known previously as Brownell–Oppenheimer variant, cerebellar ataxia is predominant and may be the only neurologic sign for several weeks (Brownell and Oppenheimer, 1965; Baiardi et al., 2017). More rarely, the disease may start with a focal neurologic deficit (like progressive hemiparesis), but also an extrapyramidal syndrome, status epilepticus, or myoclonus (Heye et al., 1990). In such cases, as well as those with prominent ataxia at onset, cognitive or behavioral changes are often only noticed later in the disease course (Mehndiratta et al., 2000; Baiardi et al., 2017). In many patients, psychiatric features may also occur early in the disease course (Table 9.2) (Brown et al., 1994; Zerr and Poser, 2002; Cordery et al., 2005; Krasnianski et al., 2017). They may comprise disorientation, psychosis, hallucinations (visual and auditory), and delusions.

Table 9.2

Neuropsychiatric symptoms and signs in sporadic Creutzfeldt–Jakob disease ($n = 30$)[a]

	% (n)
Apathy	**70** (21)
Dysphoria	**53** (16)
Appetite and eating abnormalities	**47** (14)
Agitation	**47** (14)
Hallucinations	**43** (13)
Nighttime behavior disturbances	**37** (11)
Anxiety	**37** (11)
Aberrant motor behavior	**37** (11)
Delusions	**30** (9)
Irritability	**20** (6)
Disinhibition	**13** (4)
Euphoria	**13** (4)

[a]Laura Weitz, medical thesis, CJD Surveillance Unit Göttingen, assessed these neuropsychiatric signs and symptoms using the neuropsychiatric inventory (NPI) (Cummings, 1997).

Disease evolution

With the progress of the disease, cognitive deficits increase and further neurologic signs become evident. The classic CJD symptoms and signs during disease evolution include, besides dementia, visual and/or cerebellar signs (mainly ataxia), pyramidal and/or extrapyramidal signs, myoclonus, and akinetic mutism. Patients may also develop dysarthria, loss of speech, mutism, apraxia, hallucinations, and epileptic seizures.

Advanced stages

In the advanced stage of the disease, patients lose contact with the environment, and are usually bedridden, akinetic, and mute (Otto et al., 1998). Tonus abnormalities (rigor and/or spasticity) and myoclonus are mostly present. Patients more often die within months or weeks, but they (atypical cases) may survive for years (most commonly 1–3 years). The main cause of death is pneumonia due to aspiration.

NEUROPATHOLOGIC FEATURES

Microscopic histopathologic lesions in sCJD include PrP^{TSE} aggregate deposition, which is associated with amyloid plaques in about 10% of cases, spongiform change, microglial activation, synaptic and neuronal loss, and astrocytic gliosis (Parchi et al., 2011). PrP^{TSE} deposition and microglial activation occur first, rapidly followed by spongiform change and synaptic damage, whereas astrocytic gliosis and neuronal loss develop later.

PrP^{TSE} depositions

Owing to the wide phenotypic heterogeneity of the disease a number of morphologic variants of PrP^{TSE} deposits can be detected by immunohistochemistry either isolated or in combination. Among them, the most significant patterns of PrP^{TSE} deposition that are observed in sCJD include the following:

1. Synaptic, the most common, comprises delicate, microgranular, diffuse PrP^{TSE} microdeposits which are best seen in the cerebral cortex (especially in the occipital lobe) and molecular layer of cerebellum.
2. Plaque-like consists of small, well-defined, and rounded focal PrP^{TSE} deposits, which are best visualized in the cerebral cortex, striatum, thalamus, granular layer of cerebellum, cerebellar white matter, and, occasionally, in the subcortical white matter.

3. Perivacuolar, a coarse type of staining, is often associated with large confluent vacuoles and best detected in the cerebral cortex.
4. Perineuronal, a membrane type of staining delineating the perikarya and dendrites of neurons, is best seen in the pyramidal neurons of the deep cortical layers and hippocampus.

Microglial activation

Among the glial changes, microglial activation has attracted particular interest for its possible dual, opposite effects in prion disease and, more generally, in chronic neurodegeneration. According to current evidence microglia is involved in PrP^{TSE} clearance but may also favor neuroinflammation and the development of further neurodegeneration and disease progression (Amor and Woodroofe, 2014). Studies on the timing of microglial activation in prion diseases were primarily conducted in animal models (Ransohoff and Perry, 2009). In murine models, numerous activated microglia, generated by the proliferation of the local resident cells, appear early in the disease course. In post-mortem sCJD brains, microgliosis is widespread, paralleling the spread of prions and of neurodegeneration (Franceschini et al., 2018).

Spongiform change

The vacuolar changes occurring in the neuropil of sCJD-affected brains are also significantly heterogeneous in morphology (Parchi et al., 2011; Parchi and Saverioni, 2012). Based on the mean size of vacuoles, three types of spongiform change can be recognized. Most commonly, the spongiform change consists of small, round, vacuoles of 2–5 μm in mean diameter. Typically, this type of spongiform change is found in the cerebral cortex, striatum, thalamus, and molecular layer of cerebellum. A second very distinctive form of spongiform change, which is typically observed in the cerebral cortex, mainly comprises large vacuoles of 15–20 μm in diameter that show the tendency to merge in grape-like structures. The third type of spongiform change is characterized by vacuoles of intermediate mean size. This type of spongiform change has little tendency to merge and is most commonly seen in subcortical structures, including the cerebellum. Spongiform change is an invariable finding in sCJD, although vacuole size, severity, and regional distribution may vary significantly according to the disease subtype and stage. In particular, the degree of gliosis and neuronal loss significantly affects the appearance of the spongiform change, which is ultimately substituted by the unspecific status spongiosus in case of severe neurodegeneration.

Synaptic loss

PrP^C is highly concentrated in presynaptic terminals, where it co-localizes with synaptophysin and is highly prevalent in brain structures associated with synaptic plasticity (Herms et al., 1999). Consequently, the loss of normal PrP^C function may contribute to synaptic dysfunction and ultimately to neuronal loss. A decrease in synaptic proteins, such as synapsin, SNAP-25, and synaptophysin, has been demonstrated in postmortem CJD cerebral cortex and cerebellum (Ferrer et al., 1999, 2000). However, these analyses were undertaken at a time when there was extensive neuronal death and thus severe synaptic loss would be expected. However, in an experimental transmission study involving three distinctive strains, synaptic loss was present in the hippocampus or limbic system in the absence of significant neuronal loss (Hilton et al., 2013), supporting the idea that synaptic loss may be an early pathologic event in sCJD.

Neuronal loss and astrocytic gliosis

Neuronal loss is strongly linked to disease duration, and therefore, highly variable. It may at times be difficult to assess without systematic morphometry or, on the contrary, may be extremely severe with practically no discernible neurons left in the cerebral cortex, striatum, thalamus, and granular layer of the cerebellum.

Amyloid plaques

About 10% of sCJD brains, belonging to a distinct disease subtype, have classic compact "kuru-type" amyloid plaques formed by PrP^{TSE} deposits that are visible on routine stainings. They also stain with periodic acid–Schiff and thioflavine S. Kuru plaques are most frequent in the cerebellar cortex, where they are usually confined at the border between the granular and Purkinje cell layers, but they can also occur in the cerebral cortex in cases with a prolonged clinical course.

Very rarely, amyloid plaques with "kuru-type" morphology were also seen at different subcortical white-matter sites, including the cerebellar white matter, in patients with a long disease duration and an otherwise classic sCJD subtype and therefore lacking the typical cerebellar kuru plaques described above (Kobayashi et al., 2008; Rossi et al., 2017).

Secondary tauopathy

A secondary tauopathy characterized by brain deposition of abnormal p-tau aggregates has been recently documented in sCJD. After the initial suggestion that only prion diseases associated with PrP amyloid plaques such as Gerstmann-Sträussler-Scheinker develop p-tau deposits, Reiniger et al. (2011) demonstrated that a tiny punctate, PrP-specific, p-tau immunoreactivity positively correlating with PrP^{TSE} burden is consistently found in sCJD brains, irrespective of the molecular subtype and the Alzheimer disease-related associated pathology. Consistently, in a follow-up study (Kovacs et al., 2017), these small neuritic profiles were regarded as the most frequent type of tau immunoreactivity in sCJD brains. Finally, Lattanzio et al. (2017) showed that the prion-specific secondary tauopathy especially affects the sCJD subtypes linked to the V2 strain (e.g., VV2 and MV2K; see paragraph on molecular subtypes, below) and, most significantly, that in such cases the tauopathy is severe enough to determine a significant increase in p-tau levels in the CSF.

Subtypes of sCJD and their distinctive clinicopathologic features

Current sCJD classification recognizes at least six clinicopathologic phenotypes that largely correlate at the molecular level with two PrP^{TSE} types with distinctive physicochemical properties and the genotype at *PRNP* codon 129 (Fig. 9.2) (Parchi et al., 1999a, 2009; Parchi and Saverioni, 2012). PrP^{TSE} types 1 and 2 have been originally described by Parchi et al. (1996, 1997) as two alternative forms of the proteinase K-generated, unglycosylated C-terminal cores of the PrP^{TSE} molecule, thought to reflect two major conformations of PrP^{TSE} aggregates. PrP^{TSE} type 1 has a relative electrophoretic mobility of 21 kDa and a primary proteinase K cleavage site at residue 82, while PrP^{TSE} type 2 has a relative molecular mass of 19 kDa and a primary cleavage site at residue 97 (Fig. 9.2) (Parchi et al., 2000).

The recognized subtypes of sCJD result from all possible codon 129 genotype/PrP^{TSE} type combinations (MM1, VV1, MM2, VV2, etc.), with a few exceptions: MM1 and MV1 cases were merged in one subtype (MM(V) 1) since they are phenotypically indistinguishable, whereas, on the contrary, the MM2 group was divided into two subtypes based on the very distinctive cortical and thalamic histopathology observed in the two groups (MM2-cortical or MM 2C and MM2-thalamic or MM 2T) (Table 9.3). Moreover, a variant resembling the MM1 subtype in most features but showing, as distinctive trait, the presence of widespread PrP-amyloid plaques in the white matter has been recognized and designated as p-MM1 (Kobayashi et al., 2008; Rossi et al., 2017).

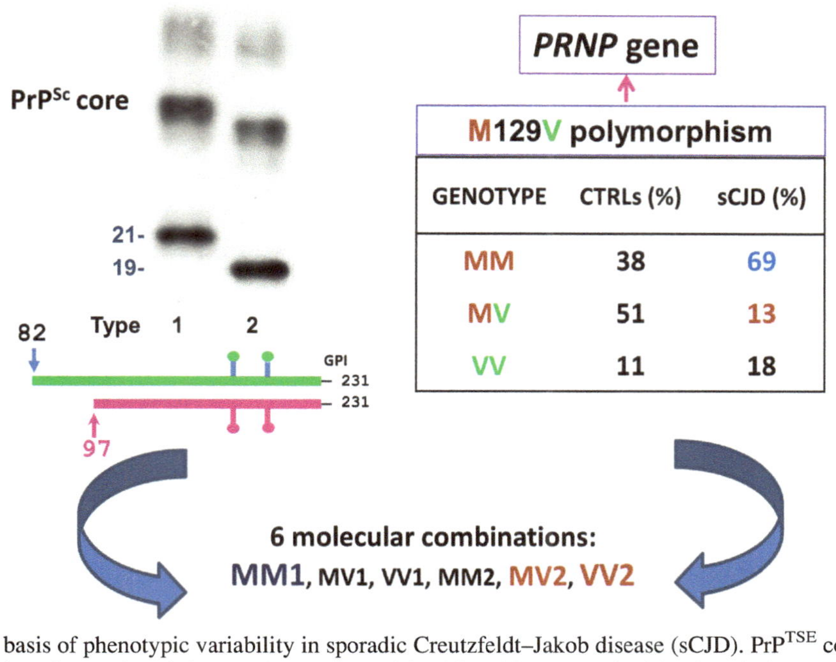

Fig. 9.2. Molecular basis of phenotypic variability in sporadic Creutzfeldt–Jakob disease (sCJD). PrP^{TSE} core fragments type 1 and type 2 differ for the primary site of cleavage by PK (in position 82 and 97, respectively). The relative percentage of codon 129 genotypes in both controls (CTRLs) and sCJD refers to the Caucasian population. The combination of each of the two PrP^{TSE} types with the three codon 129 genotypes generate six molecular groups, with MM1, VV2, and MV2 accounting for the large majority of cases.

Table 9.3

Distinctive clinical and pathological features of sporadic Creutzfeldt–Jakob disease subtypes

	Molecular disease subtype	Median age at onset (range) (years)	Median duration (range) (months)	Most prominent clinical signs/ symptoms	Distinctive histopathologic features
Frequent	MM1(V)1	68 (31–86)	4 (1–24)	Dementia, cortical anopsia, ataxia, myoclonus	Neocortex (especially in occipital lobe), striatum, thalamus, and cerebellum constantly affected "synaptic type" PrP staining
	MV2K	65 (36–83)	17 (4–48)	Ataxia, dementia, extrapyramidal	Similar to VV2 with more involvement of the cerebral cortex, amyloid kuru plaques in the cerebellum, plaque-like focal PrP deposits
	VV2	64 (40–83)	6.5 (3–18)	Prominent ataxia, late dementia	Prominent pathology in cerebellum and subcortical areas, late cortical involvement, plaque-like and perineuronal PrP staining
Rare	MM2T	52 (26–71)	16 (8–36)	Ataxia, diplopia, psychiatric signs, sleep loss, late cognitive impairment	Atrophy of the thalamus and inferior olive, focal spongiosis limited to the cerebral cortex
	MM2C	64 (49–77)	16 (9–36)	Progressive dementia for several months	Spongiosis with large confluent vacuoles; perivacuolar PrP staining
	VV1	44 (19–55)	21 (17–42)	Dementia at onset, later ataxia and extrapyramidal	Severe pathology in the cerebral cortex and striatum with sparing of brainstem nuclei and cerebellum
	p-MM1[a]	58 (48–70)	22 (13–38)	Progressive dementia and neurologic signs for several months	Moderate to severe pathology. MM1-like lesion profile. Widespread PrP amyloid plaques in subcortical and deep nuclei white matter

[a]p-, with PrP amyloid plaques in white matter.
From: Parchi et al. (1999a, 2009); Zerr et al. (2000a); Meissner et al. (2005); Krasnianski et al. (2006a, b); Rossi et al. (2017).

The main clinical and pathologic features of sCJD subtypes are summarized in Table 9.3.

GENERAL FEATURES

Discriminating clinical characteristics among molecular sCJD subtypes include age at onset, disease duration and frequency, and evolution of symptoms and signs (Parchi et al., 1999b; Zerr et al., 2000b). The classic disease subtype, MM(V)1, begins at a median age of 68 years (31–86 years), which is similar to the median age at onset of sCJD MM2C (67 years: range 49–75 years) and only slightly higher than those of the VV2 (64 years: range 40–83 years) and MV2K (64 years: range 36–83 years). In contrast, patients with the rarer VV1 and MM 2T are characterized by a significantly younger age at onset (44 years: range 19–55 and 52 years: range 26–71 years, respectively). The reasons for this variable age at onset among subtypes are still the subject of speculation.

The median disease duration reported for all forms of sCJD is around 6 months (Zerr et al., 2000b); it is, however, strongly influenced by disease subtype. The shortest median disease duration, well below 1 year, is shown by MM(V)1 and VV2 patients, whereas those belonging to all other subtypes have a median disease duration between 1 and 2 years (Table 9.3) (Parchi et al., 1999a;

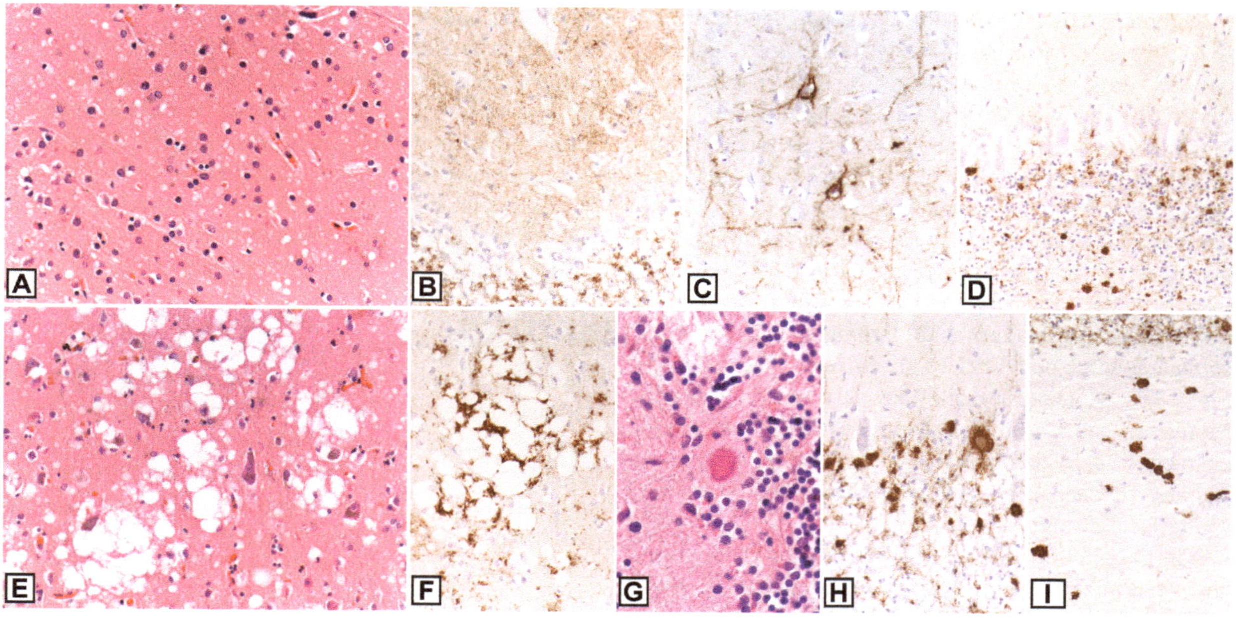

Fig. 9.3. Distinctive histopathologic features of sporadic Creutzfeldt–Jakob disease (sCJD). (**A**) Typical spongiform change characterized by small, fine, microvacuoles in the neuropil of sCJD MM1 (hematoxylin and eosin (H&E) stain, occipital cortex). (**B**) Synaptic pattern of PrP deposition in cerebellum of sCJD MM1. A delicate diffuse staining is seen in the molecular layer while in the granular cell layers the cerebellar glomeruli are stained. (**C**) Perineuronal PrP^{TSE} staining in the deep cortical layers of sCJD VV2. (**D**) Plaque-like PrP deposits in the granular layer of the cerebellum in sCJD VV2. These plaque-like deposits are not visible on routine H&E or periodic acid–Schiff-stained sections. Spongiform changes characterized by relatively large confluent vacuoles (**E**) (H&E stain), with perivacuolar PrP^{TSE} staining (**F**) as typically seen in MM 2C sCJD. Typically, dense, coarse deposits of PrP are seen surrounding confluent vacuoles (**F**). (**G**) Unicentric amyloid plaque of the kuru type in the cerebellar granular layer in sCJD MV 2K (H&E stain). Plaque-like PrP deposits in the granular and molecular layers of cerebellum (**H**) and cerebellar white matter (**I**) in sCJD MV 2K. (Adapted from Parchi and Saverioni, 2012).

Zerr et al., 2000b). The core clinical characteristics and neuropathologic features of the sCJD subtypes are given below (Table 9.3).

Common subtypes

MM(V)1

The most common MM(V)1 type, so-called classic form of CJD, comprises about 65% of all cases and can occur either in a pure form or associated with focal PrP^{TSE} type 2 deposition and MM2C features (see paragraph on mixed types).

Symptoms and signs at onset, often already multisystemic at this early stage, may vary and include cognitive decline in most cases and visual signs of central origin, language dysfunction, ataxia, myoclonus or other involuntary movements, each occurring in about one-fourth/one-third of patients in various combinations (Parchi et al., 1999a; Zerr et al., 2000b). Neurologic signs are unilateral at onset in about 25% of cases. The histopathology in this CJD type includes the classic type of spongiform change with small (2–10 μm) round to oval vacuoles, predominantly located in the neuropil (Fig. 9.3A). In the cerebral neocortex, vacuolation is seen in all layers and is often more prominent in the occipital lobe. The striatum and, to a lesser extent, the thalamus are also invariably affected, whereas the hippocampus and brainstem are remarkably spared. In the cerebellum spongiform change is limited to the molecular layer, and a focal distribution is often observed. Immumohistochemistry shows a synaptic type of PrP^{TSE} staining, which is best seen in the cerebral cortex, and cerebellum (Fig. 9.3B), and less consistently, in the basal ganglia and thalamus (Parchi et al., 2012).

VV2

This phenotype comprises about 15–20% of sCJD cases. The clinical phenotype is characterized by an early onset of cerebellar symptoms and signs, which invariably occur within 2 months from disease onset. Early manifestations also include oculomotor abnormalities, memory loss, behavioral disturbances, and signs of peripheral nervous system or medullary involvement. In contrast, cognitive decline other than memory impairment and myoclonus are late features, with dementia occurring after at least 4 months of clinical course (Baiardi et al., 2017).

Pathologically, VV2 subjects show moderate to severe spongiform change and gliosis with variable neuronal loss in the gray matter of limbic structures, striatum, thalamus, hypothalamus, cerebellum, and brainstem. In contrast, the neocortex is relatively spared, especially in cases with a rapid course (i.e., less than 6 months). The spongiform change in the cortex is often laminar and mainly involves the deep layers. Immunostaining is characterized by the presence of focal plaque-like PrP deposits (Fig. 9.3D). Another distinctive immunostaining feature is the strong reaction around some neuronal perikarya (e.g., perineuronal staining: Fig. 9.3C), while the neuropil shows the synaptic pattern. Moreover, cases with less than 1 year of duration are characterized by laminar distribution of the immunostaining in deep cortical layers corresponding to the spongiform change.

The distribution of PrP^{TSE}, like that of the spongiform change, is affected by the duration of the disease. In cases of less than 5 months' duration, PrP^{TSE} is present in relatively large and similar amounts throughout the brain, except for the neocortex, where it is present in limited amounts. This distribution is, therefore, quite different from that of MM1 subjects in which PrP^{TSE} is most abundant in the neocortex. In cases of over 1 year's duration PrP^{TSE} also markedly increases in the neocortex so that it becomes homogeneously distributed in most gray-matter regions (Baiardi et al., 2017).

MV2K

This phenotype affects about 10% of cases, and is also known as the kuru plaque variant. This subtype shows significant similarities with the VV2 phenotype, but is characterized by a significantly lower progression rate. The relatively prolonged disease duration and diverse symptomatology especially at onset are, indeed, remarkable features (Parchi et al., 1999a, 2009; Krasnianski et al., 2006b). Dementia is the first clinical sign in about half of cases. However, the disease can also start with ataxia or extrapyramidal signs.

The distinctive pathologic features of this type are cerebellar kuru plaques (Fig. 9.3G), while other pathologic changes are similar to VV2 with more consistent plaque-like deposits (Fig. 9.3H and I).

Rare subtypes

VV1

The VV1 type represents the rarest subtype, with a frequency of about 1%. Most reported patients are male of relatively young age (Parchi et al., 1999a; Meissner et al., 2005). The clinical disease typically starts with psychiatric or cognitive abnormalities. Later in the course, extrapyramidal signs and ataxia develop, while myoclonus is less frequent. The pathology in these subjects predominantly affects the corticostriatal regions, while other subcortical structures, including the cerebellum, are relatively spared. PrP immunohistochemistry shows a faint punctuate staining in the cerebral cortex, despite the severe spongiform change.

MM2T

This rare disease subtype is also known as sporadic familial insomnia (Parchi et al., 1999a, b; Meissner et al., 2005; Puoti et al., 2012) (described in detail in Chapter 15). Clinically, insomnia with inability to initiate and maintain sleep, frequent arousals, and enacted dreams can be a peculiar symptom of this phenotype, although it is not invariably detected. The clinical presentation is heterogeneous, but most often includes cognitive impairment and ataxia, whereas psychiatric and visual signs are less common and dysautonomia is rare. At early stages, sleep abnormalities are not commonly reported but they are also rarely specifically investigated by polysomnography. Other motor signs, including diplopia, dysarthria, dysphagia, and pyramidal signs, may also be part of the clinical phenotype. Myoclonus, spontaneous and evoked, is also typically present. Neuropathologically, there is prominent atrophy of the thalamus and inferior olive with only minor pathologic changes in other areas of the brain. Spongiform change may be absent or virtually limited to the cerebral cortex. Unique among sCJD subtypes is also the relative preservation of the striatum. PrP^{TSE} immunohistochemistry may be positive only in the cerebral cortex where the most significant PrP^{TSE} accumulation is found.

MM2C

The cortical variant of MM2 subtype is characterized by progressive dementia and disturbances of higher cognitive function, high frequency of aphasia and apraxia, and late myoclonus (Parchi et al., 1999b; Krasnianski et al., 2006a). The lesion profile of MM2C subjects is similar to that of the MM1 or MV1 group, with the exception of the cerebellum that lacks significant spongiform change despite the relatively long duration of symptoms. Moreover, the spongiform change typically consists of large and coarse vacuoles (Fig. 9.3E). PrP immunohistochemistry shows a coarse pattern of staining (Fig. 9.3F), which is often called perivacuolar because of its prevalent localization at the rim of the large vacuoles (Parchi et al., 2012).

p-MM1

The existence of an additional rare disease subtype, occurring in approximately 0.5% of sCJD cases, has been recently established (Kobayashi et al., 2008; Rossi et al., 2017). The novel histotype largely overlaps with sCJD MM1 but shows, as a very distinctive feature, PrP-amyloid plaques of kuru type in both subcortical and deep nuclei white matter. Moreover, the presence of amyloid plaques in p-CJD MM1 correlates with a slower clinical progression in comparison to typical MM1. Notably, p-CJD MM1 shares both PrP^{TSE} and transmission properties with classic CJD MM1, pointing to a host-dependent factor as the cause of the distinctive amyloid plaques (Rossi et al., 2017).

sCJD types with "mixed" molecular and pathologic features

PrP^{TSE} types 1 and 2 have also been found to co-occur in the same brain in about 35% of cases (Parchi et al., 2009). Although co-occurrence was detected in all codon 129 genotypes, PrP^{TSE} types 1 and 2 co-occurred more frequently in MM (43%) than in MV (23%) or VV (15%) subjects. The overall results indicated that the deposition of either type 1 or 2, when concurrent, is not random and always characterized by the coexistence of phenotypic features already described for the "pure" subtypes.

Type MM(V)1 + 2C

The variant MM/MV1 + 2C is by far the most common mixed type of sCJD. As many as 43% of all MM cases turned out to be mixed MM1 + 2C cases on very close inspection (Parchi et al., 2009). This includes cases in which the large and confluent vacuoles are only found in very restricted regions of the cerebral cortex or the thalamus, making the demonstration of PrP^{TSE} type 1 and 2 co-occurrence by Western blot very difficult (Notari et al., 2007). Given the rarity of the other mixed phenotypes, this is the only subtype in which clinical correlations were drawn. It was found that both disease duration and frequency of symptoms at onset in MM(V) 1 + 2C subjects vary according to the relative load of the two protein types. Thus, while the clinical phenotype in MM(V) 1 + 2C with a focal PrP^{TSE} type 2 deposition (with up to five brain regions involved) does not significantly differ from those of the MM(V)1 phenotype, the disease duration becomes significantly longer and cerebellar signs less frequent at onset with increasing type 2 load (Parchi et al., 2009).

Similarly, the histopathology in this variant shows varying relative amounts of features previously described in the pure MM(V)1 and MM(V)2C subtypes. More precisely, this type is characterized by confluent foci of spongiform change with large vacuoles interspersed with classic microvacuolation, and by a mixed synaptic/perivacuolar or coarse pattern of PrP deposition.

Type VV2+1

At variance with patients carrying the M allele, the occurrence of mixed phenotypic features in VV cases is essentially based on the demonstration of PrP^{TSE} types 1 and 2 coexistence by immunoblotting. Indeed, the lesion profile and pattern of PrP staining in the rare VV2 + 1 type show features that are largely overlapping with those of typical VV2 sCJD cases (Parchi et al., 2009).

Other subtypes

Two additional rare mixed phenotypes that are both associated with PrP^{TSE} type 2 and therefore only identifiable histopathologically include sCD MV 2K+2C and MM 2T+2C (Parchi et al., 2009; Parchi and Saverioni, 2012).

Molecular basis of phenotypic variability and prion strains

The phenotypic heterogeneity of sCJD and other prion diseases is related to both prion strains and host genetic factors. Prion strains are defined as animal or human "isolates" that, after inoculation into syngenic hosts, cause diseases with distinct characteristics, such as incubation period, pattern of PrP^{TSE} distribution, and regional severity of neuropathologic changes. It is currently largely believed that biologic diversity of prion strains is enciphered in distinct PrP^{TSE} conformers forming distinct ordered aggregates. Conversely, the MV polymorphic codon 129 in the *PRNP* gene is by far the most significant identified host genetic factor influencing CJD susceptibility and phenotypic expression even independently from prion strain. Current evidence indicates that five out of six sCJD subtypes (MM1, MM2C, MM2T, VV1, and VV2) behave as distinct prion strains after serial transmission into animal models. As the only exception, the VV2 and MV2K variants showed the same transmission properties, indicating a host–genotype (codon 129) effect (Bishop et al., 2010; Kobayashi et al., 2010; Parchi et al., 2010; Moda et al., 2012). Interestingly, the CJD strain isolated from sCJD VV2 and MV2K, currently designated as V2, has been causally linked to the kuru epidemic as well to many iatrogenic cases of CJD secondary to contaminated growth hormone or dura mater grafts (Parchi et al., 2010; Kobayashi et al., 2014; Takeuchi et al., 2016; Ritchie et al., 2017). Intriguingly, at variance with sCJD, in these acquired forms of CJD the V2 strains affect subjects carrying all three codon 129 genotypes, including the MM. Thus, the identification of the V2 strain in CJD patients carrying MM at codon 129 may be considered evidence for an acquired CJD etiology (Kobayashi et al., 2014).

From the results summarized above human strains appear in excess with respect to PrP^{TSE} types 1 and 2 dichotomy (i.e., five strains vs. two protein types), which, according to the prion theory, would indicate that PrP^{TSE} types 1 and 2 are heterogeneous species. Evidence from a number of recent studies at least partially supports this contention. Using standardized high buffer strength for brain homogenization, proteinase K digestion at pH 6.9 with a high enzyme concentration, and long-running gels, Notari et al. (2004) characterized an additional PrP^{TSE} band with an electrophoretic mobility, of approximately 20 kDa, which is intermediate between types 1 and 2 and specifically associated with sCJD MV2K. Other studies focusing on truncated PrP^{TSE} C-terminal fragments of about 12 and 13 kDa (PrP-CTF12/13) showed that these fragments also contribute to generate subtype-specific proteinase K-resistant PrP^{TSE} profiles in sCJD (Capellari et al., 2000; Zou et al., 2003; Notari et al., 2008).

PrP^{TSE} from different CJD subtypes can also be typed through its glycoform ratio, that is, the ratio between the three differently glycosylated isoforms of the abnormal protein (e.g., diglycosylated, monoglycosylated, and unglycosylated). Although the PrP^{TSE} glycotype in sCJD is most often characterized by an overrepresentation of the monoglycosylated form, there are also strain-specific significant differences in the relative abundance of the diglycosylated form among disease subtypes (Parchi et al., 1999a). Interestingly, the relative amount of both diglycosylated PrP^{TSE} and CTF13 appears to correlate with the degree of PrP^{TSE} sensitivity to proteinase K digestion, although in opposite directions. Indeed, PrP^{TSE} in sCJD VV2 shows the highest resistance to proteinase K digestion, the most abundant diglycosylated band and no detectable CTF13, whereas, in contrast, PrP^{TSE} in VV1 is the most sensitive to proteases, has the lowest diglycosylated form and the highest amount of PrP-CTF13 (Saverioni et al., 2013). Taken together, these data suggest that each sCJD subtype can be associated with a specific "profile" of PrP^{TSE} based on glycotype and size of abnormal PrP fragments, possibly reflecting subtype-specific structural characteristics of the abnormal protein aggregate, including glycosylation, that also determine the frangibility of the PrP^{TSE} aggregate and its resistance to protease digestion.

In the early 2000s the description and characterization of a proteinase K-sensitive form of PrP^{TSE} ($sPrP^{TSE}$), which, like PrP^{C}, is fully degraded at a relatively low proteinase K activity, seemed to open a potential new perspective to the study of PrP^{TSE} properties and their relationship to prion strains (Tzaban et al., 2002; Pastrana et al., 2006). Pursuing some findings obtained in experimental models of prion disease (Safar et al., 1998), suggesting a relationship between $sPrP^{TSE}/rPrP^{TSE}$ ratio and strain-specific properties such as incubation time, Safar et al. (2005) reported that $sPrP^{TSE}$ represents an invariable and quantitatively significant component of prions, contributing up to 90% of the whole PrP^{TSE} signal in sCJD. Moreover, they described an inverse correlation between the relative amount of $sPrP^{TSE}$ and subtype-specific properties such as the clinical duration of the disease (Kim et al., 2011).

More recently, Saverioni et al. (2013) also looked for $sPrP^{TSE}$ in purified detergent-insoluble PrP^{TSE} across the whole spectrum of sCJD prions. At variance with Safar et al. (2005), their results showed that $sPrP^{TSE}$ always (i.e., in all CJD strains) represents a relatively minor component of abnormal PrP not exceeding 10% of total detergent-insoluble PrP^{TSE}. Thus, this significant discrepancy, which may in part depend on methodologic aspects or data interpretation, needs to be further explored and explained.

The conformational stability of PrP^{TSE} aggregates in sCJD subtypes has also been recently studied using different experimental procedures. Guanidine hydrochloride-induced unfolding, the most commonly used approach, has been variably measured by: (1) the extent of exposure of a conformational epitope that is hidden in the native conformation (conformation-dependent immunoassay); (2) the progressive loss of proteinase K resistance (conformational stability assay); or (3) the increase in solubility of PrP^{TSE} (stability and solubility assay) (Safar et al., 1998; Peretz et al., 2001; Pirisinu et al., 2010).

In the few studies performed to date in sCJD, MM1 PrP^{TSE} was shown to be more stable than MM 2C PrP^{TSE} by both conformational stability assay and stability and solubility assay (Cali et al., 2006; Choi et al., 2010; Pirisinu et al., 2010). Similarly, based on hydrogen/deuterium exchange coupled with mass spectrometry, Safar et al. (2015) demonstrated that MM1 and MM2C PrP^{TSE} differ in their structural organization, both at the level of the polypeptide backbone as well as the quaternary packing arrangements.

Finally, in a recent study, Cescatti et al. (2016) obtained similar denaturation curves among the six sCJD subtypes analyzed by conformational stability assay, indicating that guanidine hydrochloride does not significantly perturb the strain-specific structural organization of PrP^{TSE}. Cescatti et al. (2016) also studied the effect of heating (in the presence of sodium dodecyl sulfate) on PrP^{TSE} aggregates. At variance with the negative results obtained with guanidine hydrochloride, the effect of temperature on PrP^{TSE} solubilization varied significantly according to the sCJD variant. The calculated T_{50} was lowest for VV1, MM2T, and MM2C ($T_{50} < 55°C$) and highest for MM1 and VV2, and MV 2K ($T_{50} > 80°C$). Interestingly, since the most thermostable prion protein types were those associated with the most prevalent phenotypes and most rapidly and efficiently transmitting strains (MM1 and VV2), the results suggest a direct correlation between strain replication efficiency and thermostability of prion protein aggregates.

CLINICAL DIAGNOSTIC INVESTIGATIONS

Electroencephalogram (EEG)

Characteristic EEG changes in CJD, characterized by periodic bi- and triphasic sharp-wave complexes (PSWCs) were first described in the middle of the 20th century (Levy et al., 1986). Since then, PSWCs have been considered an important clue in support of the clinical diagnosis of the disease. PSWCs can be detected as early as the third week after disease onset, but, in general, they are not an early finding in sCJD. Indeed, PSWCs occur after 2–3 months of clinical progression in most cases.

Objective criteria of EEG assessment have been suggested (Steinhoff et al., 1996). The low diagnostic sensitivity of EEG PSWCs detection, which is around 64%, is due to the fact that PSWCs are seen in the middle and late disease stages with a relatively high frequency in sCJD MM(V)1, and only rarely and at an advanced clinical stage in the other subtypes.

Another drawback associated with EEG recording is that the specificity of this investigation is also relatively low, given the incidence of at least 11% false-positive results among clinically suspected sCJD patients (Steinhoff et al., 1996). The list of possible differential diagnoses for diseases associated with PSWCs is comprehensive and includes a variety of encephalites, metabolic encephalopathies, lithium intoxication, hepatic encephalopathy, hyperammonemia, hypoglycemia, multiple cerebral abscesses, electrolyte imbalance, intracerebral lymphoma, Alzheimer disease, dementia with Lewy bodies, and Binswanger disease (Will, 1991; Steinhoff et al., 1996; Haik et al., 2000; Tschampa et al., 2001; Yemisci et al., 2003).

In summary, all the above-listed characteristics make the EEG the least significant among the diagnostic investigations currently available to the clinician in support of the clinical diagnosis of sCJD.

Magnetic resonance imaging

MRI has played an important role in the clinical diagnosis of CJD since the late 1980s (Collie et al., 2001). The application of modern techniques, such as fluid-attenuated inversion recovery (FLAIR) and diffusion-weighted imaging (DWI) since the late 1990s (Bahn et al., 1997; Bahn and Parchi, 1999; Schröter et al., 2000, Kallenberg et al., 2006) has significantly increased the diagnostic value of brain MRI (Tschampa et al., 2005; Young et al., 2005), allowing a better detection of signal abnormalities in comparison to T2- and proton density (PD)-weighted imaging either in basal ganglia or cerebral cortex (or both), reaching 92–96% sensitivity in sCJD patients, according to most recent studies (Schröter et al., 2000; Shiga et al., 2004; Young et al., 2005; Collins et al., 2006; Lodi et al., 2009; Vitali et al., 2011; Carswell et al., 2012; Grau-Rivera et al., 2016; Fragoso et al., 2017; Gaudino et al., 2017). The changes, which are highly characteristic for the disease, are also associated with a relatively high diagnostic specificity of 88–94% (Meissner et al., 2004; Shiga et al., 2004; Tschampa et al., 2005; Young et al., 2005; Vitali et al., 2011).

Evidence indicates that DWI is more sensitive also against FLAIR for the detection of signal abnormalities in CJD, especially in the cerebral cortex (Pereira, 2002; Shiga et al., 2004; Ukisu et al., 2005; Hyare et al., 2010; Riva-Amarante et al., 2011; Satoh et al., 2011; Vitali et al., 2011) (Fig. 9.4). Furthermore, DWI was shown to best detect the signal hyperintensities in the early disease stage (Shiga et al., 2004; Tomita et al., 2004; Alvarez et al., 2005), which likely reflects the spongiform change being the main cause of DWI hyperintensities in sCJD (Manners et al., 2009).

Using DWI or FLAIR imaging, the CJD-associated signal abnormalities are, overall, detected more frequently in the cerebral cortex than in basal ganglia or other brain regions (Tschampa et al., 2007). In 68% the cortical ribbon was affected in combination with subcortical structures, whereas in 24–42% the signal was limited to the cerebral cortex (Shiga et al., 2004; Young et al., 2005).

Besides the cerebral cortex and basal ganglia, the signal increase in CJD may affect the hippocampus, thalamus, and mesencephalon, while it is hardly detected in the cerebellum, despite the frequent cerebellar tropism of human prions (Blasco Olcina et al., 2001; Meissner et al., 2009; Parchi and Saverioni, 2012). This is most likely due to the complexity of the cerebellar anatomy and the fact that spongiform change in CJD is limited to the very thin molecular layer.

Only limited data are available on serial MRI assessments in CJD. Signal intensity usually increases as

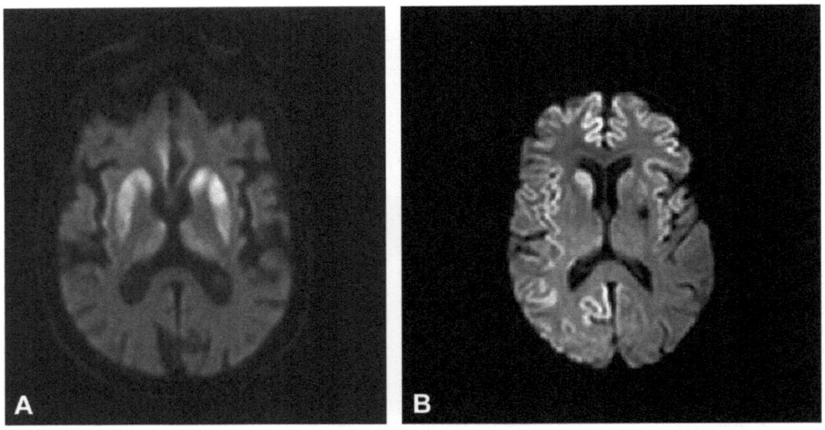

Fig. 9.4. Brain diffusion-weighted imaging (DWI) magnetic resonance in sporadic Creutzfeldt–Jakob disease (sCJD). (**A**) Hyperintense basal ganglia in DWI in a patient with sCJD MV 2K. (**B**) Hyperintense basal ganglia and cortex in DWI in a patient with sCJD MM1.

disease progresses and becomes more widespread, involving additional brain regions (Matoba et al., 2001; Tribl et al., 2002; Arruda et al., 2004; Ukisu et al., 2005; Eisenmenger et al., 2016). In some patients, only cortical signal alterations are found in the early disease stage, followed by basal ganglia hyperintensity at a later stage (Demaerel et al., 1999; Kropp et al., 2000; Tribl et al., 2002; Satoh et al., 2007). However, even the opposite spread can be observed, especially in disease subtypes such as VV2 with an "ascending" progression of histopathologic changes from subcortical areas to the cerebral cortex (Baiardi et al., 2017). Indeed, the regional profile of MRI signal changes and its evolution during the disease course, reflecting the underlying heterogeneity of lesion profiles that is observed neuropathologically among sCJD subtypes, may contribute to distinguishing them at clinical stages (Meissner et al., 2009; Zerr et al., 2009; Bekiesinska-Figatowska et al., 2012; Caobelli et al., 2015; Baiardi et al., 2016, 2017).

CEREBROSPINAL FLUID ANALYSIS

CSF analysis plays an important role in the clinical diagnosis of CJD to exclude an inflammatory disease on the one hand and to consolidate the clinical diagnosis on the other. Brain-derived CSF protein assays serving as surrogate markers for neuronal damage have provided, along with DW MRI, the main support for the clinical diagnosis of sCJD in the past 15–20 years. More recently, the development of an in vitro amplification system for the detection of aggregated PrP^{TSE} in human CSF has contributed the most significant innovation in the field with a high potential for the improvement of the premortem in vivo diagnosis of CJD.

Routine CSF parameters

Routine analyses of CSF samples from patients with CJD is usually unrevealing (Brown et al., 1994; Jacobi et al., 2005; Green et al., 2007). CSF invariably lacks even a mild pleiocytosis, whereas a slight unspecific increase in total protein is observed in about one-third of cases. Finally, oligoclonal bands can be occasionally found in some patients (Olsson, 1980; Jones et al., 1985; Brown et al., 1994; Jacobi et al., 2005).

Surrogate markers: 14-3-3, tau and other proteins

The family of 14-3-3 proteins was one of the earliest CSF biomarkers reaching an impact on the clinical diagnosis of sCJD (Harrington et al., 1986; Hsich et al., 1996; Zerr et al., 1996, 1998; Chohan et al., 2010; Satoh et al., 2010; Coulthart et al., 2011; Matsui et al., 2011; Muayqil et al., 2012; Leitao et al., 2016; Schmitz et al., 2016b). These are a group of cytosolic polypeptides with regulatory functions, which are released in the CSF during neuronal damage. As a consequence, not only CJD but also other pathologic conditions characterized by a rapid course and neuronal damage, such as stroke, inflammation, paraneoplastic syndromes, tumor, epileptic fits and atypical, rapidly evolving nonprion neurodegenerative dementias may yield a (false) positive test (Zerr et al., 1998; Chitravas et al., 2011; Lattanzio et al., 2017). The detection of abnormal 14-3-3 protein levels is helpful for the differential diagnosis. Several studies demonstrated an 85–95% diagnostic sensitivity and a 74–96% specificity for the 14-3-3 assay, with the wide span of calculated specificity significantly depending on the type of non-CJD population analyzed (Rosenmann et al., 1997;

Table 9.4

Sensitivity[a] of various cerebrospinal fluid assays for brain-derived proteins in sporadic Creutzfeldt–Jakob disease (sCJD)

	14-3-3 % (positive/all)	t-tau % (positive/all)	S100b % (positive/all)	NSE % (positive/all)
sCJD	**84.7** (1475/1740)	**86.9** (958/1102)	**82** (483/589)	**73** (379/517)

[a]Values for 14-3-3 and t-tau represent the sum of those reported in Sanchez-Juan et al. (2006) and Lattanzio et al. (2017). Those for S100b and NSE are from Sanchez-Juan et al. (2006).
NSE, neuron-specific enolase.

Zerr et al., 1997, 1998, 2000a; Lemstra et al., 2000; Aksamit et al., 2001; Brandel et al., 2001; Green et al., 2001, 2007; Sanchez-Valle et al., 2002; Castellani et al., 2004; Collins et al., 2006; Sanchez-Juan et al., 2006; Satoh et al., 2006; Shiga et al., 2006; Koscova et al., 2016; Fourier et al., 2017; Lattanzio et al., 2017). Indeed, the specificity of this test increases significantly if cases with a positive standard MRI showing distinct (non-CJD) pathology and/or those showing an inflammatory pattern in the CSF are excluded. Thus, 14-3-3 CSF detection represents a strong supportive diagnostic tool in the appropriate clinical context. The sensitivity of the test may vary depending on the composition of the sCJD population, given that the assay has a significantly lower sensitivity for sCJD subtypes associated with PrP^{TSE} type 2 and a relatively long disease duration (e.g., MV2K, MM2C, and MM2T) (Table 9.4) (Collins et al., 2000; Zerr et al., 2000a; Castellani et al., 2004; Krasnianski et al., 2006a; Lattanzio et al., 2017; Llorens et al., 2017b).

Serial testing of 14-3-3 during the disease course by means of repeated lumbar punctures demonstrated a substantial increase in sensitivity and specificity (Giraud et al., 2002; Sanchez-Juan et al., 2006, 2007). While in CJD there is usually a further increase in 14-3-3 levels as the disease progresses, patients with acute neuronal damage often show the opposite (Sanchez-Juan et al., 2007).

Besides 14-3-3, the microtubule-associated protein tau is also largely used as a surrogate CSF marker for the premortem diagnosis of sCJD, having shown comparable sensitivity and specificity to 14-3-3 (Otto et al., 2002; Riemenschneider et al., 2003; Sanchez-Juan et al., 2006; Hamlin et al., 2012; Karch et al., 2016; Leitao et al., 2016; Abu Rumeileh et al., 2017; Lattanzio et al., 2017). Furthermore, some studies have also underlined the diagnostic value of the ratio between phosphorylated tau and total tau protein (p-tau/t-tau) in the differential diagnosis between sCJD and Alzheimer disease or between sCJD and large clinically unselected populations of patients with dementia (Riemenschneider et al., 2003; Blennow et al., 2005; Buerger et al., 2006; Goodall et al., 2006; Satoh et al., 2006; Bahl et al., 2009; Skillback et al., 2014; Dorey et al., 2015; Abu Rumeileh et al., 2017; Lattanzio et al., 2017). Similarly to 14-3-3, the levels of both t-tau and p-tau also vary significantly according to the molecular disease subtype (Wang et al. 2010; van Harten et al., 2011; Skillback et al., 2014; Gmitterova et al., 2016; Lattanzio et al., 2017).

Additional CSF brain proteins that have been investigated for their potential diagnostic value in CJD include neuron-specific enolase (Sanchez-Juan et al., 2006, 2007; Satoh et al., 2007; Bahl et al., 2009; Forner et al., 2015), amyloid β 1–40, 1–42 (Wiltfang et al., 2003; Mollenhauer et al., 2011; Varges et al., 2011; Lattanzio et al., 2017), S100B (Mollenhauer et al., 2003; Van Everbroeck et al., 2003; Sanchez-Juan et al., 2006, 2007; Coulthart et al., 2011), and alpha-synuclein (Kasai et al., 2014; Llorens et al., 2017a, b).

PrP-amyloid aggregation assays (RT-QuIC)

The recent development of the real-time quaking-induced conversion (RT-QuIC) assay (details in Chapter 19), an in vitro fluorimetric assay which is able to indirectly detect very low amounts of PrP^{TSE} aggregates, based on the capacity of PrP^{TSE} to induce recombinant (rec-) PrP conversion and aggregation, has provided a very promising tool to improve the early diagnosis of human prion diseases (Wilham et al., 2010). By exploiting the self-replicating (seeding) power of pathogenic PrP^{TSE}, RT-QuIC ultrasensitively detects limited amounts of abnormal protein in CSF and other tissue samples. Results obtained in several laboratories with the first generation of this assay, which mainly uses a full-length (23–231) hamster recombinant prion protein ($rPrP^{sen}$) as substrate, demonstrated 79–86% sensitivity and 99–100% specificity (Atarashi et al., 2011; McGuire et al., 2012; Cramm et al., 2015; Lattanzio et al., 2017). Furthermore, a high reproducibility of the assay in the interlaboratory setting and across various CSF storage conditions, such as short-term CSF storage at different temperatures, long-term storage, repeated freezing and thawing cycles, has also been demonstrated (Cramm et al., 2016; McGuire et al., 2016, Schmitz et al., 2016a).

Orru et al. (2015) have recently introduced an improved, second-generation RT-QuIC for CSF (IQ-CSF) assay that uses a truncated form of hamster recombinant PrP ($rPrP^{sen}$, amino acids 90–231) as a substrate and other experimental conditions. Initial evaluation of the IQ-CSF assay indicated greater analytic and diagnostic sensitivity, and markedly shorter testing times (Bongianni et al., 2017; Foutz et al., 2017; Groveman et al., 2017; Franceschini et al., 2017). Given the huge diagnostic and analytic potential of the technique, future studies should aim to develop a type-specific RT-QuIC to discriminate the molecular subtypes of sCJD cases in vitam to bring the epidemiologic surveillance of sCJD to the next level.

CLINICAL DIAGNOSIS

The clinical diagnosis of CJD is based on the combination of clinical signs and results of diagnostic investigations (Fig. 9.5 and Table 9.5), the latter demonstrating heterogeneous sensitivity across molecular disease subtypes. For example, the sensitivity of detection of PSWCs in the EEG is very high in the classic MM1 subtype, but very low in all the others. On the other hand, MRI, by revealing a typical, almost subtype-specific, lesion pattern such as a high signal intensity in the basal ganglia and thalamus in VV2, a prominent signal

Diagnostic criteria for surveillance of sporadic CJD from 1 January 2017

1.1 **DEFINITE**

Progressive neurological syndrome **AND**

Neuropathologically **or** immunohistochemically **or** biochemically confirmed

1.2 **PROBABLE**

1.2.1 I + two of II and typical EEG*

OR 1.2.2 I + two of II and typical MRI brain scan **

OR 1.2.3 I + two of II and positive CSF 14-3-3

OR 1.2.4 Progressive neurological syndrome and positive RT-QuIC in CSF or other tissues

1.3 **POSSIBLE**

I + two of II + duration < 2 years

I Rapidly progressive cognitive impairment

II A Myoclonus

B Visual or cerebellar problems

C Pyramidal or extrapyramidal features

D Akinetic mutism

*Generalized periodic complexes

**High signal in caudate/putamen on MRI brain scan or at least two cortical regions (temporal, parietal, occipital) either on DWI or FLAIR

Fig. 9.5. Diagnostic criteria for surveillance of sporadic Creutzfeldt–Jakob disease from 1 January 2017. CSF, cerebrospinal fluid; DWI, diffusion-weighted imaging; EEG, electroencephalogram; FLAIR, fluid-attenuated inversion recovery; MRI, magnetic resonance imaging; RT-QuIC, real-time quaking-induced conversion assay.

Table 9.5

Performance of diagnostic tests in sporadic Creutzfeldt–Jakob disease (sCJD) subtypes (according to literature and own data)

				MM2				
			MM1/MV1[a]	Cortical	Thalamic	MV2K	VV1	VV2
EEG	PSWCs		+	–	–	–	–	–
CSF	14-3-3[b]		+	(+)	–	(+)	+	+
MRI	Basal ganglia		+	(+)	–	+	(+)	+
	Cortex		+	+	–	+	+	(+)
	Thalamus	Hyperintensity	(+)		–	+	–	+
		Pulvinar sign[c]				(+)	–	–
	Hippocampus		(+)	(+)	–	(+)	+	(+)
SPECT PET	Hypoperfusion/ hypometabolism in various areas		+	+	+	+	+	?

[a]Corresponds to classic sCJD with a rapid disease course.
[b]14-3-3 protein in CSF may be negative in up to 30% of MV2K and MM2C cases.
[c]The "pulvinar sign" is defined as hyperintensity of the pulvinar compared to the anterior putamen.
+ common; (+) less frequent; – rare; ? no data. CSF, cerebrospinal fluid; EEG, electroencephalogram; MRI, magnetic resonance imaging; PET, positron emission tomography; PSWCs, periodic sharp-wave complexes; SPECT, single-photon emission computed tomography.

hyperintensity in MM2C or a marked asymmetry in MM1, provides the most information in such cases. Finally, CSF assays have a lower sensitivity in atypical subtypes such as MV2K, MM2C, and MM2T. Thus, clinical parameters, diagnostic investigations, as well as codon 129 genotyping all need to be taken into account to achieve the most accurate clinical diagnosis (Meissner et al., 2005; Zerr et al., 2009; Parchi and Capellari, 2013).

CONCLUSIONS

The diagnosis of sCJD has significantly improved in recent years with the advent of refined brain-imaging techniques and the development of specific CSF assays. These diagnostic investigations, combined with improved knowledge about the disease phenotypic spectrum, have also significantly increased the potential for a subtype-specific early diagnosis of sCJD, which would be facilitated by the revision of current diagnostic criteria. Despite these significant advances, however, no safe effective therapies currently exist for CJD. Besides the search for an effective pharmaceutical agent, future studies should aim to further define the molecular basis of prion strains and their distinct cellular targeting and the origin of sCJD which all appear central to the understanding of prion disease and possibly other protein misfolding disorders.

References

Abu Rumeileh S, Lattanzio F, Stanzani Maserati M et al. (2017). Diagnostic accuracy of a combined analysis of cerebrospinal fluid t-PrP, t-tau, p-tau, and Abeta42 in the differential diagnosis of Creutzfeldt-Jakob disease from Alzheimer's disease with emphasis on atypical disease variants. J Alzheimers Dis 55: 1471–1480.

Aksamit Jr AJ, Preissner CM, Homburger HA (2001). Quantitation of 14-3-3 and neuron-specific enolase proteins in CSF in Creutzfeldt-Jakob disease. Neurology 57: 728–730.

Alpérovitch A, Zerr I, Pocchiari M et al. (1999). Codon 129 prion protein genotype and sporadic Creutzfeldt-Jakob disease. Lancet 353: 1673–1674.

Alvarez FJ, Bisbe J, Bisbe V et al. (2005). Magnetic resonance imaging findings in preclinical Creutzeldt-Jakob disease. Int J Neurosci 115: 1219–1225.

Amor S, Woodroofe MN (2014). Innate and adaptive immune responses in neurodegeneration and repair. Immunology 141: 287–291.

Arruda WO, Bordignon KC, Milano JB et al. (2004). Creutzfeldt-Jakob disease, Heidenhain variant: case report with MRI (DWI) findings. Arq Neuropsiquiatr 62: 347–352.

Atarashi R, Satoh K, Sano K et al. (2011). Ultrasensitive human prion detection in cerebrospinal fluid by real-time quaking-induced conversion. Nat Med 17: 175–178.

Bahl JM, Heegaard NH, Falkenhorst G et al. (2009). The diagnostic efficiency of biomarkers in sporadic Creutzfeldt-Jakob disease compared to Alzheimer's disease. Neurobiol Aging 30: 1834–1841.

Bahn MM, Parchi P (1999). Abnormal diffusion-weighted magnetic resonance images in Creutzfeldt-Jakob disease. Arch Neurol 56: 577–583.

Bahn MM, Kido DK, Lin W et al. (1997). Brain magnetic resonance diffusion abnormalities in Creutzfeldt-Jakob disease. Arch Neurol 54: 1411–1415.

Baiardi S, Capellari S, Ladogana A et al. (2016). Revisiting the Heidenhain variant of Creutzfeldt-Jakob disease: evidence for prion type variability influencing clinical course and laboratory findings. J Alzheimers Dis 50: 465–476.

Baiardi S, Magherini A, Capellari S et al. (2017). Towards an early clinical diagnosis of sporadic CJD VV2 (ataxic type). J Neurol Neurosurg Psychiatry 88: 764–772.

Bekiesinska-Figatowska M, Kuczynska-Zardzewialy A, Pomianowska B et al. (2012). The value of magnetic resonance imaging in the early diagnosis of Creutzfeldt-Jakob disease - own experience. Pol J Radiol 77: 63–67.

Bishop MT, Will RG, Manson JC (2010). Defining sporadic Creutzfeldt-Jakob disease strains and their transmission properties. Proc Natl Acad Sci U S A 107: 12005–12010.

Blasco Olcina R, Yaya Huaman R, Garces Sanchez M et al. (2001). Creutzfeldt-Jakob disease with unilateral onset: clinical profile and neuroimaging. Neurologia 16: 381–384.

Blennow K, Johansson A, Zetterberg H (2005). Diagnostic value of 14-3-3beta immunoblot and T-tau/P-tau ratio in clinically suspected Creutzfeldt-Jakob disease. Int J Mol Med 16: 1147–1149.

Boesenberg C, Schulz-Schaeffer WJ, Meissner B et al. (2005). Clinical course in young patients with sporadic Creutzfeldt-Jakob disease. Ann Neurol 58: 533–543.

Bongianni M, Orru C, Groveman BR et al. (2017). Diagnosis of human prion disease using real-time quaking-induced conversion testing of olfactory mucosa and cerebrospinal fluid samples. JAMA Neurol 74: 155–162.

Brandel JP, Delasnene-Laupretre N, Laplanche JL et al. (2000). Diagnosis of Creutzfeldt-Jakob disease: effect of clinical criteria on incidence estimates. Neurology 54: 1095–1099.

Brandel JP, Peoc'h K, Beaudry P et al. (2001). 14-3-3 protein cerebrospinal fluid detection in human growth hormone-treated Creutzfeldt-Jakob disease patients. Ann Neurol 49: 257–260.

Brown P, Gibbs Jr CJ, Rodgers-Johnson P et al. (1994). Human spongiform encephalopathy: the National Institutes of Health series of 300 cases of experimentally transmitted disease. Ann Neurol 35: 513–529.

Brownell B, Oppenheimer DR (1965). An ataxic form of subacute presenile polioencephalopathy (Creutzfeldt-Jakob disease). J Neurol Neurosurg Psychiatry 28: 350–361.

Buerger K, Otto M, Teipel SJ et al. (2006). Dissociation between CSF total tau and tau protein phosphorylated at threonine 231 in Creutzfeldt-Jakob disease. Neurobiol Aging 27: 10–15.

Cali I, Castellani R, Yuan J et al. (2006). Classification of sporadic Creutzfeldt-Jakob disease revisited. Brain 129: 2266–2277.

Caobelli F, Cobelli M, Pizzocaro C et al. (2015). The role of neuroimaging in evaluating patients affected by Creutzfeldt-Jakob disease: a systematic review of the literature. J Neuroimaging 25: 2–13.

Capellari S, Parchi P, Russo CM et al. (2000). Effect of the E200K mutation on prion protein metabolism. Comparative study of a cell model and human brain. Am J Pathol 157: 613–622.

Capellari S, Strammiello R, Saverioni D et al. (2011). Genetic Creutzfeldt-Jakob disease and fatal familial insomnia: insights into phenotypic variability and disease pathogenesis. Acta Neuropathol 121: 21–37.

Carswell C, Thompson A, Lukic A et al. (2012). MRI findings are often missed in the diagnosis of Creutzfeldt-Jakob disease. BMC Neurol 12: 153.

Castellani RJ, Colucci M, Xie Z et al. (2004). Sensitivity of 14-3-3 protein test varies in subtypes of sporadic Creutzfeldt-Jakob disease. Neurology 63: 436–442.

Cescatti M, Saverioni D, Capellari S et al. (2016). Analysis of conformational stability of abnormal prion protein aggregates across the spectrum of Creutzfeldt-Jakob disease prions. J Virol 90: 6244–6254.

Chitravas N, Jung RS, Kofskey DM et al. (2011). Treatable neurological disorders misdiagnosed as Creutzfeldt-Jakob disease. Ann Neurol 70: 437–444.

Chohan G, Pennington C, Mackenzie JM et al. (2010). The role of cerebrospinal fluid 14-3-3 and other proteins in the diagnosis of sporadic Creutzfeldt-Jakob disease in the UK: a 10-year review. J Neurol Neurosurg Psychiatry 81: 1243–1248.

Choi YP, Peden AH, Groner A et al. (2010). Distinct stability states of disease-associated human prion protein identified by conformation-dependent immunoassay. J Virol 84: 12030–12038.

Collie DA, Sellar RJ, Zeidler M et al. (2001). MRI of Creutzfeldt-Jakob disease: imaging features and recommended MRI protocol. Clin Radiol 56: 726–739.

Collins S, Boyd A, Fletcher A et al. (2000). Creutzfeldt-Jakob disease: diagnostic utility of 14-3-3 protein immunodetection in cerebrospinal fluid. J Clin Neurosci 7: 203–208.

Collins S, Boyd A, Lee JS et al. (2002). Creutzfeldt-Jakob disease in Australia 1970–1999. Neurology 59: 1365–1371.

Collins SJ, Sanchez-Juan P, Masters CL et al. (2006). Determinants of diagnostic investigation sensitivities across the clinical spectrum of sporadic Creutzfeldt-Jakob disease. Brain 129: 2278–2287.

Cordery RJ, Alner K, Cipolotti L et al. (2005). The neuropsychology of variant CJD: a comparative study with inherited and sporadic forms of prion disease. J Neurol Neurosurg Psychiatry 76: 330–336.

Coulthart MB, Jansen GH, Olsen E et al. (2011). Diagnostic accuracy of cerebrospinal fluid protein markers for sporadic Creutzfeldt-Jakob disease in Canada: a 6-year prospective study. BMC Neurol 11: 133.

Cousens SN, Vynnycky E, Zeidler M et al. (1997). Predicting the CJD epidemic in humans. Nature 385: 197–198.

Cramm M, Schmitz M, Karch A et al. (2015). Characteristic CSF prion seeding efficiency in humans with prion diseases. Mol Neurobiol 51: 396–405.

Cramm M, Schmitz M, Karch A et al. (2016). Stability and reproducibility underscore utility of RT-QuIC for diagnosis of Creutzfeldt-Jakob disease. Mol Neurobiol 53: 1896–1904.

Cummings J (1997). The neuropsychiatric inventory: assessing psychopahtology in dementia patients. Neurology 48 (Suppl 6): 10–16.

de Silva R (1996). Pooled plasma derivatives and Creutzfeldt-Jakob disease. Lancet 347: 967.

Demaerel P, Baert AL, Vanopdenbosch L et al. (1999). Diffusion-weighted MRI in sporadic Creutzfeldt-Jakob disease. Neurology 52: 205–208.

Dorey A, Tholance Y, Vighetto A et al. (2015). Association of cerebrospinal fluid prion protein levels and the distinction between Alzheimer disease and Creutzfeldt-Jakob disease. JAMA Neurol 72: 267–275.

Eisenmenger L, Porter MC, Carswell CJ et al. (2016). Evolution of diffusion-weighted magnetic resonance imaging signal abnormality in sporadic Creutzfeldt-Jakob disease, with histopathological correlation. JAMA Neurol 73: 76–84.

Ferrer I, Rivera R, Blanco R et al. (1999). Expression of proteins linked to exocytosis and neurotransmission in patients with Creutzfeldt-Jakob disease. Neurobiol Dis 6: 92–100.

Ferrer I, Puig B, Blanco R et al. (2000). Prion protein deposition and abnormal synaptic protein expression in the cerebellum in Creutzfeldt-Jakob disease. Neuroscience 97: 715–726.

Forner SA, Takada LT, Bettcher BM et al. (2015). Comparing CSF biomarkers and brain MRI in the diagnosis of sporadic Creutzfeldt-Jakob disease. Neurol Clin Pract 5: 116–125.

Fourier A, Dorey A, Perret-Liaudet A et al. (2017). Detection of CSF 14-3-3 protein in sporadic Creutzfeldt-Jakob disease patients using a new automated capillary Western assay. Mol Neurobiol.

Foutz A, Appleby BS, Hamlin C et al. (2017). Diagnostic and prognostic value of human prion detection in cerebrospinal fluid. Ann Neurol 81: 79–92.

Fragoso DC, Goncalves Filho AL de M et al. (2017). Imaging of Creutzfeldt-Jakob disease: imaging patterns and their differential diagnosis. Radiographics 37: 234–257.

Franceschini A, Baiardi S, Hughson AG et al. (2017). High diagnostic value of second generation CSF RT-QuIC across the wide spectrum of CJD prions. Sci Rep 7 (1): 10655.

Franceschini A, Strammiello R, Capellari S et al. (2018). Regional pattern of microgliosis in sporadic Creutzfeldt-Jakob disease in relation to phenotypic variants and disease progression. Neuropathol Appl Neurobiol. https://doi.org/10.1111/nan.12461. [Epub ahead of print].

Gaudino S, Gangemi E, Colantonio R et al. (2017). Neuroradiology of human prion diseases, diagnosis and differential diagnosis. Radiol Med 122: 369–385.

Giraud P, Biacabe A, Chazot G et al. (2002). Increased detection of 14-3-3 protein in cerebrospinal fluid in sporadic Creutzfeldt-Jakob disease during the disease course. Eur Neurol 48: 218–221.

Gmitterova K, Heinemann U, Krasnianski A et al. (2016). Cerebrospinal fluid markers in the differentiation of molecular subtypes of sporadic Creutzfeldt-Jakob disease. Eur J Neurol 23: 1126–1133.

Goodall CA, Head MW, Everington D et al. (2006). Raised CSF phospho-tau concentrations in variant Creutzfeldt-Jakob disease: diagnostic and pathological implications. J Neurol Neurosurg Psychiatry 77: 89–91.

Grau-Rivera O, Sanchez-Valle R, Bargallo N et al. (2016). Sporadic MM2-thalamic + cortical Creutzfeldt-Jakob disease: Utility of diffusion tensor imaging in the detection of cortical involvement in vivo. Neuropathology 36: 199–204.

Green AJ, Thompson EJ, Stewart GE et al. (2001). Use of 14-3-3 and other brain-specific proteins in CSF in the diagnosis of variant Creutzfeldt-Jakob disease. J Neurol Neurosurg Psychiatry 70: 744–748.

Green A, Sanchez-Juan P, Ladogana A et al. (2007). CSF analysis in patients with sporadic CJD and other transmissible spongiform encephalopathies. Eur J Neurol 14: 121–124.

Groveman BR, Orru CD, Hughson AG et al. (2017). Extended and direct evaluation of RT-QuIC assays for Creutzfeldt-Jakob disease diagnosis. Ann Clin Transl Neurol 4: 139–144.

Haik S, Brandel JP, Sazdovitch V et al. (2000). Dementia with Lewy bodies in a neuropathologic series of suspected Creutzfeldt-Jakob disease. Neurology 55: 1401–1404.

Hamlin C, Puoti G, Bern S et al. (2012). A comparison of tau and 14-3-3 protein in the diagnosis of Creutzfeldt-Jakob disease. Neurology 79: 547–552.

Harrington MG, Merrill CR, Asher DM et al. (1986). Abnormal proteins in the cerebrospinal fluid of patients with Creutzfeldt-Jakob disease. N Engl J Med 315: 279–283.

Heidenhain A (1929). Klinische und anatomische Untersuchungen über eine eigenartige organische Erkrankung des Zentralnervensystems im Praesenium. Z Ges Neurol Psychiatr 118: 49–114.

Heinemann U, Krasnianski A, Meissner B et al. (2007). Creutzfeldt-Jakob disease in Germany: a prospective 12-year surveillance. Brain 130: 1350–1359.

Herms J, Tings T, Gall S et al. (1999). Evidence of presynaptic location and function of the prion protein. J Neurosci 19: 8866–8875.

Heye N, Henkes H, Hansen M-L et al. (1990). Focal-unilateral accentuation of changes observed in the early stage of Creutzfeldt-Jakob disease. J Neurol Sci 95: 105–110.

Hilton KJ, Cunningham C, Reynolds RA et al. (2013). Early hippocampal synaptic loss precedes neuronal loss and associates with early behavioural deficits in three distinct strains of prion disease. PLoS One 8: e68062.

Hsich G, Kenney K, Gibbs CJ et al. (1996). The 14-3-3 brain protein in cerebrospinal fluid as a marker for transmissible spongifrom encephalopathies. N Engl J Med 335: 924–930.

Hyare H, Thornton J, Stevens J et al. (2010). High-b-value diffusion MR imaging and basal nuclei apparent diffusion coefficient measurements in variant and sporadic Creutzfeldt-Jakob disease. AJNR Am J Neuroradiol 31: 521–526.

Jacobi C, Arlt S, Reiber H et al. (2005). Immunoglobulins and virus-specific antibodies in patients with Creutzfeldt-Jakob disease. Acta Neurol Scand 111: 185–190.

Jones Jr HR, Hedley-Whyte ET, Freidberg SR et al. (1985). Ataxic Creutzfeldt-Jakob disease: diagnostic techniques and neuropathologic observations in early disease. Neurology 35: 254–257.

Kallenberg K, Schulz-Schaeffer WJ, Jastrow U et al. (2006). Creutzfeldt-Jakob disease: comparative analysis of MR imaging sequences. AJNR Am J Neuroradiol 27: 1459–1462.

Karch A, Koch A, Zapf A et al. (2016). Partial verification bias and incorporation bias affected accuracy estimates of diagnostic studies for biomarkers that were part of an existing composite gold standard. J Clin Epidemiol 78: 73–82.

Kasai T, Tokuda T, Ishii R et al. (2014). Increased alpha-synuclein levels in the cerebrospinal fluid of patients with Creutzfeldt-Jakob disease. J Neurol 261: 1203–1209.

Kim C, Haldiman T, Cohen Y et al. (2011). Protease-sensitive conformers in broad spectrum of distinct PrPSc structures in sporadic Creutzfeldt-Jakob disease are indicator of progression rate. PLoS Pathog 7: e1002242.

Knight R, Brazier M, Collins SJ (2004). Human prion diseases: cause, clinical and diagnostic aspects. Contrib Microbiol 11: 72–97.

Kobayashi A, Arima K, Ogawa M et al. (2008). Plaque-type deposition of prion protein in the damaged white matter of sporadic Creutzfeldt-Jakob disease MM1 patients. Acta Neuropathol 116: 561–566.

Kobayashi A, Sakuma N, Matsuura Y et al. (2010). Experimental verification of a traceback phenomenon in prion infection. J Virol 84: 3230–3238.

Kobayashi A, Matsuura Y, Mohri S et al. (2014). Distinct origins of dura mater graft-associated Creutzfeldt-Jakob disease: past and future problems. Acta Neuropathol Commun 2: 32.

Koscova S, Zakova Slivarichova D, Tomeckova I et al. (2016). Cerebrospinal fluid biomarkers in the diagnosis of Creutzfeldt-Jakob disease in Slovak patients: over 10-year period review. Mol Neurobiol 54: 5919–5927.

Kovacs GG, Kwong LK, Grossman M et al. (2017). Tauopathy with hippocampal 4-repeat tau immunoreactive spherical inclusions: a report of three cases. Brain Pathol. https://doi.org/10.1111/bpa.12482.

Krasnianski A, Meissner B, Schulz-Schaeffer W et al. (2006a). Clinical features and diagnosis of the MM2 cortical subtype of sporadic Creutzfeldt-Jakob disease. Arch Neurol 63: 876–880.

Krasnianski A, Schulz-Schaeffer WJ, Kallenberg K et al. (2006b). Clinical findings and diagnostic tests in the MV2 subtype of sporadic CJD. Brain 129: 2288–2296.

Krasnianski A, Bohling GT, Heinemann U et al. (2017). Neuropsychological symptoms in sporadic Creutzfeldt-Jakob disease patients in Germany. J Alzheimers Dis 59: 329–337.

Kropp S, Schulz-Schaeffer WJ, Finkenstaedt M et al. (1999). The Heidenhain variant of Creutzfeldt-Jakob disease. Arch Neurol 56: 55–61.

Kropp S, Finkenstaedt M, Zerr I et al. (2000). Diffusion-weighted MRI in patients with Creutzfeldt-Jakob disease. Nervenarzt 71: 91–95.

Ladogana A, Puopolo M, Croes EA et al. (2005). Mortality from Creutzfeldt-Jakob disease and related disorders in Europe, Australia, and Canada. Neurology 64: 1586–1591.

Lattanzio F, Abu-Rumeileh S, Franceschini A et al. (2017). Prion-specific and surrogate CSF biomarkers in Creutzfeldt-Jakob disease: diagnostic accuracy in relation to molecular subtypes and analysis of neuropathological correlates of p-tau and Abeta42 levels. Acta Neuropathol 133: 559–578.

Leitao MJ, Baldeiras I, Almeida MR et al. (2016). Sporadic Creutzfeldt-Jakob disease diagnostic accuracy is improved by a new CSF ELISA 14-3-3gamma assay. Neuroscience 322: 398–407.

Lemstra AW, van Meegen MT, Vreyling JP et al. (2000). 14-3-3 testing in diagnosing Creutzfeldt-Jakob disease: a prospective study in 112 patients. Neurology 55: 514–516.

Levy SR, Chiappa KH, Burke CJ et al. (1986). Early evolution and incidence of electroencephalographic abnormalities in Creutzfeldt-Jakob disease. J Clin Neurophysiol 3: 1–21.

Llorens F, Kruse N, Karch A et al. (2017a). Validation of alpha-synuclein as a CSF biomarker for sporadic Creutzfeldt-Jakob disease. Mol Neurobiol. https://doi.org/10.1007/s12035-D17-D479-5.

Llorens F, Kruse N, Schmitz M et al. (2017b). Evaluation of alpha-synuclein as a novel cerebrospinal fluid biomarker in different forms of prion diseases. Alzheimers Dement 13: 710–719.

Lodi R, Parchi P, Tonon C et al. (2009). Magnetic resonance diagnostic markers in clinically sporadic prion disease: a combined brain magnetic resonance imaging and spectroscopy study. Brain 132: 2669–2679.

Manners DN, Parchi P, Tonon C et al. (2009). Pathologic correlates of diffusion MRI changes in Creutzfeldt-Jakob disease. Neurology 72: 1425–1431.

Matoba M, Tonoma H, Miyaji H et al. (2001). Creutzfeldt-Jakob disease: serial changes on diffusion-weighted MRI. J Comput Assist Tomogr 25: 274–277.

Matsui Y, Satoh K, Miyazaki T et al. (2011). High sensitivity of an ELISA kit for detection of the gamma-isoform of 14-3-3 proteins: usefulness in laboratory diagnosis of human prion disease. BMC Neurol 11: 120.

McGuire LI, Peden AH, Orru CD et al. (2012). Real time quaking-induced conversion analysis of cerebrospinal fluid in sporadic Creutzfeldt-Jakob disease. Ann Neurol 72: 278–285.

McGuire LI, Poleggi A, Poggiolini I et al. (2016). Cerebrospinal fluid real-time quaking-induced conversion is a robust and reliable test for sporadic Creutzfeldt-Jakob disease: an international study. Ann Neurol 80: 160–165.

Mehndiratta MM, Chowdhury D, Gupta M (2000). Stroke like presentation of Creutzfeldt-Jakob disease. J Assoc Physicians India 48: 658–659.

Meissner B, Kortner K, Bartl M et al. (2004). Sporadic Creutzfeldt-Jakob disease: magnetic resonance imaging and clinical findings. Neurology 63: 450–456.

Meissner B, Westner IM, Kallenberg K et al. (2005). Sporadic Creutzfeldt-Jakob disease: clinical and diagnostic characteristics of the rare VV1 type. Neurology 65: 1544–1550.

Meissner B, Kallenberg K, Sanchez-Juan P et al. (2009). MRI and clinical syndrome in dura mater-related Creutzfeldt-Jakob disease. J Neurol 256: 355–363.

Minikel EV, Vallabh SM, Lek M et al. (2016). Quantifying prion disease penetrance using large population control cohorts. Sci Transl Med 8: 322ra9.

Moda F, Suardi S, Di Fede G et al. (2012). MM2-thalamic Creutzfeldt-Jakob disease: neuropathological, biochemical and transmission studies identify a distinctive prion strain. Brain Pathol 22: 662–669.

Mollenhauer B, Serafin S, Zerr I et al. (2003). Diagnostic problems during late course in Creutzfeldt-Jakob disease. J Neurol 250: 629–630.

Mollenhauer B, Locascio JJ, Schulz-Schaeffer W et al. (2011). Alpha-synuclein and tau concentrations in cerebrospinal fluid of patients presenting with parkinsonism: a cohort study. Lancet Neurol 10: 230–240.

Muayqil T, Gronseth G, Camicioli R (2012). Evidence-based guideline: diagnostic accuracy of CSF 14-3-3 protein in sporadic Creutzfeldt-Jakob disease: report of the guideline development subcommittee of the American Academy of Neurology. Neurology 79: 1499–1506.

Notari S, Capellari S, Giese A et al. (2004). Effects of different experimental conditions on the PrPSc core generated by protease digestion: implications for strain typing and molecular classification of CJD. J Biol Chem 279: 16797–16804.

Notari S, Capellari S, Langeveld J et al. (2007). A refined method for molecular typing reveals that co-occurrence of PrP(Sc) types in Creutzfeldt-Jakob disease is not the rule. Lab Investig 87: 1103–1112.

Notari S, Strammiello R, Capellari S et al. (2008). Characterization of truncated forms of abnormal prion protein in Creutzfeldt-Jakob disease. J Biol Chem 283: 30557–30565.

Olsson JE (1980). Brain and CSF proteins in Creutzfeldt-Jakob disease. Eur Neurol 19: 85–90.

Orru CD, Groveman BR, Hughson AG et al. (2015). Rapid and sensitive RT-QuIC detection of human Creutzfeldt-Jakob disease using cerebrospinal fluid. MBio 6.

Otto A, Zerr I, Lantsch M et al. (1998). Akinetic mutism as a classification criterion for the diagnosis of Creutzfeldt-Jakob disease. J Neurol Neurosurg Psychiatry 64: 524–528.

Otto M, Wiltfang J, Cepek L et al. (2002). Tau protein and 14-3-3 protein in the differential diagnosis of Creutzfeldt-Jakob disease. Neurology 58: 192–197.

Palmer MS, Dryden AJ, Hughes JT et al. (1991). Homozygous prion protein genotype predisposes to sporadic Creutzfeldt-Jakob disease. Nature 352: 340–342.

Parchi P, Capellari S (2013). Prion disease: diagnostic value of cerebrospinal fluid markers. Nat Rev Neurol 9: 10–11.

Parchi P, Saverioni D (2012). Molecular pathology, classification, and diagnosis of sporadic human prion disease variants. Folia Neuropathol 50: 20–45.

Parchi P, Castellani R, Capellari S et al. (1996). Molecular basis of phenotypic variability in sporadic Creutzfeldt-Jakob disease. Ann Neurol 39: 767–778.

Parchi P, Capellari S, Chen SG et al. (1997). Typing prion isoforms. Nature 386: 232–234.

Parchi P, Giese A, Capellari S et al. (1999a). Classification of sporadic Creutzfeldt-Jakob disease based on molecular and phenotypic analysis of 300 subjects. Ann Neurol 46: 224–233.

Parchi P, Capellari S, Chin S et al. (1999b). A subtype of sporadic prion disease mimicking fatal familial insomnia. Neurology 52: 1757–1763.

Parchi P, Zou W, Wang W et al. (2000). Genetic influence on the structural variations of the abnormal prion protein. Proc Natl Acad Sci U S A 97: 10168–10172.

Parchi P, Strammiello R, Notari S et al. (2009). Incidence and spectrum of sporadic Creutzfeldt-Jakob disease variants with mixed phenotype and co-occurrence of PrPSc types: an updated classification. Acta Neuropathol 118: 659–671.

Parchi P, Cescatti M, Notari S et al. (2010). Agent strain variation in human prion disease: insights from a molecular and pathological review of the National Institutes of Health series of experimentally transmitted disease. Brain 133: 3030–3042.

Parchi P, Strammiello R, Giese A et al. (2011). Phenotypic variability of sporadic human prion disease and its molecular basis: past, present, and future. Acta Neuropathol 121: 91–112.

Parchi P, de Boni L, Saverioni D et al. (2012). Consensus classification of human prion disease histotypes allows reliable identification of molecular subtypes: an inter-rater study among surveillance centres in Europe and USA. Acta Neuropathol 124: 517–529.

Pastrana MA, Sajnani G, Onisko B et al. (2006). Isolation and characterization of a proteinase K-sensitive PrPSc fraction. Biochemistry 45: 15710–15717.

Pereira E (2002). Diffusion-weighted sequence on MRI for the diagnosis of Creutzfeldt-Jakob disease. Arq Neuropsiquiatr 60: 906–908.

Peretz D, Scot MR, Groth D et al. (2001). Strain-specified relative conformational stability of the scrapie prion protein. Protein Sci 10: 854–863.

Pirisinu L, Di Bari M, Marcon S et al. (2010). A new method for the characterization of strain-specific conformational stability of protease-sensitive and protease-resistant PrPSc. PLoS One 5: e12723.

Pocchiari M, Puopolo M, Croes EA et al. (2004). Predictors of survival in sporadic Creutzfeldt-Jakob disease and other human transmissible spongiform encephalopathies. Brain (10): 2348–2359.

Puoti G, Bizzi A, Forloni G et al. (2012). Sporadic human prion diseases: molecular insights and diagnosis. Lancet Neurol 11: 618–628.

Ransohoff RM, Perry VH (2009). Microglial physiology: unique stimuli, specialized responses. Annu Rev Immunol 27: 119–145.

Reiniger L, Lukic A, Linehan J et al. (2011). Tau, prions and Abeta: the triad of neurodegeneration. Acta Neuropathol 121: 5–20.

Riemenschneider M, Wagenpfeil S, Vanderstichele H et al. (2003). Phospho-tau/total tau ratio in cerebrospinal fluid discriminates Creutzfeldt-Jakob disease from other dementias. Mol Psychiatry 8: 343–347.

Ritchie DL, Barria MA, Peden AH et al. (2017). UK iatrogenic Creutzfeldt-Jakob disease: investigating human prion transmission across genotypic barriers using human tissue-based and molecular approaches. Acta Neuropathol (4): 579–595.

Riva-Amarante E, Jimenez-Huete A, Toledano R et al. (2011). Usefulness of high b-value diffusion-weighted MRI in the diagnosis of Creutzfeldt-Jakob disease. Neurologia 26: 331–336.

Rosenmann H, Meiner Z, Kahana E et al. (1997). Detection of 14-3-3 protein in the CSF of genetic Creutzfeldt-Jakob disease. Neurology 49: 593–595.

Rossi M, Saverioni D, Di Bari M et al. (2017). Atypical Creutzfeldt-Jakob disease with PrP-amyloid plaques in white matter: molecular characterization and transmission to bank voles show the M1 strain signature. Acta Neuropathol Commun 5 (1): 87.

Safar JG, Wille H, Itri V et al. (1998). Eight prion strains have PrP(Sc) molecules with different conformations. Nat Med 4: 1157–1165.

Safar JG, Geschwind MD, Deering C et al. (2005). Diagnosis of human prion disease. Proc Natl Acad Sci U S A 102: 3501–3506.

Safar JG, Xiao X, Kabir ME et al. (2015). Structural determinants of phenotypic diversity and replication rate of human prions. PLoS Pathog 11: e1004832.

Sanchez-Juan P, Green A, Ladogana A et al. (2006). CSF tests in the differential diagnosis of Creutzfeldt-Jakob disease. Neurology 67: 637–643.

Sanchez-Juan P, Sanchez-Valle R, Green A et al. (2007). Influence of timing on CSF tests value for Creutzfeldt-Jakob disease diagnosis. J Neurol 254: 901–906.

Sanchez-Valle R, Saiz A, Graus F (2002). 14-3-3 Protein isoforms and atypical patterns of the 14-3-3 assay in the diagnosis of Creutzfeldt-Jakob disease. Neurosci Lett 320: 69–72.

Satoh K, Shirabe S, Eguchi H et al. (2006). 14-3-3 protein, total tau and phosphorylated tau in cerebrospinal fluid of patients with Creutzfeldt-Jakob disease and neurodegenerative disease in Japan. Cell Mol Neurobiol 26: 45–52.

Satoh K, Shirabe S, Tsujin A et al. (2007). Total tau protein in cerebrospinal fluid and diffusion-weighted MRI as an early diagnostic marker for Creutzfeldt-Jakob disease. Dement Geriatr Cogn Disord 24: 207–212.

Satoh K, Tobiume M, Matsui Y et al. (2010). Establishment of a standard 14-3-3 protein assay of cerebrospinal fluid as a diagnostic tool for Creutzfeldt-Jakob disease. Lab Investig 90: 1637–1644.

Satoh K, Nakaoke R, Nishiura Y et al. (2011). Early detection of sporadic CJD by diffusion-weighted MRI before the onset of symptoms. J Neurol Neurosurg Psychiatry 82: 942–943.

Saverioni D, Notari S, Capellari S et al. (2013). Analyses of protease resistance and aggregation state of abnormal prion protein across the spectrum of human prions. J Biol Chem 288: 27972–27985.

Schmitz M, Cramm M, Llorens F et al. (2016a). The real-time quaking-induced conversion assay for detection of human prion disease and study of other protein misfolding diseases. Nat Protoc 11: 2233–2242.

Schmitz M, Ebert E, Stoeck K et al. (2016b). Validation of 14-3-3 protein as a marker in sporadic Creutzfeldt-Jakob disease diagnostic. Mol Neurobiol 53: 2189–2199.

Schröter A, Zerr I, Henkel K et al. (2000). Magnetic resonance imaging in the clinical diagnosis of Creutzfeldt-Jakob disease. Arch Neurol 57: 1751–1757.

Shiga Y, Miyazawa K, Sato S et al. (2004). Diffusion-weighted MRI abnormalities as an early diagnostic marker for Creutzfeldt-Jakob disease. Neurology 63: 443–449.

Shiga Y, Wakabayashi H, Miyazawa K et al. (2006). 14-3-3 protein levels and isoform patterns in the cerebrospinal fluid of Creutzfeldt-Jakob disease patients in the progressive and terminal stages. J Clin Neurosci 13: 661–665.

Skillback T, Rosen C, Asztely F et al. (2014). Diagnostic performance of cerebrospinal fluid total tau and phosphorylated tau in Creutzfeldt-Jakob disease: results from the Swedish Mortality Registry. JAMA Neurol 71: 476–483.

Steinhoff BJ, Racker S, Herrendorf G et al. (1996). Accuracy and reliability of periodic sharp wave complexes in Creutzfeldt-Jakob disease. Arch Neurol 53: 162–166.

Takeuchi A, Kobayashi A, Parchi P et al. (2016). Distinctive properties of plaque-type dura mater graft-associated Creutzfeldt-Jakob disease in cell-protein misfolding cyclic amplification. Lab Investig 96: 581–587.

Tomita I, Sato K, Shirabe S et al. (2004). Serial diffusion-weighted MRI (DWI) in a patient with sporadic Creuztfeldt-Jakob disease. Rinsho Shinkeigaku 44: 182–186.

Tribl GG, Strasser G, Zeitlhofer J et al. (2002). Sequential MRI in a case of Creutzfeldt-Jakob disease. Neuroradiology 44: 223–226.

Tschampa HJ, Neumann M, Zerr I et al. (2001). Patients with Alzheimer's disease and dementia with Lewy bodies mistaken for Creutzfeldt-Jakob disease. J Neurol Neurosurg Psychiatry 71: 33–39.

Tschampa HJ, Kallenberg K, Urbach H et al. (2005). MRI in the diagnosis of sporadic Creutzfeldt-Jakob disease: a study on inter-observer agreement. Brain 128: 2026–2033.

Tschampa HJ, Kallenberg K, Kretzschmar HA et al. (2007). Pattern of cortical changes in sporadic Creutzfeldt-Jakob disease. Am J Neuroradiol 28: 1114–1118.

Tsuji Y, Kanamori H, Murakami G et al. (2004). Heidenhain variant of Creutzfeldt-Jakob disease: diffusion-weighted MRI and PET characteristics. J Neuroimaging 14: 63–66.

Tzaban S, Friedlander G, Schonberger O et al. (2002). Protease-sensitive scrapie prion protein in aggregates of heterogeneous sizes. Biochemistry 41: 12868–12875.

Ukisu R, Kushihashi T, Kitanosono T et al. (2005). Serial diffusion-weighted MRI of Creutzfeldt-Jakob disease. Am J Roentgenol 184: 560–566.

Van Everbroeck B, Quoilin S, Boons J et al. (2003). A prospective study of CSF markers in 250 patients with possible Creutzfeldt-Jakob disease. J Neurol Neurosurg Psychiatry 74: 1210–1214.

van Harten AC, Kester MI, Visser PJ et al. (2011). Tau and p-tau as CSF biomarkers in dementia: a meta-analysis. Clin Chem Lab Med 49: 353–366.

Varges D, Jung K, Gawinecka J et al. (2011). Amyloid-beta 1-42 levels are modified by apolipoprotein E epsilon4 in Creutzfeldt-Jakob disease in a similar manner as in Alzheimer's disease. J Alzheimers Dis 23: 717–726.

Vitali P, Maccagnano E, Caverzasi E et al. (2011). Diffusion-weighted MRI hyperintensity patterns differentiate CJD from other rapid dementias. Neurology 76: 1711–1719.

Wang GR, Gao C, Shi Q et al. (2010). Elevated levels of tau protein in cerebrospinal fluid of patients with probable Creutzfeldt-Jakob disease. Am J Med Sci 340: 291–295.

Wilham JM, Orru CD, Bessen RA et al. (2010). Rapid end-point quantitation of prion seeding activity with sensitivity comparable to bioassays. PLoS Pathog 6: e1001217.

Will RG (1991). The spongiform encephalopathies. J Neurol Neurosurg Psychiatry 54: 761–763.

Will RG, Ironside JW, Zeidler M et al. (1996). A new variant of Creutzfeldt-Jakob disease in the UK. Lancet 347: 921–925.

Will RG, Alperovitch A, Poser S et al. (1998). Descriptive epidemiology of Creutzfeldt-Jakob disease in six European countries, 1993-1995. EU Collaborative Study Group for CJD. Ann Neurol 43: 763–767.

Wiltfang J, Esselmann H, Smirnov A et al. (2003). Beta-amyloid peptides in cerebrospinal fluid of patients with Creutzfeldt-Jakob disease. Ann Neurol 54: 263–267.

Yemisci M, Gurer G, Saygi S et al. (2003). Generalised periodic epileptiform discharges: clinical features, neuroradiological evaluation and prognosis in 37 adult patients. Seizure 12: 465–472.

Young GS, Geschwind MD, Fischbein NJ et al. (2005). Diffusion-weighted and fluid-attenuated inversion recovery imaging in Creutzfeldt-Jakob disease: high sensitivity and specificity for diagnosis. AJNR Am J Neuroradiol 26: 1551–1562.

Zerr I, Poser S (2002). Clinical diagnosis and differential diagnosis of CJD and vCJD. With special emphasis on laboratory tests. APMIS 110: 88–98.

Zerr I, Bodemer M, Oto M et al. (1996). Diagnosis of Creutzfeldt-Jakob disease by two-dimensional gel electrophoresis of cerebrospinal fluid. Lancet 348: 846–849.

Zerr I, Bodemer M, Weber T (1997). The 14-3-3 brain protein and transmissible spongiform encephalopathy. N Engl J Med 336: 874. author reply 874–875.

Zerr I, Bodemer M, Gefeller O et al. (1998). Detection of 14-3-3 protein in the cerebrospinal fluid supports the diagnosis of Creutzfeldt-Jakob disease. Ann Neurol 43: 32–40.

Zerr I, Pocchiari M, Collins S et al. (2000a). Analysis of EEG and CSF 14-3-3 proteins as aids to the diagnosis of Creutzfeldt-Jakob disease. Neurology 55: 811–815.

Zerr I, Schulz-Schaeffer WJ, Giese A et al. (2000b). Current clinical diagnosis in Creutzfeldt-Jakob disease: identification of uncommon variants. Ann Neurol 48: 323–329.

Zerr I, Kallenberg K, Summers DM et al. (2009). Updated clinical diagnostic criteria for sporadic Creutzfeldt-Jakob disease. Brain 132: 2659–2668.

Zou WQ, Capellari S, Parchi P et al. (2003). Identification of novel proteinase K-resistant C-terminal fragments of PrP in Creutzfeldt-Jakob disease. J Biol Chem 278: 40429–40436.

Handbook of Clinical Neurology, Vol. 153 (3rd series)
Human Prion Diseases
M. Pocchiari and J. Manson, Editors
https://doi.org/10.1016/B978-0-444-63945-5.00010-6

Chapter 10

Variably protease-sensitive prionopathy

SILVIO NOTARI[1], BRIAN S. APPLEBY[1,2,3,4], AND PIERLUIGI GAMBETTI[1]*
[1]*Department of Pathology, Case Western Reserve University, Cleveland, OH, United States*
[2]*National Prion Disease Pathology Surveillance Center, Case Western Reserve University, Cleveland, OH, United States*
[3]*Department of Neurology, Case Western Reserve University, Cleveland, OH, United States*
[4]*Department of Psychiatry, Case Western Reserve University, Cleveland, OH, United States*

Abstract

Variably protease-sensitive prionopathy (VPSPr), originally identified in 2008, was further characterized and renamed in 2010. Thirty-seven cases of VPSPr have been reported to date, consistent with estimated prevalence of 0.7–1.7% of all sporadic prion diseases. The lack of gene mutations establishes VPSPr as a sporadic form of human prion diseases, along with sporadic Creutzfeldt–Jakob disease (sCJD) and sporadic fatal insomnia. Like sCJD, VPSPr affects patients harboring any of the three genotypes, MM, MV, and VV at the prion protein (PrP) gene polymorphic codon 129, with VPSPr VV accounting for 65% of all VPSPr cases. Distinguishing clinical features include a median 2-year duration and presentation with psychiatric signs, speech/language impairment, or cognitive decline. Neuropathology comprises moderate spongiform degeneration, PrP amyloid miniplaques, and a target-like or plaque-like PrP deposition. The abnormal PrP associated with VPSPr typically forms an electrophoretic profile of five to seven bands (according to the antibody) presenting variable protease resistance depending on the 129 genotype. The familial prion disease associated with the V180I PrP gene mutation which harbors an abnormal PrP with similar electrophoretic profile might serve as a model for VPSPr. Transmission to animals has definitively established VPSPr as a prion disease. Because of its recent identification, rarity, and the elusiveness of its abnormal PrP, VPSPr remains largely understudied.

INTRODUCTION

Variably protease-sensitive prionopathy (VPSPr) was originally described in 2008 based on a study of 11 US subjects (Gambetti et al., 2008). The identification of this rare and clinically rather indistinct novel condition, and its prompt independent validation that followed, was made possible by the existence of many national prion surveillance centers worldwide dedicated to the examination and tissue banking of prion diseases. During regular examination of acquired cases at the US National Prion Disease Pathology Surveillance Center (NPDPSC), it was noted that in rare but recurring cases, brain tissues tested positive for the presence of abnormal, disease-related prion protein (PrP^{TSE}) by immunohistochemical techniques. However, they were negative following biochemical analysis by gel electrophoresis and immunoblotting of PrP^{TSE}, a test that is typically performed following treatment with proteinase K (PK) given the common PrP^{TSE} protease resistance in prion diseases. Enhanced analyses demonstrated the presence of a peculiar form of PrP^{TSE} that was particularly sensitive to PK digestion and displayed a distinctive multiple-band profile upon immunoblotting.

Genetic analysis established that all subjects were homozygotes for the codon valine (V) at position 129 of the prion protein (PrP) gene, the site of a common and nonpathogenic methionine polymorphism, M129V (Parchi et al., 1999; Gambetti et al., 2003, 2011). Moreover, no mutation was found in and adjacent to the coding

*Correspondence to: Pierluigi Gambetti, Department of Pathology, Case Western Reserve University, Cleveland, OH, USA. E-mail: pxg13@case.edu

region of the PrP gene where genetic mutations reside in inherited prion diseases, thus defining VPSPr as a sporadic prion disease (Gambetti et al., 2003, 2008; Kong et al., 2004). A subsequent study (Zou et al., 2010) reporting 15 additional cases from the United States and Italy established that all three M129V genotypes, MM, MV, and VV, not just VV, were affected in VPSPr. This property makes VPSPr the only sporadic human prion disease that affects the three 129 genotypes besides sporadic Creutzfeldt–Jakob disease (sCJD) (Chapter 9). This second study also revealed that PrP^{TSE} resistance to PK treatment varied according to the 129 genotype. This finding led to the amendment of the disease label from the original protease-sensitive prionopathy (PSPr) in the first 2008 publication to the current VPSPr (Gambetti et al., 2008; Zou et al., 2010).

Two additional VPSPr features emerged. First, VPSPr prevalence in the three 129 genotypes was found to be MM 11%, MV 24%, VV 65% (Table 10.1), which is almost the opposite of that associated with sCJD (MM 68%, MV 16%, VV 16%) (Collins et al., 2006), indicating that the role played by the 129 genotype is different in the two diseases. Second, several VPSPr patients have a family history of cognitive impairment, which raises the possibility of a genetic component in VPSPr. Unfortunately, no genetic or neuropathologic examination has been performed on cognitively impaired relatives of VPSPr patients.

EPIDEMIOLOGY

To date, 37 cases of VPSPr have been published. They include 25 from the United States (Gambetti et al., 2008; Zou et al., 2010; Cannon et al., 2014), five from the United Kingdom (Head et al., 2009, 2010, 2013); two each from Italy and Spain (Giaccone et al., 2007; Rodríguez-Martínez et al., 2010, 2012; Zou et al., 2010), and one each from Austria, Germany, and The Netherlands (Krebs et al., 2007; Jansen et al., 2010; Assar et al., 2015). One of the US cases was diagnosed incidentally at autopsy of a 93-year-old neurologically asymptomatic individual (Ghoshal et al., 2015). As for the M129V polymorphic genotype, the 37 cases include 24 VV homozygotes, nine MV heterozygotes, and four MM homozygotes. In addition, the US NPDPSC lists a total of 57 cases of VPSPr (inclusive of the 25 published) from a total of 3279 sporadic prion disease cases, which would estimate the VPSPr prevalence at 1.7% among all sporadic prion diseases (US National Prion Disease Pathology Surveillance Center, 2017). Thirteen VPSPR cases are stored by the National CJD Surveillance and Research Unit in the United Kingdom, which by the same calculation would result in a 0.7% prevalence of VPSPr there (UK National CJD Research and Surveillance Unit, 2017). Head et al. (2013) have estimated that VPSPr accounts for one death per 4 years in the ~60 million UK population. Adding together the unpublished cases stored by the US and UK prion surveillance centers brings the total number of known VPSPr cases worldwide to at least 77. However, it is likely that VPSPr is underreported, given that in most cases it is initially misdiagnosed as one of the non-Alzheimer dementias, conditions in which autopsies are not regularly performed (Puoti et al., 2012).

DEFINITION

VPSPr is a novel sporadic prion disease, which may account for almost 2% of all sporadic prion diseases. Similar to sporadic Creutzfeldt–Jakob disease (sCJD), VPSPr affects individuals harboring each of the three genotypes at codon 129 of the PrP gene, thus segregating VPSPr into three subtypes: MM, MV, and VV. The M129V genotype slightly affects disease phenotype and PrP^{TSE} features. Overall, mean age at onset is 70 and duration 2 years. Clinical presentation often includes one or more of three sets of signs: psychiatric abnormalities, speech/language impairment, and cognitive decline (Table 10.1). Histopathologic features include moderate cortical and subcortical spongiform degeneration (SD) and miniplaques in the cerebellum, while PrP immunostaining often reveals a distinctive target-like granular pattern. Depending on the antibody used, PrP^{TSE} forms a five- or seven-band ladder-like electrophoretic profile with increasing protease resistance from VV to MM subtypes.

CLINICAL FEATURES

Demographics

VPSPr is unique given its departure from the clinical aspects typically observed in other human prion diseases. The clinical diagnosis of VPSPr is difficult because of its nonspecific clinical presentation and noncontributory diagnostic tests that are typically suggestive of prion disease.

The polymorphism at codon 129 of the PrP gene affects many aspects of this prion disease, including susceptibility to the disease, age at onset, illness duration, clinical symptoms, and diagnostic test results (Table 10.2). Contrary to sCJD, the majority of VPSPr cases are homozygous for valine at codon 129 (65%), and the minority are homozygous for methionine (11%) (Table 10.2). VPSPr is typically a mid- to late-life illness with a mean age at onset of 70 years (range 48–87 years) (Puoti et al., 2012). The presence of valine at codon 129 seemingly has a dose–effect relationship toward a younger age at onset (mean age at onset: VV = 67, MV = 74, MM = 78 years) (Table 10.2).

Table 10.1

Classification of variably protease-sensitive prionopathy

		Clinical feature			Histopathology SD[a]			PrP immunostaining pattern[a]	
129 subtype	N	Onset (years)	Course (months)	Type of presentation[b]	C. cort	BG	Cereb	C. cortex	Cereb
MM[c]	3	66 (55–78)	56 (41–78)	Parkinsonian, ataxic, cognitive	++	++	+	Granular, plaque-like of various sizes	Granular, small plaque-like
MV	9	73 ± (65–81)	37 (7–72)	Psychiatric, parkinsonian, cognitive behavioral, aphasic	+++	+++	±	Fine granular with rarer larger granule or plaque-like	Amyloid miniplaques, plaque-like, granular
VV[d]	24	64 ± (48–77)	30 (10–78)	Psychiatric, ataxic, cognitive, behavioral, spastic gate, gaze palsy				As above but forming target-like structures	

[a]Typical spongiform degeneration (SD) severity, rated relatively to the three genotypes, and typical immunostaining patterns.
[b]Often clinical presentation included two types coexisting or in rapid succession.
[c]MM group includes four cases, but the fourth was asymptomatic.
[d]Includes one case treated with doxycycline for 4 years.
BG, basal ganglia; C. cort, cerebral cortex; Cereb, cerebellum.

Table 10.2

Clinical characteristics of variable protease-sensitive prionopathy (VPSPr)

	PRNP codon 129 polymorphism			
	Met-Met	Met-Val	Val-Val	All genotypes
Mean age at onset (years, range)	78 (64–87)	74 (65–81)	67 (48–77)	70 (48–87)
Duration (months, range)	41 (10–73)	34 (7–91)	18 (10–60)	24 (7–91)
Family history of dementia	33%	0%	60%	42%
Clinical presentation	Psychiatric symptoms, aphasia, parkinsonism, ataxia	Psychiatric symptoms, cognitive impairment	Psychiatric symptoms, cognitive impairment, aphasia	Psychiatric symptoms, speech/language impairment, cognitive impairment
Advanced clinical symptoms	Cognitive impairment, aphasia, myoclonus	Ataxia, parkinsonism, ataxia	Ataxia, parkinsonism, myoclonus	Ataxia, parkinsonism, myoclonus
EEG suggestive of prion disease	50%	25%	0%	9%
CSF (14-3-3 and tau) sensitivity	50%	0%	37%	21%
Brain MRI suggestive of prion disease	0%	0%	5%	3%

CSF, cerebrospinal fluid; EEG, electroencephalogram; MRI, magnetic resonance imaging.

An important difference between VPSPr and other sporadic prion diseases is its prolonged illness duration, which likely affects clinical ascertainment of cases. The duration of VPSPr is best measured in years as opposed to months, with a mean disease duration of 2 years (Puoti et al., 2012). Cases with durations over 6 and 7 years have been described in the literature (Appleby et al., 2009; Head et al., 2013). The codon 129 polymorphism affects disease duration, with the presence of valine resulting in a shorter duration, which is the opposite of what is observed in sCJD (Table 10.2) (Parchi et al., 1999; Puoti et al., 2012). Because of the insidious onset and slower progression of clinical symptoms compared to sCJD, it is likely more difficult to accurately determine the time of disease onset in VPSPr cases.

Table 10.3

Proposed clinical criteria for variable protease-sensitive prionopathy

A. Symptoms (both 1 and 2)
   1. Cognitive impairment
   2. Two or more of the following:
      (a) Psychiatric symptoms
      (b) Parkinsonism or aphasia
      (c) Ataxia or myoclonus

B. Duration < 8 years

C. Lack of alternative etiology or phenotype divergence from other neurodegenerative atypical dementias

Clinical course

The clinical presentation and course in VPSPr can best be described as an atypical dementia and differ from the phenotype observed in most cases of sCJD. One or more of a triad of symptoms characterizes the clinical presentation of VPSPr: psychiatric symptoms, speech/language impairment, and cognitive decline (Puoti et al., 2012). Most VV and MV cases present with psychiatric symptoms, cognitive decline, and/or aphasia. Cases homozygous for methionine have initial symptoms more similar to classic sCJD with psychiatric symptoms, aphasia, parkinsonism, and ataxia. Psychiatric symptoms often include disinhibition, euphoria, impulsivity, and apathy (Zou et al., 2010). Speech and language impairments include anomic or semantic aphasia with or without dysarthria. Cognitive impairment is most often associated with frontal lobe dysfunction (e.g., dysexecutive syndrome).

Whereas the initial presentation of VPSPr is mostly characterized by cortical impairments, subcortical and cerebellar symptoms arise later in the disease course. Cognitive decline is observed in all cases at some point in the disease (Puoti et al., 2012). Parkinsonism, ataxia, and myoclonus often develop later in the disease course. Additionally, certain codon 129 polymorphisms are marked by a paucity of specific symptoms. For example, aphasia is rare in MV cases and psychiatric symptoms are rare in MM cases (Zou et al., 2010). Clinical criteria including symptoms are proposed in Table 10.3.

CLINICAL TESTS

Diagnostic workup

Many cases of sCJD do not have a classic CJD clinical phenotype, but are often ascertained during the diagnostic workup because of a test that is suggestive of prion disease (Appleby et al., 2014). Unfortunately, the typical tests used to diagnose prion disease are often unhelpful in the diagnosis of VPSPr. Hence, the ability to successfully diagnose VPSPr relies on the clinical phenotype and exclusion of other etiologies.

Electroencephalogram (EEG)

Periodic sharp-wave complexes (PSWCs) on EEG are suggestive of prion disease and are part of the World Health Organization's diagnostic criteria for sCJD (World Health Organization, 1998). The presence of PSWCs is rare in VPSPr, with an estimated overall sensitivity of 9% (Puoti et al., 2012). PSWCs have been detected in 25% of MV and 50% of MM cases. No reported VV cases have demonstrated PSWCs. Typically, EEGs are normal or demonstrate generalized slowing (Gambetti et al., 2008). In some cases, EEGs are initially normal and then progress to generalized slowing later in the disease course (Head et al., 2009; Rodríguez-Martínez et al., 2012).

Cerebrospinal fluid

The increase of certain cerebrospinal fluid (CSF) proteins can be suggestive of prion disease. Rise of 14-3-3 in CSF with a clinical duration less than 2 years is part of the World Health Organization diagnostic criteria for sCJD (World Health Organization, 1998). Unfortunately, CSF 14-3-3 protein is typically negative or weakly positive (e.g., nondiagnostic) in VPSPr (Gambetti et al., 2008; Head et al., 2009; Jansen et al., 2010; Rodríguez-Martínez et al., 2012; Assar et al., 2015). However, a study detected positive CSF 14-3-3 protein in 50% of all UK VPSPr cases (Head et al., 2013). When CSF 14-3-3 is combined with tau, diagnostic sensitivity is 21% in all VPSPr cases with differing sensitivities by codon 129 genotype (Puoti et al., 2012). No MV cases demonstrated diagnostic 14-3-3/tau levels, whereas 50% of MM and 37% of VV cases had CSF results suggestive of prion disease. In the UK series, CSF S100b was positive in 75% of cases (Head et al., 2013), though this is not a diagnostic test that is routinely used in the diagnosis of prion disease. Two VV cases of VPSPr were reported to have elevated CSF protein levels (175 mg/dL and 126 mg/dL), the significance of which is unknown (Gambetti et al., 2008). CSF from one case of VPSPr was tested with real-time quaking-induced conversion (RT-QuIC) and found to be negative (Lattanzio et al., 2017). However, using the second generation RT-QuIC (IQ-CSF) 3 out of 3 cases of VPSPr were positive (Franceschini et al., 2017).

Neuroimaging

Brain magnetic resonance imaging (MRI) is a sensitive and specific diagnostic tool for sCJD. Hyperintensity on diffusion-weighted imaging (DWI) is typically seen in the basal ganglia and/or in a gyral pattern of the cortex in sCJD (Zerr et al., 2009); however; these brain MRI findings suggestive of prion disease are typically not present in VPSPr. Only two cases to date have demonstrated brain MRI findings suggestive of prion disease, both of which were VV at codon 129 (Zou et al., 2010; Assar et al., 2015). Brain MRIs of VPSPr cases typically demonstrate diffuse cortical atrophy, with some cases showing preferential atrophy of the frontal and/or parietal lobes and the cerebellum (Gambetti et al., 2008; Rodríguez-Martínez et al., 2012; Head et al., 2013). Overall, diagnostic sensitivity of brain MRI is 3% (Puoti et al., 2012). Single-photon emission computed tomography (SPECT) has been performed in three cases of VPSPr. All cases demonstrated hypoperfusion, which was global in one case and asymmetric in two (Gambetti et al., 2008; Rodríguez-Martínez et al., 2012).

DIFFERENTIAL DIAGNOSIS

Because the clinical features of VPSPr resemble atypical dementias, these cases are most often initially misdiagnosed as non-Alzheimer disease dementias. The most common clinical misdiagnoses of VPSPr include normal-pressure hydrocephalus, dementia with Lewy bodies, and frontotemporal lobar degeneration (Gambetti et al., 2011). One can certainly understand how VPSPr may be initially misdiagnosed as an atypical dementia. The prominent symptoms of aphasia, parkinsonism, and frontal lobe syndrome are suggestive of several frontotemporal lobar degeneration subtypes, including frontotemporal dementia, primary progressive aphasia, semantic dementia, progressive supranuclear palsy, and corticobasal syndrome. The prominent parkinsonian symptoms with cognitive impairment may also be suggestive of dementia with Lewy bodies or Parkinson disease dementia. Because of the prominence of psychiatric symptoms, some cases may initially be diagnosed as having a mood disorder (Gambetti et al., 2008; Assar et al., 2015).

As diagnosis of VPSPr currently stands, it is very difficult to discern the above atypical dementias from VPSPr in the initial stages of the disease. In fact, diagnosis of prion disease is often not considered until later in the disease course (Gambetti et al., 2008). One item that may signal a diagnosis of VPSPr, as opposed to one of the above atypical dementias, is a divergence from the expected clinical course of a previously diagnosed atypical dementia. For example, ataxia would not be expected in any of the above conditions and should prompt the consideration of VPSPr as the etiology. Additionally, a faster than expected disease progression may also be suggestive of VPSPr. Aside from disease-specific modalities (e.g., amyloid imaging), neuroimaging may be misleading and lead to an initial diagnosis of frontotemporal lobar degeneration due to frontal atrophy or asymmetric hypoperfusion on SPECT.

NEUROPATHOLOGY

The common histopathologic feature to all codon 129 genotypic subtypes of VPSPr is a moderate degree of SD, which similarly affects cerebral neocortex, entorhinal cortex, basal ganglia, and thalamus, and to a lesser degree the molecular layer of the cerebellum, while typically the hippocampus is spared (Fig. 10.1) (Jansen et al., 2010; Zou et al., 2010; Head et al., 2013). The SD brain distribution is similar to, but less severe than, that of sCJDMM1 (sCJD associated with PrP MM genotype and PrP^{TSE} type 1), the most common subtype of sCJD. However, the SD vacuoles of VPSPr differ in size since they are on average 50% larger than those of sCJDMM1 (9 ± 3 vs. 6 ± 1) and spread over a larger range of sizes (Parchi et al., 1999; Zou et al., 2010); however they are smaller and not as closely clustered or confluent as the vacuoles in the sCJDMM2 subtype (Parchi et al., 1999; Zou et al., 2010).

A distinctive feature is the presence of very small prion plaques in the molecular layer of the cerebellum and, rarely, the hippocampal region that are often irregular in shape and may comprise several cores (Fig. 10.2) (Gambetti et al., 2008; Zou et al., 2010; Head et al., 2013; Cannon et al., 2014). Immunoelectron microscopic examination of cerebellar and hippocampal miniplaques demonstrated poorly demarcated structures containing clusters of PrP-labeled fibrils embedded in an amorphous matrix. These features have been interpreted as consistent with poorly formed or immature amyloid plaques (Gambetti et al., 2008; Cannon et al., 2014). In VV cases, thioflavin S and FSB (*bis*-styrylbenzenes) staining procedures confirmed the presence of amyloid in many cerebellar miniplaques, while the cerebral

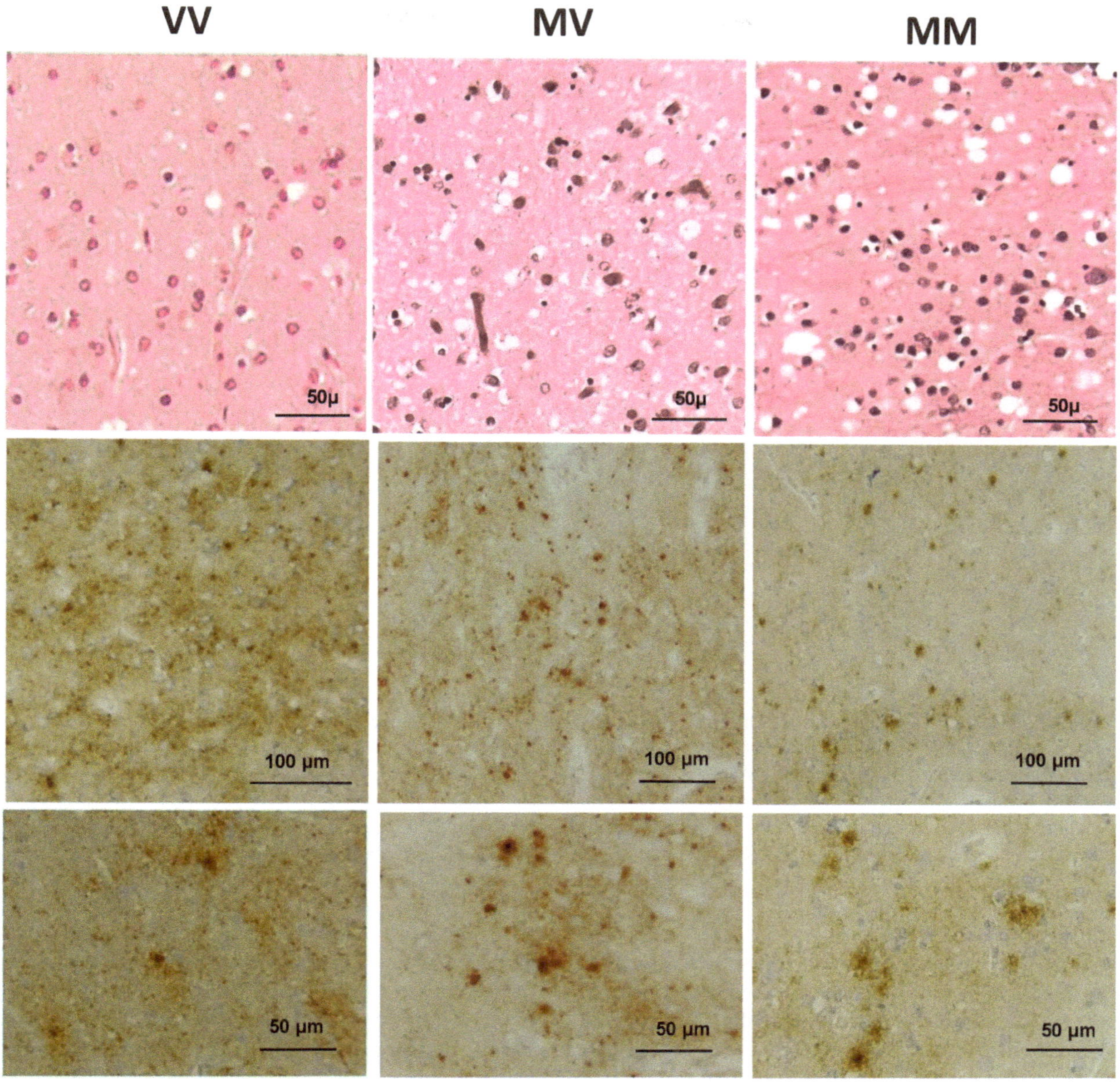

Fig. 10.1. Spongiform degeneration and prion protein (PrP) immunohistochemical pattern in the three genotypes of variably protease-sensitive prionopathy (VPSPr). Top row: mild to moderate spongiform degeneration in the three genotypes comprised of approximately 60% larger vacuoles than sporadic CJDMM1, the most common subtype of sporadic Creutzfeldt–Jakob disease. Middle and lower rows: PrP immunohistochemistry: fine granular deposits sometimes distributed in a tigroid pattern in VPSPr-129VV (VV, middle row); at higher magnification (lowest row) occasionally finer granules surround bigger ones in a target-like formation. Similar granular immunostaining in VPSPr-129MV but with less noticeable tigroid and target-like patterns (MV, middle and lowest rows). Plaque-like immunostaining in a fine granular background in VPSPr-129MM. Antibody to PrP 3F4. (Reproduced from Zou WQ, Puoti G, Xiao X, et al. (2010) Variably protease-sensitive prionopathy: a new sporadic disease of the prion protein. Ann Neurol 68: 162–172, with permission from John Wiley.)

neocortex remained seemingly negative (Flaherty et al., 2007; Puoti et al., unpublished data).

PrP immunostaining generally codistributes with SD and typically shows coarse granules in a background of a fine granular or "synaptic" pattern, often shaped as target-like formations with rounded clusters of granules surrounding a larger central one. A peculiar selective immune staining of the hippocampal molecular layer has also been noted in VV cases (Gambetti et al., 2008). In the cerebellum the pattern consists of small rounded deposits, which often show the tinctorial characteristics of real plaques and correspond to the

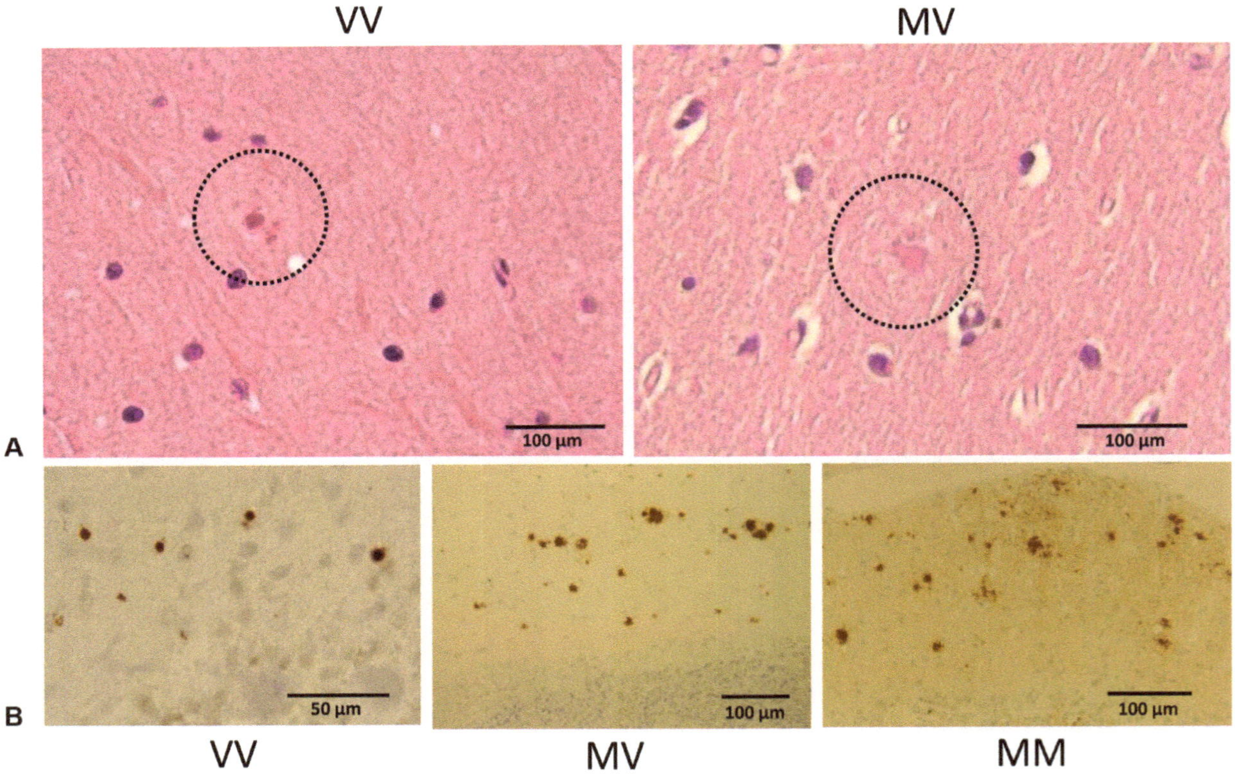

Fig. 10.2. Histopathology and prion protein (PrP) immunohistochemistry of the cerebellar molecular layer. (**A**) Miniplaques often with multiple cores in VPSPr-129VV and -129MV. (**B**) Miniplaques immunostain intensely as round, compact, and sharply bordered structures in the 129VV and 129MV VPSPr genotypes. To date cerebellar miniplaques have not been reported in VPSPr-129MM. In this condition PrP immunostaining of cerebellar molecular layer demonstrates more loose, plaque-like structures rather than plaque (**B**, MM). Antibody to PrP 3F4. (Reproduced from Zou WQ, Puoti G, Xiao X, et al. (2010) Variably protease-sensitive prionopathy: a new sporadic disease of the prion protein. Ann Neurol 68: 162–172, with permission from John Wiley.)

miniplaques described above in the cerebellar molecular layer. Other cerebellar regions are not immunostained. Miniplaques and plaque-like deposits are also seen in the dorsal parts of the midbrain (Gambetti et al., 2008).

Separating neuropathologic features of the individual subtypes of VPSPr according to the 129 genotype is challenging because the variations are not substantial and the MM and MV subtype cohorts are still relatively small. Overall, VV and MV cases seem to share more similarities between them than with the MM subtype. While all subtypes share similar SD distribution profiles and similar vacuole sizes, the severity appears to be comparably higher in the VV and MV subsets than in the MM (Fig. 10.1) (Zou et al., 2010). The immunostaining patterns in the cerebral cortex of the VV subset most often consist of the aforementioned target-like formations. This pattern seems to become less well organized and detectable in MV heterozygotes and is virtually lost in MM homozygotes, where the immunostaining pattern is primarily plaque-like (Fig. 10.1) (Giaccone et al., 2007; Rodríguez-Martínez et al., 2010; Zou et al., 2010; Head et al., 2013). Similarly, presence of PrP amyloid miniplaques, while well documented in VV and MV subsets, has not been reported in MM homozygotes (Zou et al., 2010; Head et al., 2013). Combined, these findings seem to outline a trend running from the 129VV to the 129MM subset toward the formation of PrP^{TSE} that shows an increasing propensity to aggregate and less to form amyloid. This trend would be inversely related to codon V dosage.

Another reported but little explored issue is the occurrence of co-pathologies in VPSPr. The majority of cases belonging to the three 129 genotypes harbor tau pathology preferentially in the lower medial temporal cortex, especially entorhinal and transitional cortices and hippocampal gyrus, which has been rated Braak stage 2 or higher, while the neocortex is minimally involved. Aβ plaques may also co-occur (Braak and Braak, 1995; Giaccone et al., 2007; Head et al., 2010; Rodríguez-Martínez et al., 2012). Ballooned neurons have been reported in two cases and pretangle formations have been observed in pigmented nuclei of one case (Giaccone et al., 2007; Rodriguez-Martinez et al., 2010; Cannon et al., 2014). Five cases harbored comorbidities of VPSPR and neurodegenerative diseases that included diffuse Lewy body disease (Head et al., 2010; Assar et al., 2015), argyrophilic grain disease (Giaccone et al., 2007; Rodríguez-Martínez et al., 2010), and amyotrophic lateral sclerosis (Cannon et al., 2014).

DISEASE-ASSOCIATED PRION PROTEIN

The PrP^{TSE} associated with VPSPr displays a panoply of peculiar features (Gambetti et al., 2008; Zou et al., 2010; Puoti et al., 2012). Following appropriate immunoblot procedures, PK-resistant PrP^{TSE} ($resPrP^{TSE}$) associated with VPSPr forms a distinctive ladder profile that comprises five or seven fragments (depending on the use of antibodies to the PrP N-terminus or to the C-terminus) (Fig. 10.3). The $resPrP^{TSE}$ fragments originate exclusively from the monoglycosylated and unglycosylated isoforms, which results in the lack of diglycosylated isoform in the $resPrP^{TSE}$ immunoblot profile even though this glycoform is present in the PK-untreated total PrP preparations (Gambetti et al., 2008; Zou et al., 2010).

The five PrP^{TSE} immunoblot bands demonstrated by N-terminus antibodies comprise fragments of 26, 23, 20, 17, and 7 kDa (Fig. 10.3) (Zou et al., 2010). Based on molecular weight and experiments with hydrofluoric acid to assess the presence of the glycolipid anchor, the five $resPrP^{TSE}$ fragments have been tentatively identified (Notari et al., 2008; Dagdanova et al., 2010; Notari et al., unpublished data). Fragments 26 and 20 kDa originate from the monoglycosylated and unglycosylated isoforms, following N-terminus truncation by PK treatment; the 23- and 17-kDa fragments are the anchorless counterpart of the above two fragments, and the 7 kDa is a fragment that lacks a large portion of both N-and C-termini and is unglycosylated (Fig. 10.3) (Zou et al., 2010; Pirisinu et al., 2013). These conclusions are consistent with the result of enzymatic deglycosylation, which, as expected, reduces the original five fragments to three: the 20-kDa unglycosylated fragment, its 17-kDa anchorless counterpart, and the 7-kDa internal fragment (Fig. 10.3) (Zou et al., 2010).

Antibodies to the PrP C-terminus demonstrate the presence of two additional bands: one with an electrophoretic mobility of 12–13 kDa that matches the CTF12/13, two C-terminal fragments described in all sCJD subtypes (Zou et al., 2003), and one migrating at 7 kDa. The latter, despite the similar molecular weight, must be quite different from the 7-kDa fragment detected by the N-terminal antibody and rather may be an additional C-terminal fragment extensively truncated at the N-terminus.

The peculiar lack of the PrP^{TSE} diglycosylated form has been shown to result from the presence of only the isoform monoglycosylated at residue 197 among the $resPrP^{TSE}$ fragments, while neither the isoform monoglycosylated at residue 181 nor the 181 and 197 diglycosylated isoform is converted to $resPrP^{TSE}$ (Xiao et al., 2013).

The N- and C-termini of the 7-kDa fragment have been characterized by epitope mapping (Pirisinu et al., 2013). The N-terminus appears ragged with alternative termini at residues 97, 99, and 103, while the C-terminus has been identified at residue 152. This amino acid sequence would predict a relative mass of 5–6 kDa. No similar data are available for the N-termini of the other fragments.

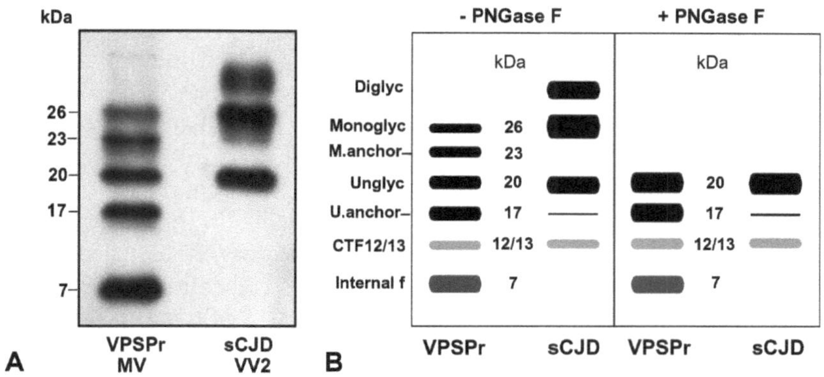

Fig. 10.3. Immunoblot of proteinase K-treated prion protein ($resPrP^{TSE}$) from VPSPr-129MV and sCJDVV2 subtype demonstrated by an N-terminus antibody and diagrammatic representation of all bands detected by antibodies to N- and C-terminus. (**A**) The immunoblot compares the five-band ladder profile formed by $resPrP^{TSE}$ associated with VPSPr with the three-band profile of a sporadic Creutzfeldt–Jakob disease subtype. Antibody 1E4. (**B**) In black: four fragments detected by antibodies to the N-terminus; In light gray: the fragment recognized by antibodies to C-terminus, the so-called CTF-12/13 (Zou et al., 2003); in deep gray: the two different fragments as for N- and C-terminus but comigrating 7-kDa fragments, one detected by antibodies to the N-terminus and the other by antibodies to C-terminus. Diglyc: diglycosylated isoform; Monoglyc: monoglycosylated; M.anchor- : presumed monoglycosylated anchorless; U.anchor- : presumed unglycosylated anchorless; Unglyc: unglycosylated.

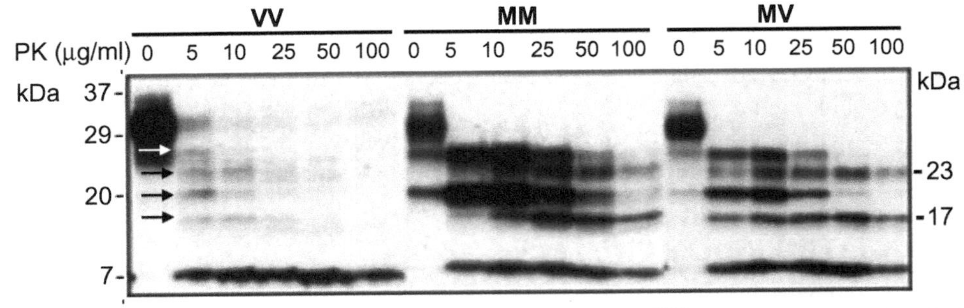

Fig. 10.4. Proteinase K (PK) titration of disease-associated prion protein (PrP^{TSE}) from VPSPr associated with the 129VV, 129MM, or 129MV genotype. Brain homogenates from 129VV, 129MM, and 129MV genotypes were treated with PK at various concentrations between 0 and 100 μg/mL and probed with 1E4. Overall, the PK resistance of the 7-kDa fragment is similarly high in all three VPSPr 129 genotypes. The other four fragments of the ladder (arrows) are definitely less PK-resistant in VPSPr-129VV than in the other two VPSPr genotypes. Besides the 7 kDa, three fragments (23, 20, and 17 kDa) in VPSPr-129MM and two (23 and 17 kDa) in -129MV are highly resistant to PK digestion. (Reproduced from Zou WQ, Puoti G, Xiao X, et al. (2010) Variably protease-sensitive prionopathy: a new sporadic disease of the prion protein. Ann Neurol 68: 162–172, with permission from John Wiley.)

Two other distinctive features of VPSPr PrP^{TSE} are amount and sensitivity to protease digestion. Analyses of the representation of total PrP^{TSE} (comprising both PK-sensitive and resistant components) carried out in VPSPr-VV have shown that total PrP^{TSE} accounts for approximately 3.5% of PrP preparations, including normal or cellular PrP (PrP^{C}) and PrP^{TSE}, about 16 times less than in the sCJDMM1 subtype (Gambetti et al., 2008). Furthermore, according to this study, 24% of the total PrP^{TSE} is PK-resistant, compared to nearly 90% in the sCJDMM1 subtype. These data explain the low amount of $resPrP^{TSE}$ in VPSPr (Gambetti et al., 2008). A compounding issue is that antibody 3F4, which is widely used to probe human PrP^{TSE} species, does not react well with some fragments of VPSPr-associated PrP^{TSE}, particularly in the VV subtype (Gambetti et al., 2008). As for the PK sensitivity of PrP^{TSE}, it is highest in the VV subtype and lower in subtypes MV and MM (Fig. 10.4). In fact, PK titration experiments showed that VPSPr MM and MV have a low PK sensitivity even compared with those of sCJD subtypes (Saverioni et al., 2013). However, PK sensitivity also varies among the five $resPrP^{TSE}$ fragments recognized by antibodies to the N-terminus. The 7-kDa fragment is the most PK-resistant across the three subtypes; it is the only highly PK-resistant fragment in VPSPr VV while two more fragments, 23 kDa and 17 kDa, show significant and similar PK resistance in the MV and MM subtypes (Fig. 10.4) (Zou et al., 2010). Notably, all these three fragments are anchorless.

Several tests performed to assess the conformational characteristics of VPSPr total PrP^{TSE} have underlined divergences with PrP^{TSE} species associated with sCJD subtypes (Gambetti et al., 2008; Pirisinu et al., 2013; Saverioni et al., 2013; Cali et al., unpublished data). First, sedimentation in sucrose gradients and fractionation by gel filtration, both of which separate PrP^{TSE} aggregates according to size (Rhodes et al., 2009), have shown that VPSPr PrP^{TSE} forms far fewer large aggregates than the PrP^{TSE} of sCJDVV1 (30% vs. 58% of total PrP^{TSE}), with few aggregates exceeding 2000 kDa. Similar data have been obtained by Saverioni and colleagues (2013) in a study comparing VPSPr with other sCJD. However, VPSPr data differ much less from those of Gerstmann–Sträussler–Scheinker (GSS) subtype carrying the A117V PrP gene mutation (GSS^{A117V}) (Gambetti et al., 2008). Moreover, the banding pattern formed on immunoblot by PrP^{TSE} collected from the fractions that contain large aggregates differed in VPSPr from that of sCJDVV1 (the sCJD subtype used in this comparative study) and, to a lesser extent, from that of GSS^{A117V}.

Second, PrP^{TSE} conformational stability has been tested with the conformational stability and solubility assay, which derives stability data by measuring the amount of the denaturing agent guanidine hydrochloride needed to solubilize 50% of native total PrP^{TSE} ($GdnHCL_{1/2}$) (Pirisinu et al., 2013). The conformational stability and solubility assay has demonstrated that PrP^{TSE} conformational stability is higher in VPSPr VV ($GdnHCL_{1/2}$ 2.18) than in the VPSPr MV and MM subtypes that have similar $GdnHCL_{1/2}$ values (1.63 and 1.67, respectively) (Pirisinu et al., 2013). Similar results have been obtained with the comparable conformational stability assay (Peretz et al., 2001; Cali et al., 2009; Cali et al., unpublished data).

The properties of the $resPrP^{TSE}$ associated with VPSPr invite two considerations. First, the lack of the 181 glycoform in VPSPr $resPrP^{TSE}$ is likely due to the incompetence of the normal 181 glycoform to adopt the $resPrP^{TSE}$ conformation characteristics of VPSPr and, therefore, to acquire PK resistance. Alternatively, it has been suggested that the 181 glycan is anomalous and hinders the conversion of the 181 glycoform to $resPrP^{TSE}$ (Nishina et al., 2006; Xiao et al., 2013). Second, the presence of both anchor-linked and anchorless conformers of the mono- and unglycosylated isoforms (fragments 26 and 23, as well as 20 and 17 kDa, respectively) exemplifies the remarkable heterogeneity of PrP^{TSE} in VPSPr, which must reflect multiple conformations. As a result of this heterogeneity, a fraction of these two isoforms is PK-resistant at the C-terminus while the other is not and becomes anchorless. Furthermore, the size of the C-terminus region that remains PK-sensitive in the two anchorless fragments differs from that of the 7-kDa fragment. Based on the relative mass and detectability with the antibody to the C-terminus, the PK-sensitive C-terminal region of the 23- and 17-kDa anchorless fragments must be small once the mass reduction due to loss of the anchor is taken into account. In contrast, according to epitope mapping data, the 7-kDa fragment is generated by PK digestion of nearly 80 C-terminus residues.

Finally, the original report of VPSPr also described the limited presence of the three-band $resPrP^{TSE}$ isoform with a $resPrP^{TSE}$ type 1 electrophoretic mobility that is typically associated with subtypes of sCJD (Gambetti et al., 2008). Significant to minimal amounts of three-band $resPrP^{TSE}$ were detected in putamen, thalamus, and substantia nigra of three out of eight cases tested (Gambetti et al., 2008). This finding indicates that the three-band $resPrP^{TSE}$ characteristic of sCJD may occasionally occur in subcortical regions of VPSPr subjects. More recently, Peden et al. (2014) and Rodríguez-Martínez et al. (2012) and their colleagues have reported the presence of sCJD $resPrP^{TSE}$ in the cerebellum of three cases of VPSPr VV. In the latter report, sCJD $resPrP^{TSE}$ was type 2, but the PrP immunostaining pattern of the cerebellum was apparently consistent with VPSPr rather than sCJDVV2, as would be expected by the presence of $resPrP^{TSE}$ type 2 in a subject harboring the VV genotype.

All of these features, but especially the number and heterogeneity of the $resPrP^{TSE}$ fragments that imply distinct conformations, currently establish $resPrP^{TSE}$ associated with VPSPr as a unique $resPrP^{TSE}$ isoform or strain among sporadic human prion diseases.

EXPERIMENTAL TRANSMISSION AND IN VITRO AMPLIFICATION

Experimental transmission

VPSPr has been experimentally transmitted to transgenic (Tg) mice in two concurrent studies (Diack et al., 2014; Notari et al., 2014a). Notari and colleagues (2014a) inoculated four lines of Tg mice expressing PrP^{C} with 129 residues M or V at levels ranging from one- to eight-fold normal human brain levels on a murine PrP^{C} null background. Brain homogenates (BH) from 12 VPSPr subjects that comprised six VV, four MV, and two MM subtypes were used as inocula. Mice of the same lines served as negative and positive controls. None of the 112 mice challenged with VPSPr BH developed clinical signs. 54% of the mice challenged with matching (i.e., having the same M or V genotype) BH from VPSPr VV or MM, showed histologic lesions that immunoreacted with PrP antibodies and 34% had positive immunoblots, further confirming the presence of PrP^{TSE} (Fig. 10.5). There appeared to be no significant variation in attack rate between high (8 ×) and intermediate (3 ×) PrP expression mice. Five of six VPSPr VV BH and one of two MM BH inoculated into 129 matching mice transmitted the disease. The non-transmissible MM BH was from a clinically asymptomatic subject diagnosed at autopsy.

No transmission occurred when the 129 genotype was mismatched (i.e., BH VV was inoculated to 129M or MM into 129V mice). Surprisingly, there was also no transmission when BH MV was inoculated to 129V or 129M mice. These findings clearly point to an amino acid sequence barrier introduced by the M129V polymorphism.

Histologic lesions of two types were observed. The first featured poorly structured and often clustered plaques, most often located at the border of the hippocampus and the overlying white matter, and occasionally in periventricular regions (Fig. 10.5). Plaques appeared to be more prevalent in mice expressing PrP^{C} 8 fold than 3 fold and to be more compact and better formed following inoculation with BH from VPSPr VV than MM (Fig. 10.5). The lesion of the second type consisted of focal SD located in the lacunosum-moleculare layer of the hippocampal formation (Fig. 10.5). Both plaques and SD areas were intensely reactive with PrP antibodies. Widespread PrP deposition was not detected in any of the mice challenged with any VPSPr BH. Immunoblot demonstrated small amounts of $resPrP^{TSE}$ forming a ladder resembling (Fig. 10.6), but apparently more PK-resistant than that associated with VPSPr, which was exclusively observed in the 8 × PrP expression 129V Tg mice. Deglycosylation reduced the bands to three that matched the electrophoretic mobility of the corresponding VPSPr bands (Fig. 10.6). No PrP^{TSE} was recovered in negative controls while all sCJD subtypes transmitted to positive controls with efficiency comparable to that reported in other studies. Surprisingly, none of the positive mice transmitted the disease on second passage.

Very similar results were obtained by Diack and coworkers (2014), following inoculation of BH from

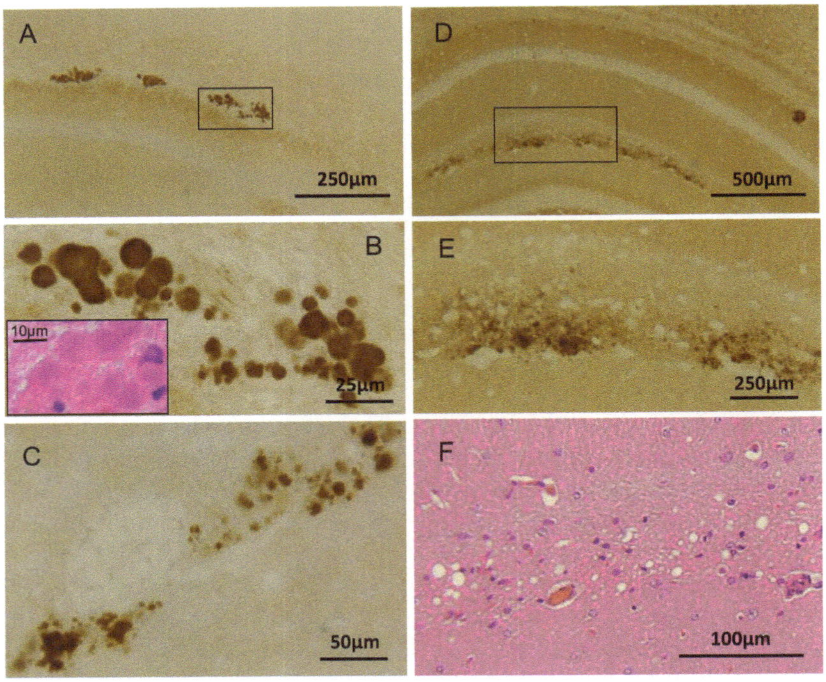

Fig. 10.5. Immunohistochemistry and histopathology brain lesions in Tg mice inoculated with variably protease-sensitive prionopathy (VPSPr) extracts. (**A**) Clusters of prion plaques typically observed at the border of hippocampus and overlying white matter (Tg(HuPrP129V)×8); box marks area shown in (**B**). (**B**) At higher magnification, plaques appear often confluent or fragmented and are intensely prion protein (PrP)-immunoreactive; at hematoxylin and eosin stain, plaques show an amorphous core lacking the spiny appearance of typical kuru plaques (inset). (**C**) In (Tg(HuPrP129M)×2) mice inoculated with VPSPr-129MM, PrP aggregates generally appear looser and form fewer well-bounded plaques. (**D–F**) Second type of lesion consisting of PrP granular deposits in the lacunosum-moleculare layer of the hippocampal formation (**D** and **E**) that codistribute with spongiform degeneration (**F**) (box in **D** marks area shown in **E**). Antibody 3F4. (Reproduced from Notari S, Xiao X, Espinosa JC, et al. (2014a) Transmission characteristics of variably protease-sensitive prionopathy. Emerg Infect Dis 20: 2006–2014.)

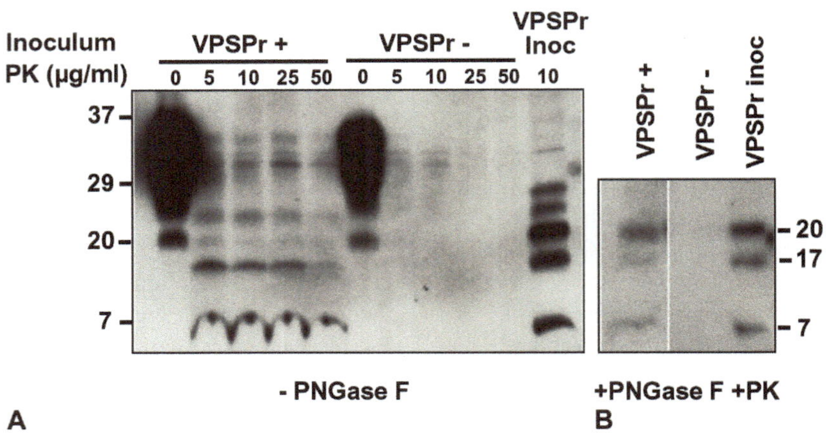

Fig. 10.6. Immunoblot of abnormal prion protein (PrP^{TSE}) recovered from brains of variably protease-sensitive prionopathy (VPSPr)-inoculated Tg mice and controls. (**A**) Extract from brains of VPSPr-inoculated mice (VPSPr+), treated with increasing amounts of proteinase K (PK) show PK-resistant PrP^{TSE} ($resPrP^{TSE}$) fragments with a ladder-like electrophoretic profile even at high concentrations of PK (50 µg/mL). Nonspecific bands are seen in negative control mice (VPSPr–). The banding pattern in VPSPr+ roughly recapitulates that of $resPrP^{TSE}$ from the VPSPr inoculum (VPSPr Inoc). (**B**) VPSPr+ extracts treated with PK (25 µg/mL) and PNGase F show three $resPrP^{TSE}$ bands migrating at ~20 kDa, ~17 kDa, and ~7 kDa that replicate those of similarly treated VPSPr inoculum (VPSPr Inoc). No bands can be detected in the negative Tg mice (VPSPr–). All preparations were run on the same gel, but unnecessary lanes were removed. Antibody 1E4. (Reproduced from Notari S, Xiao X, Espinosa JC, et al. (2014a) Transmission characteristics of variably protease-sensitive prionopathy. Emerg Infect Dis 20: 2006–2014.)

two subjects with VPSPr-VV and one with VPSPr-MV to Tg mice that were produced by gene targeting and expressed human PrP MM, MV and VV at physiologic levels. Transmission succeeded only with VPSPr-VV. Challenge of Tg mice with BH mismatched for the 129 residue also seems to support the presence of a primary structure barrier, as in the study of Notari and colleagues (2014a), although perhaps not as strict, since VPSPr VV was transmitted to 129M Tg mice, albeit to only one of 15 inoculated mice. Histologic lesions and patterns of PrP deposition were virtually identical, although lesions apparently were less frequent, presumably due to the lower PrP expression levels of the mice used in this study. Plaques were shown to contain amyloid by thioflavin S staining. No PrP^{TSE} was demonstrated by immunoblot analyses. No data were reported on second passage.

Both studies prompt several considerations. VPSPr MV failed to transmit and at present remains the only VPSPr subtype with no evidence of transmission. The lack of clinical signs in PrP^{TSE}-positive mice is likely due to the focality of the lesions and their location in relatively silent brain regions. Prion plaques similar in type and location to those described in these two studies have been observed previously in Tg and wild-type mice challenged with human BH or in vitro preparations that share the property of harboring plaques or seeding plaque formation (Piccardo et al., 2007; Asante et al., 2013; Pirisinu et al., 2016). The failure to transmit the disease upon second passage is puzzling but not unprecedented (Wadsworth et al., 2004; Piccardo et al., 2007, 2013). Based on the low amount of $resPrP^{TSE}$ in VPSPr, which indicates a low conversion efficiency, it has been proposed that due to limited amplification and propagation of the seed at first passage, along with the relative short lifespan of the mouse, the actual $resPrP^{TSE}$ concentration in the whole brain of the inoculated mouse is lower than that of the inoculum (Notari et al., 2014a). Furthermore, the failure of the second passage also suggests that there is no significant adaptation of the seed to the host during the first passage in VPSPr transmission despite the long incubation. Future studies of VPSPr transmission to more receptive hosts, such as the bank vole (Nonno et al., 2012), as well as experiments of PrP^{TSE} rescue from brains of mice used in these two studies may clarify this issue.

Nonetheless, both these studies definitively establish that VPSPr is a transmissible prion disease and further highlight the unique properties of VPSPr PrP^{TSE} among sporadic prion diseases.

In vitro amplification

The propensity of VPSPr PrP^{TSE} to convert PrP^{C} to its misfolded form was analyzed with protein misfolding cyclic amplification (PMCA) by two groups. Successful, albeit weak, amplification of VPSPr-VV PrP^{TSE} has been reported by Peden et al. (2014), using two kinds of substrate: "human PrP expressing Tg mice" and human brain. The stronger amplification was obtained with Tg mice as substrate. Additionally, in this study, a PrP^{TSE} species, described as similar to the sCJD type 2 and found in the cerebellum of two VV cases, was positively amplified with PMCA. Notari and coworkers, in a preliminary study (Gambetti et al., 2012; Notari et al., 2014b), succeeded in amplifying VPSPr PrP^{TSE} using human PrP^{C} from different Tg mice as substrate. The highest amplification was obtained using PrP^{C} 129V from Tg152 mice expressing four to eight times normal levels of PrP^{C} as substrate (Telling et al., 1995). With Tg mice expressing PrP129M or 129V at the same lower level ($2\times$) (Kong et al., 2005 and unpublished data), amplification was sensitive to the M129V polymorphism and occurred only when 129 residues matched; however these mice supported a less robust amplification. Following PK treatment, the amplified $resPrP^{TSE}$ reproduced the same electrophoretic ladder-like profile as the seed (Gambetti et al., 2012; Notari et al., 2014b).

Peden et al. (2014) also demonstrated the capacity of VPSPr to convert recPrP to its misfolded form by real-time quaking-induced conversion (RT-QuIC), another amplification technique.

These studies definitively establish the propensity of VPSPr to replicate in vitro.

ANIMAL MODELS

It has recently been found that $resPrP^{TSE}$ associated with in a familial form of CJD harboring the V180I PrP gene mutation ($fCJD^{V180I}$) displays an electrophoretic profile and antibody immunoreactivity that mimic those of VPSPr (Fig. 10.7) (Xiao et al., 2013). The electrophoretic profile, when probed with N-terminus antibodies, includes five bands that co-migrate with those of VPSPr, although show some difference in the ratios. Remarkably, as in VPSPr, both monoglycosylated at residue 181 and diglycosylated isoforms fail to convert to $resPrP^{TSE}$; thus, of the three glycoforms only the 197 monoglycosylated is converted even though total PrP from $fCJD^{V180I}$ contains both monoglycosylated and diglycosylated isoforms like VPSPr. The virtually identical mobility of the five bands supports the notion that the $resPrP^{TSE}$ fragments have common properties in the two diseases, and therefore anchorless fragments may also be present in $fCJD^{V180I}$. These striking similarities indicate that the $resPrP^{TSE}$ isoforms associated with VPSPr and $fCJD^{V180I}$ share similar conformations in spite of the different etiologies of the two diseases (genetic in $fCJD^{V180}$, sporadic in VPSPr). Because it is

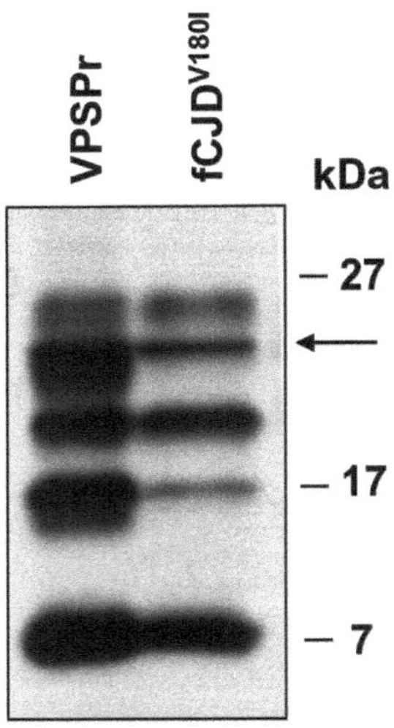

Fig. 10.7. Immunoblot of proteinase K-resistant prion protein from variably protease-sensitive prionopathy (VPSPr) and V180I brain extracts. The electrophoretic mobility of the individual bands is very similar, consistent with similar primary structure. Representation of at least two bands, monoglycosylated and unglycosylated anchorless (arrow and 17 kDa), is noticeably different. Antibody1E4.

a genetic disease, fCJD^{V180I} would lend itself better to the study of pathogenetic mechanisms and might be a valid model to shed light on VPSPr.

CONSIDERATIONS ON ETIOLOGY AND PATHOGENESIS

Because VPSPr is rare, has been identified recently, and is associated with a particularly complex PrP^{TSE} isoform, it is especially challenging to speculate on its etiology and pathogenesis. According to the current hypothesis of multiple strain formation and competitive selection of the most efficient strain (Surewicz and Apostol, 2011; Weissman et al., 2011; Gambetti, 2013), VPSPr-associated PrP^{TSE} might result from the aberrant selection of an incompetent strain. This hypothesis would be consistent with rarity, as well as inefficient conversion and propagation of the PrP^{TSE} associated with VPSPr. The selection of the VPSPr PrP^{TSE} is likely to be strongly favored by 129V allele dosage, since VV homozygotes account for 65% of all affected subjects, despite the 12% frequency of this genotype in a normal Caucasian population (Zimmermann et al., 1999). This distribution is different from that of sCJD, where MM subjects account for 68% of cases and the VV for 16% (Collins et al., 2006). This divergence implies distinct roles for the 129 genotypes in the two diseases.

VPSPr-affected subjects frequently have a positive family history that cannot be ignored. Cognitive impairment with prevalence as high as 60% has been reported in the original cohort of 11 VPSPr VV patients (Gambetti et al., 2008). Two additional VV patients had a family history of a condition similar to amyotrophic lateral sclerosis (or amyotrophic lateral sclerosis was a comorbidity (Jansen et al., 2010; Cannon et al., 2014). Since no mutation has been detected in the coding region of the PrP gene in any of VPSPr-affected subjects, the presence of a variation involving other regions of the PrP gene or other parts of the genome needs to be investigated to assess the role of a genetic component in VPSPr.

VPSPr-associated PrP^{TSE} also has unique features, including the inability to acquire resistance to proteases by the PrP glycosylated at residue 181, regardless of whether it is the mono- or diglycosylated isoform, and by part of the C-terminus. Furthermore, data from experimental transmission also indicate that, compared to most subtypes of sCJD, conversion of the host PrP^{C} and propagation of newly formed PrP^{TSE} are slow and very limited. These features need to be clarified to begin understanding the pathogenetic mechanisms that underlie VPSPr.

REFERENCES

Appleby BS, Appleby KK, Crain BJ et al. (2009). Characteristics of established and proposed sporadic Creutzfeldt–Jakob disease variants. Arch Neurol 66: 208–215.

Appleby BS, Rincon-Beardsley TD, Appleby KK et al. (2014). Initial diagnoses of patients ultimately diagnosed with prion disease. J Alzheimers Dis 42: 833–839.

Asante EA, Linehan JM, Smidak M et al. (2013). Inherited prion disease A117V is not simply a proteinopathy but produces prions transmissible to transgenic mice expressing homologous prion protein. PLoS Pathog 9: e1003643.

Assar H, Topakian R, Weis S et al. (2015). A case of variably protease-sensitive prionopathy treated with doxycycline. J Neurol Neurosurg Psychiatry 86: 816–818.

Braak H, Braak E (1995). Staging of Alzheimer's disease-related neurofibrillary changes. Neurobiol Aging 16: 271–278.

Cali I, Castellani R, Alshekhlee A et al. (2009). Co-existence of scrapie prion protein types 1 and 2 in sporadic Creutzfeldt–Jakob disease: its effect on the phenotype and prion-type characteristics. Brain 132: 2643–2658.

Cannon A, Bieniek KF, Lin WL et al. (2014). Concurrent variably protease-sensitive prionopathy and amyotrophic lateral sclerosis. Acta Neuropathol 128: 313–315.

Collins SJ, Sanchez-Juan P, Masters CL et al. (2006). Determinants of diagnostic investigation sensitivities across the clinical spectrum of sporadic Creutzfeldt–Jakob disease. Brain 129: 2278–2287.

Dagdanova A, Ilchenko S, Notari S et al. (2010). Characterization of prion protein in human urine. J Biol Chem 285: 30489–30495.

Diack AB, Ritchie DL, Peden AH et al. (2014). Variably protease-sensitive prionopathy, a unique prion variant with inefficient transmission properties. Emerg Infect Dis 20: 1969–1979.

Flaherty DP, Walsh SM, Kiyota T et al. (2007). Polyfluorinated bis-styrylbenzene beta-amyloid plaque binding ligands. J Med Chem 50: 4986–4992.

Franceschini A, Baiardi S, Hughson AG et al. (2017). High diagnostic value of second generation CSF RT-QuIC across the wide spectrum of CJD prions. Sci Rep 7: 10655.

Gambetti P (2013). Creationism and evolutionism in prions. Am J Pathol 182: 623–627.

Gambetti P, Kong Q, Zou W et al. (2003). Sporadic and familial CJD: classification and characterization. Br Med Bull 66: 213–239.

Gambetti P, Dong Z, Yuan J et al. (2008). A novel human disease with abnormal prion protein sensitive to protease. Ann Neurol 63: 697–708.

Gambetti P, Cali I, Notari S et al. (2011). Molecular biology and pathology of prion strains in sporadic human prion diseases. Acta Neuropathol 121: 79–90.

Gambetti P, Notari S, Cracco L et al. (2012). Prion strains in human prion diseases - variably protease-sensitive prionopathy compared with other sporadic prion diseases. Conference Prion 2014. Prion 6 (S): 17.

Ghoshal N, Perry A, McKeel D et al. (2015). Variably protease-sensitive prionopathy in an apparent cognitively normal 93-year-old. Alzheimer Dis Assoc Disord 29: 173–176.

Giaccone G, Di Fede G, Mangieri M et al. (2007). A novel phenotype of sporadic Creutzfeldt–Jakob disease. J Neurol Neurosurg Psychiatry 78: 1379–1382.

Head MW, Knight R, Zeidler M et al. (2009). A case of protease sensitive prionopathy in a patient in the UK. Neuropathol Appl Neurobiol 35: 628–632.

Head MW, Lowrie S, Chohan G et al. (2010). Variably protease-sensitive prionopathy in a PRNP codon 129 heterozygous UK patient with co-existing tau, α synuclein and Aβ pathology. Acta Neuropathol 120: 821–823.

Head MW, Yull HM, Ritchie DL et al. (2013). Variably protease-sensitive prionopathy in the UK: a retrospective review 1991-2008. Brain 136: 1102–1115.

Jansen C, Head MW, van Gool WA et al. (2010). The first case of protease-sensitive prionopathy (PSPr) in The Netherlands: a patient with an unusual GSS-like clinical phenotype. J Neurol Neurosurg Psychiatry 81: 1052–1055.

Kong Q, Surewicz WK, Petersen RB et al. (2004). Inherited prion diseases. In: SB Prusiner (Ed.), Prion biology and diseases, Cold Spring Harbor Laboratory Press, New York, pp. 673–775.

Kong Q, Huang S, Zou W et al. (2005). Chronic wasting disease of elk: transmissibility to humans examined by transgenic mouse models. J Neurosci 25: 7944–7949.

Krebs B, Bader B, Klehmet J et al. (2007). A novel subtype of Creutzfeldt–Jakob disease characterized by a small 6 kDa PrP fragment. Acta Neuropathol 114: 195–199.

Lattanzio F, Abu-Rumeileh S, Franceschini A et al. (2017). Prion-specific and surrogate CSF biomarkers in Creutzfeldt–Jakob disease: diagnostic accuracy in relation to molecular subtypes and analysis of neuropathological correlates of p-tau and Aβ42 levels. Acta Neuropathol 133: 559–578.

Nishina KA, Deleault NR, Mahal SP et al. (2006). The stoichiometry of host PrPC glycoforms modulates the efficiency of PrPSc formation in vitro. Biochemistry 45: 14129–14139.

Nonno R, Di Bari M, Pirisinu L et al. (2012). Variably protease-sensitive prionopathy is transmissible in bank voles. Conference Prion 2012. Prion 6 (S): 6–7.

Notari S, Strammiello R, Capellari S et al. (2008). Characterization of novel truncated forms of abnormal prion protein in Creutzfeldt–Jakob disease. J Biol Chem 283: 30557–30565.

Notari S, Xiao X, Espinosa JC et al. (2014a). Transmission characteristics of variably protease-sensitive prionopathy. Emerg Infect Dis 20: 2006–2014.

Notari S, Qing L, Kong Q et al. (2014b). New studies on the characteristics of VPSPr: PrPSc and PrPC. Conference Prion 2014. Prion 8 (S): 132.

Parchi P, Giese A, Capellari S et al. (1999). Classification of sporadic Creutzfeldt–Jakob disease based on molecular and phenotypic analysis of 300 subjects. Ann Neurol 46: 224–233.

Peden AH, Sarode DP, Mulholland CR et al. (2014). The prion protein protease sensitivity, stability and seeding activity in variably protease sensitive prionopathy brain tissue suggests molecular overlaps with sporadic Creutzfeldt–Jakob disease. Acta Neuropathol Commun 2: 152.

Peretz D, Scott MR, Groth D et al. (2001). Strain-specified relative conformational stability of the scrapie prion protein. Protein 10: 854–863.

Piccardo P, Manson JC, King D et al. (2007). Accumulation of prion protein in the brain that is not associated with transmissible disease. Proc Natl Acad Sci U S A 104: 4712–4717.

Piccardo P, King D, Telling G et al. (2013). Manson JC, Barron RM. Dissociation of prion protein amyloid seeding from transmission of a spongiform encephalopathy. J Virol 87: 12349–12356.

Pirisinu L, Di Bari MA, D'Agostino C et al. (2016). Gerstmann-Sträussler-Scheinker disease subtypes efficiently transmit in bank voles as genuine prion diseases. Sci Rep 6: 20443.

Pirisinu L, Nonno R, Esposito E et al. (2013). Small ruminant nor98 prions share biochemical features with human Gerstmann-Sträussler-Scheinker disease and variably protease-sensitive prionopathy. PLoS One 8 (6): e66405.

Puoti G, Bizzi A, Forloni G et al. (2012). Sporadic human prion diseases: molecular insights and diagnosis. Lancet Neurol 11: 618–628.

Rhodes DG, Bossio RE, Laue TM (2009). Determination of size, molecular weight, and presence of subunits. Methods Enzymol 463: 691–723.

Rodríguez-Martínez AB, Garrido JM, Zarranz JJ et al. (2010). A novel form of human disease with a protease-sensitive prion protein and heterozygosity methionine/valine at codon 129: Case report. BMC Neurol 10: 99.

Rodríguez-Martínez AB, López de Munain A, Ferrer I et al. (2012). Coexistence of protease sensitive and resistant prion protein in 129VV homozygous sporadic Creutzfeldt–Jakob disease: a case report. J Med Case Rep 6: 348.

Saverioni D, Notari S, Capellari S et al. (2013). Analyses of protease resistance and aggregation state of abnormal prion protein across the spectrum of human prions. J Biol Chem 288: 27972–27985.

Surewicz WK, Apostol MI (2011). Prion protein and its conformational conversion: a structural perspective. Top Curr Chem 305: 135–167.

Telling GC, Scott M, Mastrianni J et al. (1995). Prion propagation in mice expressing human and chimeric PrP transgenes implicates the interaction of cellular PrP with another protein. Cell 83: 79–90.

UK National CJD Research and Surveillance Unit (NCJDRSU) (2017). Creutzfeldt–Jakob disease in the UK (by calendar year), January 9 2017. Available online at http://www.cjd.ed.ac.uk/sites/default/files/figs050117.pdf. Accessed 11 May 2017.

US National Prion Disease Pathology Surveillance Center (NPDPSC) (2017). National Prion Disease Pathology Surveillance Center cases examined, February 17, 2017. Available online at http://case.edu/med/pathology/centers/npdpsc/. Accessed 11 May 2017.

Wadsworth JD, Asante EA, Desbruslais M et al. (2004). Human prion protein with valine 129 prevents expression of variant CJD phenotype. Science 306: 1793–1796.

Weissmann C, Li J, Mahal SP et al. (2011). Prions on the move. EMBO Rep 12: 1109–1117.

World Health Organization (1998). Global surveillance, diagnosis and therapy of human transmissible spongiform encephalopathies: report of a WHO consultation, World Health Organization, Geneva.

Xiao X, Yuan J, Haïk S et al. (2013). Glycoform-selective prion formation in sporadic and familial forms of prion disease. PLoS One 8 (3): e58786.

Zerr I, Kallenberg K, Summers DM et al. (2009). Updated clinical diagnostic criteria for sporadic Creutzfeldt Jakob disease. Brain 132: 2659–2668.

Zimmermann K, Turecek PL, Schwarz HP (1999). Genotyping of the prion protein gene at codon 129. Acta Neuropathol 97: 355–358.

Zou WQ, Capellari S, Parchi P et al. (2003). Identification of novel proteinase K-resistant C-terminal fragments of PrP in Creutzfeldt–Jakob disease. J Biol Chem 278: 40429–40436.

Zou WQ, Puoti G, Xiao X et al. (2010). Variably protease-sensitive prionopathy: a new sporadic disease of the prion protein. Ann Neurol 68: 162–172.

Handbook of Clinical Neurology, Vol. 153 (3rd series)
Human Prion Diseases
M. Pocchiari and J. Manson, Editors
https://doi.org/10.1016/B978-0-444-63945-5.00011-8

Chapter 11

Variant Creutzfeldt–Jakob disease

JEAN-PHILIPPE BRANDEL[1] AND RICHARD KNIGHT[2]*

[1]*Cellule nationale de référence des MCJ, Hôpital de la Salpêtrière, Paris, France*

[2]*National CJD Research and Surveillance Unit, Centre for Clinical Brain Sciences, University of Edinburgh, United Kingdom*

Abstract

Variant CJD (vCJD) was described first in the United Kingdom in 1996. It is a zoonotic form of human prion disease, originating from dietary contamination of human food with material from bovine spongiform encephalopathy (BSE)-affected cattle. It has important epidemiologic, clinical, and neuropathogic differences from other forms of human prion disease. Cases have occurred in several countries but the United Kingdom and France have been most affected. Following the decline in BSE in cattle and the dietary protective measures adopted, vCJD has become an extremely rare disease. However, important concerns remain about asymptomatic infection in human populations (especially the United Kingdom) and the possibility of human-to-human transmission via medical and surgical interventions. Definitive diagnosis depends on neuropathology, usually undertaken at autopsy, but sometimes on brain biopsy. Clinical diagnosis with a reasonable degree of likelihood is, however, possible based on the clinical features and the finding of the pulvinar sign on cerebral magnetic resonance. There are also emerging tests (including blood tests) that have promising sensitivity and specificity for vCJD. It is a progressive illness, inevitably fatal with no curative treatment.

EPIDEMIOLOG ASPECTS

From bovine spongiform encephalopathy to new variant of Creutzfeldt–Jakob disease

In 1985, a new transmissible spongiform encephalopathy (TSE), named bovine spongiform encephalopathy (BSE), was recognized in the United Kingdom (Wells et al., 1987). Pathologic examination of the brain of affected animals and inoculation of brain homogenate samples to mice confirmed that this new zoonotic disease was due to a single agent (Fraser et al., 1992). The occurrence of an encephalopathy in domestic cats in 1990 (Aldhous, 1990) and in Bovidae (nyala, greater kudu, Arabian oryx) and Felidae (cheetah, puma, ocelot) in captivity in zoos gave arguments for transmission of the agent of BSE to other species with a rupture of the species barrier and the possibility of passage to humans (Cunningham et al., 2004).

Active surveillance on human TSE was then activated in different areas in Europe and a group of countries historically concerned with Creutzfeldt–Jakob disease (CJD), EuroCJD, was created in 1992. The countries belonging to EuroCJD were Austria, France, Germany, Italy, the Netherlands, Slovakia, and the United Kingdom. The group held meetings twice a year with the aim of comparing incidences of the different forms of CJD and detecting any possible increase or emergence of novel forms. No increase in incidence was observed but, in 1995, two cases of abnormally young patients affected with CJD were reported in the United Kingdom (Bateman et al., 1995; Britton et al., 1995). The patients were two teenagers, one male and one female, of respectively 18 and 16 years old with no specific risk factor for CJD (no familial history, no mutation or insertion on the prion protein gene (*PRNP* gene) and no known risk factor for iatrogenic CJD).

*Correspondence to: Richard Knight, BA, BM BCh, FRCP(E), Centre for Clinical Brain Sciences, Chancellor's Building, Royal Infirmary of Edinburgh, 47 Little France Crescent, Edinburgh, Scotland EH16 4TJ, United Kingdom. Tel: +44-131-537-3104, E-mail: r.knight@ed.ac.uk

The increased number of CJD cases in young patients, with atypical clinical symptoms compared to sporadic CJD (sCJD), only in the United Kingdom, the most affected country with BSE, led to the announcement of the new variant of CJD (vCJD) in British Parliament on March 20th, 1996 and the beginning of the “first mad cow crisis” (the unfortunate term “mad cow disease” was coined by journalists and is disliked generally by those affected personally by the disease).

The clinical and neuropathologic data of the 10 first patients with vCJD were published in April 1996 by the five countries of the EuroCJD group using similar methodology as in epidemiologic studies (Will et al., 1996). Shortly after, a case of vCJD was reported in France (Chazot et al., 1996). Beyond the strong epidemiologic argument – occurrence of a new human TSE in the most affected country by BSE – the link between BSE and vCJD was enhanced by biologic arguments: (1) observation, in the brains of macaques intracerebrally inoculated with the agent of BSE, of florid plaques, neuropathologic stigma of vCJD (Lasmezas et al., 1996); (2) identical migration on Western blot (type 4 or 2B) of disease-related prion protein from vCJD and BSE cases (Collinge et al., 1996); and (3) the same duration of incubation and identical histologic profile in mice inoculated with homogenates of brains of patients dead from vCJD and cattle affected with BSE in favor of a unique strain responsible for both diseases (Bruce et al., 1997). The definitive proof that the same strain of prion was the origin of BSE and vCJD came later when it was observed that the transmission characteristics to wild-type mice from brain or lymphoreticular tissues of 10 vCJD or BSE were similar (Ritchie et al., 2009).

Increasing primary cases of vCJD in the United Kingdom and in other countries

From 1996 to the end of 2016, the number of vCJD cases increased in the United Kingdom and worldwide to reach a total of 231 at the end of 2016 (http://www.cjd.ac.uk/data.html). The United Kingdom remains the most affected country with a total of 178 cases, followed by France (27 cases), Spain (5 cases), Ireland and the United States (4 cases), Italy and the Netherlands (3 cases), Canada and Portugal (2 cases), and Japan, Saudi Arabia, and Taiwan (1 case). It was decided, as a rule, that the case was classified as belonging to the country of residence at the time of diagnosis and not necessarily to the country where the BSE exposure was most likely to have occurred. After epidemiologic investigation, patients with vCJD in the United Kingdom, France (with the exception of one patient who lived in the United Kingdom for more than 6 months during the period 1980–1996), Spain, Ireland, Italy, the Netherlands, Portugal, Saudi Arabia, and Taiwan were considered to have been exposed to infection locally. In contrast, among the four cases in the United States one was considered to have been exposed in Saudi Arabia, two in the United Kingdom, and one in a country where he lived before moving to the United States (Kuwait, Russia, or Lebanon) (Maheshwari et al., 2015; Coulthart et al., 2016). For the two Canadian patients, one was considered to have been exposed in the United Kingdom and the other in Saudi Arabia (Maheshwari et al., 2015; Coulthart et al., 2016). The Japanese case was attributed to an exposure during a short stay of 24 days in the United Kingdom in early 1990 just 2 years before the peak of the BSE outbreak (Shinde et al., 2009). This is the only case in which infectious exposure has been attributed to such a brief stay in the United Kingdom but the absence of other vCJD cases in Japan to date supports this interpretation.

Food contamination is the most likely cause of vCJD (Ward et al., 2006) and it was demonstrated that the origin of contaminated beef products, for countries reporting vCJD cases not linked to UK residence or stay, was more likely linked to the level of importations from the United Kingdom between 1980 and 1996 than to indigenous cases of BSE (Sanchez-Juan et al., 2007). Even in France, with over 1000 native BSE cases, imported UK beef was the major source of exposure to BSE reaching a peak in 1994, later than the United Kingdom, clearly explaining the 5-year differential between the peak of vCJD cases in the United Kingdom (2000) and France (2005) (Chadeau-Hyam and Alpérovitch, 2005; Brandel et al., 2009).

If dietary contamination is the most likely cause, it is potentially difficult to understand why the disease affects mostly young people. However two possible explanations are relevant: (1) young people were more exposed to the infectious agent because of possible different dietary habits; (2) young people are biologically more susceptible to the agent. The amount of gut-associated lymphoreticular tissue is greater in the young and they also have a higher incidence of potentially relevant infections (such as tonsillitis) that might increase susceptibility to lymphoid involvement (St. Rose et al., 2006; Donaldson et al., 2016). An alternative assumption, that the incubation period is longer at a later age, seems unlikely because there is no relation between date of onset and age.

The relatively low number of primary cases worldwide, equal to 228 at the end of 2016, is relatively reassuring and fits with the expected number produced by various statistical and modeling analyses based on the method of retro-calculation. This method relies on the fact that the number of cases of an infectious disease depends on three parameters: number of infected persons, distribution of dates of infection, and incubation duration. Most of the analyses consider that the great majority of infected persons were teenagers at the end of the 1980s and that the incubation period is 15–20 years and is independent of age. Under these hypotheses, the estimation of the total number of primary cases of vCJD in the United Kingdom was coherent for all studies, at around 500 (Cousens et al., 1997; Cooper et al., 2000; Ghani et al., 2000; d'Aignaux et al., 2001; Valleron et al., 2001).

A predictive study based on the level of consumption of beef mechanically recovered meat and head meat gave an estimated number of vCJD cases in the United Kingdom of 362 (168 for the 1940–1969 birth cohort and 194 for the post-1969 birth cohort) (Cooper and Bird, 2003). A comparable study predicted 33 cases in France (12 for the 1940–1969 birth cohort and 21 for the post-1969 birth cohort) (Chadeau-Hyam and Alpérovitch, 2005). Until 2016, all those who had died of definite or probable vCJD and who had had genetic analysis had the same methionine-methionine polymorphism at codon 129 of *PRNP* gene. However experimental transmission studies to humanized transgenic mice showed that all genotypes were susceptible to the vCJD agent with the following gradient methionine-methionine > methionine-valine >valine-valine (Bishop et al., 2006). The announcement at the end of 2016 of a case with a methionine-valine polymorphism at codon 129 increased the previously expressed concern that a second wave (in different genotypes) could lead to an increased number of primary cases. This second wave was considered possible because differential incubation periods had been observed in kuru and in the French cohort of CJD after growth hormone treatment, with the emergence of heterozygote cases after that of homozygotes (Cervenáková et al., 1998; Brandel et al., 2003). According to statistical forecasts, the number of cases linked to the second wave will be less important compared to the number of methionine-methionine cases (Valleron et al., 2006; Garske and Ghani, 2010).

Apart from *PRNP*-129, other possible genetic risk factors have been studied. In a genomewide association study, Mead et al. (2012) identified additional candidate loci that they felt merited further investigation. Other studies have found evidence to implicate a cathepsin D polymorphism, MTMR7 and PLCXD3 (Bishop et al., 2008, 2013; Sanchez-Juan et al., 2012).

Blood-contaminated cases of vCJD, asymptomatic cases, and healthy carriers

Because of the peripheral repartition of the agent of vCJD in lymphoid tissues the risk of transmission of prion infection through blood was considered. The most important studies were made on sheep because the pathogenesis of scrapie and BSE in sheep resembles that of humans with vCJD (Foster et al., 2001). In this model it was demonstrated that BSE could be transmitted by blood (Houston et al., 2000). A further study has shown a high transmission rate of 36% and relatively short incubation period, suggesting substantial infectivity titers in blood (McCutcheon et al., 2011). Because large volume of blood can be collected and processed into different components identical to those used for blood transfusion, this study also demonstrated that all blood components could be the source of transmission even after leucoreduction (McCutcheon et al., 2011). In the United Kingdom, four cases of infection by the vCJD agent have been reported in recipients of nonleuco-reduced red blood cell concentrate from donors incubating vCJD (Llewelyn et al., 2004; Peden et al., 2004; Wroe et al., 2006; Urwin et al., 2016).

Among the four probable cases of accidental vCJD contamination through blood transfusion reported so far, three patients were methionine-homozygous at codon 129 of the *PRNP* gene and showed clinical vCJD and one patient was heterozygous and showed preclinical infection only (Peden et al., 2004). This last patient died from a nonneurologic disease 5 years after receiving a blood transfusion from a vCJD-incubating donor. PrP^{TSE} 2B was detected in the lymphoid tissues but not in the central nervous system, suggesting that, at least in peripheral tissues, the vCJD agent can propagate on a codon 129 methionine-valine genetic background. A probable case of infection was reported in a patient with hemophilia treated with coagulation factor VIII manufactured from plasma of UK donors (Peden et al., 2010). This patient, heterozygous at codon 129, identified through a specific surveillance program, demonstrated no signs of vCJD or other neurologic disease during his life and was positive for the abnormal form of the prion protein for only one sample from his spleen. To date, no additional case of posttransfusional vCJD or vCJD in patients treated for hemophilia has been reported in other countries and especially in France, where three vCJD patients known to be donors of leuco-reduced blood were identified.

Unlike the other forms of prion diseases, it was demonstrated that the agent of vCJD had the property to accumulate in lymphoid tissues (Head et al., 2004a, b). In order to evaluate the prevalence of possible healthy carriers in the British population, who had the widest exposure to the BSE agent, several studies aiming at demonstrating the presence of the abnormal form of the prion protein in lymphoid tissues (appendices and tonsils) were carried out in the United Kingdom. All these studies used strictly anonymized specimens removed during routine surgery.

The more informative studies were those done on appendices. The first study found three positive appendices on 12,674 specimens from the birth cohort in which most vCJD cases have arisen (1961–1985), leading to an estimation of prevalence of healthy carriers of 237 per million or 1 per 4000, but with very wide 95% confidence intervals (Hilton et al., 2004). The second study was larger than the first one and found 16 positive samples on 32 441 from two different birth cohorts, 1961–1981 and 1941–1960. The global estimated prevalence was 493 per million (95% confidence interval 282–801) or 1 per 2000 (95% confidence interval 1/3500–1/1250) (Gill et al., 2013). The studies on frozen or paraffin-embedded tonsil tissues did not bring additional useful data for the estimation of prevalence of healthy carriers in the United Kingdom (Frosh et al., 2004; Clewley et al., 2009; de Marco et al., 2010). The genotype at codon 129 of the *PRNP* gene could be determined for 2 out of 3 patients of the first study (all valine-valine) and for all the patients of the second study (8 methionine-methionine, 4 methionine-valine, and 4 valine-valine). These results indicate that the BSE agent may infect individuals of any genotype at codon 129. Although it has been generally accepted that the finding of abnormal prion protein in lymphoreticular specimens such as the appendix indicates BSE/vCJD infection, it was thought important to confirm this.

A further UK population study was, therefore, undertaken, comparing three time/birth cohort periods: before likely dietary BSE exposure, during the accepted BSE period, and after establishment of the full UK human dietary protection measures. The full results are not yet published but positive appendices were found in all three time periods, with no statistically significant difference between them (Public Health England, 2016). This must call into question either the current assumptions made about human population BSE exposure or the acceptance that a positive result indicates BSE/vCJD infection.

PATHOLOGIC ASPECTS

Peripheral localization of PrP^{TSE}

The pathogenesis of vCJD is distinct from the other forms of human prion disease because disease-related prion protein (PrP^{TSE}) has been detected in many peripheral tissues. In humans and animals, the normal and cellular form of the prion protein (PrP^c) is expressed in high concentrations in the central nervous system but also in less abundance in extraneuronal tissues. Because the disease-related isoform, PrP^{TSE}, is derived from PrP^c, tissues that express PrP^c are most likely to support prion accumulation and the rates of normal PrP^c expression can be one of the factors that affect the development of prion diseases. The distribution of PrP^{TSE} in nonneuronal tissues depends as well on the prion strain. Multiple prion strains are recognized and are associated with distinct PrP^{TSE} types, which can be distinguished by Western blot analysis with distinct cleavage sites to proteinase K implying different PrP^{TSE} conformations and by differences in glycoform ratios of protease-digested PrP^{TSE}. The PrP^{TSE} type detected on Western blot is similar in brain in cases of vCJD and in cases of BSE and classified as type 4 or type 2B (Collinge et al., 1996; Parchi et al., 1997).

The specificities to the host play also an important role. Thus in BSE the PrP^{TSE} is mainly present in the central nervous system whereas in vCJD the replication occurs also in the peripheral tissues. The first evidence was provided by the observation of accumulation of PrP^{TSE} in tonsillar tissue obtained at necropsy of a patient who died of vCJD using both immunohistochemistry and Western blot analysis of frozen tissue with a type 4 (2B) PrP^{TSE} (Hill et al., 1997). The second was brought by detection of positive immunoreactivity for PrP^{TSE} in the cytoplasm of cells, predominantly in germinal centers of an appendix removed 8 months before the onset of vCJD in a young British patient (Hilton et al., 1998). Then, a study on necropsy tissues confirmed that lymphoid tissues (tonsil, spleen, lymph nodes) from patients with neuropathologically confirmed vCJD were constantly positive for PrP^{TSE} with immunocytochemistry and Western blot methods (Hill et al., 1997). Such accumulation of PrP^{TSE} in lymphoid tissues has never been observed in patients who have died of sporadic or genetic forms of CJD or in normal controls, leading to the possibility of using tonsil biopsy as a diagnostic test in case of suspected vCJD (Hill et al., 1997). With a highly sensitive immunoblot method, PrP^{TSE} could be uniformly detected in tonsil, spleen, and lymph node, readily in the retina and optic nerve, at very low concentration in rectum, adrenal gland, and thymus from 1–4 patients and could not be detected in other peripheral tissues, particularly in blood (buffy coat) and appendix (Wadsworth et al., 2001).

Arguments on infectivity of lymphoid tissues in vCJD have been brought by transmission experiments in wild-type mice and infectivity of tonsil and spleen could be evaluated 100–1000 times less than in brain (Bruce et al., 2001). An accumulation of PrP^{TSE} was observed in catecholaminergic neurons of the celiac, superior mesenteric, and stellate ganglia of the autonomic nervous system in vCJD (Haik et al., 2003). This accumulation was never seen in controls or patients with sporadic or iatrogenic CJD. These results and the fact that it was known that the human enteric system expresses cellular prion protein PrP (Shmakov et al., 2000) support the hypothesis of the oral route of contamination of vCJD patients and a role for sympathetic neurons system in prion propagation from the gut to the central nervous system.

By means of immunohistochemical or biochemical studies, PrP^{TSE} was also detected in one case of vCJD with a long disease duration (more than twice the usual average duration of evolution) in the dura mater, liver, pancreas, kidney, ovary, uterus, and skin, indicating that the number of organs affected in vCJD is greater than previously thought (Notari et al., 2010). This was further confirmed with the development of highly sensitive techniques of detection. By using the protein misfolding cyclic amplification (PMCA) technique to detect minute quantities of PrP^{TSE} it was possible to bring out abnormal prion protein in urine of patients with vCJD but never in patients with sporadic or genetic CJD or with other degenerative diseases (Moda et al., 2014). PrP^{TSE} was detectable only after extensive amplification, suggesting that the concentration of the infectious protein in urine is small. With the same techniques abnormal protein prion was detected in blood (notably in plasma) of patients with vCJD and not in blood of controls or patients affected by other neurodegenerative diseases or sCJD (except for one British patient) (Bougard et al., 2016; Concha-Marambio et al., 2016). Detection of abnormal prion protein was also observed in presymptomatic vCJD patients (Bougard et al., 2016).

Neuropathology

Macroscopically, cerebral cortical atrophy and cerebellar atrophy, predominant in the vermis, were identified in cases with long disease duration without other significant macroscopic abnormalities. At the microscopic level, the neuropathologic features of vCJD are those of a TSE, with spongiform changes, neuronal loss, and astrocytosis. Spongiform changes are widespread in a patchy distribution within the cerebral cortex involving all cortical layers. Confluent cortical spongiform changes are rare but most evident in the occipital and inferior frontal cortex. No spongiform changes are detected in the hippocampus, but the entorhinal cortex shows patchy microvacuolar spongiform changes. Confluent spongiform changes are always present in the caudate nucleus and putamen. Focal spongiform changes involve many of the nuclei in the anterior and medial thalamus, often in the absence of plaques. The posterior thalamic nuclei are relatively spared. Mild spongiform changes are detected in the hypothalamus, the periaqueductal gray matter in the midbrain, and in the gray matter of the pons and medulla, but not in spinal cord. In cerebellum, spongiform changes are observed throughout the hemispheres and vermis and are confluent in the molecular layer with a patchy distribution. Cerebral cortical neuronal loss is marked in the occipital lobe in all cases but more severe and widespread, with astrocytosis, in cases with a long clinical history. Even in these cases, the neuronal loss in the hippocampus remains moderate.

The basal ganglia shows variable neuronal loss, which was most evident in cases with severe and confluent spongiform change. In the medial and posterior regions of the thalamus the neuronal loss is severe with marked astrocytosis. In the midbrain, neuronal loss and astrocytosis occur in the superior periaqueductal gray matter and in the inferior colliculi. Neuronal loss and astrocytosis are observed in all layers of cerebellar cortex and are proportional to the duration of the disease. Neuronal loss and astrocytosis are not prominent in the pons, medulla, and spinal cord.

The hallmarks of vCJD are the observation of numerous large plaques with a fibrillary structure throughout the cerebral cortex, cerebellum, basal ganglia, thalamus, and hypothalamus. These plaques resemble kuru plaques with a dense eosinophilic center and pale periphery of radiating fibrils on hematoxylin and eosin stain. Many are surrounded by a zone of spongiform changes and these are called "florid plaques" (Fig. 11.1). They measure up to 150 mm. They were previously described in experimental transmission of Icelandic scrapie in mice and observed in some cases of iatrogenic CJD after dura mater graft (Kretzschmar et al., 2003). In iatrogenic cases, they are less numerous than in the vCJD cases.

Florid plaques are present in all autopsy cases but may be absent in cases with only brain biopsy. Florid plaques

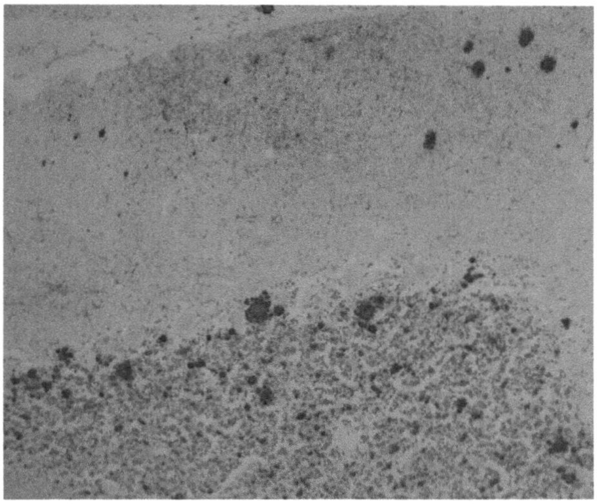

Fig. 11.1. Florid plaque in variant Creutzfeldt–Jakob disease brain. (Courtesy of Professor Colin Smith, CCBS, University of Edinburgh, United Kingdom.)

as well as smaller plaques composed of finely punctated fibrils and pericellular PrP deposition are observed in the cerebral cortex and in the molecular layer of the cerebellum. The florid plaques show strong staining on immunocytochemistry for PrP, which also reveals smaller plaques, often arranged in irregular clusters within the neuropil. These "cluster plaques" were present in all cases. In addition, there is a widespread amorphous pericellular deposition of PrP around small neurons in both cerebral and cerebellar cortex. Some PrP deposits are identified around capillaries of the cerebral and cerebellar cortex. A dense PrP synaptic accumulation is observed in the dentate fascia, subiculum, and entorhinal cortex which also contain small cluster plaques. In the basal ganglia there is a perineuronal pattern of PrP accumulation and a synaptic pattern of immunoreactivity is detected in the thalamus and hypothalamus with occasional plaques. Synaptic and perineuronal immunoreactivity is also present in the midbrain, pons, medulla, and spinal cord. Astrocytosis is well visualized on immunocytochemistry for glial fibrillary acidic protein. With this technique astrocytosis is observed in posterior thalamus, midbrain, cerebral and cerebellar cortex, often associated with severe neuronal loss.

The cases of vCJD from France and the United Kingdom are indistinguishable clinically and pathologically with totally similar brain lesion profiles and a consistent pattern of PrP^{TSE} deposition (Brandel et al., 2009). PrP^{TSE} in vCJD exhibits a peculiar profile on Western blot, with an unglycosylated band migrated at 19 kDa and a higher representation of diglycosylated PrP molecules (PrP^{TSE} 4 or 2B) (Collinge et al., 1996; Parchi et al., 1997). This biochemical signature is a useful hallmark of BSE agent replication in other species, including nonhuman primates (Hill et al., 1997; Lasmezas et al., 2005). It has been observed in all French and British patients so far (Brandel et al., 2009).

In addition, in contrast with sporadic and genetic CJD (Puoti et al., 1999; Haik et al., 2004; Head et al., 2004a, b), the same biochemical signature is detected in all brain areas studied (Brandel et al. 2009). This highly uniform biochemical and pathologic signature of vCJD is consistent with the presence of a unique infectious strain. This is reinforced by the observation of similarities in lesion profiles after transmission to wild-type mice of brain material from human vCJD patients from the United Kingdom and from four non-UK countries (Diack et al., 2012). However, experimental arguments from transmission studies are in favor of the coexistence of the predominant strain with a minor strain (Haik and Brandel, 2011). This minor strain is only revealed on transgenic mice overexpressing human M129 PrP and not on transgenic mice produced by gene targeting (Bishop et al., 2006; Beringue et al., 2008).

CLINICAL FEATURES

General description

Age

vCJD has to date affected a younger age group than is typical for sCJD. In the United Kingdom, for 178 definite or probable vCJD cases, the median age at onset was 26 years (range 12–74 years), and the median age at death was 28 years (compared with 67 and 68 years as the respective medians for sCJD) (http://www.cjd.ac.uk/data.html). The 27 definite or probable vCJD cases in France were also relatively young, although slightly older than the UK cases, with a median age at onset of 36 years (range 18–57 years). However, it is important to note that vCJD has affected older people (the oldest UK person affected was 74 years old) and other forms of prion disease may affect younger people (such as atypical sCJD and genetic prion disease).

Sex

There is no definite sex difference in vCJD cases.

Duration

This is a relatively rapidly progressive illness in terms of neurologic disease, although significantly slower in progression relative to typical sCJD. The median duration of illness in 178 definite and probable UK cases was 14 months (range 6–114 months) and 13.5 months (range 8–27 months) in French cases. In the United Kingdom, the median duration of sCJD is 4 months (range 1–74 months). Like all prion diseases, with no presently effective treatment, progression to death is the inevitable course.

General illness profile

In the discussion that follows, a general distinction is made between psychiatric features (such as depression, anxiety, and delusions) and neurologic features (such as ataxia, involuntary movements, somatosensory disturbance, cognitive impairment). It is recognized that this distinction may be slightly imprecise at times, with all features resulting from brain disease, but it has practical utility in the clinical consideration of cases and the diagnostic process.

Psychiatric features typically dominate the earlier part of the illness and may be the sole presenting feature. Characteristic specifically neurologic features include painful sensory symptoms, cerebellar ataxia, cognitive impairment, and involuntary movements (especially myoclonus).

In a detailed examination of 100 definite and probable UK cases, 63% presented with psychiatric features alone, 22% had a mixture of psychiatric and neurologic features from onset, and 15% had neurologic features that preceded psychiatric ones. The prominence of psychiatric features was reflected in specialist referral patterns: 38% of patients were referred initially to psychiatric services and 63% were referred at some point in the illness (Spencer et al., 2002).

In this detailed study, Spencer et al. (2002) divided the psychiatric and neurologic clinical features in the 100 cases into common ($\geq$ 50% of cases), less common (25–50%), and rare (<25%) and then, according to time of occurrence, into early (0–4 months of illness), later (4–6 months), and late (>6 months). On this classification, there were no common early neurologic features and only one less common early neurologic feature (that of pain). Although 57% of cases developed at least one neurologic feature within 2 months of illness onset, this was often a rather nonspecific feature and occurred in the context of a significant psychiatric presentation.

The initial clinical presentation of vCJD is rather nonspecific and many diagnoses (neurologic and psychiatric) may be considered quite reasonably in the early illness stages.

Psychiatric features

Even in the earliest reports of vCJD cases, psychiatric features were noted to be prominent clinical manifestations. Of the first 14 UK cases, all had psychiatric features and these were presenting features in 9 of them (Zeidler et al., 1997b). Depression was the commonest psychiatric diagnosis but 2 patients had first-rank symptoms of a psychotic illness. Delusions were common, but usually unsustained, typically lasting only hours or days. Five patients had auditory and eight visual hallucinations. In a later report, based on the first 33 of the 35 UK cases, 32 exhibited psychiatric symptoms in the early stages of illness and, in 31, these were the first disease manifestations – either isolated or in conjunction with other features (Will et al., 1999). For 17 of these 33 patients, a psychiatrist was the first specialist doctor involved and, in a further 8, a psychiatrist was involved after initial referral to a neurologist.

It was noted that only one of the first 14 UK cases was not seen by a psychiatrist, whereas this was true of 7 of the subsequent 19 cases, perhaps reflecting the increasing recognition of vCJD in the UK medical community (Will et al., 1999).

In this report of 33 UK cases, it was noted that abnormal neurologic signs were not always present, even when there were neurologic symptoms – in one notable case, even at 15 months after illness onset.

A report of a French case described a patient who was diagnosed with major depression and admitted after 6 months to a psychiatric unit. He subsequently developed delusions (noted to be transient, often occurring for a few hours) and auditory hallucinations. The authors noted that these features were broadly similar to those described in UK cases (Dervaux et al., 2001). In 15 reported French cases, 7 presented with psychiatric symptoms: severe depression, aggression, and delusions (Brandel et al., 2009).

A review of the standard clinical diagnostic criteria for vCJD, based on 106 definite UK cases, found that 92% had some psychiatric features in the early phase of the illness (Heath et al., 2010).

In the review of the first 100 UK cases, the reported common early psychiatric features were generally rather nonspecific: dysphoria, withdrawal/loss of interest, anxiety/aggression, and insomnia (Spencer et al., 2002). Given this, and the overall clinical description, there are two important points that need to be kept in mind. Firstly, an initial psychiatric diagnosis of, say, primary depression, may be entirely reasonable until developments make it clear that the depression is secondary to an underlying neurologic illness. Secondly, some patients do not present with psychiatric features and the initial symptoms can indeed be specifically neurologic.

The psychiatric problems and, indeed, their treatment can make the assessment of other features difficult. For example, pain may be a complaint in some depression presentations and involuntary movements may be side-effects of certain psychotropic medications.

Pain/sensory features

As stated above, in the review of the first 100 UK cases, there were no common early neurologic features and only one less common early neurologic feature: pain (Spencer et al., 2002). Sensory symptoms had been reported as significant clinical features in previous publications concerning vCJD (Zeidler et al., 1997a; Brandel et al., 2009). One paper described the sensory features in some detail, based on a review of the first 50 UK cases (Macleod et al., 2002). In this review, 64% of patients had persistent sensory symptoms and 16% did not (in 18% there were insufficient data to decide). The sensory symptoms were lateralized in nearly a third of affected cases, in keeping with a cerebral hemisphere – possibly thalamic – causation. The symptoms were varied: limb pain in 63%, cold feelings in 25%, dysesthesiae in 28%, parasthesiae in 31%, and numbness in 25% (some individuals had more than one symptom). In 32 patients with sensory symptoms, there were only 6 with definite sensory signs; however, the clinical sensory examination may well be difficult in patients with psychiatric or cognitive problems. A review of the standard clinical diagnostic criteria for vCJD, based on 106 definite UK cases, found 63% had persistent painful sensory symptoms (Heath et al., 2010).

Cerebellar features

Definitive cerebellar ataxia or features suggestive of this (such as impaired balance or coordination) are typical clinical manifestations. In the review of the first definite 106 UK cases, 97% were found to have had ataxia at some point in the illness (Heath et al., 2010). In the review of the first 100 UK cases, gait disturbance, impaired coordination, and dysarthria appeared typically at around 4–6 months of illness with specific features such as dysdiadochokinesis appearing at a median of around 6 months (Spencer et al., 2002). In a review of 162 UK cases, 93% of cases showed cerebellar signs at some point in the illness (National CJD Reseach and Surveillance Unit unpublisheddata).

Involuntary movements

As with other human prion diseases, the commonest involuntary movement seen is that of myoclonus and this is typically a later feature of the illness. In the study of the first 100 UK cases, myoclonus generally occurred around 6 months or later of illness (Spencer et al., 2002). Other movement disorders such as tremor, chorea, and dystonia are also seen and also relatively later in the illness course. In the review of 106 definite UK cases, 94% of patients had features of chorea, dystonia, or myoclonus at some point in their illness (Heath et al., 2010).

Cognitive impairment

Cognitive impairment leading to dementia is invariable but this can be difficult to assess in the earlier illness phase if there are significant psychiatric features. Typically, when cognitive features emerge, they are nonspecific ones such as poor memory and disorientation (Spencer et al., 2002).

Other features

It is not surprising that a serious progressive brain disease can produce, at some stage of the illness, a variety of clinical abnormalities other than those discussed above. However, these are generally relatively nonspecific, such as the finding of extensor plantar responses and primitive reflexes. However, a few specific points are worth mentioning. Oculomotor problems occur in around half the cases, sometimes associated with complaints of diplopia (National CJD Reseach and Surveillance Unit unpublished data). Interestingly, certain specific problems are uncommon: epileptic seizures have been documented in only 8% and typical extrapyramidal features in only around 4% of UK cases (National CJD Reseach and Surveillance Unit unpublished data).

DIAGNOSIS

General approach

The diagnosis of vCJD can be considered in four stages: (1) suspicion of the diagnosis; (2) tests to exclude other possibilities; (3) tests to support the diagnosis; (4) absolute confirmation of diagnosis.

Suspicion of the diagnosis

A suspicion of vCJD reflects two broad considerations: the clinical profile and the overall diagnostic context. With respect to the latter, it is important to note that vCJD is a very rare illness and there is a strong geographic link with most cases in the United Kingdom and France.

As with many diseases, the passage of time, with the development of the illness, may provide helpful diagnostic information.

Tests to exclude other possibilities

Clearly, the differential diagnosis in the initial stages of illness is potentially very wide. A primary psychiatric illness is a very reasonable consideration in many presentations. In addition, many, much commoner, neurologic illnesses may present with neuropsychiatric features or with cerebellar ataxia, involuntary movements, and/or cognitive impairment. The assessment of such cases requires clinical neurologic expertise. It should be noted that, aside from other psychiatric or neurologic illnesses, other forms of prion disease are important differential diagnoses (in particular, genetic prion disease and atypical sCJD). One important point is, therefore, to perform *PRNP* mutation testing, with appropriate consent. Genetic forms of prion disease may present at a relatively young age, with neuropsychiatric features and a family history may be absent. *PRNP* analysis also allows codon 129 genotyping; currently, an MV or VV genotype would make the diagnosis less likely. Additionally, atypical sCJD is an important differential diagnosis of vCJD, and atypical features are more likely in MV and VV genotype individuals. However, being non-MM cannot exclude the possibility of vCJD.

Tests to support the diagnosis

Supportive tests are discussed in detail below. However, it should be noted that certain tests (such as cerebrospinal fluid (CSF) examination or cerebral magnetic resonance (MR)) are very important in the exclusion of other

Table 11.1

Diagnostic criteria for variant Creutzfeldt–Jakob disease (CJD)

Subsection	Item	Criterion
I	A	Progressive neuropsychiatric disorder
	B	Duration of illness <6 months
	C	Routine investigations do not suggest an alternative diagnosis
	D	No history of potential iatrogenic exposure
	E	No evidence of a familial form of TSE
II	A	Early psychiatric features[a]
	B	Persistent painful sensory symptoms[b]
	C	Ataxia
	D	Myoclonus or chorea or dystonia
	E	Dementia
III	A	EEG does not show the typical appearance of sporadic CJD[c] in the early stages of illness
	B	Bilateral pulvinar high signal on MRI scan
IV		Positive tonsil biopsy[d]
Definite	IA and neuropathologic confirmation of vCJD[e]	
Probable	I and 4/5 of II and IIIA and IIIB; or I and IVA	
Possible	I and 4/5 of II and IIIA	

[a]Depression, anxiety, apathy, withdrawal, delusions.
[b]This includes frank pain and/or dysesthesia.
[c]The typical appearance of the EEG in sporadic CJD consists of generalized triphasic periodic complexes at approximately 1 per second. These may occasionally be seen in the late stages of vCJD.
[d]Tonsil biopsy is not recommended routinely, nor in cases with EEG appearances typical of sporadic CJD, but may be useful in suspect cases in which the clinical features are compatible with vCJD and MRI does not show bilateral pulvinar high signal.
[e]Spongiform change and extensive prion protein deposition with florid plaques throughout the cerebrum and cerebellum.
EEG, electroencephalography; MRI, magnetic resonance imaging; TSE, transmissible spongiform encephalopathy; vCJD _ variant Creutzfeldt–Jakob disease.

illnesses and are usually undertaken for this reason in the first instance.

Absolute confirmation of diagnosis

Presently, the only absolute confirmatory test is neuropathologic examination, which requires either a brain biopsy or examination of the brain at autopsy. It is arguable that brain biopsy is indicated only in those cases where a reasonable and potentially treatable illness cannot otherwise be excluded.

Diagnostic criteria for vCJD are used in international surveillance and research to classify cases into definite, probable, and possible categories (Table 11.1).

These criteria have been reviewed and validated in one study showing that, in terms of sensitivity, 83% of 106 definite cases would be classifiable as probable vCJD (with 6 cases classified as possible vCJD). The specificity was found to be 100%, with no autopsy/cerebral biopsy-proven non-vCJD cases being classified as probable vCJD in life (Heath et al., 2010).

It is important to note that all but one tested cases of definite and probable vCJD have been of the *PRNP*-129 MM genotype. The clinical phenotype (including investigation results) may be different in the other 129 genotypes, although there is no definite evidence for this. The single definite case of MV vCJD showed some clinical phenotypic variation from the commonest MM picture but was within the general clinical envelope of previously described vCJD cases (Mok et al., 2017). One other reported case of MV genotype met only the possible criteria for vCJD and was not clinically distinct from other vCJD cases (Kaski et al., 2009).

Cerebral MR

The cerebral MR shows characteristic changes in the majority of cases of vCJD (Fig. 11.2). The disease hallmark is the so-called pulvinar sign, consisting of high signal in the posterior thalamus. Other areas may be involved, such as the dorsomedial thalamic nuclei and the periaqueductal gray matter (Collie et al., 2001, 2003; Summers et al., 2002). It is important to note that high signal may also be seen in the caudate and putamen in vCJD (areas that are characteristically involved in sCJD), but the pulvinar sign, as defined, consists of signal intensity that is higher in the posterior thalamus than in any other area such as the anterior basal ganglia. It is also important to note that some cases of vCJD may show MR changes that are truly characteristic of sCJD (Mok et al., 2017). Cortical signal change, often seen in sCJD,

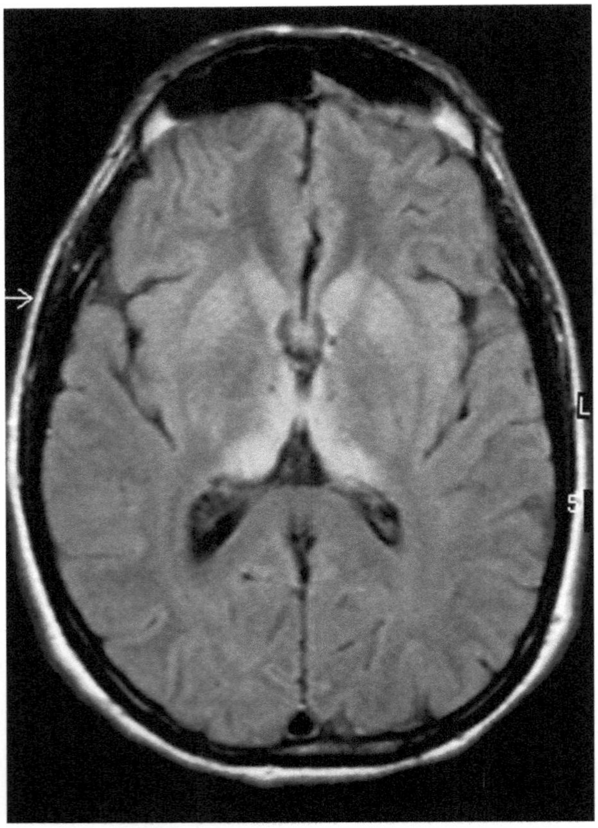

Fig. 11.2. The magnetic resonance pulvinar sign in variant Creutzfeldt–Jakob disease (vCJD). This is a fluid-attenuated inversion recovery magnetic resonance image in vCJD, showing hyperintensity in the caudate/putamen but much greater hyperintensity in the posterior and medial thalamic region (the pulvinar sign). (Courtesy of Dr David Summers, Department of Neuroradiology, Lothian University Hospitals Trust, Edinburgh.)

is not commonly seen in vCJD and cerebral atrophy is also uncommon (Summers et al., 2002; Collie et al., 2003).

For vCJD, the order of sensitivity in MR sequences is diffusion-weighted imaging > fluid-attenuated inversion recovery (FLAIR) > Proton Density (PD) > T2 > T1. In a study of 86 neuropathologically confirmed cases of vCJD, 9% of T1 images, 81% of PD images, and 100% of FLAIR images showed the characteristic pulvinar sign –though the authors state they have seen a probable case without this feature on FLAIR (Collie et al., 2003).

As the MR data are derived from clinical practice, rather than from formal, designed studies, it is difficult to comment on the evolution of any MR changes during the course of the illness. However, it is worth repeating the scan if the initial images do not show the pulvinar sign, even though it can be absent even at late disease stages (Collie et al., 2003). The pulvinar sign may also exist at the onset of the disease and then disappear (Brandel et al., 2010).

CSF examination

The examination of the CSF is an important step in the differential diagnosis as various inflammatory central nervous system diseases may present in a similar fashion to vCJD. In vCJD, the routine CSF examination is usually normal, with no pleocytosis, or shows only a relatively modest total protein elevation. CSF 14-3-3 testing is of less diagnostic utility for vCJD than sCJD as it is positive in only around 50% of cases (Green et al., 2001). CSF tau is raised in vCJD and a more sensitive indicator than 14-3-3; however its specificity is reduced by the fact that such elevations may be seen in a number of other neurodegenerative diseases (Green et al., 2001). CSF phospho-tau is elevated in vCJD CSF and to levels that are generally higher than found in sCJD, but it is uncertain as to how useful this is in distinguishing variant and sporadic forms (Goodall et al., 2006).

CSF real-time quaking-induced conversion (RT-QuIC), a very sensitive and specific test in sCJD, has, interestingly and notably, proven negative in cases of vCJD (McGuire et al., 2012, 2016; AJE Green, personal communication). This is, therefore, a potentially useful test in differentiating between cases of sporadic and variant disease.

Blood tests

Developing reliable blood tests for prion disease has proved difficult. However, there are interesting and important results that are promising for vCJD diagnosis in future cases.

Edgeworth et al. (2011) reported a test called the direct detection assay which was studied further with a reported sensitivity of around 71% for clinical vCJD and a specificity of 100% for CJD, although with occasional positive results in sCJD (Jackson et al., 2014).

More recently, two significantly more sensitive tests have been reported (Bougard et al., 2016; Concha-Marambio et al., 2016). The test described by Concha-Marambio et al. (2016) is PMCA-based and reported 100% sensitivity and 100% specificity when 14 vCJD specimens and 153 controls (including sCJD specimens) were tested. The test described by Bougard et al. (2016), also PMCA-based, reported 100% sensitivity and 100% diagnostic specificity on testing 18 vCJD samples, 67 sCJD samples, and 238 non-CJD controls. However, of the 67 sCJD samples, 1 was positive. They also reported positive results in samples taken presymptomatically from 2 vCJD cases, i.e., they confirmed positivity in preclinical as well as clinical vCJD.

Initially, there were concerns that blood tests for prion disease might be affected by the anticoagulant used in collecting the sample and the test reported by

Edgeworth is reported to require ethylenediaminetetraacetic acid blood samples. However, the tests reported by Bougard and Concha-Marambio appear to work equally well whatever anticoagulant is used. It is interesting that, while these blood tests appear to be useful specifically for vCJD, occasional positive results are seen in sCJD.

Urine tests

One study found that a PMCA-based urine test was sensitive and specific for vCJD. Thirteen of 14 vCJD samples tested were positive. Other samples from sCJD, genetic prion disease, other neurodegenerative disorders, and normal controls were negative (Moda et al., 2014). This is an interesting result on a small number of specimens tested in a single study.

Tonsil biopsy

As discussed above, abnormal prion protein is found in the lymphoreticular tissue in vCJD but not other forms of human prion disease. As a result, tonsil biopsy has become an accepted clinical diagnostic test in vCJD. Hill et al. (1999) reported a positive finding of abnormal prion protein in tonsil biopsies from 8 patients with definite or probable vCJD. A negative result cannot totally exclude vCJD but a definitely positive result has not been seen in any clinical condition other than vCJD. Since the accepted view is that lymphoreticular involvement precedes clinical illness in BSE/vCJD infection, there is one theoretical caveat: a positive tonsil biopsy could, conceivably, reflect preclinical infection rather than relevant illness; this is supported by the finding of positive results in UK general population studies (Hilton et al., 2004; Clewley et al., 2009; Gill et al., 2013). However, if a tonsil biopsy is being undertaken in the appropriate clinical illness context, a positive result is highly likely to be diagnostically relevant.

Nasal brushing

Recent reports describe the use of nasal brushing to obtain olfactory neurons with sensitive and specific detection of abnormal prion protein using RT-QuIC methodology (Orru et al., 2014; Bongianni et al., 2017). These reports concern forms of human prion disease other than vCJD (mostly sCJD); however there is no reason to believe this approach would not work also with vCJD.

EEG

The electroencephalogram (EEG) may be normal in the early stages of vCJD; with disease progression, nonspecific loss of normal background rhythms and excess slow-wave activity are seen. The typical periodic discharges found in many cases of sCJD either do not develop in vCJD or are seen only in very late, preterminal stages in some patients. In the United Kingdom, periodic discharges have not been seen in any case. In 15 French cases, 3 cases showed some periodic activity in the last stages of illness, but this activity would not have been regarded as the typical periodic EEG of sCJD according to some published criteria (Brandel et al., 2009). There are two reports of periodic EEG findings like those seen in sCJD, but they were found very late in the course of the disease (Binelli et al., 2006; Yamada, 2006).

TREATMENT AND MANAGEMENT

Specific treatment

There is no treatment that is proven to have a disease-modifying effect in vCJD. There is some evidence that the duration of illness was prolonged in a few patients treated with intraventricular pentosan polysulfate (Bone et al., 2008). However, these patients were treated in an unselected way and not in the context of a designed trial. All these patients progressed and died; only one such treated patient had an autopsy examination with no reduction of the overall neuropathologic changes in the brain (Newman et al., 2014).

A treatment trial in the United Kingdom using oral quinacrine showed no benefit in CJD patients, including 18 cases of vCJD (Collinge et al., 2009).

General management

The general management of vCJD is essentially supportive and symptomatic. Pain, depression, and agitation can be managed according to usual practice. Involuntary movements may be treated if it is felt to be clinically necessary. As patients lose mobility and the ability to care for themselves, then appropriate supportive measures need to be taken. If feeding and swallowing are impaired, then a decision needs to be taken as how best to manage the problem A nasogastric tube or percutaneous gastrostomy may be indicated though, in the insertion of the latter, there are important potential infection considerations (for example, if inserted endoscopically, the endoscope must then be deemed capable of transmitting the disease to others). Urinary incontinence and mobility problems may require urinary catheterization. Although there are important considerations concerning the potential for transmission of vCJD to others, there is no evidence to suggest that ordinary personal or clinical care contact is a risk. General universal precautions are all that are necessary. There are some publications discussing nursing aspects of prion diseases, including vCJD, and some countries have organized charitable support networks (Barnett, 2002; Weller et al., 2003; Barnett and McLean, 2005; www.cjdisa.com).

CONCLUSIONS

One important feature of prion diseases is that they vary in behavior: although scrapie in sheep does not appear to be a zoonotic risk to humans, this is not true of BSE in cattle. In addition, it may be difficult to predict the transmission characteristics and consequent public health relevance of any emerging animal prion disease; this is of particular importance given the current spread of chronic wasting disease in cervid species. The significance of precautionary protective measures is illustrated by the absence, to date, of any UK cases of vCJD in people born after 1989. A vital question about vCJD is the magnitude of asymptomatic infection in previously BSE-exposed populations and this is underlined by the present uncertainty over the meaning of the UK population appendix studies. Clinical diagnosis has been improved by the development of tests based on the specific nature of disease-related prion protein. One blood test has been found to detect presymptomatic disease, albeit in a very limited study, and this raises the possibility of screening blood donations in the future.

References

Aldhous P (1990). BSE: spongiform encephalopathy found in cat. Nature 345: 194.

Barnett F (2002). Nursing patients with variant Creutzfeldt–Jakob disease at home. Br J Community Nurs 7: 445–450.

Barnett F, McLean G (2005). Care management of Creutzfeldt–Jakob disease within the United Kingdom. J Nurs Manag 13: 111–118.

Bateman D, Hilton D, Love S et al. (1995). Sporadic Cretuzfeldt-Jakob disease in a 18-year-old in the UK. Lancet 346: 1155–1156.

Beringue V, Le Dur A, Tixador P et al. (2008). Prominent and persistent extraneural infection in human PrP transgenic mice infected with variant CJD. PLoS One 3: e1419.

Binelli S, Agazzi P, Giaccone G et al. (2006). Periodic electroencephalogram complexes in a patient with variant Creutzfeldt–Jakob disease. Ann Neurol 59: 423–427.

Bishop MT, Hart P, Aitchison L et al. (2006). Predicting susceptibility and incubation time of human-to-human transmission of vCJD. Lancet Neurol 5: 393–398.

Bishop MT, Kovacs GJ, Sanchez-Juan P et al. (2008). Cathepsin D SNP associated with increased risk of variant Creutzfeldt–Jakob Disease. BMC Medical Genetics 20089: 31.

Bishop MT, Sanchez-Juan P, Knight RS (2013). Splice site SNPs of phospholipase PLCXD3 are significantly associated with variant and sporadic Creutzfeldt–Jakob disease. BMC Med Genet 12 14 (1): 91.

Bone I, Belton L, Walker AS et al. (2008). Intraventricular pentosan polysulphate in human prion diseases: an observational study in the UK. Eur J Neurol 15: 458–464.

Bongianni M, Orru C, Groveman BR et al. (2017). Diagnosis of human prion disease using real-time quaking-induced conversion testing of olfactory mucosa and cerebrospinal fluid samples. JAMA Neurol 74: 155–162.

Bougard D, Brandel JP, Bélondrade M et al. (2016). Prion detection in the plasma of pre-symptomatic blood donors and symptomatic subjects with variant Creutzfeldt–Jakob disease. Sci Transl Med 8: 370ra182.

Brandel JP, Preece M, Brown P et al. (2003). Distribution of codon 129 genotype in human growth hormone-treated CJD patients in France and the UK. Lancet 362: 128–130.

Brandel JP, Heath CA, Head MW et al. (2009). Variant Creutzfeldt–Jakob disease in France and the United Kingdom: evidence for the same agent strain. Ann Neurol 65: 249–256.

Brandel JP, Galanaud D, Freeman L (2010). Variant or sporadic Creutzfeldt–Jakob disease? Lancet 375: 889.

Britton TC, Al-Sarraj S, Shaw C et al. (1995). Sporadic Cretuzfeldt-Jakob disease in a 16-year-old in the UK. Lancet 346: 1155.

Bruce ME, Will RG, Ironside JW (1997). Transmissions to mice indicate that 'new variant' CJD is caused by the BSE agent. Nature 389: 498–501.

Bruce ME, McConnell I, Will RG et al. (2001). Detection of variant Creutzfeldt–Jakob disease infectivity in extraneural tissues. Lancet 358: 208–209.

Cervenáková L, Goldfarb LG, Garruto R et al. (1998). Phenotype-genotype studies in kuru: implications for new variant Creutzfeldt–Jakob disease. Proc Natl Acad Sci U S A 95: 13239–13241.

Chadeau-Hyam M, Alpérovitch A (2005). Risk of variant Creutzfeldt–Jakob disease in France. Int J Epidemiol 34: 46–52.

Chazot G, Broussolle E, Lapras CL et al. (1996). New variant of Creutzfeldt–Jakob disease in a 26-year-old French man. Lancet 347: 1181.

Clewley JP, Kelly CM, Andrews N et al. (2009). Prevalence of disease related prion protein in anonymous tonsil specimens in Britain: cross sectional opportunistic survey. BMJ 338: b1442.

Collie DA, Sellar RJ, Zeidler M et al. (2001). MRI of Creutzfeldt-Jakob: imaging features and recommended MRI protocol. Clin Radiol 56: 726–739.

Collie DA, Summers DM, Sellar RJ et al. (2003). Diagnosing variant Creutzfeldt–Jakob disease with the pulvinar sign: MR imaging findings in 86 neuropathologically confirmed cases. Am J Neuroradiol 24: 1560–1569.

Collinge J, Sidle KC, Meads J et al. (1996). Molecular analysis of prion strain variation and the aetiology of 'new variant' CJD. Nature 383: 685–690.

Collinge J, Gorham M, Hudson F et al. (2009). (2009) Safety and efficacy of quinacrine in human prion disease (PRION-1 study): a patient-preference trial. Lancet Neurol 8: 334–344.

Concha-Marambio L, Pritzkow S, Moda F et al. (2016). Highly sensitive and specific detection of prions in blood of variant

Creutzfeldt–Jakob disease patients. Sci Transl Med 8: 370ra183.

Cooper JD, Bird SM (2003). Predicting incidence of variant Creutzfeldt–Jakob disease from UK dietary exposure to bovine spongiform encephalopathy for the 1940 to 1969 and post-1969 birth cohorts. Int J Epidemiol 32: 784–791.

Cooper JD, Bird SM, de Angelis D (2000). Prevalence of detectable abnormal prion protein in persons incubating vCJD: plausible incubation periods and cautious inference. J Epidemiol Biostat 5: 209–219.

Coulthart MB, Geschwind MD, Qureshi S et al. (2016). A case cluster of variant Creutzfeldt–Jakob disease linked to the kingdom of Saudi Arabia. Brain 139: 2609–2616.

Cousens SN, Vynnycky E, Zeidler M et al. (1997). Predicting the CJD epidemic in humans. Nature 385: 197–198.

Cunningham AA, Kirkwood JK, Dawson M et al. (2004). Bovine spongiform encephalopathy infectivity in greater kudu (*Tragelaphus strepsiceros*). Emerg Infect Dis 10: 1044–1049.

d'Aignaux JN, Cousens SN, Smith PG (2001). Predictability of the UK variant Creutzfeldt–Jakob disease epidemic. Science 294: 1729–1731.

de Marco MF, Linehan J, Gill ON et al. (2010). Large-scale immunohistochemical examination for lymphoreticular prion protein in tonsil specimens collected in Britain. J Pathol 222: 380–387.

Dervaux A, Vicart S, Lopes F et al. (2001). Psychiatric features of vCJD similar in France and UK. Br J Psychiatry 178: 276.

Diack AB, Ritchie D, Bishop M et al. (2012). Constant transmission properties of variant Creutzfeldt–Jakob disease in 5 countries. Emerg Infect Dis 18: 1574–1579.

Donaldson DS, Sehgal A, Rios D et al. (2016). Increased Abundance of M cells in the gut epithelium dramatically enhances oral prion disease susceptibility. PLoS Pathog 12: e1006075.

Edgeworth JA, Farmer M, Sicilia A et al. (2011). Detection of prion infection in variant Creutzfeldt-Jakob disease: a blood-based assay. Lancet 377 (9764): 487–493.

Foster JD, Parnham DW, Hunter N et al. (2001). Distribution of the prion protein in sheep terminally affected with BSE following experimental oral transmission. J Gen Virol 82: 2319–2326.

Fraser H, Bruce ME, Chree A et al. (1992). Transmission of bovine spongiform encephalopathy and scrapie to mice. J Gen Virol 73: 1891–1897.

Frosh A, Smith LC, Jackson CJ et al. (2004). Analysis of 2000 consecutive UK tonsillectomy specimens for disease-related prion protein. Lancet 364: 1260–1262.

Garske T, Ghani AC (2010). Uncertainty in the tail of the variant Creutzfeldt–Jakob disease epidemic in the UK. PLoS ONE 5: e15626.

Ghani AC, Ferguson NM, Donnelly CA et al. (2000). Predicted vCJD mortality in Great Britain. Nature 406: 583–584.

Gill ON, Spencer Y, Richard-Loendt A et al. (2013). Prevalent abnormal prion protein in human appendixes after bovine spongiform encephalopathy epizootic: large scale survey. BMJ 347: f5675.

Goodall CA, Head MW, Everington D et al. (2006). Raised CSF phospho-tau concentrations in variant Creutzfeldt–Jakob disease: diagnostic and pathological implications. J Neurol Neurosurg Psychiatry 77: 89–91.

Green AJE, Thompson EJ, Stewart GE et al. (2001). Use of 14-3-3 and other brain-specific proteins in CSF in the diagnosis of variant Creutzfeldt–Jakob disease. JNNP 70: 744–748.

Haik S, Brandel JP (2011). Biochemical and strain properties of CJD prions: complexity versus simplicity. J Neurochem 119: 251–261.

Haik S, Faucheux BA, Sazdovitch V (2003). The sympathetic nervous system is involved in variant Creutzfeldt–Jakob disease. Nat Med 9: 1121–1123.

Haik S, Peoc'h K, Brandel JP et al. (2004). Striking PrPsc heterogeneity in inherited prion diseases with the D178N mutation. Ann Neurol 56: 909–910.

Head MW, Bunn TJ, Bishop MT et al. (2004a). Prion protein heterogeneity in sporadic but not variant Creutzfeldt–Jakob disease: UK cases 1991–2002. Ann Neurol 55: 851–859.

Head MW, Ritchie D, Smith N et al. (2004b). Peripheral tissue involvement in sporadic, iatrogenic, and variant Creutzfeldt–Jakob disease: an immunohistochemical, quantitative, and biochemical study. Am J Pathol 164: 143–153.

Heath CA, Cooper SA, Murray K et al. (2010). Validation of diagnostic criteria for variant Creutzfeldt–Jakob disease. Ann Neurol 67: 761–770.

Hill AF, Desbruslais M, Joiner S et al. (1997). The same prion strain causes vCJD and BSE. Nature 389: 448–450.

Hill AF, Butterworth RJ, Joiner S et al. (1999). Investigation of variant Creutzfeldt–Jakob disease and other human prion diseases with tonsil biopsy samples. Lancet 353: 183–189.

Hilton DA, Fathers E, Edwards P et al. (1998). Prion immunoreactivity in appendix before clinical onset of variant Creutzfeldt–Jakob disease. Lancet 352: 703–704.

Hilton DA, Ghani AC, Conyers L et al. (2004). Prevalence of lymphoreticular prion protein accumulation in UK tissue samples. J Pathol 203: 733–739.

Houston F, Foster JD, Chong A et al. (2000). Transmission of BSE by blood transfusion in sheep. Lancet 356: 999–1000.

Jackson GS, Burk-Rafel J, Edgeworth JA et al. (2014). Population screening for variant CJD using a novel blood test. Diagnostic accuracy and feasibility study. JAMA Neurol 7: 421–428.

Kaski D, Mead S, Hyare H et al. (2009). Variant CJD in an individual heterozygous for PRNP codon 129. Lancet 374: 2128.

Kretzschmar HA, Sethi S, Földvári Z et al. (2003). Iatrogenic Creutzfeldt–Jakob disease with florid plaques. Brain Pathol 13: 245–249.

Lasmezas CI, Deslys JP, Demaimay R et al. (1996). BSE transmission to macaques. Nature 381: 743–744.

Lasmezas CI, Comoy E, Hawkins S et al. (2005). Risk of oral infection with bovine spongiform encephalopathy agent in primates. Lancet 365: 781–783.

Llewelyn CA, Hewitt PE, Knight RS et al. (2004). Possible transmission of variant Creutzfeldt–Jakob disease by blood transfusion. Lancet 363: 417–421.

Maheshwari A, Fischer M, Gambetti P et al. (2015). Recent US case of variant Creutzfeldt–Jakob disease – global implications. Emerg Infect Dis 21: 750–759.

Macleod MA, Stewart GE, Zeidler MI et al. (2002). Sensory features of variant Creutzfeldt–Jakob disease. J Neurol 249: 706–711.

McCutcheon S, Alejo Blanco AR, Houston EF et al. (2011). All clinically-relevant blood components transmit prion disease following a single blood transfusion: a sheep model of vCJD. PLoS One 6: e23169.

McGuire L, Peden AH, Orrú CD et al. (2012). Real time quaking-induced conversion analysis of cerebrospinal fluid in sporadic Creutzfeldt-Jakob disease. Ann Neurol 72 (2): 278–285.

McGuire L, Poleggi A, Poggiolini I et al. (2016). Cerebrospinal fluid real-time quaking-induced conversion is a robust and reliable test for sporadic Creutzfeldt-Jakob disease: An international study. Ann Neurol 80 (1): 160–165.

Mead S, Uphill J, Beck J et al. (2012). Genome-wide association study in multiple human prion diseases suggests genetic risk factors additional to PRNP. J Hum Mol Genet 21: 1897–1906.

Moda F, Gambetti P, Notari S et al. (2014). Prions in the urine of patients with variant Creutzfeldt–Jakob disease. N Engl J Med 371: 530–539.

Mok T, Jaunmuktane Z, Joiner S et al. (2017). Variant Creutzfeldt–Jakob disease in a patient with heterozygosity at PRNP codon 129. N Engl J Med 376: 292–294.

Newman PK, Todd NV, Scoones D et al. (2014). Postmortem findings in a case of variant Creutzfeldt–Jakob disease treated with intraventricular pentosan polysulfate. JNNP 85: 921–924.

Notari S, Moleres FJ, Hunter SB et al. (2010). Multiorgan detection and characterization of protease-resistant prion protein in a case of variant CJD examined in the United States. PLoS One 5: e8765.

Orru CD, Bongianni M, Tonoli G et al. (2014). A test for Creutzfeldt–Jakob disease using nasal brushings. N Engl J Med 371: 519–529.

Parchi P, Capellari S, Chen SG et al. (1997). Typing prion isoforms. Nature 386: 232–234.

Peden AH, Head MW, Ritchie DL et al. (2004). Preclinical vCJD after blood transfusion in a PRNP codon 129 heterozygous patient. Lancet 364: 527–529.

Peden A, McCardle L, Head MW et al. (2010). Variant CJD infection in the spleen of a neurologically asymptomatic UK adult patient with haemophilia. Haemophilia 16: 296–304.

Public Health England (2016). Health protection report. Summary results of the third national survey of abnormal prion prevalence in archived appendix specimens. Infection Report 10: 26.

Puoti G, Giaccone G, Rossi G et al. (1999). Sporadic Creutzfeldt–Jakob disease: co-occurrence of different types of PrP(Sc) in the same brain. Neurology 53: 2173–2176.

Ritchie DL, Boyle A, McConnell I et al. (2009). Transmissions of variant Creutzfeldt–Jakob disease from brain and lymphoreticular tissue show uniform and conserved bovine spongiform encephalopathy-related phenotypic properties on primary and secondary passage in wild-type mice. J Gen Virol 90: 3075–3082.

Sanchez-Juan P, Cousens SN, Will RG et al. (2007). Source of variant Creutzfeldt–Jakob disease outside United Kingdom. Emerg Infect Dis 13: 1166–1169.

Sanchez-Juan P, Bishop MT, Aulchenko YS et al. (2012). Genome-wide study links MTMR7 gene to variant Creutzfeldt–Jakob risk. Neurobiol Aging 33: 1487.e21–1487.e28.

Shinde A, Kunieda T, Kinoshita Y et al. (2009). The first Japanese patient with variant Creutzfeldt–Jakob disease (vCJD). Neuropathology 29: 713–719.

Shmakov AN, McLennan NF, McBride P et al. (2000). Cellular prion protein is expressed in the human enteric nervous system. Nat Med 6: 840–841.

Spencer MD, Knight RSG, Will RG (2002). First hundred cases of variant Creutzfeldt–Jakob disease: retrospective case note of early psychiatric and neurological features. BMJ 342: 1479–1482.

St. Rose SG, Hunter N, Matthews L et al. (2006). Comparative evidence for a link between Peyer's patch development and susceptibility to transmissible spongiform encephalopathies. BMC Infect Dis 6: 5.

Summers DM, Collie DA, Sellar RJ et al. (2002). The pulvinar sign and diagnosis of Creutzfeldt-Jakob disease. Neurology 59 (6): 962.

Urwin PJ, Mackenzie JM, Llewelyn CA et al. (2016). Creutzfeldt–Jakob disease and blood transfusion: updated results of the UK Transfusion Medicine Epidemiology Review Study. Vox Sang 110: 310–316.

Valleron AJ, Boelle PY, Will R et al. (2001). Estimation of epidemic size and incubation time based on age characteristics of vCJD in the United Kingdom. Science 294: 1726–1728.

Valleron AJ, Boelle PY, Chatignoux E et al. (2006). Can a second wave of new variant of the CJD be discarded in absence of observation of clinical non Met-Met cases? Rev Epidemiol Sante Publique 54: 111–115.

Wadsworth JD, Joiner S, Hill AF et al. (2001). Tissue distribution of protease resistant prion protein in variant Creutzfeldt–Jakob disease using a highly sensitive immunoblotting assay. Lancet 358: 171–180.

Ward HJ, Everington D, Cousens SN et al. (2006). Risk factors for variant Creutzfeldt–Jakob disease: a case-control study. Ann Neurol. 2006 59: 111–120.

Weller B, Knight R, Will R (2003). An overview of the care issues for Creutzfeldt–Jakob disease. Eur J Palliat Care 10: 5–8.

Wells GA, Scott AC, Johnson CT et al. (1987). A novel progressive spongiform encephalopathy in cattle. Vet Rec 121: 419–420.

Will RG, Ironside JW, Zeidler M et al. (1996). A new variant of Creutzfeldt–Jakob disease in the UK. Lancet 347: 921–925.

Will RG, Stewart G, Zeidler M et al. (1999). Psychiatric features of new variant Creutzfeldtˇ Jakob disease. Psychiatric Bull 23: 264–267.

Wroe SJ, Pal S, Siddique D et al. (2006). Clinical presentation and pre-mortem diagnosis of variant Creutzfeldt–Jakob disease associated with blood transfusion: a case report. Lancet 368: 2061–2067.

Yamada M (2006). The first Japanese case of variant Creutzfeldt–Jakob disease showing periodic electroencephalogram. Lancet 367: 874.

Zeidler M, Stewart GE, Barraclough CR et al. (1997a). New variant Creutzfeldt–Jakob disease: neurological features and diagnostic tests. Lancet 350: 903–907.

Zeidler M, Johnstone EC, Bamber RW et al. (1997b). New variant Creutzfeldt–Jakob disease: psychiatric features. Lancet 350: 908–910.

Handbook of Clinical Neurology, Vol. 153 (3rd series)
Human Prion Diseases
M. Pocchiari and J. Manson, Editors
https://doi.org/10.1016/B978-0-444-63945-5.00012-X

Chapter 12

Iatrogenic Creutzfeldt–Jakob disease

ATSUSHI KOBAYASHI[1], TETSUYUKI KITAMOTO[2], AND HIDEHIRO MIZUSAWA[3]*

[1]*Laboratory of Comparative Pathology, Graduate School of Veterinary Medicine, Hokkaido University, Kita-ku, Sapporo, Japan*

[2]*Department of Neurological Science, Tohoku University Graduate School of Medicine, Aoba-ku, Sendai, Japan*

[3]*National Center of Neurology and Psychiatry, Kodaira, Japan*

Abstract

Iatrogenic transmission of Creutzfeldt–Jakob disease (CJD) has occurred through particular medical procedures. Among them, dura mater grafts and pituitary-derived growth hormone obtained from human cadavers undiagnosed as CJD are the most frequent sources of infection. Recent advances in our knowledge about dura mater graft- and human pituitary-derived growth hormone-associated CJD patients have revealed that the combination of the infected CJD strain and the *PRNP* genotype of the patient determines their clinical, neuropathologic, and biochemical features. In this chapter, we summarize the clinical, neuropathologic, biochemical, and diagnostic features of dura mater graft- and human pituitary-derived growth hormone-associated CJD patients for the appropriate diagnosis of iatrogenic CJD.

INTRODUCTION AND BRIEF HISTORY

Iatrogenic Creutzfeldt–Jakob diseases (iCJD) represent a part of acquired prion diseases that have known sources of etiologic prions and include kuru and variant CJD as well. iCJD are defined as CJD transmitted by medical and surgical procedures.

Neurosurgical transmission was first suggested by Nevin et al. in 1960, when 3 CJD cases developed 18–24 months after neurosurgical procedures in a hospital where a few CJD patients received brain biopsy and other invasive procedures (Nevin et al., 1960). The very first case associated with a cadaveric corneal graft was reported in 1974 when the patient developed CJD 18 months after transplantation from a donor with pathologically proven CJD (Duffy et al., 1974). The second case developed CJD 30 years after transplantation and was described in 1997 (Heckmann et al., 1997). Electroencepalogram (EEG) recordings with deep needle electrodes were also reported as a transmission procedure in 2 cases of iCJD in 1977 (Bernoulli et al., 1977). This was confirmed by experimental implantation of the suspected electrodes causing CJD in a chimpanzee (Brown et al., 1992). Another case of neurosurgical transmission was reported in France in 1980 (Foncin et al., 1980).

Dura mater graft-associated iCJD (dCJD) was first reported in 1987 in the United States (CDC, 1987) and more than 200 cases have since been documented in many countries (Brown et al., 2012). Among them, more than half were registered in Japan (Sato et al., 2005; Hamaguchi et al., 2013). The number of Japanese dCJD patients reached 152 by August 2017. In other countries, the numbers of patients ranged from 1 to 14 (Clavel and Clavel, 1996; Brooke et al., 2004; Heath et al., 2006; Toovey et al., 2006; Heinemann et al., 2007; Kim et al., 2011; Brandel et al., 2013; Hall et al., 2014). The source of cadaveric dura mater in most cases when identified was Lyodura produced by B. Broun Melsungen. Two other sources include 1 case of Tutoplast dura (Hannah et al., 2001) and another case of locally produced dura.

In 1996 when the first case of variant CJD case was reported, the Japanese Government conducted a nationwide survey that unexpectedly revealed many CJD cases with cadaveric dura grafting. After two more nationwide

*Correspondence to: Hidehiro Mizusawa, National Center Hospital, National Center of Neurology and Psychiatry, 4-1-1 Ogawa-higashi-machi, Kodaira, 187–8511, Japan. Tel: +81-42-346-1780, E-mail: mizusawa@ncnp.go.jp

surveys a prospective survey was carried out for all the cases of prion diseases including dCJD (Sato et al., 2005; Nozaki et al., 2010). Analysis of the 152 dCJD cases in Japan revealed etiologic diseases, including tumor, bleeding, unruptured aneurysms, hematoma, hemifacial spasm, trigeminal neuralgia, malformation, trauma, and ossification of the posterior longitudinal ligament, as reported previously (Nozaki et al., 2010; Hamaguchi et al., 2013). Grafting was performed very frequently from 1982 to 1987 when the first case of dCJD was reported in the United States and 1N NaOH treatment had been added to the sterilization process of cadaveric dura mater (Sato et al., 2005).

In 1985, 2 CJD cases that had received human pituitary-derived growth hormone (hGH) in the United States and 1 such case in the United Kingdom were reported (Gibbs et al., 1985; Koch et al., 1985; Powel-Jackson et al., 1985). Since then, by 2012, 226 cases had accumulated from many countries, mostly in France (119 cases/1170 recipients, 10.2%), the United Kingdom (65 cases/1800 recipients, 3.6%), and the United States (29 cases/2700 recipients, 1.1%) (Brown et al., 2012). There were only one or a few cases in other countries, including New Zealand, Brazil, the Netherlands, Australia, Ireland, and Qatar.

The circumstantial evidence of cadaveric hGH transmission to humans is a unique clinical feature of patients, which include unusually young age at onset with progressive cerebellar syndrome with only delayed dementia, if any, as compared with typical sporadic CJD (sCJD) which is characterized by old age at onset with rapidly progressive dementia (Will, 2003; Rudge et al., 2015). The evidence was supported by successful transmission of CJD in a squirrel monkey with a potentially contaminated batch of hGH (Gibbs et al., 1993).

CLINICAL FEATURES

Dura mater graft-associated CJD (dCJD)

The age at onset ranged from the second to ninth decade of life with mean age at onset of 56.0 ± 14.9 years, which is more than 10 years younger than that of sCJD. The incubation time was 13.4 ± 6.7 years (1–30 years and 11 months). Neuropathologic analyses of 23 dCJD cases showed there are two types: plaque and nonplaque types (Noguchi-Shinohara et al., 2007). Plaque-type dCJD has a plaque-type deposition of abnormal prion protein (PrP^{TSE}) which sometimes resembles the florid plaques found in variant CJD (Shimizu et al., 1999). Nonplaque-type dCJD was pathologically characterized by spongiform encephalopathy similar to that of the sCJD MM/MV1 subtype. The relative frequency of plaque-type dCJD is estimated to be about 30–40% and nonplaque-type about 60–70% in Japan.

The clinical and laboratory features of plaque-type dCJD include onset with progressive gait disturbance, mainly ataxia, a relatively long clinical course, and no or late occurrence of periodic sharp-wave complexes (PSWCs) on EEG. In contrast, clinical and laboratory features of nonplaque-type dCJD are similar to those of sCJD MM/MV1 subtype. High signal intensity of diffusion-weighted imaging (DWI) on magnetic resonance imaging (MRI) and positive 14-3-3 protein of CSF are common features in both plaque and nonplaque types of dCJD. DWI high signal intensity in the thalamus may be a characteristic of plaque-type dCJD in addition to that in the striatum and cerebral cortices (Fig. 12.1). The clinical features of plaque-type dCJD are diagnostic challenge in cases with progressive ataxia in human cadaveric dura mater recipients which could be diagnosed as probable dCJD.

Human pituitary-derived growth hormone-associated CJD (hGH CJD)

The mean incubation period of all available cases was estimated to be 17 (5–42) years based on the midpoint date as the date of infection because, usually, the treatment periods ranged over many years. There are some differences among countries with many hGH CJD cases; the mean incubation period is 13 years in France, 20 years in the United Kingdom, and 22 years in the United States (Huillard d'Aignaux et al., 1999; Swerdlow et al., 2003). The shorter period in France may result from the narrower limit of infection date and is close to the 13.5 years of 4 CJD patients who received human gonadotropin in Australia. This is also similar to the 13.4 years of dCJD. A recent study on the incubation periods of UK cases related to the codon 129 polymorphism described 30.8 (26.9–32.6) years in 129 M/M homozygotes, 23.4 (9.0–36.7) years in 129 M/V heterozygotes, and 14.3 (7.7–20.2) years in 129 V/V homozygotes (Rudge et al., 2015).

Clinically, ataxic gait is the most common initial symptom followed by tremor, leg pain, daytime somnolence, dizziness, headache, myoclonus, and cognitive impairment (Will, 2003; Rudge et al., 2015). Rarely, cognitive decline appears at an early stage (Cordery et al., 2003). The leg pain includes hypersensitivity to light touch and various dysesthesia, such as itchy sensation, patchy tingling, burning, and numbness. Neurologic findings include cerebellar ataxic gait, myoclonus, cerebellar dysarthria, pyramidal tract sign, cognitive impairment, urine and fecal incontinence, and finally akinetic mutism.

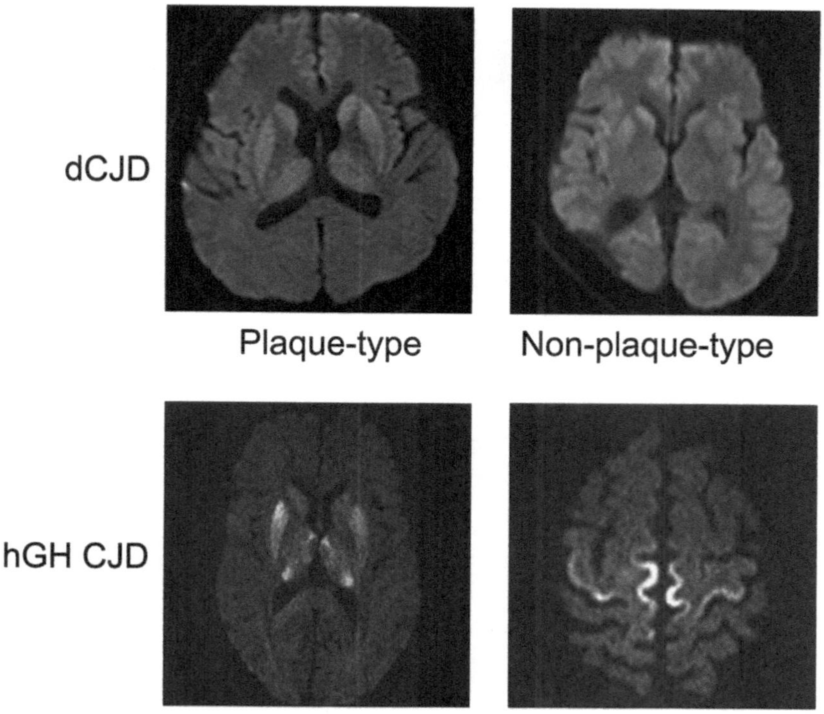

Fig. 12.1. Magnetic resonance imaging (MRI)-diffusion-weighted imaging (DWI) of dura mater graft-associated iatrogenic Creutzfeldt–Jakob disease (dCJD) and human growth hormone (hGH) CJD. More thalamic hyperintensity on MRI-DWI may be a characteristic of plaque-type dCJD. (Courtesy of Dr. Yoshihisa Watanabe.) In addition to cerebral cortical involvement, hyperintensities of the basal ganglia and thalamus in hGH CJD resemble those in plaque-type dCJD. (Courtesy of Dr. Harpreet Hyare and Dr. Peter Rudge.)

Among 21 patients, 6 showed normal EEG initially and the other 15 showed generalized slow activity. Only one of the 15 revealed short runs of PSWCs (Rudge et al., 2015). On MRI DWI, high signal intensity was observed in the thalamus, caudate nucleus, and putamen in most cases (Fig. 12.1). In the cerebral cortex, the cingulate gyrus, frontal gyrus, and cerebellum were also frequently affected and the paracentral lobule, parietal lobe, and hippocampus were less frequently involved (Lewis et al., 2006; Appleby et al., 2013; Rudge et al., 2015).

NEUROPATHOLOGIC FEATURES

dCJD

The neuropathologic features of dCJD patients are not uniform, as mentioned above. In Japan, 68% of dCJD patients show the synaptic-type deposition of PrP^{TSE} in the brain similar to that of patients with the sCJD MM/MV1 subtype, and are designated as nonplaque-type dCJD, while 32% of dCJD patients show PrP^{TSE} amyloid plaques similar to those of patients with the sCJD MV2 subtype and are designated as plaque-type dCJD (Fig. 12.2) (Takashima et al., 1997; Shimizu et al., 1999; Hoshi et al., 2000; Kimura et al., 2001; Mochizuki et al., 2003; Satoh et al., 2003; Noguchi-Shinohara et al., 2007; Yamada et al., 2009). The neuropathologic features of the nonplaque-type dCJD patients resemble those of the sCJD MM/MV1 subtype, including severe brain atrophy, spongiform changes, neuronal loss, astrocytic gliosis, and diffuse synaptic-type PrP^{TSE} deposition in the cerebral and cerebellar gray matter (Satoh et al., 2003; Yamada et al., 2009). In contrast, the neuropathologic features of plaque-type dCJD patients are characterized by mild brain atrophy, perineuronal PrP^{TSE} deposition, and PrP^{TSE} amyloid plaques, in addition to spongiform changes, neuronal loss, and gliosis (Satoh et al., 2003; Yamada et al., 2009). The PrP^{TSE} amyloid plaques are widely distributed over the cerebral gray matter, the cerebellar gray matter, and the cerebellar white matter. Some PrP^{TSE} amyloid plaques are surrounded by vacuoles, resembling the florid plaques of variant CJD (Shimizu et al., 1999; Mochizuki et al., 2003; Yamada et al., 2009). The two subgroups of dCJD have also been recognized in European countries and the United States (Lane et al., 1994; Kopp et al., 1996; Radbauer et al., 1998; Kretzschmar et al., 2003).

The reason for the existence of the two neuropathologically distinct subgroups of dCJD has remained elusive for years. However, recent advances in our knowledge of

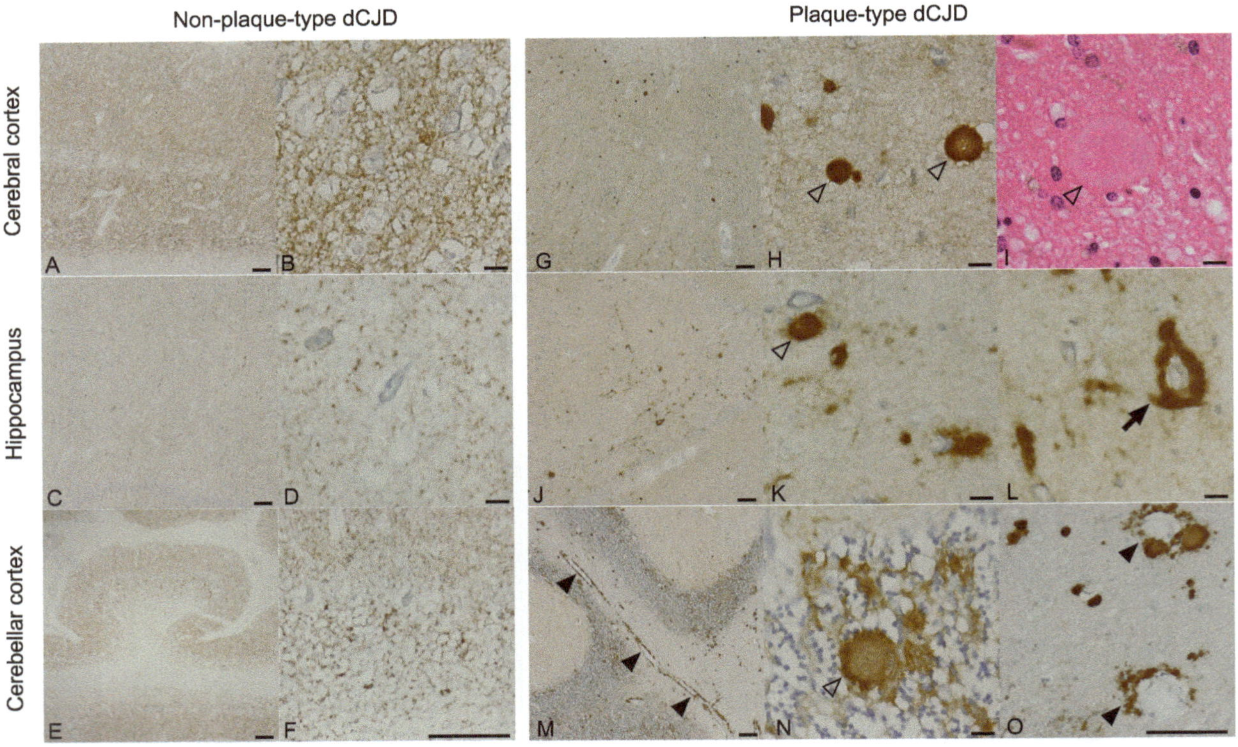

Fig. 12.2. Neuropathologic features of nonplaque-type dura mater graft-associated iatrogenic Creutzfeldt–Jakob disease (dCJD) and plaque-type dCJD. (**A–F**) Nonplaque-type dCJD patients show fine granular to diffuse synaptic-type deposition of PrP^{TSE} in the cerebral gray matter (**A**, **B**), hippocampus (**C**, **D**), and cerebellar gray matter (**E**, **F**). (**G-O**) Plaque-type dCJD patients show large PrP^{TSE} amyloid plaques (**H**, **I**, **K**, **N**: open arrowheads) and perineuronal PrP^{TSE} deposition (**L**: arrow) besides the synaptic-type PrP^{TSE} deposition (Lane et al., 1994; Kopp et al., 1996; Takashima et al., 1997; Radbauer et al., 1998; Shimizu et al., 1999; Hoshi et al., 2000; Kimura et al., 2001; Kretzschmar et al., 2003; Mochizuki et al., 2003; Satoh et al., 2003; Noguchi-Shinohara et al., 2007; Yamada et al., 2009). In the cerebellum, the formation of PrP^{TSE} amyloid plaques is most prominent in the granular cell layer (**M**, **N**). In addition, perivascular PrP^{TSE} deposition is remarkable in the cerebellar white matter (**M**, **O**: filled arrowheads). Immunohistochemical analysis of PrP (**A–H**, **J–O**); hematoxylin and eosin stain (**I**). Scale bars, 100 μm (**A**, **C**, **E**, **F**, **G**, **J**, **M**, **O**); 10 μm (**B**, **D**, **H**, **I**, **K**, **L**, **N**).

dCJD patients and those gained from experimental animal models of iCJD have raised the possibility that the distinct neuropathologic features might be caused by different sCJD strains (Kobayashi et al., 2007, 2009, 2014). To date, five sCJD strains have been proposed according to the disease phenotypes in patients and their transmission properties in transgenic mice expressing human prion protein (PrP), namely M1 (MM1/MV1 subtype, which corresponds to 40% of total sCJD cases), V1 (VV1 subtype, ~1%), M2C (MM2C subtype, ~1%), M2T (MM2T subtype, ~1%), and V2 (VV2 and MV2 subtypes, 23%) (Parchi et al., 1999, 2011; Bishop et al., 2010; Moda et al., 2012). In addition, the co-occurrence of distinct prion strains in the same patient such as M1+M2C (MM/MV1+2C subtype, which corresponds to 28% of total sCJD cases) has been recognized (Parchi et al., 2011). In experimental animal models of iCJD, infection with the M1 strain or the co-occurring M1+M2C strains caused synaptic-type PrP^{TSE} deposition in the brain similar to that of nonplaque-type dCJD patients, while infection with the V2 strain caused plaque-type PrP^{TSE} deposition similar to that of plaque-type dCJD patients (Fig. 12.3) (Kobayashi et al., 2007, 2013, 2016). Interestingly, mice inoculated with the M1 strain or the co-occurring M1 +M2C strains showed the synaptic-type PrP^{TSE} deposition regardless of their genotype at polymorphic (methionine, M or valine, V) codon 129 of the *PRNP* gene, whereas the V2 strain-inoculated mice showed various amounts of PrP^{TSE} plaques depending on their *PRNP* codon 129 genotype, i.e., mice carrying the 129 M/M genotype showed numerous PrP^{TSE} plaques but mice carrying the 129 V/V or M/V genotype showed only a small number of PrP^{TSE} plaques (Kobayashi et al., 2013, 2015a). Indeed, all plaque-type dCJD cases reported to date were 129 M/M homozygotes not only in Japan, where the vast majority of the general population are 129 M/M homozygotes, but also in European countries (Kopp et al., 1996; Kretzschmar et al., 2003; Yamada et al., 2009; Nozaki et al., 2010). Further

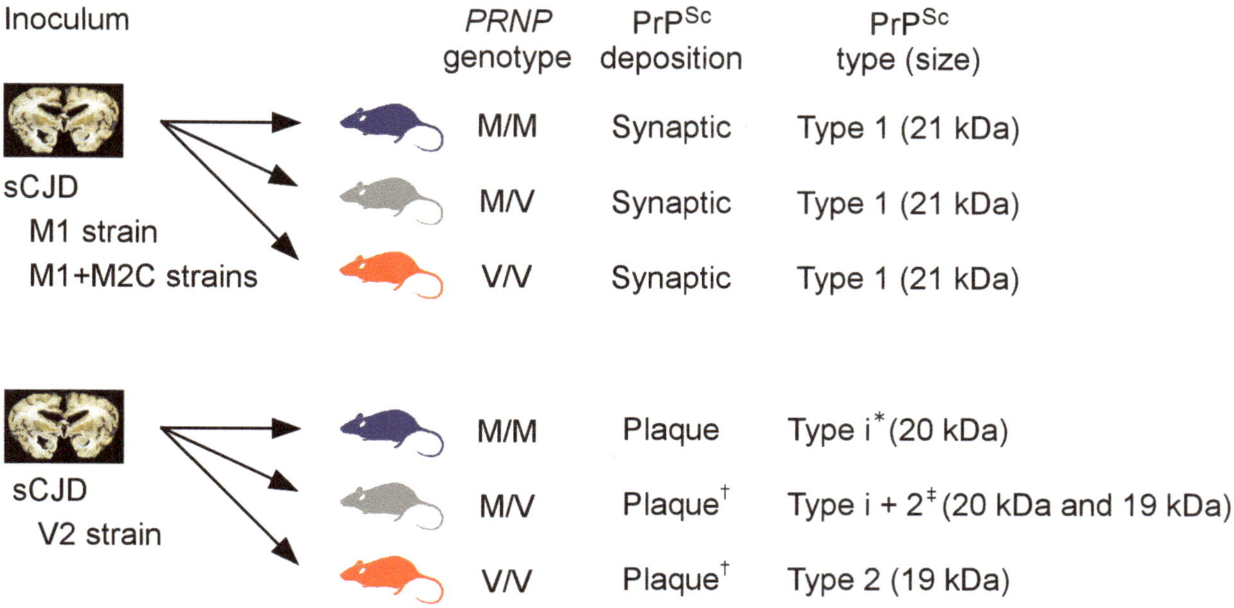

Fig. 12.3. Experimental animal models of iatrogenic Creutzfeldt–Jakob disease (CJD). To model the iatrogenic transmission of sporadic CJD (sCJD) prions, knockin mice expressing human prion protein (PrP) with the 129 M/M, M/V, or V/V genotype were intracerebrally challenged with the representative sCJD strains. Mice inoculated with the M1 sCJD strain or co-occurring M1 +M2C strains showed synaptic-type PrP^{TSE} deposition and type 1 PrP^{TSE} accumulation in the brain regardless of their *PRNP* codon 129 genotype. Meanwhile, mice inoculated with the V2 sCJD strain showed diverse neuropathologic and biochemical features depending on the codon 129 genotype (Kobayashi et al., 2007, 2013, 2016). *Intermediate-type PrP^{TSE}. †The number and distribution of PrP^{TSE} plaques were relatively limited. ‡A mixture of the intermediate-type and type 2 PrP^{TSE}.

neuropathologic analysis of dCJD patients with the 129 V/V or M/V genotype will be needed in the future to clarify whether they show the two distinct neuropathologic features similar to those of the 129 M/M patients.

Meanwhile, similarities in transmissibility to experimental animals (Kobayashi et al., 2007, 2010, 2013, 2015a) or in seeding activity in protein misfolding cyclic amplification (Takeuchi et al., 2016a) among the M1 sCJD strain, the co-occurring M1+M2C sCJD strains, and brain materials from nonplaque-type dCJD patients, or between the V2 sCJD strain and brain materials from plaque-type dCJD patients, also support the possibility that the two distinct subgroups of dCJD might be caused by infection with different sCJD strains. The similar transmissibility between the M1 sCJD strain and the co-occurring M1+M2C strains has been considered to be due to the reduced infectivity of the M2C sCJD strain (Kobayashi et al., 2013, 2016).

Furthermore, it is noteworthy that the ratio of the nonplaque-type dCJD among total dCJD cases in Japan is quite similar to the combined ratio of the sCJD MM/MV1 subtype (M1 strain) and the sCJD MM/MV1 +2C subtype (co-occurring M1+M2C strains) among total sCJD cases in Europe where the causative dura mater grafts were prepared. Meanwhile, the ratio of the plaque-type dCJD among total dCJD cases is similar to the combined ratio of the sCJD VV2 and MV2 subtypes (V2 strain) among total sCJD cases (Yamada et al., 2009; Parchi et al., 2011; Kobayashi et al., 2016). During 1983–1987, when ~80% of dCJD patients underwent dura mater transplantation, as many as 100,000 patches were used in Japan (Nakamura et al., 1999; Hamaguchi et al., 2013). Thus, a portion of these grafts might have been contaminated with more than one sCJD strain, reflecting the existing ratio of the sCJD subtypes in donors.

Taken together, accumulating evidence suggests that infection with the M1 sCJD strain or the co-occurring M1+M2C sCJD strains might be responsible for the dCJD subgroup that shows the synaptic-type PrP^{TSE} deposition, whereas infection with the V2 sCJD strain might be responsible for the dCJD subgroup that shows the plaque-type PrP^{TSE} deposition.

hGH CJD

hGH CJD patients can also be divided into two subgroups based on their neuropathologic features, presumably reflecting the neuropathologic properties of the infected sCJD strains (Cali et al., 2015), as suggested in dCJD. One subgroup showed neuropathologic features resembling those of the nonplaque-type dCJD or sCJD MM/MV1 subtype, whereas the other subgroup showed characteristic features resembling those of the plaque-type dCJD (Delisle et al., 1993;

Billette de Villemeur et al., 1994; Croes et al., 2002; Cali et al., 2015). In contrast to dCJD, however, the majority of hGH CJD cases showed the plaque-type pathology and appeared to have been caused by infection with the V2 sCJD strain (Rudge et al., 2015; Head et al., 2016; Peckeu et al., 2016; Ritchie et al., 2016). In pathologically examined French hGH CJD cases, all 129 M/M patients and half of the 129 M/V patients showed PrP^{TSE} amyloid plaques in the brain (Billette de Villemeur et al., 1994; Peckeu et al., 2016). In the UK cases, 3 out of 4 129 M/M patients and all 129 M/V patients had PrP^{TSE} amyloid plaques (Rudge et al., 2015; Moore et al., 2016; Ritchie et al., 2016). Thus, a large number of hGH CJD patients showed PrP^{TSE} amyloid plaques that were indicative of infection with the V2 sCJD strain.

In addition, although hGH CJD patients with the 129 V/V genotype lacked PrP^{TSE} amyloid plaques and showed only perineuronal and plaque-like PrP^{TSE} deposits (Peckeu et al., 2016; Ritchie et al., 2016), the scarcity of PrP^{TSE} amyloid plaques in the 129 V/V patients cannot exclude the possibility of infection with the V2 sCJD strain because the V2 sCJD strain-infected 129 V/V mice showed only a small number of PrP^{TSE} plaques compared with the 129 M/M mice in experimental transmission studies, as described above (Fig. 12.3) (Kobayashi et al., 2007, 2013, 2015a), and sCJD VV2 patients show only perineuronal and plaque-like PrP^{TSE} deposits (Parchi et al., 1999, 2011). In fact, the biochemical features of the 129 V/V hGH CJD patients (Collinge et al., 1996; Head et al., 2016; Ritchie et al., 2016) also support the possibility of infection with the V2 sCJD strain, as described below.

Furthermore, similarities in the seeding activity in protein misfolding cyclic amplification between the V2 sCJD strain and brain materials from hGH CJD patients with PrP^{TSE} amyloid plaques or plaque-like PrP^{TSE} deposits also suggested that these hGH CJD cases might have been infected with the V2 sCJD strain (Ritchie et al., 2016; Takeuchi et al., 2016b). On the other hand, the number of patients infected with the M1 sCJD strain or the co-occurring M1+M2C sCJD strains and showing only synaptic-type PrP^{TSE} deposition appeared to be limited in hGH CJD compared with dCJD (Rudge et al., 2015; Head et al., 2016; Peckeu et al., 2016; Ritchie et al., 2016).

It has been estimated that ~400,000 pituitary glands were used to treat 1848 patients from 1959 to 1985 in the United Kingdom (Swerdlow et al., 2003). UK mortality data indicate that 1 in 7000 deaths could have been due to sCJD in the 1970s (Rudge et al., 2015). Therefore, a portion of these pituitary glands are considered to have been contaminated with more than one sCJD strain, reflecting the existing ratio of the sCJD subtypes in donors, as were cadaveric dura mater grafts that caused dCJD. Nevertheless, in hGH CJD, the V2 sCJD strain-originated subgroup has been overrepresented, whereas the M1 sCJD strain-originated subgroup has been underrepresented. Since the routes of prion infection were different between hGH CJD cases and dCJD cases, i.e., intramusucular or subcutaneous administration vs. intracerebral administration, these data raise the possibility that the M1 sCJD strain might infect less efficiently than the V2 sCJD strain through peripheral routes.

Taken together, infection with the M1 sCJD strain or the co-occurring M1+M2C sCJD strains might be responsible for the hGH CJD subgroup showing the synaptic-type PrP^{TSE} deposition, whereas infection with the V2 sCJD strain might be responsible for the hGH CJD subgroup showing the plaque-type PrP^{TSE} deposition, similar to the two subgroups of dCJD. However, the proportion of the subgroup originating from the V2 sCJD strain compared to that originating from the M1 sCJD strain seems to be higher in hGH CJD than in dCJD.

BIOCHEMICAL FEATURES

dCJD

The biochemical features of dCJD patients are also variable, probably reflecting the heterogeneity of the infected sCJD strains. In Japanese dCJD patients, who were almost entirely 129 M/M homozygotes, the nonplaque-type dCJD cases had type 1 (21 kDa) PrP^{TSE} (according to Parchi's classification of PrP^{TSE}: Parchi et al., 1999), whereas the plaque-type dCJD cases had the unusual type (20 kDa) of PrP^{TSE} that were intermediate between type 1 and type 2 (19 kDa) PrP^{TSE} and were therefore designated as the intermediate type (type i PrP^{TSE}) (Fig. 12.4) (Kobayashi et al., 2007). The i PrP^{TSE} type has also been reported in a German plaque-type dCJD patient carrying the 129 M/M genotype (Kretzschmar et al., 2003). Thus, not only the neuropathologic features but also the biochemical features of dCJD patients might be determined by the infected sCJD strain. In fact, in experimental animal models of iCJD, infection with the M1 sCJD strain or the co-occurring M1+M2C sCJD strains caused type 1 PrP^{TSE} accumulation in the brain regardless of the host *PRNP* codon 129 genotype, whereas infection with the V2 sCJD strain caused type i PrP^{TSE} accumulation in the 129 M/M mice, type 2 PrP^{TSE} accumulation in the 129 V/V mice, and a mixture of type i and type 2 PrP^{TSE} accumulation in the 129 M/V mice (Fig. 12.3) (Kobayashi et al., 2007, 2013, 2016). Thus, these experimental data indicate that the dCJD subgroup originating from the M1 sCJD strain might show type 1 PrP^{TSE} accumulation regardless of the host *PRNP* codon 129 genotype, whereas that originating from the V2 sCJD strain might show type i and/or type 2 PrP^{TSE} accumulation depending on the host *PRNP*

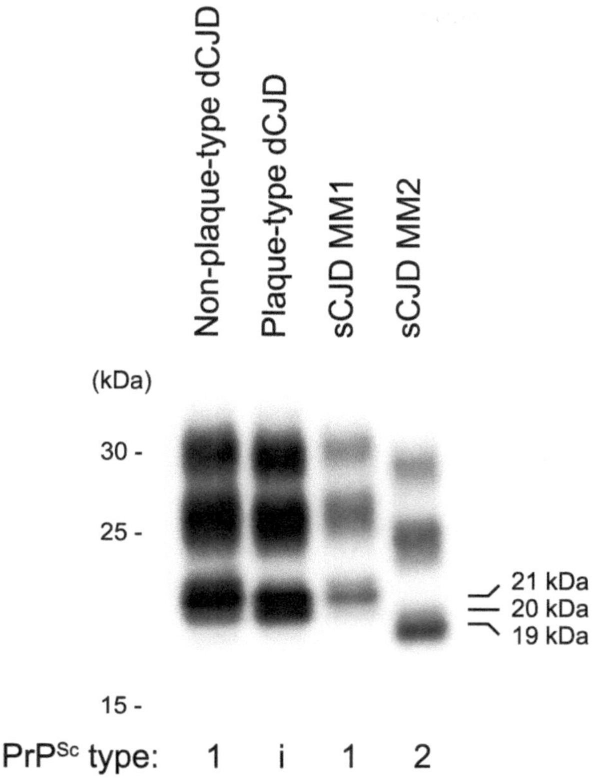

Fig. 12.4. Biochemical features of non-plaque-type dura mater graft-associated iatrogenic Creutzfeldt–Jakob disease (dCJD) and plaque-type dCJD. Western blot analysis of protease-resistant PrP^{TSE} reveals type 1 (21 kDa) PrP^{TSE} accumulation in the brain of nonplaque-type dCJD patients with the 129 M/M genotype. Meanwhile, plaque-type dCJD patients with the 129 M/M genotype show the intermediate type (type i, 20 kDa) PrP^{TSE} located between type 1 and type 2 (19 kDa) PrP^{TSE} (Kobayashi et al., 2007). *sCJD*, sporadic CJD.

codon 129 genotype. To confirm this possibility, further biochemical analysis of dCJD patients with the 129 V/V or M/V genotype will be required. At present, analysis of a limited number of nonplaque-type dCJD patients, i.e., the dCJD subgroup originating from the M1 sCJD strain, carrying the 129 V/V or M/V genotype, has shown type 1 PrP^{TSE} accumulation in the brain (Jansen et al., 2012).

hGH CJD

The biochemical features of hGH CJD patients were not investigated so much until recently compared with those of dCJD patients. It has been reported that hGH CJD patients with the 129 M/M genotype showed type 1 PrP^{TSE} accumulation, while patients with the 129 V/V or M/V genotype showed type 2 PrP^{TSE} accumulation (Collinge et al., 1996; Jansen et al., 2012; Cali et al., 2015; Rudge et al., 2015; Peckeu et al., 2016).

A recent sophisticated analysis of hGH CJD patients in the United Kingdom has shown that the biochemical features of hGH CJD patients are as variable as those of dCJD patients, reflecting the diversity of the infected sCJD strains (Ritchie et al., 2016). In the 21 UK hGH CJD cases examined, 1 129 M/M patient had type 1 PrP^{TSE}, 1 129 M/M patient had type i PrP^{TSE}, 12 129 M/V patients had a mixture of type i and type 2 PrP^{TSE}, and 7 129 V/V patients had type 2 PrP^{TSE} in the brain. The accumulation of type 1 PrP^{TSE} is indicative of infection with the M1 sCJD strain, whereas that of type i and/or type 2 PrP^{TSE} is indicative of infection with the V2 sCJD strain, as described above. Thus, the biochemical properties of the hGH CJD patients also suggest that the proportion of the subgroup originating from the V2 sCJD strain compared to that originating from the M1 sCJD strain is higher in hGH CJD than in dCJD. Of note, the 129 M/M hGH CJD patients reported to date to have had type 1 PrP^{TSE} were neuropathologically divided into two subgroups, showing the synaptic-type PrP^{TSE} deposition or PrP^{TSE} amyloid plaques (Cali et al., 2015; Rudge et al., 2015). Further studies will be required to determine whether these 129 M/M hGH patients with PrP^{TSE} amyloid plaques might have actually had type i PrP^{TSE}. It is noteworthy that type i PrP^{TSE} in plaque-type dCJD patients had long been confused with type 1 until stringent protease conditions and long gel electrophoresis were introduced for the PrP^{TSE} typing (Notari et al., 2004, 2007). In addition, analysis of the carboxyl-terminal PrP^{TSE} fragments may help to distinguish type i PrP^{TSE} from type 1 PrP^{TSE} (Kobayashi et al., 2015a).

BIOMARKERS

Several biomarkers for CSF tests are available for the clinical diagnosis of iCJD as well as sCJD. These markers include 14-3-3 protein, tau protein, and disease-associated PrP (Sanchez-Juan et al., 2006; Atarashi et al., 2011).

The sensitivity of 14-3-3 tests for the detection of dCJD is similar to that of sCJD. In Japan, the positive rates for 14-3-3 tests were 83% in dCJD and 87% in sCJD (Nozaki et al., 2010). It is noteworthy that the positive rate of the plaque-type dCJD patients (50%) was lower than that of the nonplaque-type dCJD patients (88%) (Yamada et al., 2009). The lower sensitivity of the 14-3-3 tests in Japanese plaque-type dCJD cases might be related to its lowest sensitivity in the sCJD MV2 subtype (30–76%) among the sCJD subtypes (Zerr et al., 2000; Castellani et al., 2004; Sanchez-Juan et al., 2006; Heinemann et al., 2007). Indeed, the plaque-type dCJD and sCJD MV2 subtype share common features such as slow progression of the disease, the lack or late occurrence of PSWCs on EEG, mild brain atrophy, PrP^{TSE} amyloid plaques, and type i PrP^{TSE}

accumulation in the brain (Parchi et al., 1999; Notari et al., 2004; Kobayashi et al., 2007, 2013; Noguchi-Shinohara et al., 2007; Yamada et al., 2009). Similarly, the sensitivity of the 14-3-3 tests in the hGH CJD cases in European countries appeared to be lower than that in sCJD cases. The positive rate of the 14-3-3 tests was 85% in European sCJD cases (Sanchez-Juan et al., 2006), whereas in hGH CJD cases it dropped to 43–70% (Brandel et al., 2001; Rudge et al., 2015). Since plaque-type dCJD and the majority of hGH CJD cases can be considered to have been caused by infection with the V2 sCJD strain, these data indicate that the sensitivity of 14-3-3 tests for the detection of the iCJD subgroup originating from the V2 sCJD strain might be relatively low compared with that originating from the M1 sCJD strain. To test this possibility, further studies with a larger number of iCJD patients will be needed.

Meanwhile, the sensitivity of tau tests for the detection of iCJD was also lower than that for sCJD in European countries, though it was not specified whether the iCJD cases were hGH CJD or dCJD. The positive rates of tau tests were 53% in iCJD and 86% in sCJD (Sanchez-Juan et al., 2006). Of note, the sensitivity of tau tests was also the lowest in the sCJD MV2 subtype (53%) among the sCJD subtypes (Sanchez-Juan et al., 2006). Therefore, these data may indicate that the sensitivity of the tau tests for detection of the iCJD subgroup originating from the V2 sCJD strain might also be relatively low compared with that originating from the M1 sCJD strain.

Detection of the disease-associated PrP in CSF by real-time quaking-induced conversion (RT-QuIC) has also been reported in iCJD as well as sCJD (Atarashi et al., 2011; Ritchie et al., 2016). The sensitivity of the RT-QuIC assay was not significantly different between the iCJD subgroup originating from the M1 sCJD strain and that originating from the V2 sCJD strain. This finding is compatible with reports that the sensitivity of RT-QuIC assay was not significantly different between the M1 sCJD strain and the V2 sCJD strain (Atarashi et al., 2011; McGuire et al., 2012; Peden et al., 2012). Since only a limited number of iCJD patients have so far been examined using the RT-QuIC assay, further studies will be needed to confirm the usefulness of this assay for the diagnosis of iCJD.

GENOTYPE

dCJD

There are two nonpathogenic polymorphisms in the *PRNP* gene: methionine (M) or valine (V) at codon 129, and glutamic acid (E) or lysine (K) at codon 219. In Japan, almost all dCJD patients were 129 M/M homozygotes, reflecting the predominance of this genotype in

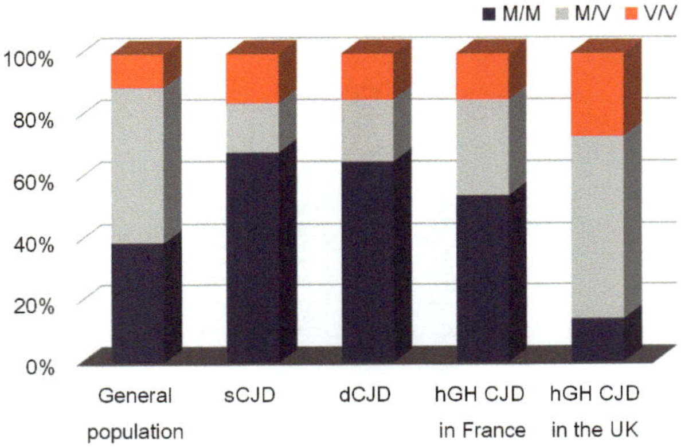

Fig. 12.5. Distribution of the genotypes at polymorphic codon 129 of the *PRNP* gene. In European sporadic Creutzfeldt–Jakob disease (sCJD) cases, 129 M/M homozygotes and 129 V/V homozygotes have been overrepresented compared with the general population (Alperovitch et al., 1999; Brandel et al., 2003). Meanwhile, 129 M/V heterozygotes have been underrepresented in European sCJD cases, suggesting protective effects of this genotype against CJD (Palmer et al., 1991; Laplanche et al., 1994; Salvatore et al., 1994; Windl et al., 1996; Kobayashi et al., 2015b). A similar genotypic distribution has been recognized in dura mater graft-associated iatrogenic CJD (dCJD) cases in countries other than Japan and human growth hormone (hGH) CJD cases in France (Brown et al., 2012). In contrast, in hGH CJD cases in the United Kingdom, 129 V/V homozygotes have been overrepresented, whereas 129 M/M homozygotes have been underrepresented (Brandel et al., 2003; Rudge et al., 2015).

the general population (Doh-ura et al., 1991; Nozaki et al., 2010; Kobayashi et al., 2015b). In dCJD patients in countries other than Japan, 129 M/M homozygotes and 129 V/V homozygotes have been overrepresented, whereas 129 M/V heterozygotes have been underrepresented (Fig. 12.5) (Brown et al., 2012). This pattern of genotypic distribution is quite similar to that of sCJD patients (Palmer et al., 1991; Laplanche et al., 1994; Salvatore et al., 1994; Windl et al., 1996). Therefore, the 129M/V heterozygosity might confer partial resistance against dCJD as well as against sCJD (Kobayashi et al, 2015b). It has not been examined so far whether the dCJD subgroup originating from the M1 sCJD strain and that originating from the V2 sCJD strain show the distinct predispositions of the *PRNP* codon 129 genotypes. It is noteworthy that 219 E/K heterozygosity is not protective against dCJD originating from the M1 sCJD strain (Kobayashi et al., 2015b), though this genotype confers resistance against the development of sCJD (Shibuya et al., 1998).

hGH CJD

In hGH CJD patients in France and the United States, 129 M/M homozygotes and 129 V/V homozygotes have been overrepresented, whereas 129 M/V heterozygotes have been underrepresented (Fig. 12.5) (Brandel et al., 2003; Brown et al., 2012). In addition, these 129M/V heterozygous patients showed significantly longer incubation periods than the homozygous patients (d'Aignaux et al., 1999). Thus, the 129M/V heterozygosity might confer partial resistance against hGH CJD, as well.

On the other hand, hGH CJD patients in the United Kingdom showed a distinct pattern in the *PRNP* genotypic distribution. In the United Kingdom, 129 V/V homozygotes have been overrepresented, whereas 129 M/M homozygotes have been underrepresented (Fig. 12.5). The reason for the different *PRNP* genotypic distribution in the United Kingdom has remained elusive. It may be explained by contamination with a high titer of the V2 sCJD strain in hGH used in the United Kingdom or by successful screening of donors particularly showing the typical CJD features, i.e., the M1 sCJD strain-associated features (Rudge et al., 2015).

Of note, both in France and the United Kingdom, hGH cases with the 129 V/V genotype occurred earlier than 129 M/M or M/V cases (Brandel et al., 2003; Brown et al., 2012; Rudge et al., 2015). In the initial study of French and UK patients, 22 or 52% were 129 V/V homozygotes (Brandel et al., 2003). However, the number of 129 V/V cases did not increase thereafter, except for one UK case, whereas the number of 129 M/M and M/V cases increased in subsequent studies (Brown et al., 2012; Rudge et al., 2015). These epidemiologic data are compatible with the experimental finding that the V2 sCJD strain-inoculated 129 V/V mice showed shorter incubation periods than the 129 M/M or M/V mice (Kobayashi et al., 2013). The effects of the *PRNP* codon 219 genotypes on the susceptibility to hGH CJD have remained unknown because the polymorphism at codon 219 is found only in Asian and Pacific populations.

CONCLUDING REMARKS

Recent progress in the study of dCJD and hGH CJD has revealed that the combination of the infected sCJD strain and the *PRNP* genotype of the patient determines the clinical, neuropathologic, and biochemical features. As the characteristic features of the V2 sCJD strain-originated subgroup could help to identify iCJD cases among presumed sporadic cases (Kobayashi et al., 2015a), the possibility of iatrogenic infection should be carefully considered in CJD patients showing atypical clinicopathologic and biochemical features.

ACKNOWLEDGMENTS

We thank Brent Bell for critical review of the manuscript. The surveillance on CJD has been supported by Grants-in-Aid from the Ministry of Health, Labor and Welfare of Japan (TK and HM), and the experimental transmission study of iCJD was supported by Grants-in-Aid from the Ministry of Health, Labor and Welfare of Japan (AK and TK), Grants-in-Aid for Scientific Research from JSPS (AK and TK), a grant from MEXT for the Joint Research Program of the Research Center for Zoonosis Control, Hokkaido University (TK), and a Grant-in-Aid for Scientific Research on Innovative Areas (Brain Protein Aging and Dementia Control) from MEXT (TK).

REFERENCES

Alperovitch A, Zerr I, Pocchiari M et al. (1999). Codon 129 prion protein genotype and sporadic Creutzfeldt–Jakob disease. Lancet 353: 1673–1674.

Appleby BS, Lu M, Bizzi A (2013). Iatrogenic Creutzfeldt–Jakob disease from commercial cadaveric human growth hormone. Emerg Infect Dis 19: 682–684.

Atarashi R, Satoh K, Sano K et al. (2011). Ultrasensitive human prion detection in cerebrospinal fluid by real-time quaking-induced conversion. Nat Med 17: 175–178.

Bernoulli C, Sigfried J, Baungarten G et al. (1977). Danger of accidental person to person transmission of Creutzfeldt–Jakob disease by surgery. Lancet 1: 478–479.

Billette de Villemeur T, Gelot A, Deslys JP et al. (1994). Iatrogenic Creutzfeldt–Jakob disease in three growth hormone recipients: a neuropathological study. Neuropathol Appl Neurobiol 20: 111–117.

Bishop MT, Will RG, Manson JC (2010). Defining sporadic Creutzfeldt–Jakob disease strains and their transmission properties. Proc Natl Acad Sci U S A 107: 12005–12010.

Brandel JP, Peoc'h K, Beaudry P et al. (2001). 14-3-3 protein cerebrospinal fluid detection in human growth hormone-treated Creutzfeldt–Jakob disease patients. Ann Neurol 49: 257–260.

Brandel J-P, Pecheu L, Haiek S (2013). The French surveillance network of Creutzfeldt–Jakob disease. Epidemiological data in France and world-wide. Transfus Clin Biol 20: 395–397.

Brandel JP, Preece M, Brown P et al. (2003). Distribution of codon 129 genotype in human growth hormone-treated CJD patients in France and the UK. Lancet 362: 128–130.

Brooke FJ, Boyd A, Klug GM et al. (2004). Lvodura use and the risk of iatrogenic Creutzfeldt–Jakob disease in Australia. Med J Aust 180: 177–181.

Brown P, Preece MA, Will RG (1992). 'Friendly fire' in medicine: hormones, homografts, and Creutzfeldt–Jakob disease. Lancet 340: 24–27.

Brown P, Brandel J-P, Sato T et al. (2012). Iatrogenic Creutzfeldt–Jakob disease, final assessment. Emerg Infect Dis 18: 901–907.

Cali I, Miller CJ, Parisi JE et al. (2015). Distinct pathological phenotypes of Creutzfeldt–Jakob disease in recipients of prion-contaminated growth hormone. Acta Neuropathol Commun 3: 37.

Castellani RJ1, Colucci M, Xie Z et al. (2004). Sensitivity of 14-3-3 protein test varies in subtypes of sporadic Creutzfeldt–Jakob disease. Neurology 63: 436–442.

CDC (1987). Epidemiologic notes and reports rapidly progressive dementia in a patient who received a cadaveric dura mater graft. MMWR 36: 49–50.

Clavel M, Clavel P (1996). Creutzfeldt–Jakob disease transmitted by dura mater graft. Eur Neurol 36: 239–240.

Collinge J, Sidle KC, Meads J et al. (1996). Molecular analysis of prion strain variation and the aetiology of 'new variant' CJD. Nature 383: 685–690.

Cordery RJ, Hall M, Cipolotti L et al. (2003). Early cognitive decline in Creutzfeldt–Jakob disease associated with human growth hormone treatment. J Neurol Neurosurg Psychiatry 74: 1412–1416.

Croes EA, Roks G, Jansen GH et al. (2002). Creutzfeldt–Jakob disease 38 years after diagnostic use of human growth hormone. J Neurol Neurosurg Psychiatry 72: 792–793.

d'Aignaux JH, Costagliola D, Maccario J et al. (1999). Incubation period of Creutzfeldt–Jakob disease in human growth hormone recipients in France. Neurology 53: 1197–1201.

Delisle MB, Fabre N, Rochiccioli P et al. (1993). Creutzfeldt–Jakob disease after treatment with human extracted growth hormone. A clinicopathological study. Rev Neurol (Paris) 149: 524–527.

Doh-ura K, Kitamoto T, Sakaki Y et al. (1991). CJD discrepancy. Nature 353: 801–802.

Duffy P, Wolf J, Collins G et al. (1974). Possible person-to-person transmission of Creutzfeldt–Jakob disease. N Engl J Med 290: 692–693.

Foncin J-F, Gaches J, Cathala F et al. (1980). Transmission iatrogene inherhumaine possible de maladie de Creutzfeldt–Jakob avec atteinte des grains de cervelet. Rev Neurol 136: 280.

Gibbs CJJ, Joy A, Heffner DOR et al. (1985). Clinical and pathological features and laboratory confirmation of Creutzfeldt–Jakob disease in a recipient of pituitary-derived human growth hormone. 313: 734–738.

Gibbs CJJ, Asher DM, Brown P et al. (1993). Creutzfeldt–Jakob disease infectivity of growth hormone derived human pituitary glands. N Engl J Med 300: 358–359.

Hall V, Brookes D, Nacul L et al. (2014). Managing the risk of iatrogenic transmission of Creutzfeldt–Jakob disease in the UK. J Hosp Infct 88: 22–27.

Hamaguchi T, Sakai K, Noguchi-Shinohara M et al. (2013). Insight into the frequent occurrence of dura mater graft-associated Creutzfeldt–Jakob disease in Japan. J Neurol Neurosurg Psychiatry 84: 1171–1175.

Hannah EL, Belay ED, Gambetti P et al. (2001). Creutzfeldt–Jakob diseaseafter receipt of a previously unimplicated brand of dura mater graft. Neurology 56: 1080–1083.

Head MW, Ritchie DL, Yull HM et al. (2016). Iatrogenic Creutzfeldt–Jakob disease in human growth hormone recipients in the United Kingdom. Prion 10: S92.

Heath CA, Barker RA, Esmonde TFG et al. (2006). Dura mater-associated Creutzfeldt–Jakob disease: experience from surveillance in the UK. J Neurol Neurosurg Psychiatry 77: 880–882.

Heckmann JG, Lang CJG, Petruch F et al. (1997). Transmission of Creutzfeldt–Jakob disease via a corneal transplant. J Neurol Neurosurg Psychiatry 62: 388–390.

Heinemann U, Krasnianski A, Meissner B et al. (2007). Creutzfeldt–Jakob disease in Germany: a prospective 12-year surveillance. Brain 130: 1350–1359.

Hoshi K, Yoshino H, Urata J et al. (2000). Creutzfeldt–Jakob disease associated with cadaveric dura mater grafts in Japan. Neurology 55: 718–721.

Huillard d'Aignaux J, Costagliola D, Maccario J (1999). Incubation period of Creutzfeldt–Jakob disease in human growth hormone recipients in France. Neurology 53: 1197–1201.

Jansen C, Parchi P, Capellari S et al. (2012). Human prion diseases in the Netherlands (1998–2009): clinical, genetic and molecular aspects. PLoS One 7: e36333.

Kim HL, Do JY, Cho HJ et al. (2011). Dura mater graft associated Creutzfeldt–Jakob disease: the first case in Korea. J Korean Med Sci 26: 1515–1517.

Kimura K, Nonaka A, Tashiro H et al. (2001). Atypical form of dura graft associated Creutzfeldt–Jakob disease: report of a postmortem case with review of the literature. J Neurol Neurosurg Psychiatry 70: 696–699.

Kobayashi A, Asano M, Mohri S et al. (2007). Cross-sequence transmission of sporadic Creutzfeldt–Jakob disease creates a new prion strain. J Biol Chem 282: 30022–30028.

Kobayashi A, Asano M, Mohri S et al. (2009). A traceback phenomenon can reveal the origin of prion infection. Neuropathology 29: 619–624.

Kobayashi A, Sakuma N, Matsuura Y et al. (2010). Experimental verification of a traceback phenomenon in prion infection. J Virol 84: 3230–3238.

Kobayashi A, Iwasaki Y, Otsuka H et al. (2013). Deciphering the pathogenesis of sporadic Creutzfeldt–Jakob disease with codon 129 M/V and type 2 abnormal prion protein. Acta Neuropathol Commun (1): 74.

Kobayashi A, Matsuura Y, Mohri S et al. (2014). Distinct origins of dura mater graft-associated Creutzfeldt–Jakob disease: past and future problems. Acta Neuropathol Commun 2: 32.

Kobayashi A, Parchi P, Yamada M et al. (2015a). Transmission properties of atypical Creutzfeldt–Jakob disease: a clue to disease etiology? J Virol 89: 3939–3946.

Kobayashi A, Teruya K, Matsuura Y et al. (2015b). The influence of PRNP polymorphisms on human prion disease susceptibility: an update. Acta Neuropathol 130: 159–170.

Kobayashi A, Matsuura Y, Iwaki T et al. (2016). Sporadic Creutzfeldt–Jakob disease MM1+2C and MM1 are identical in transmission properties. Brain Pathol 26: 95–101.

Koch TK, Berg BO, DeArmond SJ et al. (1985). Creutzfeldt–Jakob disease in a young adult with idiopathic hypopituitarism. N Engl J Med 313: 731–733.

Kopp N, Streichenberger N, Deslys JP et al. (1996). Creutzfeldt–Jakob disease in a 52-year-old woman with florid plaques. Lancet 348: 1239–1240.

Kretzschmar HA, Sethi S, Földvári Z et al. (2003). Iatrogenic Creutzfeldt–Jakob disease with florid plaques. Brain Pathol 13: 245–249.

Lane KL, Brown P, Howell DN et al. (1994). Creutzfeldt–Jakob disease in a pregnant woman with an implanted dura mater graft. Neurosurgery 34: 737–740.

Laplanche JL, Delasnerie-Lauprêtre N, Brandel JP et al. (1994). Molecular genetics of prion diseases in France. French Research Group on Epidemiology of Human Spongiform Encephalopathies. Neurology 44: 2347–2351.

Lewis AM, Yu M, DeArmond SJ (2006). Human growth hormone-related iatrogenic Creutzfeldt–Jakob disease with abnormal imaging. Arch Neurol 63: 288–290.

McGuire LI, Peden AH, Orrú CD et al. (2012). Real time quaking-induced conversion analysis of cerebrospinal fluid in sporadic Creutzfeldt–Jakob disease. Ann Neurol 72: 278–285.

Mochizuki Y, Mizutani T, Tajiri N et al. (2003). Creutzfeldt–Jakob disease with florid plaques after cadaveric dura mater graft. Neuropathology 23: 136–140.

Moda F, Suardi S, Di Fede G et al. (2012). MM2-thalamic Creutzfeldt–Jakob disease: neuropathological, biochemical and transmission studies identify a distinctive prion strain. Brain Pathol 22: 662–669.

Moore RA, Head MW, Ironside JW et al. (2016). The distribution of prion protein allotypes differs between sporadic and iatrogenic Creutzfeldt–Jakob disease patients. PLoS Pathog 12: e1005416.

Nakamura Y, Aso E, Yanagawa H (1999). Relative risk of Creutzfeldt–Jakob disease with cadaveric dura transplantation in Japan. Neurology 52: 218–220.

Nevin S, McMenemey WH, Behrman S et al. (1960). Subacute spongiform encephalopathy-a subacute form of encephalopathy attributable to vascular dysfunction (spongiform cerebral atrophy). Brain 83: 519–563.

Noguchi-Shinohara M, Hamaguchi T, Kitamoto T et al. (2007). Clinical features and diagnosis of dura mater graft associated Creutzfeldt–Jakob disease. Neurology 69: 360–367.

Notari S, Capellari S, Giese A et al. (2004). Effects of different experimental conditions on the PrPSc core generated by protease digestion: implications for strain typing and molecular classification of CJD. J Biol Chem 279: 16797–16804.

Notari S, Capellari S, Langeveld J et al. (2007). A refined method for molecular typing reveals that co-occurrence of PrP(Sc) types in Creutzfeldt-Jakob disease is not the rule. Lab Invest 87: 1103–1112.

Nozaki I, Hamaguchi T, Sanjo N et al. (2010). Prospective 10-year surveillance of human prion diseases in Japan. Brain 133: 3043–3057.

Palmer MS, Dryden AJ, Hughes JT et al. (1991). Homozygous prion protein genotype predisposes to sporadic Creutzfeldt–Jakob disease. Nature 352: 340–342.

Parchi P, Giese A, Capellari S et al. (1999). Classification of sporadic Creutzfeldt–Jakob disease based on molecular and phenotypic analysis of 300 subjects. Ann Neurol 46: 224–233.

Parchi P, Strammiello R, Giese A et al. (2011). Phenotypic variability of sporadic human prion disease and its molecular basis: past, present, and future. Acta Neuropathol 121: 91–112.

Peckeu L, Sazdovitch V, Privat N et al. (2016). Iatrogenic CJD after human GH treatment in France: effect of sex, dose and genetics on the susceptibility of a possible infection by a V2 sCJD strain. Prion 10: S96.

Peden AH, McGuire LI, Appleford NE et al. (2012). Sensitive and specific detection of sporadic Creutzfeldt–Jakob disease brain prion protein using real-time quaking-induced conversion. J Gen Virol 93: 438–449.

Powel-Jackson J Weller, RO Kennedy P et al. (1985). Creutzfeldt–Jakob disease after administration of humen growth hormone. Lancet 326: 244–246.

Radbauer C, Hainfellner JA, Gaudernak T et al. (1998). Creutzfeldt–Jakob disease in a dura transplant recipient: first observation in Austria. Wien Klin Wochenschr 110: 496–500.

Ritchie DL, Barria MA, Peden AH et al. (2016). UK Iatrogenic Creutzfeldt–Jakob disease: investigating human prion transmission across genotypic barriers using human tissue-based and molecular approaches. Acta Neuropathol 133: 579–595.

Rudge P, Jaunmuktane Z, Adlard P et al. (2015). Iatrogenic CJD due to pituitary-derived growth hormone with genetically determined incubation times of up to 40 years. Brain 138: 3386–3399.

Salvatore M, Genuardi M, Petraroli R et al. (1994). Polymorphisms of the prion protein gene in Italian patients with Creutzfeldt–Jakob disease. Hum Genet 94: 375–379.

Sanchez-Juan P, Green A, Ladogana A et al. (2006). CSF tests in the differential diagnosis of Creutzfeldt–Jakob disease. Neurology 67: 637–643.

Sato T, Masuda M, Utsumi Y et al. (2005). Dura mater related Creutzfeldt–Jakob disease in Japan: relationship between sites of grafts and clinical features. In: T Kitamoto (Ed.), Prions. Food and Drug Safety. Springer, Tokyo, pp. 31–40.

Satoh K, Muramoto T, Tanaka T et al. (2003). Association of an 11–12 kDa protease-resistant prion protein fragment with subtypes of dura graft-associated Creutzfeldt–Jakob disease and other prion diseases. J Gen Virol 84: 2885–2893.

Shibuya S, Higuchi J, Shin RW et al. (1998). Protective prion protein polymorphisms against sporadic Creutzfeldt–Jakob disease. Lancet 351: 419.

Shimizu S, Hoshi K, Muramoto T et al. (1999). Creutzfeldt–Jakob disease with florid-type plaques after cadaveric dura mater grafting. Arch Neurol 56: 357–362.

Swerdlow AJ, Higgins CD, Adlard P et al. (2003). Creutzfeldt–Jakob disease in United Kingdom patients treated with human pituitary growth hormone. Neurology 61: 783–791.

Takashima S, Tateishi J, Taguchi Y et al. (1997). Creutzfeldt–Jakob disease with florid plaques after cadaveric dural graft in a Japanese woman. Lancet 350: 865–866.

Takeuchi A, Kobayashi A, Parchi P et al. (2016a). Distinctive properties of plaque-type dura mater graft-associated Creutzfeldt–Jakob disease in cell-protein misfolding cyclic amplification. Lab Investig 96: 581–587.

Takeuchi A, Yamamoto M, Parchi P et al. (2016b). Identification of the origin of Creutzfeldt–Jakob disease after cadaveric sourced pituitary growth hormone treatment using an amplification property in protein misfolding cyclic amplification. Prion 10: S58–S59.

Toovey S, Britz M, Hewlett RH (2006). A case of dura mater graft-associated Creutzfeldt–Jakob disease in South Africa. S Afr Med J 96: 592–593.

Will RG (2003). Acquired prion disease: iatrogenic CJD, variant CJD, kuru. Br Med Bull 66: 255–265.

Windl O, Dempster M, Estibeiro JP et al. (1996). Genetic basis of Creutzfeldt–Jakob disease in the United Kingdom: a systematic analysis of predisposing mutations and allelic variation in the PRNP gene. Hum Genet 98: 259–264.

Yamada M, Noguchi-Shinohara M, Hamaguchi T et al. (2009). Dura mater graft-associated Creutzfeldt–Jakob disease in Japan: clinicopathological and molecular characterization of the two distinct subtypes. Neuropathology 29: 609–618.

Zerr I, Schulz-Schaeffer WJ, Giese A et al. (2000). Current clinical diagnosis in Creutzfeldt–Jakob disease: identification of uncommon variants. Ann Neurol 48: 323–329.

Handbook of Clinical Neurology, Vol. 153 (3rd series)
Human Prion Diseases
M. Pocchiari and J. Manson, Editors
https://doi.org/10.1016/B978-0-444-63945-5.00013-1

Chapter 13

Genetic Creutzfeldt–Jakob disease

ANNA LADOGANA[1] AND GABOR G. KOVACS[2]*
[1]*Department of Neuroscience, Istituto Superiore di Sanità, Rome, Italy*
[2]*Institute of Neurology, Medical University of Vienna and Austrian Reference Center for Human Prion Diseases, Vienna, Austria; and Hungarian Reference Center for Human Prion Diseases, Budapest, Hungary*

Abstract

Genetic Creutzfeldt–Jakob disease (CJD) is associated with mutations in the human PrP gene (*PRNP*) on chromosome 20p12-pter. Pathogenic mutations have been identified in 10–15% of all CJD patients, who often have a family history of autosomal-dominant pattern of inheritance and variable penetrance. However, the use of genetic tests implemented by surveillance networks all over the world increasingly identifies unexpectedly *PRNP* mutations in persons apparently presenting with a sporadic form of CJD. A high phenotypic variability was reported in genetic prion diseases, which partly overlap with the features of sporadic CJD. Here we review recent advances on the epidemiologic, clinical, and neuropathologic features of cases that phenotypically resemble CJD linked to point and insert mutations of the *PRNP* gene. Multidisciplinary studies are still required to understand the phenotypic spectrum, penetrance, and significance of *PRNP* mutations.

INTRODUCTION

About 10–15% of human prion diseases or transmissible spongiform encephalopathies (TSE) are linked to mutations in the prion protein gene, *PRNP*, and inherited with an autosomal-dominant pattern, though with variable penetrance (Ladogana et al., 2005a). The *PRNP* mutations consist of point mutations leading to amino acid substitution, premature stop codon, or insertion of octapeptide repeats (OPR) in the N-terminal region of the *PRNP* (Schmitz et al., 2017). The pathogenicity of some *PRNP* mutations is formally established by genetic linkage analyses (Hsiao et al, 1989; Goldfarb et al., 1992a; Poulter et al., 1992) and supported by a high penetrance in others (Minikel et al., 2016). However, genetic testing is increasingly identifying unexpected *PRNP* mutations in persons apparently affected by sporadic Creutzfeldt–Jakob disease (CJD) and for this reason the term genetic prion diseases is preferred to that of familial prion diseases (Kovacs et al., 2005b). The absence of a family history of CJD in a significant number of genetic CJD patients is either related to the low penetrance of specific mutations or to the possibility that some mutations are rare polymorphisms that increase susceptibility to prion misfolding aggregation triggered by spontaneous events or exposure to a "seeding" prion (Lloyd et al., 2013).

Historically, genetic prion diseases were classified on the basis of clinical and neuropathologic phenotypes as genetic CJD (rapidly progressive dementia associated with spongiform encephalopathy), Gerstmann–Sträussler–Scheinker (GSS) disease (encephalo(myelo) pathy with multicentric amyloid plaques (see Chapter 14), or fatal familial insomnia (FFI) (see Chapter 15) (Budka et al., 1995; WHO, 2003; Ghetti et al., 2011).

All genetic prion diseases are associated with point mutations or basepair insertions in the *PRNP* and show deposition in the brain of the abnormal, misfolded form of the host-encoded PrP, termed PrP^{TSE}. Basepair insertions in the *PRNP* may cause atypical diseases that are difficult to classify as CJD or GSS phenotype (Kovacs et al., 2002). Moreover, stop codon mutations show PrP^{TSE} cerebral amyloid angiopathy and present with

*Correspondence to: Gabor G. Kovacs, AKH4J, Währinger Gürtel 18–20, A-1090 Vienna, Austria. Tel: +43-1-40400-550570, E-mail: gabor.kovacs@meduniwien.ac.at

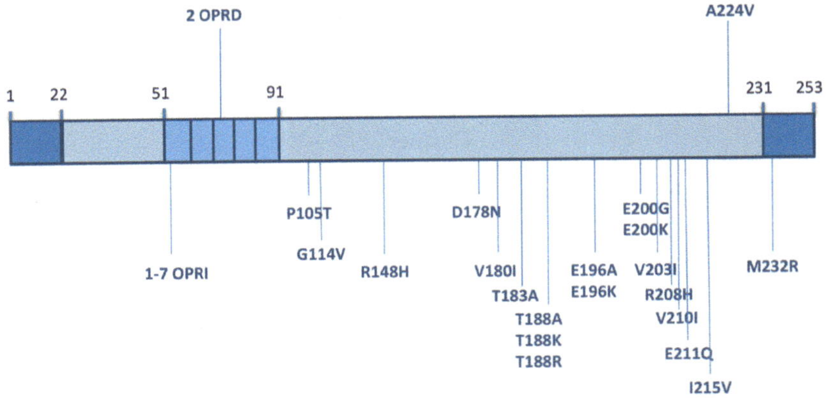

Fig. 13.1. PrP mutations linked to genetic Creutzfeldt–Jakob disease. A schematic representation of the full-length PrP is shown with the cleaved signal sequences in blue and the octapeptide region in light blue. *OPRD*, octapeptide repeat deletions; *OPRI*, octapeptide repeat insertions.

memory disturbance, disorientation, and progressive dementia (Y145X-129M), Alzheimer-type dementia (Y160X-129M), or cognitive impairment, aphasia, and myoclonus (Y226X-129V/M) (Ghetti et al., 2003). An unusual phenotype associated with Y163X genotype was recently reported (Mead et al., 2013; Mead and Reilly, 2015). This form, named PrP systemic amyloidosis, is characterized by diarrhea and autonomic neuropathy associated with PrP amyloid deposition throughout peripheral organs, including the bowel and peripheral nerves. Finally, a few *PRNP* mutations were reported in patients with or without a clinical phenotype reminiscent of CJD (e.g., S97N-129M, T193I-129M, F198V-129M, R208C-129M-E219K, K194E) (Kotta et al., 2006; Zheng et al., 2008; Takada et al., 2017). The neuropathologic phenotype and the pathogenicity of these mutations await clarification.

Most often *PRNP* mutations are associated with specific clinical and neuropathologic phenotypes. However, there is also evidence that within the same family, mutation carriers develop different clinical phenotypes (Barbanti et al., 1996; Piccardo et al., 1998; De Michele et al., 2003). A further striking example of phenotypic variability is the mutation at codon 178 (substitution of the aspartic acid with asparagine, D178N), which is associated with two different prion diseases depending on whether the mutation co-segregates with methionine (FFI) or valine (genetic CJD) at the polymorphic codon 129 (Goldfarb et al., 1992b). Thus, the polymorphic codon 129 is one of the factors that modify the characteristics of genetic prion diseases. In this chapter we focus on genetic prion diseases linked to point and insert mutations that are associated with spongiform encephalopathy that phenotypically resemble CJD (Fig. 13.1). Due to the importance of the polymorphism at codon 129, we have classified genetic CJD into haplotypes based on the *PRNP* mutation and the polymorphic codon 129 on the *PRNP* mutant allele (Table 13.1).

SURVEILLANCE, DIAGNOSTIC APPROACH, AND PATHOGENESIS

Epidemiologic and molecular studies have revealed that the incidence of genetic CJD differs from country to country (Ladogana et al., 2005a) and that the distribution and frequency of mutation in *PRNP* vary significantly between Caucasian and East Asian races (Fig. 13.2), likely due to different genetic backgrounds (Jeong and Kim, 2014). For surveillance purposes, genetic CJD cases are classified as definite when they are neuropathologically confirmed and are associated either with a pathogenic CJD-related *PRNP* mutation or with at least a first-degree relative with definite or probable prion disease. Genetic CJD cases are classified as probable when they show progressive neuropsychiatric symptoms and either carry a pathogenic CJD-related *PRNP* mutation or have a first-degree relative with definite or probable prion disease.

As for sporadic CJD, the diagnostic process for genetic CJD includes brain magnetic resonance imaging (MRI) and detection of protein 14-3-3 in the cerebrospinal fluid (CSF) (see comments below for each mutation). However, the presence of a pathogenic *PRNP* in a patient with a progressive neuropsychiatric syndrome is per se a valid support for the clinical diagnosis of prion disease. Moreover, diagnosis has been markedly improved by the novel ultrasensitive seeding assays based on amplified detection of pathologic PrP in CSF or olfactory mucosa samples (Zanusso et al., 2016; Bongianni et al., 2017) (Fig. 13.3). Finally, neuropathologic alterations are characterized by various depositions of PrP^{TSE} in the brain reminiscent of sporadic CJD (Parchi et al., 2009), although some mutation carriers show PrP immunostaining patterns that deviate from those seen in sporadic CJD (Fig. 13.4).

In genetic CJD, PrP^{TSE} deposition is likely facilitated through various mechanisms by the disease-linked mutations (Capellari et al., 2011; Giachin et al., 2013).

Table 13.1

Demographic and laboratory characteristics of genetic Creutzfeldt–Jakob disease (CJD)

PRNP haplotype		No. of published cases	Positive family history (%)	Age at onset: range (years)	Disease duration: range (months)	EEG PSWC positive/tested	14-3-3 in CSF positive/tested	CJD-typical brain MRI positive/tested	RT-QuIC CSF positive/tested	RT-QuIC OM positive/tested
P105T-129V		3	100	36–45	36–72	0/2	0/1	1/1	–	–
G114-129M		12	82	18–75	12–48	0/5	0/3	2/4	–	–
R148H-129M		4	25	53–82	2–18	1/3	1/3	1/1	–	–
D178N-129V		31	97	26–73	2–51	7/53	8/14	7/10	1/2	
V180I-129M		218	2	44–93	1–70	16/172	57/71	179/180	43/71	
V180I-129V		1	0	75	35	0/1	0/1	1/1	0/1	0/1
T183A-129M		12	100	37–49	24–108	0/7	0/1	0/2	–	–
T188A-129M		1	0	82	4	1/1	1/1	–	–	–
T188K-129M		20	35	40–80	2–13	5/17	14/18	12/19	–	–
T188R-129M		2	0	55, 66	14, 16	0/2	1/2	1/2	–	–
E196A-129M		3	0	54–76	10–22	2/3	3/3	3/3	–	–
E196K-129M		10	50	64–80	2–18	1/10	9/10	4/7	0/1	
E196K-129V		2	0	65, 71	3.5, 9	0/2	2/2	0/1	–	–
E200G-129V		1	100	57	30	0/1	–	1/1	–	–
E200K-129M	Chile	39	100	39–66	2–7	232/308	273/320	115/160	79/84	2/2
	Israel	377	100	34–84	1–111					
	EU countries, Australia, Canada	172	49.1	33–84	2–36					
	Argentina	33	60	35–80	2–18					
	Japan	63	44	31–83	1–32					
	China	24	11	42–70	2–13					
E200K-129V		3	0	47–67	3.5–6	–	4/4	–	4/4	–
V203I-129M		14	0	48–80	1–52	11/13	11/11	8/8	3/3	
V203I-129V		1	0	66	2	–	1/1	1/1	–	–
R208H-129M		12	14.3	45–74	2–28	7/11	5/9	4/9	1/1	–
R208H-129V		4	0	62–67	7–30	2/4	2/4	3/4	0/1	–
V210I-129M	EU countries, Australia, Canada	69	12.3	39–82	2-34	65/87	94/101	10/54	30/31	2/2
	Italy	210	21	24–87	1–73					

Continued

Table 13.1

Continued

V210I-129V	1	0	75	4	–	–	–	–	–
E211Q-129M	6	86	41–81	3–32	5/6	3/3	–	–	–
I215V-129M	2	100	55, 77	15, 16	2/3	1/3	0/3	–	–
A224V-129V	1	0	48	32	0/1	0/1	1/1	–	–
M232R-129M	63	3	15–82	1–78	46/61	31/43	55/60	7/9	–
M232R/V180I-129M	4	0	65–74	1–47	1/1	1/1	4/4	–	–
1 OPRI-129M	7	28.6	58–85	2–35	4/7	5/5	0/4	–	–
2 OPRI-129M	3	66.6	58–75	3–156	1/3	–	0/1	–	–
2 OPRI-129V	2	50	59, 61	120, 84	0/1	–	0/1	–	–
3 OPRI-129M	1	0	69	36	1/1	0/1	1/1	–	–
3 OPRI-129V	1	0	69	4	0/1	1/1	–	–	–
4 OPRI-129M	12	17	39–85	2–77	6/9	3/7	5/14	1/1	–
4 OPRI-129V	2	0	38, 82	4, 17	1/2	1/1	1/1	–	–
5 OPRI-129M	21	86	26–63	4–228	3/14	1/3	0/6	1/1	
6 OPRI-129M	40	100	20–49	12–252	1/26	1/5	0/16	–	–
6 OPRI-129V	5	40	33–51	3–180	0/5	–	0/5	–	–
7 OPRI-129M	9	100 (one *de-novo* insertion)	19–44	50–228	1/9	0/1	1/4	–	–
7 OPRI-129V	2	100	51, 59	7, 65	1/2	–	1/2	–	–
2-OPRD	2	50	64, 86	18, 23	1/2	1/1	0/2	–	–

CSF, cerebrospinal fluid; EEG, electroencephalogram; MRI, magnetic resonance imaging; OM, olfactory mucosa; PSWC, periodic sharp-wave complex; RT-QuIC, real-time quaking-induced conversion.

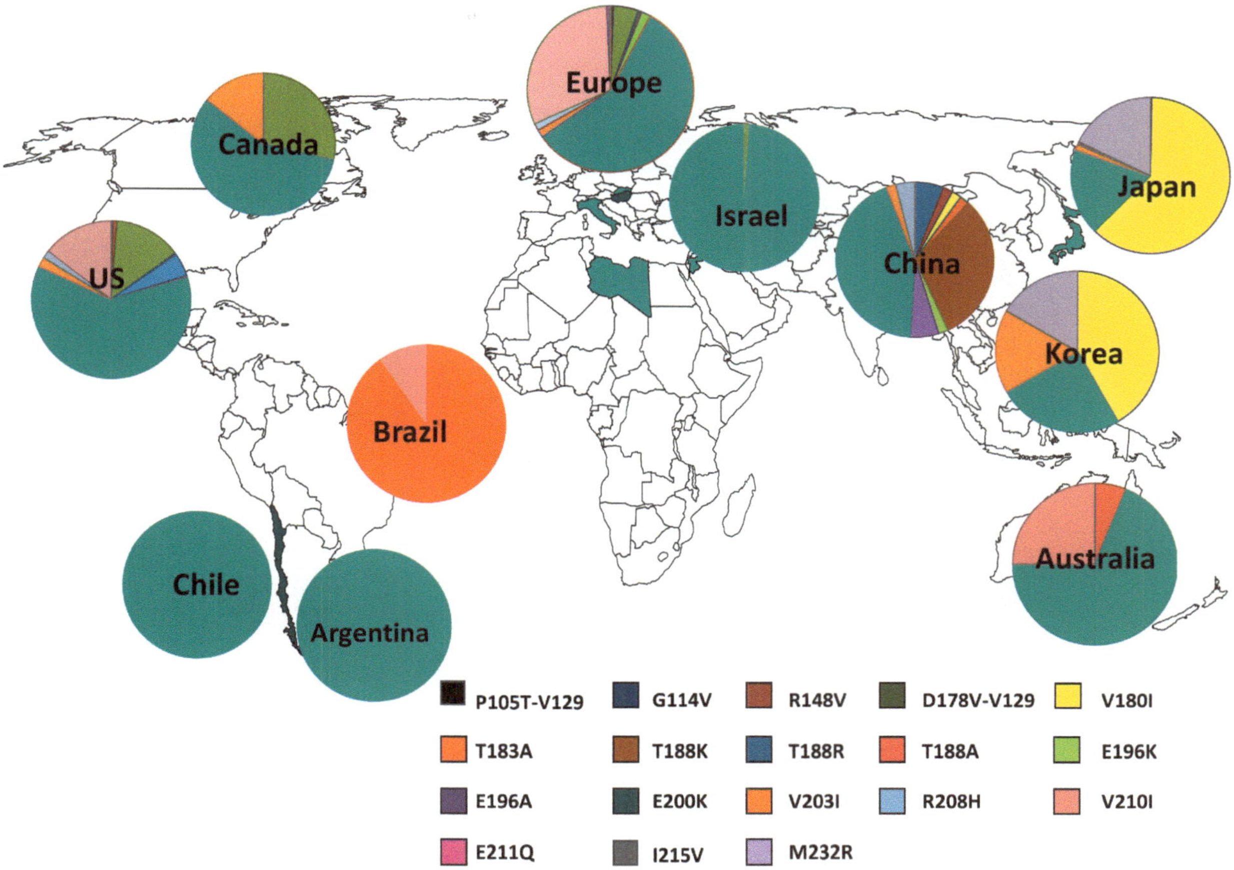

Fig. 13.2. Worldwide distribution of *PRNP* point mutations linked to genetic Creutzfeldt–Jakob disease (CJD) in countries with CJD surveillance system. The countries where geographic cluster/high incidence of E200K mutation cases was reported are colored in blue.

In some genetic CJD the conversion of PrP^{c} into PrP^{TSE} is limited to the mutant protein, while in others the PrP^{TSE} derives only from the normal or mutant protein (Cardone et al., 2014). Brain samples from CJD patients carrying different *PRNP* mutations are transmissible to laboratory animals through injection of infected tissues in wild-type (Tateishi and Kitamoto, 1995; Nonno et al., 2006) or transgenic rodents (Mastrianni et al., 2001). This feature has relevant implications for public health and strengthens the need for surveillance for the genetic forms of prion diseases. Finally, there are transgenic mouse models that recapitulate features of the corresponding human *PRNP* mutations associated with genetic CJD, such as the model for E200K genetic CJD expressing chimeric mouse/human (TgMHu2M) E199KPrP on a null or wild-type PrP background (Friedman-Levi et al., 2011).

GENOTYPES AND PHENOTYPES ASSOCIATED WITH GENETIC CJD

In the present section, we provide an overview of the clinical and pathologic phenotypes occurring in genetic CJD according to different *PRNP* mutations by the increasing order in the position of the mutated codon (Table 13.1).

P105T-129V

Epidemiology and genetics

Direct sequencing of the *PRNP* gene revealed a change of the coding sequence at codon 105 from proline (P) to threonine (T) in an index patient of a family, with at least three members showing CJD-like symptoms from Switzerland (Polymenidou et al., 2011).

Clinical phenotype

Two individuals presented with progressive dementia with gait disorder. One patient showed progressive memory decline and dementia, together with a pronounced pancerebellar syndrome and myoclonic jerks on arms and legs. The electroencephalogram (EEG) was normal and protein 14-3-3 remained undetectable in CSF. Fluid-attenuated inversion recovery (FLAIR) MRI

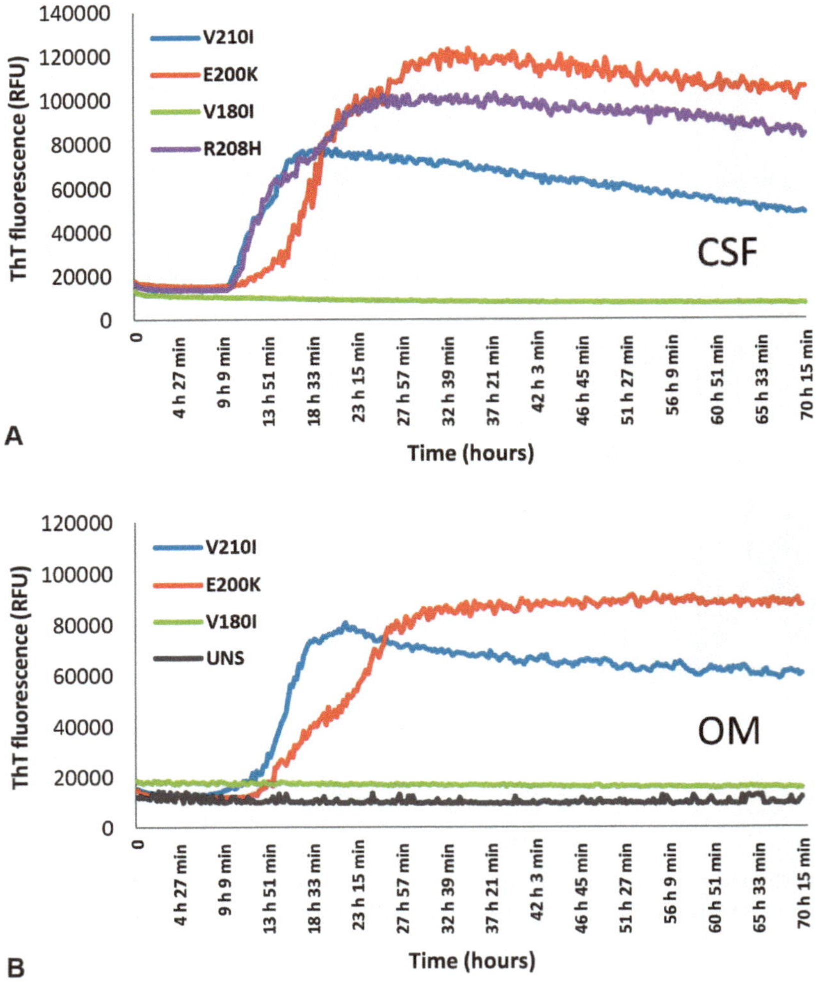

Fig. 13.3. (**A**) Real-time quaking-induced conversion (RT-QuIC) reactions seeded with 15 μL of human cerebrospinal fluid (CSF) samples from genetic Creutzfeldt–Jakob disease (CJD) cases. Each line is the mean of the fluorescence readings of four walls. (**B**) RT-QuIC reactions seeded with 2 μL of human olfactory mucosa (OM) samples (according to Bongianni et al., 2017) from genetic CJD cases. Each line is the mean of the fluorescence readings of four walls.

images showed hyperintense lesions in the cortical ribbon and thalamus (Polymenidou et al., 2011).

Neuropathology and biochemistry

Spongiform change and neuronal loss were found throughout the cerebral cortex in the single examined patient. The cerebellum was only mildly affected. Immunohistochemical staining revealed PrP^{TSE} deposits in a synaptic pattern in all cortical layers with some plaque-like deposits and unicentric PrP^{TSE} plaques in deeper cortical layers. Rare PrP^{TSE} plaques were detectable in the molecular and granular cell layer of the cerebellar cortex as well as the cerebellar white matter. The basal ganglia showed a synaptic pattern. Immunostaining for tau, beta-amyloid, ubiquitin, and alpha-synuclein revealed no additional pathology (Polymenidou et al., 2011). Proteinase K (PK)-resistant PrP (PrP^{res}) was undetectable by conventional Western blotting and barely detectable after phosphotungstate precipitation, where it displayed an atypical pattern suggestive of noncanonic conformation. Characterization of the PK-resistant bands revealed a 6-kDa unglycosylated PK-resistant fragment and two bands of high molecular weight (~15 and ~25 kDa) that were probably partially glycosylated (Polymenidou et al., 2011).

G114V-129M

Epidemiology and genetics

The glycine (G) to valine (V) change at codon 114 (G114V) was first described in a Uruguayan family in homozygosity for M or heterozygosity M/V at codon 129 in three of five affected members (Rodriguez et al., 2005). This rare mutation was also found in a Chinese family where four individuals were found

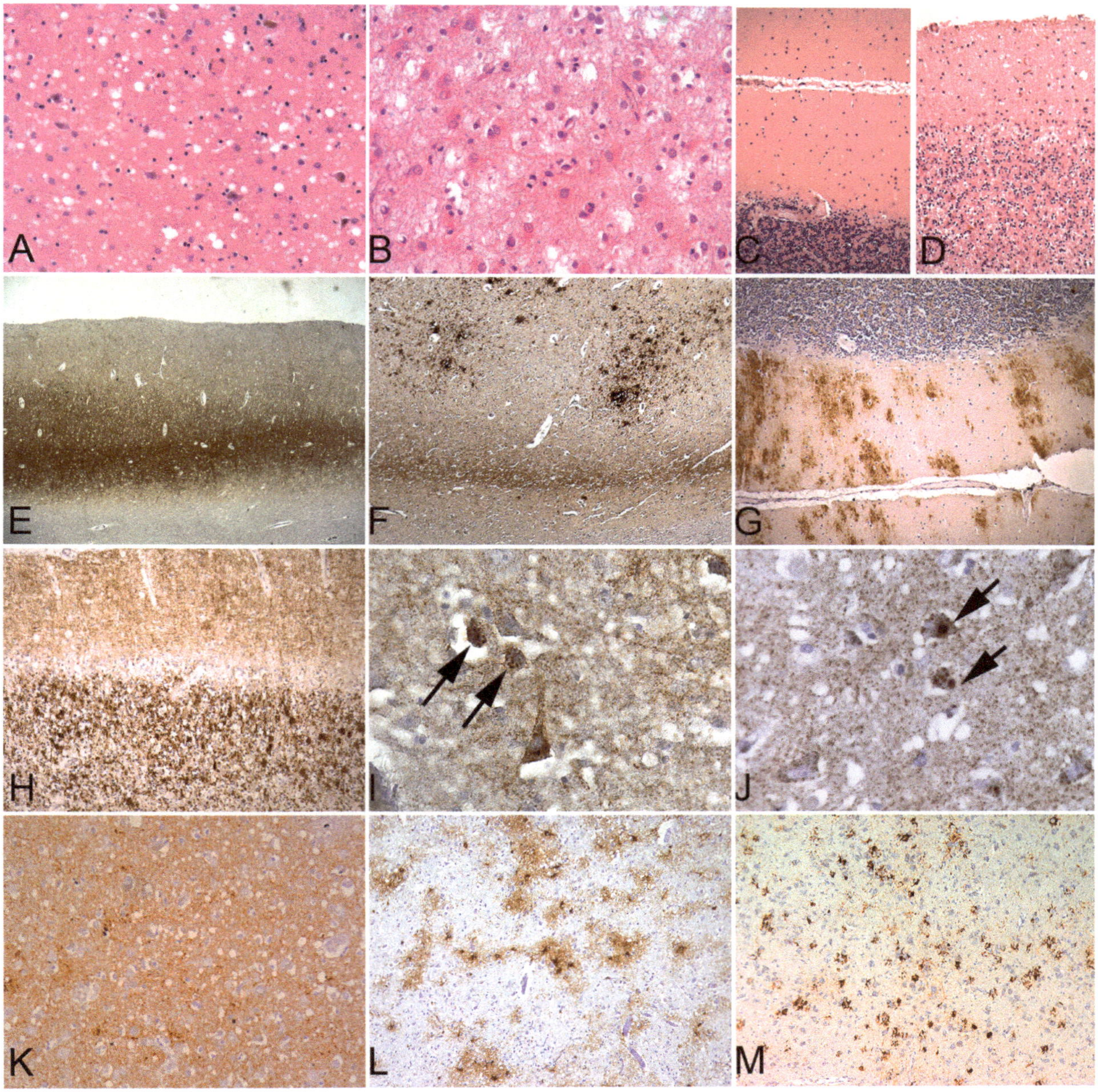

Fig. 13.4. Neuropathologic alterations in genetic Creutzfeldt–Jakob disease (CJD) as exemplified by mutations E200K (**A–J**) and V203I (**K–M**). (**A**) Characteristic spongiform change in the thalamus. (**B**) Severe astrogliosis and neuronal loss in the frontal cortex. (**C**) Some cases show preserved cerebellum. (**D**) Other cases show spongiform change in the cerebellum. (**E**) Synaptic PrP immunoreactivity predominating in the deeper layers in the frontal cortex. (**F**) Synaptic and patchy perivacuolar staining in the frontal cortex. (**G**) Characteristic stripe-like PrP immunoreactivity pattern in the cerebellum. (**H**) Synaptic and granular PrP deposits in the cerebellum. (**I**) Small intraneuronal PrP immunoreactive dots in cortical neurons (arrows). (**J**) Larger PrP inclusion body-like immunoreactivity in cortical neurons (arrows). (**K**) Diffuse synaptic PrP immunoreactivity in the temporal cortex. (**L**) Prominent phosphorylated-tau immunoreactive astrogliopathy in the same temporal cortex as shown in (**K**). (**M**) Prominent phosphorylated-tau immunoreactive astrogliopathy in the amygdala in the same case as shown in (**K**) and (**L**).

affected (Ye et al., 2008; Liu et al., 2010); mutation carriers were found in healthy members of both families at the age of 41, 44, 45, and 61 year old, suggesting an incomplete penetrance. Single cases were reported from India, Turkey, and the United States (Beck et al., 2010; Minikel et al., 2016).

Clinical features

Age at onset ranged from 18 to 28 years in the Uruguayan family and from 32 to 45 years in the Chinese one, but the Indian patient was 75 years old. Neuropsychiatric symptoms at onset, late dementia, prominent pyramidal and extrapyramidal signs, myoclonus, and long disease duration (> 1 year) characterize the clinical picture of disease. EEG and 14-3-3 test on CSF were not supportive for the diagnosis (Rodriguez et al., 2005; Shi et al., 2015), while diffusion-weighted imaging (DWI) brain MRI showed hyperintensity of the basal ganglia in 2 of 4 patients (Beck et al., 2010; Liu et al., 2010).

Neuropathology and biochemistry

Neuropathologic observation, available for only 1 patient, showed spongiform change and synaptic PrP^{TSE} immunoreactivity, as seen in sporadic CJD (Rodriguez et al., 2005; Shi et al., 2012). Western blotting for PrP^{res} in various brain regions showed a pattern similar to that observed in sporadic MM1 CJD samples (Shi et al., 2012).

R148H-129M

Epidemiology and genetics

The arginine (R) to histidine (H) change at codon 148 (R148H) in 3 M homozygous patients was reported in Germany, China, and the United States (Krebs et al., 2005; Shi et al., 2015; Takada et al., 2017), while a single-codon 129 heterozygous case was from the United States (Pastore et al., 2005). This mutation has likely a low penetrance based on the rarity of cases, their negative family history, and the presence of mutant alleles in control populations (Minikel et al., 2016).

Clinical features

Clinically, the genetic R148H CJD resembles sporadic CJD MM129 type 1 in codon 129 MM patients and sporadic CJD MV129 type 2 in the heterozygous patient.

Patients show gait impairment, rapid cognitive deterioration, psychiatric symptoms, myoclonus, and akinetic mutism.

The EEG pattern shows typical periodic activity in 1 case (Krebs et al., 2005), 14-3-3 protein in 1 case (Krebs et al., 2005), and CJD-characteristic brain MRI in 2 of 3 patients (Krebs et al., 2005; Shi et al., 2015; Takada et al., 2017).

Neuropathology and biochemistry

The neuropathologic features are reminiscent of either the MM1 (Krebs et al., 2005) or MV2 subtype (Pastore et al., 2005) of sporadic CJD. In particular, variable spongiform degeneration was seen in cerebral cortex, basal ganglia, thalamus, and cerebellum, while immunostaining for PrP^{TSE} showed a synaptic pattern with or without kuru-type plaques. These observations were supported by Western blot, which showed features similar to those observed in MM1 (Krebs et al., 2005) or MV2 sporadic CJD samples (Pastore et al., 2005).

D178N-129V

Epidemiology and genetics

The aspartic acid (D) to asparagine (N) substitution at codon 178 (D178N) was first discovered in a large Finnish family (Goldfarb et al., 1991a) described by Haltia and coworkers in 1979. Subsequently, this mutation was identified in several unrelated North American families of European descent (Brown et al, 1992a; Goldfarb et al., 1992a), in French families (Brown et al., 1991; Nieto et al., 1991; Laplanche et al., 1992), and in 2 patients of Russian or Yugoslavian Jewish origin living in Israel (Rosenmann et al., 1998). Afterward, cases were also reported in other European countries, Canada, and Japan (Kovacs et al., 2005b; Marcon et al., 2014; Minikel et al., 2016). This mutation has historic interest because it was found in the first reported CJD family (the "Backer" family) originally reported by Meggendorf in 1930 (Brown et al., 1994; Kretzschmar et al., 1995).

The D178N *PRNP* mutation has the peculiarity that its phenotypic expression is mainly modulated by the genotype at codon 129 on the mutant allele. The presence of V on the mutant allele manifests as genetic CJD, while the presence of M on the mutant allele manifests as FFI (see Chapter 15). However, a phenotypic variability was also observed in 129M/M D178N patients, who show clinical and pathologic features of CJD or FFI, suggesting that other factors play a role in determining phenotypic expression of D178N mutation (Zarranz et al., 2005).

Clinical features

Clinically, patients resemble sporadic CJD VV129 type 1 (Capellari et al., 2011) with a wide range of survival (median clinical duration of 15 months) (Kovacs et al., 2005b). Codon 129 valine homozygous patients show a shorter earlier age at onset and survival time than heterozygous patients (Goldfarb et al., 1992b; Kovacs et al., 2005b).

Clinical presentation is characterized by early cognitive impairment, usually with severe memory loss evolving over months or years, often associated with behavioral and psychiatric symptoms (Brown et al., 1992a; Rosenmann et al., 1998; Marcon et al., 2014). During the course of disease, patients develop myoclonus (74%), and cerebellar (86%), extrapyramidal (67%), pyramidal (49%), and visual signs (21%). Akinetic mutism was reported in only 1 case (Marcon et al., 2014).

EEG shows diffuse slow-wave activity but the typical periodicity was not present in most cases (Brown et al., 1992a; Marcon et al., 2014). Different studies reported brain MRI hyperintensity in basal ganglia and cortical regions between 71% and 100% and positive 14-3-3 protein test between 33% and 100%. Elevated levels of total tau were reported in some patients (Ladogana et al., 2009; Lattanzio et al., 2017). Real-time quaking-induced conversion (RT-QuIC) analysis of CSF samples revealed the presence of the pathologic prion protein in only one of the two tested cases (Lattanzio et al., 2017).

Neuropathology and biochemistry

Spongiform degeneration, neuronal loss, and reactive astrogliosis are usually prominent in these cases. In contrast to the cerebral cortex and basal ganglia, the cerebellum and brainstem are relatively spared (Capellari et al., 2011). Immunostaining for PrP^{TSE} shows a diffuse synaptic pattern predominantly in areas with prominent spongiform change. In contrast the cerebellum shows a minimal amount of PrP^{TSE} deposits. Kuru-type plaques are not reported. A panencephalopathic phenotype has been reported with the involvement of the cerebellum and presence of clusters of small focal PrP^{TSE} deposits, different from those observed in VV1 sporadic CJD (Marcon et al., 2014). The D178N-129V haplotype segregates with PrP^{res} type 1; however, the glycoform ratio is consistently dominated by the diglycosylated form, whereas the unglycosylated form is markedly underrepresented (Capellari et al., 2011).

V180I-129M and occasionally V180I-129V

Epidemiology and genetics

The valine (V) to isoleucine (I) change at codon 180 (V180I) is an extremely rare genetic CJD in Caucasian populations (Nixon et al., 2000; Kovacs et al., 2005b; Minikel et al., 2016; Takada et al., 2017), while it is the most frequent form in Japan (Nozaki et al., 2010; Minikel et al., 2016). A few cases were also described in China and South Korea (Jeong and Kim, 2014; Shi et al., 2015). The penetrance of V180I mutations is estimated to be very low, based on negative familial history for dementia in 94% of Japanese patients (Qina et al., 2014) and estimates of mutated healthy carriers in the general population (Minikel et al., 2016).

Clinical features

Clinically, patients with V180I-129M haplotype resemble sporadic CJD MM2C (Capellari et al., 2011). Affected subjects have a mean age at onset of 77.6 years (Qina et al., 2014) and a mean clinical duration of 16.4 months with a wide range of survival (Minikel et al., 2016). The polymorphism at codon 129 did not affect age at onset or disease duration (Qina et al., 2014). Clinical presentation is characterized by cognitive impairment evolving often as a slowly progressive dementia. During the course of disease, patients develop extrapyramidal (54%), psychiatric (50%), and pyramidal signs (46%), and akinetic mutism (57%) (Qina et al., 2014). Myoclonus and cerebellar signs are not so frequent and visual signs are rare. Clinical features are also similar in the few cases where the mutated allele is in *cis* with V at codon 129 (Qina et al., 2014; Pocchiari et al., 2016). EEG shows the typical periodic activity only in 9% of cases (Qina et al., 2014); brain MRI shows hyperintense signals in cortical areas or basal ganglia in 99% of cases (Qina et al., 2014); 14-3-3 protein test and elevated levels of total tau in the CSF were reported in 80% and 84% of patients, respectively (Qina et al., 2014). The RT-QuIC analysis of CSF samples revealed the presence of the pathologic prion protein in 60% of cases (Qina et al., 2014; Pocchiari et al., 2016).

Neuropathology and biochemistry

Diffuse spongiform degeneration in the cerebral cortex and basal ganglia was noted in all cases (Iwasaki et al., 2011). Involvement of the cerebellum and brainstem is mild in spite of the prolonged disease duration (Iwasaki et al., 2011). Immunostaining for PrP^{TSE} showed a synaptic-type pattern without plaque-type deposition in the cerebral neocortex in most examined cases. In 1 patient with M homozygosity at codon 129 linear-type PrP^{TSE} deposition in the CA4 and small plaque-like PrP^{TSE} deposition in the parahippocampal gyrus, striatum, and cerebellar molecular layer were also reported (Iwasaki et al., 2011). Kuru plaques were detected in a case with MV heterozygosity at codon 129 (Iwasaki et al., 1999). A case report mentioned intraneuronal deposits (Nixon et al., 2000), reminiscent of those seen in a subset of E200K genetic CJD cases (Kovacs et al., 2012). Western blot revealed type 1 or 2 PrP^{res} together with the peculiar feature of the lack of the diglycoform band (Chasseigneaux et al., 2006; Iwasaki et al., 2011).

T183A-129M

Epidemiology and genetics

The threonine (T) to alanine (A) change at codon 183 (T183A) was first found in a Brazilian family of Spanish and Italian origin in two affected members and in 12 healthy family members (Nitrini et al., 1997). The mutation was then reported in a North American patient (Capellari et al., 1999), in a German patient (Grasbon-Frodl et al., 2004) previously included in the screening for early-onset dementia (Finckh et al., 2000), and recently in a Chinese patient affected by dementia (Shi et al., 2015).

Clinical features

Age at onset is relatively early (<50 years) with a prolonged clinical course (mean duration, 4 years). Clinical signs are suggestive of a frontotemporal dementia (Nitrini et al., 1997), Alzheimer disease (Grasbon-Frodl et al., 2004), or an early-onset isolated dementia (Shi et al., 2015). Periodic discharges at EEG are not present (Nitrini et al., 1997), brain MRI is not typical for CJD (Grasbon-Frodl et al., 2004; Shi et al., 2015), and the 14-3-3 protein is negative (Shi et al., 2015).

Neuropathology and biochemistry

In the original report neuropathologic examination of 3 patients showed severe spongiform change and neuronal loss in the deep cortical layers and in the putamen. The putamen and cerebellum displayed punctuate and plaque-like prion protein immunoreactivity (Nitrini et al., 1997). Another case (associated with MM homozygosity at codon 129) showed synaptic fine granular staining pattern with perivascular accentuation in neocortical regions and the molecular and granular layers of the cerebellum. In addition, numerous "miniplaques" were noted in the molecular layer of the cerebellum (Grasbon-Frodl et al., 2004). Biochemical examination showed type 2 PrP^{res} with marked underrepresentation of diglycosylated bands (Grasbon-Frodl et al., 2004; Capellari et al., 2011).

T188K-R-A

Three different substitutions of residue 188 of the prion protein were associated with genetic CJD.

Epidemiology and genetics

The threonine (T) to lysine (K) change at codon 188 (T188K) is the most frequent mutation in this residue and the second most common form of genetic CJD in China, with 16 cases reported up to 2015 (Shi et al., 2015). It was first reported in an Austrian patient affected by dementia (Finckh et al., 2000) and in 3 German patients with methionine at codon 129 on the mutant allele (Roeber et al., 2008). This mutation was also found in healthy carriers at the age of 79 and 55 years.

The threonine (T) to arginine (R) substitution (T188R) was described in one German individual with V homozygosity at codon 129 (Windl et al., 1999; Roeber et al., 2008) and one Mexican-American individual with heterozygosity M/V at codon 129 but V in *cis* (Tartaglia et al., 2010). It was also found in two healthy individuals aged 80 (codon 129MV) and 56 (codon 129 VV) (Tartaglia et al., 2010).

The threonine (T) to alanine (A) substitution (T188A) associated with MM homozygosity at codon 129 has been described in an octogenarian patient from Australia (Collins et al., 2000) with no information on family history.

Clinical features

Genetic CJD with T188K-129M haplotype resembles sporadic CJD 129 MM type 1. The mean age at onset is 62 (Finckh et al., 2000; Roeber et al., 2008; Chen et al., 2013) with the majority of cases in the 50–59-year age group (Shi et al., 2015), with a median duration of illness of 4 months (Chen et al., 2013). Clinically the disease manifests with progressive dementia, myoclonus, and cerebellar, visual, pyramidal, and extrapyramidal signs (Roeber et al., 2008; Chen et al., 2013). The EEG shows the typical periodic activity in 12.5% of Chinese cases (Shi et al., 2015) and in the 3 German cases (Finckh et al., 2000; Roeber et al., 2008), while high signal in basal ganglia or cortices was reported in 68.8% (Shi et al., 2015). The 14-3-3 protein test sensitivity was 69% (Roeber et al., 2008; Shi et al., 2015). All cases fulfill the criteria for probable CJD.

In the T188R cases, the German case (aged 66 years and disease duration of 16 month) did not fulfill the criteria of CJD because of paucity of typical clinical signs, although the EEG showed periodic sharp-wave complexes (PSWCs) and CSF 14-3-3 test was positive (Roeber et al., 2008). The US case (aged 55 years and disease duration of 14 months) presented with behavioral changes, rapid progressive dementia, dysmetria, and myoclonus. Brain MRI showed mild diffuse cortical atrophy with restricted diffusion in the cortex and striatum; the EEG showed an unspecific slow pattern and CSF 14-3-3 was inconclusive.

The threonine (T) to alanine (A) change at codon 188 (T188A) was reported only in one 82-year-old woman with disease duration of 4 months. The EEG showed PSWC and 14-3-3 was positive (Collins et al., 2000).

Neuropathology and biochemistry

Histologic examination was reported in a single case with the T188K mutation and revealed severe spongiform changes in all layers of the cerebral cortex, status spongiosus in the entorhinal, transentorhinal, and occipital cortex, putamen, and caudate nuclei. The cerebellar cortex showed moderate spongiform changes of the molecular layer, and the brainstem was nearly free of spongiform change. Immunostaining for PrP^{TSE} revealed strong synaptic staining (Roeber et al., 2008). Western blotting of PrP^{res} showed a pattern similar to the type 1 pattern of sCJD case with an additional fragment migrating at about 17 kDa (Roeber et al., 2008).

Brain examination of cases with the T188R mutation and MV heterozygosity (with methionine on the mutated allele) showed typical spongiform encephalopathy and, in addition to the typical PrP^{TSE} synaptic staining, there were patches of plaque-like deposits throughout the cortex and subcortical structures. PrP^{res} type was compatible with the type 1 seen in sporadic CJD (Tartaglia et al., 2010).

The only examined case with the T188A mutation had a CJD pathognomonic histologic appearance, but immunohistochemical staining for PrP^{TSE} was repeatedly negative. Western immunoblot analysis for PrP^{res} was not performed (Collins et al., 2000).

E196A-129M

Epidemiology and genetics

A substitution from glutamic acid (E) to alanine (A) associated with codon 129 methionine homozygosity was reported in three unrelated Chinese patients (Zhang et al., 2014; Shi et al., 2016).

Clinical features

Progressive dementia, cerebellar symptoms, myoclonus, and akinetic mutism were described in all three individuals. CSF 14-3-3 examination was positive, while EEG revealed PSWC in 1 patient and brain MRI striatal high signal was present in the other 2 patients (Zhang et al., 2014; Shi et al., 2016).

Neuropathology and biochemistry

Because no histologic or biochemical examinations have been reported so far, the classification of these cases as genetic CJD is based only on clinical and instrumental findings.

E196K-129M and occasionally E196K-129V

Epidemiology and genetics

The glutamic acid (E) to lysine (K) change at codon 196 (E196K) and homozygosity for M at codon 129 was first described in a French woman with clinical and pathologic features of CJD (Peoc'h et al., 2000). A second case was described in a woman of Italian origin (Tumani et al., 2002), with codon 129 V homozygosity, who shared a remote history of depression with another Italian case described a few years later (Clerici et al., 2008). Seven additional cases were then reported: one from Austria (Kovacs et al., 2005b) and six from Germany (Schelzke et al., 2011). In the German patients, the mutation was associated either with codon 129 heterozygosity or homozygosity (both for M and V). More recently, other single cases from France (Béjot et al., 2010), China (Shi et al., 2011), and Italy (Minikel et al., 2016) have been reported. In some cases family history was postive or revealed dementia in relatives, while in others it was negative.

Clinical features

Clinically, genetic CJD linked to E196K mutation is characterized by a late mean age at onset (73.2 years) and a median duration of 8 months. Psychiatric symptoms were often present at onset together with cognitive impairment, while during the course of disease patients develop myoclonus, and cerebellar, pyramidal, and extrapyramidal signs. Akinetic mutism was described in the majority of patients.

EEG does not usually show the typical periodic activity and brain MRI shows hyperintensity in cortical areas or basal ganglia in about 57% of patients.

The 14-3-3 protein test was positive in all patients but 1 and elevated levels of total tau were reported in 3 patients (Clerici et al., 2008; Schelze et al., 2011).

Neuropathology and biochemistry

Histologic examination demonstrated morphologic and immunohistochemical features of CJD. Two examined cases closely resemble sporadic CJD MM/MV1 and one case sporadic CJD VV2 (Eigenbrod et al., 2011). A fourth patient (129 MM) showed only minor synaptic PrP^{TSE} deposits in the molecular layer of the cerebellum and granular cell layers together with a small number of focal plaque-like PrP^{TSE} deposits in the molecular layer (Eigenbrod et al., 2011). Western blot examination showed either type 1 or type 2 PrP^{res} pattern corresponding to the histopathologic findings, except for one case where Western blot revealed PrP^{res} type 2 in all brain samples and, in addition, PrP^{res} type 1 in the frontal and occipital cortex (Eigenbrod et al., 2011). The glycoform ratios were different from those found in sCJD cases with underrepresentation of nonglycosylated forms in all brain regions (Eigenbrod et al., 2011).

E200K-129 M and occasionally E200K-129V

Epidemiology and genetics

The glutamic acid (E) to lysine (K) substitution at codon 200 (E200K) is the most common *PRNP* mutation worldwide and the only one causing clustered cases. This mutation was first identified in a CJD family from Poland (Goldgaber et al., 1989) while the first identified cluster was reported in Slovakia (Goldfarb et al., 1990a). Shortly thereafter, Libyan Jewish patients were found to carry the same mutation (Goldfarb et al., 1990b; Hsiao et al., 1991), as did patients in Chile (Brown et al., 1992b). E200K-associated CJD was then described in Jewish families of Tunisian (Brown et al., 1991) and Greek origins (Goldfarb et al., 1990c; Larue et al., 2006), and non-Jewish population groups in Italy (D'Alessandro et al, 1998; Ladogana et al., 2005b), Spain (Coria et al., 1995), Britain (Collinge et al., 1993; Windl et al., 1996), Japan (Inoue et al., 1994), Austria (Hainfellner et al., 1996), and Argentina (Taratuto et al., 2002). A high incidence was reported in Hungary, particularly in areas with historic and geographic relations to the Slovakian population (Kovacs et al., 2005a, 2007). More recently it was reported in other European countries, Canada (Kovacs et al., 2005b), Korea (Choi et al., 2009), and China (Gao et al., 2010), expanding the worldwide distribution of this mutation. In the areas where cases are clustered, the CJD annual incidence rate is 5–154 times higher than the world average (Ladogana and Pocchiari, unpublished data; Miyakawa et al., 1998; Mitrová and Belay, 2002; Kovacs et al., 2007).

The study of ancestral origins of alleles carrying the E200K mutation demonstrated that Libyan, Tunisian, Chilean, Italian, and Spanish families share the same historic allele, suggesting that the E200K mutation may have originated from a single mutation event, perhaps in Spain, and spread to all these populations with Sephardic migrants who were expelled from Spain in the Middle Ages. Slovakian families and a family of Polish origin show another unique allele associated with the disease (Lee et al., 1999). The mutant alleles in families from Germany, Sicily, and Austria are somewhat similar to each other, but different from both Mediterranean and Eastern European alleles (the mutated allele co-segregates with valine rather than methionine at codon 129). Finally, the Japanese allele is different from any of the others. These observations led to the conclusion that independent mutational events are responsible for the distribution of the E200K mutation.

The E200K mutation shows an autosomal-dominant inheritance of disease with a variable penetrance, which means that some mutation carriers never develop CJD. The overall penetrance rate of the E200K mutation estimated by survival analysis was 59.5% in the Slovakian population (Mitrová and Belay, 2002) and 67% in the Italian cluster of Calabria (D'Alessandro et al., 1998), and reached 100% in Israeli Libyan Jews (Spudich et al., 1995).

Clinical features

Genetic CJD with E200K-129M haplotype is almost indistinguishable from sporadic CJD-MM129 type 1 (Capellari et al., 2011) apart from a younger age at onset, which is however similar in Caucasian (median 60.4 years, $n = 175$) (Kovacs et al., 2005b) and Asian patients (mean, 61.1 years, $n = 63$) (Minikel et al., 2016). The range of disease onset is between 27 and 84 years (Ladogana and Pocchiari, unpublished data; Kovacs et al., 2005b) and it is not likely influenced by codon 129 polymorphism (Kovacs et al., 2005b). The median clinical duration is 5 months in both Caucasian (Kovacs et al., 2005b) and Asian populations (Minikel et al., 2016), with a wide range of survival from 1 to 74 months (Kovacs et al., 2005b; Takada et al., 2017). The polymorphism at codon 129 influences disease duration of mutant patients, as methionine homozygous patients show a shorter survival than heterozygous ones (Pocchiari et al., 2004).

A few carriers of homozygous E200K mutation were also identified. These patients showed no significant difference in age at onset and disease duration from heterozygous ones (Simon et al., 2000).

The typical presentation of E200K-M129 CJD is a rapidly progressive dementia with gait or balance disturbances and behavioral changes (Cohen et al., 2016a). Afterward, patients usually develop myoclonus, and pyramidal or extrapyramidal signs (Meiner et al., 1997; Kovacs et al., 2011; Krasnianski et al., 2016; Takada et al., 2017). Atypical clinical presentations include peripheral neuropathy (Neufeld et al., 1992; Chapman et al., 1993; Kovacs et al., 2011), supranuclear gaze palsy (Bertoni et al., 1992; Kovacs et al., 2011), sleep disturbances (Taratuto et al., 2002), and corticobasal syndrome (Necpál et al., 2016).

The disease reported in E200K-V129 CJD patients is similar to sporadic CJD-VV129 type 2 (Hainfellner et al., 1999; Puoti et al., 2000; Baiardi et al., 2017).

Different studies reported EEG with typical periodic activity (PSWC) in 68–89% of cases (Meiner et al., 1997; Kovacs et al., 2005b; Higuma et al., 2013; Minikel et al., 2016) and FLAIR and DWI brain MRI hyperintensity in basal ganglia and cortical areas in 45–95% (Kovacs et al., 2005b; Fulbright et al., 2008; Breithaupt et al., 2013; Higuma et al., 2013; Cohen et al., 2016b), confirming that the diagnostic criteria for sporadic CJD applied also to genetic E200K patients. Hyperintensity is occasionally present in the thalamus with a pattern resembling the pulvinar sign observed in variant CJD (Kovacs et al., 2009, 2011). Asymptomatic carriers who finally convert to CJD do not show significant changes in the brain MRI scans, questioning its use in presymptomatic individuals (Cohen et al., 2015).

The 14-3-3 protein test sensitivity ranges from 77% to 89% and the total tau from 72% to 85% (Ladogana et al., 2009; Meiner et al., 2011; Breithaupt et al., 2013; Higuma et al., 2013; Shi et al., 2015; Krasnianski et al., 2016; Lattanzio et al., 2017). RT-QuIC has a sensitivity from 85% to 100% in the CSF (Higuma et al., 2013; Sano et al., 2013; Cramm et al., 2016; Lattanzio et al., 2017) and 100% in the olfactory mucosa (only 2 patients) (Bongianni et al., 2017). This positive result might open new perspectives for monitoring presymptomatic carriers.

Neuropathology and biochemistry

The classic triad of spongiform change, neuronal loss, and reactive astrocytosis is seen in E200K mutation cases. Immunostaining for PrP^{TSE} reveals diffuse/synaptic deposits, patchy aggregates in the neuropil or around vacuoles, plaques without amyloid characteristics, fine perineuronal immunodeposits, and prominent intraneuronal dots (Kovacs et al., 2011). The neuropathology of E200K mutation is similar to MM1 sporadic CJD (Fig. 13.4A, B), but there are features (Fig. 13.4C–J) not seen in sporadic CJD, including a distinct type of intraneuronal PrP^{TSE} immunoreactivity that distinguishes a subset of E200K mutation cases from sporadic CJD (Kovacs et al., 2012). These deposits are small globular darkly immunostained cytoplasmic PrP^{TSE} with a size ranging between 1.5 and 4.0 μm. In some cells, there are single large globular structures with a size (between 7.5 and 15 μm) similar to or larger than the nuclei of the neuron. These deposits are seen irrespective of codon 129 polymorphism and are clearly different from the diffuse cytoplasmic staining and punctuate staining seen in sporadic CJD, especially in VV2 and MV2 cases (Kovacs et al., 2012), but reminiscent of intraneuronal deposit observed in the V180I *PRNP* mutation with abnormally glycosylated PrP^{TSE} (Nixon et al., 2000).

A further distinct feature is the presence of a stripe-like pattern of PrP^{TSE} immunoreactivity in the cerebellar cortex that is associated with less prominent spongiform change in the molecular layer and less neuronal loss in the granular layer than cases with diffuse/synaptic PrP^{TSE} immunoreactivity involving all cerebellar layers (Jarius et al., 2003; Kovacs et al., 2011). This pattern is distinct from that seen in OPRI cases in the molecular layer of the cerebellum (King et al., 2003), similar to that reported in one case of FFI (Almer et al., 1999).

Further, distinct features in E200K mutated cases are: (1) a trend for more prominent involvement of the deeper layers irrespective of codon 129 polymorphism (a feature more characteristic of VV2 sporadic CJD); (2) a lack of amyloid kuru-type plaques in cases with MV at codon 129 even when associated with type 2 PrP^{res} (as characteristic for sporadic CJD MV2); and (3) the frequent association with other neurodegeneration-related protein deposits (Kovacs et al., 2011). Additional proteinopathies include frequent A-beta deposits, neuron-related tau pathologies, and histologic signs of Lewy body alpha-synuclein pathology (Kovacs et al., 2011). Together these lesions may lead to complex clinical symptoms (e.g., early-onset L-dopa-responsive Parkinson disease before the appearance of CJD-like clinical signs) and a rapid progressive course (Kovacs et al., 2011). These complex deposits of various misfolded proteins were not fully emphasized (Kovacs et al., 2011), likely because previous neuropathologic reports were not detailed or neuropathology differs in patients with distinct ancestral origins (Lee et al., 1999).

Western blot examination shows type 1 or type 2 PrP^{res}, including their co-occurrence in the same brain. However, distinct glycoform ratios can be recognized (Cardone et al., 1999; Hill et al., 2006; Kovacs et al., 2011).

E200G-129V

Epidemiology and genetics

The glutamate (E) to glycine (G) change at codon 200 (E200G) of *PRNP* was reported in a US patient of British descent and her asymptomatic younger sibling (Kim et al., 2013).

Clinical features

Disease onset was at 57 years old with gait problems followed by cognitive deterioration that progressed slowly over time with language and memory disturbances (Mini Mental State Examination of 25/30 at 25 months after onset). Extensive neuropsychologic testing revealed mild cognitive impairment. Cerebellar and extrapyramidal signs were observed, although no myoclonus or other involuntary movements. EEG showed bilateral slowing without typical periodic activity and brain MRI showed cortical ribboning and striatal hyperintensity on FLAIR and DWI. CSF 14-3-3 test was inconclusive, while total tau was elevated (1351 pg/mL).

Neuropathology and biochemistry

In addition to the signs of spongiform encephalopathy, immunostaining revealed PrP^{TSE} perivacuolar and diffuse finely granular synaptic staining in the cerebral cortex. Occasional larger plaque-like deposits were also seen. In addition, abundant punctate, linear, and curvilinear arrays of PrP^{TSE} in the striatum and other regions, including the hippocampus, substantia nigra, midbrain tegmentum, periaqueductal gray, and medullary inferior olivary nucleus were also reported (Kim et al., 2013). Western blot analysis showed type 2 PrP^{res} with prominent representation of diglycosylated and underrepresentation of unglycosylated species (Kim et al., 2013).

V203I-129M and occasionally V203I-129V

Epidemiology and genetics

Genetic CJD associated with the valine (V) to isoleucine (I) substitution at codon 203 (V203I) and homozygosity for M at codon 129 was first described in an Italian patient (Peoc'h et al., 2000). The mutation was then reported in France, Austria, and Canada (Kovacs et al., 2005b, 2017; Minikel et al., 2016) and in one codon

129 heterozygous patient in Italy (Cistaro et al., 2017). The mutation was also found in East Asian populations: one case in China (Shi et al., 2013), three cases in Japan, where a homozygous mutated patient was found (Komatsu et al., 2014; Minikel et al., 2016), and a V203I-129V haplotype in Korea (Jeong et al., 2010). Family history is negative in all the cases reported so far (Table 13.1).

Clinical features

Genetic CJD with V203I-129M haplotype is almost indistinguishable from sporadic CJD. The disease affects subjects with a mean age at onset of 69 years and a median clinical duration of 4 months. Clinical symptoms and signs include rapid progressive dementia, myoclonus, cerebellar, pyramidal, extrapyramidal signs, and akinetic mutism. EEG shows the typical periodic activity in the majority of cases and brain MRI hyperintensity in cortical areas or basal ganglia. The 14-3-3 protein test was positive in all cases, tau values were elevated, and RT-QuIC analysis amplified the pathologic prion protein in the CSF (Sano et al., 2013; Lattanzio et al., 2017). Brain 18F-fluorodeoxyglucose (FDG) positron emission tomography/ computed tomography showed decreased 18F-FDG uptakes bilaterally in cortical regions but also hypermetabolic aspects in left temporomesial lobe and subcortical areas (Cistaro et al., 2017).

A V203I-129V patient presented with gait disturbance followed by rapidly progressive cognitive dysfunction, extrapyramidal signs, urinary incontinence, pyramidal signs, and myoclonus (Jeong et al., 2010).

Neuropathology and biochemistry

Spongiform encephalopathy was reported in 4 cases (Jeong et al., 2010; Kovacs et al., 2017). Immunostaining for PrP^{TSE} reveals diffuse synaptic (Fig. 13.4K), perineuronal, and somatosynaptic depositions (Kovacs et al., 2017). A concomitant unusual 4R tauopathy with peculiar astrogliopathy (Fig. 13.4L, M) involving the hippocampus, amygdala, frontal and temporal cortex, and to a lesser extent, subcortical regions including basal ganglia and thalamus, was recently reported (Kovacs et al., 2017). Western blot analysis in a single patient revealed a typical PrP^{res} type 1 pattern, characterized by three bands migrating at about 30, 26, and 21 kDa together with an additional band at 17 kDa, which is different from the bands seen in most sporadic CJD cases (Jeong et al., 2010).

R208H 129M and occasionally R208H-129V

Epidemiology and genetics

The arginine (R) to histidine (H) change at codon 208 (R208H) associated with M at codon 129 was first identified in the United States in 1996 (Mastrianni et al., 1996). Since then a few cases have been described in European countries, Japan, and China (Capellari et al., 2005; Roeber et al., 2005; Basset-Leobon et al., 2006; Nozaki et al., 2010; Chen et al., 2011; Shi et al., 2015, Mitrova et al., 2015; Ladogana and Pocchiari, unpublished data). The R08H associated with V at codon 129 was identified in 4 cases in Europe (Basset-Leobon et al., 2006; Mellina et al., 2007; Matej et al., 2012; Vita et al., 2013).

Clinical features

Genetic CJD with R208H-129M haplotype is similar to sporadic CJD MM129 type 1. The mean age at onset is 64 years and median disease duration is 7 months. Clinically, the disease manifests with progressive dementia, myoclonus, and cerebellar/visual, pyramidal and extrapyramidal signs (Roeber et al., 2005; Chen et al., 2011). The EEG pattern shows the typical periodic activity in the majority of cases, while the 14-3-3 protein test is positive in 60% and brain MRI in 44% of cases.

RT-QuIC analysis amplified the pathologic prion protein in the CSF of 1 patient (Poleggi, personal communication).

The presentation of genetic CJD with R208H-129V haplotype is very close to that of sporadic CJD VV2. Mean age at onset is 64 years and median disease duration is 12.5 months. Interestingly, psychiatric symptoms at onset were described in all reported cases, while in 1 case the initial presentation was similar to progressive supranuclear palsy (Matej et al., 2012). The EEG pattern shows typical periodic activity and brain MRI is positive in 50% of cases, while the 14-3-3 protein test is positive in 75% of cases. RT-QuIC analysis did not amplify the pathologic prion protein in the CSF in the single patient tested so far (Lattanzio et al., 2017).

Neuropathology and biochemistry

Neuropathologic studies revealed spongiform encephalopathy. Immunostaining for PrP^{TSE} overlaps with that of sporadic CJD, including synaptic, perineuronal, perivacuolar, and plaque-like deposits (Mastrianni et al., 1996; Capellari et al., 2001; Roeber et al., 2005; Matej et al., 2012). Kuru-type plaques, as seen in MV2 sporadic CJD, were reported particularly in the molecular layer of the cerebellum in 1 case with VV homozygosity at codon 129 (Basset-Leobon et al., 2006). Tau pathology, mainly restricted to the temporal lobe, was also reported (Roeber et al., 2005; Matej et al., 2012), but with characteristics deviating from other tauopathies. Western blot analysis revealed type 1 PrP^{res} in 2 cases with MM homozygosity at codon 129 (Mastrianni et al., 1996; Capellari et al., 2001), and type 2A pattern in two codon 129 VV homozygous cases (Basset-Leobon et al., 2006; Matej et al., 2012). In addition, a band of 17 kDa and a glycosylation ratio differing from the ratios described in sporadic CJD have been reported in 1 case with MM at codon 129 (Roeber et al., 2005).

V210I-129 M and occasionally V210I-129V

Epidemiology and genetics

The valine (V) to isoleucine (I) substitution at codon 210 (V210I) was first identified in a CJD family from Italy (Pocchiari et al., 1993) and one from France (Ripoll et al., 1993). Then, single cases were reported in Japan, China (Furukawa et al., 1996; Shyu et al., 1996), North Africa (Mouillet-Richard et al., 1999), Brazil (Huang et al., 2001), and other European and non-European countries (Kovacs et al., 2005b; Takada et al., 2017). Its frequency, however, varies among countries. In most countries, the incidence is very low while in Italy it represents 42% of all *PRNP* mutations, mostly located in three nearby provinces of Campania and Apulia regions (Ladogana et al., 2005b). *PRNP* screening in unselected subjects reported to the Italian CJD surveillance center revealed an unexpected number of cases linked to V210I mutation with no family history of CJD. An attempt to quantify the penetrance of V210I mutation by using Bayesian analysis resulted in a lifetime risk of about 10% (Minikel et al., 2016). However, there are uncertainties on the validity of this study due to the presence of geographic clusters and the absence of allelic frequency and age distribution of the general population in these areas.

Clinical features

Similar to E200K-CJD, genetic CJD with V210I-M129 haplotype is almost indistinguishable from sporadic CJD-MM 1. The disease affects relatively young subjects with a mean age at onset of 61 years ($n = 211$), which is unaffected by the codon 129 polymorphism (Kovacs et al., 2005b; Ladogana and Pocchiari, unpublished data). The median clinical duration is 4 months with a wide range of survival (Ladogana and Pocchiari, unpublished data), which is partially influenced by the polymorphism at codon 129 with methionine homozygous showing shorter survival than heterozygous patients (Pocchiari et al., 2004).

The clinical presentation is usually characterized by cerebellar (38%, mainly as ataxic gait), cognitive (36%), and psychiatric dysfunctions (22%) (Ladogana and Pocchiari, unpublished data). During the course of the disease, patients develop dementia in 98% (in a few cases the disease progresses so rapidly that it is not possible to establish the presence of dementia), cerebellar symptoms and signs in 82%, myoclonus in 79%, extrapyramidal signs in 60%, and visual signs in 60% of cases (Ladogana and Pocchiari, unpublished data). Unusual clinical presentations include isolated visual symptoms as initial manifestation, similar to the "Heidenhain variant" of sporadic CJD (Imbriani et al., 2016) or spastic paraparesis with an early selective involvement of the corticospinal tracts, as revealed by diffusion tensor imaging (Conte et al., 2015).

Depending upon the studies, the EEG shows the typical periodic activity (PSWC) in between 44% and 79% of cases (Kovacs et al., 2005b; Breithaupt et al., 2013; Krasnianski et al., 2016). Brain MRI hyperintensity of basal ganglia and cortical areas was reported in between 15% and 37% of cases (Kovacs et al., 2005b; Krasnianski et al., 2016).

The 14-3-3 protein test is positive in 85–100% of patients while a high level of total tau is present in 100% (Ladogana et al., 2009; Krasnianski et al., 2016; Lattanzio et al., 2017). RT-QuIC analysis of CSF samples revealed the presence of the pathologic prion protein with high sensitivity (95–100%) (Conte et al., 2015; Cramm et al., 2016; Imbriani et al., 2016; Steinanacker et al., 2016; Lattanzio et al., 2017). PrP^{TSE} was also detected by RT-QuIC in the olfactory mucosa of 2 patients (Bongianni et al., 2017).

Neuropathology and biochemistry

Neuropathologic and biochemical studies, reported only in a few cases, show spongiform changes in the cerebral cortex and cerebellum and a pattern of PrP^{res} reminiscent of MM1 sporadic CJD (Pocchiari et al, 1993; Mastrianni et al., 2001; Capellari et al., 2011).

E211Q-129M

Epidemiology and genetics

Two different substitutions were found at the glutamic acid (E) residue 211 of *PRNP*: the glutamine (Q) substitution (E211Q) associated with genetic CJD, and the aspartic acid (D) substitution (E211D) associated with GSS (Peoc'h et al., 2012). This phenotypic dichotomy represents an example of great variability of clinical presentation linked to a single-residue substitution of the prion protein.

The E211Q mutation, though very rare, was reported in families with more than one member affected by CJD in France and Italy (Peoc'h et al., 2000; Ladogana et al., 2001). Eleven cases linked to this mutation have so far been recorded (Owen et al., 2014; Minikel et al., 2016).

Clinical phenotype

Genetic CJD with E211Q-129M haplotype is almost indistinguishable from sporadic CJD. The mean age at onset is 67 years with a median disease duration of

7 months. Clinical manifestations consist of rapid progressive dementia, severe cerebellar ataxia, myoclonus, akinetic mutism, and the presence of periodic synchronous discharges on EEG or positive 14-3-3 test. Brain MRI findings are not available so far.

Neuropathology and biochemistry

Spongiform change and gliosis were observed in the striatum and the isocortex in 2 cases, together with very mild synaptic deposits, especially in the cerebellar cortex (Peoc'h et al., 2012). Amyloid plaques were not observed. Western blot revealed a PrP^{res} pattern with co-occurrence of types 1 and 2A, with high prevalence of type 1 (Peoc'h et al., 2012).

I215V-129M

Epidemiology and genetics

An isoleucine to valine change at codon 215 was reported in two different families from the same geographic region of Spain (Muñoz-Nieto et al., 2013). Both patients carried M homozygosity at codon 129 and had no family history of prion disease, but an older brother of one of these two patients carrying MV heterozygosity at codon 129 developed Alzheimer disease.

Clinical phenotype

Both patients presented with a clinical phenotype of rapid progressive neuropsychiatric symptoms, one at 55 years and the other at 76 years. Disease duration was 15 and 12 months, respectively. EEG was compatible with CJD and brain MRI showed atrophy in the cortical areas. CSF 14-3-3 examination was positive in only 1 patient (76 years old). A third patient (brother of the 76-year-old case) developed slowly progressive cognitive decline without MRI and EEG features of CJD and with negative 14-3-3 examination. The duration of illness was 54 months (Muñoz-Nieto et al., 2013) and the patient had neuropathologically confirmed Alzheimer disease.

Neuropathology and biochemistry

Neuropathology was characterized by spongiform changes and neuronal loss with reactive astrocytosis compatible with prion disease. In 1 case, immunostaining for PrP^{TSE} was not performed while in the second one it gave a negative result using the 3F4 anti-PrP antibody. Western blot examination was not reported.

A224V-129V

Epidemiology and genetics

The alanine (A) to valine (V) change at codon 224 (A224V) was reported in a U.S patient with no family history for CJD (Watts et al., 2015).

Clinical phenotype

The disease was similar to the rare VV1 subtype of sporadic CJD. The patient was a 48-year-old patient with memory disturbances followed by walking and other motor problems that worsened over time. The EEG did not show typical periodic activity, while MRI showed cortical ribboning and striatal hyperintensity on FLAIR and DWI. The CSF 14-3-3 test was inconclusive, while total tau was elevated (6300 pg/mL).

Neuropathology and biochemistry

The main histopathologic features were severe degeneration and loss of neurons. Immunostaining for PrP^{TSE} revealed densely packed, finely granular deposition in the cerebral and cerebellar cortex. No neurofibrillary tangles were observed. Western blot revealed PrP^{res} consistent with type 1 (Watts et al., 2015).

M232R-129M

Epidemiology and genetics

The substitution of methionine to arginine at codon 232 (M232R) is among the most frequent mutations in the Japanese population (Nozaki et al., 2010, Minikel et al., 2016) where, in a single patient, it was also found in homozygosity (Kon et al., 2015). The mutation was also described in China (Zheng et al., 2008) and South Korea (Choi et al., 2009; Jeong and Kim, 2014), but not yet in the Caucasian population. The low frequency of family history, the occurrence of 3 cases carrying the mutation with a definite alternative diagnosis (Shiga et al., 2007), and the finding that the mutation is highly frequent in healthy individuals (Minikel et al., 2016) suggest that this amino acid substitution is either a poorly pathogenic mutation with a very low penetrance (0.1%) or a polymorphism that increases the risk of developing sporadic CJD.

A double mutation (M232R/V180I) was reported in 2 Japanese patients, 84 and 74 years old (Hitoshi et al., 1993; Nozaki et al., 2010; Koh et al., 2015).

Clinical features

Genetic CJD with M232R-129M haplotype is almost indistinguishable from sporadic CJD. The disease affects subjects with a mean age at onset of 65 years and a mean clinical duration (Japanese patients) of 9 months (n = 63), with a wide range of survival (Minikel et al., 2016). The majority of these patients show rapid progressive dementia, but there are a few patients who experience a relatively slow progression (Shiga et al., 2007).

The EEG pattern shows the typical periodic activity in 75% of cases and brain MRI the typical hyperintensity of basal nuclei and/or cortical regions in 92% (Minikel et al., 2016). The 14-3-3 protein test is positive in 72% of cases and the total tau, with a cut-off at 1260 pg/mL, has 94% sensitivity (Higuma et al., 2013). The rate of PrP^{TSE} detection by RT-QuIC test in the CSF was 78% (Higuma et al., 2013).

The double mutation M232R/V180I-129M presented with dysarthria, gait disturbance, and cognitive impairment in 1 patient, and with severe dementia, myoclonus, and akinetic mutism in the other patient.

Neuropathology and biochemistry

Histopathologic examinations show spongiform change, neuronal loss, and severe astrocytosis together with diffuse synaptic PrP^{TSE} immunoreactivity in the gray matter with no plaque-type deposition (Hoque et al., 1996). The rapid- and slow-type clinical phenotypes show distinct neuropathologic lesions. The rapid type shows neuropathologic lesions and PrP^{TSE} immunostaining patterns compatible with MM1 sporadic CJD while the slow type shows a mixed phenotype with perivacuolar PrP^{TSE} deposits as in MM2 sporadic CJD, and a PrP^{TSE} synaptic type as MM1 sporadic CJD (Shiga et al., 2007; Nozaki et al., 2010). Brain homogenates from 2 patients were successfully transmitted to experimental animals (Hoque et al., 1996).

Neuropathology was performed in only 1 case with the double mutation (M232R/V180I) and showed spongiform changes and diffuse PrP^{TSE} immunostaining. Western blot revealed type 1 PrP^{res} but with undetectable dyglicosylated band (Hitoshi et al., 1993).

Octapeptide repeat insertions

Epidemiology and genetics

Besides single-point mutations of *PRNP*, insertions of 24-basepair repeats in the OPR coding regions were described. The region of the *PRNP* between codons 51 and 91 in human normally comprises one nonapeptide and four octapeptide coding sequences (Kretzschmar et al., 1986). An insert mutation of six OPR insertions (OPRIs) was identified for the first time in a British CJD family (Owen et al., 1989). Since then, additional families have been reported from several European countries, the United States, Japan, and China, in which the affected members had insertion from 1 to 12 repeats (Goldfarb et al., 1991b; Oda et al., 1995; Capellari et al., 1997; Wang et al., 2007). Disease-associated insert mutations are stable between generations; however a de novo insert mutation in the *PRNP* was once observed (Mauro et al., 2008). Unequal crossover and recombination were proposed as the cause of extra repeat formations (Goldfarb et al., 1991b). OPRIs are classified based on the number of additional repeats (Table 13.1), even though basepair insertion of similar size may differ in both the arrangement of repeats and their sequence (Nicholl et al., 1995; Croes et al., 2004).

Clinical features

Clinical and neuropathologic heterogeneity characterizes the phenotypic expression of OPRI, including CJD, GSS, and early- and late-onset dementia (Goldfarb et al., 1992c; Laplanche et al., 1995; Pietrini et al., 2003; Croes et al., 2004). This marked heterogeneity was observed in affected members between and within families (Collinge et al., 1992; Mead et al., 2006). The major molecular determinant that likely influences the phenotype is the size of the OPRI (Croes et al., 2004), but other factors, such as the PrP^{TSE} type, the codon 129 polymorphism, and polymorphisms upstream the open reading frame of *PRNP*, may also play important roles (Poulter et al., 1992; Mead et al., 2006; Jansen et al., 2011).

Neuropathology and biochemistry

The neuropathologic features in cases with OPRI vary considerably from CJD-like, GGS-like, to other phenotypes not easily classified as either CJD or GSS. That is why it is more correct to call the OPRI-related diseases inherited prion diseases with variable phenotype unless the CJD or GSS phenotype is clearly evident. Histopathologically, the variability is mostly seen in cases with 5–7 OPRIs. Immunostaining for PrP^{TSE} shows peculiar deposits, such as linear accumulations perpendicular to the surface in the molecular layer of the cerebellum, especially in the 6-OPRI cases (King et al., 2003) and less frequently in 4- and 7-OPRI cases (Kitamoto et al., 1992; Campbell et al., 1996). This immunoreactivity is more coarse type than seen in some cases with the E200K point mutation (Jarius et al., 2003). Some cases with 6-OPRI show amyloid plaques while others show eosinophilic globular PrP^{TSE} deposits without amyloid characteristics (Gelpi et al., 2005). The rarely reported Western blots in OPRI cases are usually consistent with that seen in sporadic CJD (Capellari et al., 2011). 7-OPRI cases may show amyloid plaques and low-molecular-weight PrP^{res} fragments in Western blot as in GSS (Jansen et al., 2011).

1–4 OPRI-129M and occasionally 1–4 OPRI-129V

Patients with one to four OPRI-129M usually present with a typical CJD phenotype with rapidly progressive dementia, myoclonus, and cerebellar symptoms (Takada et al., 2017). Based on cases reported with available demographic information ($n = 23$), the mean age at onset is 61 years and the median disease duration is 6 months. EEG is typical in 48% of cases, CSF 14-3-3 protein is positive in 62%, and brain MRI shows characteristic CJD scans in 36%. In one isolated case a slowly progressive dementia was observed without other neurologic focal signs and long disease duration. These OPRIs showed low penetrance with only a few cases with dementia in the family history.

Two patients, with 2 OPRI-129V, showed an atypical CJD phenotype characterized by an early and slowly progressive dementia with or without cerebellar signs (van Harten et al., 2000; Croes et al., 2004).

5–7 OPRI

Patients with 5–7 OPRI-linked disease show different clinical phenotypes, such as typical CJD, early-onset CJD with long disease duration, Huntington disease with chorea and dystonia, or GSS-like disease. The 6-OPRI is the most frequent insertion of this group and usually presents with a progressive cortical dementia, behavioral changes that often precede cognitive deterioration, cerebellar ataxia, and pyramidal signs. Myoclonus and other involuntary movements are also frequent and occasionally epileptic seizures. EEG and brain MRI are not usually helpful for the diagnosis.

Octapeptide repeat deletions (OPRDs)

2 OPRD

Deletion of two octapeptides coupled with methionine at codon 129 was first identified in a woman of Northern European origin with no family history of neurodegenerative diseases who developed rapidly progressive dementia at age 86 and died 23 months later. Because EEG and brain MRI did not show the characteristic features of CJD and neuropathology was not performed, a diagnosis of CJD was not confirmed (Beck et al., 2001).

The 2-OPRD was also reported in a male patient, who at age 62 developed a rapid progressive dementia with seizures and myoclonus and died 18 months after onset (Capellari et al., 2002). His mother had been diagnosed with Alzheimer disease and died in her 80s. The neuropathologic and biochemical findings were similar to those reported in sporadic CJD MM type 1 (Capellari et al., 2002). Three other nonrelated patients were recently reported in the Netherlands (Minikel et al., 2016).

Finally, one OPRD was found as a rare polymorphism in several populations of different ethnic origin and is not considered to predispose to CJD or to any other type of human prion disease.

CONCLUSIONS

There are several amino acid changes and string of 8 OPRIs or OPRDs that determine prion diseases with clinical and pathologic features similar to sporadic CJD. Changes in the primary structure likely facilitate the conformational switch of PrPc into PrP^{TSE}, but it is still unclear why mutated carriers develop disease at different ages and a good proportion of them do not develop disease at all. These unsolved pathogenic issues have critical implications for giving correct information to family members about the risk of developing disease and family planning.

The proportion of genetic CJD has increased in the last years, likely because of improvement in the diagnosis of CJD and the broad availability of genetic tests, which are always recommended when there is evidence of other CJD cases in the family, but also in those patients with an unremarkable family history but who fall in the high-risk category because they are born in regions with a high incidence of genetic CJD, belong to Sephardic Jewish families, or simply have a relatively young age at onset (i.e., in the 50s). Genetic analysis requires a written informed consent from patients but, because of their severe cognitive deterioration, this is usually obtained from family members (Bechtel and Geschwind, 2013) without proper genetic counseling. In CJD, the diagnosis and results of the genetic test are usually communicated to relatives rather than to patients because they have often greatly mentally deteriorated. Learning about a fatal diagnosis is distressing for relatives and even more so when they know that the cause of the disease comes from a genetic mutation that might affect other members of the family.

In cases of rare or extremely rare mutations, medical professionals are faced with doubts about the pathogenic role of the mutation in determining CJD and this uncertainty finally impacts the correct information they communicate to relatives. It is therefore important to implement studies aiming to improve the correct penetrance of each mutation.

The genetic forms of CJD have crucial implications in clinical practice and public health. Carriers of *PRNP* mutations may harbor infectivity in tissues before the development of clinical signs and therefore they cannot donate blood or tissues and should inform health professionals before undergoing any type of surgery in order to enable correct planning of ad hoc measures for the decontamination of instruments and surgical rooms.

At-risk subjects are family members of a CJD patient who is a carrier of a pathogenic *PRNP* mutation and subjects belonging to a CJD-affected family with an unknown carrier status.

The high incidence of genetic CJD in restricted cluster areas poses further problems for the prevention of possible spread of disease by medical and surgical procedures. In Slovakia, for example, where there is a high incidence of E200K genetic CJD in a close geographic area, genetic testing of corneal donors has been introduced for the prevention of possible iatrogenic transmission (Mitrová et al., 2011).

Predictive genetic tests for healthy blood relatives should be considered after genetic counseling following international guidelines for adult-onset untreatable neurodegenerative disease (Bechtel and Geschwind, 2013; MacLeod et al., 2013). Predictive tests should not be performed on minors.

Finally, because there is as yet no effective therapy for CJD-affected patients and experimental data strongly suggest that any possible treatment should start well before the development of clinical signs (Vetrugno et al., 2015), it is reasonable to attempt preventive therapy with poorly toxic drugs (for example, doxycycline) in mutated carriers years before the presumed onset of disease (Pocchiari and Ladogana, 2015), as has been proposed for FFI (Forloni et al., 2015).

ACKNOWLEDGMENTS

We gratefully acknowledge Professor E. Kahana and Drs X.P. Dong and J. Wang for communicating their updated data on CJD surveillance in Israel and China, and A. Poleggi and M. Equestre for kindly providing data on the detection of PrP^{TSE} in the CSF and olfactory mucosa of a patient with genetic CJD using the RT-QuIC assay. We also thank C. Gasparrini for her valuable administrative support and M. Delle Femmine for the figures and editing.

References

Almer G, Hainfellner JA, Brücke T (1999). Fatal familial insomnia: a new Austrian family. Brain 122: 5–16.

Baiardi S, Magherini A, Capellari S et al. (2017). Towards an early clinical diagnosis of sporadic CJD VV2 (ataxic type). J Neurol Neurosurg Psychiatry 88: 764–772.

Barbanti P, Fabbrini G, Salvatore M et al. (1996). Polymorphism at codon 129 or codon 219 of PRNP and clinical heterogeneity in a previously unreported family with Gerstmann-Sträussler-Scheinker disease (PrP-P102L mutation). Neurology 47: 734–741.

Basset-Leobon C, Uro-Coste E, Peoc'h K et al. (2006). Familial Creutzfeldt–Jakob disease with an R208H-129V haplotype and Kuru plaques. Arch Neurol 63: 449–452.

Bechtel K, Geschwind MD (2013). Ethics in prion disease. Prog Neurobiol 110: 29–44.

Beck JA, Mead S, Campbell TA et al. (2001). Two-octapeptide repeat deletion of prion protein associated with rapidly progressive dementia. Neurology 57: 354–356.

Beck JA, Poulter M, Campbell TA et al. (2010). PRNP allelic series from 19 years of prion protein gene sequencing at the MRC Prion Unit. Hum Mutat 31: E1551–E1563.

Béjot Y, Osseby GV, Caillier M et al. (2010). Rare E196K mutation in the PRNP gene of a patient exhibiting behavioral abnormalities. Clin Neurol Neurosurg 112: 244–247.

Bertoni JM, Brown P, Goldfarb LG et al. (1992). Familial Creutzfeldt–Jakob disease (codon 200 mutation) with supranuclear palsy. JAMA 268: 2413–2415.

Bongianni M, Orrù C, Groveman BR et al. (2017). Diagnosis of human prion disease using real-time quaking-induced conversion testing of olfactory mucosa and cerebrospinal fluid samples. JAMA Neurol. 74: 1–8.

Breithaupt M, Romero C, Kallenberg K et al. (2013). Magnetic resonance imaging in E200K and V210I mutations of the prion protein gene. Alzheimer Dis Assoc Disord 27: 87–90.

Brown P, Goldfarb LG, Cathala F et al. (1991). The molecular genetics of familial Creutzfeldt–Jakob disease in France. J Neurol Sci 105: 240–246.

Brown P, Goldfarb LG, Kovanen J et al. (1992a). Phenotypic characteristics of familial Creutzfeldt–Jakob disease associated with the codon 178Asn PRNP mutation. Ann Neurol 31: 282–285.

Brown P, Galvez S, Goldfarb LG et al. (1992b). Familial Creutzfeldt–Jakob disease in Chile is associated with the codon 200 mutation of the PRNP amyloid precursor gene on chromosome 20. J Neurol Sci 112: 65–67.

Brown P, Cervenakova L, Boellaard JW et al. (1994). Identification of a PRNP gene mutation in Jakob's original Creutzfeldt–Jakob disease family. Lancet 344: 130–131.

Budka H, Aguzzi A, Brown P et al. (1995). Neuropathological diagnostic criteria for Creutzfeldt–Jakob disease (CJD) and other human spongiform encephalopathies (prion diseases). Brain Pathol 5: 459–466.

Campbell TA, Palmer MS, Will RG et al. (1996). A prion disease with a novel 96-base pair insertional mutation in the prion protein gene. Neurology 46: 761–766.

Capellari S, Vital C, Parchi P et al. (1997). Familial prion disease with a novel 144-bp insertion in the prion protein gene in a Basque family. Neurology 49: 133–141.

Capellari S, Parchi P, Bennett D et al. (1999). First North American report of the T183A mutation in the prion protein gene: clinical, pathological, and biochemical analysis of one case. Neurology 52 Supplement 2 A324.

Capellari S, Ladogana A, Volpi G et al. (2001). First report of the R208H-129MM haplotype in the prion protein gene in a European subject with CJD. Neurol Sci 22: 109.

Capellari S, Parchi P, Wolff BD et al. (2002). Creutzfeldt–Jakob disease associated with a deletion of two repeats in the prion protein gene. Neurology 59: 1628–1630.

Capellari S, Cardone F, Notari S et al. (2005). Creutzfeldt–Jakob disease associated with the R208H mutation in the prion protein gene. Neurology 64: 905–907.

Capellari S, Strammiello R, Saverioni D et al. (2011). Genetic Creutzfeldt–Jakob disease and fatal familial insomnia: insights into phenotypic variability and disease pathogenesis. Acta Neuropathol 121: 21–37.

Cardone F, Liu QG, Peraroli R et al. (1999). Prion protein glycotype analysis in familial and sporadic Creutzfeldt–Jakob disease patients. Brain Res Bull 49: 429–433.

Cardone F, Principe S, Schininà ME et al. (2014). Mutant PrPCJD prevails over wild-type PrPCJD in the brain of

V210I and R208H genetic Creutzfeldt–Jakob disease patients. Biochem Biophys Res Commun 454: 289–294.

Chapman J, Brown P, Goldfarb LG et al. (1993). Clinical heterogeneity and unusual presentations of Creutzfeldt–Jakob disease in Jewish patients with the PRNP codon 200 mutation. J Neurol Neurosurg Psychiatry 56: 1109–1112.

Chasseigneaux S, Haïk S, Laffont-Proust I et al. (2006). V180I mutation of the prion protein gene associated with atypical PrPSc glycosylation. Neurosci Lett 408: 165–169.

Chen C, Shi Q, Tian C et al. (2011). The first Chinese case of Creutzfeldt–Jakob disease patient with R208H mutation in PRNP. Prion 5: 232–234.

Chen C, Shi Q, Zhou W et al. (2013). Clinical and familial characteristics of eight Chinese patients with T188K genetic Creutzfeldt–Jakob disease. Infect Genet Evol 14: 120–124.

Choi BY, Kim SY, Seo SY et al. (2009). Mutations at codons 178, 200-129, and 232 contributed to the inherited prion diseases in Korean patients. BMC Infect Dis 9: 132.

Cistaro A, Cassalia L, Ferrara C et al. (2017). Brain 18F-FDG PET/CT findings in a case of genetic Creutzfeldt–Jakob disease due to V203I heterozygous mutation in the PRNP gene. J Neurol 264: 170–173.

Clerici F, Elia A, Girotti F et al. (2008). Atypical presentation of Creutzfeldt–Jakob disease: the first Italian case associated with E196K mutation in the PRNP gene. J Neurol Sci 275: 145–147.

Cohen OS, Chapman J, Korczyn AD et al. (2015). Familial Creutzfeldt–Jakob disease with the E200K mutation: longitudinal neuroimaging from asymptomatic to symptomatic CJD. J Neurol 262: 604–613.

Cohen OS, Kimiagar I, Korczyn AD et al. (2016a). Unusual presentations in patients with E200K familial Creutzfeldt–Jakob disease. Eur J Neurol 23: 871–877.

Cohen OS, Chapman J, Korczyn AD et al. (2016b). Clinical radiological correlation in E200K familial Creutzfeldt–Jakob disease. J Neural Transm 123: 1457–1462.

Collinge J, Brown J, Hardy J et al. (1992). Inherited prion disease with 144 base pair gene insertion. Brain 115: 687–710.

Collinge J, Palmer MS, Campbell T et al. (1993). Inherited prion disease (PrP lysine 200) in Britain: two case reports. BMJ 306: 301–302.

Collins S, Boyd A, Fletcher A et al. (2000). Novel prion protein gene mutation in an octogenarian with Creutzfeldt–Jakob disease. Arch Neurol 57: 1058–1063.

Conte F, Giordano A, Tortora F et al. (2015). Early-onset spastic paraparesis as presenting sign of familial Creutzfeldt–Jakob disease. Parkinsonism Relat Disord 21: 1479–1480.

Coria F, Quadrado N, Rubio I et al. (1995). In: Genetics of spongiform encephalopathy in Spain: preliminary data, Fifth meeting of the European Neurological Society (Munich, 17-21 June), abstract 227.

Cramm M, Schmitz M, Karch A et al. (2016). Stability and reproducibility underscore utility of RT-QuIC for diagnosis of Creutzfeldt–Jakob disease. Mol Neurobiol 53: 1896–1904.

Croes EA, Theuns J, Houwing-Duistermaat JJ et al. (2004). Octapeptide repeat insertions in the prion protein gene and early onset dementia. J Neurol Neurosurg Psychiatry 75: 1166–1170.

D'Alessandro M, Petraroli R, Ladogana A et al. (1998). High incidence of Creutzfeldt–Jakob disease in rural Calabria, Italy. Lancet 352: 1989–1990.

De Michele G, Pocchiari M, Petraroli R et al. (2003). Variable phenotype in a P102L Gerstmann-Sträussler-Scheinker Italian family. Can J Neurol Sci 30: 233–236.

Eigenbrod S, Frick P, Giese A et al. (2011). Comprehensive neuropathologic analysis of genetic prion disease associated with the E196K mutation in PRNP reveals phenotypic heterogeneity. J Neuropathol Exp Neurol 70: 192–200.

Finckh U, Muller-Thomsen T, Mann U et al. (2000). High frequency of mutations in four different disease genes in early-onset dementia. Ann NY Acad Sci 920: 100–106.

Forloni G, Tettamanti M, Lucca U et al. (2015). Preventive study in subjects at risk of fatal familial insomnia: innovative approach to rare diseases. Prion 9: 75–79.

Friedman-Levi Y, Meiner Z, Canello T et al. (2011). Fatal prion disease in a mouse model of genetic E200K Creutzfeldt–Jakob disease. PLoS Pathog 7: e1002350.

Fulbright RK, Hoffmann C, Lee H et al. (2008). MR imaging of familial Creutzfeldt-Jakob disease: a blinded and controlled study. AJNR Am J Neuroradiol 29: 1638–1643.

Furukawa H, Kitamoto T, Hashiguchi H et al. (1996). A Japanese case of Creutzfeldt–Jakob disease with a point mutation in the prion protein gene at codon 210. J Neurol Sci 141: 120–122.

Gao C, Shi Q, Zhou W et al. (2010). The first Chinese case of Creutzfeldt–Jakob disease with mutation of E200K in PRNP. Biomed Environ Sci 23: 158–160.

Gelpi E, Kovacs GG, Ströbel T et al. (2005). Prion disease with a 144 base pair insertion: unusual cerebellar prion protein immunoreactivity. Acta Neuropathol 110: 513–519.

Ghetti B, Tagliavini F, Takao M et al. (2003). Hereditary prion protein amyloidoses. Clin Lab Med 23: 65–85.

Ghetti B, Tagliavini F, Kovacs GG, Piccardo P (2011). Gerstmann-Sträussler-Scheinker disease. In: DW Dickson, RO Weller (Eds.), Neurodegeneration: the molecular pathology of dementia and movement disorders. Blackwell Publishing, Chichester, pp. 364–377.

Giachin G, Biljan I, Ilc G et al. (2013). Probing early misfolding events in prion protein mutants by NMR spectroscopy. Molecules 18: 9451–9476.

Goldfarb LG, Mitrova E, Brown P et al. (1990a). Mutation in codon 200 of scrapie amyloid protein gene in two clusters of Creutzfeldt–Jakob disease in Slovakia. Lancet 336: 514–515.

Goldfarb LG, Korczyn AD, Brown P et al. (1990b). Mutation in codon 200 of scrapie amyloid precursor gene linked to Creutzfeldt–Jakob disease in Sephardic Jews of Libyan and non-Libyan origin. Lancet 336: 637–638.

Goldfarb LG, Brown P, Goldgaber D et al. (1990c). Identical mutation in unrelated patients with Creutzfeldt–Jakob disease. Lancet 336: 174–175.

Goldfarb LG, Haltia M, Brown P et al. (1991a). New mutation in scrapie amyloid precursor gene (at codon 178) in Finnish Creutzfeldt–Jakob kindred. Lancet 337: 425.

Goldfarb LG, Brown P, McCombie WR et al. (1991b). Transmissible familial Creutzfeldt–Jakob disease associated with five, seven and eight extra octapeptide coding repeats in the PRNP gene. Proc Natl Acad Sci USA 88: 10926–10930.

Goldfarb LG, Brown P, Haltia M et al. (1992a). Creutzfeldt–Jakob disease cosegregates with the codon 178Asn PRNP mutation in families of European origin. Ann Neurol 31: 274–281.

Goldfarb LG, Petersen RB, Tabaton M et al. (1992b). Fatal familial insomnia and familial Creutzfeldt–Jakob disease: disease phenotype determined by a DNA polymorphism. Science 258: 806–808.

Goldfarb LG, Brown P, Vrbovska A et al. (1992c). An insert mutation in the chromosome 20 amyloid precursor gene in a Gerstmann-Sträussler-Scheinker family. J Neurol Sci 111: 189–194.

Goldgaber D, Goldfarb LG, Brown P et al. (1989). Mutations in familial Creutzfeldt–Jakob disease and Gerstmann-Straussler-Scheinker's syndrome. Exp Neurol 106: 204–206.

Grasbon-Frodl E, Lorenz H, Mann U et al. (2004). Loss of glycosylation associated with the T183A mutation in human prion disease. Acta Neuropathol 108: 476–484.

Hainfellner JA, Jellinger K, Diringer H et al. (1996). Creutzfeldt–Jakob disease in Austria Wien Klin Wochenschr 108: 759–763.

Hainfellner JA, Parchi P, Kitamoto T et al. (1999). A novel phenotype in familial Creutzfeldt–Jakob disease: prion protein gene E200K mutation coupled with valine at codon 129 and type 2 protease resistant prion protein. Ann Neurol 45: 812–816.

Haltia M, Kovanen J, Van Crevel H et al. (1979). Familial Creutzfeldt–Jakob disease. J Neurol Sci 42: 381–389.

Higuma M, Sanjo N, Satoh K et al. (2013). Relationships between clinicopathological features and cerebrospinal fluid biomarkers in Japanese patients with genetic prion diseases. PLoS One 8: e60003.

Hill AF, Joiner S, Beck JA et al. (2006). Distinct glycoform ratios of protease resistant prion protein associated with PRNP point mutations. Brain 129: 676–685.

Hitoshi S, Nagura H, Yamanouchi H et al. (1993). Double mutations at codon 180 and codon 232 of the PRNP gene in an apparently sporadic case of Creutzfeldt–Jakob disease. J Neurol Sci 120: 208–212.

Hoque MZ, Kitamoto T, Furukawa H et al. (1996). Mutation in the prion protein gene at codon 232 in Japanese patients with Creutzfeldt–Jakob disease: a clinicopathological, immunohistochemical and transmission study. Acta Neuropathol 92: 441–446.

Hsiao K, Baker HF, Crow TJ et al. (1989). Linkage of a prion protein missense variant to Gerstmann-Straussler syndrome. Nature 338: 342–345.

Hsiao K, Meiner Z, Kahana E et al. (1991). Mutation of the prion protein in Libyan Jews with Creutzfeldt–Jakob disease. N Engl J Med 324: 1091–1097.

Huang N, Marie SK, Kok F et al. (2001). Familial Creutzfeldt–Jakob disease associated with a point mutation at codon 210 of the prion protein gene. Arq Neuropsiquiatr 59: 932–935.

Imbriani P, Marfia GA, Marciani MG et al. (2016). Heidenhain variant in two patients with inherited V210I Creutzfeldt–Jakob disease. Int J Neurosci 126: 381–383.

Inoue I, Kitamoto T, Doh-ura K et al. (1994). Japanese family with Creutzfeldt–Jakob disease with codon 200 point mutation of the prion protein gene. Neurology 44: 299–301.

Iwasaki Y, Sone M, Kato T et al. (1999). Clinicopathological characteristics of Creutzfeldt–Jakob disease with a PrP V180I mutation and M129V polymorphism on different alleles. Rinsho Shinkeigaku 39: 800–806.

Iwasaki Y, Mori K, Ito M et al. (2011). An autopsied case of V180I Creutzfeldt–Jakob disease presenting with panencephalopathic-type pathology and a characteristic prion protein type. Neuropathology 31: 540–548.

Jansen C, Voet W, Head MW et al. (2011). A novel seven-octapeptide repeat insertion in the prion protein gene (PRNP) in a Dutch pedigree with Gerstmann-Straussler-Scheinker disease phenotype: comparison with similar cases from the literature. Acta Neuropathol 121: 59–68.

Jarius C, Kovacs GG, Belay G et al. (2003). Distinctive cerebellar immunoreactivity for the prion protein in familial (E200K) Creutzfeldt–Jakob disease. Acta Neuropathol 105: 449–454.

Jeong BH, Kim YS (2014). Genetic studies in human prion diseases. J Korean Med Sci 29: 623–632.

Jeong BH, Jeon YC, Lee YJ et al. (2010). Creutzfeldt–Jakob disease with the V203I mutation and M129V polymorphism of the prion protein gene (PRNP) and a 17 kDa prion protein fragment. Neuropathol Appl Neurobiol 36: 558–563.

Kim MO, Cali I, Oehler A et al. (2013). Genetic CJD with a novel E200G mutation in the prion protein gene and comparison with E200K mutation cases. Acta Neuropathol Commun 1: 80.

King A, Doey L, Rossor M et al. (2003). Phenotypic variability in the brain of a family with a prion disease characterized by a 144-base pair insertion in the prion protein gene. Neuropathol Appl Neurobiol 29: 98–105.

Kitamoto T, Doh-ura K, Muramoto T et al. (1992). The primary structure of the prion protein influences the distribution of abnormal prion protein in the central nervous system. Am J Pathol 141: 271–277.

Koh K, Takaki R, Miwa M et al. (2015). A case of Creutzfeldt–Jakob disease with a double mutation (V180I/M232R) in the PRNP gene. Rinsho Shinkeigaku 55: 424–427.

Komatsu J, Sakai K, Hamaguchi T et al. (2014). Creutzfeldt–Jakob disease associated with a V203I homozygous mutation in the prion protein gene. Prion 8: 336–338.

Kon T, Miki Y, Arai A et al. (2015). Creutzfeldt–Jakob disease with homozygous M232R mutation: A case report. J Neurol Sci 352: 108–109.

Kovacs GG, Trabattoni G, Hainfellner JA et al. (2002). Mutations of the prion protein gene phenotypic spectrum. J Neurol 249: 1567–1582.

Kovacs GG, László L, Bakos A et al. (2005a). Increased incidence of genetic human prion disease in Hungary. Neurology 65: 1666–1669.

Kovacs GG, Puopolo M, Ladogana A et al. (2005b). Genetic prion disease: the EUROCJD experience. Hum Genet 118: 166.

Kovacs GG, Bakos A, Mitrova E et al. (2007). Human prion diseases: the Hungarian experience. Ideggyogy Sz 60: 447–452.

Kovacs GG, Horvath S, Ströbel T et al. (2009). Genetic Creutzfeldt–Jakob disease mimicking variant Creutzfeldt–Jakob disease. J Neurol Neurosurg Psychiatry 80: 1410–1411.

Kovacs GG, Seguin J, Quadrio I et al. (2011). Genetic Creutzfeldt–Jakob disease associated with the E200K mutation: characterization of a complex proteinopathy. Acta Neuropathol 121: 39–57.

Kovacs GG, Molnár K, Keller E et al. (2012). Intraneuronal immunoreactivity for the prion protein distinguishes a subset of E200K genetic from sporadic Creutzfeldt–Jakob disease. J Neuropathol Exp Neurol 71: 223–232.

Kovacs GG, Rahimi J, Ströbel T et al. (2017). Tau pathology in Creutzfeldt–Jakob disease revisited. Brain Pathology 27: 332–344.

Kotta K, Paspaltsis I, Bostantjopoulou S et al. (2006). Novel mutation of the PRNP gene of a clinical CJD case. BMC Infect Dis 6: 169.

Krasnianski A, Heinemann U, Ponto C et al. (2016). Clinical findings and diagnosis in genetic prion diseases in Germany. Eur J Epidemiol 31: 187–196.

Krebs B, Lederer RM, Windl O et al. (2005). Creutzfeldt–Jakob disease associated with an R148H mutation of the prion protein gene. Neurogenetics 6: 97–100.

Kretzschmar HA, Stowring LE, Westaway D et al. (1986). Molecular cloning of a human prion protein cDNA. DNA 5: 315–324.

Kretzschmar HA, Neumann M, Stavrou D (1995). Codon 178 mutation of the human prion protein gene in a German family (Backer family): sequencing data from 72-year-old celloidin-embedded brain tissue. Acta Neuropathol 89: 96–98.

Ladogana A, Almonti S, Petraroli R et al. (2001). Mutation of the PRNP gene at codon 211 in familial Creutzfelt-Jakob disease. American Journal of Medical Genetics 103: 133–137.

Ladogana A, Puopolo M, Croes EA et al. (2005a). Mortality from Creutzfeldt–Jakob disease and related disorders in Europe, Australia, and Canada. Neurology 64: 1586–1591.

Ladogana A, Puopolo M, Poleggi A et al. (2005b). High incidence of genetic human transmissible spongiform encephalopathies in Italy. Neurology 64: 1592–1597.

Ladogana A, Sanchez-Juan P, Mitrová E et al. (2009). Cerebrospinal fluid biomarkers in human genetic transmissible spongiform encephalopathies. J Neurol 256: 1620–1628.

Laplanche JL, Chatelain J, Thomas S et al. (1992). Uncommon phenotype for a codon 178 mutation of the human PrP gene. Ann Neurol 31: 345.

Laplanche JL, Delasnerie-Lauprêtre N, Brandel JP et al. (1995). Two novel insertions in the prion protein gene in patients with late-onset dementia. Hum Mol Genet 4: 1109–1111.

Larue S, Verreault S, Gould P et al. (2006). A case of familial Creutzfeldt–Jakob disease presenting with dry cough. Can J Neurol Sci 33: 243–245.

Lattanzio F, Abu-Rumeileh S, Franceschini A et al. (2017). Prion-specific and surrogate CSF biomarkers in Creutzfeldt–Jakob disease: diagnostic accuracy in relation to molecular subtypes and analysis of neuropathological correlates of p-tau and Aβ42 levels. Acta Neuropathol 133: 559–578.

Lee HS, Sambuughin N, Cervenakova L et al. (1999). Ancestral origins and worldwide distribution of the PRNP 200K mutation causing familial Creutzfeldt–Jakob disease. Am J Hum Genet 64: 1063–1070.

Liu Z, Jia L, Piao Y et al. (2010). Creutzfeldt–Jakob disease with PRNP G114V mutation in a Chinese family. Acta Neurol Scand 121: 377–383.

Lloyd SE, Mead S, Collinge J (2013). Genetics of prion diseases. Curr Opin Genet Dev 23: 345–351.

MacLeod R, Tibben A, Frontali M et al. (2013). Editorial Committee and Working Group 'Genetic Testing Counselling' of the European Huntington Disease Network. Recommendations for the predictive genetic test in Huntington's disease. Clin Genet 83: 221–231.

Marcon G, Indaco A, Di Fede G et al. (2014). Panencephalopathic Creutzfeldt–Jakob Disease with distinct pattern of prion protein deposition in a patient with D178N mutation and homozygosity for valine at codon 129 of the prion protein gene. Brain Pathology 24: 148–151.

Mastrianni JA, Iannicola C, Myers RM et al. (1996). Mutation of the prion protein gene at codon 208 in familial Creutzfeldt–Jakob disease. Neurology 47: 1305–1312.

Mastrianni JA, Capellari S, Telling GC et al. (2001). Inherited prion disease caused by the V210I mutation: transmission to transgenic mice. Neurology 57: 2198–2205.

Matej R, Kovacs GG, Johanidesova S et al. (2012). Genetic Creutzfeldt–Jakob disease with R208H mutation presenting as progressive supranuclear palsy. Mov Disord 27: 476–479.

Mauro C, Giaccone G, Piscosquito G et al. (2008). A novel insertional mutation in the prion protein gene: clinical and bio-molecular findings. J Neurol Neurosurg Psychiatry 79: 1395–1398.

Mead S, Reilly MM (2015). A new prion disease: relationship with central and peripheral amyloidoses. Nat Rev Neurol 11: 90–97.

Mead S, Poulter M, Beck J et al. (2006). Inherited prion disease with six octapeptide repeat insertional mutation – molecular analysis of phenotypic heterogeneity. Brain 129: 2297–2317.

Mead S, Gandhi S, Beck J et al. (2013). A novel prion disease associated with diarrhea and autonomic neuropathy. N Engl J Med 369: 1904–1914.

Meiner Z, Gabizon R, Prusiner SB (1997). Familial Creutzfeldt–Jakob disease. Codon 200 prion disease in Libyan Jews. Medicine (Baltimore) 76: 227–237.

Meiner Z, Kahana E, Baitcher F et al. (2011). Tau and 14-3-3 of genetic and sporadic Creutzfeldt–Jakob disease patients in Israel. J Neurol 258: 255–262.

Mellina V, Equestre M, Poleggi A et al. (2007). Creutzfeldt Jakob disease associated with the R208H-129V haplotype in the protein gene. P04.108, p121. Prion 2007, Edinburgh, 26-28 September 2007.

Minikel EV, Vallabh SM, Lek M et al. (2016). Quantifying prion disease penetrance using large population control cohorts. Sci Transl Med. 8: 322ra9.

Mitrová E, Belay G (2002). Creutzfeldt–Jakob disease with E200K mutation in Slovakia: characterization and development. Acta Virol 46: 31–39.

Mitrová E, Cernák A, Slivarichová D et al. (2011). Experience with preventive genetic testing of corneal donors in Slovakia. Cornea 30: 987–990.

Mitrova E, Belay G, Slivarichova-Zakova D et al. (2015). The first case of genetic Creutzfeldt–Jakob disease with the rare mutation R208H, methionine/valine heterozygous at codon 129 of the prion protein gene. Clinical Medicine Journal 1: 101–105.

Miyakawa T, Inoue K, Iseki E et al. (1998). Japanese Creutzfeldt–Jakob disease patients exhibiting high incidence of the E200K PRNP mutation and located in the basin of a river. Neurol Res 20: 684–688.

Mouillet-Richard S, Teil C, Lenne M et al. (1999). Mutation at codon 210 (V210I) of the prion protein gene in a North African patient with Creutzfeldt–Jakob disease. J Neurol Sci 168: 141–144.

Muñoz-Nieto M, Ramonet N, López-Gastón JI et al. (2013). A novel mutation I215V in the PRNP gene associated with Creutzfeldt–Jakob and Alzheimer's diseases in three patients with divergent clinical phenotypes. J Neurol 260: 77–84.

Necpál J, Stelzer M, Koščová S et al. (2016). A corticobasal syndrome variant of familial Creutzfeldt–Jakob disease with stroke-like onset. Case Rep Neurol Med 2016: 4167391.

Neufeld MY, Josiphov J, Korczyn AD (1992). Demyelinating peripheral neuropathy in Creutzfeldt–Jakob disease. Muscle Nerve 15: 1234–1239.

Nicholl D, Windl O, de Silva R et al. (1995). Inherited Creutzfeldt–Jakob disease in a British family associated with a novel 144 base pair insertion of the prion protein gene. J Neurol Neurosurg Psychiatry 58: 65–69.

Nieto A, Goldfarb LG, Brown P et al. (1991). Codon 178 mutation in ethnically diverse Creutzfeldt–Jakob disease families. Lancet 337: 622–623.

Nitrini R, Rosemberg S, Passos-Bueno MR et al. (1997). Familial spongiform encephalopathy associated with a novel prion protein gene mutation. Ann Neurol 42: 138–146.

Nixon R, Camicioli R, Cervenakova L et al. (2000). The PRNP-V180I mutation is associated with abnormally glycosylated PrPCJD and intracellular PrP accumulations. In: XIVth International Congress of Neuropathology, Brain Pathology, Birmingham, UK, p. 670.

Nonno R, Di Bari MA, Cardone F et al. (2006). Efficient transmission and characterization of Creutzfeldt–Jakob disease strains in bank voles. PLoS Pathog 2: e12.

Nozaki I, Hamaguchi T, Sanjo N et al. (2010). Prospective 10-year surveillance of human prion diseases in Japan. Brain 133: 3043–3057.

Oda T, Kitamoto T, Tateishi J et al. (1995). Prion disease with 144 base pair insertion in a Japanese family line. Acta Neuropathol 90: 80–86.

Owen F, Poulter M, Lofthouse R et al. (1989). Insertion in prion protein gene in familial Creutzfeldt–Jakob disease. Lancet 1: 51–52.

Owen J, Beck J, Campbell T et al. (2014). Predictive testing for inherited prion disease: report of 22 years experience. Eur J Hum Genet 22: 1351–1356.

Parchi P, Strammiello R, Notari S et al. (2009). Incidence and spectrum of sporadic Creutzfeldt- Jakob disease variants with mixed phenotype and co-occurrence of PrPSc types: an updated classification. Acta Neuropathol 118: 659–671.

Pastore M, Chin SS, Bell KL et al. (2005). Creutzfeldt–Jakob disease (CJD) with a mutation at codon 148 of prion protein gene: relationship with sporadic CJD. Am J Pathol 167: 1729–1738.

Peoc'h K, Manivet P, Beaudry P et al. (2000). Identification of three novel mutations (E196K, V203I, E211Q) in the prion protein gene (PRNP) in inherited prion diseases with Creutzfeldt–Jakob disease phenotype. Hum Mutat 15: 482.

Peoc'h K, Levavasseur E, Delmont E et al. (2012). Substitutions at residue 211 in the prion protein drive a switch between CJD and GSS syndrome, a new mechanism governing inherited neurodegenerative disorders. Hum Mol Genet 2: 5417–5428.

Piccardo P, Dlouhy SR, Lievens PM et al. (1998). Phenotypic variability of Gerstmann-Sträussler-Scheinker disease is associated with prion protein heterogeneity. J Neuropathol Exp Neurol 57: 979–988.

Pietrini V, Puoti G, Limido L et al. (2003). Creutzfeldt–Jakob disease with a novel extra-repeat insertional mutation in the PRNP gene. Neurology 61: 1288–1291.

Pocchiari M, Ladogana A (2015). Rethinking of doxycycline therapy in Creutzfeldt–Jakob disease. J Neurol Neurosurg Psychiatry 86: 705.

Pocchiari M, Salvatore M, Cutruzzola F et al. (1993). A new point mutation of the prion protein gene in Creutzfeldt–Jakob disease. Ann Neurol 34: 802–807.

Pocchiari M, Puopolo M, Croes EA et al. (2004). Predictors of survival in sporadic Creutzfeldt–Jakob disease and other human transmissible spongiform encephalopathies. Brain 127: 2348–2359.

Pocchiari M, Colaizzo E, Tiple D et al. (2016). The first Italian case of Creutzfeldt–Jakob disease with V180I mutation in the PrP gene (PRNP) Prion 10 Supplement: 1 abstract: P-141: S110–S110.

Polymenidou M, Prokop S, Jung HH et al. (2011). Atypical prion protein conformation in familial prion disease with PRNP P105T mutation. Brain Pathol 21: 209–214.

Poulter M, Baker HF, Frith CD et al. (1992). Inherited prion disease with 144 base pair gene insertion (1. Genealogical and molecular studies). Brain 115: 675–685.

Puoti G, Rossi G, Giaccone G et al. (2000). Polymorphism at codon 129 of PRNP affects the phenotypic expression of Creutzfeldt–Jakob disease linked to E200K mutation. Ann Neurol 48: 269–270.

Qina T, Sanjo N, Hizume M et al. (2014). Clinical features of genetic Creutzfeldt–Jakob disease with V180I mutation in the prion protein gene. BMJ Open 4: e004968.

Ripoll L, Laplanche JL, Salzmann M et al. (1993). A new point mutation in the prion protein gene at codon 210 in Creutzfeldt–Jakob disease. Neurology 43: 1934–1938.

Rodriguez MM, Peoc'h K, Haïk S et al. (2005). A novel mutation (G114V) in the prion protein gene in a family with inherited prion disease. Neurology 64: 1455–1457.

Roeber S, Krebs B, Neumann M et al. (2005). Creutzfeldt–Jakob disease in a patient with an R208H mutation of the prion protein gene (PRNP) and a 17-kDa prion protein fragment. Acta Neuropathol 109: 443–448.

Roeber S, Grasbon-Frodl EM, Windl O et al. (2008). Evidence for a pathogenic role of different mutations at codon 188 of PRNP. PLoS ONE 3: e2147.

Rosenmann H, Vardi J, Finkelstein Y et al. (1998). Identification in Israel of 2 Jewish Creutzfeld-Jakob disease patients with a 178 mutation at their PrP gene. Acta Neurol Scand 97: 184–187.

Sano K, Satoh K, Atarashi R et al. (2013). Early detection of abnormal prion protein in genetic human prion diseases now possible using real-time QUIC assay. PLoS ONE 8: e54915.

Schelzke G, Eigenbrod S, Romero C et al. (2011). Genetic prion disease with codon 196 PRNP mutation: clinical and pathological findings. Neurobiol Aging 32: 756.

Schmitz M, Dittmar K, Llorens F et al. (2017). Hereditary human prion diseases: an update. Mol Neurobiol. 54: 4138–4149.

Shi Q, Chen C, Song XN et al. (2011). A Chinese Creutzfeldt–Jakob disease patient with E196K mutation in PRNP. Prion 5: 117–120.

Shi Q, Zhang BY, Gao C et al. (2012). The diversities of PrP (Sc) distributions and pathologic changes in various brain regions from a Chinese patient with G114V genetic CJD. Neuropathology 32: 51–59.

Shi Q, Chen C, Wang XJ et al. (2013). Rare V203I mutation in the PRNP gene of a Chinese patient with Creutzfeldt–Jakob disease. Prion 7: 259–262.

Shi Q, Zhou W, Chen C et al. (2015). The features of genetic prion diseases based on Chinese surveillance program. PLoS ONE 10: e0139552.

Shi Q, Zhou W, Chen C et al. (2016). Rare E196A mutation in PRNP gene of 3 Chinese patients with Creutzfeldt-Jacob disease. Prion 10: 331–337.

Shiga Y, Satoh K, Kitamoto T et al. (2007). Two different clinical phenotypes of Creutzfeldt–Jakob disease with a M232R substitution. J Neurol 254: 1509–1517.

Shyu WC, Hsu YD, Kao MC et al. (1996). Panencephalitic Creutzfeldt–Jakob disease in a Chinese family. Unusual presentation with PrP codon 210 mutation and identification by PCR-SSCP. J Neurol Sci 143: 176–180.

Simon ES, Kahana E, Chapman J et al. (2000). Creutzfeldt–Jakob disease profile in patients homozygous for the PRNP E200K mutation. Ann Neurol 47: 257–260.

Spudich S, Mastrianni JA, Wrensch M et al. (1995). Complete penetrance of Creutzfeldt–Jakob disease in Libyan Jews carrying the E200K mutation in the prion protein gene. Mol Med 1: 607–613.

Takada LT, Kim MO, Cleveland RW et al. (2017). Genetic prion disease: experience of a rapidly progressive dementia center in the United States and a review of the literature. Am J Med Genet B Neuropsychiatr Genet 174: 36–69.

Taratuto AL, Piccardo P, Reich EG et al. (2002). Insomnia associated with thalamic involvement in E200K Creutzfeldt–Jakob disease. Neurology 58: 362–367.

Tartaglia MC, Thai JN, See T et al. (2010). Pathologic evidence that the T188R mutation in PRNP is associated with prion disease. J Neuropathol Exp Neurol 69: 1220–1227.

Tateishi J, Kitamoto T (1995). Inherited prion diseases and transmission to rodents. Brain Pathol 5: 53–59.

Tumani H, Windl O, Kretzschmar HA et al. (2002). Clinically atypical CJD: diagnostic relevance of cerebrospinal fluid markers and molecular genetic analysis? Dtsch Med Wochenschr 127: 318–320.

van Harten B, van Gool WA, Van Langen IM et al. (2000). A new mutation in the prion protein gene: A patient with dementia and white matter changes. Neurology 55: 1055–1057.

Vetrugno V, Puopolo M, Cardone F et al. (2015). The future for treating Creutzfeldt–Jakob disease. Expert Opinion on Orphan Drugs 3: 57–74.

Vita MG, Gaudino S, Di Giuda D et al. (2013). R208H-129VV haplotype in the prion protein gene: phenotype and neuroimaging of a patient with genetic Creutzfeldt–Jakob disease. J Neurol 260: 2650–2652.

Wang XF, Guo YJ, Zhang BY et al. (2007). Creutzfeldt–Jakob disease in a Chinese patient with a novel seven extra-repeat insertion in PRNP. J Neurol Neurosurg Psychiatry 78: 201–203.

Watts JC, Giles K, Serban A et al. (2015). Modulation of Creutzfeldt–Jakob disease prion propagation by the A224V mutation. Ann Neurol 78: 540–553.

WHO (2003). WHO manual for surveillance of human transmissible spongiform encephalopathies including variant Creutzfeldt–Jakob disease, WHO, Geneva, pp. 1–90.

Windl O, Dempster M, Estibeiro JP et al. (1996). Genetic basis of Creutzfeldt–Jakob disease in the United Kingdom: a systematic analysis of predisposing mutations and allelic variation in the PRNP gene. Hum Genet 98: 259–264.

Windl O, Giese A, Schulz-Schaeffer W et al. (1999). Molecular genetics of human prion diseases in Germany. Hum Genet 105: 244–252.

Ye J, Han J, Shi Q et al. (2008). Human prion disease with a G114V mutation and epidemiological studies in a Chinese family: a case series. J Med Case Rep 2: 331.

Zanusso G, Monaco S, Pocchiari M et al. (2016). Advanced tests for early and accurate diagnosis of Creutzfeldt–Jakob disease. Nat Rev Neurol 12: 325–333.

Zarranz JJ, Digon A, Atares B et al. (2005). Phenotypic variability in familial prion diseases due to the D178N mutation. J Neurol Neurosurg Psychiatry 76: 1491–1496.

Zhang H, Wang M, Wu L et al. (2014). Novel prion protein gene mutation at codon 196 (E196A) in a septuagenarian with Creutzfeldt–Jakob disease. Clin Neurosci 21: 175–178.

Zheng L, Longfei J, Jing Y et al. (2008). PRNP mutations in a series of apparently sporadic neurodegenerative dementias in China. Am J Med Genet B Neuropsychiatr Genet 147B: 938–944.

Handbook of Clinical Neurology, Vol. 153 (3rd series)
Human Prion Diseases
M. Pocchiari and J. Manson, Editors
https://doi.org/10.1016/B978-0-444-63945-5.00014-3

Chapter 14

Dominantly inherited prion protein cerebral amyloidoses – a modern view of Gerstmann–Sträussler–Scheinker

BERNARDINO GHETTI[1]*, PEDRO PICCARDO[2], AND GIANLUIGI ZANUSSO[3]

[1]*Department of Pathology and Laboratory Medicine, Indiana University School of Medicine, Indianapolis, IN, United States*

[2]*The Roslin Institute and Royal (Dick) School of Veterinary Studies, University of Edinburgh, Roslin, Midlothian, United Kingdom*

[3]*Department of Neurosciences, Biomedicine and Movement Sciences, University of Verona, Verona, Italy*

Abstract

Among genetically determined neurodegenerative diseases, the dominantly inherited prion protein cerebral amyloidoses are characterized by deposition of amyloid in cerebral parenchyma or blood vessels. Among them, Gerstmann–Sträussler–Scheinker disease has been the first to be described. Their clinical, neuropathologic, and molecular phenotypes are distinct from those observed in Creutzfeldt–Jakob disease (CJD) and related spongiform encephalopathies. It is not understood why specific mutations in the prion protein gene (*PRNP*) cause cerebral amyloidosis and others cause CJD. A significant neurobiologic event in these amyloidoses is the frequent coexistence of prion amyloid with tau neurofibrillary pathology, a phenomenon suggesting that similar pathogenetic mechanisms may be shared among different diseases in the sequence of events occurring in the cascade from amyloid formation to tau aggregation. This chapter describes the clinical, neuropathologic, and biochemical phenotypes associated with each of the *PRNP* mutations causing an inherited cerebral amyloidosis and emphasizes the variability of phenotypes.

INTRODUCTION

The eponymous name Gerstmann–Sträussler–Scheinker (GSS) disease, introduced in the literature by Schlote et al. (1980), originates from the names of the authors of the scientific report, describing the neuropathologic features of a patient from the Austrian family "H" (Gerstmann et al., 1936). A dominantly inherited neurologic disorder had affected multiple generations of the "H" kindred and in 1912, 1928, and 1936, the main characteristics of the disease's clinical and pathologic phenotypes had been described in two affected family members (Dimitz, 1913; Gerstmann, 1928; Gerstmann et al., 1936). Cerebellar ataxia, dysdiadochokinesia, as well as action and intention tremor were the initial symptoms. With progression of the disease, the patients became unable to walk, stand, or sit upright; they had a disturbance of speech, swallowing difficulties, lateral and vertical gaze nystagmus, and bilateral Babinski signs. They had behavioral and mood alterations as well as a cognitive decline. At the macroscopic examination of the brain, atrophy of the cerebral hemispheres and the cerebellar vermis were described. The histologic analysis revealed the presence of focal deposits of an amorphous substance in the cerebral cortex, basal ganglia, and cerebellum. These deposits had single or multiple cores and, although morphologically different from the senile plaques found in Alzheimer disease, similarities with the senile plaques were noted (Gerstmann et al., 1936). The neuropathology of four additional family members was reported: one case by von Braunmühl in 1954 and three by Seitelberger in 1962. Seitelberger emphasized both the presence of mild to moderate spongiform changes as well as the morphologic similarity of the focal deposits to the plaques occurring in the prion disease known as kuru (Seitelberger, 1962, 1981).

*Correspondence to: Bernardino Ghetti, MD, Indiana University School of Medicine, Department of Pathology and Laboratory Medicine, 635 Barnhill Drive, MS A138, Indianapolis IN 46202, United States. Tel: +1-317-274-7818, E-mail: bghetti@iupui.edu

Masters et al. (1981) studied the clinicopathologic data from hereditary syndromes, similar to that reported in Austrian family "H," and carried out experimental studies, inoculating brain tissue from affected individuals of some of these kindreds into primates. Two main facts emerged: (1) amyloid deposits are a constant pathologic feature, but spongiform changes are not always present; and (2) a spongiform encephalopathy developed in the recipient animals, following brain tissue inoculation. These results were seminal in establishing a possible pathogenetic link between a dominantly inherited neurodegenerative cerebral amyloidosis and Creutzfeldt–Jakob disease (CJD).

In 1985, a GSS-like dominantly inherited disease was described in members of a large Indiana kindred; the condition was clinically characterized by ataxia, parkinsonism, and dementia. Neuropathologic studies revealed numerous multicentric amyloid plaques in the parenchyma of the cerebrum and cerebellum (Azzarelli et al., 1985). However, a unique and previously unrecognized neuropathologic feature was the coexistence of amyloid deposits and neurofibrillary tangles in the cerebral cortex and subcortical nuclei. The neurofibrillary tangles were made of paired helical filaments that, in pictures obtained by transmission electron microscopy, appeared identical to those seen in Alzheimer disease.

In 1987, amyloid plaques, from an individual with a GSS-like disorder, were immunolabeled using antibodies raised against PrP and in 1988, the coexistence between prion protein (PrP)-immunopositive amyloid plaques and tau-immunopositive neurofibrillary tangles was demonstrated in the brain tissue of affected individuals from the Indiana kindred (Kitamoto et al., 1987; Ghetti et al., 1988, 1989).

In 1989, a missense mutation at codon 102 of the *PRNP* gene was first reported to be associated with GSS and, in 1991, the same mutation was also found in affected members of the "H" family (Hsiao et al., 1989; Kretzschmar et al., 1991). By 1995, the pedigree of the "H" family included 221 family members, with 20 having been affected by the disease (Hainfellner et al., 1995).

In 1991, an insert of eight extra copies of a repeating octapeptide coding sequence was identified in the *PRNP* region between codons 51 and 91, in individuals affected by a GSS-like hereditary syndrome (Goldfarb et al., 1991). This was the first instance of an insertion mutation, rather than a point mutation, being associated with clinical and neuropathologic changes seen in a GSS-like disorder. A primate, inoculated with a tissue homogenate obtained postmortem from brain of one of the affected individuals, developed a spongiform encephalopathy (Goldfarb et al., 1991).

In 1992, the disease-causing gene in individuals of the Indiana kindred was mapped and a missense mutation at codon 198 of *PRNP* was found in all affected individuals (Dlouhy et al., 1992; Hsiao et al., 1992).

In 1996, the first case of a unique, previously unrecognized, novel and peculiar PrP amyloidosis was reported (Ghetti et al., 1996b). The patient, who carried a nonsense mutation at codon 145 of *PRNP*, presented with an Alzheimer disease-like symptomatology. Neuropathologically, a PrP cerebral amyloid angiopathy (PrP-CAA) coexisted with numerous tau-immunopositive neurofibrillary tangles.

Thus, PrP amyloidosis appears to be a central unifying pathologic event in a clinically heterogeneous group of dominantly inherited prion diseases that, from the neuropsychiatric and neuropathologic points of view, differs substantially from the group of prion diseases, that are characterized predominantly by the presence of a spongiform encephalopathy. For this reason, we choose to group under the broader term of dominantly inherited PrP cerebral amyloidoses those syndromes that have the following characteristics: (1) one of the following types of *PRNP* mutations: missense, insertion, nonsense, and deletion; (2) PrP parenchymal or vascular amyloid in the central nervous system; (3) variable clinical phenotype, that may be characterized by one of the following: (1) ataxia and personality disorder, similar to that described by Gerstmann et al. in the "H". family, often accompanied by pyramidal and parkinsonian signs; (2) psychosis followed by neurologic and cognitive decline; (3) Alzheimer disease-like dementia; (4) frontotemporal dementia.

In the GSS phenotype, associated with missense mutations, the neurologic symptoms start, in most cases, between the third and the sixth decades of life; they may be preceded by apathy and depression. The disease duration ranges from a few months to 15 years (Ghetti et al., 2011).

In the cases with six or more octapeptide repeat insertions, the neurologic phenotype is predominantly characterized by cognitive and behavioral changes consistent with frontotemporal dementia, language dysfunction, and gait ataxia as well as clinical or electrophysiologic evidence of epileptiform activity. Symptoms start, in most cases, between the third and fifth decades of life. The disease duration ranges from 1 to 7 years (Schmitz et al., 2017).

The clinical phenotype associated with nonsense (stop codon) mutations is predominantly characterized by cognitive and behavioral changes, consistent with those seen in Alzheimer disease (Ghetti et al., 1996b; Jayadev et al., 2011; Mead et al., 2013). Onset of chronic diarrhea and autonomic failure may precede the

Alzheimer-like syndrome. The disease may last as long as 7 years.

The signs and symptoms of dominantly inherited PrP cerebral amyloidoses may vary in onset and combination. The pathologic features may vary according to *PRNP* mutation and variability occurs in the neuropathology that accompanies PrP amyloid deposits. The neuropathologic phenotype is characterized by parenchymal or vascular amyloidosis, which may be accompanied by tau neurofibrillary tangles or, less frequently, by spongiform changes. The dominantly inherited PrP cerebral amyloidoses may be subdivided into the following four neuropathologic subgroups, characterized by: (1) parenchymal PrP amyloid and prominent spongiform changes; (2) parenchymal PrP amyloid and minimal or no spongiform changes; (3) parenchymal PrP amyloid coexisting with severe tau neurofibrillary pathology, and absent or minimal spongiform changes; and (4) vascular PrP-CAA coexisting with severe neurofibrillary pathology. The lesions of these dominantly inherited PrP cerebral amyloidoses are most numerous in the cerebral cortex, basal ganglia, and cerebellar cortex.

EPIDEMIOLOGY

Incidence and prevalence

The incidence of the dominantly inherited PrP cerebral amyloidoses is not fully known, since familial clusters are not systematically recognized and reported. Hereditary cerebral PrP amyloidoses associated with the GSS phenotypes have been reported in Argentina (Riudavets et al., 2014; Saenz-Farret et al., 2016), Australia (Panegyres et al., 2001), Austria (Hainfellner et al., 1995), Brazil (Smid et al., 2017), Canada (Hudson et al., 1983), China and Taiwan (Wang et al., 2006; Chi et al., 2010), Denmark (Bergstrom et al., 2009), France (Tranchant et al., 1992; Laplanche et al., 1999), Germany (Windl et al., 1999), Hungary (Majtenyi et al., 2000), India (Rogaeva et al., 2006), Indonesia (Rowe et al., 2007), Ireland (Mallucci et al., 1999), Israel (Goldhammer et al., 1993), Italy (De Michele et al., 2003), Japan (Kitamoto et al., 1993), South Korea (Park et al., 2010), Netherlands (Jansen et al., 2011), Poland (Zimowski et al., 2012), Russia and Slovenia (Kojovic et al., 2011), Spain (Alzualde et al., 2010), Switzerland (Polymenidou et al., 2011), the United Kingdom (Adam et al., 1982), and the United States (Mastrianni et al., 1995).

Distribution and frequency of *PRNP* mutations associated with GSS appear to be distinct between Caucasians and East Asians. The most common mutation in Caucasian and East Asian patients is P102L, while the mutation P105L is most frequently reported in East Asian populations, especially Japanese. The mutation A117V has been reported only in Caucasians (Chen and Dong, 2016). From a review of the literature, it is estimated that a total of approximately 390 cases of GSS have been reported, including 248 carrying the P102L mutation (Kim et al., 2017; Takada et al., 2017). GSS is probably underdiagnosed due to variability of its clinical phenotype, which may present with ataxia, spastic parapesis, parkinsonism, amyotrophy, or dementia.

Age and gender distribution

The onset of clinical signs and symptoms may occur from late in the second decade to early in the eighth decade of life, with a duration ranging from a few months to over 15 years. This disease occurs equally in males and females.

GENETICS

The dominantly inherited PrP cerebral amyloidoses are genetically transmitted with a penetrance of almost 100%. Early linkage analysis studies helped to established the relationship between GSS and mutations in the *PRNP* gene. *PRNP* is located on the short arm of chromosome 20 and encodes for PrP (Hsiao et al., 1989; Dlouhy et al., 1992; Prusiner, 1999; Collinge, 2001). Currently, at least 24 missense and nonsense mutations in the *PRNP* gene are known to be associated with hereditary cerebral PrP amyloidoses, including 19 missense mutations associated with a GSS-like phenotype and five nonsense (stop codon) mutations, mostly associated with a PrP-CAA. A two-basepair deletion at codon 178 results in a premature stop codon mutation at codon 203 (Honda et al., 2016). Furthermore, hereditary PrP cerebral amyloidosis is also seen in association with insertional mutations of 144, 168, 192, 216, and 288 additional basepair repeats in the octapeptide repeat region or a 24-basepair repeat insertional mutation between codon 129 and 130 (Hinnell et al., 2011) (Fig. 14.1 and Tables 14.1 and 14.2).

Commonly, in prion diseases the haplotype is defined by a *PRNP* mutation in combination with the genotype at codon 129; the latter codes for methionine or valine. Genetic mutation in *PRNP* and polymorphisms at codon 129; in the *PRNP* may be a modifier of the clinical and pathologic characteristics (Dlouhy et al., 1992; Prusiner, 1999; Collinge, 2001). Polymorphism at codon 219 may also modify the phenotype (Furukawa et al., 1995).

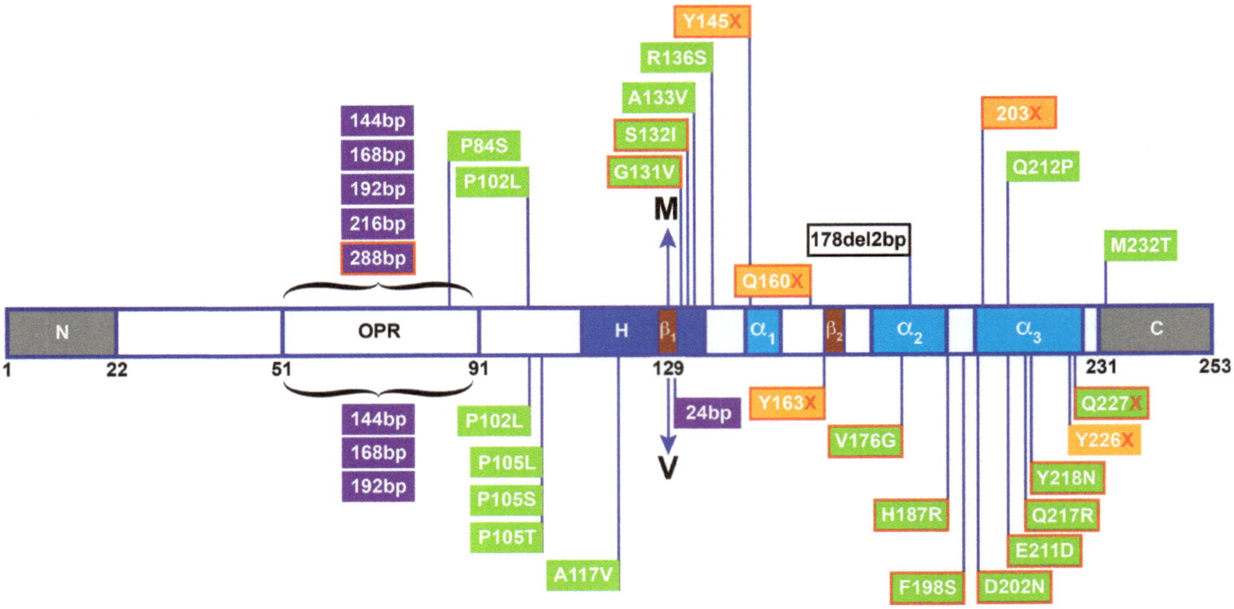

Fig. 14.1. Mutations associated with dominantly inherited prion protein amyloidosis. Green boxes indicate missense mutations associated with Gerstmann–Sträussler–Scheinker phenotype. Orange boxes indicate nonsense mutations associated with prion protein cerebral amyloid angiopathy phenotype. Violet boxes indicate insertion mutations associated with variable phenotype. White box indicates a deletion mutation resulting in a stop codon. Boxes with red margin indicate the presence of tau pathology.

Table 14.1

Haplotypes, nucleotide and amino acid changes, and number of cases

	Nucleotide change		Amino acid change		
Mutation	Normal	Disease	Normal	Disease	Number ofcases
P84S-129M	CCT	TCT	Pro	Ser	1
P102L-129M	CCG	CTG	Pro	Leu	>248
P102L-129M-219K	CCG	CTG	Pro	Leu	1
P102L-129V	CCG	CTG	Pro	Leu	2
P105L-129V	CCA	CTA	Pro	Leu	14
P105S-129V	CCA	TCA	Pro	Ser	1
P105T-129V	CCC	ACC	Pro	Thr	7
A117V-129V	GCA	GTG	Ala	Val	40
G131V-129M	GGA	GTA	Gly	Val	3
S132I-129M	AGT	ATT	Ser	Ile	2
A133V-129M-219K	GCC	GTC	Ala	Val	1
R136S-129M	Not available	Not available	Arg	Ser	Not available
V176G-129V	GTG	GGG	Val	Gly	1
H187R-129V	CAC	CGC	His	Arg	7
F198S-129V	TTC	TCC	Phe	Ser	30
D202N-129V	GAC	AAC	Asp	Asn	2
E211D-129V	GAG	GAC	Glu	Asp	1
Q212P-129M	CAG	CCG	Gln	Pro	2
Q217R-129V	CAG	CGG	Gln	Arg	7
Y218N-129V	TAC	AAC	Tyr	Asn	1
Q227X-129V	CAG	TAG	Gln	stop	1
M232T-129M	ATG	ACG	Met	Thr	1
Y145X-129M	TAT	TAG	Tyr	stop	1
Q160X-129M	CAA	TAA	Tyr	stop	3
Y163X-129V	TAC	TAG	Tyr	stop	1
Y226X-129V	TAC	TAA	Tyr	stop	1

Table 14.2

Neuropathologic phenotypes and *PRNP* mutations

PRNP mutation	Spongiform encephalopathy	PrP amyloid	Tau pathology	PrP Western blot
P84S-129M	No	Plaques focal	Not reported	Low-molecular-weight bands
P102L-129M	Two types: yes/no	Plaques widespread	Not consistently present	Low molecular-weight bands
P102L-129M-219K	No	None	Not reported	PrP27-30 and low-molecular-weight bands or low molecular-weight bands
P102L-129V	No	Plaques widespread	Not reported	Not reported
P105L-129V	No	Plaques widespread	Not consistently present	Low-molecular-weight bands
P105S-129V	Yes	Plaques widespread	Not reported	No low-molecular-weight bands
P105T-129V	Yes	Plaques focal	Not reported	High and low-molecular-weight bands
A117V-129V	No	Plaques widespread	Not consistently present	Low-molecular-weight bands
G131V-129M	No	Plaques widespread	Tau deposits in neuronal perikarya	Low-molecular-weight bands
S132I-129M	No	Plaques widespread	Tau deposits in neuronal perikarya	Low-molecular-weight bands
A133V-129M-219K	Yes	Cerebellum	Not reported	Not reported
R136S-129M	Not reported	Not reported	Not reported	Not reported
V176G-129V	Yes	Plaques widespread	Tau deposits in neuronal perikarya	Low-molecular-weight bands
H187R-129V	No	Plaques widespread	Tau deposits in neuronal perikarya	Low-molecular-weight bands
F198S-129V	No	Plaques widespread	Tau deposits in neuronal perikarya	Low-molecular-weight bands
E211D-129V	Yes	Plaques widespread	Tau deposits in neuronal perikarya	Low-molecular-weight bands
D202N-129V	No	Plaques widespread	Tau deposits in neuronal perikarya	Low-molecular-weight bands
Q212P-129M	No	Plaques widespread	Not tau deposits in neuronal perikarya	Low-molecular-weight bands
Q217R-129V	No	Plaques widespread	Tau deposits in neuronal perikarya	Low-molecular-weight bands
Y218N-129V	No	Plaques widespread	Tau deposits in neuronal perikarya	Low-molecular-weight bands
Q227X-129V	No	Plaques widespread	Tau deposits in neuronal perikarya	Not reported
M232T-129M	Not reported	Plaques widespread	Not reported	Not reported
Y145X-129M	No	Angiopathy	Tau deposits in neuronal perikarya	Low-molecular-weight bands
Q160X-129M	No	Plaques and angiopathy	Tau deposits in neuronal perikarya	Low-molecular-weight bands
Y163X-129V	No	Angiopathy	Tau deposits in neuronal perikarya	Not reported
Y226X-129V	No	Angiopathy	Dot-like deposits	Not reported

Continued

Table 14.2

Continued

PRNP mutation	Spongiform encephalopathy	PrP amyloid	Tau pathology	PrP Western blot
Q227X-129V	Yes	Plaques widespread	Tau deposits in neuronal perikarya	Low-molecular-weight bands
24 bpi-129V	Yes	Plaques widespread	Tau deposits in neuronal perikarya	Not reported
144 bpi-129V	Yes	Plaques widespread	Not present	PrP27-30
168 bpi-129M	Yes	Plaques focal	Not reported	Not reported
168 bpi-129V	Yes	Plaques widespread	Not consistently present	PrP27-30
192 bpi-129M	Yes	Plaques focal	Not reported	Not reported
192 bpi-129V	Yes	Plaques widespread	Not present	Not reported
216 bpi-129M	Yes	Plaques focal	Not reported	Not reported
288 bpi-129M	Yes	Plaques widespread	Tau deposits in neuronal perikarya	Not reported
178del2bp-129M	Yes	Plaques widespread	Tau deposits in neuronal perikarya	Low-molecular-weight bands

THE DOMINANTLY INHERITED PRION PROTEIN CEREBRAL AMYLOIDOSES

The initial phases of the psychiatric and neurologic manifestations of the dominantly inherited PrP cerebral amyloidoses will require future detailed studies. An early molecular diagnosis of *PRNP* mutations along with the knowledge of biomarker alterations and structural modifications as seen by imaging will allow researchers to carefully identify the psychiatric symptoms that precede neurologic manifestations. Psychiatric symptoms in early stages of disease have been described in dominantly inherited PrP cerebral amyloidoses that are associated with insertional mutations and missense mutations. Furthermore, it remais to be determined if specific *PRNP* mutations can also affect any central nervous system developmental stages.

Due to the wide spectrum of clinical and neuropathologic characteristics, it is useful to describe individually the phenotypic characteristics associated with each of the *PRNP* mutations. In dominantly inherited PrP cerebral amyloidoses, the most common neuropathologic features are PrP amyloid plaques and diffuse deposits, moderate to severe neuronal loss and glial proliferation in the cerebral cortex, deep gray nuclei, and cerebellar cortex. Parenchymal PrP amyloid deposits are birefringent after Congo red stain and strongly fluorescent in thioflavin S preparations. On electron microscopy, the amyloid is composed of bundles of fibrils radiating out from a central core, each fibril measuring 8–10nm in diameter. The core of the amyloid plaque is immunoreactive to antibodies raised against the midregion of PrP, but nonreactive or weakly reactive to antibodies raised against the amino- and carboxy-terminal regions of PrP. In contrast, there is immunopositivity to antibodies raised against the amino and carboxy-terminal regions of PrP in the area surrounding the amyloid core. Nonfibrillar PrP deposits appear as diffusely immunolabeled areas in the neuropil (Ghetti et al., 1995, 1996a).

The biochemical features of pathologic PrP in dominantly inherited PrP cerebral amyloidoses are unique and distinctive from other human prion disorders. These consist in the detection of pathognomonic C- and N-terminally truncated PrP fragments, also named PrP internal fragments (PrP^{IF}), resistant to protease treatment and absent in large series of CJD (Tagliavini et al., 1991; Ghetti et al., 1996a; Piccardo et al., 1996, 1998; Zanusso et al., 2014) (Fig. 14.2).

These PrP^{IF} are detected in untreated brain extracts but are consistently enriched following proteinase K (PK) treatment. The biochemical characterization of pathologic PrP has been carried out in most hereditary PrP cerebral amyloidosis associated with PrP mutations and the biochemical PrP patterns correlate with the clinical and pathologic phenotypes. We describe biochemical PrP patterns associated with each mutation and, for simplicity, we represent only the resulting monomers.

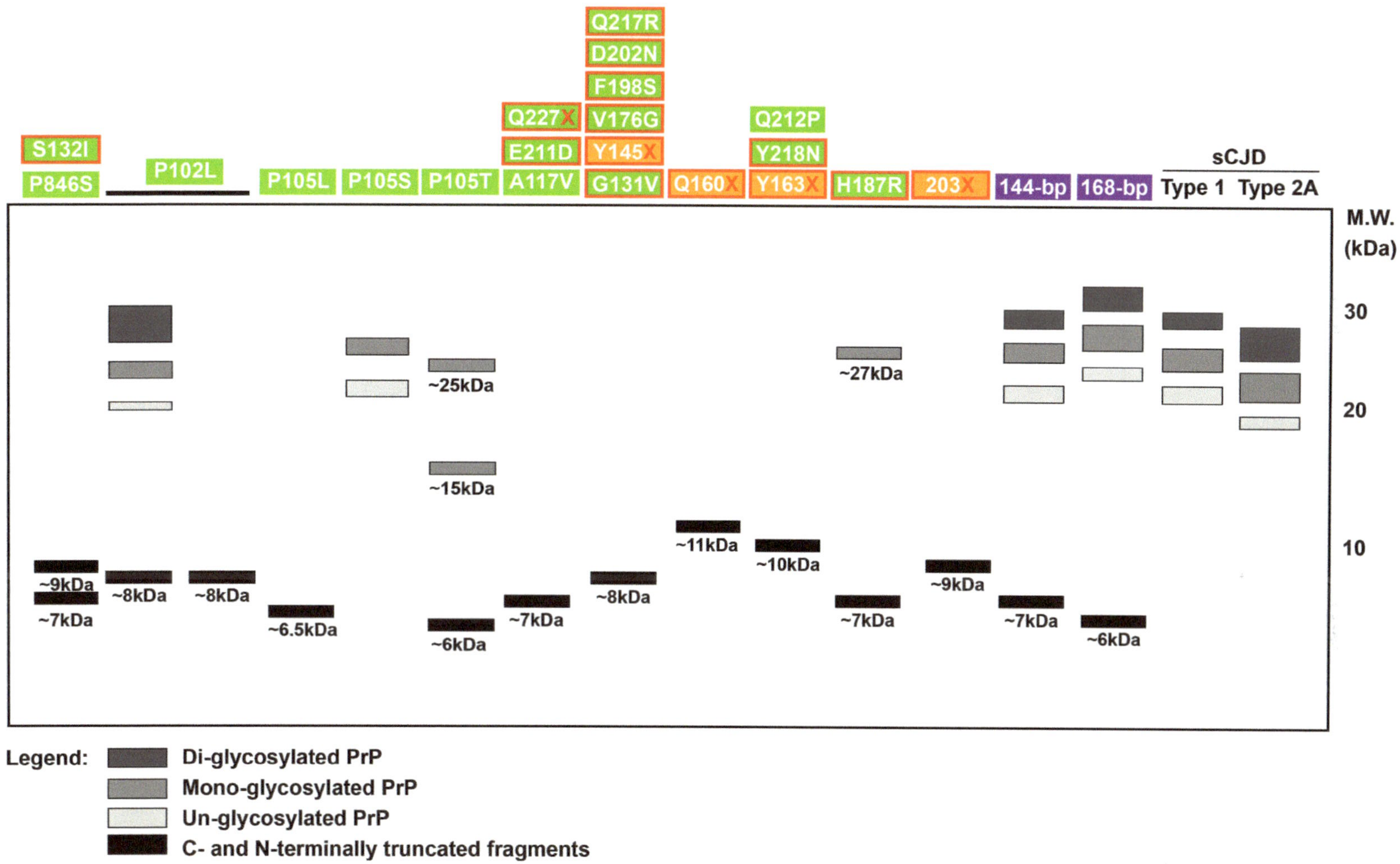

Fig. 14.2. Schematic summary of prion protein (*PrP*) bands as obtained by Western blot analysis from brain homogenates of human cases affected by dominantly inherited PrP amyloidoses. *sCJD*, sporadic Creutzfeldt–Jakob disease.

DOMINANTLY INHERITED PRION PROTEIN CEREBRAL AMYLOIDOSES

Gerstmann–Sträussler–Scheinker disease and variants previously grouped under the GSS eponym

The neurologic signs and symptoms have been described in more detail than the psychiatric symptoms; the latter may precede and accompany the initial phase of the disorder. Progressive cerebellar ataxia and pyramidal signs, followed by dementia, are the cardinal features; however, additional signs and symptoms may be seen in the hereditary PrP cerebral amyloidosis of this group (Ghetti et al., 1995; Gambetti et al., 1999). Phenotypic heterogeneity exists both within and between families with the same mutation. Following the discovery of numerous *PRNP* mutations associated with hereditary PrP cerebral amyloidosis, a haplotype-specific pattern of clinical presentation has been observed.

The neuropathologic phenotypes associated with these forms vary substantially, not only in morphologic characteristics, but also in severity; however, the main histologic feature is the presence of amyloid plaques in the parenchyma of the cerebrum and cerebellum. These plaques are the result of the deposition of PrP fragments. Furthermore, mild to severe cerebral and cerebellar atrophy is present, frequently with degeneration of the pyramidal tract. Phenotypic heterogeneity is observed most often between haplotypes, but it is also seen within individuals with the same haplotype (Ghetti et al., 1995, 1996a; Webb et al., 2008).

Pioneering studies on PrP biochemical patterns had been carried out in A117V, F198S, and Q217R, from purified amyloid preparations. PrP aggregates obtained by in vitro proteolysis contained 7–8-kDa PrP fragments, mainly deriving from mutant PrP alleles (Tagliavini et al., 1991, 1994, 2001; Piccardo et al., 1996, 1998).

P84S-129V

Clinical phenotype

In the seventh decade of life, a Caucasian male had a rapid neurologic and cognitive decline, involving memory, language, visual perception, and limb ataxia. The condition was diagnosed as Alzheimer disease. He died 2 years after the onset of symptoms (Jones et al., 2014).

Neuropathology

Multicentric plaques made of PrP amyloid were present in the cerebral cortex, basal ganglia, thalamus, and cerebellum, and occasionally in the white matter. Small PrP deposits were also observed in the brainstem and spinal cord. Patchy spongiform changes were present in the molecular layer of the cerebellum (Jones et al., 2014).

Biochemistry

Western blot analysis of homogenates of frontal and temporal cortex showed two low-molecular-mass PK-resistant PrP (PrP^{res}) bands in the 7- and 9-kDa range (Fig. 14.2).

P102L-129M

Clinical phenotype

The P102L-129M mutation coupled with methionine at residue 129 is the most common haplotype associated with GSS. Clinical symptoms start in the third to sixth decades of life, with a disease duration of a few months to 6 years. P102L mutation carriers who are MM homozygotes at codon 129 have an earlier onset than MV heterozygotes. Apolipoprotein E (*ApoE*) ε4 carriers appear to have a delayed age of onset.

Two distinct phenotypes can be observed. One is characterized by a progressive cerebellar syndrome with ataxia, dysarthria, and incoordination of saccadic movements, frequently accompanied by pyramidal and pseudobulbar signs. Behavioral and cognitive dysfunction may be present at the onset or follow the initial neurologic dysfunction. Amyotrophy and an electromyographic pattern of denervation may be seen early in the course of the disease. The other phenotype is characterized by a very rapid disease course ranging from 5 to 9 months with a clinical picture indistinguishable from that of CJD (Ghetti et al., 2011). In such cases, myoclonus and pseudoperiodic sharp-wave discharges on the electroencephalogram (EEG) are observed. Hyperthermia, tachycardia, and hyperhidrosis may occur due to sympathetic hyperactivity. Dementia or akinetic mutism is present in the late stages.

Computed tomography (CT) and magnetic resonance imaging (MRI) (Fig. 14.3) may show cerebral and cerebellar atrophy; single-photon emission computed tomography (SPECT) may reveal hypoperfusion of the frontal cortex and cerebellum (Webb et al., 2008). PrP amyloid cannot be detected by [^{11}C]PiB positron emission tomography (PET) imaging (Deters et al., 2016).

Neuropathology

The P102L-129M haplotype may be associated with two distinct neuropathologic phenotypes that can be seen in different patients of the same family, as reported also in the "H" family (Hainfellner et al., 1995). The two phenotypes differ regarding the presence or absence of spongiform degeneration of gray-matter structures.

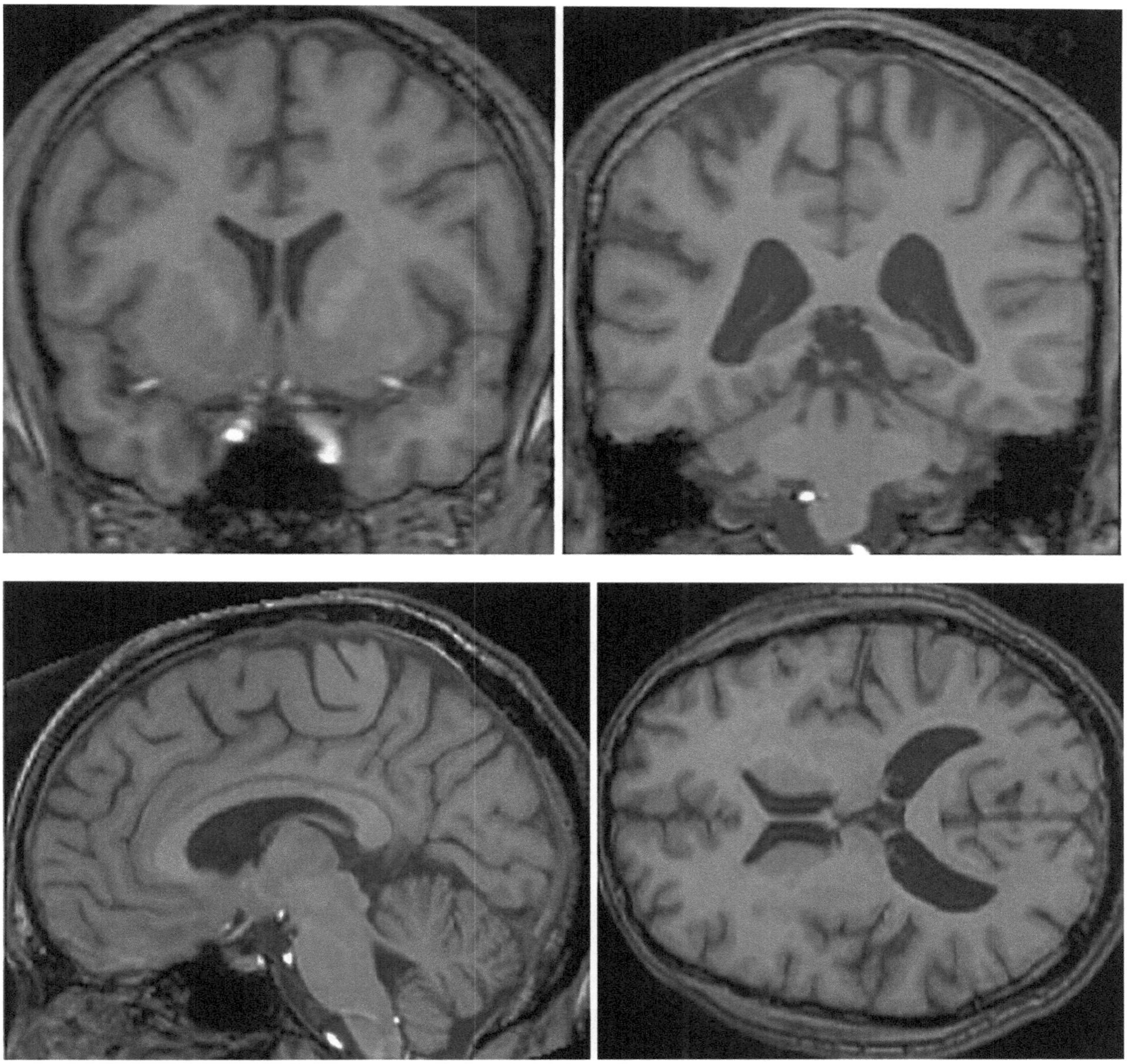

Fig. 14.3. Magnetic resonance imaging scans of a patient with Gerstmann–Sträussler–Scheinker disease, associated with a P102L-129M mutation. Ventricular dilatation and cerebral atrophy are evident.

Thus, the most frequently observed phenotype is characterized by the presence of unicentric or multicentric plaques made of PrP amyloid coexisting with a severe spongiform degeneration. A less frequently observed phenotype is characterized by the presence of exclusively unicentric or multicentric plaques made of PrP amyloid. Unicentric or multicentric plaques are most numerous in the molecular layer of the cerebellum; however, they may also be present throughout the gray matter of the cerebrum. PrP amyloid plaques as well as PrP diffuse plaques are accompanied by a severe astrocytic proliferation. Neuronal loss is observed in association with both phenotypes; however, it is most severe when there is spongiform degeneration (Gerstmann et al., 1936; Gambetti et al., 1999; Ghetti et al., 2011) (Figs 14.4–14.6).

Biochemistry

The biochemical pattern of PrP^{res} is characterized by two distinct phenotypes, one consisting in the co-presence of the 21-kDa C-terminal fragment and the 8-kDa PrP^{IF} and another with PrP^{IF} only. The first biochemical phenotype is observed in individuals who develop a CJD-like disease while the second occurs in those with a GSS-like progressive neurodegenerative disorder (Piccardo et al., 1998). It should be mentioned that the

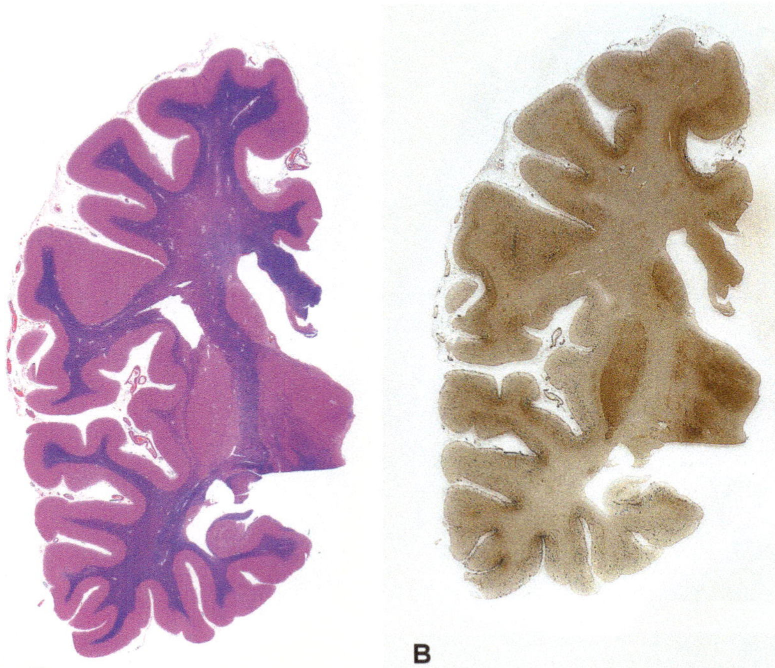

Fig. 14.4. Coronal sections of a cerebral hemisphere of a patient with Gerstmann–Sträussler–Scheinker disease, associated with a P102L-129M mutation. (**A**) Atrophy of the frontal and temporal lobes as well as loss of myelin stain in the white matter is noted. (**B**) Prion protein immunoreactivity is present in the cerebral cortex, caudate nucleus, putamen, and thalamus.

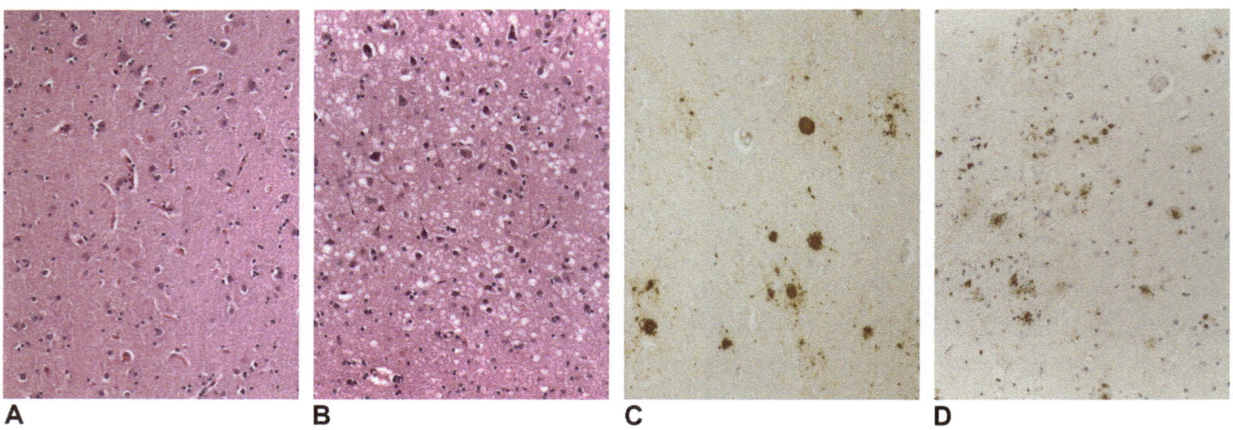

Fig. 14.5. Cerebral cortex of a patient with Gerstmann–Sträussler–Scheinker disease, associated with a P102L-129M mutation. (**A**) No spongiform changes are present. Multiple eosinophilic amyloid plaques are scattered in the neuropil. (**B**) Spongiform changes are present. Eosinophilic amyloid plaques are seen in the neuropil. (**C**) Prion protein plaques and diffuse deposits are shown by immunohistochemistry in the case with no spongiform changes. (**D**) Prion protein plaques and diffuse deposits are shown by immunohistochemistry in the case with spongiform changes.

glycotype of 21-kDa PrP^{res} is similar to that observed in sporadic CJD, except for a diglycosylated-dominant profile (Parchi et al., 1998). Protein sequencing analysis showed that the 21-kDa fragment is cleaved at N-terminal residues 78 and 82 while the 8-kDa peptide demonstrated N-terminal cleavage sites at residues 74, 78, 80, and 82 and multiple C-terminus ending points spanning positions 147–153. Both fragments originated exclusively from the mutated allele (Parchi et al., 1998) (Fig. 14.2).

P102L-129V

Clinical phenotype

The clinical phenotype is characterized by apathy and depression, seizures, cerebellar ataxia, dysarthria, and

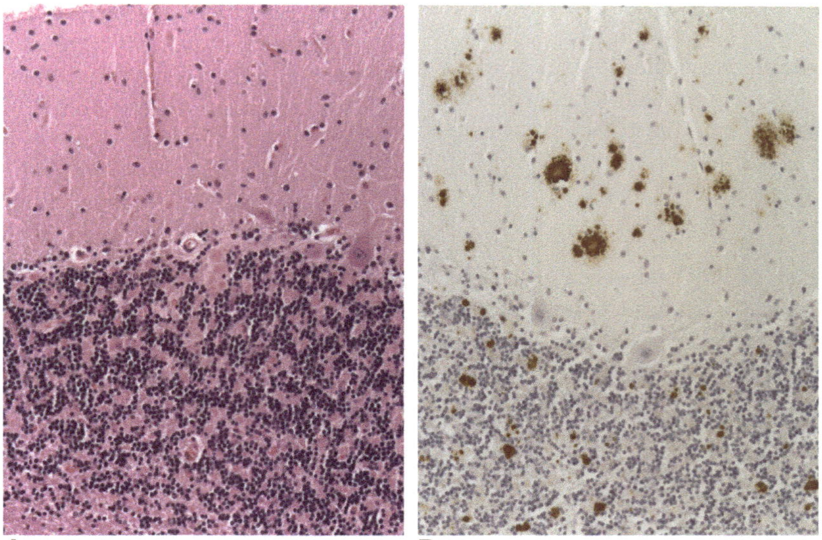

Fig. 14.6. Cerebellar cortex of a patient with Gerstmann–Sträussler–Scheinker disease, associated with a P102L-129 M mutation. (**A**) No spongiform changes are present. Multiple eosinophilic amyloid plaques are present in the molecular and granule cell layers. (**B**) Unicentric and multicentric prion protein plaques are shown by immunohistochemistry.

numbness of the lower extremities. The duration of the illness varies between 4 and 12 years (Young et al., 1997; Bianca et al., 2003). Dementia was not reported in either of the observed patients.

Neuropathology

In the corticospinal, spinocerebellar, and gracile tracts there is a moderate to severe loss of fibers. PrP amyloid plaques are frequently seen in the cerebellar cortex and to a lesser extent in the neocortex. Diffuse PrP deposits are present in the substantia gelatinosa within the dorsal horn of the spinal cord. No spongiform degeneration is seen (Young et al., 1997).

Biochemistry

The biochemical PrP pattern has not been reported (Fig. 14.2).

P105L-129V

Clinical phenotype

The majority of cases belong to Japanese families. The neurologic symptoms may be preceded by psychiatric abnormalities. The first manifestations, that dominate the clinical picture, are a spastic gait, hyperreflexia, and the Babinski sign (Kitamoto et al., 1993; Yamada et al., 1999). Fine finger tremor, rigidity of limbs, parkinsonism, and ataxia are not uncommon. A report of a single case associated with memory disturbance, dysarthria, extrapyramidal signs, and ataxic gait without spasticity widens the clinical spectrum (Iwasaki et al., 2009). In the late stages, paraparesis progresses to tetraparesis as emotional incontinence and dementia dominate. EEG studies do not describe pseudoperiodic sharp-wave discharges. MRI shows hypointensity of the striatum. Electromyography (EMG) may show denervation, while evoked potentials reveal conduction delays in the posterior funiculus and pyramidal tract. The age at onset of the neurologic signs is in the fourth and fifth decades of life; the duration of the disease ranges from 6 to 12 years (Kitamoto et al., 1993; Yamada et al., 1999).

Neuropathology

PrP amyloid plaques and diffuse deposits are frequent in the cerebral, but rare in the cerebellar, cortex. PrP burden in the precentral gyrus, striatum, and thalamus is most severe. Spongiform changes are not present. Neurofibrillary tangles have been reported in some cases (Kitamoto et al., 1993). Axonal loss occurs in the pyramidal tracts.

Biochemistry

Immunoblot analysis showed an N- and C-terminally truncated PK-resistant PrP migrating at 6 kDa (Yamada et al., 1999) (Fig. 14.2).

P105S-129V

Clinical phenotype

In a single case, the onset was at 30 years of age. Clinical signs and symptoms included withdrawal, poor personal care, receptive and expressive aphasia, and parkinsonism. The duration of illness was 10 years (Tunnell et al., 2008).

Neuropathology

In addition to spongiform encephalopathy, large multicentric amyloid plaques were present in the neocortex, hippocampus, and cerebellum. Tau pathology was not observed (Tunnell et al., 2008).

Biochemistry

The biochemical pattern of PrP^{res} consisted of the presence of two N-terminally truncated fragments of ~21 and 26 kDa representing the unglycosylated and monoglycosylated isoforms. A similar pattern of incomplete PrP glycosylation was also observed in association with PrP mutations T183A and V180I, that are located close to the glycosylation sites and have a genetically determined CJD disease phenotype (Tunnell et al., 2008) (Fig. 14.2).

P105T-129V

Clinical phenotype

In the fourth decade of life, a male had a progressive memory loss and cerebellar ataxia. The neurologic signs progressed toward a pancerebellar syndrome with ataxia and myoclonic jerks. By [F-18]fluorodeoxyglucose (FDG), there was hypometabolism in the left cerebral hemisphere. Hyperintense signal in the cerebral cortex and thalamus on fluid-attenuated inversion recovery (FLAIR) and diffusion-weighted imaging (DWI) was present. In the late stage, the patient was wheelchair-bound and had severe dementia. Death occurred 6 years after the onset of symptoms. The father had died affected by a similar disorder (Polymenidou et al., 2011). The same mutation has been reported in six members of a family from East Indian origin, including a 13-year-old child (Rogaeva et al., 2006).

Neuropathology

Unicentric plaques made of PrP-amyloid were present in the deep cortical layers as well as spongiform changes and a dense PrP synaptic-like pattern.

Biochemistry

Western blot analysis of PK-treated brain homogenates showed a 6-kDa unglycosylated PK-resistant fragment and two bands of approximately 15 and 25 kDa (Fig. 14.2).

A117V-129V

Clinical phenotype

The mutation has been reported in France, Germany, Hungary, England, Ireland, the United States, and, recently, in Argentina (Saenz-Farret et al., 2016). The two Argentinian patients were siblings; they also had a heterozygous variant of uncertain pathogenic significance at codon 165 (R165H), in addition to the A117V-129V mutation. Various clinical phenotypes may be associated with the A117V-129V haplotype (Nochlin et al., 1989; Mallucci et al., 1999). Behavioral and personality disturbances, such as mood swings, aggressive behavior, and paranoia, frequently present long before neurologic signs and symptoms. In some individuals, extrapyramidal signs with parkinsonian features occur early in the course of the disease. Pyramidal signs, amyotrophy, myoclonus, emotional lability, and a pseudobulbar syndrome may follow. In the Argentinian siblings, presenting symptoms were upper-limb paresthesias, frequent falls, and right hemiparesis, followed by dysphagia, dysarthria, and myoclonic jerks. Ocular examination revealed a difficulty in initiating saccades.

Phenotypic variability among affected individuals may occur within the affected members of a single family. No pseudoperiodic sharp-wave discharges are seen on EEG. Results from CT scans vary from normality to moderate cerebral atrophy. Cerebrocortical atrophy, severe loss of white matter, and enlargement of the lateral ventricles are detected on MRI (Fig. 14.7). A decreased FDG uptake in the cortex and subcortical nuclei is evident on PET. The age at onset of clinical signs is in the second to seventh decade of life; duration ranges from 1 to 11 years.

Neuropathology

Cerebral atrophy is seen in some cases. Throughout the cerebral cortex, basal ganglia, and thalamus there are variable amounts of PrP amyloid plaques and diffuse deposits. In the cerebellum, plaques may be absent or present in variable amounts. Pyramidal tract degeneration may be present. Spongiform degeneration may be focally present. Neuronal loss may be severe in the substantia nigra. Neurofibrillary tangles have been described in individuals with a long disease duration (Nochlin et al., 1989) (Figs 14.8–14.10).

Biochemistry

Following PK digestion, PrP^{res} is composed of N- and C-terminally truncated peptides migrating at 7 and 14 kDa with other minor bands at higher molecular weights. The 7-kDa band represents the PrP^{res} monomeric form, while the other band is a dimer and multimers incomptetely solubilized. Fragments of 7 kDa had been sequenced showing N- and C-terminal ragged ends spanning from G86 and G90 and ending with R148, E152, and D153 (Tagliavini et al., 2001) (Fig. 14.2).

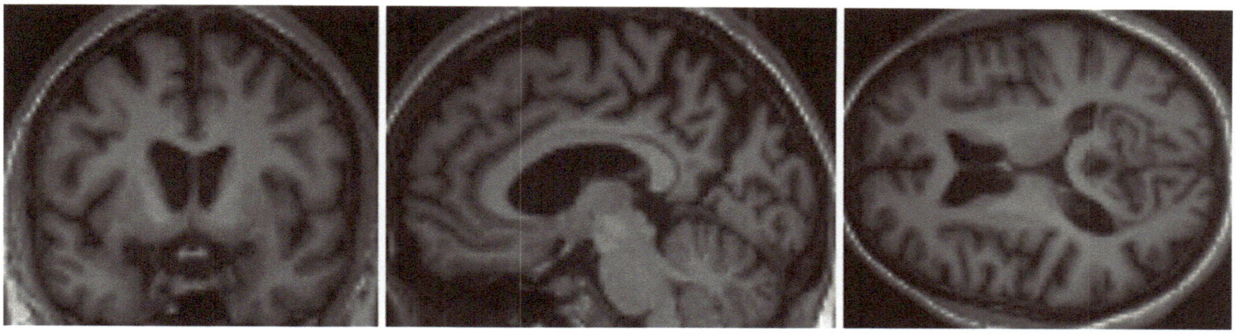

Fig. 14.7. Magnetic resonance imaging scans of a patient with Gerstmann–Sträussler–Scheinker disease, associated with an A117V-129V mutation. Ventricular dilatation and cerebral atrophy are evident.

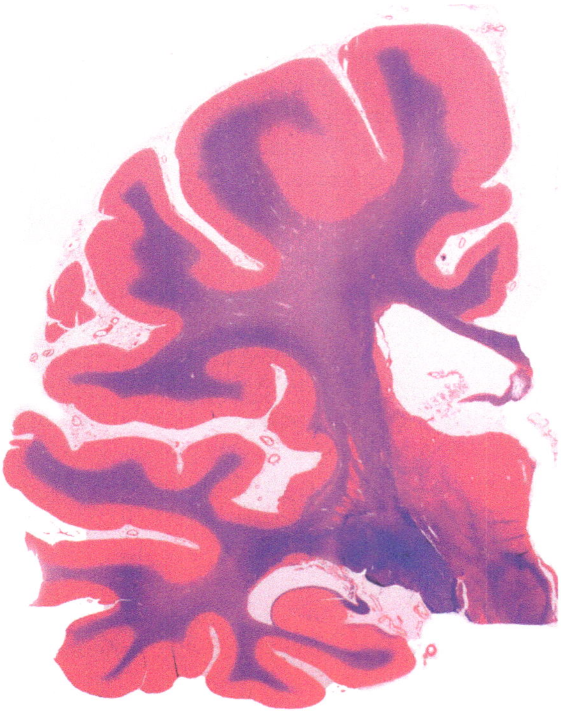

Fig. 14.8. Coronal sections of a cerebral hemisphere of a patient with Gerstmann–Sträussler–Scheinker disease, associated with an A117V-129V mutation. Atrophy of the frontal and temporal lobes as well as loss of myelin stain in the white matter is present.

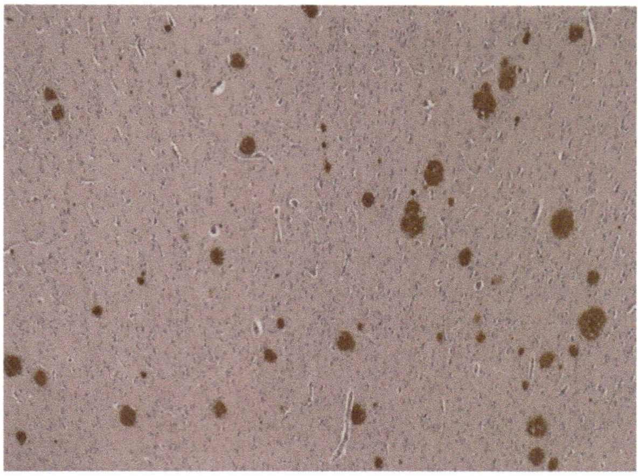

Fig. 14.9. Cerebral cortex of a patient with Gerstmann–Sträussler–Scheinker GSS, associated with an A117V-129V mutation. No spongiform changes are present. Multiple well-circumscribed scattered prion protein plaques of different dimension are shown by immunohistochemistry.

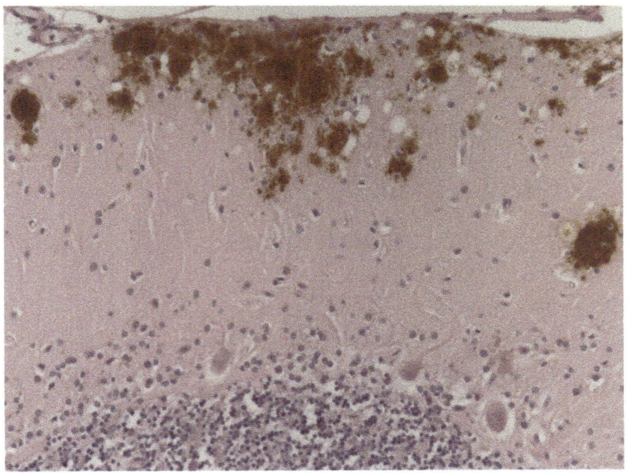

Fig. 14.10. Molecular layer of the cerebellar cortex from a patient with Gerstmann–Sträussler–Scheinker disease, associated with an A117V-129V mutation. Prion protein plaques and diffuse deposits are shown by immunohistochemistry. Mild spongiform changes are present.

G131V-129M

Clinical phenotype

Changes in personality, decrease in cognitive performance, apraxia, tremor, and increased deep tendon reflexes are the presenting signs. MRI images show cerebral and cerebellar atrophy. EEGs do not show pseudoperiodic sharp waves. In the late stages, dementia becomes progressively more severe and ataxia develops. The clinical onset is in the fifth decade of life and the disease has a duration of 9 years (Panegyres et al., 2001).

Neuropathology

PrP amyloid plaques and diffuse deposits are seen in the cortex and subcortical nuclei as well as in the cerebellum. Neurofibrillary tangles are seen in the Ammon's horn and in the entorhinal cortex. No spongiform degeneration is seen (Panegyres et al., 2001).

Biochemistry

Immunoblot analysis of PK-treated brain homogenates demonstrated four bands of 8, 18, 26, and 31 kDa (Panegyres et al., 2001) (Fig. 14.2).

S132I-129M

Clinical phenotype

The clinical phenotype is characterized by progressive cognitive decline in one family member (18 months' duration of illness) and progressive ataxia with dementia in another (7 years' duration). The clinical onset was at 39 and 62 years of age (Hilton et al., 2009).

Neuropathology

Amyloid plaques were observed in the neocortex, basal ganglia, thalamus, and cerebellum. A moderate tau pathology coexisted with PrP plaques (Hilton et al., 2009).

Biochemistry

Western blot analysis of PK-treated brain homogenate showed two small internal fragments of 7 and 9 kDa lacking the N- and C-terminus (Hilton et al., 2009) (Fig. 14.2).

A133V-129M-219K

Clinical phenotype

Clinical presentation was characterized by supranuclear palsy-like syndrome in a 62-year-old patient with 4 months' duration (Rowe et al., 2007).

Neuropathology

PrP amyloid plaques were confined to the cerebellum. Spongiform encephalopathy is observed in other regions (Rowe et al., 2007).

Biochemistry

It is not reported.

R136S-129M

Clinical and neuropathologic phenotypes are not described in detail (Head et al., 2015).

V176G-129V

Clinical phenotype

In the seventh decade of life, a female, who had been estranged from her family members, had progressive memory loss, dysphasia, behavioral changes, cerebellar ataxia with bilateral intention tremor, hyperreflexia, and myoclonus following a surgical procedure. Death occurred 1 month after surgery (Simpson et al., 2013).

Neuropathology

Unicentric and multicentric plaques made of PrP amyloid were present in the deep cortical layers. Spongiform changes in cerebral and cerebellar cortices and basal ganglia were mild. Tau-immunoreactive neurons were present in the hippocampus.

Biochemistry

A PrP^{Pres} main fragment with an approximate molecular mass of 8 kDa was detected. Peptide mapping using a series of anti-PrP monoclonal antibodies predicted that this fragment resulted from PrP cleavage around residues 60 and 140. Slower-migrating bands were also observed resulting from incomplete 8-kDa fragment solubilization (Simpson et al., 2013) (Fig. 14.2).

H187R-129V

Clinical phenotype

The clinical phenotype is characterized by progressive cognitive impairment, cerebellar ataxia, and dysarthria followed by myoclonus, seizures, and occasionally pyramidal and extrapyramidal signs. The initial symptoms may vary, even within members of the same family.

Neuroimaging shows severe, widespread atrophy of the cerebrum and cerebellum. The age at onset is in the third to six decade of life with a duration of 3–18 years (Cervenakova et al., 1999; Butefisch et al., 2000; Hall et al., 2005; Colucci et al., 2006).

Neuropathology

Spongiform degeneration has not been reported. Diffuse atrophy and gliosis are most evident in the subcortical white matter. In the hippocampus and cerebellum there are PrP diffuse deposits and amyloid plaques while in the neocortex mostly diffuse deposits are found. The PrP deposits have a round or elongated, "curly" appearance.

Neurofibrillary tangles may be found in the hippocampus (Colucci et al., 2006).

Biochemistry

Biochemical analysis showed two main PK-resistant internal fragments of 7 and 14 kDa representing the monomer and the dimer respectively. An additional band was detected at 27 kDa, not observed in association with other mutations. N-terminus sequence of 14- and 7-kDa fragments had been determined showing N-terminal ragged ends spanning from G82 to W99 (Colucci et al., 2006) (Fig. 14.2).

F198S-129V

Clinical phenotype

Eye movement abnormalities and mild memory impairment may be the earliest detectable neurologic and cognitive manifestations. These may be preceded by a psychotic depression. The clinical phenotype is characterized by clumsiness in walking followed by ataxia, dysarthria, mild tremor, rigidity, bradykinesia, as well as a gradual loss of short-term memory, and progressive cognitive impairment evolving into dementia (Farlow et al., 1989; Unverzagt et al., 1997). In the early stages, MRI studies show cerebellar atrophy (Fig. 14.11).

The symptoms may progress slowly over a 5-year period or rapidly over as little as 1 year. The age at onset of clinical signs ranges from late in the fourth decade to early in the eighth decade of life. Patients homozygous for valine at codon 129 have clinical signs more than 10 years earlier, on average, than heterozygous patients (Dlouhy et al., 1992). The duration of the disease ranges from 2 to 15 years. Sequential follow-up MRI scans revealed progressive atrophy of the cerebral cortex and of the cerebellum (Fig. 14.11). Reduced metabolism was demonstrared by [F-18]FDG PET. [F-18]FDDNP binding was evident in the cerebral cortex, basal ganglia, and cerebellum. Basal ganglia involvement could be observed in mutation carriers years before the onset of neurologic symptoms; however, the significance of this finding is not clear (Kepe et al., 2010). Two mutation carriers had hyperintense signal in limbic, neocortical, and subcortical regions on FLAIR and DWI (Vitali et al., 2011). [F-18]FDG PET and structural MRI demonstrated a reduced metabolism and mild atrophy, respectively, in the same regions of symptomatic individuals (Kepe et al., 2010). Currently, no PET ligand is available to demonstrate specifically PrP deposits. [C11]PiB, which is selective for Aβ deposits, showed no signal in asymptomatic and symptomatic individuals who were *PRNP* F198S mutation carriers (Deters et al., 2016).

[^{18}F]flortaucipir PET scans showed uptake in the basal ganglia, frontal gyri, cingulate gyrus, sensorimotor cortex, and insula compared to cognitively normal older adults. The topography of tau deposition in areas indicated by [^{18}F]flortaucipir PET was confirmed by immunohistochemistry in a patient who expired 9 months after the [^{18}F]flortaucipir PET. The distribution of tau differs significantly from that observed in Alzheimer disease (Risacher et al., 2018).

Neuropathology

Numerous PrP deposits, in the form of PrP amyloid and diffuse plaques, coexisting with severe tau neurofibrillary pathology, including neurofibrillary tangles and neuropil threads, are the distinctive elements of the neuropathologic phenotype (Figs 14.12 and 14.13) (Ghetti et al., 1989). The PrP deposition is the most severe reported among all dominantly inherited PrP cerebral amyloidosis. The gray structures of the cerebrum, cerebellum, and brainstem contain PrP amyloid and diffuse plaques (Figs 14.14 and 14.15). The amyloid plaques have single or multiple cores, and therefore are referred to as unicentric and multicentric plaques (Fig. 14.16). The burden of PrP amyloid is highest in layers 1, 4,

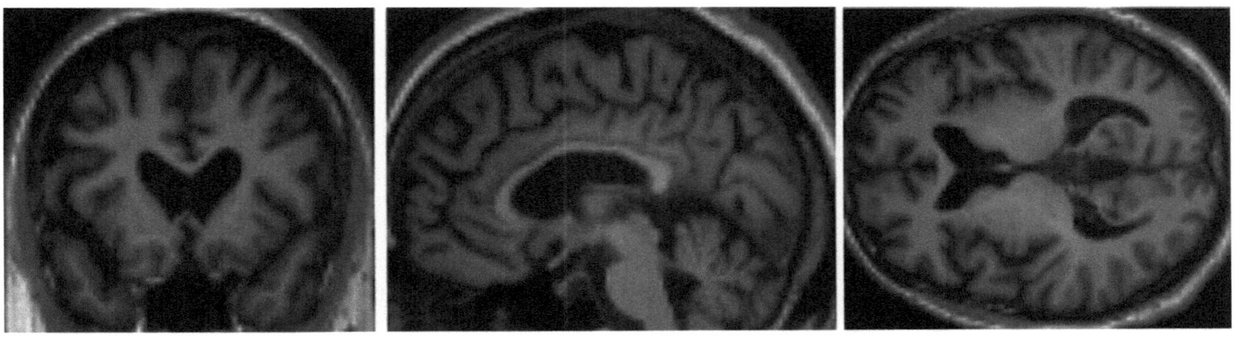

Fig. 14.11. Magnetic resonance imaging scans of a patient with Gerstmann–Sträussler–Scheinker disease, associated with a mutation in F198S-129V show cerebral and cerebellar atrophy. In the cerebral hemispheres, ventricular dilatation, loss of white matter, and atrophy of the cortex and of the corpus callosum are evident.

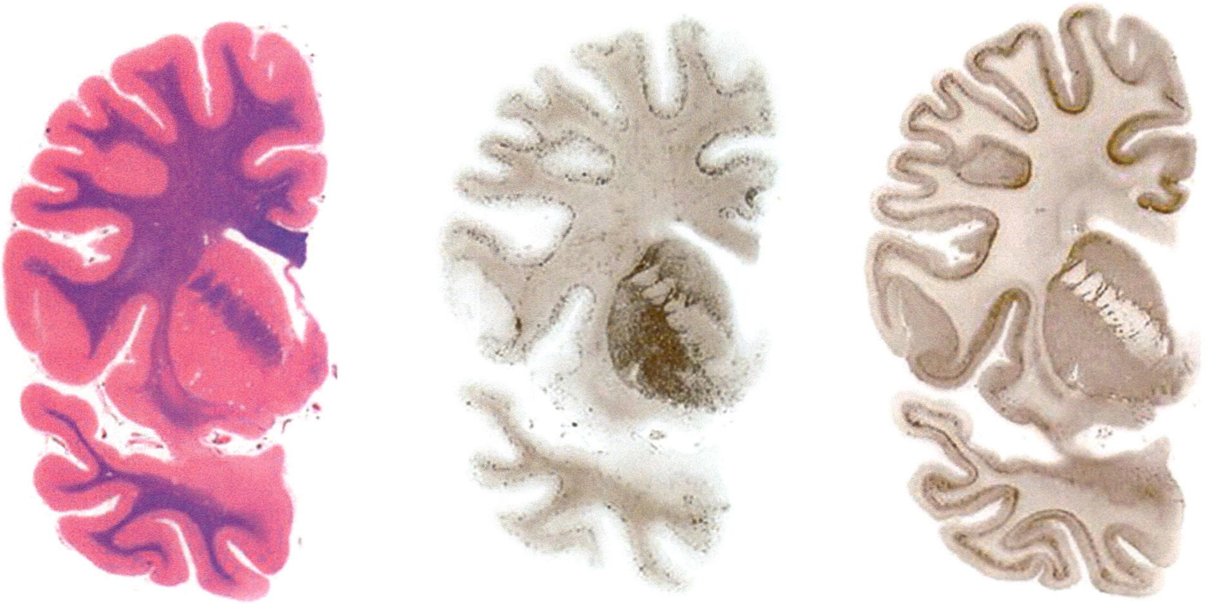

Fig. 14.12. Coronal sections of a cerebral hemisphere of a patient with Gerstmann–Sträussler–Scheinker disease, associated with an F198S-129 V mutation. (**A**) Mild atrophy of the frontal and temporal lobes as well as mild loss of myelin stain in the white matter are noted. (**B**) Prion protein immunoreactivity is present in the cerebral cortex, caudate nucleus, putamen. (**C**) Tau immunoreactivity is present in the cerebral cortex, caudate nucleus, putamen, and thalamus.

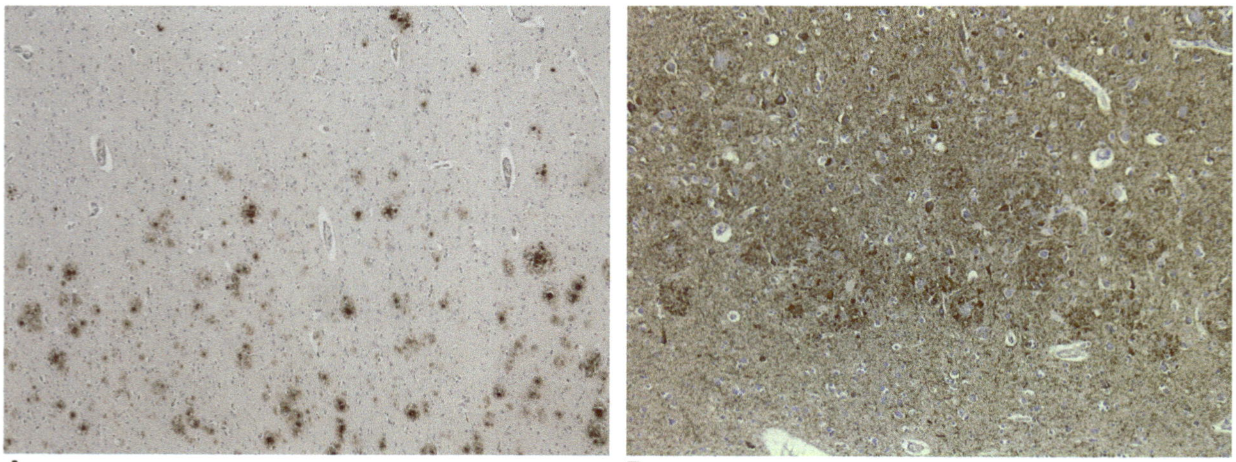

Fig. 14.13. Serial sections of cerebral cortex from a patient with Gerstmann–Sträussler–Scheinker disease, associated with an F198S-129 V mutation. (**A**) No spongiform changes are present. Numerous scattered prion protein diffuse deposits, unicentric plaques, and multicentric plaques of different dimension are shown by immunohistochemistry. (**B**) Severe tau pathology is shown by immunohistochemistry. Tau deposits are seen in the perikarya of neurons, in neuropil threads, and in the processes surrounding the plaques.

5, and 6 of the frontal, insular, temporal, and parietal cortices. In the hippocampus, the stratum lacunosum moleculare of the CA1 sector and the subiculum are similarly affected. Astrocytes, astrocytic processes, and microglial cells surround the cores of the plaque. In the neocortex, amyloid cores may appear morphologically similar to the neuritic plaques of Alzheimer disease, due to the association with tau-immunolabeled or silver-stained neurites. Neurofibrillary tangles and neuropil threads are found in the anatomic regions where PrP deposits are present. In the neocortex of some affected individuals, α-synuclein

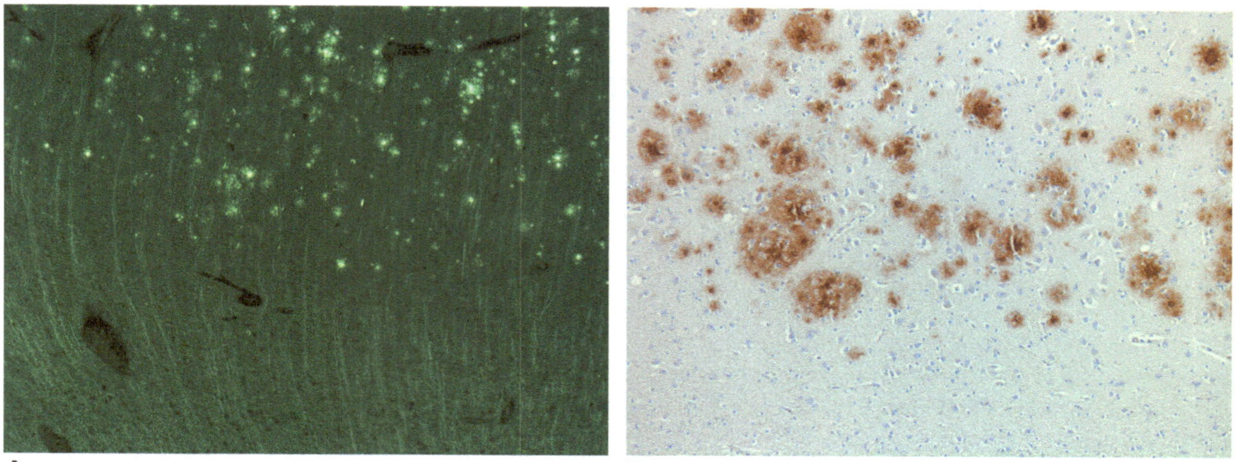

A B

Fig. 14.14. Serial sections of cerebral cortex from a patient with Gerstmann–Sträussler–Scheinker disease, associated with an F198S-129 V mutation. (**A**) Numerous fluorescent amyloid unicentric plaques and multicentric plaques in the lower cortical layers are present among bundles of myelinated axons. (**B**) Numerous unicentric and multicentric prion protein amyloid plaques in the lower cortical layers are shown by immunohistochemistry.

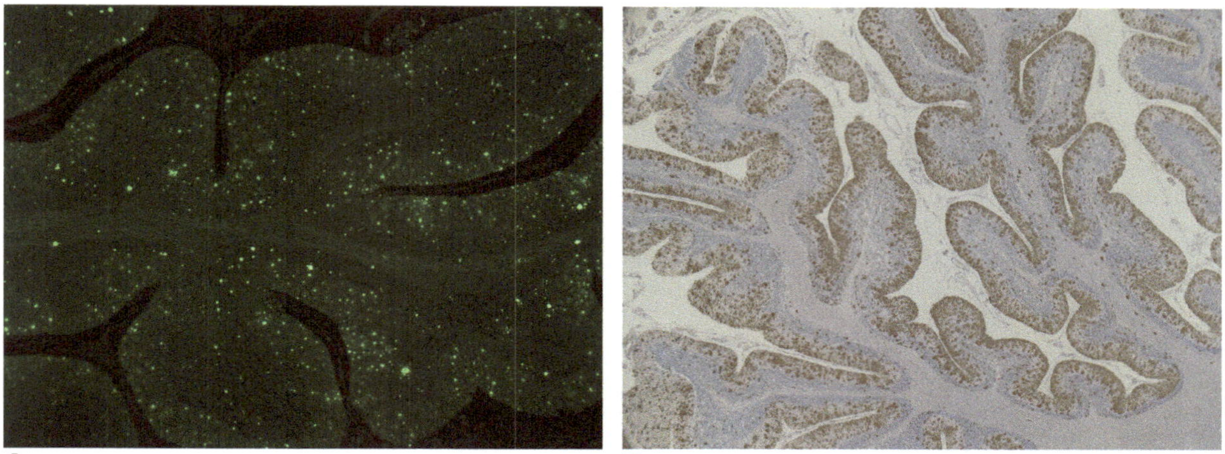

A B

Fig. 14.15. Cerebellar cortex from a patient with Gerstmann–Sträussler–Scheinker disease, associated with an F198S-129 V mutation. (**A**) Numerous fluorescent amyloid unicentric and multicentric plaques are present in the molecular layer; few plaques are also present in the granule cell layer and in the white matter. (**B**) Numerous prion protein amyloid plaques in the lower cortical layers are shown by immunohistochemistry.

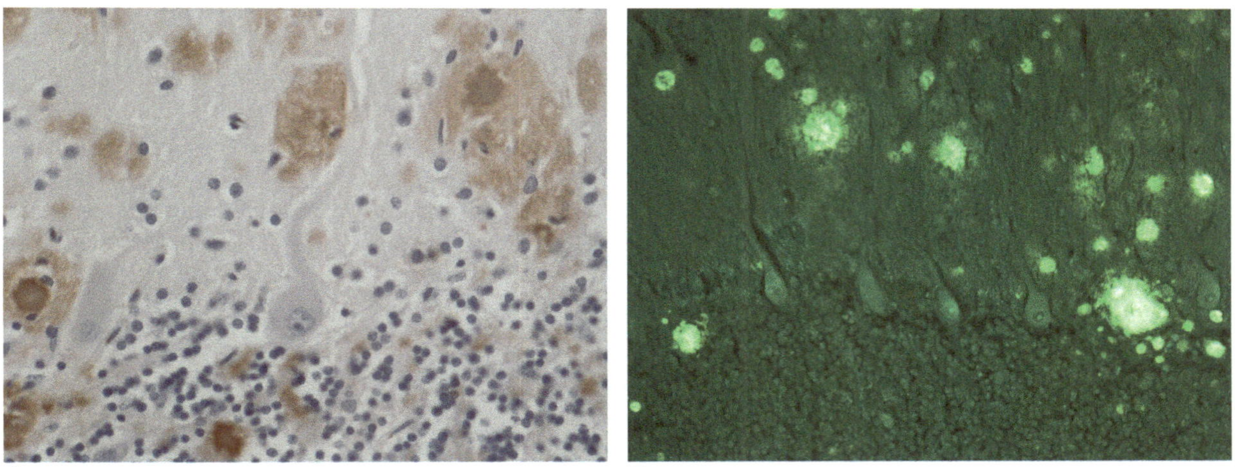

A B

Fig. 14.16. Cerebellar cortex from a patient with Gerstmann–Sträussler–Scheinker disease, associated with an F198S-129 V mutation. (**A**) Fluorescent amyloid plaques are shown at high magnification. (**B**) Prion protein amyloid plaques and diffuse deposits are shown by immunohistochemistry.

immunopositive Lewy bodies were seen. Iron deposits in the globus pallidus, striatum, red nucleus, and substantia nigra are seen. Spongiform changes are rarely observed (Ghetti et al., 1995, 1996a).

Biochemistry

Biochemical analysis of F198S PK digested brain homogenates generated three prominent bands migrating at 27–29, 18–19, and 8 kDa. However, the slower-migrating band corresponding to 8-kDa monomer. Previous studies have shown that in F198S PrP amyloid is composed of two internal fragment of 11 and 7 kDa spanning residues 58–150 and 81–150, respectively (Tagliavini et al., 1991; Piccardo et al., 1996; Zanusso et al., 2014) (Fig. 14.2).

D202N-129V

Clinical phenotype

The clinical phenotype is characterized by axial akinetic rigidity, gait and postural disturbances, backward falls, impairment of downgaze, moderate dementia, and hyperreflexia, with onset in the eighth decade of life and up to a 6-year duration. Atrophy of the frontal and temporal lobes, midbrain, and cerebellar vermis is demonstrated by MRI (Piccardo et al., 1998).

Neuropathology

PrP-immunopositive deposits are observed in the neocortex, hippocampus, basal ganglia, amygdala, cerebellar cortex, dentate nucleus, substantia nigra, and inferior olivary nucleus. Tau-immunopositive neurons, neuropil threads, and neurofibrillary tangles are diffuse in all gray-matter structures, and most severe in the neocortex, hippocampus, striatum, and midbrain. No spongiform degeneration is observed (Piccardo et al., 1998).

Biochemistry

The biochemical pattern of PrP^{res} is similar to the one reported in GSS F198S (Piccardo et al., 1998) (Fig. 14.2).

E211D-129V

Clinical phenotype

Three females in two generations of a family had onset of clinical signs in the sixth and seventh decades of life. Two of them died 3 years and one 13 years after onset. Their neuropsychiatric syndrome was characterized by cerebellar ataxia, myoclonic jerks of upper limbs, frontal dementia, and visuospatial apraxia. Cerebellar atrophy was shown by a CT scan (Peoc'h et al., 2012).

Neuropathology

Only one patient was examined post mortem. A severe burden of PrP amyloid plaques in the cerebral cortex, caudate nucleus, and cerebellar cortex was seen. Neurofibrillary tangles and dystrophic neurites were numerous.

Biochemistry

Western blot pattern of PrP^{res} was characterized by the presence of a C- and N-terminal truncated 7-kDa fragment, as also observed in A117V and Q227X mutations.

Q212P-129M

Clinical phenotype

Gradual incoordination and slurring of speech, followed by dysarthria and ataxia, but not dementia, have been reported. Onset late in the sixth decade and a duration of 8 years have been recorded (Piccardo et al., 1998).

Neuropathology

PrP amyloid burden is mild throughout the central nervous system as compared to that seen in other forms of dominantly inherited PrP cerebral amyloidoses. No spongiform degeneration is seen (Piccardo et al., 1998). In the spinal cord, degeneration of myelinated fibers of the anterior and lateral corticospinal tracts has been described.

Biochemistry

Biochemically, in GSS Q212P PrP^{res} is characterized by a prominent band of 10 kDa and by a minor band of 20 kDa. These correspond to the monomer and the dimer of PrP^{res} internal fragment (Piccardo et al., 1998) (Fig. 14.2).

Q217R-129V

Clinical phenotype

Neurologic signs may be preceded by episodes of mania or depression, followed by gradual memory loss, progressive gait disturbances, parkinsonism, and dementia. Onset of clinical signs varies from the fifth to seventh decade; they may last 2–6 years (Hsiao et al., 1992; Ghetti et al., 1994).

Neuropathology

This neuropathologic phenotype is similar to that associated with the F198S-129V haplotype, with severe PrP amyloid plaque burden, no spongiform degeneration, but numerous neurofibrillary tangles in the cerebral cortex, amygdala, substantia innominata, and thalamus.

In a single case, Lewy bodies have been found in the substantia nigra (Ghetti et al., 1994).

Biochemistry

In GSS Q217R, the biochemical pattern of PrP^{res} overlaps with the one reported in GSS F198S (Piccardo et al., 1998) (Fig. 14.2).

Y218N-129V

Clinical phenotype

The age at onset is in the sixth or seventh decade of life. Memory and language impairment is an early manifestation of the disease. SPECT in the early stages showed asymmetric bifrontal and parieto-occipital hypoperfusion, more pronounced in the left hemisphere. In the late stages, there is severe global deterioration. Aphasia and myclonus are described. No ataxia or motor impairment is observed, even in advanced stages. The duration of the symptomatology is 5–6 years (Alzualde et al., 2010).

Neuropathology

Diffuse unicentric and multicentric PrP amyloid deposits are present in the cerebral and cerebellar cortices. These lesions coexist with tau-immunopositive neurofibrillary tangles and dystrophic neurites in the cerebral cortex and hippocampus (Alzualde et al., 2010).

Biochemistry

PrP^{res} is characterized by a lower band of 10 kDa and by other bands migrating at 20 and 30 kDa were not recognized by antibodies directed to the N- and C- termini. This PrP^{res} pattern is similar to that observed in association with the Q212P mutation (Alzualde et al., 2010) (Fig. 14.2).

Q227X-129V

Clinical phenotype

A slowly progressive hypokinetic rigid syndrome with cognitive decline, starting late in the fourth decade of life, evolves into a syndrome characterized by aphasia, memory disturbances, personality changes, and epileptic seizures with no ataxia or pyramidal signs. Duration of illness is reported to be 6 years (Jansen et al., 2010).

Neuropathology

Numerous multicentric and unicentric plaques in the cerebral cortex predominate in the frontal and temporal cortices, subcortical nuclei and hippocampus, with the cerebellum being relatively spared. Tau-immunopositive neurofibrillary tangles, neuropil threads, and dystrophic neurites are numerous in the neocortex (Jansen et al., 2010).

Biochemistry

The biochemical pattern of PrP^{res} is very similar to the one reported in GSS F198S (Jansen et al., 2010).

M232T-129M

Clinical phenotype

Cerebellar signs and spastic paraparesis are the initial symptoms followed by dementia. The age at onset is in the fifth decade and the duration is 6 years (Liberski et al., 2000).

Neuropathology

PrP amyloid plaques and diffuse deposits are seen in the neocortex, subcortical nuclei, and cerebellum. It is unclear whether spongiform changes are present (Liberski et al., 2000).

Biochemistry

The biochemical pattern of PrP^{res} has not been described.

DOMINANTLY INHERITED PRION PROTEIN CEREBRAL AMYLOIDOSES

Prion protein cerebral amyloid angiopathy variant

Y145X-129M

Clinical phenotype

The clinical phenotype is characterized by memory disturbance, disorientation, and progressive dementia. The EEG does not show pseudoperiodic sharp waves. The age at onset is in the fourth decade and the duration is 21 years (Ghetti et al., 1996b).

Neuropathology

The cerebral and cerebellar hemispheres are atrophic, with a severe neuronal loss and gliosis. PrP amyloid angiopathy involves the walls of small and medium-sized parenchymal and leptomeningeal blood vessels, with PrP amyloid fibrils being adjacent to and within the vessel walls (Fig. 14.17). Neurofibrillary tangles, neuropil threads, and dystrophic neurites are decorated by phosphorylation-dependent and phosphorylation-independent tau antibodies. Tau pathology coexists with the PrP amyloid angiopathy (Fig. 14.18). Thioflavin S fluoresence reveals both neurofibrillary tangles and amyloid angiopathy (Fig. 14.19).There are no spongiform changes (Ghetti et al., 1996a, b).

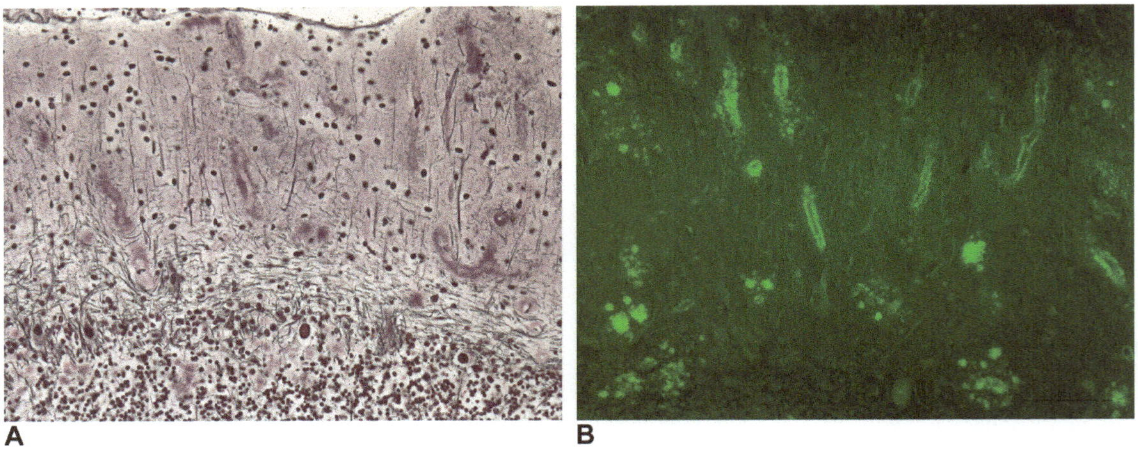

Fig. 14.17. Cerebellar cortex from a patient with prion protein cerebral amyloid angiopathy, associated with a Y145X-129M mutation. (A) Blood vessels with amyloid angiopathy are shown using the Bodian's silver stain. No spongiform changes are present. Loss of Purkinje cells is evident. (B) Fluorescent blood vessels with amyloid angiopathy are shown using the thioflavin S method.

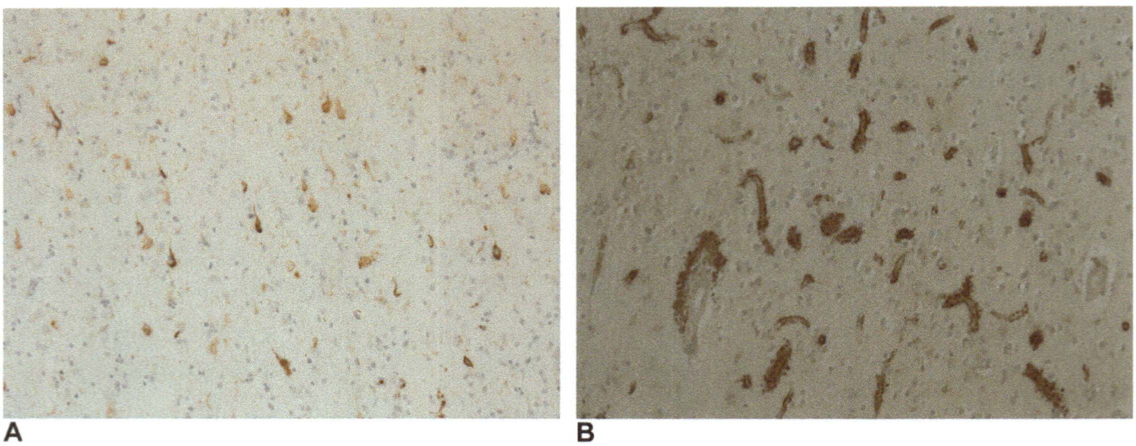

Fig. 14.18. Cerebral cortex from a patient with prion protein cerebral amyloid angiopathy, associated with a Y145X-129M mutation. (A) Tau pathology is shown by immunohistochemistry. Tau deposits are seen in the perikarya of neurons. No spongiform changes are present. (B) Blood vessels with prion protein amyloid angiopathy are shown by immunohistochemistry.

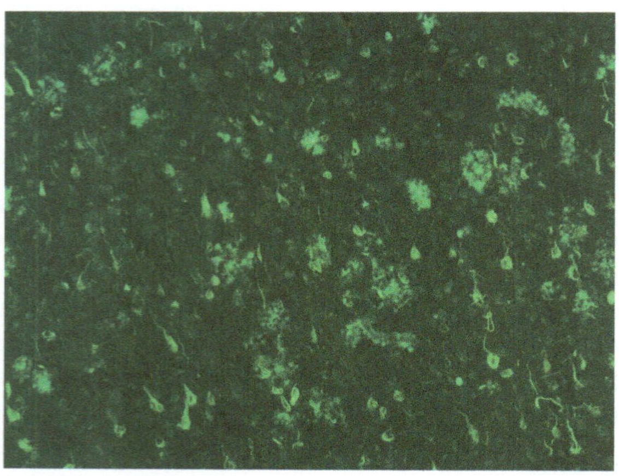

Fig. 14.19. Cerebral cortex from a patient with prion protein cerebral amyloid angiopathy, associated with a Y145X-129M mutation. Fluorescent blood neurofibrillary tangles and blood vessels with amyloid angiopathy are shown using the thioflavin S method.

Biochemistry

The biochemical pattern of PrP^{res} is characterized by a main internal fragment of 8 kDa similar to that reported for other mutations associated with a GSS-like phenotype (Zanusso et al., 2014) (Fig. 14.2).

Q160X-129M

Clinical phenotype

A progressive memory impairment leading to severe dementia, clinically similar to Alzheimer disease or frontotemporal dementia, has been reported in different families. The disease starts in the fourth or fifth decade of life and has an 8-year duration (Jayadev et al., 2011). In addition to the dementia, gastrointestinal symptoms and peripheral neuropathy are caused by PrP deposition outside the central nervous system (Fong et al., 2017).

Neuropathology

Neuropathologic studies in two patients revealed extensive limbic and neocortical tau-immunopositive neurofibrillary tangles and neurites, made of paired helical filaments. The core of the neuritic plaques is immunolabeled with antibodies again PrP. No immunopositive Aβ is present (Jayadev et al., 2011).

Biochemistry

Western blot analysis is characterized by a PK-resistant prominent band of 11 kDa in addition to a smear of higher-molecular-weight bands. The smaller fragments likely derive from mutated allele (Jayadev et al., 2011) (Fig. 14.2).

Y163X-129V

Clinical phenotype

The clinical phenotype is characterized by autonomic failure, predominantly axonal sensory peripheral neuropathy and late-onset cognitive decline. Gastrointestinal symptoms have also been reported (Mead et al., 2013).

Neuropathology

There is extensive parenchymal and vascular PrP deposition with widespread neurofibrillary tangle formation. PrP deposits were noted in the duodenum as well.

Biochemistry

Immunoblot analysis of PK-treated brain homogenates showed a prominent fragment of 10 kDa while additional slower-migrating bands correspond to stable oligomers resistant to detergent solubilization (Mead et al., 2013) (Fig. 14.2).

Y226X-129V

Clinical phenotype

The phenotype is characterized initially by cognitive impairment and aphasia. Myoclonic jerks were noted in the late stages of the disease. MRI showed hyperintensity in the white matter, while EEG revealed periodic synchronous wave complexes. The age at onset was 55 years and the duration was 2½ years (Jansen et al., 2010).

Neuropathology

Neuropathology is characterized by diffuse amyloid angiopathy involving small to medium-sized arteries and arterioles of the cerebral and cerebellar cortex and leptomeninges. Amyloid deposition also involved the capillaries. There were focal tau-immunoreactive dot-like deposits, but neurofibrillary tangles were not present (Jansen et al., 2010).

Biochemistry

The biochemical pattern of PrP^{res} has not been reported.

DOMINANTLY INHERITED PRION PROTEIN CEREBRAL AMYLOIDOSES: VARIABLE PHENOTYPES

Insertional mutations in the octapeptide repeat region

Ins 144bp-120V, Ins 168bp-129M, Ins 192bp-129V, Ins 216bp-129M, and Ins 288bp-120M

Clinical phenotype

The phenotypes associated with the insertional mutations are highly variable; however, individuals with 6–12 additional repeats have a dominantly inherited PrP cerebral amyloidosis, clinically characterized by mental deterioration accompanied by cerebellar and extrapyramidal signs. These individuals often lack the pseudoperiodic sharp-wave complexes on EEG examination and may have prominent psychiatric features. It appears that the age at onset and duration of the disease may be related to the number of inserted repeats. These specific mutations are associated with age at onset in the third to sixth decade of life and a disease duration of 5 months to 13 years (Goldfarb et al., 1992; Duchen et al., 1993; Krasemann et al., 1995; van Gool et al., 1995; Gambetti et al., 1999; Ironside et al., 2008; Kumar et al., 2011; Vital et al., 2011; Head et al., 2015).

Neuropathology

Cerebral and cerebellar atrophy with neuronal loss, gliosis, and spongiform changes have been reported in individuals carrying insertional mutations of 144, 168, 192, 216, and 288 bp. A distinct change is the presence of unicentric and multicentric PrP amyloid plaques as well as PrP diffuse deposits in the cerebral gray matter and in the cerebellum. Tau pathology has been reported in the form of dot-like deposits. In individuals carrying the 288-bp insertion numerous PrP amyloid multicentric plaques were present in the cerebral and cerebellar gray matter. In the neocortex numerous tau-positive neurofibrillary tangles and neuropil threads were present (Gambetti et al., 1999; Ghetti and Gambetti, 1999).

Biochemistry

Western blot analysis of PrP^{res} in 168 bp is characterized by the typical three bands observed in sporadic CJD corresponding to the di-, mono-, and unglycosylated isoforms. However, in 168 bp the unglycosylated PrP^{res} band migrates 2 kDa slower than type 1 PrP^{res}. An additional small PrP^{res} fragment of 8 kDa is observed identical to that found in GSS P102L (Jansen et al., 2011) (Fig. 14.2).

Insertional mutation between codon 129 and 130

Ins 24bp-129V

Clinical phenotype

In the fourth decade of life, cognitive decline and epilepsy are the presenting symptoms (Hinnell et al., 2011). The disease progresses with abnormalities of ocular movements, personality changes, disinhibition, deficit in executive functions, and dysdiadochokinesia. MRI revealed mild diffuse cerebral cortical atrophy and mild cerebellar atrophy.

Neuropathology

Neuropathologically neuronal loss, multicentric plaques, microspongiosis were observed.

Biochemistry

Biochemistry is not known.

Deletion mutation

178del2bp-129M

Clinical phenotype

This deletion results in a premature stop codon mutation at residue 203 (203X) of the PrP (Honda et al., 2016). Clinically, symptoms begin in the third decade of life with autonomic dysfunction, and mild cognitive impairment; gastrointestinal and genitourinary systems are also affected.

Neuropathology

Neuropathology shows PrP deposits adjacent to blood vessels and parenchyma of cerebrum and cerebellum. Neurofibrillary tangles were also present in the neocortex and hippocampus. Multiple peripheral organs had deposits of PrP.

Biochemistry

Western blot analysis after PK treatment showed a prominent fragment of 9 kDa as well as an upper smear of incompletely solubilized tissue (Honda et al., 2016) (Fig. 14.2).

DIFFERENTIAL DIAGNOSIS OF DOMINANTLY INHERITED PRION PROTEIN CEREBRAL AMYLOIDOSES

Clinically, dominantly inherited PrP cerebral amyloidoses may mimic several neurodegenerative diseases, including olivopontocerebellar atrophy, spinocerebellar ataxia, Parkinson disease, progressive supranuclear palsy, amyotrophic lateral sclerosis, Huntington disease, Alzheimer disease, or frontotemporal dementia.

Conventional MRI examination is not diagnostic since the lesion patterns observed in dominantly inherited PrP cerebral amyloidoses are comparable to those seen in other neurodegenerative disorders, such as, for example, a marked atrophy of the cerebral cortex, cerebellar vermis, and hemispheres, and of the brainstem. P105S-129V mutation should be considered in the presence of a hyperintense signal of the caudate and putamen, and of the cerebral cortex in DWI . In addition, MRI in patients with the P102L mutation might show a widespread cerebral cortical hyperintensity, involving caudate nuclei in DWI, as also observed in sporadic CJD, or more rarely, an involvement of bilateral pulvinar, as in variant CJD (Kanata et al., 2008). Cerebrospinal fluid surrogate biomarkers, such as 14.3.3 or tau protein levels, are helpful in determining the rate of disease progression, but are not diagnostic.

Among the most reliable diagnostic tools developed in recent years for prion diseases is the real-time quaking-induced conversion (RT-QuIC) assay. This assay has been highly effective in detecting prion-seeding activity in cerebrospinal fluid and olfactory epithelium of patients with sporadic and genetic CJD. In GSS mutations, CSF had been tested in P102L mutation, showing a positive result in 90% of patients (Sano et al., 2013) and in 50% of olfactory mucosa (OM) samples (Bongianni et al., 2017). RT-QuIC was positive in the cerebrospinal fluid of a single case of D202N mutation and in another with an insertion of eight repeats and negative in a A117V case (Franceschini et al., 2017). However, the number of samples tested is too low to draw any conclusions about test sensitivity. RT-QuIC has been shown to efficiently amplify brain homogenate from A117V, F198S, and H187R mutations by using PrP bank vole as amplification substrate, but no data are available from cerebrospinal fluid or other biologic fluids in patients (Orrù et al., 2015).

For a neuropathologic diagnosis, PrP immunohistochemistry is essential to separate GSS from other nonprion diseases associated with amyloid deposition in the central nervous system. A differential diagnosis between GSS associated with the P102L-129M haplotype and some forms of CJD, including variant CJD, may be difficult if carried out only using PrP immunohistochemistry. As mentioned above, Western blot analysis is essential to differentiate the biochemical pattern of PrP^{res} associated with GSS mutations from the various forms of CJD. When a dominantly inherited PrP cerebral amyloidosis is clinically suspected, molecular genetic analyses are the final step.

PATHOGENESIS OF THE DOMINANTLY INHERITED PRION PROTEIN CEREBRAL AMYLOIDOSES

The pathogenesis of dominantly inherited PrP cerebral amyloidoses remains largely unknown and, in particular, a unique feature is that distinct mutations in *PRNP* cause PrP to acquire an abnormal conformation, resulting in the formation of protease-resistant amino- and carboxy-terminal-truncated PrP peptides that have high fibrillogenic properties. These truncated peptides are mainly composed of mutated PrP, and accumulate extracellularly, leading to the formation of amyloid deposits in brain tissue and/or vessel walls. In vitro studies have shown that synthetic peptides corresponding to the PrP fragments extracted from brain tissue are readily assembled into amyloid fibrils (Tagliavini et al., 1993).

It has been proposed that a PrP pathogenic mechanism is a toxic gain of function secondary to the misfolding of mutated PrP. However, such a mechanism might not apply to all mutant PrP species, since some mutations had little effect on the stability and folding kinetics of PrP (Swietnicki et al., 1998). In P102L, it has been reported that wild-type PrP is also involved in disease propagation, but with a different distribution from that of PrP P102L, explaining the multiple disease phenotypes associated with P102L mutation (Wadsworth et al., 2006).

Patients with dominantly inherited PrP cerebral amyloidoses accumulate PrP, forming deposits with and without amyloid properties. The contribution of both types of deposits to the pathogenesis of these complex diseases remains unknown. To address this issue, Chesebro et al. (2010) developed a mouse model in which, in contrast to normal PrP, the expression of the transgene array results in the formation of a PrP species that is not anchored to the outer cell membrane. Transgenic mice, expressing anchorless PrP inoculated with a mouse-adapted TSE agent, developed an amyloid angiopathy in the absence of spongiform degeneration, a pathology that is highly different from that seen in wild-type mice. Therefore, the topology of PrP appears to modulate the kinetics of PrP deposition as well as the neuropathologic phenotype (Chesebro et al., 2010).

Two *PRNP* mutations associated with GSS variants have been modeled in transgenic mice (Hsiao et al., 1990; Manson et al., 1999; Yang et al., 2009). Overexpression of both PrP P102L and PrP A117V resulted in a neurologic disease in mice characterized histopathologically by variable spongiform degeneration of the brain and PrP-containing amyloid plaques (Hsiao et al., 1990; Yang et al., 2009). In contrast, mice expressing wild-type levels of PrP P102L expressed in "knockin" transgenic mouse model remained disease-free during their normal lifespan (Manson et al., 1999). The data suggest that expression of mutant PrP might not always be associated with infectivity.

To further address this issue, bioassays using brain extracts from two patients with phenotypically different forms of GSS P102L (one with and one without spongiform degeneration) were inoculated into "knockin" transgenic PrP P102L mice. Efficient transmission of a spongiform encephalopathy was seen only using extracts obtained from the patient with spongiform degeneration. Extracts from a patient without spongiform degeneration led to inefficient transmission of disease and the accumulation of PrP amyloid. In conclusion, these experiments suggest that amyloid formation may be caused by PrP misfolding and aggregation in the absence of an infectious TSE agent (Piccardo et al., 2007).

Recently, it has been demonstrated that F198S and A117V mutations associated with an 8-kDa PrP^{Sc} fragment were successfully transmitted to bank voles, inducing a prion disease characterized by a spongiform encephalopathy. These findings indicate that the 8-kDa fragment retains infectivity (Pirisinu et al., 2016).

A distinct neuropathologic finding in many of the dominantly inherited PrP amyloidoses is the presence of tau pathology. When tau coexists with PrP amyloid deposits, neuronal parykaria and neuronal processes, but not glial cells, appear to contain abnormal tau. Tau is present in neurons as neurofibrillary tangles or as a diffuse tau immunopositivity. The currently available data indicate that, in PrP amyloidosis, 3R/4R tau is present, as in Alzheimer disease. The atomic structure of neurofibrillary tangles has been revealed by cryoelectron microscopy in Alzheimer disease (Fitzpatrick et al., 2017). Similar studies are urgently needed to determine whether in PrP amyloidoses 3R/4R tau is consistently present. The pathogenic role of mutated PrP in inducing tau hyperphosphorylation remains unclear.

REFERENCES

Adam J, Crow TJ, Duchen LW et al. (1982). Familial cerebral amyloidosis and spongiform encephalopathy. J Neurol Neurosurg Psychiatry 45: 37–45.

Alzualde A, Indakoetxea B, Ferrer I et al. (2010). A novel PRNP Y218N mutation in Gerstmann–Sträussler–Scheinker disease with neurofibrillary degeneration. J Neuropathol Exp Neurol 69: 789–800.

Azzarelli B, Muller J, Ghetti B et al. (1985). Cerebellar plaques in familial Alzheimer's disease (Gerstmann–Sträussler–Scheinker variant?). Acta Neuropathol 65: 235–246.

Bergstrom AL, Heegaard PM, Dyrbye H et al. (2009). Localization of disease-related PrP in Danish patients with different subtypes of prion disease. Clin Neuropathol 28: 321–332.

Bianca M, Bianca S, Vecchio I et al. (2003). Gerstmann–Sträussler–Scheinker disease with P102L-V129 mutation: a case with psychiatric manifestations at onset. Ann Genet 46: 467–469.

Bongianni M, Orru C, Groveman BR et al. (2017). Diagnosis of human prion disease using real-time quaking-induced conversion testing of olfactory mucosa and cerebrospinal fluid samples. JAMA Neurol 74: 155–162.

Butefisch CM, Gambetti P, Cervenakova L et al. (2000). Inherited prion encephalopathy associated with the novel PRNP H187R mutation: a clinical study. Neurology 55: 517–522.

Cervenakova L, Buetefisch C, Lee HS et al. (1999). Novel PRNP sequence variant associated with familial encephalopathy. Am J Med Genet 88: 653–656.

Chen C, Dong XP (2016). Epidemiological characteristics of human prion diseases. Infect Dis Poverty 5: 47.

Chesebro B, Race B, Meade-White K et al. (2010). Fatal transmissible amyloid encephalopathy: a new type of prion disease associated with lack of prion protein membrane anchoring. PLoS Pathog 6: e1000800.

Chi NF, Lee YC, Lu YC et al. (2010). Transmissible spongiform encephalopathies with P102L mutation of PRNP manifesting different phenotypes: clinical, neuroimaging, and electrophysiological studies in Chinese kindred in Taiwan. J Neurol 257: 191–197.

Collinge J (2001). Prion diseases of humans and animals: their causes and molecular basis. Annu Rev Neurosci 24: 519–550.

Colucci M, Moleres F, Xie Z et al. (2006). Gerstmann–Sträussler–Scheinker: a new phenotype with 'curly' PrP deposits. J Neuropathol Exp Neurol 65: 642–651.

De Michele G, Pocchiari M, Petraroli R et al. (2003). Variable phenotype in a P102L Gerstmann–Sträussler–Scheinker Italian family. Can J Neurol Sci 30: 233–236.

Deters KD, Risacher SL, Yoder KK et al. (2016). [(11)C]PiB PET in Gerstmann–Sträussler–Scheinker disease. Am J Nucl Med Mol Imaging 6: 84–93.

Dimitz L (1913). Bericht des Vereines für Psychiatrie und Neurologie in Wien. Jahrb Psychiatr Neurol 384.

Dlouhy S, Hsiao K, Farlow M et al. (1992). Linkage of the Indiana kindred of Gerstmann–Sträussler–Scheinker disease to the prion protein gene. Nat Genet 1: 64–67.

Duchen L, Poulter M, Harding A (1993). Dementia associated with a 216 base pair insertion in the prion protein gene. Clinical and neuropathological features. Brain 116: 555–567.

Farlow M, Yee R, Dlouhy S et al. (1989). Gerstmann–Sträussler–Scheinker disease. I. Extending the clinical spectrum. Neurology 39: 1446–1452.

Fitzpatrick AWP, Falcon B, He S et al. (2017). Cryo-EM structures of tau filaments from Alzheimer's disease. Nature 547: 185–190.

Fong J, Rojas J, Bang J et al. (2017). Genetic prion disease caused by PRNP Q160X mutation presenting with an orbitofrontal syndrome, cyclic diarrhea, and peripheral neuropathy. J Alzheimers Dis 55: 249–258.

Franceschini A, Baiardi S, Hughson AG et al. (2017). High diagnostic value of second generation CSF RT-QuIC across the wide spectrum of CJD prions. Sci Rep 7: 10655.

Furukawa H, Kitamoto T, Tanaka Y et al. (1995). New variant prion protein in a Japanese family with Gerstmann-Sträussler syndrome. Brain Res Mol Brain Res 30: 385–388.

Gambetti P, Petersen C, Parchi P et al. (1999). Inherited prion diseases. In: SB Prusiner (Ed.), Prion biology and diseases, Cold Spring Harbor Laboratory Press, Cold Spring Harbor, NY.

Gerstmann J (1928). Über ein noch nicht beschriebenes Reflexphanomen bei einer Erkrankung des zerebellaren Systems. Wien Med Wochenschr: 906–908.

Gerstmann J, Sträussler E, Scheinker I (1936). Über eine eigenartige hereditär-familiäre Erkrankung des Zentralnervensystems. Zugleich ein Beitrag zur Frage des vorzeitigen lokalen Alterns Z Gesamt. Neurol Psychiat: 736–762.

Ghetti B, Gambetti P (1999). Human prion diseases. In: M Mattson (Ed.), Advances in cell aging and gerontology, vol. 3: genetic aberrancies and neurodegenerative disorders Greenwich, Jai Press, CT.

Ghetti B, Tagliavini F, Masters C et al. (1988). Gerstmann–Sträussler–Scheinker disease. II. Neurofibrillary tangles and plaques with PrP-amyloid coexist in an affected family. Neurology 38 (Suppl 1): 266.

Ghetti B, Tagliavini F, Masters C et al. (1989). Gerstmann–Sträussler–Scheinker disease. II. Neurofibrillary tangles and plaques with PrP-amyloid coexist in an affected family. Neurology 39: 1453–1461.

Ghetti B, Tagliavini F, Giaccone G et al. (1994). Familial Gerstmann–Sträussler–Scheinker disease with neurofibrillary tangles. Mol Neurobiol 8: 41–48.

Ghetti B, Dlouhy SR, Giaccone G et al. (1995). Gerstmann–Sträussler–Scheinker disease and the Indiana kindred. Brain Pathol 5: 61–75.

Ghetti B, Piccardo P, Frangione B et al. (1996a). Prion protein amyloidosis. Brain Pathol 6: 127–145.

Ghetti B, Piccardo P, Spillantini M et al. (1996b). Vascular variant of prion protein cerebral amyloidosis with tau-positive neurofibrillary tangles: the phenotype of the stop codon 145 mutation in PRNP. Proc Natl Acad Sci U S A 93: 744–748.

Ghetti B, Tagliavini F, Kovacs G et al. (2011). Gerstmann Sträussler Scheinker disease. In: D Dickson, R Weller (Eds.), Neurodegneration: the molecular pathology of dementia and movement disorders, 2nd edn, Blackwell Publishing, Hoboken, NJ.

Goldfarb L, Brown P, McCombie W et al. (1991). Transmissible familial Creutzfeldt-Jakob disease associated with five, seven, and eight extra octapeptide coding repeats in the PRNP gene. Proc Natl Acad Sci U S A 88: 10926–10930.

Goldfarb LG, Brown P, Vrbovska A et al. (1992). An insert mutation in the chromosome 20 amyloid precursor gene in a Gerstmann–Sträussler–Scheinker family. J Neurol Sci 111: 189–194.

Goldhammer Y, Gabizon R, Meiner Z et al. (1993). An Israeli family with Gerstmann–Sträussler–Scheinker disease manifesting the codon 102 mutation in the prion protein gene. Neurology 43: 2718–2719.

Hainfellner JA, Brantner-Inthaler S, Cervenakova L et al. (1995). The original Gerstmann–Sträussler–Scheinker family of Austria: divergent clinicopathological phenotypes but constant PrP genotype. Brain Pathol 5: 201–211.

Hall DA, Leehey MA, Filley CM et al. (2005). PRNP H187R mutation associated with neuropsychiatric disorders in childhood and dementia. Neurology 64: 1304–1306.

Head M, Ironside J, Ghetti B et al. (2015). Prion diseases. In: J Ironside. A Perry (Eds.), Greenfield's neuropathology, 9th edn, CRC Press, Taylor & Francis Group, Boca Raton.

Hilton D, Head M, Singh V et al. (2009). Familial prion disease with a novel serine to isoleucine mutation at codon 132 of prion protein gene (PRNP). Neuropathol Appl Neurobiol 35: 111–115.

Hinnell C, Coulthart MB, Jansen GH et al. (2011). Gerstmann–Sträussler–Scheinker disease due to a novel prion protein gene mutation. Neurology 76: 485–487.

Honda H, Matsuzono K, Fushimi S et al. (2016). C-terminal-deleted prion protein fragment is a major accumulated component of systemic PrP deposits in hereditary prion disease with a 2-Bp (CT) deletion in PRNP codon 178. J Neuropathol Exp Neurol 75: 1008–1019.

Hsiao K, Baker H, Crow T et al. (1989). Linkage of a prion protein missense variant to Gerstmann-Sträussler syndrome. Nature 338: 342–345.

Hsiao K, Scott M, Foster D et al. (1990). Spontaneous neurodegeneration in transgenic mice with mutant prion protein. Science 250: 1587–1590.

Hsiao K, Dlouhy S, Farlow M et al. (1992). Mutant prion proteins in Gerstmann–Sträussler–Scheinker disease with neurofibrillary tangles. Nat Genet 1: 68–71.

Hudson AJ, Farrell MA, Kalnins R et al. (1983). Gerstmann–Sträussler–Scheinker disease with coincidental familial onset. Ann Neurol 14: 670–678.

Ironside J, Ghetti B, Head MW et al. (2008). Prion diseases. In: S Love, D Louis, D Ellison (Eds.), Greenfield's neuropathology, 8th edn. Hodder (Arnold), London.

Iwasaki Y, Kizawa M, Hori N et al. (2009). A case of Gerstmann–Sträussler–Scheinker syndrome with the P105L prion protein gene mutation presenting with ataxia and extrapyramidal signs without spastic paraparesis. Clin Neurol Neurosurg 111: 606–609.

Jansen C, Parchi P, Capellari S et al. (2010). Prion protein amyloidosis with divergent phenotype associated with two novel nonsense mutations in PRNP. Acta Neuropathol 119: 189–197.

Jansen C, Voet W, Head M et al. (2011). A novel seven-octapeptide repeat insertion in the prion protein gene (PRNP) in a Dutch pedigree with Gerstmann–Sträussler–Scheinker disease phenotype: comparison with similar cases from the literature. Acta Neuropathol 121: 59–68.

Jayadev S, Nochlin D, Poorkaj P et al. (2011). Familial prion disease with Alzheimer disease-like tau pathology and clinical phenotype. Ann Neurol 69: 712–720.

Jones M, Odunsi S, du Plessis D et al. (2014). Gerstmann–Sträussler–Scheinker disease: novel PRNP mutation and VGKC-complex antibodies. Neurology 82: 2107–2111.

Kanata A, Saigoh K, Mitsui Y et al. (2008). Case of Gerstmann–Sträussler–Scheinker syndrome (GSS-P102L) mimicking variant Creuzfeld-Jakob disease in clinical manifestation and MRI findings. Rinsho Shinkeigaku 48: 179–183.

Kepe V, Ghetti B, Farlow M et al. (2010). PET of brain prion protein amyloid in Gerstmann–Sträussler–Scheinker disease. Brain Pathol 20: 419–430.

Kim M, Takada L, Wong K et al. (2017). Genetic PrP prion diseases. In: Cold Spring Harb Perspect Bio, pii: a033134. doi: 110.1101/cshperspect.a033134.

Kitamoto T, Ogomori K, Tateishi J et al. (1987). Formic acid pretreatment enhances immunostaining of cerebral and systemic amyloids. Lab Investig 57: 230–236.

Kitamoto T, Amano N, Terao Y et al. (1993). A new inherited prion disease (PrP-P105L mutation) showing spastic paraparesis. Ann Neurol 34: 808–813.

Kojovic M, Glavac D, Ozek B et al. (2011). De novo P102L mutation in a patient with Gerstmann–Sträussler–Scheinker disease. Eur J Neurol 18: e152–e153.

Krasemann S, Zerr I, Weber T et al. (1995). Prion disease associated with a novel nine octapeptide repeat insertion in the PRNP gene. Brain Res Mol Brain Res 34: 173–176.

Kretzschmar H, Honold G, Seitelberger F et al. (1991). Prion protein mutation in family first reported by Gerstmann, Sträussler, and Scheinker. Lancet 337: 1160.

Kumar N, Boeve B, Boot B et al. (2011). Clinical characterization of a kindred with a novel 12-octapeptide repeat insertion in the prion protein gene. Arch Neurol 68: 1165–1170.

Laplanche J, Hachimi K, Durieux I et al. (1999). Prominent psychiatric features and early onset in an inherited prion disease with a new insertional mutation in the prion protein gene. Brain 122: 2375–2386.

Liberski P, Bratosiewicz J, Barcikowska M et al. (2000). A case of sporadic Creutzfeldt-Jakob disease with a Gerstmann–Sträussler–Scheinker phenotype but no alterations in the PRNP gene. Acta Neuropathol 100: 233–234.

Majtenyi C, Brown P, Cervenakova L et al. (2000). A three-sister sibship of Gerstmann–Sträussler–Scheinker disease with a CJD phenotype. Neurology 54: 2133–2137.

Mallucci G, Campbell T, Dickinson A et al. (1999). Inherited prion disease with an alanine to valine mutation at codon 117 in the prion protein gene. Brain 122: 1823–1837.

Manson J, Jamieson E, Baybutt H et al. (1999). A single amino acid alteration (101L) introduced into murine PrP dramatically alters incubation time of transmissible spongiform encephalopathy. EMBO J 18: 6855–6864.

Masters C, Gajdusek D, Gibbs CJ (1981). Creutzfeldt-Jakob disease virus isolations from the Gerstmann-Sträussler syndrome with an analysis of the various forms of amyloid plaque deposition in the virus-induced spongiform encephalopathies. Brain 104: 559–588.

Mastrianni JA, Curtis MT, Oberholtzer JC et al. (1995). Prion disease (PrP-A117V) presenting with ataxia instead of dementia. Neurology 45: 2042–2050.

Mead S, Gandhi S, Beck J et al. (2013). A novel prion disease associated with diarrhea and autonomic neuropathy. N Engl J Med 369: 1904–1914.

Nochlin D, Sumi S, Bird T et al. (1989). Familial dementia with PrP-positive amyloid plaques: a variant of Gerstmann-Sträussler syndrome. Neurology 39: 910–918.

Orrù CD, Groveman BR, Raymond LD et al. (2015). Bank Vole Prion Protein As an Apparently Universal Substrate for RT-QuIC-Based Detection and Discrimination of Prion Strains. PLoS Pathog 11: e1004983.

Panegyres P, Toufexis K, Kakulas B et al. (2001). A new PRNP mutation (G131V) associated with Gerstmann–Sträussler–Scheinker disease. Arch Neurol 58: 1899–1902.

Parchi P, Chen S, Brown P et al. (1998). Different patterns of truncated prion protein fragments correlate with distinct phenotypes in P102L Gerstmann–Sträussler–Scheinker disease. Proc Natl Acad Sci U S A 95: 8322–8327.

Park MJ, Jo HY, Cheon SM et al. (2010). A case of Gerstmann–Sträussler–Scheinker disease. J Clin Neurol 6: 46–50.

Peoc'h K, Levavasseur E, Delmont E et al. (2012). Substitutions at residue 211 in the prion protein drive a switch between CJD and GSS syndrome, a new mechanism governing inherited neurodegenerative disorders. Hum Mol Genet 21: 5417–5428.

Piccardo P, Seiler C, Dlouhy S et al. (1996). Proteinase-K-resistant prion protein isoforms in Gerstmann–Sträussler–Scheinker disease (Indiana kindred). J Neuropathol Exp Neurol 55: 1157–1163.

Piccardo P, Dlouhy S, Lievens P et al. (1998). Phenotypic variability of Gerstmann–Sträussler–Scheinker disease is associated with prion protein heterogeneity. J Neuropathol Exp Neurol 57: 979–988.

Piccardo P, Manson J, King D et al. (2007). Accumulation of prion protein in the brain that is not associated with transmissible disease. Proc Natl Acad Sci U S A 104: 4712–4717.

Pirisinu L, Di Bari MA, D'Agostino C et al. (2016). Gerstmann–Sträussler–Scheinker disease subtypes efficiently transmit in bank voles as genuine prion diseases. Sci Rep 6: 20443.

Polymenidou M, Prokop S, Jung HH et al. (2011). Atypical prion protein conformation in familial prion disease with PRNP P105T mutation. Brain Pathol 21: 209–214.

Prusiner S (1999). An introduction to prion biology and diseases. In: SB Prusiner (Ed.), Prion biology and diseases, Cold Spring Harbor Laboratory Press, Cold Spring Harbor, NY.

Risacher S, Farlow M, Bateman D et al. (2018). Detection of tau in Gerstmann-Sträussler-Scheinker disease (PRNP F198S) by [18F]Flortaucipir PET. Acta Neuropathol Commun (in press).

Riudavets MA, Sraka MA, Schultz M et al. (2014). Gerstmann–Sträussler–Scheinker syndrome with variable phenotype in a new kindred with PRNP-P102L mutation. Brain Pathol 24: 142–147.

Rogaeva E, Zadikoff C, Ponesse J et al. (2006). Childhood onset in familial prion disease with a novel mutation in the PRNP gene. Arch Neurol 63: 1016–1021.

Rowe D, Lewis V, Needham M et al. (2007). Novel prion protein gene mutation presenting with subacute PSP-like syndrome. Neurology 68: 868–870.

Saenz-Farret M, Ramirez-Gomez CC, Araoz-Olivos N et al. (2016). Gerstmann–Sträussler–Scheinker syndrome in an Argentinean family due to mutationat codon 117 of the prion protein gene (PrPA117V). J Neurol Sci 364: 50–52.

Sano K, Satoh K, Atarashi R et al. (2013). Early detection of abnormal prion protein in genetic human prion diseases now possible using real-time QUIC assay. PLoS One 8: e54915.

Schlote W, Boellaard JW, Schumm F et al. (1980). Gerstmann–Sträussler–Scheinker's disease. Electron-microscopic observations on a brain biopsy. Acta Neuropathol 52: 203–211.

Schmitz M, Dittmar K, Llorens F et al. (2017). Hereditary human prion diseases: an update. Mol Neurobiol 54: 4138–4149.

Seitelberger F (1962). Unusual familial-hereditary disease of the central nervous system in a Lower Austrian family (with a contribution to comparative neuropathology of kuru). Wien Klin Wochenschr 74: 687–691.

Seitelberger F (1981). Sträussler's disease. Acta Neuropathol Suppl 7: 341–343.

Simpson M, Johanssen V, Boyd A et al. (2013). Unusual clinical and molecular-pathological profile of Gerstmann–Sträussler–Scheinker disease associated with a novel PRNP mutation (V176G). JAMA Neurol 70: 1180–1185.

Smid J, Studart A, Landemberger M et al. (2017). High phenotypic variability in Gerstmann–Sträussler–Scheinker disease. Arq Neuropsiquiatr 75: 331–338.

Swietnicki W, Petersen R, Gambetti P et al. (1998). Familial mutations and the thermodynamic stability of the recombinant human prion protein. J Biol Chem 273: 31048–31052.

Tagliavini F, Prelli F, Ghiso J et al. (1991). Amyloid protein of Gerstmann–Sträussler–Scheinker disease (Indiana kindred) is an 11 kd fragment of prion protein with an N-terminal glycine at codon 58. EMBO J 10: 513–519.

Tagliavini F, Prelli F, Verga L et al. (1993). Synthetic peptides homologous to prion protein residues 106-147 form amyloid-like fibrils in vitro. Proc Natl Acad Sci U S A 90: 9678–9682.

Tagliavini F, Prelli F, Porro M et al. (1994). Amyloid fibrils in Gerstmann–Sträussler–Scheinker disease (Indiana and Swedish kindreds) express only PrP peptides encoded by the mutant allele. Cell 79: 695–703.

Tagliavini F, Lievens P, Tranchant C et al. (2001). A 7-kDa prion protein (PrP) fragment, an integral component of the PrP region required for infectivity, is the major amyloid protein in Gerstmann–Sträussler–Scheinker disease A117V. J Biol Chem 276: 6009–6015.

Takada LT, Kim MO, Cleveland RW et al. (2017). Genetic prion disease: experience of a rapidly progressive dementia center in the United States and a review of the literature. Am J Med Genet B Neuropsychiatr Genet 174: 36–69.

Tranchant C, Doh-ura K, Warter J et al. (1992). Gerstmann–Sträussler–Scheinker disease in an Alsatian family: clinical and genetic studies. J Neurol Neurosurg Psychiatry 55: 185–187.

Tunnell E, Wollman R, Mallik S et al. (2008). A novel PRNP-P105S mutation associated with atypical prion disease and a rare PrPSc conformation. Neurology 71: 1431–1438.

Unverzagt FW, Farlow MR, Norton J et al. (1997). Neuropsychological function in patients with Gerstmann–Sträussler–Scheinker disease from the Indiana kindred (F198S). J Int Neuropsychol Soc 3: 169–178.

van Gool WA, Hensels GW, Hoogerwaard EM et al. (1995). Hypokinesia and presenile dementia in a Dutch family with a novel insertion in the prion protein gene. Brain 118: 1565–1571.

Vital A, Laplanche JL, Bastard JR et al. (2011). A case of Gerstmann–Sträussler–Scheinker disease with a novel six octapeptide repeat insertion. Neuropathol Appl Neurobiol 37: 554–559.

Vitali P, Maccagnano E, Caverzasi E et al. (2011). Diffusion-weighted MRI hyperintensity patterns differentiate CJD from other rapid dementias. Neurology 76: 1711–1719.

Von Braunmühl A (1954). [An unusual hereditary familial disease of the central nervous system.]. Arch Psychiatr Nervenkr Z Gesamte Neurol Psychiatr 191: 419–449.

Wadsworth JD, Joiner S, Linehan JM et al. (2006). Phenotypic heterogeneity in inherited prion disease (P102L) is associated with differential propagation of protease-resistant wild-type and mutant prion protein. Brain 129: 1557–1569.

Wang Y, Qiao XY, Zhao CB et al. (2006). Report on the first Chinese family with Gerstmann–Sträussler–Scheinker disease manifesting the codon 102 mutation in the prion protein gene. Neuropathology 26: 429–432.

Webb T, Poulter M, Beck J et al. (2008). Phenotypic heterogeneity and genetic modification of P102L inherited prion disease in an international series. Brain 131: 2632–2646.

Windl O, Giese A, Schulz-Schaeffer W et al. (1999). Molecular genetics of human prion diseases in Germany. Hum Genet 105: 244–252.

Yamada M, Itoh Y, Inaba A et al. (1999). An inherited prion disease with a PrP P105L mutation: clinicopathologic and PrP heterogeneity. Neurology 53: 181–188.

Yang W, Cook J, Rassbach B et al. (2009). A new transgenic mouse model of Gerstmann–Sträussler–Scheinker syndrome caused by the A117V mutation of PRNP. J Neurosci 29: 10072–10080.

Young K, Clark H, Piccardo P et al. (1997). Gerstmann–Sträussler–Scheinker disease with the PRNP P102L mutation and valine at codon 129. Brain Res Mol Brain Res 44: 147–150.

Zanusso G, Fiorini M, Ferrari S et al. (2014). Gerstmann–Sträussler–Scheinker disease and "anchorless prion protein" mice share prion conformational properties diverging from sporadic Creutzfeldt-Jakob disease. J Biol Chem 289: 4870–4881.

Zimowski J, Kulczycki J, Lojkowska W et al. (2012). Hereditary form of prion disease in Poland. Neurol Neurochir Pol 46: 509–518.

Handbook of Clinical Neurology, Vol. 153 (3rd series)
Human Prion Diseases
M. Pocchiari and J. Manson, Editors
https://doi.org/10.1016/B978-0-444-63945-5.00015-5

Chapter 15

Fatal familial insomnia and sporadic fatal insomnia

LAURA CRACCO[1], BRIAN S. APPLEBY[2,3,4], AND PIERLUIGI GAMBETTI[1,*,†]
[1]*Department of Pathology, Case Western Reserve University, Cleveland, OH, United States*
[2]*National Prion Disease Pathology Surveillance Center, Case Western Reserve University, Cleveland, OH, United States*
[3]*Department of Neurology, Case Western Reserve University, Cleveland, OH, United States*
[4]*Department of Psychiatry, Case Western Reserve University, Cleveland, OH, United States*

Abstract

Fatal familial insomnia (FFI) and sporadic fatal insomnia (sFI), or thalamic form of sporadic Creutzfeldt–Jakob disease MM2 (sCJDMM2T), are prion diseases originally named and characterized in 1992 and 1999, respectively. FFI is genetically determined and linked to a D178N mutation coupled with the M129 genotype in the prion protein gene (*PRNP*) at chromosome 20. sFI is a phenocopy of FFI and likely its sporadic form. Both diseases are primarily characterized by progressive sleep impairment, disturbances of autonomic nervous system, and motor signs associated with severe loss of nerve cells in medial thalamic nuclei. Both diseases harbor an abnormal disease-associated prion protein isoform, resistant to proteases with relative mass of 19 kDa identified as resPrP^{TSE} type 2. To date at least 70 kindreds affected by FFI with 198 members and 18 unrelated carriers along with 25 typical cases of sFI have been published. The D178N-129M mutation is thought to cause FFI by destabilizing the mutated prion protein and facilitating its conversion to PrP^{TSE}. The thalamus is the brain region first affected. A similar mechanism triggered spontaneously may underlie sFI.

FATAL FAMILIAL INSOMNIA

History

Severe thalamic atrophy as a distinct clinical and pathologic entity has been reported from at least 1939 (Stern, 1939). In his review *Jakob-Creutzfeldt Disease* in 1968, Kirschbaum introduced the *thalamic* subgroup comprising five previously published cases (Stern, 1939; Poursines et al., 1953; Schulman, 1956; Garcin et al., 1962, 1963; McMenemey et al., 1965). In 1975 and 1983, Martin and colleagues proposed a classification of *Thalamic degenerations or Thalamic dementias* in three groups according to whether the thalamic degeneration is: (1) associated with minimal or no extrathalamic pathology; (2) a component of *multiple system atrophy*; or (3) associated with significant amounts of gliosis and spongiform degeneration in the cerebral cortex and, therefore, belonging to the group of transmissible spongiform encephalopathies or prion diseases (Martin, 1975; Martin et al., 1983; see Manetto et al., 1992; Petersen et al., 1992; Parchi et al., 1999a for review).

In 1986, Lugaresi et al. reported in detail and named *Fatal Familial Insomnia* (FFI), an inherited condition characterized by severe and progressive sleep impairment, dysautonomia, and motor signs associated with severe atrophy of the anterior and medial dorsal thalamic nuclei. The proband, a 53-year-old man, experienced a progressive reduction of nocturnal sleep associated with progressive dysfunction of the autonomic system with pyrexia, diaphoresis, and sphincter dysfunction over several months. Nocturnal sleep became disturbed by increasing movements and enacted dreams. Motor signs

†"To Professor Elio Lugaresi, the mentor who critically shaped my early professional life, the collaborator who initiated all this work and a precious friend throughout" Pierluigi.

*Correspondence to: Dr. Pierluigi Gambetti, Case Western Reserve University, Institute of Pathology, 2085 Adelbert Road, 4th floor, room 419, Cleveland OH 44106, United States. E-mail: pxg13@case.edu

with tremor, dysarthria, clumsy gait, and myoclonus became more pronounced and memory deficit ensued. The patient progressed into stupor, became comatose, and expired 9 months after clinical onset.

Electroencephalographic (EEG) and polysomnographic (PSG) studies revealed that wakefulness alternated with periods of desynchronization of electric activity with features of the abnormal rapid eye movement (REM) stage, which corresponded to the dreaming episodes. Physiologic EEG patterns of sleep, like spindles, K complexes, and delta activity, were not observed, nor were periodic or pseudoperiodic slow-wave activities characteristic of Creutzfeldt–Jakob disease (CJD) seen. Neurovegetative tests were consistent with autonomic failure, while the assessment of the neuroendocrine system revealed that, although capable of responding to stimuli, it failed to maintain normal hormone levels, which were low and showed no circadian rhythms. No cognitive impairment was revealed in neuropsychologic testing, even 7 months after disease onset. The patient did not respond to various pharmacologic attempts to improve his sleep disorder. Remarkably, while the barbiturate Pentothal and diazepam, a benzodiazepine, had no effect, the benzodiazepine receptor antagonist flumazenil could reverse the stupor state of the patient and establish a better-organized EEG background activity, albeit temporarily (Whitwam and Amrein, 1995). Clinical and EEG findings obtained from the proband were confirmed in four affected relatives.

Neuropathologic examination carried out on the proband and one of his sisters revealed 80–96% loss of large neurons in the anterior and medial dorsal thalamic nuclei with reactive astrogliosis. Possible atrophy was also noted in the inferior olivary nucleus. No spongiform degeneration nor other significant lesions were detected (Lugaresi et al., 1986).

In the same year as Lugaresi and colleagues, Little and coworkers (1986) reported a kindred malady under the label of *Familial myoclonic dementia masquerading as Creutzfeldt-Jakob disease*, also characterized by a thalamic pathology very similar to that described by Lugaresi et al. and lacking significant spongiform degeneration. Although several patients had cognitive impairment and motor signs, 6 of the 7 patients examined also had either somnolence or insomnia. The failure to demonstrate the presence of abnormal, disease-related prion protein (PrP^{TSE}) in tissue and to transmit the disease to primates, along with the lack of spongiform degeneration and of EEG signs, led to the exclusion of the diagnosis of familial CJD (fCJD) and to the addition of this kindred to the group of *thalamic dementias* (Martin, 1975; see Kong et al., 2004, for review).

The study of additional cases from the original kindred published by Lugaresi and coworkers, which had longer disease durations, revealed the presence of foci of typical spongiform degeneration. This observation led to the demonstration in 1992 that FFI is linked to the substitution of the 178 aspartic acid for asparagine (D178N mutation) in the PrP gene and it harbors PrP^{TSE}. These findings conclusively established FFI as a new phenotype in familial human prion diseases (Manetto et al., 1992; Medori et al., 1992b).

Concomitantly, a study from another group reported linkage of the D178N mutation to a CJD-like phenotype ($fCJD^{D178N}$) (Goldfarb et al., 1991, 1992a; Brown et al., 1992). This finding, that implied the linkage of the D178N mutation to two distinct phenotypes, FFI and CJD, stimulated a second genetic study. Analyses of several FFI and CJD-like affected families demonstrated that the methionine (M)-valine (V) polymorphism, a common feature of codon 129 of the human PrP gene, was the switch that determined the two phenotypes linked to the D178N mutation. Thus, the coupling of the D178N mutated codon with codon 129M results in FFI, while the CJD phenotype requires coupling with codon 129V (Goldfarb et al., 1992b). Furthermore, the obligated presence of codons 129M and 129V on the mutated alleles in FFI and $fCJD^{D178N}$, respectively, combined with the presence of either 129M or 129V in normal alleles resulted in the presence of two genetically distinct subsets of patients in both diseases: the 129MM and 129VV homozygotes in FFI and $fCJD^{D178N}$, respectively, and the 129MV heterozygotes in both diseases (Goldfarb et al., 1992b). It was shown that duration of the clinical disease, as well as other clinical and histopathologic features, differs between homozygous and heterozygous patient populations in FFI (Goldfarb et al., 1992b; Parchi et al., 1995; Gambetti et al., 2003a, b; Pocchiari et al., 2004; Cortelli et al., 2014; Krasnianski et al., 2014; Llorens et al., 2017).

Definition

FFI is a genetically determined prion disease linked to the D178N pathogenic mutation coupled with the polymorphic M codon at position 129 (Goldfarb et al., 1992b; Medori et al., 1992b). FFI typically presents between the ages of 40 and 60 and has a variable duration of several months to a few years. Decreased and disturbed sleep with somnolence, demonstrated either clinically or via sleep studies, and dysfunction of the autonomic system, later accompanied by motor and eventually cognitive signs, are typical clinical features. The thalamus appears to be the earliest and most severely affected brain structure, since it shows decreased metabolism by positron emission tomography (PET) even in the preclinical stage, and severe atrophy is invariably observed at autopsy examination. Clinical and histopathologic features may vary between 129 homozygous (MM) and heterozygous (MV) patients. No treatment is currently available.

Epidemiology

To date, at least 70 kindreds, 18 unrelated carriers with no available pedigree, and 198 kindred members are known to carry the D178N-129M allele linked to FFI worldwide (Table 15.1). Overall, considering also the unrelated carriers as kindreds, 26 kindreds were reported in China, 16 in Germany, 12 in Spain, eight in Italy, six in France, five in the United States, three in Japan and Australia, and two in the United Kingdom and South Korea. Austria related one kindred, as well as Brazil, Canada, Macedonia, and the Netherlands. These data seem to indicate that, considering their population size, Germany and Spain have the highest prevalence of FFI.

It is noteworthy that a 2004 review (Kong et al., 2004) reported 24 kindreds of FFI and six unrelated carriers for a total of 57 individuals which originated from 10 countries. Fourteen years later the number of FFI kindreds and unrelated carriers has almost tripled and the countries of origin of these cases have risen to 15. The relatively high prevalence of FFI in countries such as Germany and Spain along with the finding that over half of the FFI kindreds worldwide reside in Western Europe raise the issue of the mutational events leading to this relatively high prevalence of FFI. Two studies address this issue. In a study of 38 FFI subjects from Spain, Germany, and Italy, Rodríguez-Martínez and colleagues (2008) detected two independent mutational events shared by all the subjects. In contrast, in two other studies Dagvadorj et al. (2002) and Lee and Goldfarb (2008), upon analyses of subjects belonging to 13 FFI and $fCJD^{D178N}$ families, and two unrelated D178N-129V carriers from several European countries, Canada and the United States, reported that the D178N mutation originated independently in each kindred and unrelated carrier examined.

Clinical features

Demographics

FFI typically presents between the fourth and sixth decade of life, most often between the ages of 51 and 60 years (Table 15.2) (Pocchiari et al., 2004; Sikorska and Liberski, 2012). Although PrP codon 129 genotype has not been shown to affect age at disease onset (Gambetti et al., 2003a), it influences survival time, which overall typically is slightly longer than 1 year, ranging from 8 to 72 months with a mean duration of 15.6 ± 2.2 months (Pocchiari et al., 2004; Sikorska and Liberski, 2012). However, in 129MM homozygous patients disease duration is shorter (mean = 11 ± 4 months) compared to 129MV heterozygotes (mean = 23 ± 19 months) (Gambetti et al., 2003a). The reported shorter survival times in China and Japan (8.2 and 10.6 months respectively) compared to Western countries, despite greater utilization of life-prolonging care, are likely to be related to the prevalence of the 129MM genotype in Asian countries (Gao et al., 2011; Nagoshi et al., 2011; Chen et al., 2013).

Signs and symptoms

The clinical presentation of FFI is also affected by the PrP genotype at the polymorphic codon 129 (Table 15.3). In 129 homozygotes, the earliest symptoms are usually sleep and vegetative disturbances, compared to heterozygotes that typically also show visual symptoms and ataxia (Krasnianski et al., 2014). Throughout the disease course homozygotes tend to have more prominent insomnia, myoclonus, autonomic dysfunction, spatial disorientation, hallucinations, and weight loss (Gambetti et al., 2003a; Krasnianski et al., 2014) while heterozygotes are more likely to demonstrate ataxia, dysarthria, seizures, and bulbar symptoms. Even gait characteristics appear to be affected by codon 129 genotype since homozygotes demonstrate a cautious gait with difficulties in turning and tandem gait whereas heterozygotes experience worsening of equilibrium with latero/retropulsion (Cortelli et al., 2014).

Overall, the clinical phenomenology of FFI can be divided into three categories: (1) sleep disorder; (2) autonomic symptoms; and (3) classic prion disease symptoms. Disruption of sleep is generally an early symptom, especially in 129MM patients, and often includes progressive reduction of sleep time and quality of sleep with relative preservation of light or low-stage sleep (Guaraldi et al., 2011; Sikorska and Liberski, 2012). Severe and persistent insomnia is associated with motor overactivation, and sympathetic activation that results in episodes of dream enactment that often consist of stereotyped movements of daily activities that can be recalled upon awakening. These episodes, which have been defined as agrypnia excitata with oneiric stupor, are longer and nearly continuous compared to other REM sleep behavior disorders, which are generally shorter and episodic. Importantly, symptoms related to sleep must be elicited as they may not be reported spontaneously by the patient and/or family.

Autonomic symptoms are a classic finding of FFI and include hypertension, tachycardia, hyperhidrosis, hyperpyrexia, impotence, lacrimation, and salivation (Gambetti et al., 2003a; Sikorska and Liberski, 2012). Psychiatric symptoms are common (87% of patients) in FFI and may also be due to autonomic dysfunction given persistent elevated plasma catecholamine and cortisol

Table 15.1

Published fatal familial insomnia (FFI) kindreds, confirmed members, and unrelated carriers, listed by country of residence

Publication[a]	Kindred[b]	Members[c]	Country
Silburn et al. (1996)[d]	1	8	Australia
McLean et al. (1997)[d]	1	≥4	
Chang et al. (2011)[e]	1	1	
Almer et al. (1999)	1	4	Austria
Pedroso et al. (2013)[f]	1	1	Brazil
Spacey et al. (2004)[g]	1	2	Canada
Yu et al. (2007)	1	9	China
Shi et al. (2010)	1	11	
Zhang et al. (2010)	1	2	
Shi et al. (2012)	6 (2)	10	
Peng et al. (2015)	1	2	
Sun et al. (2015)	1	1	
Lu et al. (2017)	1	3	
Wu et al. (2017)	3 (1)	7	
Sun et al. (2017)	1	2	
Chen et al. (2018)	4 (3)	≥6	
Julien et al. (1990)	1	≥5	France
Colombier et al. (1997)	1	2	
Marcaud et al. (2003)	1	1	
Dauvilliers et al. (2004)	1	1	
Dimitri et al. (2006)	(1)	0	
Haïk et al. (2008)	1	1	
Kretzschmar et al. (1998)	4 (4)	4	Germany
Harder et al. (1999)[h]	1	≥9	
Bär et al. (2002)	(1)	0	
Wermke et al. (2006)	1	1	
Thomas et al. (2006)	(1)	0	
Friedrich et al. (2008)	(1)	0	
Synofzik et al. (2009)	1	2	
Froböse et al. (2012)	1	1	
Rupprecht et al. (2013)	1	1	
Lugaresi et al. (1986)[i]	1	≥35	Italy
Medori et al. (1992a)[i]	1	2	
Parchi et al. (1995)[i]	(1)	0	
Cortelli et al. (1997)[i]	1	1	
Padovani et al. (1998)	1	2	
Rossi et al. (1998)	1	1	
Raggi et al. (2009)	1	1	
Baldin et al. (2009)[j,k]	1	1	
Nagayama et al. (1996)	(1)	0	Japan
Taniwaki et al. (2000)	1	2	
Saitoh et al. (2010)	1	2	
Guerreiro et al. (2009)	1	1	Macedonia
Choi et al. (2009)	(1)	0	South Korea
Lee et al. (2014)	1	3	
Tabernero et al. (2000)	1	2	Spain
Zarranz et al. (2005a)	≥7	≥14	
Gistau et al. (2006)	1	2	
Iriarte et al. (2007)	1	2	
Oliveros et al. (2009)	(1)	0	
Casas-Mendez et al. (2011)	1	3	
Jansen et al. (2011)[l]	1	1	Netherlands
Will et al. (1998)	2	2	United Kingdom
Little et al. (1986)[m]	1	≥7	United States
Petersen et al. (1992)[m]	1	2	

Table 15.1

Continued

Publication[a]	Kindred[b]	Members[c]	Country
Bosque et al. (1992)[k]	1	3	
Brown et al. (1998)[m]	1	≥3	
Schenkein and Montagna (2006)	1	5	

[a]For practical reasons only the first detailed description of the kindred is reported.
[b]In parentheses mutation carrier with no FFI pedigree (unrelated carrier).
[c]Kindred members with confirmed D178N-129M mutation and/or neuropathologic features of FFI.
[d]Irish–Danish and Irish descent, respectively.
[e]Immigrated from Vietnam.
[f]Portuguese descent.
[g]Chinese descent.
[h]Kindred comprised of three branches identified as A, B, C with ≥3, ≥5, and 1 subjects, respectively.
[i]FFI-1 (with French members, (Rancurel et al., 1994)), FFI-2, FFI-10, FFI-3, respectively.
[j]Immigrated from Morocco.
[k]D178N allele with 24-bp deletion.
[l]Immigrated from Egypt.
[m]British, German, and English descent, respectively.
Table generated from retrievable data including publications and personal communications with authors.

Table 15.2

Clinical characteristics of fatal familial insomnia

Age at onset (years)	Mean = 46 (range 18–74)
Disease duration (months)	Mean = 16 (range 8–72)
Common symptoms	Sleep disturbance, disorientation, cognitive impairment, weight loss, ataxia, autonomic symptoms, visual disturbances
Polysomnogram	Reduction in sleep spindles, K-complexes, slow-wave sleep, REM sleep, and total sleep time
Electroencephalogram	Rarely demonstrate periodic sharp-wave complexes
CSF biomarkers	14-3-3 and tau are typically negative, RT-QuIC is positive in more than 80% of cases
Brain MRI	Hyperintensity on diffusion-weighted imaging is typically absent, but has been reported in some cases
Brain FDG-PET/ SPECT	Early thalamic hypometabolism/ hypoperfusion that may spread to other areas of the brain as the disease progresses

CSF, cerebrospinal fluid; FDG-PET, fluorodeoxyglucose positron emission tomography; MRI, magnetic resonance imaging; REM, rapid eye movement; RT-QuIC, real-time quaking-induced conversion; SPECT, single-photon emission computed tomography.

levels (Portaluppi et al., 1994). Hallucinations are reported in over half of patients and are often associated with personality change, depression, anxiety, aggressiveness, disinhibition, and listlessness (Krasnianski et al., 2014). Dysautonomia may be related to sympathetic overactivity as no pressor response is seen in patients who are given intravenous norepinephrine. FFI patients also experience little to no sedative effect and catecholamines remain elevated when they are given clonidine (Cortelli et al., 1991). Patients likely succumb to metabolic exhaustion given that motor activity is increased by 80% and 24-hour energy expenditure is elevated by 60% (Plazzi et al., 1997).

Classic symptoms of CJD are also observed in FFI, albeit they usually occur later in the disease course (Sikorska and Liberski, 2012). The cognitive impairment reported by FFI patients differs from that of classic dementia often observed in other prion diseases since it consists of an alteration in level of alertness and vigilance. It includes early impairment in attention, working memory, impaired temporal ordering of events, and the aforementioned progressive dream-like state (Gallassi et al., 1996), features that are not typically seen in other cortical or subcortical dementias. Pyramidal symptoms may include brisk tendon reflexes and Babinski's sign (Gambetti et al., 2003a). Gait disorders tend to present about 5 months into the disease and can occur with dysarthria (Sikorska and Liberski, 2012; Cortelli et al., 2014). Visual symptoms and myoclonus also occur as they do in CJD, but generally later in the disease course (Krasnianski et al., 2014).

To help assist with the diagnosis, Krasnianski and colleagues (2014) have developed an algorithm for diagnosing FFI. Patients with suspected FFI must have an organic sleep disturbance that is either clinically apparent or observed via PSG. They must also display at least two "CJD-like symptoms/signs," including psychiatric

Table 15.3

Clinical disease progression of fatal familial insomnia

Codon 129 polymorphism	Disease stage	Typical symptoms
MM	Mild	Sleep disturbances and autonomic symptoms
	Moderate	Bulbar and visual symptoms, cognitive impairment, hallucinations
	Severe	Ataxia, dysarthria, myoclonus, pyramidal symptoms
MV	Mild	Sleep disturbances, visual changes, ataxia
	Moderate	Bulbar symptoms, cognitive impairment, autonomic symptoms
	Severe	Myoclonus, hallucinations, dysarthria, pyramidal symptoms

Table 15.4

Diagnostic criteria for fatal familial insomnia (FFI)

Definitive diagnosis	Presence of D178N-129M mutation in a symptomatic patient
Probable clinical diagnosis	A. Organic sleep disturbance, either clinically or via polysomnogram
	B. At least two “prion-like” signs/symptoms:
	a. Psychiatric symptoms such as personality change, anxiety, depression, aggressiveness, disinhibition, or hallucinations
	b. Ataxia
	c. Visual symptoms
	d. Myoclonus
	e. Cognitive changes
	C. At least one FFI-specific symptom
	a. Weight loss of > 10 kg over 6-month duration
	b. Autonomic symptoms such as tachycardia, hypertension, hyperthermia, or hyperhidrosis
	c. Husky voice
Suggestive diagnostic tests	A. Loss of sleep architecture on polysomnogram
	B. Hypometabolism/hypoperfusion in the thalami on brain FDG-PET or SPECT scan
	C. Positive RT-QuIC in CSF or olfactory epithelium in patients with FFI phenotype

CSF, cerebrospinal fluid; FDG-PET, fluorodeoxyglucose positron emission tomography; RT-QuIC, real-time quaking-induced conversion; SPECT, single-photon emission computed tomography.

symptoms (e.g., visual hallucinations, personality change, depression, anxiety, aggressiveness, disinhibition, and listlessness), ataxia, visual changes, myoclonus, and cognitive impairment. Thirdly, suspected patients must demonstrate at least one “relatively disease-specific symptom/sign” such as weight loss of at least 10 kg over 6 months, vegetative symptoms (aka autonomic symptoms) (e.g., hyperhidrosis, hypertension, tachycardia, obstipation, and hyperthermia), and husky voice. Diagnostic criteria for FFI are listed in Table 15.4.

Differential diagnosis

Diagnosing FFI clinically can be difficult due to its relative clinical heterogeneity. Obtaining a family history and focusing on sleep symptoms of related family members are helpful since the identification of the PrP gene D178N-129M can provide diagnosis at an early stage of the disease. From a purely clinical perspective, the presence of the agrypnia excitata syndrome can mimic delirium tremens and Morvan’s fibrillary chorea (Montagna et al., 2003). The autonomic dysfunction can be severe enough to cause other conditions like posterior reversible encephalopathy syndrome that may mask the underlying cause (Froböse et al., 2014). Additionally, other genetic prion diseases may sometimes resemble FFI (Appleby et al., 2010). As with any rapidly progressive neurodegenerative condition, reversible causes like *N*-methyl-D-aspartate receptor encephalitis should be considered (Marques et al., 2014). Prominent symptoms of disturbance of consciousness and visual hallucinations may suggest a diagnosis of dementia with Lewy bodies. FFI may also be initially misdiagnosed as a psychiatric disorder (e.g., posttraumatic stress disorder or primary psychosis) due to prominent early psychiatric symptoms.

Diagnosis tests

In addition to the demonstration of the disease causing PrP gene allele D178N-129M, which would definitively establish the diagnosis, three tests – PSG, brain imaging, and the test commonly performed in cerebrospinal fluid (CSF), named real-time quaking-induced conversion (RT-QuIC) – are especially helpful in the clinical diagnosis of FFI.

Polysomnography and electroencephalography

PSG is often helpful from the early stages of the clinical disease, even in the absence of overt clinical signs of insomnia, and should be considered in the presence of other signs even when insomnia is not reported (Cortelli et al., 2006). PSG typically shows progressive deterioration of sleep architecture, including reduction in sleep spindles, K complexes, and total sleep time (Montagna et al., 2003). Slow-wave sleep is usually affected first, followed by reduction of REM sleep. The 129MV genotype patients generally have less severe sleep findings (Gambetti et al., 2003a). No PSG alterations have been found in asymptomatic mutation carriers (Ferrillo et al., 2001). Periodic sharp-wave complexes (PSWCs), which are included in the diagnostic criteria for sporadic CJD (sCJD), often are not observed in FFI (Kovacs et al., 2005; Chen et al., 2013; Chen et al., 2018). EEGs typically demonstrate generalized slowing that may include scattered PSWCs in patients with myoclonus and prolonged disease duration (Gambetti et al., 2003a).

Cerebrospinal fluid markers

Of the CSF biomarkers used in the diagnosis of prion diseases, like 14-3-3, S100b, neuron-specific enolase, and tau, the recently introduced RT-QuIC, which is based on the direct detection of PrP^{TSE}, has emerged as the most powerful and reliable test. In a study of 12 FFI subjects, CSF RT-QuIC was positive in 83% of cases (Sano et al., 2013) although in a later study by Franceschini et al. (Franceschini et al., 2017), 2/2 FFI cases demonstrated negative RT-QuIC results. FFI also demonstrated the longest RT-QuIC lag time indicating low amount or rate of conversion of normal PrP to PrP^{TSE} compared to fCJD and sCJD (Cramm et al., 2015). RT-QuIC can also detect prion-seeding activity in the olfactory mucosa of FFI patients (Redaelli et al., 2017). Other commonly used CSF tests in prion disease, such as 14-3-3 and tau, demonstrate very low sensitivity (Ladogana et al., 2009; Chen et al., 2018).

Neuroimaging

Brain magnetic resonance imaging (MRI) is often unhelpful in the diagnosis of FFI. Twelve cases of FFI were all reported negative (Chen et al., 2013), while MRI-positive FFI cases remain isolated observations (Ortega-Cubero et al., 2013; Takada et al., 2017; Chen et al., 2018). Other neuroimaging modalities, such as fluorodeoxyglucose FDG-PET) and single-photon emission computed tomography (SPECT) are very valuable in FFI. FDG-PET has demonstrated significant decreased metabolism in the thalamus and cingulate cortex in very early stages of the disease (Cortelli et al., 1997; Mastrianni et al., 1999; Harder et al., 2004; Ortega-Cubero et al., 2013; Prieto et al., 2015) (Fig. 15.1). Hypometabolism spreads to other brain regions as the disease progresses. FFI 129MV patients show more widespread hypometabolism (Gambetti et al., 2003a). SPECT imaging has also demonstrated a dramatic decrease in dopamine and serotonin transporters in the thalamic and hypothalamic region in 2 FFI patients (Klöppel et al., 2002).

In a study conducted by Cortelli and colleagues (2006), prospective brain FDG-PET scans and PSGs

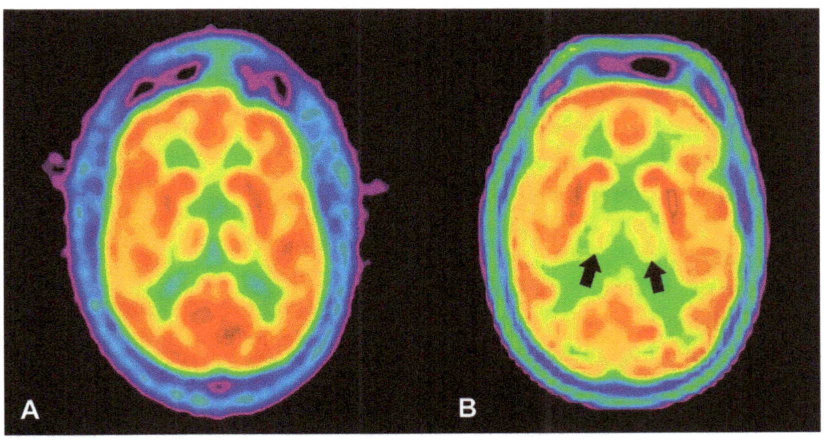

Fig. 15.1. Positron emission tomography image of brain regional metabolism determined with fluorodeoxyglucose (FDG-PET). (**A**) Control; (**B**) Fatal familial insomnia patient. Arrows demarcate hypometabolism (denoted by exclusive presence of yellow color) in the thalamus typically observed in fatal familial insomnia at early stages. Lighter colors (e.g., yellow) in brain FDG-PET scans represent hypometabolism.

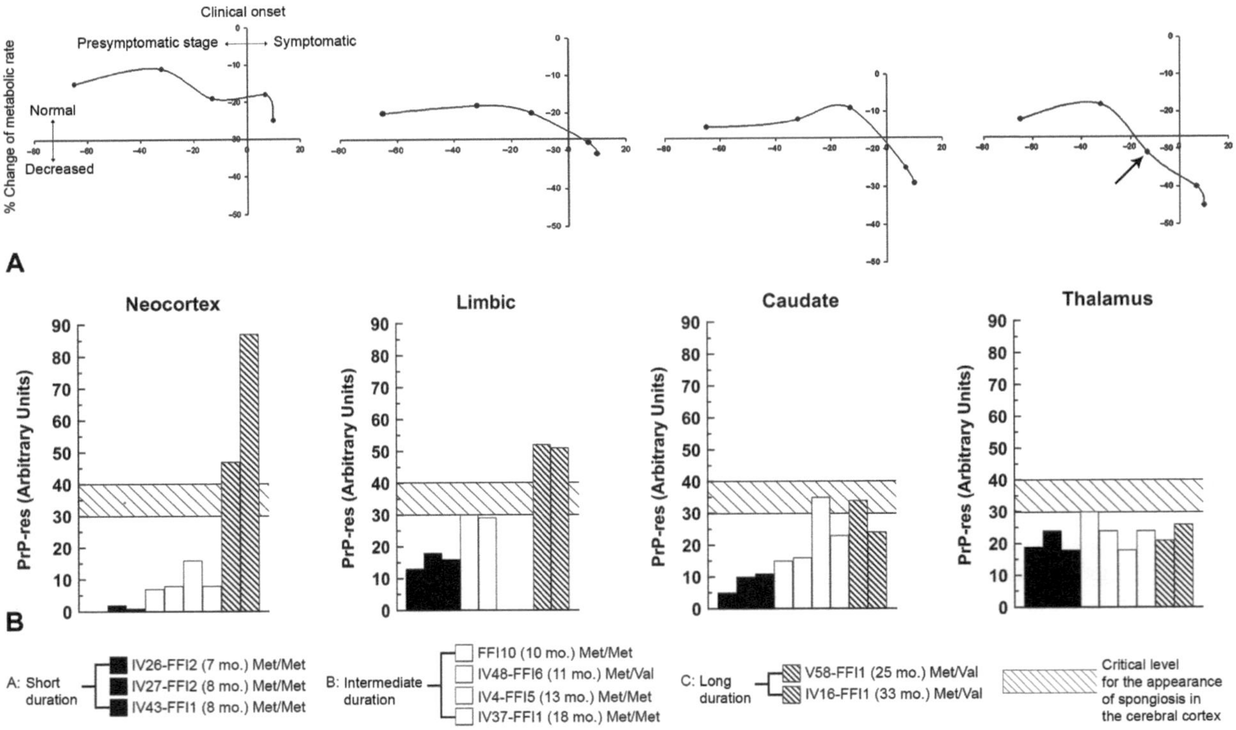

Fig. 15.2. Serial fluorodeoxyglucose positron emission tomography of regional cerebral metabolism of glucose (rCMRglu) and quantitative autopsy determinations of protease-resistant prion protein (resPrP^{TSE}) in fatal familial insomnia (FFI)-affected subjects. (**A**) rCMRglu in indicated brain regions of a FFI mutation carrier at 65, 32, 13 months before and 7 and 10 months after the clinical onset of FFI; each dot along the curve represents a relative value; numbers in *x*-axis indicate days before and after clinical onset, which is identified by 0 at the intersection with the *y*-axis; numbers in *y*-axis refer to metabolic values; values below the *x*-axis are significantly decreased. Arrow: thalamic hypometabolism detected 13 months before the clinical onset. (**B**) Relative amounts of resPrP^{TSE} in indicated regions related to disease durations of 7–33 months in 9 FFI subjects. Both (**A**) and (**B**) sets of data point to the thalamus as the site of early resPrP^{TSE} accumulation and where resPrP^{TSE} steady state is attained, while resPrP^{TSE} accumulation is late in the cerebral cortex reaching significant levels, presumably needed to cause spongiform degeneration, only after long disease duration (see Parchi et al., 1995; Cortelli et al., 2006 for details). Statistics: thalamus: not significant; caudate: short vs. long duration $p < 0.01$; limbic cortex: short vs. intermediate and vs. long $p < 0.01$–0.001; neocortex all three durations $p < 0.001$–0.0001 (Student's *t*-test). (Modified from Cortelli P, Perani D, Montagna P, et al. (2006) Pre-symptomatic diagnosis in fatal familial insomnia: serial neurophysiological and 18FDG-PET studies. Brain 129: 668–675, with permission from Oxford University Press and from Parchi P, Castellani R, Cortelli P, et al. (1995) Regional distribution of protease-resistant prion protein in fatal familial insomnia. Ann Neurol 38: 21–29, with permission from John Wiley.)

were conducted on known FFI mutation carriers, non-mutation carriers from the same family, and controls. In 1 of the 4 mutation carriers who became symptomatic during the study, focal thalamic hypometabolism was detected on an FDG-PET scan performed 13 months prior to symptom onset (Fig. 15.2A). Although the macrostructure of sleep was normal at this time, spectral analysis detected reduction of the sigma band on EEG that is associated with corticothalamic synchronization. These two findings in a presymptomatic FFI mutation carrier provide strong evidence that disease pathology starts in the thalamus. The results of this study also suggest that brain FDG-PET and spectral analysis of EEG in asymptomatic mutation carriers may be used as a biomarker to assist with predicting age at disease onset as well as to assess response to potential treatments.

Therapeutics

As with all human prion diseases, there is no currently available treatment or cure. FFI is further complicated by the fact that its symptoms are difficult to treat. FFI responds poorly to typical symptomatic treatment of insomnia such as sedatives and benzodiazepines (Julien et al., 1998; Will et al., 1998). There is one case report of improved sleep with the use of the melatonergic antidepressant agomelatine (Froböse et al., 2012). There is also an ongoing preventative trial using doxycycline 100 mg/day in patients carrying the FFI mutation, the results of which will not be known for some time (Forloni et al., 2015). Mounting evidence indicates that treatment efficacy is likely to be directly related to how early in the course of the disease the treatment is started. It is encouraging that the PET study by Cortelli et al. (2006) and the diagnosis by olfactory mucosa examination by Redaelli et al. (2017) raise the possibility of preclinical diagnosis in FFI. If a treatment becomes available, FFI could potentially be treated preventively before any clinical signs become detectable.

Neuropathology

There is wide consensus that the neuropathologic features of FFI are well characterized and consistent in the majority of cases (Manetto et al., 1992; Parchi et al., 1995; Reder et al., 1995; Almer et al., 1999; Llorens et al., 2016, 2017). However, especially in 129MV heterozygous patients, the histopathology may be more widespread regarding the atrophy of thalamic nuclei and spongiform degeneration (Parchi et al., 1995; Zarranz et al., 2005b; Llorens et al., 2017). It is currently unclear whether these histopathologic variations are linked to 129MV heterozygosity, to disease duration (which is longer on average than it is in 129MM homozygous patients), or to both (Goldfarb et al., 1992b; Manetto et al., 1992; Parchi et al., 1995, 2000a). It is likely that the 129MV heterozygosity plays a role in this setting since the presence of valine may destabilize the phenotype, as is the case in sCJD patients with 129MV genotype and PrP^{TSE} type 2 (Parchi et al., 2009).

In subjects with short disease duration (approximately $\leq$ 10 months), the essential lesion is severe loss of neurons (up to 80–90%) with prominent astrogliosis but no spongiform degeneration affecting anterior (A) and medial dorsal (MD) nuclei of the thalamus, along with variable astrogliosis and neuronal depletion in the inferior olive (Fig. 15.3A). Occasionally, mild focal spongiform degeneration in the entorhinal cortex and subiculum may be present (Little et al., 1986; Manetto et al., 1992; Parchi et al., 1995; Reder et al., 1995; Almer et al., 1999; Llorens et al., 2017). With longer disease duration, neuronal loss and gliosis with no spongiform degeneration may expand to other thalamic nuclei, most often to ventral lateral and pulvinar nuclei, while increasing spongiform degeneration and gliosis are found in the cerebral cortex, eventually affecting all lobes and occasionally the neostriatum. In at least 2 heterozygous cases, spongiform degeneration is made of large and often confluent vacuoles similar to those observed in sCJD associated with 129MM homozygosity and PrP^{TSE} type 2 (sCJDMM2) (Fig. 15.4B) (Manetto et al., 1992; Kretzschmar et al., 1998; Parchi et al., 1999b). Cerebellar atrophy with loss of Purkinje cells and astrogliosis associated with the presence of "torpedo" formations may also be observed (Manetto et al., 1992; Parchi et al., 1995; Almer et al., 1999).

Immunohistochemistry for PrP is often negative, especially in A and MD thalamic nuclei. However, even in the absence of spongiform degeneration, there may be areas of punctate immunostaining and presence of small polymorphic deposits (Fig. 15.4A). In the presence of spongiform degeneration, the immunostaining is granular and occasionally perivacuolar, but definitely different from the

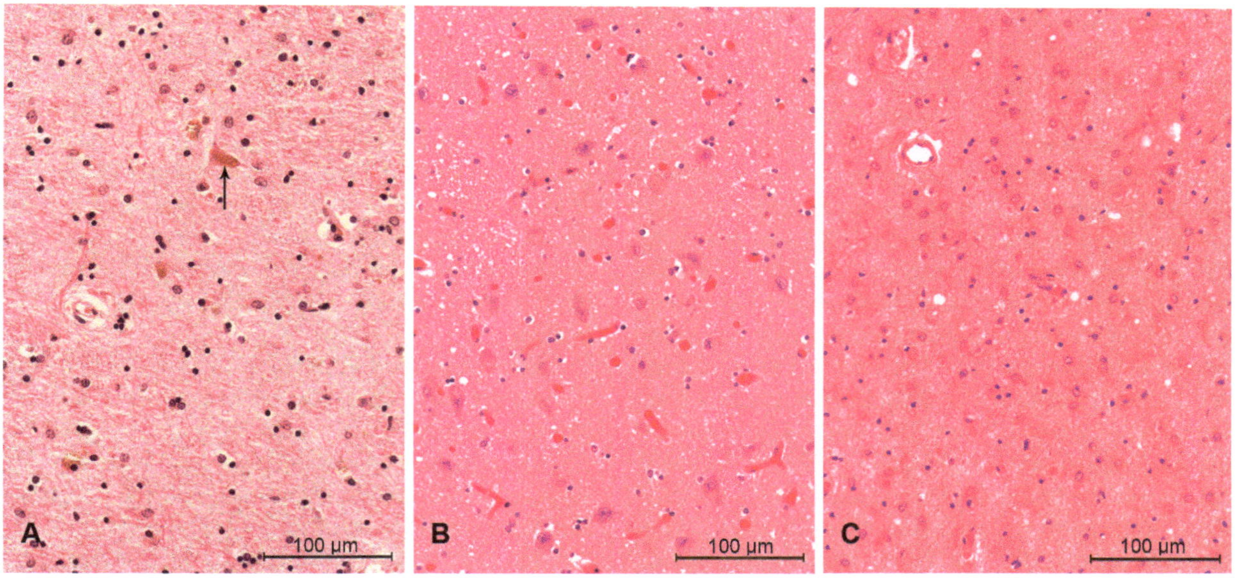

Fig. 15.3. Microphotographs of mediodorsal thalamic nucleus in fatal familial insomnia (FFI), normal control, and sporadic fatal insomnia (sFI). Severe neuronal depletion with reactive astrogliosis with no appreciable spongiform degeneration is demonstrated in FFI (**A**) and sFI (**C**) compared with the control (**B**). Reactive astrogliosis is more noticeable in sFI than in FFI. Arrow: abnormal neuron. (**A–C**) Hematoxylin and eosin.

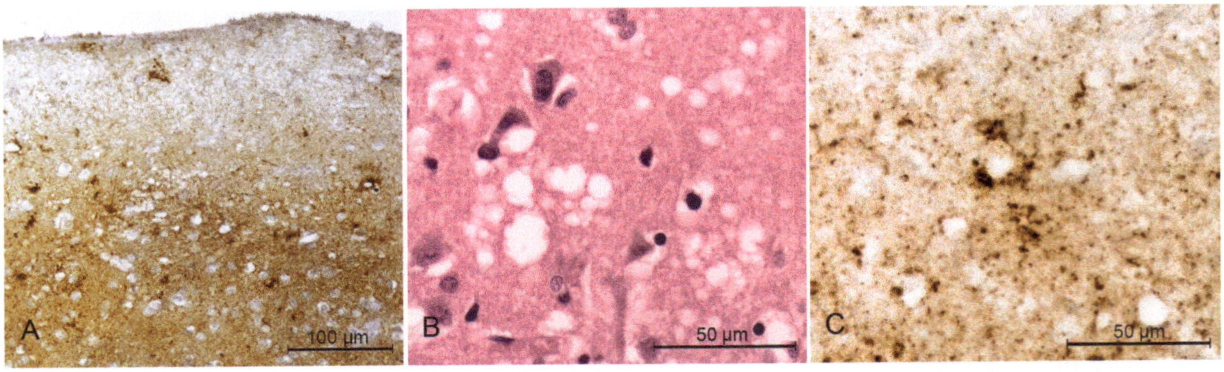

Fig. 15.4. Microphotographs of fatal familial insomnia cerebral cortex. (**A**) PrP immunostaining of the molecular and external granular layers in an area with no spongiform degeneration showing small irregular aggregates. (**B**) Spongiform degeneration with large clustered vacuoles in cerebral cortex similar to that of sporadic Creutzfeldt–Jakob disease MM2 but associated with a different PrP immunostaining pattern, made of granular deposits occasionally surrounding vacuoles (**C**). (**A** and **C**) Antibody to PrP 3F4; (**B**) Hematoxylin and eosin.

immune staining pattern of sCJDMM2, despite the similarity of the spongiform degeneration type in the two diseases (Fig. 15.4C). Prominent patchy or strip-like PrP immunostaining pattern in the cerebellar cortex has been observed in at least 2 cases (Almer et al., 1999; Zarranz et al., 2005b). Apoptosis, microglial activation, and inflammatory response, especially in severely affected thalamic nuclei, also contribute to the histopathologic features (Dorandeu et al., 1998; Llorens et al., 2016).

The homogeneity and specificity of the FFI histopathologic phenotype, comprising thalamic atrophy associated with variable but generally limited or no spongiform degeneration, have been challenged. McLean et al. (1997) and Zarranz et al. (2005a, b) have briefly described 2 subjects carrying a reliably proven D178N, 129MM genotype, who show widespread spongiform degeneration but apparently lack thalamic atrophy. Conversely, severe thalamic atrophy, although accompanied by co-localized spongiform degeneration, has been observed in 2 cases carrying the glutamic acid-to-lysine mutation at codon 200 (E200K) associated with 129MM genotype (Chapman et al., 1994; Taratuto et al., 2002). Clinically, both E200K subjects had insomnia, and the PSG recording obtained in 1 case was indistinguishable from the PSG described in FFI (Chapman et al., 1994; Taratuto et al., 2002). Remarkably, however, immunoblotting and N-terminus amino acid sequencing by Taratuto and collaborators (2002) definitively determined the presence of proteinase K (PK)-resistant PrP^{TSE} ($resPrP^{TSE}$) type 1 in one of the E200K, 129MM cases, while $resPrP^{TSE}$ in FFI is consistently type 2; see also General characteristics, below. Unfortunately, none of these analyses were performed for the other two D178N, 129MM cases mentioned above nor for the other E200K, 129MM case (Chapman et al., 1994; McLean et al., 1997; Zarranz et al., 2005b). The rarity of these atypical cases raises the possibility that the D178N-129M and E200K-129M pathogenic alleles are occasionally associated with cases that escape the typical phenotype associated with these two mutations to adopt, at least partially, the phenotype of the other mutated genotype (see also Pathogenetic hypothesis, below). Furthermore, in a clinical study of 7 symptomatic carriers of the D178N mutation MM homozygous at codon 129, Chen et al. (Chen et al., 2018) stated that four carriers "were more likely the CJD phenotype". However, they reported that all 7 patients had sleep disturbances and autonomic symptoms, and that the two tested cases had both positive, apparently FFI-like, polysomnography while none had an EEG typical of CJD and one only had a CJD typical MRI. Additionally, speculations on alternative phenotypes of FFI should be cautious when the case studied lacks of PSG analysis and autopsy (Guerreiro et al., 2009). As previously stated, definitive disease phenotype determination requires at least a polysomnographic recording and autopsy examination since thalamic atrophy is often undetectable by MRI and CT imaging.

The proposal that FFI and $fCJD^{D178N}$ are "extremes of a spectrum rather than discrete and separate entities" ignores a large body of evidence, based on direct PrP^{TSE} studies, experimental transmission, and modeling, that supports the distinct strain properties of the PrP^{TSE} species associated with FFI and $fCJD^{D178N}$ (Monari et al., 1994; Petersen et al., 1996; Telling et al., 1996; McLean et al., 1997; Parchi et al., 2000b; Apetri et al., 2005; Zarranz et al., 2005b; Guerreiro et al., 2009; Lee et al., 2010; Chiesa et al., 2016; Chen et al., 2018; see also Structure, below).

Disease-associated prion protein

General characteristics

The abnormal prion protein, PrP^{TSE}, associated with FFI is type 2B. According to the classification originally proposed by Parchi et al. (1996, 1997, 1999b), most human PrP^{TSE} species can be separated into two groups identified as types 1 and 2, based on the electrophoretic relative mass of the unglycosylated form generated following digestion of total PrP with PK to detect $resPrP^{TSE}$. In $resPrP^{TSE}$ type 2, the relative mass of the unglycosylated form is approximately 19 kDa while the matching $resPrP^{TSE}$ type 1 has a relative mass of approximately 21 kDa. The letter B identifies the ratio of the three $resPrP^{TSE}$ glycoforms, which includes diglycosylated, monoglycosylated, and unglycosylated conformers (Parchi et al., 1997). In FFI the glycoform ratio is dominated by the diglycosylated isoform, while the unglycosylated is the least represented (Monari et al., 1994; Parchi et al., 1995).

Currently PrP^{TSE} types 1 and 2 are viewed as two families of prion strains segregated by their distinct conformations (Monari et al., 1994; Parchi et al., 2000b; Safar et al., 2015). Indeed, PrP^{TSE} types 1 and 2 are consistently associated with distinct disease phenotypes (Gambetti et al., 2003a, 2011). The typing of the PrP^{TSE} associated with FFI has been further confirmed by amino acid sequencing of $resPrP^{TSE}$ (performed in heterozygotes because of the inadequate amount of $resPrP^{TSE}$ for purification in homozygotes), which has shown that the $resPrP^{TSE}$ N-terminus is at residue serine 97 as expected, given the electrophoretic mobility of 19 kDa of $resPrP^{TSE}$ type 2 (Parchi et al., 2000b). Furthermore, the N-terminus of the FFI-associated $resPrP^{TSE}$ is minimally ragged compared to the PrP^{TSE} harbored in sCJD with 129 MV heterozygosis and PrP^{TSE} type 2 (sCJDMV2). This finding indicates that PrP^{TSE} in FFI is more homogeneous than in the matching sCJD subtype, allowing a more precise cleavage by PK (Parchi et al., 2000b).

$resPrP^{TSE}$ amount and distribution

The amount and distribution of $resPrP^{TSE}$ in FFI, as determined by quantitative immunoblotting of tissue extracts from various brain regions, exhibit a characteristic profile shared with sporadic fatal insomnia (sFI) and distinct from that of sCJD subtypes (Fig. 15.5) (Parchi et al., 2000a). The amount of $resPrP^{TSE}$ is also directly related to disease duration (Fig. 15.2B) (Parchi et al., 1995, 1999a, 2000a). Up to 8 months duration, $resPrP^{TSE}$ is undetectable in the neocortex and barely detectable elsewhere with the relatively largest amount located in entorhinal cortex (Parchi et al., 1995; Padovani et al., 1998). At 10 months from onset, $resPrP^{TSE}$ can be demonstrated in the neocortex, where it progressively increases until it reaches the highest levels of all other brain regions (Parchi et al., 1995). Nevertheless, even in the case with the longest duration examined in the study by Parchi and coworkers (1995) (33 months), $resPrP^{TSE}$ amounts in the frontal cortex and MD thalamic nucleus, respectively, remain over 6 and 20 times smaller than the matching amounts in sCJDMM1, the archetype of sCJD that is associated with 129MM homozygosity and PrP^{TSE} type 1.

The low amounts of $resPrP^{TSE}$ are consistent with the finding that in FFI (and $fCJD^{D178N}$), unlike other PrP gene mutations where the normal or wild-type PrP (PrP^{C}) is also converted to $resPrP^{TSE}$, all of the PrP^{TSE}, including detergent-insoluble and PK-resistant fractions, originates exclusively from the mutated allele in both 129 homozygous and heterozygous forms (Chen et al., 1997). Furthermore, only approximately 17% or less of total D178N mutated PrP (PrP^{D178N}) is converted to $resPrP^{TSE}$ (Chen et al., 1997; Llorens et al., 2016). However, the amount of the detergent-insoluble and PK-sensitive component of total PrP^{TSE} has not been rigorously assessed in FFI. Furthermore, presence of small amounts of PrP oligomers has been recently reported in the thalamus (Llorens et al., 2016).

Structure

Riek et al. (1998) have shown that in PrP^{C} aspartic acid at position 178 (D178) is linked by hydrogen bonds to the side chains of residues arginine 164 (R164) on one side, and to the side chains of tyrosine 128 (Y128) on the other; the latter is sequentially adjacent to the M129V polymorphic site. This strategic location raises the possibility that the D178N mutation selectively affects the entire hydrogen bonding network of the region in ways that differ according to the residue, M or V, in position 129. This chain of events would impose on PrP^{TSE} distinct conformations in FFI and $fCJD^{D178N}$ (Riek et al., 1998).

This hypothesis has been supported and expanded in subsequent studies (see van der Kamp and Daggett, 2009, for review). Apetri and colleagues (2005) have shown in recombinant PrP (recPrP) that the presence of the D178N mutation facilitates conformational conversion to oligomeric β-sheet-rich forms and that D178N mutated amyloid fibrils formed *in vitro* by recPrP differ in the secondary structure from the fibrils formed by wild-type recPrP. Furthermore, the conversion to oligomeric β-sheet-rich forms is faster in the D178N-129M recPrP than in the D178N-129V isoform while the M129V polymorphism has no effect on the conversion of wild-type recPrP (Apetri et al., 2005). The destabilizing effect of the D178N mutation inducing conformational conversion has been attributed to various events, such as abolition of the salt bridges between D178 and R164, interference with the adjacent disulfide

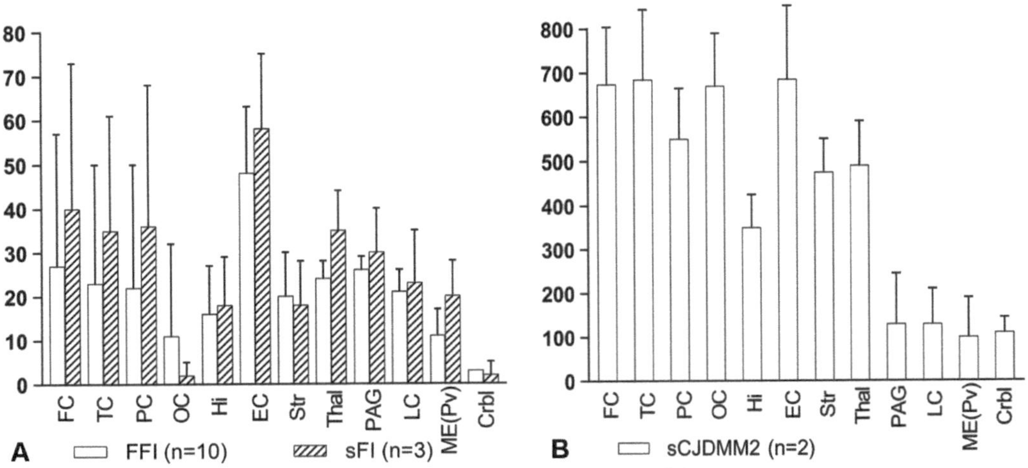

Fig. 15.5. Regional brain distribution of protease-resistant prion protein (resPrP^{TSE}) in fatal familial insomnia (FFI), sporadic fatal insomnia (sFI) and sporadic Creutzfeldt–Jakob disease (sCJD) MM2 (sCJDMM2). (**A**) Comparative analysis of resPrP^{TSE} distribution in FFI and sFI reveals a similar profile with consistently higher resPrP^{TSE} amounts in sFI than in FFI. Standard deviations are much higher in the cerebral cortex of the FFI and sFI due to the disease duration impact on resPrP^{TSE} deposition. (**B**) The profile of sCJDMM2, of which sFI is considered a variant, shows a different profile with 10–20 times higher amounts of resPrP^{TSE}. Data are presented in arbitrary units (mean ± standard deviation) as percentage of the highest value obtained by densitometry in FFI subjects (see Parchi et al., 2000a, for details). *Crbl*, cerebellum; *EC*, entorhinal cortex; *FC*, frontal cortex; *Hi*, CA1 region of hippocampus; *LC*, locus coeruleus; *ME(Pv)*, medulla (periventricular gray); *OC*, occipital cortex; *PAG*, midbrain periventricular gray; *PC*, parietal cortex; *Str*, neostriatum (caudatus and putamen); *TC*, temporal cortex; Thal, thalamus (mediodorsal nucleus). (Modified from Parchi P, Capellari S, Gambetti P (2000a) Intracerebral distribution of the abnormal isoform of the prion protein in sporadic Creutzfeldt–Jakob disease and fatal insomnia. Microsc Res Tech 50: 16–25, with permission from John Wiley.)

bond, and weakening of the hydrogen bond with Y128 (Swietnicki et al., 1998; Alonso et al., 2001).

More recently, significant conformational variations among recPrP isoforms, including wild-type, D178N-129M, and D178N-129V, were further confirmed by structure determinations on crystal structures of human recPrP^{D178N} and on PrP^{D177N,128M} and PrP^{D177N,128V} obtained from transgenic (Tg) mice carrying the corresponding haplotypes (Lee et al., 2010; Tapella et al., 2013). These studies further support the notion that, owing to its strategic location, the D178N mutation lowers the stability, alters the structure, and favors the aggregation of PrP by a process that is influenced by the M129V polymorphism and results in two sets of structures linked to 129M and 129V, respectively. Although based largely on *in vitro* data, this notion is in agreement with the segregation of FFI and fCJD^{D178N} into two distinct phenotypes based on clinical neuropathologic and PrP^{TSE} features (Goldfarb et al., 1992b).

Experimental animal transmission and *in vitro* amplification

Experimental animal transmission

After several failed attempts (Little et al., 1986; Brown et al., 1994, 1995), FFI was successfully transmitted to wild-type mice (Tateishi et al., 1995) and to Tg mice (Collinge et al., 1995), although in the second study no PrP^{TSE} was demonstrated despite the presence of spongiform degeneration in the cortex and white matter. In 1996, Telling et al. transmitted a number of FFI cases, including homozygotes (129MM) and heterozygotes (129MV) as well as homozygotes affected by fCJD$^{E200K\text{-}129M}$. Transmission of fCJD$^{D178N\text{-}129V}$, the fCJD phenotype that shares the D178N mutation with FFI, failed probably because of the inoculum-host V to M heterogeneity at the 129 residue. Hosts in this study were PrP murine/human chimeric Tg mice in which the murine 96-167 PrP amino acid sequence was replaced by the matching human sequence containing the 129M residue (Tg(MHu2M) mice) (Telling et al., 1994).

Subsequently, another human/murine chimera was also inoculated with similar results (Korth et al., 2003). Three of the four FFI cases tested, including two FFI-129MM and one -129MV, transmitted the disease following inoculation of frontal cortex and thalamus, but not of cerebellum homogenates (Telling et al., 1996). Furthermore, the incubation period was reduced by 30–50% from first to second passage (Korth et al., 2003). Histopathology and PrP^{TSE} distribution markedly differed in FFI and fCJD^{E200K}-inoculated mice. Furthermore, Tg mice challenged with FFI and fCJD^{E200K} reproduced PrP^{TSE} type 2 and type 1, respectively, despite the lack in these mice of the genetic mutations (D178N and E200K) linked to the two diseases. This remarkable finding provided the first substantial evidence that all the information to reproduce the specific conformation of

PrP^{TSE} or prion strain, as is the case with PrP^{TSE} types 1 and 2, is encrypted in the PrP^{TSE} itself, which may be reproduced with no genetic intervention. More recently, transmission of a 27-month duration FFI-129MV case to wild-type mice has been described (Sasaki et al., 2005).

In vitro amplification

PrP amplification is commonly achieved using protein misfolding cyclic amplification (PMCA) technology (Saborio et al., 2001). PMCA can efficiently replicate, and increase exponentially, even minute amounts of PrP^{TSE}, commonly referred to as seed, through the conversion to PrP^{TSE} of PrP^{C} provided as substrate. Barria et al. (2014) first amplified PrP^{TSE} from FFI brains, reproducing the PrP^{TSE} type 2 pattern as in FFI. Amplification of the murine PrP^{TSE} homologue, harboring the D177N mutation coupled with either a 128M or 128V residue (murine homologues of human D178N-129M or -129V) using murine PrP^{TSE} as seed has been reported by Bouybayoune et al. (2015), while recently Redaelli et al. (2017) introduced a novel clinical diagnostic test for FFI by using PMCA (as well as RT-QuIC) to amplify PrP^{TSE} from FFI autopsy tissue as well as from olfactory mucosa harvested from live patients (see Chapter 19). Unseeded PMCA to verify the spontaneous misfolding of mutant recombinant PrP produced contrasting results depending on the use of murine vs human (mutant) recPrP (Noble et al., 2015; Elezgarai et al., 2017).

Cell models

Lehmann and Harris (1996) first used metabolic labeling to model FFI in Chinese hamster ovary cells, following transfection of the D177N-128M murine PrP construct (as well as other mutated PrP constructs). Approximately 80% of the murine D177N-128M mutated PrP was found to be detergent-insoluble and 15% PK-resistant. Furthermore, the mutated PrP remained associated with the cell plasma membrane following cleavage of the glycosylphosphatidylinositol anchor linking PrP to the membrane, a defining feature of PrP^{TSE} (Caughey et al., 1989; Borchelt et al., 1990). Although variations were found among the various mutant models examined, PrP^{TSE} type 2, as well as the glycoform ratio characteristic of FFI, were not reproduced.

Different findings were reported by Petersen and coworkers (1996) in a similar study of mutated PrP in human neuroblastoma cells M-17 transfected with a construct harboring the D178N-129M or D178N-129V haplotype modeling FFI and $fCJD^{D178N}$, respectively. Mutated PrP harboring either one of the two 129 M or V residue was progressively reduced during processing through the secretory pathway in a way that was inversely related to the degree of glycosylation. This outcome resulted in preferential underrepresentation of the unglycosylated form that barely reached the cell surface and was more prominent in the FFI cell model than in the $fCJD^{D178N}$ one. This explains the underrepresentation of the unglycosylated form in PK-resistant PrP from FFI and $fCJD^{D178N}$ and suggests that it occurs before the PrP to PrP^{TSE} conversion. No PK-resistant or abnormally membrane-bound mutated PrPs were found.

Impaired transport and delivery to the surface were also observed in a morphologic study of cultured cells using D177N-128M mutated PrP chimeric with the insertion of green fluorescence protein (Ivanova et al., 2001).

In a series of studies Ma, Lindquist, and collaborators (Ma and Lindquist, 2001, 2002; Ma et al., 2002) have examined metabolic processing, including the role of the quality control system and proteosomal degradation of wild-type and D177N mutated PrP species in murine NT-2 neuroblastoma cells and COS (monkey kidney) cells. The D177N mutation was found to increase misfolding and instability of mutated PrP, which was routed through the quality control system, transported to the cytosol, and degraded in the proteasome. Inhibition of proteosomal degradation resulted in accumulation of mutated $resPrP^{TSE}$ in the cytosol, which was cytotoxic (Ma et al., 2002). Retrotranslocation of mutated PrP and formation of PrP^{TSE} with ensuing cytosolic toxicity have been strongly challenged in several similar investigations (Drisaldi et al., 2003; Roucou et al., 2003; Fioriti et al., 2005; Ashok and Hegde, 2009). Fioriti and colleagues (2005) proposed the alternative pathway where misfolded PrP^{D177N} (and other mutated PrP) is trafficked to the Golgi apparatus and directed to the endosome-lysosome compartment where conversion to PrP^{TSE} may occur. As expected, mistargeting of PrP^{D177N} resulted in its underrepresentation at the cell surface that was more prominent in the D177N-128V than in D177N-128M mutated PrP (Fioriti et al., 2005).

Complex effects of D177N-128M PrP on cell metabolism have also been reported by Massignan et al. (2010).

Animal models

Three murine models of FFI have been generated. Jackson et al. (2009), using a knock-in approach, introduced the D177N mutation (the murine homologue for the human D178N), along with two M substitutions at positions 108 and 111 of the amino acid sequence, for the stated purpose of rendering the carriers resistant to laboratory pre-existing infectious prions and generating a site recognized by the potent antibody to PrP 3F4. Mutated PrP (but not PrP from appropriate controls) was recovered in lower amounts and showed underrepresentation of the unglycosylated isoform, similar to human FFI and cell models, and appeared to be trafficked through the secretory pathway (Petersen et al., 1996).

FFI mice showed behavioral and body temperature patterns consistent with sleep deprivation after 6 months of age, but life expectancy was not shortened. Generalized brain atrophy associated with neuronal loss and astrogliosis in the thalamus and cerebellum was reported in 12–20-month-old mice, while PrP immunohistochemistry was negative. A small amount of resPrP^{TSE} was detected in 24-month-old mice. Following passage of brain homogenates from affected animals, mice from different lines showed clinical and neuropathologic abnormalities, but presence of resPrP^{TSE} was never observed.

Overall the Tg mouse generated in this study seemingly expresses FFI-like mutated PrP with characteristics similar to those of D178N/D177N mutated PrP generated in cell models. However, the validity of this Tg mouse as a model of FFI is questionable on the following grounds: (1) presence of two other substitutions in the construct; (2) lack of morphometric analyses to demonstrate preferential thalamic pathology; (3) absence of convincing evidence supporting resPrP^{TSE} presence; and (4) failure of disease transmission.

The Tg mice developed by Bouybayoune et al. (Bouybayoune et al., 2015; Chiesa et al., 2016) express murine D177N-128M (TgFFI) or -128V PrP (TgCJD) with or without an epitope tag for the 3F4 antibody. The unglycosylated isoform was underrepresented in both PrPFFI and PrPCJD, which also were insoluble and mildly resistant to PK. Following PK digestion, the resPrP^{TSE} was type 2 in both mutated PrP species, matching FFI PrP^{TSE} but not the PrP^{TSE} associated with fCJD^{D178N}. Clinically, sleep was reduced and disrupted in FFI mice in a way that was reminiscent of sleep impairment of FFI, while TgCJD mice had a different sleep pattern, characterized by partial preservation of the sleep–wake cycle (Dossena et al., 2008). Motor and cognitive impairments were also observed. Imaging and histopathology of TgFFI revealed thalamic and cerebellar atrophy, and deposition of PK-resistant PrP was reported by immunostaining; ultrastructural anomalies of the Golgi apparatus with a distinct pattern of PrP accumulation were observed in TgFFI, whereas analysis of TgCJD revealed that the mutant protein was retained mostly in the endoplasmic reticulum. Transmission attempts to a variety of mice, as well as *in vitro* replication with PMCA, failed to reveal prion infectivity. In conclusion, clinical and electrophysiologic parameters define the TgFFI mouse developed by Bouybayoune and colleagues as a good model for the FFI sleep disorder. However, immunoblotting, neuropathologic, and immunohistochemical studies do not convey convincing similarity with human FFI. The wide use of the 12B2 antibody, highly reactive to PrP^{TSE} type 1 but not type 2 present in FFI, also is unclear.

Watts et al. (2016) have generated Tg mice lines expressing bank vole PrP (BvPrP) with isoleucine at polymorphic codon 109 (BvPrPI109) harboring the D178N mutation (along with Tg lines expressing other mutated or wild-type BvPrPI109). All these Tg mice spontaneously developed a prion disease. Although Tg D178N mice yielded less mutated BvPrP due to a more rapid turnover, they became symptomatic earlier. In symptomatic animals, PK digestion of the D178N mutated BvPrP generated an ~8 kDa fragment, which likely resulted from a C-terminal cleavage. However, the ~8 kDa fragment appears to be nonspecific since a similar fragment was recovered from Tg-expressing wild-type BvPrP, as well as other mutated BvPrP. Histopathologic and PrP immunohistochemical features of Tg D178N mice differed from those observed in Tg mice expressing wild-type BvPrP, but had no resemblance to FFI lesions in type or distribution. Upon inoculation, the D178N mutated PrP transmitted a similar prion disease in a variety of mice expressing mutated and wild-type BvPrP, as well as mouse PrP. No clinical data are reported. These data indicate that, in contrast to the previous FFI models, the FFI Bv mouse does not reproduce any of the characteristics of FFI, but it does generate a D178N mutated PrP that is PK-resistant, as well as highly pathogenic and infectious. Finally, an FFI model using Tg *Drosophila melanogaster* expressing hamster or mouse PrP carrying the equivalent of human D178N mutation recently developed generated a neurotoxic phenotype (Thackray et al., 2017).

Considerations on etiology and pathogenesis

Data from PrP molecular structure, cell metabolism, and processing of the D178N mutant protein indicate that the D178N exchange is well positioned to impact the structural stability of mutated PrP. The instability results in rapid turnover of D178N PrP that brings about an abnormal distribution of D178N PrP within the cell and its underrepresentation at the cell surface, which is likely to be its critical destination (Petersen et al., 1996; Harris, 1999; Ma and Lindquist, 2001; Linden et al., 2008). Within this scenario, it is conceivable that with time mutant PrP adopts a prion-like conformation that escapes detection or breakdown by protein homeostasis mechanisms and initiates templated conversion of non-prion-like mutated PrP, triggering the prion disease (Dubnikov and Cohen, 2017). The initial adoption of the prion-like conformation must be common and consistent given the high penetrance of the D178N mutation and the relative uniformity of the FFI phenotype (Minikel et al., 2016). It seems unlikely that the D178N PrP is pathogenic before adopting the prion-like conformation since, if this were the case, mutation carriers would display at least some sign of illness, a notion which is not supported by current data (Ferrillo et al., 2001; Cortelli et al., 2006).

Whether this initial conversion is widespread or initially impacts only a specific brain region is not known. However, data obtained from two sets of studies, although basic, allow a few considerations. The first study deals with the longitudinal evaluation of brain regional metabolism by FDG-PET in FFI mutation carriers from the presymptomatic to the terminal stage of the disease (Fig. 15.2A) (Cortelli et al., 2006). In the second study the amount and distribution of resPrP^{TSE} were analyzed at autopsy in FFI-affected subjects with different disease durations ranging from 7 to 33 months (Fig. 15.2B) (Parchi et al., 1995, 2000a). Combined, the data obtained from these two studies point to the thalamus as the first brain region impacted by the disease process, likely because it is the site of initial of PrP^{TSE} formation or where PrP^{TSE} is more toxic. Indeed, the thalamus is the first region showing FDG-PET hypometabolism at least 13 months before clinical onset of the disease and virtually the only brain structure affected in short-duration cases (Fig. 15.2) (Parchi et al., 1995; Cortelli et al., 2006).

FDG-PET data indicate that, after clinical onset, the disease process spreads rapidly but orderly, involving basal ganglia, limbic cortex, and neocortex, while continuing to progress rapidly in the thalamus, which exhibits the most severe hypometabolism. Pairing FDG-PET data with postmortem analysis of resPrP^{TSE} relative amounts related to disease duration indicates a steady state of resPrP^{TSE} in thalamus, a progressive increase possibly reaching a plateau in basal ganglia and limbic cortex, and a late appearance along with apparently continuing increase in cerebral neocortex (Fig. 15.2) (Parchi et al., 1995, 2000a). Furthermore, in the cerebral cortex, spongiform degeneration seems to be directly related to the amount of resPrP^{TSE}.

These sets of data leave several questions unanswered. For example, PrP^{TSE}, although in small amounts, might cause functional (not structural) undetectable damage to critical cell populations, such as the brainstem. Such outcomes could explain the limited brain lesions at death in cases with short disease duration. How these data fit the hypothesis that prion propagation and toxicity stages are uncoupled and that neurotoxic and propagating PrP^{TSE} species are distinct is unclear (Sandberg et al., 2011). Although quantitative data indicate that in FFI resPrP^{TSE} reaches a plateau in the thalamus, they suggest that, at least in the cortex, metabolic and structural damage occur while propagation is still ongoing. Should this be the case, propagation and toxic phases would be concurrent rather than uncoupled.

SPORADIC FATAL INSOMNIA

Introduction

Sporadic Fatal Insomnia (sFI) shares many clinical and histopathologic features with FFI, to such an extent that it may be defined as a FFI phenocopy, hence its sporadic form. However, the sFI clinical and histopathologic phenotype appears to be more variable than that of the FFI variant linked to the 129 homozygous genotype. This outcome is predictable since the specific FFI mutation D178N is likely to impose more constraints on the initial spontaneous conversion to a prion-like conformation of the mutated PrP compared to the presumably idiopathic conversion and subsequent selection process of wild-type PrP (Collinge and Clarke, 2007; Collinge, 2010; Li et al., 2010; Imberdis and Harris, 2016). Although the phenotypic similarities to FFI outweigh the features shared with any of the sCJD subtypes, also after experimental transmission (Mastrianni et al., 1999; Krasnianski et al., 2014), sFI is often referred to as the thalamic form of sCJDMM2 (Moda et al., 2012; Parchi and Saverioni, 2012; Hayashi et al., 2015; Iwasaki, 2017).

Epidemiology

Thirty-two individual cases of sFI, examined at autopsy and proven to harbor PrP^{TSE}, have been reported worldwide to date. Japan contributed 13 cases, the United States 12, Italy 4, Spain 2, and the United Kingdom 1. In all but 1 case, the presence of resPrP^{TSE} was also proven by Western blot, which showed resPrP^{TSE} type 2 in 29 cases and type 1 and type 1+2 in 1 case each. Based on type, degree, and distribution of tissue lesions along with the resPrP^{TSE} features, sFI-affected subjects have been segregated as typical and atypical (Table 15.5).

The 25 cases classified as typical showed a consistently severe thalamic and olivary atrophy, while spongiform degeneration varied widely in severity and could be lacking. resPrP^{TSE} type 2 was reported in all cases but 1, where presence of PrP^{TSE} was demonstrated by immunohistochemistry (Scaravilli et al., 2000). Grau-Rivera et al. (2016) and Hamaguchi et al. (2005) and their colleagues defined two of their cases as a mix of sCJDMM2-thalamic (sCJDMM2T) and -cortical (sCJDMM2C) forms, essentially based on the presence of widespread spongiform degeneration similar to that of sCJDMM2 (Table 15.5, Hamaguchi et al., case 3, 2005; Grau-Rivera et al., 2016). Eleven of the typical cases were from the United States, 9 from Japan, 3 from Italy, and 1 from Spain and the United Kingdom.

Seven cases were defined as atypical for several reasons, including: (1) inadequate evidence supporting the predominance of the thalamic and olivary atrophy with presence of resPrP^{TSE} predominantly of type 1 in 1 case

Table 15.5

Published cases of sFI listed in order of disease duration with semiquantitative estimates of tissue lesions and segregated into typical and atypical forms[a]

		Spongiform degeneration			Neuronal depletion and astrogliosis					PrP^{TSE}
Reference (case #)	Course (months)	NeoCort.	NeoStriat.	Cerebel.	NeoCort.	NeoStriat.	Cerebel.	Med.Thal. N.	Olive	IHC
Typical										
Cracco et al. (2017) (2)	**12**	0	0	0	0	1	2.5	3.5	3.5	0
Hamaguchi et al. (2005) (8)	**13**	0	NA	NA	NA	2	1.5	3	3	0
Hamaguchi et al. (2005),[f] (3)	**14**	3	NA	NA	NA	2	1.5	3	3	3
Parchi et al. (1999a) (2)	**15**	1	0	0	0	0	1[e]	3	3	0
Parchi et al. (1999a) (4)	**15**	1	0	0	0.5	0	0.5[e]	2.5	2.5	0
Mastrianni et al. (1999)	**16**	0	0	0	NA	1.5	2	3	3	NA
Hayashi et al. (2015)	**16**	1	NA	0	0	0	1	3	3	1
Parchi et al. (1999a) (5)	**17**	1	0	0	0.5	0	0.5[e]	3	2	1.5
Parchi et al. (1999a) (1)	**18**	1	0	0	0.5	0.5	2[e]	3	3	1.5
Moody et al. (2011)	**22**	2	1	1	2	1	1	3	3	3
Parchi et al. (1999a) (3)	**24**	1	0	0	0.5	0.5	1[e]	3	3	2
Capellari et al. (2008)	**24**	2	0	0	NA	NA	NA	3	3	NA
Grau-Rivera et al. (2016)[f]	**24**	2	0	0	NA	NA	2	3	3	2
Hamaguchi et al. (2005) (7)	**25**	2	NA	NA	NA	2	1.5	3	3	2
Cracco et al. (2017) (1)	**25**	1	1	0	0.5	0.5	1	3.5	3.5	2
Cracco et al. (2017) (3)	**25**	1	0	0	0	1	2	3.5	2.5	1.5
Moda et al. (2012) (2)	**26**	2.5	NA	1	2	2	2	3	3	3
Scaravilli et al. (2000)[h]	**27**	0	0	0	2	2	2	3	3	2
Moda et al. (2012) (1)	**28**	2	NA	2	2	NA	2	3	3	1.5
Hamaguchi et al. (2005) (4)	**30**	2	NA	NA	NA	2	1.5	3	3	2
Iwasaki et al. (2006) (21)	**30**	3[c]	NA	2	1	NA	2	3	3	3
Iwasaki et al. (2006) (22)	**32**	3[d]	NA	2	1	NA	2	3	3	3
Blase et al. (2014)	**35**	2.5	NA	NA	1	NA	NA	3	3	2
Kawasaki et al. (1997)[i]	**53**	2.5	2	0	2[b]	2	2	3	3	0
Yamashita et al. (2001)[j]	**73**	2	0	0	2	2	1	4	3	2.5

Atypical[k]		Atypical neuropathologic features
Iwasaki et al. (2017)[g]	**5**	SD with "moderate" neuronal loss and reactive astrogliosis in medial thalamus. $resPrP^{TSE}$ type 1–2 with 1 > 2
Priano et al. (2009)	**10**	Status post intraventricular catheter insertion; severe neuronal loss also in neostriatum; $resPrP^{TSE}$ type 1
Mehta et al. (2008)	**18**	Severe cerebellar atrophy
Fernández-Vega et al. (2015)	**27**	Inadequate documentation of predominant thalamic-olivary neuronal loss and astrogliosis without SD
Piao et al. (2005)	**29**	SD with relative preservation of neurons in mediodorsal thalamic nucleus
Hirose et al. (2006)	**30**	Significant parenchymal rarefaction with macrophage presence in "medial thalamic nucleus"
Saito et al. (2011)[f]	**32**	"Severe" parenchymal rarefaction with macrophage proliferation in "medial thalamus"

[a]Semiquantitative estimates are based on the interpretation of descriptions and/or microphotographs provided in the individual publications.
[b]Ballooned neurons.
[c]Fine vacuoles.
[d]Mixed large and small vacuoles.
[e]Torpedoes.
[f,g]Defined as sCJDMM2-cortical + thalamic-type and sCJDMM1 + MM2 cortical with thalamic-type mixed form, respectively, in the original publications.
[h]South African subject diagnosed in the United Kingdom.
[i]Hamaguchi et al., case 5, 2005.
[j]Hamaguchi et al., case 6, 2005.
[k]Cases not used because considered atypical or not adequately documented.
SD and atrophy grading: 0 = none; 1 = minimal; 2 = mild or focal; 3 = severe or widespread; 4 = individual affected nuclei no longer recognizable because of very severe atrophy.
Cerebel: cerebellum; IHC: immunostaining/immunohistochemistry; Med.Thal.N: medial thalamic nuclei; NA: not applicable; NeoCort: neocortex; NeoStriat: neostriatum; PrP^{TSE}: abnormal prion protein; $resPrP^{TSE}$: portion of abnormal prion protein resistant to proteinase K digestion; SD: spongiform degeneration.

(Piao et al., 2005; Fernández-Vega et al., 2015; Iwasaki et al., 2017); (2) occurrence of potentially causative other pathologies along with resPrP^{TSE} type 1 (Priano et al., 2009); (3) co-occurrence of severe cerebellar atrophy of undetermined cause (Mehta et al., 2008); and (4) atypical thalamic atrophy with presence of macrophages (Hirose et al., 2006; Saito et al., 2011) (Table 15.5). Western blot analysis demonstrated the presence of type 2 resPrP^{TSE} in 5 cases, while type 1 and type 1+2 resPrP^{TSE} were found in 2 cases. Four cases were from Japan, and 1 each from Italy, Spain, and the United States.

The National Prion Disease Pathology Surveillance Center acquired 33 cases of sFI (21 unpublished) from 1997 to date, which would account for 0.9% of all cases of sporadic human prion diseases (http://case.edu/med/pathology/centers/npdpsc/pdf/web-table.pdf; reviewed on 16 Feb. 2018).

Clinical features

Signs and symptoms

Many symptoms of sFI overlap with those observed in FFI. Most patients present with cognitive decline and/or ataxia (42%), while 29% have insomnia at presentation (Puoti et al., 2012) (Table 15.6). At later stages, cognitive impairment, ataxia, insomnia and/or psychiatric symptoms, and myoclonus are common. Similar to FFI, many patients experience psychomotor hyperactivity and autonomic dysfunction (Sikorska and Liberski, 2012). Despite its name, insomnia has not been a prominent symptom in many cases of sFI unless it is specifically investigated with the patient and family members (Moda et al., 2012). Symptoms observed in atypical parkinsonian syndromes, such as oculomotor symptoms, dyskinesia, and parkinsonism, are often present in sFI at presentation (Parchi et al., 1999b; Cracco et al., 2017).

Table 15.6

Clinical characteristics of sporadic fatal insomnia

Age at onset (years)	Mean = 46 (range = 13–74)
Disease duration (months)	Mean = 24 (10–73)
Common symptoms	Sleep disturbance, cognitive impairment, psychiatric symptoms, ataxia, myoclonus
Polysomnogram	Reduction in sleep spindles, K-complexes, slow-wave sleep, REM sleep, and total sleep time
Electroencephalogram	Generalized slowing without periodic sharp-wave complexes
CSF biomarkers	14-3-3 and tau are usually negative, RT-QuIC is positive in about half of cases
Brain MRI	Hyperintensity on diffusion-weighted imaging typically absent, but has been reported in some cases
Brain FDG-PET/ SPECT	Early thalamic hypometabolism or hypoperfusion that may spread to other areas of the brain as disease progresses

CSF, cerebrospinal fluid; FDG-PET, fluorodeoxyglucose positron emission tomography; MRI, magnetic resonance imaging; REM, rapid eye movement; RT-QuIC, real-time quaking-induced conversion; SPECT, single-photon emission computed tomography.

Differential diagnosis

The differential diagnosis of sFI is similar to that of FFI. Treatable etiologies such as autoimmune encephalitis and paraneoplastic syndromes should always be considered (Mehta et al., 2008; Marques et al., 2014). Atypical movement disorders such as progressive supranuclear palsy and spinocerebellar degeneration should also be considered in addition to degenerative dementias like frontotemporal lobar degeneration and Alzheimer's disease (Hamaguchi et al., 2005; Hirose et al., 2006; Hayashi et al., 2016). We propose diagnostic clinical criteria in Table 15.7.

Table 15.7

Proposed clinical criteria for sporadic fatal insomnia (must meet A through D)

A. Symptoms (must meet 1 through 3)	1. Cognitive impairment 2. Sleep disturbance and/or psychiatric symptoms 3. Two or more typical CJD symptoms: (a) Ataxia or dysarthria (b) Visual changes (c) Pyramidal symptoms (d) Extrapyramidal symptoms (e) Myoclonus
B. Diagnostic test results (one or more)	1. Reduced sleep architecture (e.g., sleep spindles, K-complexes) on polysomnogram 2. Thalamic hypometabolism on brain FDG-PET 3. Thalamic hypoperfusion on brain SPECT
C. Lack of alternative etiology	
D. Negative for *PRNP* mutation	

CJD, Creutzfeldt–Jakob disease; FDG-PET, fluorodeoxyglucose positron emission tomography; SPECT, single-photon emission computed tomography.

Diagnostic tests

Polysomnography and electroencephalography

PSG and EEG features in sFI mimic those observed in FFI. PSG recordings are generally indistinguishable in the two diseases, which are characterized by the reduction of sleep-related EEG activities like K complexes and sleep spindles (Gambetti et al., 2003a). Importantly, all 8 sFI cases with PSG data reported in the literature demonstrated findings similar to FFI (Scaravilli et al., 2000; Capellari et al., 2008; Priano et al., 2009; Puoti et al., 2012; Grau-Rivera et al., 2016; Megelin et al., 2017). EEGs demonstrate nonspecific slowing without the PSWCs seen in CJD (Parchi et al., 1999b).

CSF markers

Elevated 14-3-3 protein levels are rarely found in sFI (Hamaguchi et al., 2005). The sensitivity of 14-3-3 with tau in sFI is about 8% (Puoti et al., 2012). RT-QuIC has been positive in four of eight reported sFI cases (Foutz et al., 2017; Lattanzio et al., 2017; Franceschini et al., 2017).

Neuroimaging

Similar to FFI, typical sCJD MRI findings are not often observed in sFI (Hamaguchi et al., 2005). Diffusion-weighted imaging hyperintensity has been reported in 8% of cases in one study (Puoti et al., 2012), while some cases exhibited cortical and cerebellar atrophy (Mehta et al., 2008). Brain FDG-PET and SPECT imaging typically show hypometabolism or hypoperfusion in the thalami and cerebral cortex (Hamaguchi et al., 2005; Hayashi et al., 2015).

Neuropathology

Typical cases

A review of the 32 cases published since the first report in 1997 indicates that currently the histopathologic diagnosis of sFI typically rests on four basic features: (1) severe depletion of neurons accompanied by marked astroglial reaction in thalamic nuclei, especially the anterior, medial dorsal, and pulvinar, with no associated spongiform degeneration; (2) variable atrophy of the inferior olives; (3) presence of PrP^{TSE} of type 2A; and (4) exclusion of pathogenic mutations in the PrP gene (Table 15.5). The thalamic atrophy consists of profound loss of neurons with robust astroglial reaction (Fig. 15.3C). The severity of the neuronal depopulation in the absence of spongiform degeneration in the thalamus distinguishes sFI from the generally mild neuronal loss with spongiform degeneration often observed in sCJD subtypes. Furthermore, the neuropil of the affected thalamic nuclei, neuronal depletion and reactive gliosis notwithstanding, is remarkably well preserved and compact, possibly because of relative preservation of crossing fibers as in FFI (Lugaresi et al., 1986). Besides lacking spongiform degeneration, atrophic thalamic nuclei should neither show conspicuous rarefaction nor contain a significant number of macrophages. The neuronal depletion and astrogliosis of the inferior olive are more variable and moderate atrophy has been reported (cases 4 and 5 of Parchi et al., 1999a; case 3 of Cracco et al., 2017).

Spongiform degeneration is not a required component but is observed to a variable extent in the majority of the cases (21 of 25 typical cases). It most often affects the cerebral neocortex and entorhinal cortex and is frequently formed by large and confluent vacuoles like those associated with sCJDMM2 (Fig. 15.6A) (Grau-Rivera et al., 2016). However, spongiform degeneration made of fine vacuoles has also been occasionally reported (Moody et al., 2011). To a lesser degree, spongiform degeneration may be found in the molecular layer of the cerebellum and in the neostriatum. Ballooned neurons have also been observed (Kawasaki et al., 1997).

The proof of PrP^{TSE} presence is critical since non-prion conditions mimicking sFI and FFI have been reported under the label of thalamic dementias (Petersen et al., 1992; Kovacs et al., 2013). In 18 of the 23 typical sFI cases in which it was tested, PrP^{TSE} presence was demonstrated by immunohistochemistry. Positive PrP immunostaining is favored by the presence of spongiform degeneration. In locations free of spongiform degeneration, PrP immunostaining may be inconspicuous, limited to a few foci often in subpial cortical regions forming a punctate or synaptic pattern with occasional presence of small polymorphic aggregates similar to those observed in FFI (Fig. 15.4A) (Moda et al., 2012; Blase et al., 2014). In the presence of spongiform degeneration, the immunostaining pattern mimics that of sCJDMM2 and exhibits perivacuolar deposition and aggregate formation, as well as plaque-like pattern in the cerebellum (Fig. 15.6B) (Parchi et al., 1999a; Blase et al., 2014). The staining pattern is punctate or "synaptic" in the presence of spongiform degeneration with fine vacuoles. Both atrophic thalamic nuclei and inferior olives immunostain weakly or not at all. Immunostains for activated astrocytes and microglia are also positive (Moda et al., 2012). The review of the 25 typical cases of various disease duration seems to support a direct relation between severity of spongiform degeneration and disease duration (Table 15.5).

Two cases harboring typical thalamic and olivary pathology have been labeled by the authors as mixed

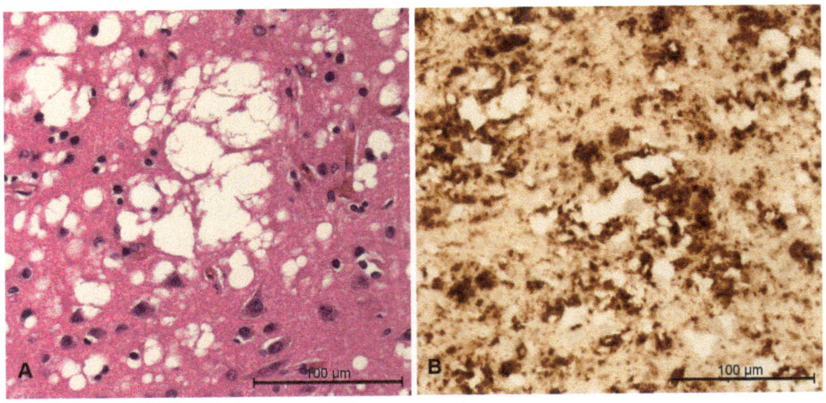

Fig. 15.6. Microphotographs of sporadic fatal insomnia (sFI) cerebral cortex. (**A**) Considerable spongiform degeneration with large, clustered vacuoles, which strongly immunostain with an antibody to PrP (**B**); both spongiform degeneration and immunostaining pattern are similar to those of sporadic Creutzfeldt–Jakob disease MM2. (**A**) Hematoxylin and eosin; (**B**) Antibody to PrP 3F4.

form of sFI (identified as sCJDMM2T) and sCJDMM2 (identified as sCJDMM2C) based on the presence of abundant spongiform degeneration (Hamaguchi et al., case 3, 2005; Grau-Rivera et al., 2016). Grau-Rivera and colleagues (2016) refer to the spongiform degeneration in their descriptions and illustrations as focal, Hamaguchi and colleagues (2005) as marked. A "mixed sCJDMM2C-T" case is also mentioned by Parchi et al. (2009). However, presence of "moderate," "significant," and "severe" spongiform degeneration has been reported in several sFI cases considered to be typical (Parchi et al., 1999a; Moda et al., 2012; Blase et al., 2014). Validation of an sFI variant based on the extent of spongiform degeneration seems premature without quantitative assessment of spongiform degeneration or rigorous comparative studies of PrP^{TSE} characteristics in typical and mixed sFI variants (also see below).

Disease-associated prion protein

General characteristics

The $resPrP^{TSE}$ conformer associated with sFI is commonly defined as type 2A, where the 2 indicates the electrophoretic relative mass of 19 kDa of the unglycosylated $resPrP^{TSE}$ form, and A identifies a ratio of the three PrP^{TSE} glycoforms distinguished by overrepresentation of the monoglycosylated form (Parchi et al., 1997; Cracco et al., 2017). The amount of $resPrP^{TSE}$ in sFI can be very low, requiring efficient electrophoretic and immunoblotting procedures. Studies of $resPrP^{TSE}$ amounts and brain distribution reveal great similarity with FFI (Fig. 15.5A) (Parchi et al., 2000a). The cerebral neocortices (occipital cortex excluded), entorhinal cortex, and hypothalamus are regions that yield relatively higher amounts, the MD and A thalamic nuclei show intermediate amounts, while the occipital cortex and cerebellum display the lowest (Parchi et al., 1999a, 2000a). A very large recovery of $resPrP^{TSE}$ from the thalamus has also been reported (Mastrianni et al., 1999). On ordinary immunoblotting, $resPrP^{TSE}$ differs in sFI and FFI only in the glycoform ratio that in FFI is characterized by overrepresentation of the diglycosylated form (ratio B) (Parchi et al., 1999a).

Distinctive features

The well-established finding that sFI and sCJDMM2 share the 129MM genotype and PrP^{TSE} type, but have quite different disease phenotypes, challenges the hypothesis that the pairing of 129 genotype and PrP^{TSE} type is the determinant of PrP^{TSE} conformational properties or strain, which then shapes the phenotype in sporadic prion diseases (Parchi et al., 1999b; Gambetti et al., 2003a, 2011). A detailed comparative study employing several conformational tests has demonstrated major variations between sFI and sCJDMM2 PrP^{TSE} species, affecting almost exclusively the detergent-insoluble but PK-sensitive component of total PrP^{TSE} (Cracco et al., 2017). Properties of this component, including glycoform ratios, two-dimensional electrophoretic profiles, and aggregation patterns, differ in the two diseases (Fig. 15.7). In contrast, the higher stability in sFI was the only significant variation between the two diseases uncovered for $resPrP^{TSE}$ (Cracco et al., 2017), but not by Cescatti et al. (Cescatti et al., 2016); however, the latter authors were unable to detect significant conformational diversity even between PrP^{TSE} associated to sCJDMM1 and sCJDMM2 by conformational stability assay while PrP^{TSE} type 1 and 2

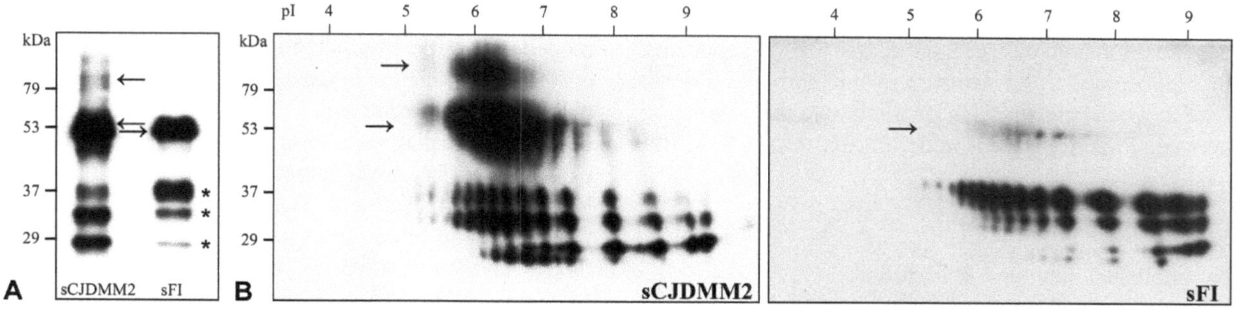

Fig. 15.7. One- and two-dimensional (1-D and 2-D) immunoblots of full-length total PrP^{TSE} immunoprecipitated from sporadic Creutzfeldt–Jakob disease MM2 (sCJDMM2) and sporadic fatal insomnia (sFI). (**A**) The 1-D immunoblot shows high-molecular-weight bands (arrows) especially prominent in sCJDMM2 preparations, in addition to the three typical PrP^{TSE} glycoforms (*) that differ in the two diseases. (**B**) In 2-D immunoblots, spots corresponding to the high-molecular-weight PrP^{TSE} components are dramatically represented in sCJDMM2 and barely detectable in sFI (arrows); glycoform ratios, number of spots, and isoelectric points differ between sCJDMM2 and sFI total PrP^{TSE} (see Cracco et al., 2017, for details). Immunoprecipitation was carried out upon sodium phosphotungstate precipitation with the antibody 8B4 to PrP N-terminus (Li et al., 2000). (Modified from Cracco L, Notari S, Cali I, et al. (2017) Novel strain properties distinguishing sporadic prion diseases sharing prion protein genotype and prion type. Sci Rep 7: 38280.)

diversity has been confirmed by various methods in several studies (Cali et al., 2009; Pirisinu et al., 2010; Kim et al., 2011; Safar et al., 2015). Combined, all these findings support the notion that sFI and sCJDMM2 harbor distinct prion strains even though they share the 129 genotype and PrP^{TSE} type, and that the diversity resides predominantly in the PK-sensitive component of PrP^{TSE}. Similar conclusions were reached in another study, although using different procedures (Saverioni et al., 2013).

Experimental animal transmission and *in vitro* amplification

Experimental animal transmission

Mastrianni et al. (1999) and Korth and colleagues (2003) have transmitted sFI and FFI to two lines of Tg chimeric mice expressing the murine PrP harboring the human PrP 96-167 sequence either intact or following the insertion of mouse PrP residues 165V and 167 glutamine (167Q). A third Tg line expressing human PrP129M was also used. All Tg mice of the first line became symptomatic 180 and 221 days after being inoculated with sFI thalamus and cerebral cortex extracts, respectively (Mastrianni et al., 1999). Spongiform degeneration and reactive astrogliosis were most prominent in the thalamus and deep cerebral neocortex (Mastrianni et al., 1999). On histoblots, $resPrP^{TSE}$ was observed mostly in the thalamus, and immunoblots demonstrated $resPrP^{TSE}$ type 2 (Mastrianni et al., 1999; Korth et al., 2003). Furthermore, all these findings matched those obtained from the same Tg lines following inoculation with FFI brain extracts (Telling et al., 1996; Korth et al., 2003). Remarkably, comparative analysis of the incubation among the different Tg lines following inoculation of brain extracts from several human prion diseases showed that FFI and sFI maintained the same pattern of incubation periods, which diverged from those of sporadic prion diseases, including sCJDMM2 (Korth et al., 2003). Combined, these findings indicate that prion strains associated with sFI and FFI are similar and differ from the sCJDMM2 strain (Mastrianni et al., 1999; Korth et al., 2003).

A knock-in murine/human chimeric mouse expressing human PrP with mouse PrP residues at the C-terminus (region 215–231) was used by Taguchi et al. (2003) to transmit sFI (identified as MM2-T-sCJD), using frontal cortex extracts from 2 sFI cases along with additional subtypes of sporadic and familial prion diseases. After 386–575-day incubation periods, 3 of the 11 sFI inoculated Tg mice exhibited widespread punctate or granular PrP^{TSE} deposits codistributed with spongiform degeneration that were shared by Tg mice challenged with other prion disease tissues. However, sFI-inoculated mice, unlike other mice, harbored typical $resPrP^{TSE}$ type 2.

Moda and coworkers (2012) have used the intracerebral and intraperitoneal route combined to inoculate cerebral cortex extracts from their case 2 of sFI (identified as MM2-thalamic sCJD) (Table 15.5) and one of sCJDMM2 (MM2-cortical sCJD) to gene-targeted Tg mice expressing human PrP-129M. Major variations emerged between sFI- and sCJDMM2-challenged Tg mice: sFI-mice developed neurologic signs 535 days after inoculation with a 93% attack rate and succumbed at 557 days, whereas sCJDMM2-mice remained asymptomatic up to 650 days post inoculation. Furthermore, while no pathology nor PrP^{TSE} was demonstrated in the sCJDMM2-mice, the sFI-mice showed spongiform degeneration with punctate and coarse PrP^{TSE} deposition in hippocampus and neocortex, and harbored PrP^{TSE} type 2. These transmission data reiterate the distinction between the prion strains underling sFI and sCJDMM2.

In vitro amplification

No published data have been found.

Pathogenetic hypothesis

In inherited diseases, the presence of pathogenic mutations establishes a firm etiology that helps understand the pathogenic events leading to the disease phenotype. In sporadic diseases, the process is much more challenging, as data on the "spontaneous" initial formation of PrP^{TSE} are limited. Current hypotheses on formation and selection of pathogenic prion strains posit the initial formation of a spectrum of conformers, which then undergo a selection leading to the predominance of a single strain (Collinge, 2010; Weissmann et al., 2011; Makarava et al., 2016). However, the selection process may occasionally vary, allowing the selection of a rarer strain (Collinge and Clarke, 2007; Collinge, 2010; Surewicz and Apostol, 2011; Gambetti, 2013). In sporadic prion diseases affecting 129MM homozygotes, approximately 86% of the cases are exclusively or predominantly associated with PrP^{TSE} type 1 and develop an sCJDMM1 phenotype, while the remaining 14% of cases harboring PrP^{TSE} type 2 segregate as approximately 12% sCJDMM2 and 1–2% sFI (Collins et al., 2006; Cracco et al., 2017) (unpublished data). Applying notions of strain formation to sporadic human prion diseases, it has been speculated that the 129MM genotype strongly favors selection of the PrP^{TSE} type 1 conformer while type 2 would be the result of a variant selection. It is conceivable that the PrP^{TSE} type 2 selection leads to the common emergence of PrP^{TSE} of the sCJDMM2 strain and rarely to the PrP^{TSE} strain linked to sFI, which must bear considerable similarities with the FFI strain (Cracco et al., 2017). This scenario might help explain the rarity and distinctive features of sFI compared to other sporadic prion diseases.

CONCLUSIONS AND FUTURE DEVELOPMENTS

FFI and sFI have well-established genetic, clinical, and histopathologic features. Basic biochemical characteristics of the mutated PrP and of the disease-associated PrP (PrP^{TSE}), including propensity to transmit experimentally and the features of the transmitted disease, have also been examined. However, FFI and sFI, as with other neurodegenerative diseases, suffer from the lack of an accurate animal model and an effective treatment. Accurate disease modeling is critical to determine the mode and locale of onset and propagation of the disease process at the molecular level. As for treatment, a first step is the development of noninvasive diagnostic tests that are reliable even at the early and possibly presymptomatic stages of the disease. It is conceivable that current diagnostic tests based on amplification of molecular amounts of PrP^{TSE} in peripheral tissues and body fluids (Moda et al., 2014; Concha-Marambio et al., 2016; Bongianni et al., 2017; Orrú et al., 2017), along with PET or SPECT, could be further refined and made widely acceptable. Treatments, which have been tested experimentally with limited success and new ones being developed, are likely to be more effective in stopping the disease process if applied at early or preclinical disease stages, as demonstrated experimentally following intraperitoneal infection (Sigurdsson et al., 2003). The development of more effective drugs combined with routine early diagnosis might deliver effective treatments to prion and other neurodegenerative diseases in the not too distant future.

ACKNOWLEDGMENTS

We are grateful to Drs. Mark Cohen (National Prion Disease Pathology Surveillance Center (NPDPSC), Case Western Reserve University, United States), Pietro Cortelli (University of Bologna, Italy), Xiao-Ping Dong (Chinese Center for Disease Control and Prevention, China), Jorge Iriarte (University of Navarra, Spain), Yi Li (Shandong University, China), Piero Parchi (University of Bologna, Italy), and Robert G. Will (University of Edinburgh, United Kingdom) for their invaluable cooperation. We also thank Dr. Ignazio Cali (Case Western Reserve University, United States) and the NPDPSC (Case Western Reserve University, United States), especially mses. Katie Glisic, Diane Kofskey, Miriam Warren, and Mr. Aaron Foutz provided skillful technical assistance.

This review was supported by National Institutes of Health Grants R01 NS083687 and P01 AI106705, and The Charles S. Britton Fund (to PG).

References

Almer G, Hainfellner JA, Brucke T et al. (1999). Fatal familial insomnia: a new Austrian family. Brain 122: 5–16.

Alonso DO, DeArmond SJ, Cohen FE et al. (2001). Mapping the early steps in the pH-induced conformational conversion of the prion protein. Proc Natl Acad Sci U S A 98: 2985–2989.

Apetri AC, Vanik DL, Surewicz WK (2005). Polymorphism at residue 129 modulates the conformational conversion of the D178N variant of human prion protein 90–231. Biochemistry 44: 15880–15888.

Appleby BS, Appleby KK, Hall RC et al. (2010). D178N, 129Val and N171S, 129Val genotype in a family with Creutzfeldt–Jakob disease. Dement Geriatr Cogn Disord 30: 424–431.

Ashok A, Hegde RS (2009). Selective processing and metabolism of disease-causing mutant prion proteins. PLoS Pathog 5: e1000479.

Baldin E, Capellari S, Provini F et al. (2009). A case of fatal familial insomnia in Africa. J Neurol 256: 1778–1779.

Bär KJ, Häger F, Nenadic I et al. (2002). Serial positron emission tomographic findings in an atypical presentation of fatal familial insomnia. Arch Neurol 59: 1815–1818.

Barria MA, Peden AH, Knight RS et al. (2014). Amplification of PrPSc from fatal familial insomnia brain tissue using wild-type human PrPC brain substrate. Prion 8: 113.

Blase JL, Cracco L, Schonberger LB et al. (2014). Sporadic fatal insomnia in an adolescent. Pediatrics 133: e766–770.

Bongianni M, Orru C, Groveman BR et al. (2017). Diagnosis of human prion disease using real-time quaking-induced conversion testing of olfactory mucosa and cerebrospinal fluid samples. JAMA Neurol 74: 155–162.

Borchelt DR, Scott M, Taraboulos A et al. (1990). Scrapie and cellular prion proteins differ in their kinetics of synthesis and topology in cultured cells. J Cell Biol 110: 743–752.

Bosque PJ, Vnencak-Jones CL, Johnson MD et al. (1992). A PrP gene codon 178 base substitution and a 24-bp interstitial deletion in familial Creutzfeldt–Jakob disease. Neurology 42: 1864–1870.

Bouybayoune I, Mantovani S, Del Gallo F et al. (2015). Transgenic fatal familial insomnia mice indicate prion infectivity-independent mechanisms of pathogenesis and phenotypic expression of disease. PLoS Pathog 11: e1004796.

Brown P, Goldfarb LG, Kovanen J et al. (1992). Phenotypic characteristics of familial Creutzfeldt–Jakob disease associated with the codon 178Asn PRNP mutation. Ann Neurol 31: 282–285.

Brown P, Gibbs Jr CJ, Rodgers-Johnson P et al. (1994). Human spongiform encephalopathy: the National Institutes of Health series of 300 cases of experimentally transmitted disease. Ann Neurol 35: 513–529.

Brown P, Kenney K, Little B et al. (1995). Intracerebral distribution of infectious amyloid protein in spongiform encephalopathy. Ann Neurol 38: 245–253.

Brown P, Cervenakova L, Powers JM (1998). FFI cases from the United States, Australia, and Japan. Brain Pathol 8: 567–570.

Cali I, Castellani R, Alshekhlee A et al. (2009). Co-existence of scrapie prion protein types 1 and 2 in sporadic Creutzfeldt-Jakob disease: its effect on the phenotype and prion-type characteristics. Brain 132: 2643–2658.

Capellari S, Parchi P, Cortelli P et al. (2008). Sporadic fatal insomnia in a fatal familial insomnia pedigree. Neurology 70: 884–885.

Casas-Mendez LF, Lujan M, Vigil L et al. (2011). Biot's breathing in a woman with fatal familial insomnia: is there a role for noninvasive ventilation? J Clin Sleep Med 7: 89–91.

Caughey B, Race RE, Ernst D et al. (1989). Prion protein biosynthesis in scrapie-infected and uninfected neuroblastoma cells. J Virol 63: 175–181.

Cescatti M, Saverioni D, Capellari S et al. (2016). Analysis of conformational stability of abnormal prion protein aggregates across the spectrum of Creutzfeldt-Jakob disease prions. J Virol 90: 6244–6254.

Chang FC, Berman Y, Buckland ME et al. (2011). Genetic prion disease-associated myelodysplasia and SIADH in siblings. Eur J Neurol 18: e149–150.

Chapman J, Ben-Israel J, Goldhammer Y et al. (1994). The risk of developing Creutzfeldt–Jakob disease in subjects with the PRNP gene codon 200 point mutation. Neurology 44: 1683–1686.

Chen SG, Parchi P, Brown P et al. (1997). Allelic origin of the abnormal prion protein isoform in familial prion diseases. Nat Med 3: 1009–1015.

Chen C, Wang JC, Shi Q et al. (2013). Analyses of the survival time and the influencing factors of chinese patients with prion diseases based on the surveillance data from 2008-2011. PLoS One 8: e62553.

Chen S, He S, Shi XH et al. (2018). The clinical features in Chinese patients with PRNP D178N mutation. Acta Neurol Scand. PMID: 29569252. https://doi.org/10.1111/ane.12924.

Chiesa R, Restelli E, Comerio L et al. (2016). Transgenic mice recapitulate the phenotypic heterogeneity of genetic prion diseases without developing prion infectivity: role of intracellular PrP retention in neurotoxicity. Prion 10: 93–102.

Choi BY, Kim SY, Seo SY et al. (2009). Mutations at codons 178, 200-129, and 232 contributed to the inherited prion diseases in Korean patients. BMC Infect Dis 9: 132.

Collinge J (2010). Medicine. Prion strain mutation and selection Science 328: 1111–1112.

Collinge J, Clarke AR (2007). A general model of prion strains and their pathogenicity. Science 318: 930–936.

Collinge J, Palmer MS, Sidle KC et al. (1995). Transmission of fatal familial insomnia to laboratory animals. Lancet 346: 569–570.

Collins SJ, Sanchez-Juan P, Masters CL et al. (2006). Determinants of diagnostic investigation sensitivities across the clinical spectrum of sporadic Creutzfeldt–Jakob disease. Brain 129: 2278–2287.

Colombier C, Geraud G, Delisle MB et al. (1997). Fatal familial insomnia: phenotypic changes determined by polymorphism of the codon 129. Rev Neurol (Paris) 153: 239–243.

Concha-Marambio L, Pritzkow S, Moda F et al. (2016). Detection of prions in blood from patients with variant Creutzfeldt–Jakob disease. Sci Transl Med 8: 370ra183.

Cortelli P, Parchi P, Contin M et al. (1991). Cardiovascular dysautonomia in fatal familial insomnia. Clin Auton Res 1: 15–21.

Cortelli P, Perani D, Parchi P et al. (1997). Cerebral metabolism in fatal familial insomnia: relation to duration, neuropathology, and distribution of protease-resistant prion protein. Neurology 49: 126–133.

Cortelli P, Perani D, Montagna P et al. (2006). Presymptomatic diagnosis in fatal familial insomnia: serial neurophysiological and 18FDG-PET studies. Brain 129: 668–675.

Cortelli P, Fabbri M, Calandra-Buonaura G et al. (2014). Gait disorders in fatal familial insomnia. Mov Disord 29: 420–424.

Cracco L, Notari S, Cali I et al. (2017). Novel strain properties distinguishing sporadic prion diseases sharing prion protein genotype and prion type. Sci Rep 7: 38280.

Cramm M, Schmitz M, Karch A et al. (2015). Characteristic CSF prion seeding efficiency in humans with prion diseases. Mol Neurobiol 51: 396–405.

Dagvadorj A, Petersen RB, Lee HS et al. (2002). Spontaneous mutations in the prion protein gene causing transmissible spongiform encephalopathy. Ann Neurol 52: 355–359.

Dauvilliers Y, Cervena K, Carlander B et al. (2004). Dissociation in circadian rhythms in a pseudohypersomnia form of fatal familial insomnia. Neurology 63: 2416–2418.

Dimitri D, Jehel L, Durr A et al. (2006). Fatal familial insomnia presenting as psychosis in an 18-year-old man. Neurology 67: 363–364.

Dorandeu A, Wingertsmann L, Chretien F et al. (1998). Neuronal apoptosis in fatal familial insomnia. Brain Pathol 8: 531–537.

Dossena S, Imeri L, Mangieri M et al. (2008). Mutant prion protein expression causes motor and memory deficits and abnormal sleep patterns in a transgenic mouse model. Neuron 60: 598–609.

Drisaldi B, Stewart RS, Adles C et al. (2003). Mutant PrP is delayed in its exit from the endoplasmic reticulum, but neither wild-type nor mutant PrP undergoes retrotranslocation prior to proteasomal degradation. J Biol Chem 278: 21732–21743.

Dubnikov T, Cohen E (2017). The emerging roles of early protein folding events in the secretory pathway in the development of neurodegenerative maladies. Front Neurosci 11: 48.

Elezgarai SR, Fernandez-Borges N, Erana H et al. (2017). Generation of a new infectious recombinant prion: a model to understand Gerstmann-Straussler-Scheinker syndrome. Sci Rep 7: 9584.

Fernández-Vega I, Ruiz-Ojeda J, Juste RA et al. (2015). Coexistence of mixed phenotype Creutzfeldt–Jakob disease, Lewy body disease and argyrophilic grain disease plus histological features of possible Alzheimer's disease: a multi-protein disorder in an autopsy case. Neuropathology 35: 56–63.

Ferrillo F, Plazzi G, Nobili L et al. (2001). Absence of sleep EEG markers in fatal familial insomnia healthy carriers: a spectral analysis study. Clin Neurophysiol 112: 1888–1892.

Fioriti L, Dossena S, Stewart LR et al. (2005). Cytosolic prion protein (PrP) is not toxic in N2a cells and primary neurons expressing pathogenic PrP mutations. J Biol Chem 280: 11320–11328.

Forloni G, Tettamanti M, Lucca U et al. (2015). Preventive study in subjects at risk of fatal familial insomnia: innovative approach to rare diseases. Prion 9: 75–79.

Foutz A, Appleby BS, Hamlin C et al. (2017). Diagnostic and prognostic value of human prion detection in cerebrospinal fluid. Ann Neurol 81: 79–92.

Franceschini A, Baiardi S, Hughson AG et al. (2017). High diagnostic value of second generation CSF RT-QuIC across the wide spectrum of CJD prions. Sci Rep 7: 10655. PMID: 28878311. https://doi.org/10.1038/s41598-017-10922-w.

Friedrich M, Körte R, Portero C et al. (2008). Fatal familial insomnia – a rare differential diagnosis in dementia. Fortschr Neurol Psychiatr 76: 36–40.

Froböse T, Slawik H, Schreiner R et al. (2012). Agomelatine improves sleep in a patient with fatal familial insomnia. Pharmacopsychiatry 45: 34–36.

Froböse T, Förstl H, Förschler A (2014). Fatal familial insomnia (FFI) complicated by posterior reversible encephalopathy syndrome (PRES). Clin Neuroradiol 24: 289–291.

Gallassi R, Morreale A, Montagna P et al. (1996). Fatal familial insomnia: behavioral and cognitive features. Neurology 46: 935–939.

Gambetti P (2013). Creationism and evolutionism in prions. Am J Pathol 182: 623–627.

Gambetti P, Kong Q, Zou W et al. (2003a). Sporadic and familial CJD: classification and characterisation. Br Med Bull 66: 213–239.

Gambetti P, Parchi P, Chen SG (2003b). Hereditary Creutzfeldt–Jakob disease and fatal familial insomnia. Clin Lab Med 23: 43–64.

Gambetti P, Cali I, Notari S et al. (2011). Molecular biology and pathology of prion strains in sporadic human prion diseases. Acta Neuropathol 121: 79–90.

Gao C, Shi Q, Tian C et al. (2011). The epidemiological, clinical, and laboratory features of sporadic Creutzfeldt–Jakob disease patients in China: surveillance data from 2006 to 2010. PLoS One 6: e24231.

Garcin R, Brion S, Khochneviss A (1962). Le syndrome de Creutzfeldt–Jakob et les syndromes cortico-striés du presenium. Rev Neurol 106: 506.

Garcin R, Brion S, Khochneviss A (1963). Le syndrome de Creutzfeldt–Jakob et les syndromes cortico-striés du presenium (à l'occasion de 5 observations anatomo-cliniques). Rev Neurol 109: 419.

Gistau VS, Pintor L, Matrai S et al. (2006). Fatal familial insomnia. Psychosomatics 47: 527–528.

Goldfarb LG, Haltia M, Brown P et al. (1991). New mutation in scrapie amyloid precursor gene (at codon 178) in Finnish Creutzfeldt–Jakob kindred. Lancet 337: 425.

Goldfarb LG, Brown P, Haltia M et al. (1992a). Creutzfeldt–Jakob disease cosegregates with the codon 178Asn PRNP mutation in families of European origin. Ann Neurol 31: 274–281.

Goldfarb LG, Petersen RB, Tabaton M et al. (1992b). Fatal familial insomnia and familial Creutzfeldt–Jakob disease: disease phenotype determined by a DNA polymorphism. Science 258: 806–808.

Grau-Rivera O, Sánchez-Valle R, Bargalló N et al. (2016). Sporadic MM2-thalamic + cortical Creutzfeldt–Jakob disease: utility of diffusion tensor imaging in the detection of cortical involvement in vivo. Neuropathology 36: 199–204.

Guaraldi P, Calandra-Buonaura G, Terlizzi R et al. (2011). Oneiric stupor: the peculiar behaviour of agrypnia excitata. Sleep Med 12 Suppl 2: S64–67.

Guerreiro RJ, Vaskov T, Crews C et al. (2009). A case of dementia with PRNP D178Ncis-129M and no insomnia. Alzheimer Dis Assoc Disord 23: 415–417.

Haïk S, Galanaud D, Linguraru MG et al. (2008). In vivo detection of thalamic gliosis: a pathoradiologic demonstration in familial fatal insomnia. Arch Neurol 65: 545–549.

Hamaguchi T, Kitamoto T, Sato T et al. (2005). Clinical diagnosis of MM2-type sporadic Creutzfeldt–Jakob disease. Neurology 64: 643–648.

Harder A, Jendroska K, Kreuz F et al. (1999). Novel twelve-generation kindred of fatal familial insomnia from germany representing the entire spectrum of disease expression. Am J Med Genet 87: 311–316.

Harder A, Gregor A, Wirth T et al. (2004). Early age of onset in fatal familial insomnia. Two novel cases and review of the literature. J Neurol 251: 715–724.

Harris DA (1999). Cellular biology of prion diseases. Clin Microbiol Rev 12: 429–444.

Hayashi Y, Iwasaki Y, Yoshikura N et al. (2015). Decreased regional cerebral blood flow in the bilateral thalami and medulla oblongata determined by an easy Z-score (eZIS) analysis of (99m)Tc-ECD-SPECT images in a case of MM2-thalamic-type sporadic Creutzfeldt–Jakob disease. J Neurol Sci 358: 447–452.

Hayashi Y, Iwasaki Y, Takekoshi A et al. (2016). An autopsy-verified case of FTLD-TDP type A with upper motor neuron-predominant motor neuron disease mimicking MM2-thalamic-type sporadic Creutzfeldt–Jakob disease. Prion 10: 492–501.

Hirose K, Iwasaki Y, Izumi M et al. (2006). MM2-thalamic-type sporadic Creutzfeldt–Jakob disease with widespread neocortical pathology. Acta Neuropathol 112: 503–511.

Imberdis T, Harris DA (2016). Synthetic prions provide clues for understanding prion diseases. Am J Pathol 186: 761–764.

Iriarte J, Ayuso T, Echavarri C et al. (2007). Agrypnia excitata in fatal familial insomnia. A video-polygraphic study. Neurology 69: 607–608.

Ivanova L, Barmada S, Kummer T et al. (2001). Mutant prion proteins are partially retained in the endoplasmic reticulum. J Biol Chem 276: 42409–42421.

Iwasaki Y (2017). Creutzfeldt–Jakob disease. Neuropathology 37: 174–188.

Iwasaki Y, Yoshida M, Hashizume Y et al. (2006). Clinicopathologic characteristics of sporadic Japanese Creutzfeldt–Jakob disease classified according to prion protein gene polymorphism and prion protein type. Acta Neuropathol 112: 561–571.

Iwasaki Y, Mori K, Ito M et al. (2017). An autopsied case of MM1 + MM2-cortical with thalamic-type sporadic Creutzfeldt–Jakob disease presenting with hyperintensities on diffusion-weighted MRI before clinical onset. Neuropathology 37: 78–85.

Jackson WS, Borkowski AW, Faas H et al. (2009). Spontaneous generation of prion infectivity in fatal familial insomnia knockin mice. Neuron 63: 438–450.

Jansen C, Parchi P, Jelles B et al. (2011). The first case of fatal familial insomnia (FFI) in the Netherlands: a patient from Egyptian descent with concurrent four repeat tau deposits. Neuropathol Appl Neurobiol 37: 549–553.

Julien J, Vital C, Deleplanque B et al. (1990). Subacute familial thalamic atrophy. Memory disorders and complete insomnia. Rev Neurol (Paris) 146: 173–178.

Julien J, Vital C, Delisle MB et al. (1998). The French FFI cases. Brain Pathol 8: 555–558.

Kawasaki K, Wakabayashi K, Kawakami A et al. (1997). Thalamic form of Creutzfeldt–Jakob disease or fatal insomnia? Report of a sporadic case with normal prion protein genotype. Acta Neuropathol 93: 317–322.

Kim C, Haldiman T, Cohen Y et al. (2011). Protease-sensitive conformers in broad spectrum of distinct PrPSc structures in sporadic Creutzfeldt-Jakob disease are indicator of progression rate. PLoS Pathog 7: e1002242.

Kirschbaum WR (1968). Jakob-Creutzfeldt disease, Elsevier, New York.

Klöppel S, Pirker W, Brücke T et al. (2002). Beta-CIT SPECT demonstrates reduced availability of serotonin transporters in patients with Fatal Familial Insomnia. J Neural Transm (Vienna) 109: 1105–1110.

Kong Q, Surewicz WK, Petersen RB et al. (2004). Inherited prion diseases. In: SB Prusiner (Ed.), Prion Biology and Diseases, 2nd edition, Cold Springs Harbor Laboratory Press, New York, NY p. 673.

Korth C, Kaneko K, Groth D et al. (2003). Abbreviated incubation times for human prions in mice expressing a chimeric mouse-human prion protein transgene. Proc Natl Acad Sci U S A 100: 4784–4789.

Kovacs GG, Puopolo M, Ladogana A et al. (2005). Genetic prion disease: the EUROCJD experience. Hum Genet 118: 166–174.

Kovacs GG, Peden A, Weis S et al. (2013). Rapidly progressive dementia with thalamic degeneration and peculiar cortical prion protein immunoreactivity, but absence of proteinase K resistant PrP: a new disease entity? Acta Neuropathol Commun 1: 72.

Krasnianski A, Sanchez Juan P, Ponto C et al. (2014). A proposal of new diagnostic pathway for fatal familial insomnia. J Neurol Neurosurg Psychiatry 85: 654–659.

Kretzschmar H, Giese A, Zerr I et al. (1998). The German FFI cases. Brain Pathol 8: 559–561.

Ladogana A, Sanchez-Juan P, Mitrova E et al. (2009). Cerebrospinal fluid biomarkers in human genetic transmissible spongiform encephalopathies. J Neurol 256: 1620–1628.

Lattanzio F, Abu-Rumeileh S, Franceschini A et al. (2017). Prion-specific and surrogate CSF biomarkers in Creutzfeldt–Jakob disease: diagnostic accuracy in relation to molecular subtypes and analysis of neuropathological correlates of p-tau and Abeta42 levels. Acta Neuropathol 133: 559–578.

Lee HS, Goldfarb LG (2008). Global distribution of fatal familial insomnia: founder or recurrent mutations. Neurogenetics 9: 301–302. author reply 303–304.

Lee S, Antony L, Hartmann R et al. (2010). Conformational diversity in prion protein variants influences intermolecular beta-sheet formation. EMBO J 29: 251–262.

Lee MJ, Shin J, Chung EJ et al. (2014). Midbrain hypometabolism in fatal familial insomnia: a case report and a statistical parametric mapping analysis of a Korean family. Case Rep Neurol 6: 243–250.

Lehmann S, Harris DA (1996). Mutant and infectious prion proteins display common biochemical properties in cultured cells. J Biol Chem 271: 1633–1637.

Li R, Liu T, Wong BS et al. (2000). Identification of an epitope in the C terminus of normal prion protein whose expression is modulated by binding events in the. N terminus J Mol Biol 301: 567–573.

Li J, Browning S, Mahal SP et al. (2010). Darwinian evolution of prions in cell culture. Science 327: 869–872.

Linden R, Martins VR, Prado MA et al. (2008). Physiology of the prion protein. Physiol Rev 88: 673–728.

Little BW, Brown PW, Rodgers-Johnson P et al. (1986). Familial myoclonic dementia masquerading as Creutzfeldt–Jakob disease. Ann Neurol 20: 231–239.

Llorens F, Thune K, Schmitz M et al. (2016). Identification of new molecular alterations in fatal familial insomnia. Hum Mol Genet 25: 2417–2436.

Llorens F, Zarranz JJ, Fischer A et al. (2017). Fatal familial insomnia: clinical aspects and molecular alterations. Curr Neurol Neurosci Rep 17: 30.

Lu T, Pan Y, Peng L et al. (2017). Fatal familial insomnia with abnormal signals on routine MRI: a case report and literature review. BMC Neurol 17: 104.

Lugaresi E, Medori R, Montagna P et al. (1986). Fatal familial insomnia and dysautonomia with selective degeneration of thalamic nuclei. N Engl J Med 315: 997–1003.

Ma J, Lindquist S (2001). Wild-type PrP and a mutant associated with prion disease are subject to retrograde transport and proteasome degradation. Proc Natl Acad Sci U S A 98: 14955–14960.

Ma J, Lindquist S (2002). Conversion of PrP to a self-perpetuating PrPSc-like conformation in the cytosol. Science 298: 1785–1788.

Ma J, Wollmann R, Lindquist S (2002). Neurotoxicity and neurodegeneration when PrP accumulates in the cytosol. Science 298: 1781–1785.

Makarava N, Savtchenko R, Alexeeva I et al. (2016). New molecular insight into mechanism of evolution of mammalian synthetic prions. Am J Pathol 186: 1006–1014.

Manetto V, Medori R, Cortelli P et al. (1992). Fatal familial insomnia: clinical and pathologic study of five new cases. Neurology 42: 312–319.

Marcaud V, Laplanche JL, Defontaines B et al. (2003). Usefulness of molecular genetic analysis of the PRNP gene in patients with cerebellar ataxia: a new case of fatal familial insomnia. Rev Neurol (Paris) 159: 199–202.

Marques IB, Teotónio R, Cunha C et al. (2014). Anti-NMDA receptor encephalitis presenting with total insomnia – a case report. J Neurol Sci 336: 276–280.

Martin JJ (1975). Thalamic degeneration. In: PJ Vinken, GW Bruyn (Eds.), Handbook of clinical neurology. Amsterdam, North-Holland.

Martin JJ, Yap M, Nei IP et al. (1983). Selective thalamic degeneration – report of a case with memory and mental disturbances. Clin Neuropathol 2: 156–162.

Massignan T, Biasini E, Lauranzano E et al. (2010). Mutant prion protein expression is associated with an alteration of the Rab GDP dissociation inhibitor alpha (GDI)/Rab11 pathway. Mol Cell Proteomics 9: 611–622.

Mastrianni JA, Nixon R, Layzer R et al. (1999). Prion protein conformation in a patient with sporadic fatal insomnia. N Engl J Med 340: 1630–1638.

McLean CA, Storey E, Gardner RJ et al. (1997). The D178N (cis-129M) "fatal familial insomnia" mutation associated with diverse clinicopathologic phenotypes in an Australian kindred. Neurology 49: 552–558.

McMenemey WH, Grant HC, Behrman S (1965). Two examples of presenile dementia (Pick's disease and Stern-Garcin syndrome) with a history of trauma. Arch Psychiatr Nervenkr (1970) 207: 128–140.

Medori R, Montagna P, Tritschler HJ et al. (1992a). Fatal familial insomnia: a second kindred with mutation of prion protein gene at codon 178. Neurology 42: 669–670.

Medori R, Tritschler HJ, LeBlanc A et al. (1992b). Fatal familial insomnia, a prion disease with a mutation at codon 178 of the prion protein gene. N Engl J Med 326: 444–449.

Megelin T, Thomas B, Ferrer X et al. (2017). Fatal familial insomnia: a video-polysomnographic case report. Sleep Med 33: 165–166.

Mehta LR, Huddleston BJ, Skalabrin EJ et al. (2008). Sporadic fatal insomnia masquerading as a paraneoplastic cerebellar syndrome. Arch Neurol 65: 971–973.

Minikel EV, Vallabh SM, Lek M et al. (2016). Quantifying prion disease penetrance using large population control cohorts. Sci Transl Med 8: 322ra329.

Moda F, Suardi S, Di Fede G et al. (2012). MM2-thalamic Creutzfeldt–Jakob disease: neuropathological, biochemical and transmission studies identify a distinctive prion strain. Brain Pathol 22: 662–669.

Moda F, Gambetti P, Notari S et al. (2014). Prions in the urine of patients with variant Creutzfeldt–Jakob disease. N Engl J Med 371: 530–539.

Monari L, Chen SG, Brown P et al. (1994). Fatal familial insomnia and familial Creutzfeldt–Jakob disease: different prion proteins determined by a DNA polymorphism. Proc Natl Acad Sci U S A 91: 2839–2842.

Montagna P, Gambetti P, Cortelli P et al. (2003). Familial and sporadic fatal insomnia. Lancet Neurol 2: 167–176.

Moody KM, Schonberger LB, Maddox RA et al. (2011). Sporadic fatal insomnia in a young woman: a diagnostic challenge: case report. BMC Neurol 11: 136.

Nagayama M, Shinohara Y, Furukawa H et al. (1996). Fatal familial insomnia with a mutation at codon 178 of the prion protein gene: first report from Japan. Neurology 47: 1313–1316.

Nagoshi K, Sadakane A, Nakamura Y et al. (2011). Duration of prion disease is longer in Japan than in other countries. J Epidemiol 21: 255–262.

Noble GP, Walsh DJ, Miller MB et al. (2015). Requirements for mutant and wild-type prion protein misfolding in vitro. Biochemistry 54: 1180–1187.

Oliveros RG, Saracibar N, Gutierrez M et al. (2009). Catatonia due to a prion familial disease. Schizophr Res 108: 309–310.

Orrú CD, Yuan J, Appleby BS et al. (2017). Prion seeding activity and infectivity in skin samples from patients with sporadic Creutzfeldt-Jakob disease. Sci Transl Med 9.

Ortega-Cubero S, Luquín MR, Domínguez I et al. (2013). Structural and functional neuroimaging in human prion diseases. Neurologia 28: 299–308.

Padovani A, D'Alessandro M, Parchi P et al. (1998). Fatal familial insomnia in a new Italian kindred. Neurology 51: 1491–1494.

Parchi P, Saverioni D (2012). Molecular pathology, classification, and diagnosis of sporadic human prion disease variants. Folia Neuropathol 50: 20–45.

Parchi P, Castellani R, Cortelli P et al. (1995). Regional distribution of protease-resistant prion protein in fatal familial insomnia. Ann Neurol 38: 21–29.

Parchi P, Castellani R, Capellari S et al. (1996). Molecular basis of phenotypic variability in sporadic Creutzfeldt–Jakob disease. Ann Neurol 39: 767–778.

Parchi P, Capellari S, Chen SG et al. (1997). Typing prion isoforms. Nature 386: 232–234.

Parchi P, Capellari S, Chin S et al. (1999a). A subtype of sporadic prion disease mimicking fatal familial insomnia. Neurology 52: 1757–1763.

Parchi P, Giese A, Capellari S et al. (1999b). Classification of sporadic Creutzfeldt–Jakob disease based on molecular and phenotypic analysis of 300 subjects. Ann Neurol 46: 224–233.

Parchi P, Capellari S, Gambetti P (2000a). Intracerebral distribution of the abnormal isoform of the prion protein in sporadic Creutzfeldt–Jakob disease and fatal insomnia. Microsc Res Tech 50: 16–25.

Parchi P, Zou W, Wang W et al. (2000b). Genetic influence on the structural variations of the abnormal prion protein. Proc Natl Acad Sci U S A 97: 10168–10172.

Parchi P, Strammiello R, Notari S et al. (2009). Incidence and spectrum of sporadic Creutzfeldt–Jakob disease variants with mixed phenotype and co-occurrence of PrPSc types: an updated classification. Acta Neuropathol 118: 659–671.

Pedroso JL, Pinto WB, Souza PV et al. (2013). Complex movement disorders in fatal familial insomnia: a clinical and genetic discussion. Neurology 81: 1098–1099.

Peng B, Zhang S, Dong H et al. (2015). Clinical, histopathological and genetic studies in a case of fatal familial insomnia with review of the literature. Int J Clin Exp Pathol 8: 10171–10177.

Petersen RB, Tabaton M, Berg L et al. (1992). Analysis of the prion protein gene in thalamic dementia. Neurology 42: 1859–1863.

Petersen RB, Parchi P, Richardson SL et al. (1996). Effect of the D178N mutation and the codon 129 polymorphism on the metabolism of the prion protein. J Biol Chem 271: 12661–12668.

Piao YS, Kakita A, Watanabe H et al. (2005). Sporadic fatal insomnia with spongiform degeneration in the thalamus and widespread PrPSc deposits in the brain. Neuropathology 25: 144–149.

Pirisinu L, Di Bari M, Marcon S et al. (2010). A new method for the characterization of strain-specific conformational stability of protease-sensitive and protease-resistant PrPSc. PLoS One 5: e12723.

Plazzi G, Schutz Y, Cortelli P et al. (1997). Motor overactivity and loss of motor circadian rhythm in fatal familial insomnia: an actigraphic study. Sleep 20: 739–742.

Pocchiari M, Puopolo M, Croes EA et al. (2004). Predictors of survival in sporadic Creutzfeldt–Jakob disease and other human transmissible spongiform encephalopathies. Brain 127: 2348–2359.

Portaluppi F, Cortelli P, Avoni P et al. (1994). Diurnal blood pressure variation and hormonal correlates in fatal familial insomnia. Hypertension 23: 569–576.

Poursines Y, Boudouresques J, Roger J (1953). Diffuse atrophic degenerative process, predominantly of the thalamus and corpus striatum; variable extrapyramidal and psychic semeiology; subacute evolution with terminal dementia. Rev Neurol (Paris) 89: 266–271.

Priano L, Giaccone G, Mangieri M et al. (2009). An atypical case of sporadic fatal insomnia. J Neurol Neurosurg Psychiatry 80: 924–927.

Prieto E, Dominguez-Prado I, Riverol M et al. (2015). Metabolic patterns in prion diseases: an FDG PET voxel-based analysis. Eur J Nucl Med Mol Imaging 42: 1522–1529.

Puoti G, Bizzi A, Forloni G et al. (2012). Sporadic human prion diseases: molecular insights and diagnosis. Lancet Neurol 11: 618–628.

Raggi A, Perani D, Giaccone G et al. (2009). The behavioural features of fatal familial insomnia: a new Italian case with pathological verification. Sleep Med 10: 581–585.

Rancurel G, Garma L, Hauw JJ et al. (1994). Familial thalamic degeneration with fatal insomnia: clinicopathological and polygraphic data on a French member of Lugaresi's Italian family. In: C Guilleminault, E Lugaresi, P Montagna et al. (Eds.), Fatal familial insomnia. Inherited prion diseases, sleep and the thalamus. Raven Press, New York, pp. 15–25.

Redaelli V, Bistaffa E, Zanusso G et al. (2017). Detection of prion seeding activity in the olfactory mucosa of patients with fatal familial insomnia. Sci Rep 7: 46269.

Reder AT, Mednick AS, Brown P et al. (1995). Clinical and genetic studies of fatal familial insomnia. Neurology 45: 1068–1075.

Riek R, Wider G, Billeter M et al. (1998). Prion protein NMR structure and familial human spongiform encephalopathies. Proc Natl Acad Sci U S A 95: 11667–11672.

Rodríguez-Martínez AB, Alfonso-Sánchez MA, Peña JA et al. (2008). Molecular evidence of founder effects of fatal familial insomnia through SNP haplotypes around the D178N mutation. Neurogenetics 9: 109–118.

Rossi G, Macchi G, Porro M et al. (1998). Fatal familial insomnia: genetic, neuropathologic, and biochemical study of a patient from a new Italian kindred. Neurology 50: 688–692.

Roucou X, Guo Q, Zhang Y et al. (2003). Cytosolic prion protein is not toxic and protects against Bax-mediated cell death in human primary neurons. J Biol Chem 278: 40877–40881.

Rupprecht S, Grimm A, Schultze T et al. (2013). Does the clinical phenotype of fatal familial insomnia depend on PRNP codon 129 methionine-valine polymorphism? J Clin Sleep Med 9: 1343–1345.

Saborio GP, Permanne B, Soto C (2001). Sensitive detection of pathological prion protein by cyclic amplification of protein misfolding. Nature 411: 810–813.

Safar JG, Xiao X, Kabir ME et al. (2015). Structural determinants of phenotypic diversity and replication rate of human prions. PLoS Pathog 11: e1004832.

Saito Y, Iwasaki Y, Aiba I et al. (2011). An autopsy case of MM2-cortical + thalamic-type sporadic Creutzfeldt–Jakob disease. Neuropathology 31: 523–530.

Saitoh Y, Ogawa M, Naito Y et al. (2010). Discordant clinicopathologic phenotypes in a Japanese kindred of fatal familial insomnia. Neurology 74: 86–89.

Sandberg MK, Al-Doujaily H, Sharps B et al. (2011). Prion propagation and toxicity in vivo occur in two distinct mechanistic phases. Nature 470: 540–542.

Sano K, Satoh K, Atarashi R et al. (2013). Early detection of abnormal prion protein in genetic human prion diseases now possible using real-time QUIC assay. PLoS One 8: e54915.

Sasaki K, Doh-ura K, Wakisaka Y et al. (2005). Fatal familial insomnia with an unusual prion protein deposition pattern: an autopsy report with an experimental transmission study. Neuropathol Appl Neurobiol 31: 80–87.

Saverioni D, Notari S, Capellari S et al. (2013). Analyses of protease resistance and aggregation state of abnormal prion protein across the spectrum of human prions. J Biol Chem 288: 27972–27985.

Scaravilli F, Cordery RJ, Kretzschmar H et al. (2000). Sporadic fatal insomnia: a case study. Ann Neurol 48: 665–668.

Schenkein J, Montagna P (2006). Self-management of fatal familial insomnia. Part 2: case report. MedGenMed 8: 66.

Schulman S (1956). Bilateral symmetrical degeneration of the thalamus. J Neuropathol Exp Neurol (Proceedings of Am Assoc of Neuropathol) 15: 208.

Shi XH, Han J, Zhang J et al. (2010). Clinical, histopathological and genetic studies in a family with fatal familial insomnia. Infect Genet Evol 10: 292–297.

Shi Q, Chen C, Gao C et al. (2012). Clinical and familial characteristics of ten Chinese patients with fatal family insomnia. Biomed Environ Sci 25: 471–475.

Sigurdsson EM, Brown DR, Alim MA et al. (2003). Copper chelation delays the onset of prion disease. J Biol Chem 278: 46199–46202.

Sikorska B, Liberski PP (2012). Human prion diseases: from kuru to variant Creutzfeldt–Jakob disease. Subcell Biochem 65: 457–496.

Silburn P, Cervenakova L, Varghese P et al. (1996). Fatal familial insomnia: a seventh family. Neurology 47: 1326–1328.

Spacey SD, Pastore M, McGillivray B et al. (2004). Fatal familial insomnia: the first account in a family of Chinese descent. Arch Neurol 61: 122–125.

Stern K (1939). Severe dementia associated with bilateral symmetrical degeneration of the thalamus. Brain 62: 157.

Sun C, Xia W, Liu Y et al. (2017). Agrypnia excitata and obstructive apnea in a patient with fatal familial insomnia from China: A case report. Medicine (Baltimore) 96: e8951.

Sun L, Li X, Lin X et al. (2015). Familial fatal insomnia with atypical clinical features in a patient with D178N mutation and homozygosity for Met at codon 129 of the prion protein gene. Prion 9: 228–235.

Surewicz WK, Apostol MI (2011). Prion protein and its conformational conversion: a structural perspective. Top Curr Chem 305: 135–167.

Swietnicki W, Petersen RB, Gambetti P et al. (1998). Familial mutations and the thermodynamic stability of the recombinant human prion protein. J Biol Chem 273: 31048–31052.

Synofzik M, Bauer P, Schols L (2009). Prion mutation D178N with highly variable disease onset and phenotype. J Neurol Neurosurg Psychiatry 80: 345–346.

Tabernero C, Polo JM, Sevillano MD et al. (2000). Fatal familial insomnia: clinical, neuropathological, and genetic description of a Spanish family. J Neurol Neurosurg Psychiatry 68: 774–777.

Taguchi Y, Mohri S, Ironside JW et al. (2003). Humanized knock-in mice expressing chimeric prion protein showed varied susceptibility to different human prions. Am J Pathol 163: 2585–2593.

Takada LT, Kim MO, Cleveland RW et al. (2017). Genetic prion disease: experience of a rapidly progressive dementia center in the United States and a review of the literature. Am J Med Genet B Neuropsychiatr Genet 174: 36–69.

Taniwaki Y, Hara H, Doh-Ura K et al. (2000). Familial Creutzfeldt–Jakob disease with D178N-129M mutation of PRNP presenting as cerebellar ataxia without insomnia. J Neurol Neurosurg Psychiatry 68: 388.

Tapella L, Stravalaci M, Bastone A et al. (2013). Epitope scanning indicates structural differences in brain-derived monomeric and aggregated mutant prion proteins related to genetic prion diseases. Biochem J 454: 417–425.

Taratuto AL, Piccardo P, Reich EG et al. (2002). Insomnia associated with thalamic involvement in E200K Creutzfeldt–Jakob disease. Neurology 58: 362–367.

Tateishi J, Brown P, Kitamoto T et al. (1995). First experimental transmission of fatal familial insomnia. Nature 376: 434–435.

Telling GC, Scott M, Hsiao KK et al. (1994). Transmission of Creutzfeldt–Jakob disease from humans to transgenic mice expressing chimeric human-mouse prion protein. Proc Natl Acad Sci U S A 91: 9936–9940.

Telling GC, Parchi P, DeArmond SJ et al. (1996). Evidence for the conformation of the pathologic isoform of the prion protein enciphering and propagating prion diversity. Science 274: 2079–2082.

Thackray AM, Cardova A, Wolf H et al. (2017). Genetic human prion disease modelled in PrP transgenic Drosophila. Biochem J 474: 3253–3267.

Thomas AV, Klein JC, Brockhaus-Dumke A et al. (2006). Fatal familial insomnia: case presentation and discussion of typical clinical and imaging findings. Nervenarzt 77: 711–715.

van der Kamp MW, Daggett V (2009). The consequences of pathogenic mutations to the human prion protein. Protein Eng Des Sel 22: 461–468.

Watts JC, Giles K, Bourkas ME et al. (2016). Towards authentic transgenic mouse models of heritable PrP prion diseases. Acta Neuropathol 132: 593–610.

Weissmann C, Li J, Mahal SP et al. (2011). Prions on the move. EMBO Rep 12: 1109–1117.

Wermke M, Teipel S, Fuchsberger T et al. (2006). Frontal diaschisis in a German case of fatal familial insomnia. J Neurol 253: 1510–1512.

Whitwam JG, Amrein R (1995). Pharmacology of flumazenil. Acta Anaesthesiol Scand Suppl 108: 3–14.

Will RG, Campbell MJ, Moss TH et al. (1998). FFI cases from the United Kingdom. Brain Pathol 8: 562–563.

Wu L, Lu H, Wang X et al. (2017). Clinical Features and Sleep Analysis of Chinese Patients with Fatal Familial Insomnia. Sci Rep 7: 3625.

Yamashita M, Yamamoto T, Nishinaka K et al. (2001). Severe brain atrophy in a case of thalamic variant of sporadic CJD with plaque-like PrP deposition. Neuropathology 21: 138–143.

Yu S, Zhang Y, Li S et al. (2007). Early onset fatal familial insomnia with rapid progression in a Chinese family line. J Neurol 254: 1300–1301.

Zarranz JJ, Digon A, Atares B et al. (2005a). Familial prion diseases in the Basque country (Spain). Neuroepidemiology 24: 103–109.

Zarranz JJ, Digon A, Atares B et al. (2005b). Phenotypic variability in familial prion diseases due to the D178N mutation. J Neurol Neurosurg Psychiatry 76: 1491–1496.

Zhang B, Hao YL, Jia FJ et al. (2010). Fatal familial insomnia: a middle-age-onset Chinese family kindred. Sleep Med 11: 498–499.

Section IV

Prion-like mechanisms in other neurodegenerative diseases

Handbook of Clinical Neurology, Vol. 153 (3rd series)
Human Prion Diseases
M. Pocchiari and J. Manson, Editors
https://doi.org/10.1016/B978-0-444-63945-5.00016-7

Chapter 16

Prion-like mechanisms in Alzheimer disease

LARY C. WALKER*
Department of Neurology and Yerkes National Primate Research Center, Emory University, Atlanta, GA, United States

Abstract

Senile plaques and neurofibrillary tangles are the principal histopathologic hallmarks of Alzheimer disease. The essential constituents of these lesions are structurally abnormal variants of normally generated proteins: Aβ protein in plaques and tau protein in tangles. At the molecular level, both proteins in a pathogenic state share key properties with classic prions, i.e., they consist of alternatively folded, β-sheet-rich forms of the proteins that autopropagate by the seeded corruption and self-assembly of like proteins. Other similarities with prions include the ability to manifest as polymorphic and polyfunctional strains, resistance to chemical and enzymatic destruction, and the ability to spread within the brain and from the periphery to the brain. In Alzheimer disease, current evidence indicates that the pathogenic cascade follows from the endogenous, sequential corruption of Aβ and then tau. Therapeutic options include reducing the production or multimerization of the proteins, uncoupling the Aβ–tauopathy connection, or promoting the inactivation or removal of anomalous assemblies from the brain. Although aberrant Aβ appears to be the prime mover of Alzheimer disease pathogenesis, once set in motion by Aβ, the prion-like propagation of tauopathy may proceed independently of Aβ; if so, Aβ might be solely targeted as an early preventive measure, but optimal treatment of Alzheimer disease at later stages of the cascade could require intervention in both pathways.

ALZHEIMER DISEASE

Epidemiology, signs, and symptoms

One of the most feared hazards of growing old is the profound deterioration of mental faculties known as dementia. More than 50 different conditions are associated with dementia (Vonsattel and Hedley-White, 2001), but of these, Alzheimer disease (AD) is the most common, with a worldwide prevalence in 2010 of approximately 35 million people (Dartigues, 2009; Holtzman et al., 2011; Reitz et al., 2011). The incidence and prevalence of AD double every 5 years between the ages of 65 and 95 (Kawas and Katzman, 1999). As the average life expectancy of populations grows in many parts of the world, and in the absence of an effective prevention or treatment, as many as 115 million people are expected to have AD in the year 2050 (Dartigues, 2009). The social and economic costs of the disease will rise accordingly (Wimo et al., 2013), with an ever greater burden of caring for afflicted persons falling on younger generations. Disease-modifying treatments are urgently needed, but these can only emerge from a deep understanding of AD itself. A defining pathologic feature of AD is the abnormal accumulation in the brain of two proteins, Aβ and tau; recent evidence shows that this process is initiated and sustained by a prion-like mechanism of seeded protein aggregation.

Symptomatically, AD typically begins with the gradual onset of mild cognitive impairment, progressing inexorably to dementia with an average clinical duration of 7–10 years (Holtzman et al., 2011) (although the time course is variable). The signs and symptoms shown by individual patients also can vary substantially, but the diagnosis of AD is established by the universal presence of core attributes, specifically progressive dementia in the context of characteristic lesions in the brain: senile (Aβ) plaques and neurofibrillary (tau) tangles.

*Correspondence to: Lary C. Walker, Department of Neurology, Emory University, 505M Whitehead Building, 615 Michael Street, Atlanta GA 30322, United States. Tel: +1 404-727-7779, E-mail: lary.walker@emory.edu

Dementia can be defined as "a decline from a person's previously established level of intellectual function that is sufficient to interfere with the everyday performance of that individual" (Holtzman et al., 2011). Based on the criteria set forth in the fifth edition of the *Diagnostic and Statistical Manual of Mental Disorders* (DSM-5: American Psychiatric Association, 2013), dementia due to AD is defined as "the insidious onset and gradual progression of substantial impairment in learning and memory and at least one other cognitive domain (complex attention, executive function, language, perceptual-motor, or social cognition) that interferes with independence in everyday activities" (Walker and Jucker, 2017). An important feature of these definitions is that the impairments are substantial, and thus become incapacitating even under ordinary circumstances.

Differential diagnosis and biomarkers

Until recently, senile plaques and neurofibrillary tangles could only be identified by microscopic analysis of brain samples, but increasingly sensitive and specific diagnostic tests are emerging that enable the detection of proteopathic abnormalities in living subjects. These include radiolabeled imaging agents for Aβ and tau in the brain, and assays for quantitation of the proteins in cerebrospinal fluid (CSF) (Lewczuk et al., 2015; Olsson et al., 2016; Villemagne et al., 2017). Investigations of these biomarkers indicate that the disease process begins two decades or more before the onset of demonstrable cognitive impairment (Jack et al., 2010; Jack and Holtzman, 2013). In addition, the presence of genetic risk factors such as the ε4 allele of apolipoprotein E (*APOEε4*) can reinforce the in-life diagnosis of AD.

It is important to place AD in the context of other brain changes that impair intellectual capacities in the elderly. In younger patients with autosomal-dominant causes of AD (below), the disease is relatively unambiguous histopathologically, i.e., lesions other than plaques and tangles are rare. With advancing age, additional disorders are increasingly likely to contribute to dementia, including cerebrovascular disease, hippocampal sclerosis, and cerebral proteopathies such as α-synucleinopathy, TDP-43 proteopathy, and others (Vonsattel and Hedley-White, 2001; Nelson et al., 2012). These maladies can cause dementia on their own, but they also sometimes coexist with AD, complicating diagnosis, exacerbating the clinical course, and likely diminishing the effectiveness of treatments directed at only one of the conditions. In addition, potentially reversible causes of a dementia-like state must be ruled out, such as depression, infections, drugs and drug interactions, thyroid dysfunction, tumors, and vitamin B_{12} deficiency, as intervention in these instances might at least partially restore cognitive function (Tripathi and Vibha, 2009; Holtzman et al., 2011).

Genetics

The probability of developing AD is influenced by certain genetic risk factors, which include rare causative, autosomal-dominant mutations with essentially complete penetrance, as well as diverse genetic polymorphisms that modulate risk to varying degrees (Tanzi, 2012; Wingo et al., 2012). Autosomal-dominant mutations associated with AD all occur in the genes that code for the Aβ precursor protein (APP) or for presenilin-1 or presenilin-2 (the presenilins being key components of intramembranous protease complexes that liberate Aβ from APP (Hardy, 2006; Holtzman et al., 2011)). The gene encoding APP is on chromosome 21, and the genes encoding presenilin-1 and presenilin-2 are on chromosomes 14 and 1, respectively.

AD-linked mutations in the presenilins and in the APP regions flanking Aβ alter the processing of APP, but mutations within the Aβ segment of APP often modify its potential to aggregate and its tissue-specificity (Holtzman et al., 2011; Haass et al., 2012). An unusual variant in the APP gene that results in an alanine to threonine substitution at position 2 of Aβ reduces the production (Jonsson et al., 2012) and aggregation proclivity (Benilova et al., 2014) of Aβ, thereby lowering the risk of AD (Jonsson et al., 2012). In contrast, an alanine to valine replacement at this position increases the production and aggregability of Aβ, causing an autosomal-recessive type of AD (Di Fede et al., 2009) with unusual neuropathologic features (Giaccone et al., 2010). Furthermore, because most patients with Down syndrome (trisomy 21) have an extra copy of the APP gene on chromosome 21, they are at greatly increased risk of developing AD as they age (Head et al., 2016). Together, these genetic data consistently implicate Aβ in the ontogeny of heredofamilial forms of AD.

Dominant and recessive genetic causes account for less than 1% of all AD cases (Holtzman et al., 2011). How, then, are genetics linked to idiopathic AD? A study of twins in Sweden indicated that the heritability for AD is as high as 79% (Gatz et al., 2006), although most of the implicated polymorphisms individually have only a slight influence on risk (Humphries and Kohli, 2014). An exception is the gene that encodes apolipoprotein E (ApoE) (Yu et al., 2014), a protein that mediates lipid transport throughout the body and is the major apolipoprotein in the brain (Chouraki and Seshadri, 2014). The three major protein isoforms of ApoE in human populations are ApoE2, ApoE3, and ApoE4. The most frequent isoform is ApoE3 (~78%), followed by ApoE4

(~14%) and ApoE2 (~8%) (Liu et al., 2013). Bearers of the *APOEε4* allele have an allele dose-dependent increase in the risk of AD, with heterozygotes having a two- to fivefold increase in risk, and homozygotes a 12–15-fold increase (Chouraki and Seshadri, 2014). The mechanism by which *APOEε4* predisposes carriers to AD is probably multifaceted (Potter and Wisniewski, 2012; Yu et al., 2014; Huang et al., 2017), but it is known that bearers of *APOEε4* begin to accumulate Aβ in the brain at least a decade earlier in life than do nonbearers (Warzok et al., 1998; Walker et al., 2000; Resnick et al., 2015). Thus, *APOEε4*, like the known dominant and recessive genetic risk factors (above), appears to augment the probability of developing AD by advancing the onset of the Aβ cascade. Indeed, all known AD-linked mutations affect the production, removal, trafficking, or tendency to aggregate of Aβ (Hardy and Selkoe, 2002).

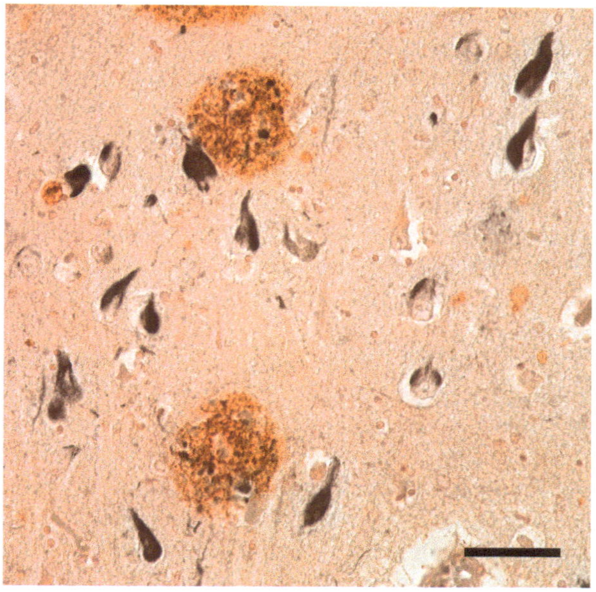

Fig. 16.1. The canonic neuropathologic features of Alzheimer disease include senile (Aβ) plaques (reddish brown) and neurofibrillary (tau) tangles (black). Aβ was immunostained with rabbit polyclonal antibody R398 to Aβ42, and tau was immunostained with mouse monoclonal antibody MC1 to paired helical filaments. CA1 field of the hippocampus. Bar = 50 μm.

Other risk factors

In addition to the genetic risk factors for AD, numerous environmental and endogenous risk factors have been identified. These include advancing age, traumatic brain injury, diabetes and metabolic disorders, inflammation, vascular disorders, gender, and lifestyle (Holtzman et al., 2011; Killin et al., 2016; Lafortune et al., 2016; Pike, 2017). In some instances these should be considered as risk factors for dementia, broadly defined, rather than for AD per se. For example, multiple small infarcts might raise the likelihood of dementia independently of AD, or they may advance the onset of dementia in people who also are incubating AD pathology in the brain.

THE NEUROPATHOLOGY OF AD IN THE CONTEXT OF THE PRION PARADIGM

Amyloid

As in the case of most proteopathies, the proteins that are implicated in the development of AD are structurally abnormal manifestations of proteins that are normally generated by cells. The abnormalities often involve an altered three-dimensional architecture (misfolding), which can be promoted by amino acid substitutions, posttranslational modifications, sequence expansions or truncations, and such characteristics of the local milieu as temperature and pH (Eisenberg and Jucker, 2012). In addition, factors that increase the concentration of certain proteins (e.g., by raising their production or impairing their removal/degradation) can elevate the risk of disease (Jucker and Walker, 2013).

A frequent indication that a protein is structurally corrupted at the molecular level is its enhanced tendency to form amyloid. In general, amyloid is a state in which a protein accumulates in tissues as masses of ~10-nm-diameter fibrils with a characteristic cross-β X-ray diffraction pattern and cross-polarization-induced birefringence after staining with the dye Congo red (Sipe et al., 2016), indicative of increased β-sheet molecular structure (Eisenberg and Jucker, 2012). In some biologic circumstances the amyloid state is functionally advantageous, particularly in prokaryotes (Fowler et al., 2007; Greenwald and Riek, 2010) (amyloid-like fibrils consisting of stacked, cross-α helices have been identified in the bacterium *Staphylococcus aureus* (Tayeb-Fligelman et al., 2017), but α-helix-based amyloid has not been described in eukaryotes). In mammals, amyloid is often pathogenic; more than 30 different amyloidoses have been reported (Sipe et al., 2016), many of which occur outside the central nervous system (Westermark et al., 2017).

Within the brain, it is not uncommon to find some degree of Aβ amyloidosis and tauopathy in the elderly; in those with dementia, abundant Aβ plaques and tau tangles are the two types of amyloid that are pathognomonic for AD (Holtzman et al., 2011; Nelson et al., 2012) (Fig. 16.1). The formation of amyloid by Aβ and tau is an obvious sign of a proteopathic process, but small oligomeric assemblies may actually be the more toxic form of the proteins (Lambert et al., 1998; Haass and Selkoe, 2007; Gerson and Kayed, 2016; Yang, 2017). Aβ in the amyloid state is virtually always present in AD, but an instructive exception is a rare hereditary type of AD caused by a mutation that changes glutamate to glycine at position 22 of Aβ (E22G; the "arctic" mutation). This mutation results in early-onset AD in which Aβ plaques lack the prototypical amyloid cores (Kalimo et al., 2013), indicating that "amyloid" in the strict sense is not required to drive the Aβ cascade. Similarly, even though misfolded prion protein (PrP) has an enhanced ability to form amyloid, PrP amyloid per se is not obligatory for the expression of prion disease (DeArmond and Prusiner, 1995).

This point bears emphasis because of the unproductive controversy (Drachman, 2014) that still bedevils the "amyloid cascade hypothesis" (aka the "amyloid hypothesis") of AD (Hardy and Selkoe, 2002; Selkoe and Hardy, 2016). The "amyloid" in the original formulation of this concept refers to β-amyloid (i.e., Aβ in a β-sheet-rich, polymerized state). There can be little doubt that Aβ is a driving force in the genesis of AD (Jack et al., 2010; Selkoe, 2011; Bateman et al., 2012; Walker and Jucker, 2015), or that β-amyloid accumulation per se is detrimental to cognition, particularly when embodied as neuritic plaques (Nelson et al., 2012). However, tauopathy is an essential downstream consequence that correlates more strongly with the degree of dementia than does the number of Aβ plaques (Wilcock and Esiri, 1982; Crystal et al., 1988; Bierer et al., 1995). This apparent inconsistency mainly reflects the importance of tauopathy for the clinical expression of the disease, but it does not invalidate the instigating role of multimeric Aβ in AD. A review of published work by the Alzheimer's Disease Neuroimaging Initiative concluded that "CSF biomarkers are consistent with disease trajectories predicted by β-amyloid cascade … and tau-mediated neurodegeneration hypotheses for AD" (Weiner et al., 2013). Because tau and Aβ both self-aggregate by the templated corruption of like proteins by misfolded seeds, once tauopathy is set in motion, it is possible that the two proteopathies progress along separate paths, both temporally and spatially.

The tau protein normally is involved in the stabilization of cellular microtubules (Spillantini and Goedert, 2013). In AD and other tauopathies, tau misfolds and becomes hyperphosphorylated; like Aβ, the altered tau molecules aggregate to form soluble oligomers and long, β-sheet-rich polymers that have the characteristics that define amyloid. The tau fibrils bundle together as neurofibrillary tangles in neurons (Fig. 16.1), although tauopathy also can afflict glial cells (Kovacs, 2015).

Tauopathy occurs in association with many brain disorders besides AD (Nelson et al., 2012). The primary tauopathies are disorders in which tau aggregation is the major abnormality (Spillantini and Goedert, 2013; Crary et al., 2014; Kovacs, 2015); in many conditions however, tauopathy is secondary to various types of injury or stress to the brain (Nelson et al., 2012). In human prion diseases, tauopathy is variable in appearance and degree (DeArmond et al., 2004; Kovacs et al., 2017), and in instances where it is relatively prominent (such as Gerstmann–Sträussler–Scheinker disease and variant Creutzfeldt–Jakob disease (CJD)) the cytology and anatomic distribution often differ from those seen in AD (Giaccone et al., 2008; Kovacs et al., 2017).

The extended neuropathology of AD

In addition to the canonic lesions that define AD – Aβ plaques and tau tangles – other changes are present in the brain that complicate the disease phenotype. One is the accumulation of Aβ in and around the walls of cerebral blood vessels, a condition known as Aβ-type cerebral amyloid angiopathy (Aβ-CAA). Aβ-CAA weakens the vascular wall and elevates the risk of intracranial hemorrhage (Biffi and Greenberg, 2011). Like Aβ plaques and tauopathy, Aβ-CAA is not specific to AD, and its prevalence increases with advancing age (Revesz et al., 2003; Biffi and Greenberg, 2011). However, some degree of Aβ-CAA is almost always present in AD (Attems and Jellinger, 2014; Vinters, 2015; Kapasi and Schneider, 2016), and it is severe in around 25% of cases (Charidimou et al., 2012). The factors that drive the inconsistent occurrence of Aβ-CAA in different people remain uncertain.

Other alterations are found to variable extents among end-stage AD cases, and most of these anomalies lack diagnostic specificity for the disease. Macroscopically, loss of brain tissue and concomitant expansion of the ventricles are common, but this varies among regions and among patients (Hauw and Duyckaerts, 2001). Evidence of inflammation includes reactive microglia and astrocytes, especially in association with Aβ plaques, as well as increased inflammatory mediators such as cytokines (Duyckaerts et al., 2009). Granulovacuolar degeneration, perisomatic granules, and Hirano bodies may be present (Duyckaerts et al., 2009), but their significance for AD per se is uncertain. Many different neuronal systems are compromised in AD (Mann and Yates, 1986; Hauw and Duyckaerts, 2001), some more markedly than others, and synapses are regionally depleted (Terry et al., 1999; Duyckaerts et al., 2009). In some cases of AD, spongiform change is evident that, though generally less severe, can resemble that seen in CJD (Smith et al., 1987; Sherzai et al., 2013) (Fig. 16.2). As noted above, other neurodegenerative conditions might be present in the brain along with the lesions of AD, particularly in older patients.

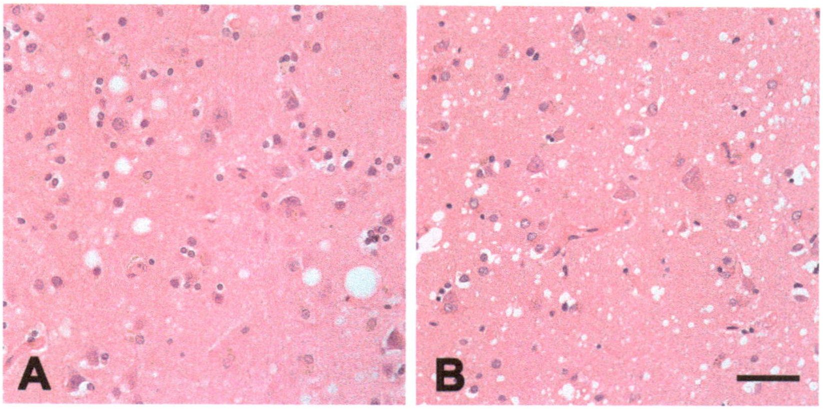

Fig. 16.2. Spongiform change (vacuoles, seen in these micrographs as white holes) in the neocortex of an Alzheimer disease patient (**A**) and in a patient with Creutzfeldt–Jakob disease (**B**). Spongiform change is not unique to prion diseases, but it is less common in Alzheimer disease, and when it occurs it is generally mild (Smith et al., 1987; Sherzai et al., 2013). Hematoxylin and eosin stain. Bar = 50 μm.

Regardless of the complexity of damage to the brain, the essential and unifying feature of AD is the obligatory presence of aggregated Aβ and tau proteins. For this reason, extensive research has been directed toward determining how the proteins misfold, self-assemble, and propagate their pathogenic features, a process that shares important commonalities with the molecular pathogenesis of prion diseases (Walker and LeVine, 2000; Walker et al., 2006, 2016; Jucker and Walker, 2013; Prusiner, 2013; Goedert, 2015; Walker and Jucker, 2015).

THE PRION-LIKE PROPERTIES OF AGGREGATED Aβ

The idea that AD might arise by a pathogenic mechanism similar to that of prion diseases has a fairly long history (Farquhar and Gajdusek, 1981; Prusiner, 1984). Based on their success in transmitting kuru and CJD to nonhuman primates (Gajdusek et al., 1966, 1968; Gibbs et al., 1968), and on the hypothesis that a "slow virus" might be involved in other neurodegenerative disorders (Gajdusek, 1977), D. Carleton Gajdusek's group attempted to experimentally transmit AD to several species of nonhuman primates via intracerebral injection of AD brain homogenates. They tentatively reported that the attempt was unsuccessful (Goudsmit et al., 1980). In Great Britain, Ridley and Baker et al. (1994) undertook similar transmission experiments in marmosets (*Callithrix jacchus*). After an incubation period of more than 5 years, they detected a significant increase in the senile plaque load of the host animals. The causative agent, however, remained uncertain.

When transgenic mouse models expressing human-type APP became available, experiments were initiated to explicitly test the hypothesis that Aβ can be induced to aggregate in the living brain by a prion-like mechanism (Kane et al., 2000). These studies showed that Aβ plaques and CAA are seedable by brain extracts from AD patients, but not by extracts derived from control brains that were devoid of aggregated Aβ (Kane et al., 2000; Walker et al., 2002; Meyer-Luehmann et al., 2006) (Fig. 16.3). AD brain extracts infused into the brains of wild-type mice (which express an aggregation-resistant sequence of Aβ) did not yield Aβ deposits.

Subsequent experiments showed unequivocally that the active agent is aggregated Aβ, and that the ability of Aβ to seed as well as the characteristics of the resulting deposits are governed by both the agent and the host (Meyer-Luehmann et al., 2006). These findings have been confirmed and extended by other laboratories (Watts et al., 2011, 2014; Morales et al., 2012, 2015a; Stohr et al., 2012, 2014; Duran-Aniotz et al., 2013, 2014; Burwinkel et al., 2018), and the collective experiments have established that the molecular features of Aβ seeds are essentially the same as those that define the pathogenicity of prions (Jucker and Walker, 2013; Morales et al., 2015b; Walker and Jucker, 2015; Walker et al., 2016). Key commonalities between Aβ seeds and PrP-prions are summarized as follows:

1. The active seeding agent is a form of the protein itself. In addition to brain extracts from AD patients, extracts from APP-transgenic mice (Meyer-Luehmann et al., 2006) and aged monkeys (Rosen et al., 2016) can seed Aβ deposition as long as aggregated Aβ is present in the donor brain. The degree of Aβ seeding is directly related to the concentration of Aβ in the brain extract (Meyer-Luehmann et al., 2006; Fritschi et al., 2014b), and even extremely

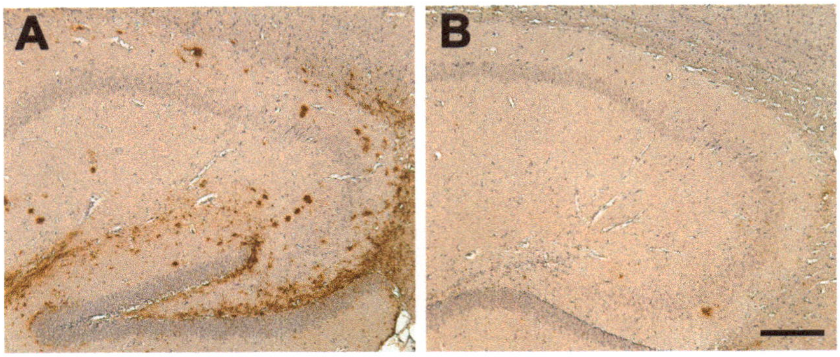

Fig. 16.3. Seeded Aβ deposition (brown) in the hippocampus of an 8-month-old TG2576 Aβ-precursor protein-transgenic mouse (sagittal sections; rostral is to the right). The hippocampus of one hemisphere (**A**) was injected 5 months earlier with clarified cortical extract from an Alzheimer disease case, and the contralateral hippocampus (**B**) received a similar amount of control brain extract lacking aggregated Aβ. The induced deposits emerge histologically in this model after around 2–3 months, and increase thereafter. Sections were incubated with polyclonal antibody R398 to Aβ42. Hematoxylin counterstain (blue). Bar = 200 μm.

small amounts of Aβ seeds are capable of stimulating aggregation in the brain (Fritschi et al., 2014b; Morales et al., 2015a). Immunodepletion of Aβ from the donor extract prior to injection nullifies the seeding effect (Meyer-Luehmann et al., 2006; Duran-Aniotz et al., 2014). Synthetic, pre-aggregated Aβ is capable of seeding deposition in vivo (Stohr et al., 2012), albeit relatively weakly (see below).

2. Aβ seeds are rich in β-sheet secondary structure. Amyloid fibrils of all types, including Aβ-amyloid and PrP-amyloid, are rich in β-sheets in which the individual β-strands run approximately perpendicular to the long axis of the fibrils (Eisenberg and Jucker, 2012). In vitro studies by Lansbury and colleagues demonstrated that pre-aggregated, β-sheet-rich seeds of synthetic Aβ efficiently induce monomeric Aβ to acquire β-sheet and assemble into amyloid (Harper and Lansbury, 1997). In addition, in vivo seeding experiments have shown that denaturation of Aβ-seed-rich brain extracts with formic acid (which disrupts the three-dimensional architecture of proteins) negates the ability of the extracts to induce plaque formation (Meyer-Luehmann et al., 2006).
3. Misfolded Aβ can manifest as structurally and functionally variant strains. In the canonic (PrP) prion diseases, prion traits and the host response vary in ways that suggest alternative structural and functional "strains" of the agent. Strain differences, in turn, have been linked to dissimilarities in PrP amino acid sequence, protease sensitivity, resistance to denaturants, and glycosylation patterns (McKintosh et al., 2003; Weissmann, 2004; Wiseman et al., 2015). However, a critical factor governing prion infectivity and disease phenotype is the molecular conformation of pathogenic PrP (PrP^{TSE} or PrP^{Sc}) (Peretz et al., 2002; Tanaka et al., 2006; Gambetti et al., 2011). Distinct prion strains often yield characteristic patterns of lesion structure and distribution in the brain (Peretz et al., 2002; DeArmond et al., 2004). An important indication that variant CJD (the human prionosis that is linked to bovine spongiform encephalopathy) is caused by a novel prion strain was the discovery of atypical lesions termed florid plaques in affected humans (Ironside et al., 2000).

As in the case of PrP-prions, Aβ can fold into strain-like variants both in vitro (Petkova et al., 2005; Nilsson et al., 2007; Yagi et al., 2007; Paravastu et al., 2008; Meinhardt et al., 2009; Kodali et al., 2010; Miller et al., 2010; Agopian and Guo, 2012; Spirig et al., 2014; Tycko, 2015, 2016) and in vivo (Meyer-Luehmann et al., 2006; Rosen et al., 2010, 2011; Heilbronner et al., 2013; Lu et al., 2013; Stohr et al., 2014; Watts et al., 2014; Cohen et al., 2015; Condello et al., 2018; Rasmussen et al., 2017). Cerebral Aβ assemblies in humans with AD vary in terms of plaque morphology (Wisniewski et al., 1989; Thal et al., 2006), ligand-binding characteristics (Rosen et al., 2010; Condello et al., 2018; Rasmussen et al., 2017), solid-state nuclear magnetic resonance features (Qiang et al., 2017), as well as conformational stability and other biophysical characteristics (Cohen et al., 2015). Interestingly, Aβ extracted from the autopsied brains of nondemented elderly subjects exhibits molecular-level features that differ in some ways from AD-derived Aβ (Piccini et al., 2005; Portelius et al., 2015). Whether these differences are indicative of fundamentally distinctive strains of Aβ, or whether they reflect early versus late stages in the pathogenesis of AD, is not certain.

Experimental studies in transgenic mice have shown that strain-like features of aggregated Aβ can be transferred from donor to host by exogenous seeding. Specifically, in the absence of seeding, APP23 mice and APP/PS1 mice develop Aβ plaques with different morphologies and ratios of the 40- and 42-amino acid lengths of Aβ (Aβ40 and Aβ42); when Aβ seeds from one transgenic mouse model were infused intracerebrally into the other, the plaque morphology (Meyer-Luehmann et al., 2006), spectral signature of bound conformation-sensitive thiophene ligands, and the Aβ40:42 ratio (Heilbronner et al., 2013) were influenced both by the source of the seeds and the type of murine host. In addition, strain-like features of Aβ from human AD cases can be at least partially replicated in mouse models (Rasmussen et al., 2017; Condello et al., 2018).

4. Aβ seeds vary in size and sensitivity to proteinase K. Infectious PrP prions exist in a wide range of sizes, the most potent of which are small and soluble (Silveira et al., 2005). Similarly, Aβ seeds can range from large fibrils to small, oligomeric seeds with high biologic potency (Langer et al., 2011). Large Aβ seeds are relatively resistant to inactivation by proteinase K, whereas – like PrP prions – oligomeric Aβ seeds are readily inactivated by the enzyme (Langer et al., 2011).

5. Some Aβ seeds are durable. When Aβ-rich brain extracts are boiled for 5 minutes prior to infusion into host mice, a significant fraction of bioactive Aβ seeds remain (Meyer-Luehmann et al., 2006). In addition, similar to PrP prions, Aβ seeds retain their potency in donor brain tissue that has been in formaldehyde for years (Fritschi et al., 2014a). Aβ seeds also are durable within the living brain; they retain some bioactivity (albeit with progressively diminishing potency) for at least 6 months after infusion into the brains of mice engineered to lack APP, and which therefore are incapable of replicating Aβ in any form (Ye et al., 2015a). Analogously, PrP prions have been reported to persist in the brains of PrP-deficient mice for up to 600 days (Diack et al., 2016). Likewise, AA amyloidosis in systemic organs can be promoted by fibrillar AA seeds (amyloid-enhancing factor) that persist in mice for at least 6 months (Lundmark et al., 2002). The endurance of some proteopathic seeds may result from their ability to adopt the highly stable, β-sheet-rich amyloid state (see above).

6. Aβ seeds spread systematically within the brain. As with PrP prions (Fraser, 1982; Buyukmihci et al., 1983; Kimberlin and Walker, 1986; Liberski et al., 2012; Rangel et al., 2014) and other proteopathic seeds (Clavaguera et al., 2009, 2013; Ahmed et al., 2014; Iba et al., 2015; Boluda et al., 2015; Hock and Polymenidou, 2016; Rey et al., 2016), Aβ seeds introduced into one part of the brain induce protein aggregation that spreads systematically to interconnected regions (Hamaguchi et al., 2012; Ye et al., 2015b). In APP-transgenic mouse models, Aβ seeds injected into the peritoneal cavity (Eisele et al., 2010, 2014) or intravenously (Burwinkel et al., 2018) travel to the brain, where many of the induced deposits are associated with cerebral blood vessels.

   The cellular mechanisms involved in the trafficking of Aβ seeds remain uncertain. Extracellular, soluble Aβ is taken up by cultured cells and concentrated in the acidic environment of endosomes/lysosomes, where the Aβ assembles into higher-molecular-weight seeds (Hu et al., 2009). Oligomeric Aβ seeds have been described that are bound to intracellular membranes and that strongly stimulate Aβ aggregation in vitro and in vivo (Marzesco et al., 2016). In cell culture experiments, Aβ seeds were demonstrated to spread by transfer from neuron to neuron (Nath et al., 2012; Domert et al., 2014), and neuroanatomic patterns of deposition are consistent with spread along neuronal pathways (Hamaguchi et al., 2012; Ronnback et al., 2012; Ye et al., 2015b) by active cellular transport and/or diffusion (Eisele and Duyckaerts, 2016). In addition, there is evidence that macrophages can phagocytose and translocate Aβ seeds (Eisele et al., 2014; Cintron et al., 2015).

   Small, cell-derived extracellular vesicles such as exosomes have been linked to the transmissibility of PrP-prions (Fevrier et al., 2004; Properzi et al., 2015; Guo et al., 2016a). Extracellular vesicles also have been suggested to ferry Aβ between cells (Rajendran et al., 2006), although their influence on the pathogenesis of AD – positive or negative – remains uncertain (Joshi et al., 2015).

7. Aβ aggregation can be instigated de novo. PrP prions induce prion disease in animals that are unlikely to have acquired the disease without exposure to exogenous prions. In contrast, many of the experiments showing seeding of Aβ have been undertaken in transgenic mouse models that, with age, eventually develop Aβ plaques and CAA spontaneously. To determine whether Aβ deposition can be seeded in normally resistant animals, Aβ-seed-rich brain extracts were injected intracerebrally into transgenic rodent models that do not generate Aβ lesions within their average lifespans; these studies indicate that Aβ deposition is inducible de novo, and in this paradigm is not simply an acceleration of an ongoing process (Morales et al., 2012; Rosen et al., 2012).

8. Aβ proteopathy is serially transmissible. Similar to PrP-prions, different strains of Aβ seeds can be successively transmitted from the initially seeded mice to subsequent hosts (Watts et al., 2014).

PRION-LIKE PROPERTIES OF Aβ: OPEN QUESTIONS

Pure, pre-aggregated synthetic Aβ is able to seed deposition in vivo, but synthetic Aβ seeds are much weaker than are Aβ seeds derived from the brain (Stohr et al., 2012). Correspondingly, generating infectious prions from purified, recombinant PrP has long been a challenge (Legname et al., 2004). Both Aβ seeds and PrP prions thus are most potent when they are generated within living tissues. The infectivity of recombinant PrP-prions can be augmented by adding certain cofactors to the medium during aggregation (Wang et al., 2010; Deleault et al., 2012; Zhang et al., 2014). It is possible that specific cofactors also are required to optimize the bioactivity of Aβ seeds in vivo. The lipid environment, for instance, influences the pathobiology of Aβ (Morgado and Garvey, 2015), and lipids are essential for the high-affinity binding of the β-amyloid imaging agent Pittsburgh compound B to cerebral Aβ (Matveev et al., 2014). Potent, in vivo active Aβ seeds recently have been generated by the seeded conversion of synthetic Aβ in a hippocampal slice culture model (Novotny et al., 2016). Clarifying the conditions that influence protein aggregation, seeding, and toxicity in living systems could disclose new therapeutic objectives for multiple proteopathies. Insights might also emerge from an analysis of senescent nonhuman primates which, despite substantial accumulation of human sequence Aβ with age, exhibit neither significant tauopathy nor dementia (Rosen et al., 2016). A possible parallel in the prion field is the dissociation of PrP amyloid seeding and transmission of spongiform encephalopathy in a mouse model (Piccardo et al., 2013).

Another open question is why the Aβ that is present in the CSF of AD patients only weakly seeds the aggregation of synthetic Aβ in vitro, and fails to seed deposition in the brains of APP-transgenic mice, even at Aβ concentrations that exceed the levels in brain extracts by a factor of 10 (Fritschi et al., 2014b). The reasons for the poor seeding efficiency of CSF Aβ are unknown, but the Aβ assemblies in CSF were found to be smaller and mostly devoid of N-terminally truncated variants compared to brain-derived Aβ (Fritschi et al., 2014b). Additionally, other substances in the CSF, such as cystatin C (Kaeser et al., 2007), might interfere with the seeding capacity of multimeric Aβ.

Finally, in an intriguing intersection of disease-related proteins, the normal, cellular form of the prion protein (PrP^{C}) was discovered to be a cell surface receptor for oligomeric Aβ (Salazar and Strittmatter, 2016). The implications of the Aβ–PrP interaction for AD appear to be complex, as its impact on Aβ toxicity or aggregation may be either deleterious (Um et al., 2012; Rushworth et al., 2013; Hu et al., 2014; Lauren, 2014) or beneficial (when it occurs in extracellular vesicles (Falker et al., 2016) or between Aβ and soluble (glycophosphatidylinositol anchor-free) PrP (Nieznanski et al., 2012)).

THE PRION-LIKE PROPERTIES OF AGGREGATED TAU

At the ultrastructural level, neurofibrillary tangles in AD consist predominantly of characteristic paired helical filaments (Crowther, 1991) that result from the ectopic polymerization of hyperphosphorylated tau protein (Lee et al., 2001; Spillantini and Goedert, 2013). Tau hyperphosphorylation is thought to be an early stage in the formation of tangles (although it can occur as a reversible phenomenon under such conditions as fetal development, hibernation, and hypothermia: Spillantini and Goedert, 2013).

Considerable evidence now supports the inclusion of tauopathy among the disorders that share a prion-like mechanism of pathogenesis. Similar to in vivo Aβ seeding, the accumulation of hyperphosphorylated tau is inducible in the brains of tau-transgenic host mice by infusion of aggregated tau seeds (Clavaguera et al., 2009, 2015; Guo and Lee, 2011; Holmes et al., 2014; Peeraer et al., 2015; Polanco et al., 2016; Gerson et al., 2016; Takeda et al., 2016). The ensuing tauopathy spreads systematically from the site of injection to axonally connected regions of the brain (Clavaguera et al., 2009, 2013; Ahmed et al., 2014; Stancu et al., 2015; Narasimhan et al., 2017), consistent with the uptake, transport, and discharge of tau seeds by neurons (Frost et al., 2009; Wu et al., 2013; Sanders et al., 2014). Neuronal activity augments the release of tau from cells in vitro, and also increases the amount of tauopathy in vivo (Wu et al., 2016). Additionally, tau antisense oligonucleotides decrease tau expression and pathology in mouse models, and also reverse pathologic tau seeding (DeVos et al., 2017). Like Aβ proteopathy and prion disease, tauopathy can be induced in the brain by tau seeds that have been infused into the peritoneal cavity (Clavaguera et al., 2014), and bioactive tau seeds exist in a range of sizes (Lasagna-Reeves et al., 2012; Mirbaha et al., 2015; Gerson et al., 2016; Jackson et al., 2016).

Brain extracts from donors with clinicopathologically distinct human tauopathies induce tau lesions in host mice that resemble the lesions in the corresponding human disorders (Clavaguera et al., 2013; Sanders et al., 2014; Boluda et al., 2015; Narasimhan et al., 2017), indicating that tau, like Aβ and PrP, can misfold into replicable proteopathic strains (Sanders et al., 2014). At the cellular level, multimeric tau is taken up by a heparan sulfate proteoglycan-associated mechanism

(Holmes et al., 2013), and the aggregates enter cells via macropinocytosis (Holmes et al., 2013; Falcon et al., 2015). Tau strains instigate distinct regional and cellular patterns of inclusions, and the strains can be reliably propagated in cell cultures (Kaufman et al., 2016). The bioactivity of tau strains in HEK cells was shown to be governed by the isoform composition (3-repeat and/or 4-repeat) of the tau seeds along with the isoform expression by the host cells (Woerman et al., 2016). Tau seeds are present in the human brain early in the development of tauopathy, and possibly prior to the histologic appearance of hyperphosphorylated tau within neurons (Furman et al., 2017).

Tau seeding differs from Aβ seeding in that tauopathy is readily inducible by AD brain extracts in nontransgenic (wild-type) mice (Audouard et al., 2016; Guo et al., 2016b). In addition, recombinant tau fibrils can fairly efficiently instigate tauopathy in tau-transgenic mice (Lasagna-Reeves et al., 2012; Clavaguera et al., 2013; Iba et al., 2013; Peeraer et al., 2015), although the potency of recombinant tau is less than that of tau that originates in brain samples (Falcon et al., 2015). Recombinant tau fibrils did not seed tauopathy in wild-type mice, possibly due to distinct conformational differences between artificially assembled fibrils and those generated in the brain (Guo et al., 2016b).

In the CSF of AD patients and transgenic mice expressing human-type tau, seed-competent tau is present that can stimulate tauopathy in cultured cells (Takeda et al., 2016), and some tau seeds in AD CSF appear to be associated with extracellular vesicles (Wang et al., 2017). The seeding capability of CSF tau in vivo, however, has not been reported; because CSF Aβ does not readily seed plaques or CAA in APP-transgenic mice (Fritschi et al., 2014b) (see above), a similar analysis of in vivo tau seeding by CSF from patients with AD (and other tauopathies) in the appropriate models could be informative.

These experiments collectively underscore the prion-like molecular properties of aggregated tau, but current evidence indicates that tauopathy, like Aβ-proteopathy, is not infectious in the customary sense of being facilely transmissible from one organism to another (Walker and Jucker, 2015). Rather, in AD, the process of tau misfolding and propagation takes place entirely within the affected organism. To model the endogenous emergence and spread of tauopathy, genetically modified mice were studied in which the expression of a disease-associated human tau transgene is restricted principally to projection neurons of the entorhinal cortex (de Calignon et al., 2012; Liu et al., 2012). The mice developed tauopathy initially in the entorhinal cortex, as expected, but with passing time the abnormalities successively emerged in axonally connected brain areas (de Calignon et al., 2012; Liu et al., 2012). Subsequent studies have found that the tau transgene is weakly expressed in other brain regions, which could influence the pattern of lesion progression (Yetman et al., 2016). However, when considered in light of the orderly neuroanatomic localization of tau lesions in interconnected brain regions in AD (Saper et al., 1987; Arnold et al., 1991; Braak and Braak, 1995), the experiments in mouse models implicate neuronal transport and cytotic mechanisms in the propagation of tau seeds within the nervous system. This possibility is indirectly supported by evidence for the neuronal trafficking of Aβ seeds, PrP prions, and other proteopathic seeds, as described above. Furthermore, in vivo imaging studies of the regional accumulation of pathogenic proteins in relation to the connectedness of the affected areas implicate the connectome in the systematic spread of seeds in AD and other neurodegenerative disorders (Bero et al., 2011; Zhou et al., 2012; Iturria-Medina et al., 2014; Raj et al., 2015).

PRION-LIKE SEEDING AND AD PATHOLOGY IN HUMANS

Between 1958 and 1985, approximately 30,000 children received a series of injections of cadaver-derived human growth hormone (c-hGH), in most instances to correct a deficiency in growth (Will, 2003; Brown et al., 2012). To obtain sufficient hormone for treatment, human pituitary glands were collected at autopsy, pooled into large batches, homogenized, and the c-hGH chemically extracted for injection. The treatment successfully stimulated growth, but years after treatment had ceased, a small percentage of the c-hGH recipients developed CJD (Brown et al., 2012). Subsequent studies have confirmed that the growth hormone was contaminated with PrP prions, which presumably originated from pituitaries inadvertently obtained from patients who had died with prion disease (Jucker and Walker, 2015). In 1985, cadaver-derived hGH was replaced by recombinant growth hormone, thereby effectively eliminating the possibility that the therapeutic agent would be contaminated by prions (Brown et al., 2012).

Hypothesizing that pituitaries collected from AD patients were likely to be included in the batches for hormone extraction, Jaunmuktane et al. (2015) sought evidence of AD-like pathology in 8 c-hGH recipients who had died of prion disease approximately 30 years after treatment. The cases ranged from 36 to 51 years of age at death – well before the lesions of idiopathic AD usually are evident – and they lacked the major genetic risk factors that would have predisposed them to early-onset AD. Along with the neurodegenerative changes typical of CJD, 4 of the subjects had extensive Aβ deposition in the brain in the form of both Aβ plaques and CAA, and 2 others had sparse Aβ deposits. Such Alzheimer-like Aβ-pathology was not present in control patients

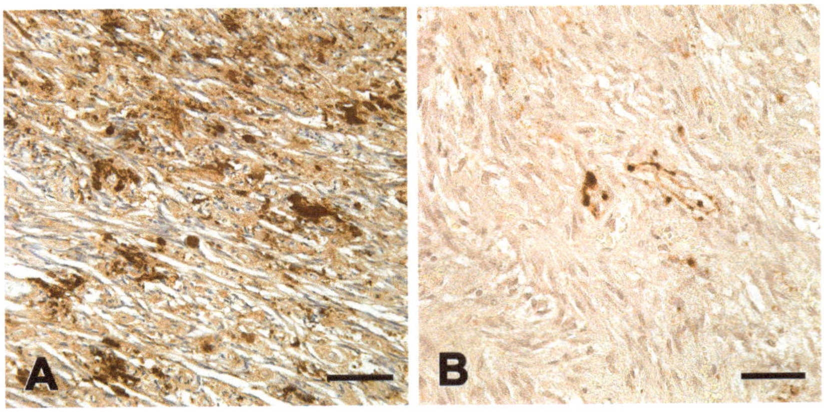

Fig. 16.4. Immunoreactive deposits (brown) of aggregated Aβ (**A**) and hyperphosphorylated tau (**B**) in the posterior lobe of the pituitary gland from a patient who had died with Alzheimer disease. Aβ was detected with antibody 82E1 to the N-terminal segment of Aβ, and tau was detected with antibody CP13 to an epitope around phosphoserine 202. The accumulation of Aβ and tau is generally mild in the pituitary. Hematoxylin counterstain (blue). Bars = 100 μm in (**A**) and 50 μm in (**B**).

of similar age who had died of other (non-c-hGH-related) prion diseases. In addition, the frequent presence of Aβ-CAA is reminiscent of the increased vascular Aβ deposition seen in APP-transgenic mice following peripheral administration of Aβ seeds (Eisele et al., 2010, 2014; Burwinkel et al., 2018).

Significant Aβ deposition also has been reported in the brains of patients who died of CJD years after receiving PrP prion-contaminated dura mater transplants (Frontzek et al., 2016; Hamaguchi et al., 2016) or in c-hGH recipients who died of causes other than CJD (Ritchie et al., 2017). The most parsimonious explanation for the presence of Aβ proteopathy in the recipients of human-derived biologics is that some batches of growth hormone and dura mater were contaminated with Aβ seeds in tissues originating from AD (or incipient AD) donors. This possibility is supported by evidence that some pituitary glands from AD patients (Irwin et al., 2013) (Fig. 16.4A) and also samples from implicated c-hGH (Duyckaerts et al., 2018) and dura mater (Kovacs et al., 2016) contain Aβ.

In light of experimental work on Aβ seeding in vivo (above), it is likely that a prion-like seeding mechanism underlies the development of Aβ plaques and Aβ-CAA in recipients of c-hGH and dura mater transplants. Surprisingly, few of these iatrogenic CJD patients also had evidence of significant tauopathy (Jaunmuktane et al., 2015; Kovacs et al., 2016; Duyckaerts et al., 2018). Mild tauopathy is present in AD-derived pituitaries (Hashizume et al., 2011; Irwin et al., 2013) (Fig. 16.4B), and, as discussed above, tauopathy is directly seedable by aggregated tau in experimental models. Some c-hGH samples have been found to contain tau (Duyckaerts et al., 2018). Furthermore, experimental studies show that tau polymerization can be cross-seeded by aggregated Aβ (Vasconcelos et al., 2016) and that tauopathy is augmented by Aβ plaques in vivo (Pooler et al., 2015; Li et al., 2016).

Whether the Aβ-positive recipients of c-hGH or dura transplants would have manifested the full AD phenotype had they lived longer cannot be known. An analysis of pituitary hormone recipients in the United States suggests that they are not more likely to develop AD than those in the general population (Irwin et al., 2013). However, longer-term follow-up and investigation of c-hGH recipients in other countries, particularly where the processing of the hormone differed from that in the United States (Brown et al., 2012), will be necessary to fully gauge the transmission risk of nonprion proteopathies in these instances.

CONCLUSIONS

The seeded propagation of misfolded Aβ is an early and obligatory occurrence in the cascade of events leading to the dementia of AD, but tauopathy is a critical downstream consequence that strongly impairs brain function. Both proteins have been shown to misfold, self-assemble, and convey their abnormal properties to like proteins by a prion-like molecular mechanism. Therapeutic strategies for AD stemming from the prion paradigm include impeding the production or multimerization of the proteins, uncoupling the pathogenic link between abnormal Aβ and tau, and promoting the elimination of the seeds from the brain. Because Aβ proteopathy and tauopathy each propagate by a prion-like mechanism of homologous protein corruption, it is likely that, once set in motion, the two pathologic processes advance more or less independently. If so, targeting Aβ should suffice for early prevention, but late-stage therapeutics will need to impede both branches of the cascade to be optimally effective. Another practical implication of the prion-like properties of misfolded Aβ and tau is to reinforce the importance of pristine instruments in neurosurgery. Finally, recognition of the prevalence of prionic mechanisms in neurodegenerative diseases could serve to integrate research efforts on these intractable disorders conceptually, experimentally, and therapeutically.

ACKNOWLEDGMENTS

I gratefully acknowledge insightful discussions with Mathias Jucker and the members of his laboratory in Tuebingen, and with David Lynn, Yury Chernoff, Anil Mehta, and Harry LeVine. This work was supported in part by National Institutes of Health grants P50 AG025688, RR00165, and OD11132, and the Alexander von Humboldt Foundation.

References

Agopian A, Guo Z (2012). Structural origin of polymorphism of Alzheimer's amyloid beta-fibrils. Biochem J 447: 43–50.

Ahmed Z, Cooper J, Murray TK et al. (2014). A novel in vivo model of tau propagation with rapid and progressive neurofibrillary tangle pathology: the pattern of spread is determined by connectivity, not proximity. Acta Neuropathol 127: 667–683.

American Psychiatric Association (2013). Diagnostic and statistical manual of mental disorders, fifth edition (DSM-5), American Psychiatric Press, Washington, DC.

Arnold SE, Hyman BT, Flory J et al. (1991). The topographical and neuroanatomical distribution of neurofibrillary tangles and neuritic plaques in the cerebral cortex of patients with Alzheimer's disease. Cereb Cortex 1: 103–116.

Attems J, Jellinger KA (2014). The overlap between vascular disease and Alzheimer's disease – lessons from pathology. BMC Med 12: 206.

Audouard E, Houben S, Masaracchia C et al. (2016). High-molecular-weight paired helical filaments from Alzheimer brain induces seeding of wild-type mouse tau into an argyrophilic 4R tau pathology in vivo. Am J Pathol 186: 2709–2722.

Baker HF, Ridley RM, Duchen LW et al. (1994). Induction of beta (A4)-amyloid in primates by injection of Alzheimer's disease brain homogenate. Comparison with transmission of spongiform encephalopathy. Mol Neurobiol 8: 25–39.

Bateman RJ, Xiong C, Benzinger TL et al. (2012). Clinical and biomarker changes in dominantly inherited Alzheimer's disease. N Engl J Med 367: 795–804.

Benilova I, Gallardo R, Ungureanu AA et al. (2014). The Alzheimer disease protective mutation A2T modulates kinetic and thermodynamic properties of amyloid-beta (Abeta) aggregation. J Biol Chem 289: 30977–30989.

Bero AW, Yan P, Roh JH et al. (2011). Neuronal activity regulates the regional vulnerability to amyloid-beta deposition. Nat Neurosci 14: 750–756.

Bierer LM, Hof PR, Purohit DP et al. (1995). Neocortical neurofibrillary tangles correlate with dementia severity in Alzheimer's disease. Arch Neurol 52: 81–88.

Biffi A, Greenberg SM (2011). Cerebral amyloid angiopathy: a systematic review. J Clin Neurol 7: 1–9.

Boluda S, Iba M, Zhang B et al. (2015). Differential induction and spread of tau pathology in young PS19 tau transgenic mice following intracerebral injections of pathological tau from Alzheimer's disease or corticobasal degeneration brains. Acta Neuropathol 129: 221–237.

Braak H, Braak E (1995). Staging of Alzheimer's disease-related neurofibrillary changes. Neurobiol Aging 16: 271–278; discussion 278–284.

Brown P, Brandel JP, Sato T et al. (2012). Iatrogenic Creutzfeldt-Jakob disease, final assessment. Emerg Infect Dis 18: 901–907.

Burwinkel M, Lutzenberger M, Heppner FL et al. (2018). Intravenous injection of beta-amyloid seeds promotes cerebral amyloid angiopathy (CAA). Acta Neuropathol Commun 6 (1): 23. https://doi.org/10.1186/s40478-018-0511-7. PMID: 29506560.

Buyukmihci N, Goehring-Harmon F, Marsh RF (1983). Neural pathogenesis of experimental scrapie after intraocular inoculation of hamsters. Exp Neurol 81: 396–406.

Charidimou A, Gang Q, Werring DJ (2012). Sporadic cerebral amyloid angiopathy revisited: recent insights into pathophysiology and clinical spectrum. J Neurol Neurosurg Psychiatry 83: 124–137.

Chouraki V, Seshadri S (2014). Genetics of Alzheimer's disease. Adv Genet 87: 245–294.

Cintron AF, Dalal NV, Dooyema J et al. (2015). Transport of cargo from periphery to brain by circulating monocytes. Brain Res 1622: 328–338.

Clavaguera F, Bolmont T, Crowther RA et al. (2009). Transmission and spreading of tauopathy in transgenic mouse brain. Nat Cell Biol 11: 909–913.

Clavaguera F, Akatsu H, Fraser G et al. (2013). Brain homogenates from human tauopathies induce tau inclusions in mouse brain. Proc Natl Acad Sci U S A 110: 9535–9540.

Clavaguera F, Hench J, Lavenir I et al. (2014). Peripheral administration of tau aggregates triggers intracerebral tauopathy in transgenic mice. Acta Neuropathol 127: 299–301.

Clavaguera F, Hench J, Goedert M et al. (2015). Invited review: prion-like transmission and spreading of tau pathology. Neuropathol Appl Neurobiol 41: 47–58.

Cohen ML, Kim C, Haldiman T et al. (2015). Rapidly progressive Alzheimer's disease features distinct structures of amyloid-beta. Brain 138: 1009–1022.

Condello C, Lemmin T, Stöhr J et al. (2018). Structural heterogeneity and intersubject variability of Aβ in familial and sporadic Alzheimer's disease. Proc Natl Acad Sci U S A 115 (4): E782–E791. https://doi.org/10.1073/pnas.1714966115. [Epub 2018 Jan 8]. PMID: 29311311.

Crary JF, Trojanowski JQ, Schneider JA et al. (2014). Primary age-related tauopathy (PART): a common pathology associated with human aging. Acta Neuropathol 128: 755–766.

Crowther RA (1991). Straight and paired helical filaments in Alzheimer disease have a common structural unit. Proc Natl Acad Sci U S A 88: 2288–2292.

Crystal H, Dickson D, Fuld P et al. (1988). Clinico-pathologic studies in dementia: nondemented subjects with pathologically confirmed Alzheimer's disease. Neurology 38: 1682–1687.

Dartigues JF (2009). Alzheimer's disease: a global challenge for the 21st century. Lancet Neurol 8: 1082–1083.

DeArmond SJ, Prusiner SB (1995). Etiology and pathogenesis of prion diseases. Am J Pathol 146: 785–811.

DeArmond SJ, Ironside JW, Bouzamondo-Bernstein E et al. (2004). Neuropathology of prion diseases. In: SB Prusiner (Ed.), Prion biology and diseases. Cold Spring Harbor Laboratory Press, Cold Spring Harbor, NY.

de Calignon A, Polydoro M, Suarez-Calvet M et al. (2012). Propagation of tau pathology in a model of early Alzheimer's disease. Neuron 73: 685–697.

Deleault NR, Piro JR, Walsh DJ et al. (2012). Isolation of phosphatidylethanolamine as a solitary cofactor for prion formation in the absence of nucleic acids. Proc Natl Acad Sci U S A 109: 8546–8551.

DeVos SL, Miller RL, Schoch KM et al. (2017). Tau reduction prevents neuronal loss and reverses pathological tau deposition and seeding in mice with tauopathy. Sci Transl Med: 9.

Diack AB, Alibhai JD, Barron R et al. (2016). Insights into mechanisms of chronic neurodegeneration. Int J Mol Sci: 17.

Di Fede G, Catania M, Morbin M et al. (2009). A recessive mutation in the APP gene with dominant-negative effect on amyloidogenesis. Science 323: 1473–1477.

Domert J, Rao SB, Agholme L et al. (2014). Spreading of amyloid-beta peptides via neuritic cell-to-cell transfer is dependent on insufficient cellular clearance. Neurobiol Dis 65: 82–92.

Drachman DA (2014). The amyloid hypothesis, time to move on: Amyloid is the downstream result, not cause, of Alzheimer's disease. Alzheimers Dement 10: 372–380.

Duran-Aniotz C, Morales R, Moreno-Gonzalez I et al. (2013). Brains from non-Alzheimer's individuals containing amyloid deposits accelerate Abeta deposition in vivo. Acta Neuropathol Commun 1: 76.

Duran-Aniotz C, Morales R, Moreno-Gonzalez I et al. (2014). Aggregate-depleted brain fails to induce Abeta deposition in a mouse model of Alzheimer's disease. PLoS One 9: e89014.

Duyckaerts C, Delatour B, Potier MC (2009). Classification and basic pathology of Alzheimer disease. Acta Neuropathol 118: 5–36.

Duyckaerts C, Sazdovitch V, Ando K et al. (2018). Neuropathology of iatrogenic Creutzfeldt-Jakob disease and immunoassay of French cadaver-sourced growth hormone batches suggest possible transmission of tauopathy and long incubation periods for the transmission of Abeta pathology. Acta Neuropathol 135 (2): 201–212. https://doi.org/10.1007/s00401-017-1791-x. [Epub 2017 Nov 22]. PMID: 29209767.

Eisele YS, Duyckaerts C (2016). Propagation of Ass pathology: hypotheses, discoveries, and yet unresolved questions from experimental and human brain studies. Acta Neuropathol 131: 5–25.

Eisele YS, Obermuller U, Heilbronner G et al. (2010). Peripherally applied Abeta-containing inoculates induce cerebral beta-amyloidosis. Science 330: 980–982.

Eisele YS, Fritschi SK, Hamaguchi T et al. (2014). Multiple factors contribute to the peripheral induction of cerebral beta-amyloidosis. J Neurosci 34: 10264–10273.

Eisenberg D, Jucker M (2012). The amyloid state of proteins in human diseases. Cell 148: 1188–1203.

Falcon B, Cavallini A, Angers R et al. (2015). Conformation determines the seeding potencies of native and recombinant Tau aggregates. J Biol Chem 290: 1049–1065.

Falker C, Hartmann A, Guett I et al. (2016). Exosomal cellular prion protein drives fibrillization of amyloid beta and counteracts amyloid beta-mediated neurotoxicity. J Neurochem 137: 88–100.

Farquhar J, Gajdusek DC (1981). Kuru: early letters and field notes from the collection of D, Raven Press, Carleton Gajdusek. New York.

Fevrier B, Vilette D, Archer F et al. (2004). Cells release prions in association with exosomes. Proc Natl Acad Sci U S A 101: 9683–9688.

Fowler DM, Koulov AV, Balch WE et al. (2007). Functional amyloid – from bacteria to humans. Trends Biochem Sci 32: 217–224.

Fraser H (1982). Neuronal spread of scrapie agent and targeting of lesions within the retino-tectal pathway. Nature 295: 149–150.

Fritschi SK, Cintron A, Ye L et al. (2014a). Abeta seeds resist inactivation by formaldehyde. Acta Neuropathol 128: 477–484.

Fritschi SK, Langer F, Kaeser SA et al. (2014b). Highly potent soluble amyloid-beta seeds in human Alzheimer brain but not cerebrospinal fluid. Brain 137: 2909–2915.

Frontzek K, Lutz MI, Aguzzi A et al. (2016). Amyloid-beta pathology and cerebral amyloid angiopathy are frequent in iatrogenic Creutzfeldt-Jakob disease after dural grafting. Swiss Med Wkly w14287: 146.

Frost B, Jacks RL, Diamond MI (2009). Propagation of tau misfolding from the outside to the inside of a cell. J Biol Chem 284: 12845–12852.

Furman JL, Vaquer-Alicea J, White CL (2017). Widespread tau seeding activity at early Braak stages. Acta Neuropathol 133: 91–100.

Gajdusek DC (1977). Unconventional viruses and the origin and disappearance of kuru. Science 197: 943–960.

Gajdusek DC, Gibbs CJ, Alpers M (1966). Experimental transmission of a kuru-like syndrome to chimpanzees. Nature 209: 794–796.

Gajdusek DC, Gibbs Jr CJ, Asher DM et al. (1968). Transmission of experimental kuru to the spider monkey (*Ateles geoffreyi*). Science 162: 693–694.

Gambetti P, Cali I, Notari S et al. (2011). Molecular biology and pathology of prion strains in sporadic human prion diseases. Acta Neuropathol 121: 79–90.

Gatz M, Reynolds CA, Fratiglioni L et al. (2006). Role of genes and environments for explaining Alzheimer disease. Arch Gen Psychiatry 63: 168–174.

Gerson J, Kayed R (2016). Therapeutic approaches targeting pathological tau aggregates. Curr Pharm Des 22: 4028–4039.

Gerson J, Castillo-Carranza DL, Sengupta U et al. (2016). Tau oligomers derived from traumatic brain injury cause cognitive impairment and accelerate onset of pathology in Htau mice. J Neurotrauma 33: 2034–2043.

Giaccone G, Mangieri M, Capobianco R et al. (2008). Tauopathy in human and experimental variant Creutzfeldt-Jakob disease. Neurobiol Aging 29: 1864–1873.

Giaccone G, Morbin M, Moda F et al. (2010). Neuropathology of the recessive A673V APP mutation: Alzheimer disease with distinctive features. Acta Neuropathol 120: 803–812.

Gibbs Jr CJ, Gajdusek DC, Asher DM et al. (1968). Creutzfeldt-Jakob disease (spongiform encephalopathy): transmission to the chimpanzee. Science 161: 388–389.

Goedert M (2015). Neurodegeneration. Alzheimer's and Parkinson's diseases: the prion concept in relation to assembled Abeta, tau, and alpha-synuclein. Science 349: 1255555.

Goudsmit J, Morrow CH, Asher DM et al. (1980). Evidence for and against the transmissibility of Alzheimer disease. Neurology 30: 945–950.

Greenwald J, Riek R (2010). Biology of amyloid: structure, function, and regulation. Structure 18: 1244–1260.

Guo JL, Lee VM (2011). Seeding of normal tau by pathological tau conformers drives pathogenesis of Alzheimer-like tangles. J Biol Chem 286: 15317–15331.

Guo BB, Bellingham SA, Hill AF (2016a). Stimulating the release of exosomes increases the intercellular transfer of prions. J Biol Chem 291: 5128–5137.

Guo JL, Narasimhan S, Changolkar L et al. (2016b). Unique pathological tau conformers from Alzheimer's brains transmit tau pathology in nontransgenic mice. J Exp Med 213: 2635–2654.

Haass C, Selkoe DJ (2007). Soluble protein oligomers in neurodegeneration: lessons from the Alzheimer's amyloid beta-peptide. Nat Rev Mol Cell Biol 8: 101–112.

Haass C, Kaether C, Thinakaran G et al. (2012). Trafficking and proteolytic processing of APP. Cold Spring Harb Perspect Med 2: a006270.

Hamaguchi T, Eisele YS, Varvel NH et al. (2012). The presence of Abeta seeds, and not age per se, is critical to the initiation of Abeta deposition in the brain. Acta Neuropathol 123: 31–37.

Hamaguchi T, Taniguchi Y, Sakai K et al. (2016). Significant association of cadaveric dura mater grafting with subpial Abeta deposition and meningeal amyloid angiopathy. Acta Neuropathol 132: 313–315.

Hardy J (2006). A hundred years of Alzheimer's disease research. Neuron 52: 3–13.

Hardy J, Selkoe DJ (2002). The amyloid hypothesis of Alzheimer's disease: progress and problems on the road to therapeutics. Science 297: 353–356.

Harper JD, Lansbury Jr PT (1997). Models of amyloid seeding in Alzheimer's disease and scrapie: mechanistic truths and physiological consequences of the time-dependent solubility of amyloid proteins. Annu Rev Biochem 66: 385–407.

Hashizume M, Takagi J, Kanehira T et al. (2011). Histologic study of age-related change in the posterior pituitary gland focusing on abnormal deposition of tau protein. Pathol Int 61: 13–18.

Hauw JJ, Duyckaerts C (2001). Alzheimer's disease. In: S Duckett, JC De La Torre (Eds.), Pathology of the aging human nervous system, 2nd edn. Oxford University Press, Oxford.

Head E, Lott IT, Wilcock DM et al. (2016). Aging in Down syndrome and the development of Alzheimer's disease neuropathology. Curr Alzheimer Res 13: 18–29.

Heilbronner G, Eisele YS, Langer F et al. (2013). Seeded strain-like transmission of beta-amyloid morphotypes in APP transgenic mice. EMBO Rep 14: 1017–1022.

Hock EM, Polymenidou M (2016). Prion-like propagation as a pathogenic principle in frontotemporal dementia. J Neurochem 138 Suppl 1: 163–183.

Holmes BB, DeVos SL, Kfoury N et al. (2013). Heparan sulfate proteoglycans mediate internalization and propagation of specific proteopathic seeds. Proc Natl Acad Sci U S A 110: E3138–E3147.

Holmes BB, Furman JL, Mahan TE et al. (2014). Proteopathic tau seeding predicts tauopathy in vivo. Proc Natl Acad Sci U S A 111: E4376–E4385.

Holtzman DM, Morris JC, Goate AM (2011). Alzheimer's disease: the challenge of the second century. Sci Transl Med 3: 77sr71.

Hu X, Crick SL, Bu G et al. (2009). Amyloid seeds formed by cellular uptake, concentration, and aggregation of the amyloid-beta peptide. Proc Natl Acad Sci U S A 106: 20324–20329.

Hu NW, Nicoll AJ, Zhang D et al. (2014). mGlu5 receptors and cellular prion protein mediate amyloid-beta-facilitated synaptic long-term depression in vivo. Nat Commun 5: 3374.

Huang YA, Zhou B, Wernig M et al. (2017). ApoE2, ApoE3, and ApoE4 differentially stimulate APP transcription and Abeta secretion. Cell 168: 427–441.

Humphries C, Kohli MA (2014). Rare variants and transcriptomics in Alzheimer disease. Curr Genet Med Rep 2: 75–84.

Iba M, Guo JL, McBride JD et al. (2013). Synthetic tau fibrils mediate transmission of neurofibrillary tangles in a transgenic mouse model of Alzheimer's-like tauopathy. J Neurosci 33: 1024–1037.

Iba M, McBride JD, Guo JL et al. (2015). Tau pathology spread in PS19 tau transgenic mice following locus coeruleus (LC) injections of synthetic tau fibrils is determined by the LC's afferent and efferent connections. Acta Neuropathol 130: 349–362.

Ironside JW, Head MW, Bell JE et al. (2000). Laboratory diagnosis of variant Creutzfeldt-Jakob disease. Histopathology 37: 1–9.

Irwin DJ, Abrams JY, Schonberger LB et al. (2013). Evaluation of potential infectivity of Alzheimer and Parkinson disease proteins in recipients of cadaver-derived human growth hormone. JAMA Neurol 70: 462–468.

Iturria-Medina Y, Sotero RC, Toussaint PJ et al. (2014). Epidemic spreading model to characterize misfolded proteins propagation in aging and associated neurodegenerative disorders. PLoS Comput Biol 10: e1003956.

Jack Jr CR, Holtzman DM (2013). Biomarker modeling of Alzheimer's disease. Neuron 80: 1347–1358.

Jack Jr CR, Knopman DS, Jagust WJ et al. (2010). Hypothetical model of dynamic biomarkers of the Alzheimer's pathological cascade. Lancet Neurol 9: 119–128.

Jackson SJ, Kerridge C, Cooper J et al. (2016). Short fibrils constitute the major species of seed-competent tau in the brains of mice transgenic for human P301S tau. J Neurosci 36: 762–772.

Jaunmuktane Z, Mead S, Ellis M et al. (2015). Evidence for human transmission of amyloid-beta pathology and cerebral amyloid angiopathy. Nature 525: 247–250.

Jonsson T, Atwal JK, Steinberg S et al. (2012). A mutation in APP protects against Alzheimer's disease and age-related cognitive decline. Nature 488: 96–99.

Joshi P, Benussi L, Furlan R et al. (2015). Extracellular vesicles in Alzheimer's disease: friends or foes? Focus on abeta-vesicle interaction. Int J Mol Sci 16: 4800–4813.

Jucker M, Walker LC (2013). Self-propagation of pathogenic protein aggregates in neurodegenerative diseases. Nature 501: 45–51.

Jucker M, Walker LC (2015). Neurodegeneration: amyloid-beta pathology induced in humans. Nature 525: 193–194.

Kaeser SA, Herzig MC, Coomaraswamy J et al. (2007). Cystatin C modulates cerebral beta-amyloidosis. Nat Genet 39: 1437–1439.

Kalimo H, Lalowski M, Bogdanovic N et al. (2013). The arctic AbetaPP mutation leads to Alzheimer's disease pathology with highly variable topographic deposition of differentially truncated Abeta. Acta Neuropathol Commun 1: 60.

Kane MD, Lipinski WJ, Callahan MJ et al. (2000). Evidence for seeding of beta-amyloid by intracerebral infusion of Alzheimer brain extracts in beta -amyloid precursor protein-transgenic mice. J Neurosci 20: 3606–3611.

Kapasi A, Schneider JA (2016). Vascular contributions to cognitive impairment, clinical Alzheimer's disease, and dementia in older persons. Biochim Biophys Acta 1862: 878–886.

Kaufman SK, Sanders DW, Thomas TL et al. (2016). Tau prion strains dictate patterns of cell pathology, progression rate, and regional vulnerability in vivo. Neuron 92: 796–812.

Kawas CH, Katzman R (1999). Epidemiology of dementia and Alzheimer disease. In: RD Terry, R Katzman, KL Bick et al. (Eds.), Alzheimer disease, Lippincott Williams and Wilkins, Philadelphia.

Killin LO, Starr JM, Shiue IJ et al. (2016). Environmental risk factors for dementia: a systematic review. BMC Geriatr 16: 175.

Kimberlin RH, Walker CA (1986). Pathogenesis of scrapie (strain 263K) in hamsters infected intracerebrally, intraperitoneally or intraocularly. J Gen Virol 67: 255–263.

Kodali R, Williams AD, Chemuru S et al. (2010). Abeta(1-40) forms five distinct amyloid structures whose beta-sheet contents and fibril stabilities are correlated. J Mol Biol 401: 503–517.

Kovacs GG (2015). Invited review: neuropathology of tauopathies: principles and practice. Neuropathol Appl Neurobiol 41: 3–23.

Kovacs GG, Lutz MI, Ricken G et al. (2016). Dura mater is a potential source of Abeta seeds. Acta Neuropathol 131: 911–923.

Kovacs GG, Rahimi J, Strobel T et al. (2017). Tau pathology in Creutzfeldt-Jakob disease revisited. Brain Pathol 27: 332–344.

Lafortune L, Martin S, Kelly S et al. (2016). Behavioural risk factors in mid-life associated with successful ageing, disability, dementia and frailty in later life: a rapid systematic review. PLoS One 11: e0144405.

Lambert MP, Barlow AK, Chromy BA et al. (1998). Diffusible, nonfibrillar ligands derived from Abeta1-42 are potent central nervous system neurotoxins. Proc Natl Acad Sci U S A 95: 6448–6453.

Langer F, Eisele YS, Fritschi SK et al. (2011). Soluble Abeta seeds are potent inducers of cerebral beta-amyloid deposition. J Neurosci 31: 14488–14495.

Lasagna-Reeves CA, Castillo-Carranza DL, Sengupta U et al. (2012). Alzheimer brain-derived tau oligomers propagate pathology from endogenous tau. Sci Rep 2: 700.

Lauren J (2014). Cellular prion protein as a therapeutic target in Alzheimer's disease. J Alzheimers Dis 38: 227–244.

Lee VM-Y, Goedert M, Trojanowski JQ (2001). Neurodegenerative tauopathies. Annual Review of Neuroscience 24: 1121–1159.

Legname G, Baskakov IV, Nguyen HO et al. (2004). Synthetic mammalian prions. Science 305: 673–676.

Lewczuk P, Mroczko B, Fagan A et al. (2015). Biomarkers of Alzheimer's disease and mild cognitive impairment: a current perspective. Adv Med Sci 60: 76–82.

Li T, Braunstein KE, Zhang J et al. (2016). The neuritic plaque facilitates pathological conversion of tau in an Alzheimer's disease mouse model. Nat Commun 7: 12082.

Liberski PP, Hainfellner JA, Sikorska B et al. (2012). Prion protein (PrP) deposits in the tectum of experimental Gerstmann-Straussler-Scheinker disease following intraocular inoculation. Folia Neuropathol 50: 85–88.

Liu L, Drouet V, Wu JW et al. (2012). Trans-synaptic spread of tau pathology in vivo. PLoS One 7: e31302.

Liu CC, Kanekiyo T, Xu H et al. (2013). Apolipoprotein E and Alzheimer disease: risk, mechanisms and therapy. Nat Rev Neurol 9: 106–118.

Lu JX, Qiang W, Yau WM et al. (2013). Molecular structure of beta-amyloid fibrils in Alzheimer's disease brain tissue. Cell 154: 1257–1268.

Lundmark K, Westermark GT, Nystrom S et al. (2002). Transmissibility of systemic amyloidosis by a prion-like mechanism. Proc Natl Acad Sci U S A 99: 6979–6984.

Mann DM, Yates PO (1986). Neurotransmitter deficits in Alzheimer's disease and in other dementing disorders. Hum Neurobiol 5: 147–158.

Marzesco AM, Flotenmeyer M, Buhler A et al. (2016). Highly potent intracellular membrane-associated Abeta seeds. Sci Rep 6: 28125.

Matveev SV, Spielmann HP, Metts BM et al. (2014). A distinct subfraction of Abeta is responsible for the high-affinity Pittsburgh compound B-binding site in Alzheimer's disease brain. J Neurochem 131: 356–368.

McKintosh E, Tabrizi SJ, Collinge J (2003). Prion diseases. J Neurovirol 9: 183–193.

Meinhardt J, Sachse C, Hortschansky P et al. (2009). Abeta (1-40) fibril polymorphism implies diverse interaction patterns in amyloid fibrils. J Mol Biol 386: 869–877.

Meyer-Luehmann M, Coomaraswamy J, Bolmont T et al. (2006). Exogenous induction of cerebral β-amyloidogenesis is governed by agent and host. Science 313: 1781–1784.

Miller Y, Ma B, Nussinov R (2010). Polymorphism in Alzheimer Abeta amyloid organization reflects conformational selection in a rugged energy landscape. Chem Rev 110: 4820–4838.

Mirbaha H, Holmes BB, Sanders DW et al. (2015). Tau trimers are the minimal propagation unit spontaneously internalized to seed intracellular aggregation. J Biol Chem 290: 14893–14903.

Morales R, Duran-Aniotz C, Castilla J et al. (2012). De novo induction of amyloid-beta deposition in vivo. Mol Psychiatry 17: 1347–1353.

Morales R, Bravo-Alegria J, Duran-Aniotz C et al. (2015a). Titration of biologically active amyloid-beta seeds in a transgenic mouse model of Alzheimer's disease. Sci Rep 5: 9349.

Morales R, Callegari K, Soto C (2015b). Prion-like features of misfolded Abeta and tau aggregates. Virus Res 207: 106–112.

Morgado I, Garvey M (2015). Lipids in amyloid-beta processing, aggregation, and toxicity. Adv Exp Med Biol 855: 67–94.

Narasimhan S, Guo JL, Changolkar L et al. (2017). Pathological tau strains from human brains recapitulate the diversity of tauopathies in nontransgenic mouse brain. J Neurosci 37 (47): 11406–11423. https://doi.org/10.1523/JNEUROSCI.1230-17.2017. [Epub 2017 Oct 20]. PMID: 29054878.

Nath S, Agholme L, Kurudenkandy FR et al. (2012). Spreading of neurodegenerative pathology via neuron-to-neuron transmission of beta-amyloid. J Neurosci 32: 8767–8777.

Nelson PT, Alafuzoff I, Bigio EH et al. (2012). Correlation of Alzheimer disease neuropathologic changes with cognitive status: a review of the literature. J Neuropathol Exp Neurol 71: 362–381.

Nieznanski K, Choi JK, Chen S et al. (2012). Soluble prion protein inhibits amyloid-beta (Abeta) fibrillization and toxicity. J Biol Chem 287: 33104–33108.

Nilsson KP, Aslund A, Berg I et al. (2007). Imaging distinct conformational states of amyloid-beta fibrils in Alzheimer's disease using novel luminescent probes. ACS Chem Biol 2: 553–560.

Novotny R, Langer F, Mahler J et al. (2016). Conversion of synthetic abeta to in vivo active seeds and amyloid plaque formation in a hippocampal slice culture model. J Neurosci 36: 5084–5093.

Olsson B, Lautner R, Andreasson U et al. (2016). CSF and blood biomarkers for the diagnosis of Alzheimer's disease: a systematic review and meta-analysis. Lancet Neurol 15: 673–684.

Paravastu AK, Leapman RD, Yau WM et al. (2008). Molecular structural basis for polymorphism in Alzheimer's beta-amyloid fibrils. Proc Natl Acad Sci U S A 105: 18349–18354.

Peeraer E, Bottelbergs A, Van Kolen K et al. (2015). Intracerebral injection of preformed synthetic tau fibrils initiates widespread tauopathy and neuronal loss in the brains of tau transgenic mice. Neurobiol Dis 73: 83–95.

Peretz D, Williamson RA, Legname G et al. (2002). A change in the conformation of prions accompanies the emergence of a new prion strain. Neuron 34: 921–932.

Petkova AT, Leapman RD, Guo Z et al. (2005). Self-propagating, molecular-level polymorphism in Alzheimer's beta-amyloid fibrils. Science 307: 262–265.

Piccardo P, King D, Telling G et al. (2013). Dissociation of prion protein amyloid seeding from transmission of a spongiform encephalopathy. J Virol 87: 12349–12356.

Piccini A, Russo C, Gliozzi A et al. (2005). Beta-amyloid is different in normal aging and in Alzheimer disease. J Biol Chem 34: 186–192.

Pike CJ (2017). Sex and the development of Alzheimer's disease. J Neurosci Res 95: 671–680.

Polanco JC, Scicluna BJ, Hill AF et al. (2016). Extracellular vesicles isolated from the brains of rTg4510 mice seed tau protein aggregation in a threshold-dependent manner. J Biol Chem 291: 12445–12466.

Pooler AM, Polydoro M, Maury EA et al. (2015). Amyloid accelerates tau propagation and toxicity in a model of early Alzheimer's disease. Acta Neuropathol Commun 3: 14.

Portelius E, Lashley T, Westerlund A et al. (2015). Brain amyloid-beta fragment signatures in pathological ageing and Alzheimer's disease by hybrid immunoprecipitation mass spectrometry. Neurodegener Dis 15: 50–57.

Potter H, Wisniewski T (2012). Apolipoprotein e: essential catalyst of the Alzheimer amyloid cascade. Int J Alzheimers Dis 2012: 489428.

Properzi F, Logozzi M, Abdel-Haq H et al. (2015). Detection of exosomal prions in blood by immunochemistry techniques. J Gen Virol 96: 1969–1974.

Prusiner SB (1984). Some speculations about prions, amyloid, and Alzheimer's disease. N Engl J Med 310: 661–663.

Prusiner SB (2013). Biology and genetics of prions causing neurodegeneration. Annu Rev Genet 47: 601–623.

Qiang W, Yau WM, Lu JX et al. (2017). Structural variation in amyloid-beta fibrils from Alzheimer's disease clinical subtypes. Nature 541: 217–221.

Raj A, LoCastro E, Kuceyeski A et al. (2015). Network diffusion model of progression predicts longitudinal patterns of atrophy and metabolism in Alzheimer's disease. Cell Rep: pii: S2211-1247(14)01063-8.

Rajendran L, Honsho M, Zahn TR et al. (2006). Alzheimer's disease beta-amyloid peptides are released in association with exosomes. Proc Natl Acad Sci U S A 103: 11172–11177.

Rangel A, Race B, Phillips K et al. (2014). Distinct patterns of spread of prion infection in brains of mice expressing anchorless or anchored forms of prion protein. Acta Neuropathol Commun 2: 8.

Rasmussen J, Mahler J, Beschorner N et al. (2017). Amyloid polymorphisms constitute distinct clouds of conformational variants in different etiological subtypes of Alzheimer's disease.

Proc Natl Acad Sci U S A 114 (49): 13018–13023. https://doi.org/10.1073/pnas.1713215114. [Epub 2017 Nov 20]. PMID: 29158413.

Reitz C, Brayne C, Mayeux R (2011). Epidemiology of Alzheimer disease. Nat Rev Neurol 7: 137–152.

Resnick SM, Bilgel M, Moghekar A et al. (2015). Changes in Abeta biomarkers and associations with APOE genotype in 2 longitudinal cohorts. Neurobiol Aging 36: 2333–2339.

Revesz T, Ghiso J, Lashley T et al. (2003). Cerebral amyloid angiopathies: a pathologic, biochemical, and genetic view. J Neuropathol Exp Neurol 62: 885–898.

Rey NL, Steiner JA, Maroof N et al. (2016). Widespread trans-neuronal propagation of alpha-synucleinopathy triggered in olfactory bulb mimics prodromal Parkinson's disease. J Exp Med 213: 1759–1778.

Ritchie DL, Adlard P, Peden AH et al. (2017). Amyloid-β accumulation in the CNS in human growth hormone recipients in the UK. Acta Neuropathol 134: 221–240.

Ronnback A, Sagelius H, Bergstedt KD et al. (2012). Amyloid neuropathology in the single Arctic APP transgenic model affects interconnected brain regions. Neurobiol Aging 33 (831): e811–839.

Rosen RF, Ciliax BJ, Wingo TS et al. (2010). Deficient high-affinity binding of Pittsburgh compound B in a case of Alzheimer's disease. Acta Neuropathol 119: 221–233.

Rosen RF, Walker LC, Levine H (2011). PIB binding in aged primate brain: enrichment of high-affinity sites in humans with Alzheimer's disease. Neurobiol Aging 32: 223–234.

Rosen RF, Fritz JJ, Dooyema J et al. (2012). Exogenous seeding of cerebral beta-amyloid deposition in betaAPP-transgenic rats. J Neurochem 120: 660–666.

Rosen RF, Tomidokoro Y, Farberg AS et al. (2016). Comparative pathobiology of beta-amyloid and the unique susceptibility of humans to Alzheimer's disease. Neurobiol Aging 44: 185–196.

Rushworth JV, Griffiths HH, Watt NT et al. (2013). Prion protein-mediated toxicity of amyloid-beta oligomers requires lipid rafts and the transmembrane LRP1. J Biol Chem 288: 8935–8951.

Salazar SV, Strittmatter SM (2016). Cellular prion protein as a receptor for amyloid-beta oligomers in Alzheimer's disease. Biochem Biophys Res Commun 291: 17112–17121.

Sanders DW, Kaufman SK, DeVos SL et al. (2014). Distinct tau prion strains propagate in cells and mice and define different tauopathies. Neuron 82: 1271–1288.

Saper CB, Wainer BH, German DC (1987). Axonal and trans-neuronal transport in the transmission of neurological disease: potential role in system degenerations, including Alzheimer's disease. Neuroscience 23: 389–398.

Selkoe DJ (2011). Resolving controversies on the path to Alzheimer's therapeutics. Nat Med 17: 1060–1065.

Selkoe DJ, Hardy J (2016). The amyloid hypothesis of Alzheimer's disease at 25 years. EMBO Mol Med 8: 595–608.

Sherzai A, Edland SD, Masliah E et al. (2013). Spongiform change in dementia with Lewy bodies and Alzheimer disease. Alzheimer Dis Assoc Disord 27: 157–161.

Silveira JR, Raymond GJ, Hughson AG et al. (2005). The most infectious prion protein particles. Nature 437: 257–261.

Sipe JD, Benson MD, Buxbaum JN et al. (2016). Amyloid fibril proteins and amyloidosis: chemical identification and clinical classification International Society of Amyloidosis 2016 Nomenclature Guidelines. Amyloid 23: 209–213.

Smith TW, Anwer U, DeGirolami U et al. (1987). Vacuolar change in Alzheimer's disease. Arch Neurol 44: 1225–1228.

Spillantini MG, Goedert M (2013). Tau pathology and neurodegeneration. Lancet Neurol 12: 609–622.

Spirig T, Ovchinnikova O, Vagt T et al. (2014). Direct evidence for self-propagation of different amyloid-beta fibril conformations. Neurodegener Dis 14: 151–159.

Stancu IC, Vasconcelos B, Ris L et al. (2015). Templated misfolding of Tau by prion-like seeding along neuronal connections impairs neuronal network function and associated behavioral outcomes in Tau transgenic mice. Acta Neuropathol 129: 875–894.

Stohr J, Watts JC, Mensinger ZL et al. (2012). Purified and synthetic Alzheimer's amyloid beta (Abeta) prions. Proc Natl Acad Sci U S A 109: 11025–11030.

Stohr J, Condello C, Watts JC et al. (2014). Distinct synthetic Abeta prion strains producing different amyloid deposits in bigenic mice. Proc Natl Acad Sci U S A 111: 10329–10334.

Takeda S, Commins C, DeVos SL et al. (2016). Seed-competent HMW tau species accumulates in the cerebrospinal fluid of Alzheimer's disease mouse model and human patients. Ann Neurol 80: 355–367.

Tanaka M, Collins SR, Toyama BH et al. (2006). The physical basis of how prion conformations determine strain phenotypes. Nature 442: 585–589.

Tanzi RE (2012). The genetics of Alzheimer disease. Cold Spring Harb Perspect Med 2.

Tayeb-Fligelman E, Tabachnikov O, Moshe A et al. (2017). The cytotoxic *Staphylococcus aureus* PSMalpha3 reveals a cross-alpha amyloid-like fibril. Science 355: 831–833.

Terry RD, Masliah E, Hansen LA (1999). The neuropathology of Alzheimer disease and the structural basis of cognitive alterations. In: RD Terry, R Katzman, KL Bick et al. (Eds.), Alzheimer disease, 2nd edn. Lippincott Williams and Wilkins, Philadelphia.

Thal DR, Capetillo-Zarate E, Del Tredici K et al. (2006). The development of amyloid beta protein deposits in the aged brain. Sci Aging Knowledge Environ 2006: re1.

Tripathi M, Vibha D (2009). Reversible dementias. Indian J Psychiatry 51 (Suppl 1): S52–55.

Tycko R (2015). Amyloid polymorphism: structural basis and neurobiological relevance. Neuron 86: 632–645.

Tycko R (2016). Alzheimer's disease: structure of aggregates revealed. Nature 537: 492–493.

Um JW, Nygaard HB, Heiss JK et al. (2012). Alzheimer amyloid-beta oligomer bound to postsynaptic prion protein activates Fyn to impair neurons. Nat Neurosci 15: 1227–1235.

Vasconcelos B, Stancu IC, Buist A et al. (2016). Heterotypic seeding of tau fibrillization by pre-aggregated Abeta provides potent seeds for prion-like seeding and propagation of tau-pathology in vivo. Acta Neuropathol 131: 549–569.

Villemagne VL, Dore V, Bourgeat P et al. (2017). Abeta-amyloid and tau imaging in dementia. Semin Nucl Med 47: 75–88.

Vinters HV (2015). Emerging concepts in Alzheimer's disease. Annu Rev Pathol 10: 291–319.

Vonsattel JP, Hedley-White ET (2001). Dementia, Oxford University Press, Pathology of the aging human nervous system. New York.

Walker LC, Jucker M (2015). Neurodegenerative diseases: expanding the prion concept. Annu Rev Neurosci 38: 87–103.

Walker LC, Jucker M (2017). The exceptional vulnerability of humans to Alzheimer's disease. Trends Mol Med 23: 534–545.

Walker LC, LeVine H (2000). The cerebral proteopathies: neurodegenerative disorders of protein conformation and assembly. Mol Neurobiol 21: 83–95.

Walker LC, Pahnke J, Madauss M et al. (2000). Apolipoprotein E4 promotes the early deposition of Abeta42 and then Abeta40 in the elderly. Acta Neuropathol 100: 36–42.

Walker LC, Callahan MJ, Bian F et al. (2002). Exogenous induction of cerebral beta-amyloidosis in betaAPP-transgenic mice. Peptides 23: 1241–1247.

Walker LC, Levine H (2006). Inducible proteopathies. Trends Neurosci 29: 438–443.

Walker LC, Schelle J, Jucker M (2016). The prion-like properties of amyloid-beta assemblies: implications for Alzheimer's disease. Cold Spring Harb Perspect Med 6.

Wang F, Wang X, Yuan CG et al. (2010). Generating a prion with bacterially expressed recombinant prion protein. Science 327: 1132–1135.

Wang Y, Balaji V, Kaniyappan S et al. (2017). The release and trans-synaptic transmission of tau via exosomes. Mol Neurodegener 12: 5.

Warzok RW, Kessler C, Apel G et al. (1998). Apolipoprotein E4 promotes incipient Alzheimer pathology in the elderly. Alzheimer Dis Assoc Disord 12: 33–39.

Watts JC, Giles K, Grillo SK et al. (2011). Bioluminescence imaging of Abeta deposition in bigenic mouse models of Alzheimer's disease. Proc Natl Acad Sci U S A 108: 2528–2533.

Watts JC, Condello C, Stohr J et al. (2014). Serial propagation of distinct strains of Abeta prions from Alzheimer's disease patients. Proc Natl Acad Sci U S A 111: 10323–10328.

Weiner MW, Veitch DP, Aisen PS et al. (2013). The Alzheimer's Disease Neuroimaging Initiative: a review of papers published since its inception. Alzheimers Dement 9: e111–194.

Weissmann C (2004). The state of the prion. Nat Rev Microbiol 2: 861–871.

Westermark GT, Fandrich M, Lundmark K et al. (2017). Noncerebral amyloidoses: aspects on seeding, cross-seeding, and transmission. Cold Spring Harb Perspect Med: pii a024323.

Wilcock GK, Esiri MM (1982). Plaques, tangles and dementia. A quantitative study. J Neurol Sci 56: 343–356.

Will RG (2003). Acquired prion disease: iatrogenic CJD, variant CJD, kuru. Br Med Bull 66: 255–265.

Wimo A, Jonsson L, Bond J et al. (2013). The worldwide economic impact of dementia 2010. Alzheimers Dement 9: 1–11: e13.

Wingo TS, Lah JJ, Levey AI et al. (2012). Autosomal recessive causes likely in early-onset Alzheimer disease. Arch Neurol 69: 59–64.

Wiseman FK, Cancellotti E, Piccardo P et al. (2015). The glycosylation status of PrPC is a key factor in determining transmissible spongiform encephalopathy transmission between species. J Virol 89: 4738–4747.

Wisniewski HM, Bancher C, Barcikowska M et al. (1989). Spectrum of morphological appearance of amyloid deposits in Alzheimer's disease. Acta Neuropathol 78: 337–347.

Woerman AL, Aoyagi A, Patel S et al. (2016). Tau prions from Alzheimer's disease and chronic traumatic encephalopathy patients propagate in cultured cells. Proc Natl Acad Sci U S A 113: E8187–E8196.

Wu JW, Herman M, Liu L et al. (2013). Small misfolded tau species are internalized via bulk endocytosis and anterogradely and retrogradely transported in neurons. J Biol Chem 288: 1856–1870.

Wu JW, Hussaini SA, Bastille IM et al. (2016). Neuronal activity enhances tau propagation and tau pathology in vivo. Nat Neurosci 19: 1085–1092.

Yagi H, Ban T, Morigaki K et al. (2007). Visualization and classification of amyloid beta supramolecular assemblies. Biochemistry 46: 15009–15017.

Yang T, Li S, Xu H et al. (2017). Large soluble oligomers of amyloid β-protein from Alzheimer brain are far less neuroactive than the smaller oligomers to which they dissociate. J Neurosci 37 (1): 152–163. https://doi.org/10.1523/JNEUROSCI.1698-16.2016. PMID: 28053038.

Ye L, Fritschi SK, Schelle J et al. (2015a). Persistence of Abeta seeds in APP null mouse brain. Nat Neurosci 18: 1559–1561.

Ye L, Hamaguchi T, Fritschi SK et al. (2015b). Progression of seed-induced Abeta deposition within the limbic connectome. Brain Pathol 25: 743–752.

Yetman MJ, Lillehaug S, Bjaalie JG et al. (2016). Transgene expression in the Nop-tTA driver line is not inherently restricted to the entorhinal cortex. Brain Struct Funct 221: 2231–2249.

Yu JT, Tan L, Hardy J (2014). Apolipoprotein E in Alzheimer's disease: an update. Annu Rev Neurosci 37: 79–100.

Zhang Y, Wang F, Wang X et al. (2014). Comparison of 2 synthetically generated recombinant prions. Prion 8.

Zhou J, Gennatas ED, Kramer JH et al. (2012). Predicting regional neurodegeneration from the healthy brain functional connectome. Neuron 73: 1216–1227.

Handbook of Clinical Neurology, Vol. 153 (3rd series)
Human Prion Diseases
M. Pocchiari and J. Manson, Editors
https://doi.org/10.1016/B978-0-444-63945-5.00017-9

Chapter 17

Prion-like propagation of pathology in Parkinson disease

LAURA VOLPICELLI-DALEY[1] AND PATRIK BRUNDIN[2]*

[1] *Center for Neurodegeneration and Experimental Therapeutics, Department of Neurology, University of Alabama at Birmingham, Birmingham, AL, United States*

[2] *Van Andel Research Institute, Center for Neurodegenerative Science, Grand Rapids, MI, United States*

Abstract

Over 100 years ago, Lewy bodies and Lewy neurites were defined as a pathologic hallmark of Parkinson disease. Eighty years later, α-synuclein was found to be the primary component of these inclusions. Emerging evidence suggests that α-synuclein pathology propagates across interconnected networks throughout the nervous system in a prion-like manner. Pathologic α-synuclein seeds aggregation of native α-synuclein, resulting in the formation of insoluble inclusions. These seeds can propagate within the neuron and to interconnected neurons, resulting in the spread of pathology throughout the brain. Here, we discuss how the findings that α-synuclein pathology spreads throughout the nervous system has revolutionized our understanding about Parkinson disease pathogenesis and resulted in the development of novel therapeutic strategies to halt disease progression.

INTRODUCTION

More than 10 million people worldwide suffer Parkinson disease (PD). This neurodegenerative disorder is classically defined by its motor symptoms, including tremor at rest, rigidity, slowness of movement, and postural instability. Research and observations presented during the past decade have led to the realization, however, that PD also leads to several nonmotor symptoms. They include depression, cognitive decline, anxiety, sleep behavior disorder, constipation, and hyposmia, which collectively represent a significant source of morbidity. More recently, it has become apparent that the clinical diagnosis is preceded, typically for 5–15 years, by a "prodromal" phase when nonmotor symptoms are evident, but the classic motor deficits have yet to appear.

Pharmacologic therapies that counteract the loss of the nigrostriatal dopamine are initially effective at alleviating the motor symptoms. However, these treatments do little to reduce the nonmotor symptoms and do not prevent the progression of the disease. Eventually, patients experience less effective alleviation of motor symptoms on dopaminergic therapies, and the therapeutic benefits are limited by the emergence of side-effects that include drug-induced dyskinesias. In advanced disease, falls and the development of dementia are significant sources of caregiver burden and they are frequently the reasons for institutionalization. Thus, a major unmet medical need is the prevention of disease progression.

Pathologically, PD is characterized by loss of dopamine neurons in the substantia nigra pars compacta and proteinaceous inclusions called Lewy bodies and Lewy neurites that are present in numerous brain regions, which, as is described in more detail later, engage an increasing number of brain regions as the disease progresses. These inclusions were first described by Friedrich Heinrich Lewy in 1912, but it was unclear what they were made up of, and therefore their importance in PD was not fully realized until 85 years later (Spillantini et al., 1997; Goedert et al., 2017). Thus, 20 years ago, the discoveries that Lewy bodies are composed mostly of the protein, α-synuclein, and that missense mutations in α-synuclein cause PD opened up the PD field to understanding underlying pathogenic

*Correspondence to: Patrik Brundin, Van Andel Research Institute, 333 Bostwick Ave NE, Grand Rapids MI 49503, United States. E-mail: Patrik.Brundin@vai.org

mechanisms (Polymeropoulos et al., 1997; Spillantini et al., 1997, 1998).

The use of α-synuclein antibodies has facilitated the identification of Lewy pathology not only in the substantia nigra pars compacta, where they are associated with the loss of dopamine neurons, but also in several other tissues. Indeed, Lewy bodies and Lewy neurites are also found in several other brain regions and in the peripheral nervous system, and this Lewy pathology likely contributes to the nonmotor symptoms of PD. Based on the systematic analyses of numerous autopsies, it has also been suggested that Lewy pathology progressively involves more regions of the nervous system as the disease advances (Braak et al., 2003c). Some of these postmortem findings indicate that the olfactory bulb and the enteric nervous system are among the first areas affected by Lewy pathology and that gradually regions that are anatomically interconnected become engaged.

Around a decade ago, it was suggested that the gradual increase in Lewy pathology, during the progression of PD, is due to prion-like propagation of α-synuclein aggregates. In this review, we will discuss: (1) evidence from human patients and animal models that pathogenic α-synuclein spreads in a prion-like manner; (2) how pathologic α-synuclein templates conversion of normal α-synuclein to form amyloid inclusions; (3) the potential triggers that cause α-synuclein to misfold; (4) the cellular mechanisms of propagation; and (5) how the prion-like hypothesis informs novel therapeutic strategies.

EVIDENCE FOR PD AS A PRION-LIKE DISEASE

Studies that examine Lewy pathology from postmortem brains from PD patients from early stages of the disease to those with advanced stages of the disease, as well as people not diagnosed with a clinical syndrome but who display so-called "incidental" Lewy body disease, show that Lewy pathology is first found in the olfactory bulb and enteric nervous system (Braak et al., 2003c). In the mildest, "stage 1" cases, Lewy bodies and Lewy neurites are apparent only in the dorsal IX/X motor nucleus and the anterior olfactory nucleus. At stage 2, Lewy bodies and Lewy neurites appear in the raphe nucleus and locus coeruleus. It is not until stage 3 that Lewy bodies and Lewy neurites are found in the substantia nigra pars compacta, particularly the posterolateral subnucleus. By stage 4, Lewy bodies and Lewy neurites are found in the CA2 region of the hippocampus and the temporal mesocortex. By stages 5 and 6, Lewy bodies and Lewy neurites localize to higher-order primary sensory and motor cortices.

Appearance of inclusions coincides with onset of symptoms; the olfactory bulb is one of the earliest sites of inclusion formation and impaired olfaction is one of the earliest symptoms of PD, appearance of inclusions in the substantia nigra pars compacta coincides with the onset of motor symptoms, and appearance of inclusions in the temporal cortex coincides with cognitive decline.

The most relevant and important findings of this study are that Lewy bodies and Lewy neurites do not seem to appear in the nervous system at random; their appearance follows a predictable topographic pattern across connected neuronal networks. There are two major possible explanations that currently are being considered. First, there is selective vulnerability to the underlying disease process in the different brain regions, explaining why they are affected at progressive stages of the disease. Alternatively, there is a transmissible agent that moves between the affected brain regions. In their original publications, Braak and colleagues (2003a) favored the idea that there was a transmissible agent that was transported between anatomically connected regions and caused the aggregation of α-synuclein. They speculated if this might be a "neurotropic virus," although in one paper they took the idea one step further and considered the possibility that the transmissible agent might even be "prion" (Braak et al., 2003a).

Another staging system was developed that, in addition to PD patients and incidental Lewy body disease cases, also included cases with dementia with Lewy bodies (DLB) and Alzheimer disease with sparse, predominantly limbic Lewy bodies (Beach et al., 2009). This staging system was developed because, when an attempt was made to classify all of these cases according to the Braak staging system or the DLB consortium staging system, up to 50% of cases could not be classified. According to this classification, stage I is olfactory bulb-predominant Lewy pathology. From here the staging diverges to stage IIa, which is brainstem-predominant pathology, or stage IIb in which most pathology is found in the limbic system. In stage III, the abundance of Lewy pathology in the brainstem and limbic region is equivalent, and in stage IV, cortical areas are involved. It has been hypothesized if a Lewy pathology travels from stage I to stage IIa, PD develops, and if Lewy pathology progresses from stage I to stage IIb, DLB develops (Beach et al., 2009).

Overall, both of the aforementioned staging systems demonstrate that Lewy pathology appears in a predictable topographic manner across connected neuronal networks. It is important to consider that it is possible that not all synucleinopathies initiate in either the olfactory bulb or vagal nerve. There may be neuron-intrinsic (so-called "cell-autonomous") mechanisms within brain regions that cause α-synuclein to convert from a normal to abnormal, pathologic conformation. The observation that the affected brain regions are connected by long neural pathways (in particular unmyelinated fibers), as opposed to the nearest cells, makes it a compelling notion that the disease process spreads along axons. That said, not until the most recent decade has robust evidence emerged from several laboratory studies showing that misfolded variants of α-synuclein may indeed be the spreading agent.

EVIDENCE FOR PD AS A PRION-LIKE DISEASE

An important advance in the understanding of PD pathogenesis and mechanisms that might contribute to disease progression is the emergence of evidence that α-synuclein aggregates can spread from one cell to another in prion-like manner. According to the prion hypothesis, small amounts of fibrillar α-synuclein act as seeds which can trigger the conversion of normal, soluble α-synuclein into insoluble α-synuclein Lewy bodies and Lewy neurites. These seeds can be released from neurons and taken up by neighboring neurons, thus inducing the spread of pathologic α-synuclein throughout the nervous system. The first clinical evidence to support this was that α-synuclein was found in human cerebrospinal fluid, suggesting that it can be released into the extracellular space (El-Agnaf et al., 2003). In addition, studies on fetal nigral grafts placed in the striatum of PD patients, who died over one decade after the surgery, showed that a subset of the pigmented neurons inside the grafts contained Lewy bodies (Kordower et al., 2008a, b; Li et al., 2008, 2010; Kurowska et al., 2011). When these findings were reported in 2008, it was proposed that the grafted neurons developed Lewy bodies as a consequence of prion-like transfer of misfolded α-synuclein originating in the host brains (Brundin et al., 2008). Notably, at the time of death, over two decades had passed since the patients had been clinically diagnosed with PD, and therefore the synucleinopathy was already widespread in the brains of the graft recipients.

In vitro cell culture models support that α-synuclein pathology can spread in a prion-like manner. It was found that α-synuclein is secreted from cultured neurons into the surrounding medium (El-Agnaf et al., 2003; Lee et al., 2005). Further studies characterized some of the regulation of α-synuclein release from cultured neurons, and went on to suggest that such extracellular α-synuclein might be taken up by surrounding neurons and trigger the activation of glia (Lee et al., 2010). However, these studies did not examine the conformation of α-synuclein released from the neurons, which is critical, because it is likely the β-sheet conformation that acts as a seed to initiate conversion of normal α-synuclein to form abnormal inclusions.

The first evidence that amyloid fibrils of α-synuclein can seed corruption of normal α-synuclein to form phosphorylated, insoluble inclusions came from studies in which fibrils generated from recombinant protein were added to HEK293 or SH-SY5Y cells stably overexpressing α-synuclein (Luk et al., 2009; Nonaka et al., 2010). These findings provided a critical proof of concept that pathogenic templating of α-synuclein could occur. However, seeding in the cultured cells required the use of a transfection reagent (e.g., cationic lipid, Bioporter) to introduce the fibrils to the cells and induce efficient seeding. Therefore, it was surprising when a subsequent study demonstrated that fibrils can simply be added to primary neurons in a dish without any reagent and that these fibrils induced the endogenous α-synuclein to form inclusions and cause neuronal dysfunction (Volpicelli-Daley et al., 2011) (Fig. 17.1). This study in cultured primary neurons was the first demonstration that fibrillar seeds can corrupt endogenous proteins. In addition, the findings suggest that concentrated α-synuclein in neuronal presynaptic terminals is required for an efficient seeding to occur. This study also demonstrated when fibrils were added to cultured neurons from α-synuclein knockout mice, no pathology or phenotypes were triggered indicating, consistent with the prion-like hypothesis, that endogenous α-synuclein needs to be present for the propagation and seeding events to take place.

The first animal models of cell-to-cell transfer of α-synuclein focused on neural transplantation paradigms. Using species-specific antibodies, it was shown that rodent neural cells grafted into adult rodent brains, which overexpressed human α-synuclein, contained human α-synuclein (Desplats et al., 2009; Hansen et al., 2011; Kordower et al., 2011). These findings demonstrated that host brain-derived α-synuclein can be taken up by grafted neurons, akin to what was suggested to have occurred in the grafted PD patients that had been analyzed a few years earlier. Subsequently, it was reported that fibrils of recombinant α-synuclein, when injected in the rodent or primate brain, induce formation of inclusions from endogenous α-synuclein (Luk et al., 2012a, b; Masuda-Suzukake et al., 2014; Paumier et al., 2015; Shimozawa et al., 2017). Importantly, injection of fibrils into the striatum, for example, primarily induces inclusion formation in neurons that directly project to the site of injection site, such as the substantia nigra pars compacta, amygdala, and cortex. Sparse aggregates also appear in neuron populations that do not project directly to the injection site, such as the olfactory bulb and hippocampus (Luk et al., 2012b; Masuda-Suzukake et al., 2013, 2014). Formation of α-synuclein

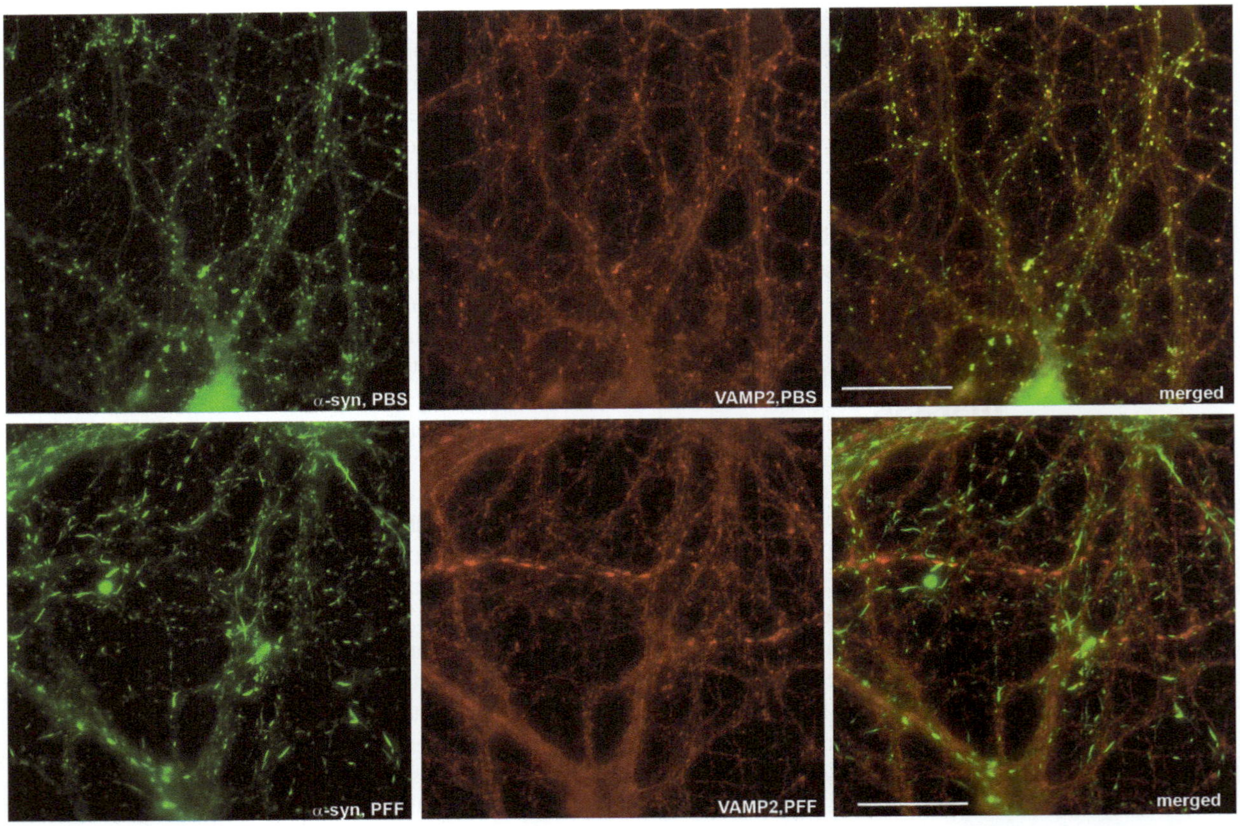

Fig. 17.1. Redistribution of α-synuclein from the presynaptic terminal to Lewy neurite-like inclusions. Primary hippocampal neurons were exposed to preformed fibrils (PFF) of α-synuclein and fixed 14 days later. Immunofluorescence was performed using an antibody to total α-synuclein (green, top panels), phospho-Ser129-α-synuclein (green, bottom panels), or VAMP2 to show presynaptic terminals. In control, phosphate-buffered saline (PBS)-exposed neurons, total α-synuclein localizes to small puncta that colocalize with VAMP2 at the presynaptic terminal. After exposure to PFF, α-synuclein localizes to serpentine-like inclusions that resemble Lewy neurites found in Parkinson disease brains and shows minimal localization to the presynaptic terminal.

inclusions in the substantia nigra leads to death of dopamine neurons, demonstrating two cardinal features of PD neuropathology, namely Lewy-like aggregates and the death of nigral neurons. As a consequence of the nigral pathology, the rodent develops motor deficits (Luk et al., 2012b; Paumier et al., 2015). Interestingly, hind limb intramuscular injection of α-synuclein fibrils in young mice expressing human wild-type or A53T synuclein produces inclusions in the central nervous system, demonstrating that pathology can spread from inoculation of peripheral sites with abnormal α-synuclein (Sacino et al., 2014).

Because olfactory bulb pathology is a feature of several synucleinopathies, recent studies have highlighted how α-synuclein fibrils injected into the olfactory bulb of wild-type mice can trigger a slowly progressing (described up to 1 year) α-synucleinopathy throughout the olfactory system and interconnected brain regions (Rey et al., 2013, 2016) (Fig. 17.2). The α-synuclein pathology eventually involves over 40 brain structures, some of which are located two or more synapses away from the injection site, and include brainstem regions such as the substantia nigra, locus coeruleus, and raphe nuclei. Mice with this progressive pathology also exhibit gradual development of olfactory deficits (Rey et al., 2018). The olfactory model is particularly interesting in the context of prodromal PD, because it replicates the olfactory deficits; α-synuclein aggregates in olfactory brain structures, in animals where very early and sparse signs of Lewy pathology, but no neurodegeneration, are observed in the substantia nigra.

Injected brain extracts from old and symptomatic α-synuclein transgenic mice can accelerate the development of Lewy-like pathology and symptoms in younger mice from the same transgenic lines (Mougenot et al., 2012). Along similar lines, but of greater clinical relevance, purified extracts of α-synuclein aggregates derived from PD or DLB brains induce inclusion formation in wild-type mice, mice heterozygous for mutant human α-synuclein, and macaque primates

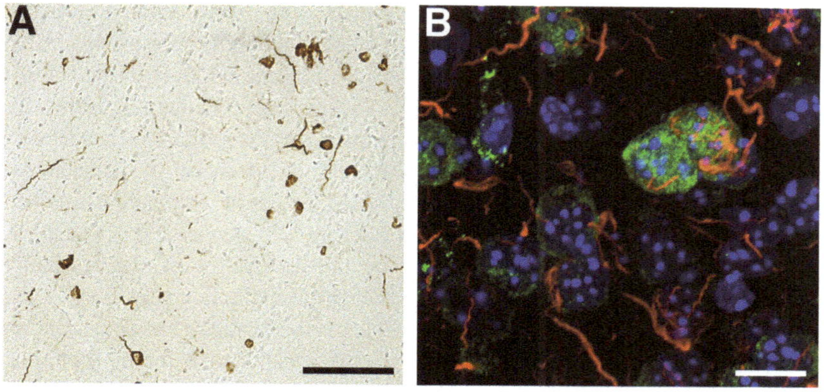

Fig. 17.2. α-Synuclein pathology in mouse model of prodromal Parkinson disease. (**A**) Mice were injected with mouse preformed fibrils (PFF) of α-synuclein unilaterally into the olfactory bulb, and perfused 12 months later for immunohistochemistry. Phospho-Ser129-α-synuclein inclusions can be seen in the piriform cortex. There are abundant inclusions with the appearance of Lewy neurites and inclusions in the soma. Scale bar = 100 μm. (**B**) Mice were injected with mouse PFF of α-synuclein unilaterally into the olfactory bulb, and were perfused 1 month later. Abundant phospho-Ser129-α-synuclein inclusions (red) can be seen in the anterior olfactory nucleus. Lewy neurite-like inclusions are apparent, as well as inclusions juxtaposed to the nucleus (NeuN, green and DAPI, blue).

(Masuda-Suzukake et al., 2013; Recasens et al., 2014). Interestingly, brain extracts from patients with multiple systems atrophy (MSA) are suggested to be more efficient, than those from PD brains, at inducing pathologic aggregates when injected into experimental animals (Watts et al., 2013; Prusiner et al., 2015). MSA is a synucleinopathy similar to PD, but unlike PD, in which inclusions are intraneuronal, α-synuclein aggregates are found primarily in oligodendrocytes. MSA is typically more rapidly progressing than PD, with a life expectancy of about 9 years compared to 20 years for PD. Also of interest, oligodendrocytes express lower, albeit not negligible, levels of α-synuclein (Djelloul et al., 2015), and it is possible that the inclusions in the oligodendrocytes are a consequence of small α-synuclein seeds propagating from neurons. It is interesting to speculate that inclusions derived from brain extracts from patients with distinct synucleinopathies (PD, DLB, or MSA) might be more or less potent due to possible structural differences in the aggregates. However, before such a conclusion can be made, it will be necessary to quantify the concentration of different types of α-synuclein assemblies in these extracts, and determine if preliminary reports of differences in seeding capacity are simply due to higher concentrations of α-synuclein aggregates in some disorders compared to others. It has not yet been possible to define precisely which molecular species of α-synuclein that most efficiently seeds aggregation of native α-synuclein. It remains possible that several different molecular forms of α-synuclein are approximately equipotent as nucleating agents, but that they are more or less likely to be taken up by the different types of cells that are present in the brain.

α-SYNUCLEIN MISFOLDING AND PERMISSIVE TEMPLATING

α-Synuclein can exist as an amphipathic α-helix, likely as a tetramer or multimer, an unfolded/disorded conformation, or β-sheet, fibrillar conformation. Unfolded α-synuclein can become misfolded and interact with other α-synuclein molecules to form multimers with β-sheet structure. These multimers build to form amyloid fibrils which are the hallmark of Lewy bodies and Lewy neurites. Either fragments of these fibrils or smaller β-sheet oligomers then act as a seed or "nucleus" to recruit monomeric α-synuclein to misfold and associate into pathogenic fibrils. It has been suggested that α-synuclein that has adopted an α-helical conformation and is associated with membranes does not convert to amyloid fibrils. The cytosolic, disordered conformation of α-synuclein, however, is susceptible to forming β-sheets that stack to form amyloid fibrils (Burre et al., 2015). The amyloid fibril form is the lowest energy conformation for α-synuclein. Missense mutations in α-synuclein that cause PD (A30P, A53T, E46K, H50Q, and G51D) reduce its association as a native multimeric α-helix complex, and increase its propensity to adopt a monomeric form (Dettmer et al., 2015). Reduced association of α-synuclein with membranes increases aggregate formation.

Other studies show that α-synuclein may aggregate while associated with membranes, but the composition of the membrane and the extent to which the central hydrophobic within the NAC domain of α-synuclein is exposed appears to determine its propensity to aggregate (Galvagnion et al., 2015; Ysselstein et al., 2015;

Galvagnion, 2017). For example, familial mutations of α-synuclein cause dissociation of the central hyrdrophobic region and increase aggregation at the membrane. Thus, within a neuron, α-synuclein likely exists in equilibrium between an α-helical/multimeric form and an unfolded from, and some factors induce misfolding, shifting α-synuclein to a β-sheet, aggregate prone conformation. These aggregates then amplify within the neuron, and it is suggested that they are released under certain conditions, allowing the cell-to-cell propagation process to ensue.

While it is clear that misfolded seeds can template α-synuclein pathology, it is unclear what factors initiate the abnormal conversion of α-synuclein to pathologic aggregates (Fig. 17.3). As mentioned above, an extremely small proportion of PD patients carry one of the six known missense mutations in the α-synuclein gene, *SNCA*. These mutations can reduce its normal α-helical/tetrameric conformation, and also influence membrane association (Burre et al., 2015; Dettmer et al., 2015; Ysselstein et al., 2015).

Duplication, triplication, and polymorphisms of the α-synuclein gene also cause a neurologic syndrome that includes PD-like features. A modest, 1.5–2-fold, increase in α-synuclein expression, as demonstrated with *SNCA* duplication, may increase levels of unfolded α-synuclein that is more easily converted into the abnormal β-sheet, aggregated conformation (Farrer et al., 2004; Miller et al., 2004; Devine et al., 2011). Certain single-nucleotide polymorphisms which are associated with a slight increase in PD are located close to *SNCA*, and studies in cultured neurons suggest that a polymorphism located in a distal enhancer of *SNCA* can lead to a small (1.06-times) increase in neuronal α-synuclein levels (Soldner et al., 2016). Levels of α-synuclein also increase in normal aging (Chu and Kordower, 2007), and this has been suggested to be due to decline of the lysosomal-autophagy system which normally degrades α-synuclein (Chu et al., 2009). These observations are consistent with the fact that age is the greatest risk factor for the development of PD. Recent work suggests that increased expression of α-synuclein in neurons might be a protective response to viral or bacterial exposure (Beatman et al., 2015; Tomlinson et al., 2017). It is conceivable that increased α-synuclein expression due to exposure to a foreign microbe increases the likelihood that α-synuclein aggregates in neurons (Fig. 17.3).

Defects in the proteostasis machinery, beyond that seen in normal aging and mentioned above, could also influence α-synuclein levels and prevent degradation of aggregates. For example, α-synuclein probably toggles between normal, unfolded, and misfolded conformations, but the misfolded conformations are efficiently cleared by the proteosome, or the autophagosome/lysosome machinery. In addition to changes occurring during normal aging, many genes shown to cause

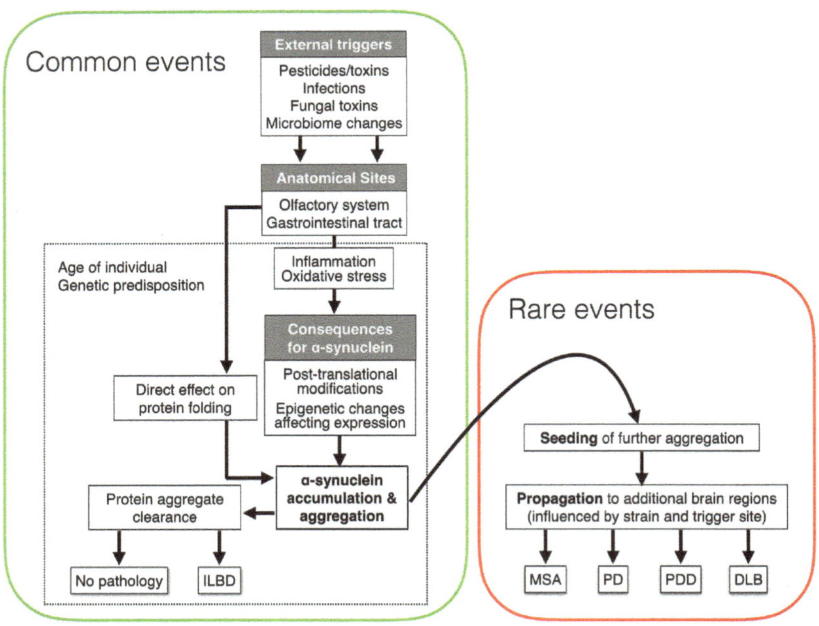

Fig. 17.3. A schematic of events leading to formation of pathologic α-synuclein aggregates and their propagation throughout the nervous system. Events that we postulate can occur frequently and in large numbers of normal individuals are depicted in the green box, whereas events with rare occurrences, and associated with the development of α-synucleinpathies, are in the red box. DLB, dementia with Lewy bodies; ILBD, incidental Lewy body disease; MSA, multiple system atrophy; PD, Parkinson disease; PDD, Parkinson disease dementia.

relatively rare inherited forms of PD play a role in protein degradation pathways such as leucine rich-repeat kinase 2, glucocerebrosidase, lysosomal type 5 P-type ATPase, and Rab7L1 (Alegre-Abarrategui et al., 2009; Mazzulli et al., 2011; Dehay et al., 2012; Usenovic et al., 2012; MacLeod et al., 2013; Orenstein et al., 2013). Thus dysfunction in these proteins could lead to an abnormal accumulation of α-synuclein and the formation of α-synuclein aggregates. Indeed, it was recently shown that neuronal expression of the disease mutant G2019S-LRRK2 slightly increases total levels of α-synuclein (Volpicelli-Daley et al., 2016), which could be due to increases in translation of α-synuclein, or impaired chaperone-mediated autophagy.

Damage to mitochondria can induce formation of pathologic α-synuclein aggregates. The pesticide rotenone inhibits complex I of mitochondria and produces reactive oxidative species (Greenamyre et al., 1992). Oxidatively modified α-synuclein is more prone to aggregation (Souza et al., 2000) (Fig. 17.3). Epidemiologic evidence indicates that pesticide exposure increases the risk of developing PD (Paul et al., 2016). Because α-synuclein pathology appears to initiate in the gut and olfactory bulb, it has been hypothesized that exposure of olfactory epithelia or enteric mucosa to pesticides and toxins may increase production of reactive oxygen species, possibly triggering inflammation and initiating abnormal conversion of α-synuclein (Rey et al., 2018).

A recent study showed that the gut microbiome can influence α-synuclein aggregation, providing further support that extrinsic factors in peripheral tissues might contribute to the abnormal conversion of α-synuclein and represent a starting point from which misfolded α-synuclein can propagate throughout the nervous system (Sampson et al., 2016). One of the earliest signs of PD is constipation and dysbiosis (Verbaan et al., 2007; Sharon et al., 2016; Houser and Tansey, 2017). Indeed, PD patients frequently exhibit intestinal inflammation (Devos et al., 2013) and demonstrate unique microbial signatures compared to control people (Scheperjans et al., 2015; Bedarf et al., 2017). Aggregates of α-synuclein appear in the enteric nervous system and vagal nerve early in the disease, in some cases 20 years before the diagnosis of PD (Braak et al., 2003b; Shannon et al., 2012; Stokholm et al., 2016). Vagotomized individuals have been suggested to have reduced risk for PD (Svensson et al., 2015; Liu et al., 2017). It is possible that inflammation in the gut, viral diseases such as hepatitis (Pakpoor et al., 2017), or exposure to toxins could cause the release of factors, e.g., short-chain fatty acids, that could somehow influence aggregation of the nervous system (Fig. 17.3). It is also interesting to speculate that many individuals harbor α-synuclein aggregates in their enteric nervous system, but that the cellular degradation machinery prevents accumulation of these aggregates.

Genetic susceptibility factors, gastrointestinal disease states could reduce lysosomal function, causing an accumulation of α-synuclein aggregates that travel the long distance along the vagal nerve, resulting in Lewy pathology in the dorsal IX/X motor nucleus (considered one of the first sites affected by α-synuclein aggregates; see above). Once present in the dorsal IX/X motor nucleus, the Lewy pathology can propagate to the locus coeruleus, substantia nigra pars compacta, and beyond, to cause PD. It is important to emphasize that the hypothesis that the gut is a starting point for PD pathology does not exclude that the olfactory system is also an initiation site for α-synuclein aggregation. Indeed, it is conceivable that different individuals who develop PD will in some cases exhibit pathology first in the olfactory bulb, while others show changes in the gut, and some might have simultaneous development of α-synuclein aggregates both in the olfactory and enteric pathways (e.g., due to an environmental insult affecting both locations) (Fig. 17.3).

α-SYNUCLEIN PATHOGENIC STRAINS

In transmissible spongiform encephalopathies or prion diseases, normal cellular prion protein Prp^{C} is converted into a pathogenic form, PrP^{TSE}, which forms β-sheet, detergent-insoluble aggregates that are protease-resistant. Different conformations of PrP^{TSE} produce different lesion profiles in distinct brain regions with different clinical phenotypes. They include Creutzfeldt–Jakob disease, Gerstmann–Straussler–Scheinker syndrome, fatal familial insomnia, and kuru. Furthermore, PrP^{TSE} from these different diseases show distinct biochemical and morphological conformations which could account for the different disease manifestations (Collinge and Clarke, 2007).

It has been hypothesized that α-synuclein can form aggregates with distinct pathologic conformations, giving rise to the different synucleinopathies. Patients with DLB present with dementia and hallucinations, but also develop motor symptoms similar to PD in a later phase. Some PD patients progress to develop dementia relatively soon after diagnosis of the motor syndrome, and are then classified as PD dementia (PDD), a condition which is virtually indistinguishable from DLB. The presence of neurocognitive symptoms is more likely when Lewy bodies are abundant in limbic and cortical brain regions (Dickson et al., 2009). The fact that PD, PDD, and DLB all involve α-synuclein aggregates and yet have distinct neuropathologic profiles and functional deficits adds fuel to the idea that different strains of α-synuclein aggregates may exist and underpin the differences.

The notion that differences in α-synuclein aggregates are important does not, however, stop with PD, PDD, and DLB. For example, as mentioned above, MSA is characterized by α-synuclein aggregates primarily in oligodendrocytes called glial cytoplasmic inclusions (Papp et al., 1989), although neuronal inclusions can also be found in MSA. Unlike PD and DLB, in which inclusions are found only in the cytoplasm, inclusions are found in the nucleus and cytoplasm in MSA. Little is known about the structural characteristics of α-synuclein aggregates in MSA, and how they differ from PD, PDD, and DLB. As previously mentioned, brain homogenates prepared from PD and MSA brains differ in their capacity to trigger synucleinopathy in experimental settings (Watts et al., 2013; Prusiner et al., 2015), suggesting that α-synuclein aggregates from MSA brains may represent a distinct strain from those found in PD.

While the evidence for strains in α-synucleinopathies is not nearly as advanced as studies of prion diseases, it appears that different "strains" of relevance to PD and MSA can be created artificially. Natively unfolded α-synuclein can adopt different folding conformations that act as templates to recruit additional monomers, leading to assembly and elongation of fibrillar assemblies with distinct conformations. For example, by varying the assembly conditions by altering the buffer, salt, or pH, α-synuclein can generate fibrils with a classic cylindric shape, or a flat, ribbon shape as demonstrated by electron microscopy (Bousset et al., 2013). The features of these distinct assemblies faithfully propagate in vitro and in cultured cells. The classic fibrillar α-synuclein appears to be more toxic to dopamine neurons when injected into the rat substantia nigra pars compacta, whereas the ribbons are unique in that they seed α-synuclein aggregate formation in both neurons and oligodendrocytes, which appears to be relevant to MSA (Peelaerts et al., 2015). Despite the aggregates taking on unique and complex three-dimensional structures, complementary primary amino acid structure is still critical for cross-seeding of distinct assemblies. As an excellent example, even though human and mouse α-synuclein share 95% amino acid identity, human fibrils are not as efficient as seeding mouse monomers, or vice versa (Luk et al., 2016).

Patients with different α-synuclein point mutations also exhibit distinct clinical PD profiles, and it can be speculated that this is related to the preferred pathogenic conformation that the mutant protein adopts. For example, patients with the G51D α-synuclein mutation can have a very early onset of the disease (as early as 19 years old), severe dementia, hallucinations, and psychiatric disturbances, and can exhibit α-synuclein inclusions in both neurons and oligodendrocytes (Kiely et al., 2013). Thus, single amino acid substitutions could change the structural properties of the α-synuclein assemblies that could cause distinct disease phenotypes.

Interestingly, α-synuclein fibrils appear to be able to convert from a strain that cannot induce tau aggregation into a strain that can seed tau aggregate formation (Guo et al., 2013). In test tube experiments, α-synuclein fibrils are generated in phosphate-buffered saline (PBS) from recombinant α-synuclein, 5% of these fibrils are added to a new fibrillization reaction with monomer, and this process is repeated several times. The distinct conformers of α-synuclein show different electrophoretic mobility after proteinase K digestion. These findings suggest that, in the brain, repeated α-synuclein fibrillization as it passes from neuron to neuron may cause a conversion to a form that is able to induce tau aggregation. Aberrant α-synuclein aggregation could lead to a more generalized disruption of protein-folding homeostasis, triggering aggregation of tau, as has been shown for polyglutamine repeat expansion diseases (Gidalevitz et al., 2006).

Often in neurodegenerative disease, different protein aggregates can occur at the same time. For example, 50% of Alzheimer disease patients, a disease characterized by Aβ plaques and neurofibrillary tangles composed of tau, display α-synuclein inclusions, primarily in the amygdala (Hamilton, 2000). PDD and DLB patients often display neurofibrillary tangles (Irwin et al., 2017). Tau is a microtubule-associated protein that is the primary component of neurofibrillary tangles. *MAPT* (the gene locus encoding tau) consistently produces a strong signal in genomewide association studies of PD patients, although the contribution of tau to PD is unknown (Satake et al., 2009; Simon-Sanchez et al., 2009; Edwards et al., 2010). Tau colocalizes with α-synuclein in Lewy bodies in PD and DLB brains. While phospho-immunoreactive tau inclusions are present in sporadic PD, they are more abundant in familial PD patients with missense α-synuclein mutations (Duda et al., 2002; Ishizawa et al., 2003; Fujishiro et al., 2013). Phopsho-tau-immunoreactive inclusions can be found in multiple brain regions, including the amygdala, nucleus basalis of Meynert, striatum, hippocampus, cortex, and brainstem (Fujishiro et al., 2013). The presence of both α-synuclein and tau aggregates, particularly in the cortex, correlates with development of PD dementia (Irwin et al., 2012). The findings that different conformations of misfolded α-synuclein trigger tau aggregation and others do not suggest these differences could contribute to why some patients develop dementia whereas others do not.

Further experiments, which compare the biochemical and morphologic differences among aggregates from different synucleinopathies and their seeding capacities, are required to clarify if distinct α-synuclein strains exist. It is unknown whether different conformations of α-synuclein contribute to the distinct clinical and histologic phenotypes of different synucleinopathies or whether posttranslational modifications, such as phosphorylation, ubiquitination, nitration, or sumoylation, are crucial contributors to the differences in pathology induced by MSA and PD brain tissues (Giasson et al., 2000; Fujiwara et al., 2002; Tofaris et al., 2003; Kim et al., 2011; Krumova et al., 2011; Vicente Miranda et al., 2017).

It is also conceivable that, even within one disorder (e.g., PD), different types of α-synuclein conformations preferentially populate different brain regions, e.g., basal ganglia versus neocortex, and that this is due to how different α-synuclein assemblies interact with varying forms of lipids (which can show differential levels between brain regions). In the brainstem, Lewy bodies in neuronal soma exhibit a dense core surrounded by a halo. By contrast, in neocortex the Lewy bodies are spheroid, have more diffuse contours, and do not display a compact halo. These neocortical α-synuclein aggregates have been suggested to represent a less mature form of Lewy bodies (Kosaka, 1978). In neurites, Lewy pathology can appear as long serpentine inclusions. Small proteinase K aggregates are also abundant in the cortex of DLB patients (Kramer and Schulz-Schaeffer, 2007). It is not clear yet which form of aggregates is more toxic – it may be that the less dense inclusions and aggregates represent the toxic species and the dense, thioflavin T-positive, Lewy bodies are inert. The existence of different strains of α-synuclein aggregates also opens up the possibility that they govern which type (e.g. PD, PDD, DLB, or MSA) of synucleinopathy develops. In line with this idea, the initial misfolding event (e.g., occurring in the olfactory bulb or enteric nervous system) could play a key role in influencing the type of α-synuclein pathology that propagates throughout the nervous system, and with which speed it will progress (Fig. 17.3).

POTENTIAL CELLULAR MECHANISMS OF PROPAGATION

There remain many outstanding questions as to how Lewy pathology propagates across the nervous system. In this section, we discuss the cellular mechanisms that might underlie cell-to-cell transfer of α-synuclein oligomers and fibrils. The pathogenic α-synuclein conformers must be released from the neuron, taken up by neighboring neurons, and escape into the cytosol where they seed conversion of endogenous α-synuclein to an abnormal aggregate-prone form. Recent data suggest how α-synuclein aggregates might be taken up by neurons. Fibrillar α-synuclein binds to heparin sulfate proteoglycans (HSPGs) and stimulates uptake by macropinocytosis in a manner independent of dynamin (Holmes et al., 2013). Heparin, which blocks binding to HSPGs, and chlorate, which blocks sulfation, inhibit the uptake of α-synuclein fibrils. The receptor, lymphocyte-activation gene 3 (LAG3), a member of the immunoglobulin superfamily, selectively binds α-synuclein fibrils and mediates their uptake (Mao et al., 2016). Antibodies to LAG3 or gene knockout of LAG3 prevent α-synuclein fibril-induced seeding of inclusions and protect against dopamine neuron loss when fibrils are injected into the striatum. It will be of great interest to learn whether neurexin or amyloid precursor-like protein, which also selectively bind fibrillar α-synuclein and are highly enriched in the brain, also facilitate propagation of α-synuclein pathology. The realization that some of the molecular pathways that mediate uptake of pathogenic α-synuclein assemblies exhibit a degree of specificity opens up the exciting possibility that the uptake process might be targeted therapeutically with small molecules.

How α-synuclein aggregates are released from the neuron remains a partial mystery. As mentioned before, α-synuclein is found in the cerebrospinal fluid (El-Agnaf et al., 2003). Both monomeric and aggregated α-synuclein can be released from neurons (Alvarez-Erviti et al., 2011; Danzer et al., 2012). α-Synuclein has been detected in exosomes and in nonexosome, soluble fractions from the conditioned media of "neuronotypic" cells, although the amount of α-synuclein associated with the exosomes appears to be relatively low (Danzer et al., 2012). Aggregates have been detected in exosomes and association of α-synuclein with cell-derived exosomes or artificial exosomes (containing the key lipids, but lacking exosomal proteins) may even accelerate pathogenic aggregation (Grey et al., 2015). Monomeric and oligomeric α-synuclein associates with exosomes, but to date, no fibrillar α-synuclein has been detected on or inside exosomes (Brahic et al., 2016).

Exosomes are small vesicles that reside inside multivesicular bodies (MVBs) that are released when the MVBs fuse with the plasma membrane. Given that α-synuclein aggregates in the neuron are cytosolic, they would have to somehow bind the limiting membrane of the MVBs and be internalized into the internal vesicles. Thus, α-synuclein aggregates would be inside the internal vesicles and would remain inside the vesicles when they are released into the extracellular space (Danzer et al., 2012). Because peripheral administration of antibodies to α-synuclein can prevent propagation of pathology in experimental models (Masliah et al., 2005; Tran et al., 2014; Spencer et al., 2017), this means the antibodies have to interact with and bind α-synuclein extracellularly, implying that exosomal release may not be the only mechanism for the extracellular spread of α-synuclein aggregates. Recently, tunneling nanotubes were shown to be a mechanism by which neurons share aggregates α-synuclein (Abounit et al., 2016). A final, as yet to be demonstrated, mechanism is that the α-synuclein fibrils permeabilize the plasma membrane directly to gain access to the extracellular space.

Another mystery is related to how imported α-synuclein gains access to the endogenous α-synuclein of a recipient cell. After endocytosis, either by a receptor-mediated mechanism or by a general macropinocytosis mechanism, fibrillar α-synuclein must penetrate the endosomal membrane to gain access to the cytoplasm, where it can seed conversion of endogenous α-synuclein. The most compelling findings are that, upon entry into cells, α-synuclein aggregates can rupture endosomes and lysosomes, and thereby directly enter the cytosol in a manner similar to the mechanism used by some viruses (Freeman et al., 2013; Flavin et al., 2017).

POTENTIAL FOR THERAPEUTICS THAT TARGET THE PRION-LIKE PROCESS

The prion-like hypothesis for α-synucleinopathies has led to the development of novel therapeutic strategies for preventing disease progression. Because α-synuclein is released into the extracellular space under certain conditions, it can be targeted by antibodies. The interest in developing immunotherapy to target α-synuclein has been around for over a decade (Masliah et al., 2005), but this research field really took off dramatically in the wake of studies demonstrating cell-to-cell transfer of the pathogenic protein. Experiments performed in rodent models of α-synucleinopathy support that antibodies targeting α-synuclein can prevent the progression of disease pathology and reduce associated behavioral phenotypes (Masliah et al., 2005; Games et al., 2014; Tran et al., 2014; Christiansen et al., 2016; Spencer et al., 2017).

Immunotherapy can be divided into two different strategies: passive immunotherapy or active immunotherapy. With passive immunotherapy, antibodies to α-synuclein are generated in the laboratory and then administered to the patient. One of these antibodies, which targets the C-terminus of α-synuclein, PRX002/RG7935, was recently demonstrated by the Prothena Corporation to have an acceptable safety and tolerability profile in a phase Ib double-blind placebo-controlled dose study (Schenk et al., 2017). Biogen also initiated a phase I clinical trial on an antibody, BIIB054, which targets human α-synuclein and was isolated from a B-cell library from elderly healthy subjects based on findings that α-synuclein antibodies or autoantibodies exist in healthy individuals and those with PD (Papachroni et al., 2007; Neff et al., 2008). By contrast, AFFiRiS has utilized an active immunotherapy approach in which patients are immunized with "AFFITOPES" or small peptides that mimic α-synuclein, in order to generate a B-cell response and antibodies to α-synuclein. AFFiRiS has completed a phase Ib trial showing that the vaccinations are safe and tolerable.

For all immunotherapies targeting α-synuclein, a potential drawback of the approach is that it might be detrimental to deplete normal, α-helical α-synuclein which has been shown to regulate presynaptic vesicle endo/exocytosis. In addition, because α-synuclein is a cytosolic protein, there may be cell intrinsic mechanisms that cause α-synuclein to convert to an abnormal conformation, and extracellular antibodies may not be able to access these molecules and prevent this conversion. That said, the realization that pathologic α-synuclein can be found in the extracellular space means that the idea of generating antibodies that only access this compartment is still viable. The specific epitopes that the antibodies are directed against, and the type of conformations that allow these epitopes to be exposed, are likely to be crucial factors. For example, antibodies that selectively recognize β-sheet, fibrillar α-synuclein may be more effective with fewer potential side-effects than antibodies against the monomeric protein. In fact, AbbVie and Bioarctic Neuroscience also recently joined in a collaboration to develop a novel antibody, BAN0805, which targets a "toxic" form of α-synuclein (http://www.bioarctic.se/news/-bioarctic-enters-into-collaboration-with-abbvie-for-parkinsons-disease-research). The emerging concept of different strains of α-synuclein aggregates (see detailed discussion above), however, might mean that there will be a need to have tailor-made, patient-specific antibodies depending on the type of α-synuclein fibrils that dominate in the brain in that particular patient. As we learn more about α-synuclein aggregates and the effects of immunotherapies in experimental models and from clinical trials, it will become apparent if this therapeutic approach will require a personalized "precision medicine" strategy.

Treatments to prevent α-synuclein aggregation or disrupt aggregates are in clinical trials as well. Neuropore has completed a phase I clinical trial of its compound, NPT200-11, which may prevent accumulation of oligomeric α-synuclein within membranes (Wrasidlo et al., 2016). Proclara Biosciences has a compound, NPT088, in a phase Ib clinical trial for Alzheimer disease. This compound utilizes a general amyloid interaction motif to target multiple amyloid domains. The goal is to inhibit aggregation of multiple proteins implicated in neurodegenerative disease, including amyloid β, tau, prion, transthyretin, and α-synuclein. However, recent studies of the NACore domain of α-synuclein using microelectron diffraction and nanocrystals has revealed crucial differences in the α-synuclein amyloid domain from amyloid fibrils formed by other proteins, such as the

11-amino-acid width of the zipper, which is larger, and the inclusion of water molecules within the interface (Rodriguez et al., 2015). Thus, it is possible that not all amyloid domains are created equal and a generic amyloid-targeting compound may not be effective for all neurodegenerative diseases.

Antisense oligonucleotides (ASOs) to reduce levels of α-synuclein may provide an alternate strategy to prevent pathologic templating of α-synuclein amyloid fibrils. ASOs have recently emerged as promising strategies to treat neurodegenerative diseases (Ottesen, 2017). ASOs are single-stranded synthetic nucleic acids that bind target mRNA via Watson–Crick basepairing, resulting in degradation of target mRNA by RNAse H, a ubiquitously expressed mammalian enzyme. Phosphorothioate-modified deoxynucleotide (DNA) and 2'-*O*-methoxyethyl sugar modifications enable ASOs to be water-soluble, resistant to exonucleases, and diffusible, and exhibit dose-dependent activity in vitro and in vivo (Bennett and Swayze, 2010). Importantly, ASOs can be targeted directly to the brain by intracerebroventricular injections and thus bypass adverse effects in the systemic organs.

As mentioned above, slightly increased cytoplasmic levels of α-synuclein may facilitate the conversion of α-synuclein from a disordered protein to form β-sheets and amyloid. Thus, slight reductions in α-synuclein may prevent it from forming inclusions. However, it is important to point out that absence of the *SNCA* gene or RNAi to knockdown levels of α-synuclein in the rodent brain causes a reductions in total dopamine levels in the striatum, which could cause adverse events in PD patients who already have low levels of dopamine (Zharikov et al., 2015). Thus, the concentrations of the ASOs would have to be carefully titrated.

The findings that cell surface receptors such as LAG3 can selectively bind to fibrillar but not monomeric α-synuclein provides a potentially novel therapeutic strategy (Mao et al., 2016). Inhibitors of the LAG3 and α-synuclein interactions could also be designed that could inhibit uptake and seeding of pathologic α-synuclein fibrils. Likely other receptors that mediate the uptake and spread of α-synuclein pathology will be identified that can also be targeted. Another potentially interesting strategy is inferred by the binding of α-synuclein with heparin sulfate glucosaminoglycans to prevent uptake of seeds (Holmes et al., 2013).

Recently, combination therapeutic approaches to treating neurodegenerative diseases have received attention. As mentioned above, inflammation may contribute to the aggregation of α-synuclein, neuron death, and progression of the disease. In turn, α-synuclein aggregates may stimulate proinflammatory response, causing a vicious cycle that amplifies the disease process. Neuroinflammation is widespread in brains of PD (McGeer et al., 1988; Brochard et al., 2009). In addition, the HLA-DR (MHC-II) gene locus is one of the top genetic links to PD in genomewide association studies, suggesting that the immune system plays a role in PD (Hamza et al., 2010). Extracellular α-synuclein binds to Toll-like receptor 2 on microglia and activates inflammatory responses (Kim et al., 2013). Activated monocytes in the brain may internalize and process released α-synuclein, and influence its spread throughout the nervous system (Lee et al., 2008). Targeting inflammation can be neuroprotective in mouse models of PD (Harms et al., 2013; Qin et al., 2016). Thus, both preventing α-synuclein aggregation and propagation in addition to inhibiting proinflammatory cascades may be the most effective strategy for modifying disease progression. AstraZeneca has completed a phase II clinical trial on AZD3241 in patients with PD (Jucaite et al., 2015). AD3241 inhibits myeloperoxidase, which is a reactive oxygen-generating enzyme expressed by microglia.

CONCLUDING REMARKS

The goal of current PD therapeutics is to prevent the progression of the disease. The evidence that pathogenic α-synuclein spreads throughout the nervous system in a prion-like manner has opened up wide avenues for novel therapeutic strategies. Current strategies already in preclinical development include preventing the abnormal conversion of α-synuclein, or immunotherapy to block the spread of extracellular pathogenic seeds. Emerging basic science research is honing in on the molecular and cellular mechanisms that increase the likelihood of α-synuclein to convert to an abnormal, aggregation-prone conformation, and on how these aggregates can propagate within the cell, to neighboring neurons and from one brain region to another. This research will be critical for identifying novel therapeutic targets and to understand if halting propagation of pathologic α-synuclein is sufficient to stop disease progression. Other factors may also contribute to disease progression, such as inflammation and metabolic failure in remaining neurons. Perhaps combination therapies that target both misfolded α-synuclein and impaired metabolic pathways will prove to be the most beneficial (Ghosh et al., 2016; Valera and Masliah, 2016).

ACKNOWLEDGMENTS

We thank Dr. Nolwen Rey for providing images for Figure 17.2, and Dr. Nolwen Rey, Dr. Martha Galvis Escobar, Dr. Jennifer Steiner and Dr. Sonia George for input and feedback on Figure 17.3. L. Volpicelli-Daley reports grants from the Department of Defense, Neurotoxin Exposure Treatment Parkinson's Disease, and the Michael J. Fox Foundation. P. Brundin acknowledges support from the Van Andel Research Institute. P. Brundin also reports grants from the Michael J. Fox Foundation, National Institutes of Health, Department of Defense, and Cure Parkinson's Trust.

References

Abounit S, Bousset L, Loria F et al. (2016). Tunneling nanotubes spread fibrillar alpha-synuclein by intercellular trafficking of lysosomes. EMBO J 35: 2120–2138.

Alegre-Abarrategui J, Christian H, Lufino MM et al. (2009). LRRK2 regulates autophagic activity and localizes to specific membrane microdomains in a novel human genomic reporter cellular model. Human Molecular Genetics 18: 4022–4034.

Alvarez-Erviti L, Seow Y, Schapira AH et al. (2011). Lysosomal dysfunction increases exosome-mediated alpha-synuclein release and transmission. Neurobiol Dis 42: 360–367.

Beach TG, Adler CH, Lue L et al. (2009). Unified staging system for Lewy body disorders: correlation with nigrostriatal degeneration, cognitive impairment and motor dysfunction. Acta Neuropathol 117: 613–634.

Beatman EL, Massey A, Shives KD et al. (2015). Alpha-synuclein expression restricts RNA viral infections in the brain. Journal of Virology 90: 2767–2782.

Bedarf JR, Hildebrand F, Coelho LP et al. (2017). Functional implications of microbial and viral gut metagenome changes in early stage L-DOPA-naive Parkinson's disease patients. Genome Medicine 9: 39.

Bennett CF, Swayze EE (2010). RNA targeting therapeutics: molecular mechanisms of antisense oligonucleotides as a therapeutic platform. Annual Review of Pharmacology and Toxicology 50: 259–293.

Bousset L, Pieri L, Ruiz-Arlandis G et al. (2013). Structural and functional characterization of two alpha-synuclein strains. Nat Commun 4: 2575.

Braak H, Rub U, Gai WP et al. (2003a). Idiopathic Parkinson's disease: possible routes by which vulnerable neuronal types may be subject to neuroinvasion by an unknown pathogen. Journal of Neural Transmission 110: 517–536.

Braak H, Rub U, Gai WP et al. (2003b). Idiopathic Parkinson's disease: possible routes by which vulnerable neuronal types may be subject to neuroinvasion by an unknown pathogen. J Neural Transm 110: 517–536.

Braak H, Del Tredici K, Rub U et al. (2003c). Staging of brain pathology related to sporadic Parkinson's disease. Neurobiol Aging 24: 197–211.

Brahic M, Bousset L, Bieri G et al. (2016). Axonal transport and secretion of fibrillar forms of alpha-synuclein, Abeta42 peptide and HTTExon 1. Acta Neuropathol 131: 539–548.

Brochard V, Combadiere B, Prigent A et al. (2009). Infiltration of CD4+ lymphocytes into the brain contributes to neurodegeneration in a mouse model of Parkinson disease. The Journal of Clinical Investigation 119: 182–192.

Brundin P, Li JY, Holton JL et al. (2008). Research in motion: the enigma of Parkinson's disease pathology spread. Nature Reviews Neuroscience 9: 741–745.

Burre J, Sharma M, Sudhof TC (2015). Definition of a molecular pathway mediating alpha-synuclein neurotoxicity. J Neurosci 35: 5221–5232.

Christiansen JR, Olesen MN, Otzen DE et al. (2016). Alpha-synuclein vaccination modulates regulatory T cell activation and microglia in the absence of brain pathology. Journal of Neuroinflammation 13: 74.

Chu Y, Kordower JH (2007). Age-associated increases of alpha-synuclein in monkeys and humans are associated with nigrostriatal dopamine depletion: is this the target for Parkinson's disease? Neurobiol Dis 25: 134–149.

Chu Y, Dodiya H, Aebischer P et al. (2009). Alterations in lysosomal and proteasomal markers in Parkinson's disease: relationship to alpha-synuclein inclusions. Neurobiol Dis 35: 385–398.

Collinge J, Clarke AR (2007). A general model of prion strains and their pathogenicity. Science 318: 930–936.

Danzer KM, Kranich LR, Ruf WP et al. (2012). Exosomal cell-to-cell transmission of alpha synuclein oligomers. Mol Neurodegener 7: 42.

Dehay B, Ramirez A, Martinez-Vicente M et al. (2012). Loss of P-type ATPase ATP13A2/PARK9 function induces general lysosomal deficiency and leads to Parkinson disease neurodegeneration. Proc Natl Acad Sci U S A 109: 9611–9616.

Desplats P, Lee HJ, Bae EJ et al. (2009). Inclusion formation and neuronal cell death through neuron-to-neuron transmission of alpha-synuclein. Proc Natl Acad Sci U S A 106: 13010–13015.

Dettmer U, Newman AJ, Soldner F et al. (2015). Parkinson-causing alpha-synuclein missense mutations shift native tetramers to monomers as a mechanism for disease initiation. Nat Commun 6: 7314.

Devine MJ, Ryten M, Vodicka P et al. (2011). Parkinson's disease induced pluripotent stem cells with triplication of the alpha-synuclein locus. Nat Commun 2: 440.

Devos D, Lebouvier T, Lardeux B et al. (2013). Colonic inflammation in Parkinson's disease. Neurobiol Dis 50: 42–48.

Dickson DW, Braak H, Duda JE et al. (2009). Neuropathological assessment of Parkinson's disease: refining the diagnostic criteria. Lancet Neurol 8: 1150–1157.

Djelloul M, Holmqvist S, Boza-Serrano A et al. (2015). Alpha-synuclein expression in the oligodendrocyte lineage: an in vitro and in vivo study using rodent and human models. Stem Cell Reports 5: 174–184.

Duda JE, Giasson BI, Mabon ME et al. (2002). Concurrence of alpha-synuclein and tau brain pathology in the Contursi kindred. Acta Neuropathol 104: 7–11.

Edwards TL, Scott WK, Almonte C et al. (2010). Genome-wide association study confirms SNPs in SNCA and the MAPT region as common risk factors for Parkinson disease. Ann Hum Genet 74: 97–109.

El-Agnaf OM, Salem SA, Paleologou KE et al. (2003). Alpha-synuclein implicated in Parkinson's disease is present in extracellular biological fluids, including human plasma. FASEB Journal 17: 1945–1947.

Farrer M, Kachergus J, Forno L et al. (2004). Comparison of kindreds with parkinsonism and alpha-synuclein genomic multiplications. Ann Neurol 55: 174–179.

Flavin WP, Bousset L, Green ZC et al. (2017). Endocytic vesicle rupture is a conserved mechanism of cellular invasion by amyloid proteins. Acta Neuropathol. https://doi.org/10.1007/s00401-017-1722-x.

Freeman D, Cedillos R, Choyke S et al. (2013). Alpha-synuclein induces lysosomal rupture and cathepsin dependent reactive oxygen species following endocytosis. PLoS One 8: e62143.

Fujishiro H, Imamura AY, Lin WL et al. (2013). Diversity of pathological features other than Lewy bodies in familial Parkinson's disease due to SNCA mutations. American Journal of Neurodegenerative Disease 2: 266–275.

Fujiwara H, Hasegawa M, Dohmae N et al. (2002). Alpha-synuclein is phosphorylated in synucleinopathy lesions. Nat Cell Biol 4: 160–164.

Galvagnion C (2017). The role of lipids interacting with a-synuclein in the pathogenesis of Parkinson's disease. Journal of Parkinson's Disease 7: 433–450.

Galvagnion C, Buell AK, Meisl G et al. (2015). Lipid vesicles trigger alpha-synuclein aggregation by stimulating primary nucleation. Nature Chemical Biology 11: 229–234.

Games D, Valera E, Spencer B et al. (2014). Reducing C-terminal-truncated alpha-synuclein by immunotherapy attenuates neurodegeneration and propagation in Parkinson's disease-like models. J Neurosci 34: 9441–9454.

Ghosh A, Tyson T, George S et al. (2016). Mitochondrial pyruvate carrier regulates autophagy, inflammation, and neurodegeneration in experimental models of Parkinson's disease. Science Translational Medicine 8: 368ra174.

Giasson BI, Duda JE, Murray IV et al. (2000). Oxidative damage linked to neurodegeneration by selective alpha-synuclein nitration in synucleinopathy lesions. Science 290: 985–989.

Gidalevitz T, Ben-Zvi A, Ho KH et al. (2006). Progressive disruption of cellular protein folding in models of polyglutamine diseases. Science 311: 1471–1474.

Goedert M, Jakes R, Spillantini MG (2017). The synucleinopathies: twenty years on. J Parkinsons Dis 7: S53–S71.

Greenamyre JT, Higgins DS, Eller RV (1992). Quantitative autoradiography of dihydrorotenone binding to complex I of the electron transport chain. J Neurochem 59: 746–749.

Grey M, Dunning CJ, Gaspar R et al. (2015). Acceleration of alpha-synuclein aggregation by exosomes. J Biol Chem 290: 2969–2982.

Guo JL, Covell DJ, Daniels JP et al. (2013). Distinct alpha-synuclein strains differentially promote tau inclusions in neurons. Cell 154: 103–117.

Hamilton RL (2000). Lewy bodies in Alzheimer's disease: a neuropathological review of 145 cases using alpha-synuclein immunohistochemistry. Brain Pathology 10: 378–384.

Hamza TH, Zabetian CP, Tenesa A et al. (2010). Common genetic variation in the HLA region is associated with late-onset sporadic Parkinson's disease. Nat Genet 42: 781–785.

Hansen C, Angot E, Bergstrom AL et al. (2011). Alpha-synuclein propagates from mouse brain to grafted dopaminergic neurons and seeds aggregation in cultured human cells. The Journal of Clinical Investigation 121: 715–725.

Harms AS, Cao S, Rowse AL et al. (2013). MHCII is required for alpha-synuclein-induced activation of microglia, CD4 T cell proliferation, and dopaminergic neurodegeneration. J Neurosci 33: 9592–9600.

Holmes BB, DeVos SL, Kfoury N et al. (2013). Heparan sulfate proteoglycans mediate internalization and propagation of specific proteopathic seeds. Proc Natl Acad Sci U S A 110: E3138–3147.

Houser MC, Tansey MG (2017). The gut-brain axis: is intestinal inflammation a silent driver of Parkinson's disease pathogenesis? In: npj Parkinson's Disease 3.

Irwin DJ, White MT, Toledo JB et al. (2012). Neuropathologic substrates of Parkinson disease dementia. Ann Neurol 72: 587–598.

Irwin DJ, Grossman M, Weintraub D et al. (2017). Neuropathological and genetic correlates of survival and dementia onset in synucleinopathies: a retrospective analysis. Lancet Neurol 16: 55–65.

Ishizawa T, Mattila P, Davies P et al. (2003). Colocalization of tau and alpha-synuclein epitopes in Lewy bodies. J Neuropathol Exp Neurol 62: 389–397.

Jucaite A, Svenningsson P, Rinne JO et al. (2015). Effect of the myeloperoxidase inhibitor AZD3241 on microglia: a PET study in Parkinson's disease. Brain 138: 2687–2700.

Kiely AP, Asi YT, Kara E et al. (2013). Alpha-synucleinopathy associated with G51D SNCA mutation: a link between Parkinson's disease and multiple system atrophy? Acta Neuropathol 125: 753–769.

Kim YM, Jang WH, Quezado MM et al. (2011). Proteasome inhibition induces alpha-synuclein SUMOylation and aggregate formation. J Neurol Sci 307: 157–161.

Kim C, Ho DH, Suk JE et al. (2013). Neuron-released oligomeric alpha-synuclein is an endogenous agonist of TLR2 for paracrine activation of microglia. Nat Commun 4: 1562.

Kordower JH, Chu Y, Hauser RA et al. (2008a). Lewy body-like pathology in long-term embryonic nigral transplants in Parkinson's disease. Nat Med 14: 504–506.

Kordower JH, Chu Y, Hauser RA et al. (2008b). Transplanted dopaminergic neurons develop PD pathologic changes: a second case report. Mov Disord 23: 2303–2306.

Kordower JH, Dodiya HB, Kordower AM et al. (2011). Transfer of host-derived alpha synuclein to grafted dopaminergic neurons in rat. Neurobiol Dis 43: 552–557.

Kosaka K (1978). Lewy bodies in cerebral cortex, report of three cases. Acta Neuropathol 42: 127–134.

Kramer ML, Schulz-Schaeffer WJ (2007). Presynaptic alpha-synuclein aggregates, not Lewy bodies, cause neurodegeneration in dementia with Lewy bodies. J Neurosci 27: 1405–1410.

Krumova P, Meulmeester E, Garrido M et al. (2011). Sumoylation inhibits alpha-synuclein aggregation and toxicity. J Cell Biol 194: 49–60.

Kurowska Z, Englund E, Widner H et al. (2011). Signs of degeneration in 12-22-year old grafts of mesencephalic dopamine neurons in patients with Parkinson's disease. J Parkinsons Dis 1: 83–92.

Lee HJ, Patel S, Lee SJ (2005). Intravesicular localization and exocytosis of alpha-synuclein and its aggregates. J Neurosci 25: 6016–6024.

Lee HJ, Suk JE, Bae EJ et al. (2008). Clearance and deposition of extracellular alpha-synuclein aggregates in microglia. Biochemical and Biophysical Research Communications 372: 423–428.

Lee HJ, Suk JE, Patrick C et al. (2010). Direct transfer of alpha-synuclein from neuron to astroglia causes inflammatory responses in synucleinopathies. J Biol Chem 285: 9262–9272.

Li JY, Englund E, Holton JL et al. (2008). Lewy bodies in grafted neurons in subjects with Parkinson's disease suggest host-to-graft disease propagation. Nat Med 14: 501–503.

Li JY, Englund E, Widner H et al. (2010). Characterization of Lewy body pathology in 12- and 16-year-old intrastriatal mesencephalic grafts surviving in a patient with Parkinson's disease. Mov Disord 25: 1091–1096.

Liu B, Fang F, Pedersen NL et al. (2017). Vagotomy and Parkinson disease: a Swedish register-based matched-cohort study. Neurology 88: 1996–2002.

Luk KC, Song C, O'Brien P et al. (2009). Exogenous alpha-synuclein fibrils seed the formation of Lewy body-like intracellular inclusions in cultured cells. Proc Natl Acad Sci U S A 106: 20051–20056.

Luk KC, Kehm VM, Zhang B et al. (2012a). Intracerebral inoculation of pathological alpha-synuclein initiates a rapidly progressive neurodegenerative alpha-synucleinopathy in mice. The Journal of Experimental Medicine 209: 975–986.

Luk KC, Kehm V, Carroll J et al. (2012b). Pathological alpha-synuclein transmission initiates Parkinson-like neurodegeneration in nontransgenic mice. Science 338: 949–953.

Luk KC, Covell DJ, Kehm VM et al. (2016). Molecular and biological compatibility with host alpha-synuclein influences fibril pathogenicity. Cell Rep 16: 3373–3387.

MacLeod DA, Rhinn H, Kuwahara T et al. (2013). RAB7L1 interacts with LRRK2 to modify intraneuronal protein sorting and Parkinson's disease risk. Neuron 77: 425–439.

Mao X, Tianhao Ou M, Karuppagounder SS et al. (2016). Pathological alpha-synuclein transmission initiated by binding lymphocyte-activation gene 3. Science 353: aah3374.

Masliah E, Rockenstein E, Adame A et al. (2005). Effects of alpha-synuclein immunization in a mouse model of Parkinson's disease. Neuron 46: 857–868.

Masuda-Suzukake M, Nonaka T, Hosokawa M et al. (2013). Prion-like spreading of pathological alpha-synuclein in brain. Brain 136: 1128–1138.

Masuda-Suzukake M, Nonaka T, Hosokawa M et al. (2014). Pathological alpha-synuclein propagates through neural networks. Acta Neuropathologica Communications 2: 88.

Mazzulli JR, Xu YH, Sun Y et al. (2011). Gaucher disease glucocerebrosidase and alpha-synuclein form a bidirectional pathogenic loop in synucleinopathies. Cell 146: 37–52.

McGeer PL, Itagaki S, Boyes BE et al. (1988). Reactive microglia are positive for HLA-DR in the substantia nigra of Parkinson's and Alzheimer's disease brains. Neurology 38: 1285–1291.

Miller DW, Hague SM, Clarimon J et al. (2004). Alpha-synuclein in blood and brain from familial Parkinson disease with SNCA locus triplication. Neurology 62: 1835–1838.

Mougenot A-L, Nicot S, Bencsik A et al. (2012). Prion-like acceleration of a synucleinopathy in a transgenic mouse model. Neurobiol Aging 33: 2225–2228.

Neff F, Wei X, Nolker C et al. (2008). Immunotherapy and naturally occurring autoantibodies in neurodegenerative disorders. Autoimmunity Reviews 7: 501–507.

Nonaka T, Watanabe ST, Iwatsubo T et al. (2010). Seeded aggregation and toxicity of α-synuclein and tau: cellular models of neurodegenerative diseases. J Biol Chem 285: 34885–34898.

Orenstein SJ, Kuo SH, Tasset I et al. (2013). Interplay of LRRK2 with chaperone-mediated autophagy. Nature Neuroscience 16: 394–406.

Ottesen EW (2017). ISS-N1 makes the first FDA-approved drug for spinal muscular atrophy. Translational Neuroscience 8: 1–6.

Pakpoor J, Noyce A, Goldacre R et al. (2017). Viral hepatitis and Parkinson disease: a national record-linkage study. Neurology 88: 1630–1633.

Papachroni KK, Ninkina N, Papapanagiotou A et al. (2007). Autoantibodies to alpha-synuclein in inherited Parkinson's disease. J Neurochem 101: 749–756.

Papp MI, Kahn JE, Lantos PL (1989). Glial cytoplasmic inclusions in the CNS of patients with multiple system atrophy (striatonigral degeneration, olivopontocerebellar atrophy and Shy-Drager syndrome). J Neurol Sci 94: 79–100.

Paul KC, Sinsheimer JS, Rhodes SL et al. (2016). Organophosphate pesticide exposures, nitric oxide synthase gene variants, and gene-pesticide interactions in a case-control study of Parkinson's disease, California (USA). Environmental Health Perspectives 124: 570–577.

Paumier KL, Luk KC, Manfredsson FP et al. (2015). Intrastriatal injection of pre-formed mouse alpha-synuclein fibrils into rats triggers alpha-synuclein pathology and bilateral nigrostriatal degeneration. Neurobiol Dis 82: 185–199.

Peelaerts W, Bousset L, Van der Perren A et al. (2015). Alpha-synuclein strains cause distinct synucleinopathies after local and systemic administration. Nature 522: 340–344.

Polymeropoulos MH, Lavedan C, Leroy E et al. (1997). Mutation in the alpha-synuclein gene identified in families with Parkinson's disease. Science 276: 2045–2047.

Prusiner SB, Woerman AL, Mordes DA et al. (2015). Evidence for alpha-synuclein prions causing multiple system atrophy in humans with parkinsonism. Proc Natl Acad Sci U S A 112: E5308–E5317.

Qin H, Buckley JA, Li X et al. (2016). Inhibition of the JAK/STAT pathway protects against alpha-synuclein-induced neuroinflammation and dopaminergic neurodegeneration. J Neurosci 36: 5144–5159.

Recasens A, Dehay B, Bove J et al. (2014). Lewy body extracts from Parkinson disease brains trigger alpha-synuclein pathology and neurodegeneration in mice and monkeys. Ann Neurol 75: 351–362.

Rey NL, Petit GH, Bousset L et al. (2013). Transfer of human alpha-synuclein from the olfactory bulb to interconnected brain regions in mice. Acta Neuropathol 126: 555–573.

Rey NL, Steiner JA, Maroof N et al. (2016). Widespread trans-neuronal propagation of alpha-synucleinopathy triggered in olfactory bulb mimics prodromal Parkinson's disease. The Journal of Experimental Medicine 213: 1759–1778.

Rey NL, Wesson DW, Brundin P (2018). The olfactory bulb as the entry site for prion-like propagation in neurodegenerative diseases. Neurobiol Dis 109: 226–248.

Rodriguez JA, Ivanova MI, Sawaya MR et al. (2015). Structure of the toxic core of alpha-synuclein from invisible crystals. Nature 525: 486–490.

Sacino AN, Brooks M, Thomas MA et al. (2014). Intramuscular injection of alpha-synuclein induces CNS alpha-synuclein pathology and a rapid-onset motor phenotype in transgenic mice. Proc Natl Acad Sci U S A 111: 10732–10737.

Sampson TR, Debelius JW, Thron T et al. (2016). Gut microbiota regulate motor deficits and neuroinflammation in a model of Parkinson's disease. Cell 167: 1469–1480 e1412.

Satake W, Nakabayashi Y, Mizuta I et al. (2009). Genome-wide association study identifies common variants at four loci as genetic risk factors for Parkinson's disease. Nat Genet 41: 1303–1307.

Schenk DB, Koller M, Ness DK et al. (2017). First-in-human assessment of PRX002, an anti-alpha-synuclein monoclonal antibody, in healthy volunteers. Mov Disord 32: 211–218.

Scheperjans F, Aho V, Pereira PA et al. (2015). Gut microbiota are related to Parkinson's disease and clinical phenotype. Mov Disord 30: 350–358.

Shannon KM, Keshavarzian A, Dodiya HB et al. (2012). Is alpha-synuclein in the colon a biomarker for premotor Parkinson's disease? Evidence from 3 cases. Mov Disord 27: 716–719.

Sharon G, Sampson TR, Geschwind DH et al. (2016). The central nervous system and the gut microbiome. Cell 167: 915–932.

Shimozawa A, Ono M, Takahara D et al. (2017). Propagation of pathological alpha-synuclein in marmoset brain. Acta Neuropathologica Communications 5: 12.

Simon-Sanchez J, Schulte C, Bras JM et al. (2009). Genome-wide association study reveals genetic risk underlying Parkinson's disease. Nat Genet 41: 1308–1312.

Soldner F, Stelzer Y, Shivalila CS et al. (2016). Parkinson-associated risk variant in distal enhancer of alpha-synuclein modulates target gene expression. Nature 533: 95–99.

Souza JM, Giasson BI, Chen Q et al. (2000). Dityrosine cross-linking promotes formation of stable alpha-synuclein polymers. Implication of nitrative and oxidative stress in the pathogenesis of neurodegenerative synucleinopathies. J Biol Chem 275: 18344–18349.

Spencer B, Valera E, Rockenstein E et al. (2017). Anti-alpha-synuclein immunotherapy reduces alpha-synuclein propagation in the axon and degeneration in a combined viral vector and transgenic model of synucleinopathy. Acta Neuropathologica Communications 5: 7.

Spillantini MG, Schmidt ML, Lee VM et al. (1997). Alpha-synuclein in Lewy bodies. Nature 388: 839–840.

Spillantini MG, Crowther RA, Jakes R et al. (1998). Alpha-synuclein in filamentous inclusions of Lewy bodies from Parkinson's disease and dementia with Lewy bodies. Proc Natl Acad Sci U S A 95: 6469–6473.

Stokholm MG, Danielsen EH, Hamilton-Dutoit SJ et al. (2016). Pathological alpha-synuclein in gastrointestinal tissues from prodromal Parkinson disease patients. Ann Neurol 79: 940–949.

Svensson E, Horvath-Puho E, Thomsen RW et al. (2015). Vagotomy and subsequent risk of Parkinson's disease. Ann Neurol 78: 522–529.

Tofaris GK, Razzaq A, Ghetti B et al. (2003). Ubiquitination of alpha-synuclein in Lewy bodies is a pathological event not associated with impairment of proteasome function. J Biol Chem 278: 44405–44411.

Tomlinson JJ, Shutinoski B, Dong L et al. (2017). Holocranohistochemistry enables the visualization of alpha-synuclein expression in the murine olfactory system and discovery of its systemic anti-microbial effects. Journal of Neural Transmission 124: 721–738.

Tran HT, Chung CH, Iba M et al. (2014). Alpha-synuclein immunotherapy blocks uptake and templated propagation of misfolded alpha-synuclein and neurodegeneration. Cell Rep 7: 2054–2065.

Usenovic M, Tresse E, Mazzulli JR et al. (2012). Deficiency of ATP13A2 leads to lysosomal dysfunction, alpha-synuclein accumulation, and neurotoxicity. J Neurosci 32: 4240–4246.

Valera E, Masliah E (2016). Combination therapies: the next logical step for the treatment of synucleinopathies? Mov Disord 31: 225–234.

Verbaan D, Marinus J, Visser M et al. (2007). Patient-reported autonomic symptoms in Parkinson disease. Neurology 69: 333–341.

Vicente Miranda H, Szego EM, Oliveira LMA et al. (2017). Glycation potentiates alpha-synuclein-associated neurodegeneration in synucleinopathies. Brain 140: 1399–1419.

Volpicelli-Daley LA, Luk KC, Patel TP et al. (2011). Exogenous alpha-synuclein fibrils induce Lewy body pathology leading to synaptic dysfunction and neuron death. Neuron 72: 57–71.

Volpicelli-Daley LA, Abdelmotilib H, Liu Z et al. (2016). G2019S-LRRK2 expression augments alpha-synuclein sequestration into inclusions in neurons. J Neurosci 36: 7415–7427.

Watts JC, Giles K, Oehler A et al. (2013). Transmission of multiple system atrophy prions to transgenic mice. Proc Natl Acad Sci U S A 110: 19555–19560.

Wrasidlo W, Tsigelny IF, Price DL et al. (2016). A de novo compound targeting alpha-synuclein improves deficits in models of Parkinson's disease. Brain 139: 3217–3236.

Ysselstein D, Joshi M, Mishra V et al. (2015). Effects of impaired membrane interactions on alpha-synuclein aggregation and neurotoxicity. Neurobiol Dis 79: 150–163.

Zharikov AD, Cannon JR, Tapias V et al. (2015). shRNA targeting alpha-synuclein prevents neurodegeneration in a Parkinson's disease model. The Journal of Clinical Investigation 125: 2721–2735.

Handbook of Clinical Neurology, Vol. 153 (3rd series)
Human Prion Diseases
M. Pocchiari and J. Manson, Editors
https://doi.org/10.1016/B978-0-444-63945-5.00018-0

Chapter 18

Prion-like mechanisms in amyotrophic lateral sclerosis

JACOB I. AYERS[1] AND NEIL R. CASHMAN[2]*

[1]*Department of Neuroscience, Center for Translational Research in Neurodegenerative Disease (CTRND), University of Florida, Gainesville, FL, United States*

[2]*Department of Medicine, Centre for Brain Health, University of British Columbia, Vancouver, BC, Canada*

Abstract

The prion hypothesis – a protein conformation capable of replicating without a nucleic acid genome – was heretical at the time of its discovery. However, the characteristics of the disease-misfolded prion protein and its ability to transmit disease, replicate, and spread are now widely accepted throughout the scientific community. In fact, in the last decade a wealth of evidence has emerged supporting similar properties observed for many of the misfolded proteins implicated in other neurodegenerative diseases, such as Alzheimer disease, Parkinson disease, tauopathies, and as described in this chapter, amyotrophic lateral sclerosis (ALS). Multiple studies have now demonstrated the ability for superoxide dismutase-1, 43-kDa transactive response (TAR) DNA-binding protein, fused-in sarcoma, and most recently, C9orf72-encoded polypeptides to display properties similar to those of prions. The majority of these are cell-free and in vitro assays, while superoxide dismutase-1 remains the only ALS-linked protein to demonstrate several prion-like properties in vivo. In this chapter, we provide an introduction to ALS and review the recent literature linking several proteins implicated in the familial forms of the disease to properties of the prion protein.

INTRODUCTION

Amyotrophic lateral sclerosis (ALS) is a devastating and ultimately fatal disease characterized by progressive paralysis caused by the degeneration of both upper and lower motor neurons in the brain, brainstem, and spinal cord. It is considered an orphan disease with an incidence of 1–2 individuals diagnosed per 100,000 each year and a prevalence of only about 5 cases per 100,000, revealing the rapidity of the disease, which in about 80% of cases is fatal within 3–5 years after diagnosis (Al-Chalabi and Hardiman, 2013). The mean age of disease onset is 55 years of age, but varies dramatically, with some cases beginning in an individual's 20s or as late as their 80s. This large variability in disease characteristics is also observed in the degree of upper vs. lower motor neuron involvement, and where the symptoms first manifest themselves (e.g., arm(s), leg(s), or bulbar) (Grad et al., 2016). Limb or bulbar muscle weakness usually begins focally before progressively spreading throughout the entire voluntary motor system, with typically late involvement of respiratory muscles. Although historically believed to cause a pure motor system degeneration, within the last 20 years clinical evidence has demonstrated cognitive impairment and a strong overlap of symptomology with frontotemporal degeneration (FTD), a disease caused by neuronal degeneration in the frontal and temporal lobes (Goldstein and Abrahams, 2013). The cognitive deficits can have a substantial negative impact on the disease phenotype and this is correlated with a decreased survival rate in patients (Olney et al., 2005).

Approximately 10% of ALS cases occur in multiple individuals within a family (familial ALS, or fALS), while the majority of cases present without any evidence of inheritance and are termed sporadic ALS (sALS). Clinically, fALS and sALS are essentially indistinguishable from one another. Mutations in the gene encoding

*Correspondence to: Neil Cashman, MD, Djavad Mowafaghian Centre for Brain Health, 2215 Wesbrook Mall, Vancouver, BC, V6T 1Z3, Canada. Tel: +1-604-822-2135, E-mail: neil.cashman@vch.ca

SOD1 were the first to be identified as a hereditary cause of ALS in 1993 (Rosen et al., 1993), and since then, mutations in more than 50 other genes have been implicated in ALS pathogenesis. However, many of these have yet to be completely validated. Genes that have consistently revealed linkage to a significant percentage of fALS cases include those encoding the 43-kDa transactive response (TAR) DNA-binding protein (TDP-43), fused-in sarcoma/translocated in liposarcoma (FUS/TLS), ubiquilin-2, senataxin, and *C9ORF72* (http://alsod.iop.kcl.ac.uk/). Although mutations within these genes cause a disease clinically and pathologically consistent with the ALS syndrome, the wild-type (WT) proteins encoded by these mutation-validated genes have a diverse set of functions, including transcription control and splicing regulation via RNA binding, proteostasis and protein quality control, and cytoskeleton support and axon development. For this reason, some believe that there is a common, as of yet unknown, pathogenic mechanism underlying all ALS.

Prion diseases consist of a number of human and animal diseases characterized by widespread neuronal loss and spongiosis in the central nervous system (CNS). These diseases are caused by the infectious prion protein, an abnormal isoform of the host-encoded normal cellular prion protein. At the time of its discovery, and for decades thereafter, the prion protein was believed to be unique in its engagement in the templated propagation mechanism of prion infectivity. More recently, a wealth of research supports the notion that other diseases caused by misfolded proteins share characteristics with prion diseases, including Alzheimer disease, Parkinson disease, Huntington disease, and ALS, among others (Guest et al., 2011) (Table 18.1). Some of the proteins implicated in these diseases undergo a gain of toxic properties and demonstrate the ability for conformational templating, cell-to-cell and neuroanatomic spread, and to exist in conformationally distinct species or "strains" (Clavaguera et al., 2009; Jucker and Walker, 2013; Sacino et al., 2013; Sanders et al., 2014; Watts et al., 2014; Peelaerts et al., 2015).

MISFOLDED PROTEINS IN ALS

SOD1

The copper zinc superoxide dismutase-1 (SOD1) protein is an antioxidant enzyme that functions in the disproportionation of highly reactive superoxide to generate hydrogen peroxide and dioxygen. SOD1 exists as an extremely stable homodimer in which each subunit contains one copper and one zinc ion along with an intrasubunit disulfide bond (Parge et al., 1992; Ogihara et al., 1996). It is an abundant protein, localized primarily in the cytosol (Crapo et al., 1992), but has also been observed within the mitochondrial intermembrane space (Field et al., 2003). *SOD1* was the first dominantly inherited gene described to have a role in ALS pathogenesis (Rosen et al., 1993) and now accounts for approximately 10–20% of all fALS cases.

Currently, there are more than 180 mutations identified in the *SOD1* gene, which span the entire length of the 153-amino-acid protein (http://alsod.iop.kcl.ac.uk/). Although all of these mutations have not been investigated, in those examined to date, the SOD1 mutation increases the propensity for the protein to adopt misfolded conformers that acquire detergent-insolubility akin to aggregates (Bruijn et al., 1998; Johnston et al., 2000; Karch et al., 2009; Prudencio et al., 2010; Wang et al., 2003). It was initially believed that the conformational change of SOD1 led to a loss of enzymatic activity and contributed to its toxicity; however, subsequent studies indicated the SOD1 dismutase activity did not correlate with disease severity (Cleveland et al., 1995). Additionally, transgenic mouse models overexpressing fALS-linked SOD1 mutants developed an ALS-like paralytic disease, despite expressing endogenous mouse SOD1, while mice lacking SOD1 exhibited no ALS-like phenotype (Borchelt et al., 1994; Gurney et al., 1994; Bruijn et al., 1998).

Although SOD1 has been the best studied of all the ALS-causing proteins, the mechanism of motor neuron loss and disease has yet to be elucidated. It is still an unresolved question as to why the motor neurons are so vulnerable, as the pathogenesis is mediated in large part by noncell autonomous mechanisms, involving other types of neurons and glial cells (Boillée et al., 2006a; Ilieva et al., 2009). Possible mechanisms of toxicity to the motor neurons include glutamate excitotoxicity (Rothstein et al., 1995; Howland et al., 2002), impairment in the protein quality control mechanisms leading to endoplasmic reticulum stress (Urushitani et al., 2002; Kabashi and Durham, 2006; Atkin et al., 2008; Saxena et al., 2009), non cell autonomous effects on glial cells and oligodendrocytes (Boillée et al., 2006b; Yamanaka et al., 2008; Kang et al., 2013), and disorganization of the axonal cytoskeleton and disruption of axonal transport (Williamson and Cleveland, 1999), among others. Even though these mechanisms are all likely to participate in ALS pathogenesis, there is no consensus on which of these processes may initiate the primary toxic cascade, and which ones may be a secondary consequent effect.

TDP43

TDP-43 is encoded by the *TARDBP* gene, which is a highly conserved and ubiquitously expressed protein localized primarily within the nucleus, and functions in

Table 18.1

Prion-like properties of amyotrophic lateral sclerosis-linked proteins

	Seeded aggregation			Spread		Inducible MND in mice			
Protein	Cell-free	Cell culture	In vivo	Cell-culture	In vivo	Recombinant protein	Murine tissue homogenates	Human tissue homogenates	Strain properties
SOD1	Chattopadhyay et al. (2008); Furukawa et al. (2008); Chia et al. (2010)	Grad et al. (2011, 2014); Münch et al. (2011)	Ayers et al. (2014a)	Grad et al. (2011, 2014); Münch et al. (2011)	Ayers et al. (2016b)	Ayers et al. (2016a)	Ayers et al. (2014a); Bidhendi et al. (2016)	n.d.	Ayers et al. (2016a); Bidhendi et al. (2016)
TDP-43	Furukawa et al. (2011)	Furukawa et al. (2011); Nonaka et al. (2013)	n.d.	Nonaka et al. (2013); Feiler et al. (2015)	n.d.	n.d.	n.d.	n.d.	Hasegawa et al. (2011)
FUS/TLS	Nomura et al. (2014)	n.d.	n.d.	n.d.	n.d.	n.d.	n.d.	n.d.	n.d.
C9orf72	n.d.	n.d.	n.d.	Westergard et al. (2016)	n.d.	n.d.	n.d.	n.d.	n.d.

MND, motor neuron disease; n.d., not done.

transcription and RNA splicing regulation (Johnson et al., 2009; Lagier-Tourenne et al., 2010). It contains two RNA recognition motifs involved in its binding of nucleic acid, an N-terminal ubiquitin-like domain, a nuclear localization signal and nuclear export signal, and a C-terminal glycine-rich domain, important in protein–protein interactions.

One pathologic feature common among both the sporadic and inherited forms of ALS is the accumulation of ubiquitinated protein inclusions that appear in both upper and lower motor neurons and in some glial cells. Similar inclusions are observed in the brains of frontotemporal lobar degeneration with ubiquitin-positive inclusions (FTLD-U) and it was revealed that TDP-43 was the major component of these inclusions in both ALS and FTLD-U (Neumann et al., 2006). Normally nuclear TDP-43 is found redistributed to these ubiquitinated inclusions in the cytoplasm of neurons and glial cells in ~95% of sporadic ALS cases (Arai et al., 2006; Neumann et al., 2006). Interestingly, the nucleus of many of these cells containing cytoplasmic TDP-43 inclusions are depleted of nuclear TDP-43, indicating that one potential pathogenic mechanism may be the loss of TDP-43 function in the nucleus (Neumann et al., 2006; Giordana et al., 2010). However, in ~5% of fALS cases and ~1% of sALS cases with no known family history, mutations in the *TARDBP* gene are detected.

There are now more than 50 mutations identified responsible for TDP-43 linked disease, that are predominantly clustered in the C-terminal region of the protein, which contains a glycine-rich domain referred to as a low-complexity domain (http://alsod.iop.kcl.ac.uk/) (Lagier-Tourenne et al., 2010; Ling et al., 2013). Pathologic inclusions of the protein are ubiquitinated and phosphorylated and are abnormally cleaved, producing C-terminal fragments (CTFs). The mislocalization of TDP-43 from the nucleus to the cytoplasm and its subsequent aggregation suggest a potential loss of function and/or gain of function as possible disease mechanisms (Arai et al., 2006; Neumann et al., 2006).

FUS/TLS

Shortly after the identification of TDP-43 mutations in cases of ALS, mutations in another ribonucleoprotein, FUS/TLS, was discovered as a cause of ~4% of fALS patients and rarely in sALS patients without a known familial history (Kwiatkowski et al., 2009; Vance et al., 2009). The 526-amino-acid protein has a single RNA recognition motif, an N-terminal domain enriched in glutamine, glycine, serine, and tyrosine residues, an arginine-glycine-glycine-rich region, and a glycine-rich region (Iko et al., 2004; Lagier-Tourenne et al., 2010). It also contains both a nuclear export signal and at the extreme C-terminal end of the protein a nuclear localization signal, which, along with the glycine-rich domain, are where the majority of the mutations (predominantly frameshift deletions) have been identified. Like TDP-43, mutations in FUS result in the mislocalization of the protein out of the nucleus and into the cytoplasm to form inclusions in both neurons and glia. Although the FUS inclusions are immunoreactive to ubiquitin and p62, indicating an involvement of the protein quality control mechanisms, there is no association between FUS and TDP-43 pathology in ALS, suggesting separate neurodegenerative mechanisms. The mechanism(s) involved in ALS pathogenesis caused by FUS mutations are not well understood but evidence for both a gain of toxic and loss of normal properties have been hypothesized (Sun et al., 2015).

C9orf72

In 2011, two independent groups reported an intronic hexanucleotide GGGGCC (G_4C_2) repeat expansion within the first intron of the *C9ORF72* gene associated with ALS and FTD patients (DeJesus-Hernandez et al., 2011; Renton et al., 2011). It is now considered the most frequent genetic cause of ALS with ~40% of fALS and 5–20% of sALS patients carrying this expansion (Reisin, 2012). Similar to other repeat expansion diseases, the size of the repeat has been found to be inversely correlated with disease duration in FTD but not ALS (Suh et al., 2015). While it is generally observed that G_4C_2 repeats of less than 30 do not cause disease, there is a large variability in the length of repeats found in those ALS and FTD patients, ranging from a few hundred to a few thousand. The normal function of the C9orf72 protein is not yet known, but recent data have indicated a potential role in cellular trafficking and revealed a differentially expressed in normal and neoplastic cells domain, suggesting it may function as a GDP-GTP nucleotide exchange factor (Farg et al., 2014; Levine et al., 2013).

Three mechanisms are proposed to account for the neurodegeneration caused by the repeat expansion: a loss of C9orf72 function (DeJesus-Hernandez et al., 2011), the production of toxic dipeptide repeat proteins via repeat-associated non-ATG translation (Zu et al., 2013), and a gain of toxic function through the formation of expanded toxic RNA species and/or transcription inhibition by forming DNA/RNA hybrids (DeJesus-Hernandez et al., 2011; Gendron et al., 2014). As this expansion is a newly discovered cause of disease, there is currently considerable research directed at which of these mechanisms are the main driving force behind the neurodegenerative process. Although the consequences of dipeptide repeat protein formation and its role in disease are unclear (Mackenzie et al., 2015), a recent report has provided evidence for cell-to-cell transmission via exosome-dependent and exosome-independent pathways in vitro (Westergard et al., 2016).

AGGREGATION AND SELF-PROPAGATION OF ALS-ASSOCIATED PROTEINS

Propagation and seeding of SOD1

Research into the properties of the prion protein and its associated disorders revealed unique properties of the infectious agent that had never before been observed for a mammalian protein, and questioned the central dogma of infectious agents; that replication required a nucleic acid genome. The most profound, and at the time controversial, finding was that of the "protein-only" hypothesis, which states that the infectious agent responsible for these diseases, PrP^{TSE}, is produced via a conformational change of the normal isoform of the prion protein into the misfolded, pathogenic isoform (Griffith, 1967). Additionally, the hypothesis postulates that the infectious prion protein replicates by an "autocatalytic" conformational conversion of the normal isoform to its pathogenic isoform (Griffith, 1967; Prusiner, 1982; Weissmann, 1991). This seminal discovery and subsequent studies in the prion field have led to a rethinking of neurodegenerative disorders and the pathogenic mechanisms involved, and have also provided a blueprint to follow when studying these diseases.

The prion protein is hypothesized to aggregate via a multistep process, referred to as template-dependent polymerization. This process is initiated through a rate-limiting nucleation step in which PrP^{TSE} "seeds" are produced. These crystal-like seeds will then rapidly elongate to form progressively larger aggregates and amyloid fibril structures. Support for this hypothesis came from cell-free experiments in which it was revealed that the normal cellular PrP^{C} could be converted into PrP^{TSE} initially through incubation in nonphysiologic conditions, and more recently by incubation while undergoing rounds of sonication or shaking, which act to continually break up these amyloid structures and thereby create more seeds (Kocisko et al., 1994; Saborio et al., 2001; Atarashi et al., 2008).

WT SOD1 is an extremely stable protein due to its intrasubunit disulfide bond, its ability to bind zinc and copper, and its dimeric nature. Removing any of these features causes SOD1 to destabilize and misfold. Studies using recombinant, apo (metal-free) SOD1 have revealed that, under destabilizing conditions such as high temperature, the presence of trifluoroethanol, or low pH, SOD1 is capable of forming detergent-insoluble amyloid fibrils that bind amyloid-specific dyes (Stathopulos et al., 2003; Furukawa et al., 2008).

Additionally, it was discovered that the spontaneous formation of both WT and mutant SOD1 fibrils can be enhanced when incubated at 37°C, with constant shaking, and mild denaturing conditions (Chattopadhyay et al., 2008; Chia et al., 2010). This in vitro cell-free assay allowed researchers to better examine some of the conditions responsible for inducing SOD1 aggregates. Using this assay, Chattopadhyay et al. (2008) revealed that just a small amount of disulfide-reduced apo SOD1 containing a mutation was capable of rapidly inducing fibrillation of the relatively stable apo WT SOD1. The kinetics of these fibrillation assays mirrored those of the prion protein, and strongly supported the idea that SOD1 aggregates to form fibrils by nucleation-dependent polymerization.

This assay was then exploited to investigate the source of the SOD1 fibril "seeds." To start to investigate the in vivo relevance of the assay, Chia et al. (2010) used spinal homogenates from several lines of transgenic mice overexpressing mutant SOD1 as their seed source to test the induction of fibril formation. It was observed that these homogenates were capable of inducing the aggregation and fibrillation of recombinant WT and mutant SOD1 when incubated in mild destabilizing conditions. These studies provided new insights into ALS disease mechanisms by revealing seeding characteristics strikingly similar to those observed for the prion protein. Additionally, they provided a potential explanation for the spread of disease throughout the CNS.

The first demonstrations for SOD1 seeding and aggregation of SOD1 in living cells were achieved through the exogenous administration of SOD1 aggregates to cell lines overexpressing soluble, nonaggregated SOD1. Both mutant and WT SOD1 aggregates were shown to be efficiently taken up into neuroblastoma cell lines by lipid raft-dependent macropinocytosis (Münch et al., 2011; Grad et al., 2014). In one study it was demonstrated that the aggregates, once inside the cells, were capable of nucleating the aggregation of the highly expressed cytosolic SOD1, causing it to become detergent-insoluble, and furthermore creating a self-perpetuating cascade of SOD1 misfolding (Münch et al., 2011). This seeding effect was persistent, as SOD1 aggregates were constantly being released and taken up by nearby cells. Although this study demonstrated a prion-like seeding characteristic of SOD1, it was reliant on overexpression of mutant SOD1 (Münch et al., 2011).

Another study demonstrated a similar phenomenon, albeit in cells expressing endogenous WT SOD1, a novel finding and one that implicates misfolding of WT SOD1 as a pathogenic cause for sporadic cases of ALS (discussed in detail below) (Grad et al., 2011). When cells were transiently transfected with various mutant SOD1 constructs, misfolding and aggregation of WT SOD1 were observed along with the acquisition of biochemical features similar to those of mutant SOD1 (Grad et al., 2011). Interestingly, the conversion of WT SOD1 by mutant SOD1 required tryptophan at position 32 for both species of SOD1, suggesting a homophilic intermolecular interaction was key to the misfolding reaction (Grad et al., 2011). Additionally, it was later demonstrated by these authors that the induced WT SOD1 aggregates were capable of seeding nearby cells through release of aggregates from dying cells or through exosome release (Grad et al., 2014; Silverman et al., 2016). These studies revealed the ability for misfolded SOD1 to act as a seed that was capable of inducing a conformational change of soluble, normally folded SOD1, and that these seeds could be released and taken up by nearby cells.

The next obvious step in demonstrating the prion-like nature of SOD1 was to determine its ability to seed and transmit disease in vivo. Research into the transmissibility of prion diseases revealed the high titer of infectious prion molecules in homogenates prepared from the brains of prion-infected mice, and researchers demonstrated this by passaging these homogenates into various animal models. One such study exploring a prion mutant known to cause a hereditary prion disease utilized a line of mice expressing levels of the mutant transgene at such low levels that disease never developed during the lifespan of the mice; therefore, this model was "primed" to develop a prion disease (Hsiao et al., 1994). Upon injection of brain homogenates prepared from a diseased mouse line expressing high levels of the transgene into the brains of the low-expressing line, the authors revealed the induction of prion disease (Hsiao et al., 1994). This study demonstrated the utility of using a "primed" animal model that expresses a mutant transgene just below the threshold level needed to induce disease for use in disease transmission experiments.

Ayers and colleagues (2014a) utilized this paradigm in an attempt to identify a permissive model for disease transmission using spinal cord homogenates from transgenic lines of mice that succumbed to motor neuron disease (MND). Through these studies, they identified a transgenic mouse model expressing the G85R mutation of SOD1 fused to yellow fluorescent protein (mice referred to as G85R-SOD1:YFP), that, when bred as heterozygous mice, never developed MND (J. Wang et al., 2009; Ayers et al., 2014a). The authors demonstrated that, when spinal cord homogenates prepared from paralyzed mice overexpressing mutant versions of SOD1 were injected into the spinal cords of G85R-SOD1:YFP mice on the day they were born (P0), the mice went on to develop MND with abundant YFP inclusions within their spinal cords and brainstem (Ayers et al., 2014a). The authors had previously tried to identify other lines of mice permissive to MND transmission, including those expressing G93A and G37R SOD1 mutations, along with a line overexpressing the WT SOD1 protein or WT SOD1 fused to YFP (WT-SOD1: YFP), but initially the G85R-SOD1:YFP mouse model was the only SOD1 transgenic mouse line they identified that developed MND using this experimental paradigm (Ayers et al., 2014a). This brought into question the effect of the bulky YFP tag fused to the c-terminal end of SOD1 on transmissibility and aggregation; however, more recently, the authors and others have revealed the successful transmission of MND in an untagged G85R mouse model, as well as two additional models expressing SOD1 truncations (Ayers et al., 2016a; Bidhendi et al., 2016).

Although these studies successfully demonstrated the transmissibility and pathogenicity of SOD1 in vivo, the spinal cord homogenates used as inoculum in these experiments contain many other factors, including immunomodulatory cytokines and chemokines that could impact disease induction. To determine if SOD1 itself was indeed the seeding factor in these experiments, studies were undertaken using in vitro aggregated, recombinant WT SOD1 (Ayers et al., 2016a). Following injection in spinal cords of P0 G85R-SOD1:YFP mice, MND was induced along with robust SOD1:YFP spinal cord inclusion pathology. Interestingly, the SOD1 pathology of the inclusions induced by WT SOD1 aggregates differed significantly from those induced following the homogenate injections, suggesting not only templated misfolding, but also the existence of SOD1 strains (discussed in later sections) (Ayers et al., 2016a). These studies leave little doubt as to the transmissibility and seeding capability of SOD1 in vivo.

TDP-43 and FUS

As mentioned above, the C-terminal region of TDP-43 contains the majority of the clinically relevant mutations that cause ALS, and also appears to be critical to the aggregation of the protein. In tissue from ALS and FTLD-TDP patients, protease-resistant CTFs are found, similar to the protease-resistant core of the prion protein (Arai et al., 2006; Neumann et al., 2006; Igaz et al., 2008). Studies on these fragments revealed that they contained a primarily β-sheet-rich conformation, and that N-terminally TDP-43 that consists only of the CTF showed an increased ability to aggregate in cultured cells and cell-free assays (Johnson et al., 2009; Guo et al., 2011). The inherent propensity for this region to aggregate is attributed to a stretch of glutamine/asparganine (Q/N) residues found in this region. The Q/N domain has been found in a number of other aggregation-prone proteins, including FUS, and is referred to as the prion-like domain, due to its presence in the Sup35 yeast prion domain (Alberti et al., 2009; Cushman et al., 2010).

Similar to those studies investigating the in vitro seeding characteristics of SOD1, studies in cell culture with various constructs of TDP-43 have revealed a seeding ability. Furukawa et al. (2011) were the first to demonstrate this property by demonstrating that recombinant WT and detergent-insoluble aggregates of TDP-43 can be internalized by human embryonic kidney cells (HEK293) and seed the fibrillization of endogenous TDP-43. Although the induced inclusions lacked several properties commonly associated with TDP-43 pathology observed in disease, such as phosphorylation and truncation creating the CTF, they were found to be ubiquitinated and detergent-insoluble (Furukawa et al., 2011). Subsequent studies by Nonaka et al. (2013) then demonstrated the ability for aggregated TDP-43 isolated from the brains of ALS and FTLD-TDP patients to induce ubiquitinated and phosphorylated TDP-43 cytoplasmic aggregates when administered to a neuronal cell line overexpressing an N-terminal hemagglutinin-tagged TDP-43. Lysates from these cells containing induced aggregates were also able to induce TDP-43 inclusions when re-administered to naïve cells (Nonaka et al., 2013; Hanspal et al., 2017). Although a handful of mouse models have been created that express human TDP-43, there have been no demonstrations of TDP-43 disease transmission in vivo (Nonaka et al., 2013).

SPREADING OF ALS SYMPTOMS AND PATHOLOGY

For classic prions, it is well established that the infectious agent is capable of spreading throughout the CNS via neuroanatomic pathway connections. The first evidence of this came about through intraocular inoculation of homogenates in mice, in which the temporal and spatial accumulation of spongiosis was found to be consistent with axonal transport along the retinotectal pathway (Fraser, 1982). This characteristic is a hallmark of prion diseases and one that is suggested to play a role in other neurodegenerative disorders caused by the accumulation of toxic proteins, such as α-synuclein in Parkinson disease (Sacino et al., 2013, 2014; Peelaerts et al., 2015), and tau in Alzheimer disease (Clavaguera et al., 2009; Sanders et al., 2014).

ALS is an extremely heterogeneous disease in which initial symptoms can appear in almost any motor group caused by degeneration of upper motor neurons and lower motor neurons. For instance, limb-onset ALS is caused by degeneration of the motor neurons controlling the upper or lower extremities, whereas bulbar-onset ALS is caused by degeneration of the motor neurons controlling speech and swallowing. One of the characteristics of muscle weakness in ALS is that it begins focally before spreading to adjacent muscles, and that within the region where symptoms first began, motor symptoms are minor at first before steadily worsening over time (Ravits, 2014; Grad et al., 2016).

Another observation is that the spread of symptoms appears to occur contiguously in the CNS. For instance, if weakness first appears in one leg, symptoms likely spread to the contralateral leg, consistent with the connectivity of motor neurons in the spinal cord. On the other hand, spread of symptoms from the leg to the ipsilateral arm is consistent with the neuroanatomy of the cerebral motor cortex, suggestive of upper motor neuron degeneration (Ravits, 2014). Lastly, it has been observed that the speed at which symptoms spread between muscle groups helps to establish the length of time a patient will live with the disease (Ravits, 2014).

Multiple mechanisms of spread have been observed and hypothesized for the progression of disease in CNS disorders, including both propagative and nonpropagative mechanisms (Kanouchi et al., 2012). In cases of fALS, every motor neuron and glial cell contains a clinically relevant ALS-causing mutation, thereby allowing the onset of symptoms to appear in almost any muscle group. It is believed that protein inclusions first appear and affect motor neurons once a certain threshold in that particular cell is reached, but why this appears to occur in one focal region within the CNS, causing the focality of clinical onset, is unknown. It is a question that plagues most neurodegenerative disorders: what is the trigger that begins the pathogenic cascade of events? Whatever the trigger may be for ALS (environmental or biologic), the clinical symptoms of the disease argue for a propagative mechanism of spread for the toxic agent (although alternate explanations, such as selective vulnerability, have been proposed) (Engelender and Isacson, 2017; Surmeier et al., 2017). This could include a contiguous cell-to-cell spread and/or a noncontiguous spread of infectivity via neuroanatomic transport or dissemination by the cerebrospinal fluid or blood (Kanouchi et al., 2012; Ravits, 2014). These scenarios are not mutually exclusive and both could contribute to the widespread pathology observed in ALS.

As mentioned above, SOD1 transmission experiments in cultured cells demonstrated the ability for SOD1 to induce and propagate misfolding to nearby cells (Grad et al., 2011, 2014; Münch and Bertolotti, 2011). Based on similar properties of the infectious prion agent and several other neurodegenerative proteins in cell culture, the intercellular transmission of SOD1 misfolding could be due to the exit of an SOD1-inducing species by one or more of the following mechanisms: (1) release of SOD1 due to cell death; (2) release of SOD1-carrying extracellular vesicles; or (3) exit and passage of SOD1 through direct cell-to-cell tunneling nanotubes. Conversely, SOD1 can be taken up into cells by: (1) endocytosis (directly or receptor-mediated) or (2) fusion of extracellular vesicles to the plasma membrane (Fig. 18.1). Multiple research groups have identified macropinocytosis, a form of endocytosis that mediates a nonselective uptake of molecules, as a mechanism of uptake of SOD1 species in the media of cultured cells (Münch and Bertolotti, 2011; Grad et al., 2014). This finding was accomplished by using inhibitors to various endocytic mechanisms of cellular entry and revealed that uptake of SOD1 was clathrin and dynamin-independent (Münch and Bertolotti, 2011; Grad et al., 2014). Although there is evidence for this mechanism in cultured cells, there are no in vivo data demonstrating the importance of macropinocytosis.

The majority of data surrounding the release of SOD1 has focused on exosomes, which are secreted, membrane-bound multivesicular endosomes that form inside cells and are 50–150 nm in diameter. These extracellular vesicles are seen to be secreted from a variety of cells in the CNS, including neurons, astrocytes, microglia, and oligodendrocytes, and can carry a variety of cargos such as nucleic acids and proteins (Raposo and Stoorvogel, 2013). They have garnered much attention recently, as they have been implicated in the spread of misfolded proteins involved in neurodegenerative diseases, including prion diseases (Fevrier et al., 2004; Perez-Gonzalez et al., 2012). In regard to ALS, SOD1 has been reported to be a component of exosomes from mammalian cells (Kim et al., 2013). In neuronal cell lines and primary astrocytic cultures overexpressing SOD1, exosomes are observed to be released carrying both WT and mutant versions of SOD1 (Gomes et al., 2007; Basso et al., 2013). In fact, SOD1-containing exosomes released from astrocytes were found to efficiently transfer the packaged SOD1 to motor neurons and contribute to their cell death (Basso et al., 2013). Although the mechanism(s) of toxicity is unknown, studies reveal that newly acquired exosomal SOD1 is capable of seeding and/or inducing SOD1 misfolding in the recipient cells (Grad et al., 2014). Further supporting the idea of cell-to-cell transfer of misfolded SOD1 and its ability to seed, this study also demonstrated that conformation-specific antibodies can block transmission of these SOD1 seeds (Grad et al., 2014). Interestingly, overexpression of mutant SOD1 actually impairs its own secretion from cells (Turner et al., 2005). Limited studies have also revealed potential mechanisms involved in the in vitro spread of TDP-43 aggregates, including via exosomes (Nonaka et al., 2013; Ding et al., 2015) and tunneling nanotubes (Ding et al., 2015). Although there are conflicting reports of the role of SOD1 dissemination via exosomes and the in vivo relevance has yet to be studied,

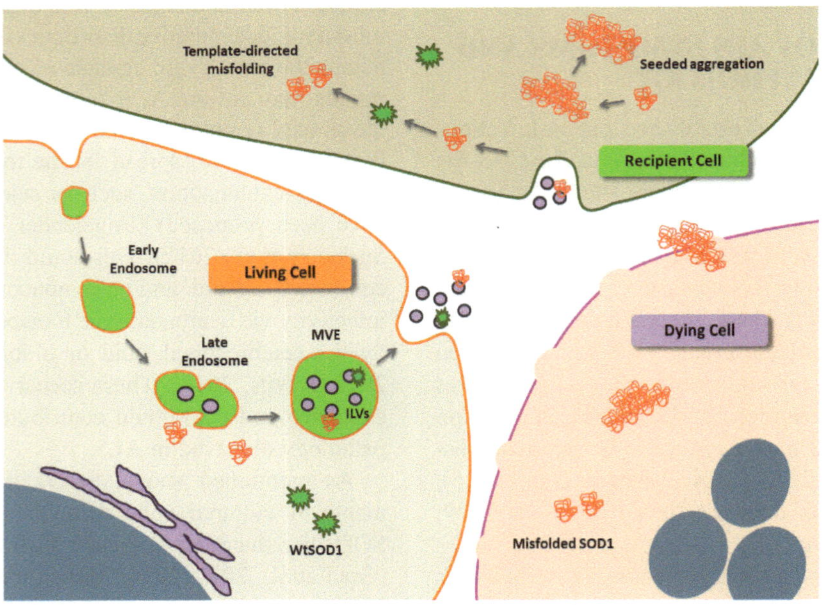

Fig. 18.1. Intercellular transmission of SOD1 misfolding. Misfolded SOD1 is packaged into intraluminal vesicles (ILVs) within the late endosome (multivesicular endosome (MVE)) and secreted into the extracellular space as exosomes. Exosomes can be taken up by neighboring cells via endocytosis. Within the recipient cell, the misfolded SOD1 species can template the misfolding of normally folded wild-type SOD1 (WtSOD1). Dead or dying cells can release SOD1 aggregates, which can be taken up by recipient cells via macropinocytosis. Seeded aggregation ensues when the aggregate recruits additional misfolded proteins to enlarge the aggregate. (Reproduced from Silverman JM, Fernando SM, Grad LI, et al. (2016) Disease mechanisms in ALS: misfolded SOD1 transferred through exosome-dependent and exosome-independent pathways. Cell Mol Neurobiol 36: 377–381.)

this mechanism deserves more attention as it could be a therapeutic target to prevent the spread of ALS pathology.

Based on the spread of clinical symptoms in ALS, it seems highly likely that the transport of toxic factors may be occurring through direct neuroanatomic transport. One technique used in the prion field to demonstrate this mechanism of spread utilized injection of the infectious agent within the sciatic nerve (Bartz et al., 2002; Ayers et al., 2009). The advantage of this injection paradigm is that it presents the injected agent to a defined and localized group of motor neurons within the lumbar spinal cord, thereby allowing for the determination of transport by examining the spatial and temporal accumulation of pathology (Bartz et al., 2002, 2007; Ayers et al., 2009). Using this experimental model, Ayers et al. (2009) unilaterally injected spinal cord homogenates from diseased SOD1 transgenic mice into the sciatic nerve of the permissive G85R-SOD1:YFP mouse model (Ayers et al., 2016b). The injections induced paralysis in the mice, beginning in the ipsilateral hind limb before spreading to the contralateral limb, similar to spread of symptoms in human ALS (Ayers et al., 2016b). This phenotype was accompanied with a spreading SOD1 and glial pathology that began focally in the lumbar spinal cord and progressed over time rostrally up the spinal cord (Ayers et al., 2016b). An important finding from this study was that deposition in the brainstem preceded deposition in the cervical spinal cord (Ayers et al., 2016b). Furthermore, though the deposition in the brain and brainstem was limited in paralyzed mice, the neuronal populations that developed SOD1 pathology had direct synaptic connections with the lumbar spinal cord (Ayers et al., 2016b). Within a given region of the CNS where pathology was observed, it was shown that pathology increased in abundance over time. This study demonstrates the ability for SOD1 pathology to spread in a predictable pattern similar to that observed for the infectious prion protein. It also implicates a role for both cell-to-cell spread and transsynaptic transport of a SOD1 pathology-inducing factor, which may be SOD1 itself.

EXISTENCE OF ALS-INDUCING PROTEIN STRAINS

During the early years of prion research it was believed that the infectious agent was a slow-acting virus (Gajdusek, 1977). Although heretical at its time, it was later revealed that the agent contains no nucleic acid and exists as an abnormal conformer of a normal, host-encoded protein (Prusiner, 1982). One reason that the hypothesis of a protein-only infectious agent was not well accepted at the time was because a variety of prion isolates displayed distinct and highly reproducible incubation periods and patterns of neuropathology, strongly reminiscent of viral strains specified by genomic polymorphisms. Through biochemical examination of the structure of various prion isolates it was determined that the tertiary structural differences of the prion molecules correlated with the heritable traits (Bessen and Marsh, 1994; Telling et al., 1996; Caughey et al., 1998). In additional studies of human prion diseases, it was determined that rare mutations could dictate the particular form of expressed familial prion disease, accompanied by distinct clinical presentations, disease course, and biochemical properties of the disease-associated prion protein (Goldfarb et al., 1992; Kovács et al., 2002). It is now widely accepted that the mutation-specific phenotypes are due to prion strains, or distinct tertiary conformations of the prion protein that "encipher" the disease-specific information (Peretz et al., 2001). This concept presages the impact that distinct protein conformers can have on the pathogenesis of neurodegenerative diseases caused by misfolded proteins.

SOD1-linked fALS is a heterogeneous disease phenotypically, with diverse clinical symptoms referable to upper or lower motor neurons, with a large variability in disease duration (1–20+ years) and age of onset (25–70 years of age) (Grad et al., 2016). However, the diversity in disease duration is not uniformly distributed, but rather shows significant association with the particular SOD1 mutation (Prudencio et al., 2009b). Similar to the impacts in disease pathogenesis from mutations in the gene encoding the prion protein, it seems reasonable to surmise that mutations in the *SOD1* gene, and the slight variation they engender in its tertiary structure (Furukawa et al., 2010; Chan et al., 2013), could allow SOD1 to impart strain-like effects on the phenotype of ALS.

To address this, Bidhendi et al. prepared homogenates from two lines of SOD1 transgenic mice, those expressing the G85R-SOD1 mutation and those expressing D90A-SOD1 (Bergh et al., 2015; Bidhendi et al., 2016). Both of these mouse models develop MND, and upon analysis of the G85R and D90A aggregates, distinct structural characteristics, molecular properties, and growth kinetics were observed (Bergh et al., 2015). Based on these differences, two discrete SOD1 strains (A and B) were hypothesized to exist in the homogenates (Bergh et al., 2015). Using a panel of polyclonal rabbit antibodies spanning the length of SOD1, it was also observed that when these two SOD1 strains were inoculated into an MND-inducible SOD1 transgenic mouse model expressing the G85R mutation, the induced SOD1 inclusions displayed two different immunoreactive profiles that matched those of the SOD1 strain inoculated (Bidhendi et al., 2016). These observations reveal the ability for the G85R-SOD1 protein to adopt different conformations and strongly support the hypothesis that the induction of SOD1 misfolding and aggregation occurs through conformational templating, similar to prion strains.

Similar findings implicating SOD1 strains were observed by Ayers et al. (2014a, b) in transmission studies using the transgenic mouse model expressing YFP tagged G85R-SOD1. Following injection with various inocula, including homogenates prepared from paralyzed SOD1-overexpressing mice and recombinant WT SOD1 fibrils, they found the induction of distinct SOD1:YFP pathologies dependent on the injected material. For example, homogenates from sick G93A-SOD1 mice induced round punctate G85R-SOD1:YFP inclusions, whereas recombinant WT SOD1 fibrils induced fibrillar inclusions with distinct skein-like inclusions within cell bodies (Fig. 18.2). Furthermore, when second passages were performed, using spinal cord homogenates from the MND-induced G85R-SOD1:YFP animals back into naïve G85R-SOD1:YFP mice, it was observed that the pathology induced was the same as the original inoculum (Fig. 18.2).

Ayers and colleagues (2014b) also demonstrated that, upon primary passage of inocula in G85R-SOD1:YFP mice, distinct incubation periods were observed, which upon second passage in naïve G85R-SOD1:YFP mice all resulted in an increased penetrance and decrease in the incubation periods by roughly 50%. In the prion field, this is referred to as "host adaptation" and is believed to be the result of a greater similarity in conformations between the inducing seed and host target upon successive passages (Bruce et al., 1994). These results provide additional support for the ability of SOD1 to undergo conformation-dependent templated propagation, and provide further evidence for the existence of SOD1 strains (Ayers et al., 2014b). Additionally, these studies provide further data demonstrating similarities between SOD1 and the prion protein, and indicate that the SOD1 protein is capable of a heritable conformational conversion through direct templating.

In regard to TDP-43 strain properties, evidence exists suggesting that TDP-43 inclusions found in FTLD-TDP are composed of distinct conformations that correlate with different pathologic subtypes on neuropathologic assessment (Mackenzie et al., 2011; Tsuji et al., 2012).

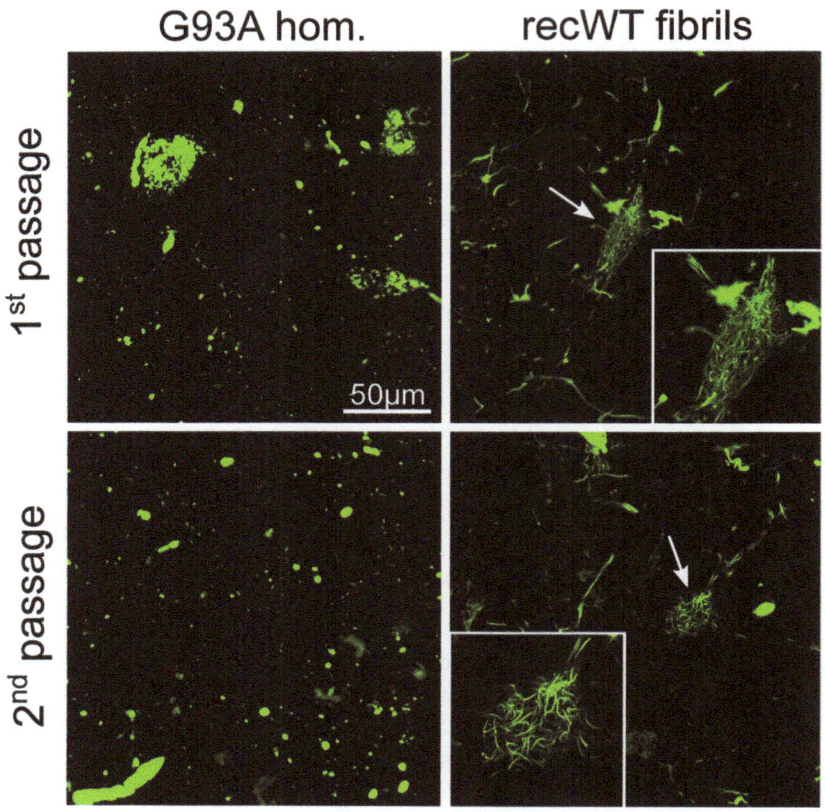

Fig. 18.2. Distinct pathologies of G85R-SOD1:YFP inclusions suggest SOD1 prion-like properties. Images of spinal cord from diseased mice injected with either first or second passages of the indicated homogenates. WT SOD1 fibrils produced distinct skein-like inclusions (arrows and insets). (Reproduced from Ayers J, Fromholt S, Koch M, et al. (2014a) Experimental transmissibility of mutant SOD1 motor neuron disease. Acta Neuropathol 128, 791–803.)

Four discrete subtypes have been posited (A–D) based on the predominant form of TDP-43 neuropathology, which correspond with the particular cause of FTLD-TDP and also the neuroanatomic location of the deposits (Mackenzie et al., 2011; Tsuji et al., 2012). For instance, type A neuropathology typically occurs in patients with behavioral FTD and those with mutations in the gene encoding progranulin, and presents with abundant dystrophic neurites and TDP-43 neuronal cytoplasmic inclusions, whereas type B occurs in patients with ALS and FTD and presents with TDP-43 cytoplasmic inclusions within all cortical layers with few dystrophic neurites. In addition to the pathologic variations observed, biochemical studies demonstrated that the C-terminal fragments of TDP-43 showed different mobility banding patterns when analyzed by immunoblotting, which correlated with the neuropathologic subtypes (Hasegawa et al., 2011). These findings suggest that different conformations or strains of misfolded TDP-43 could engender distinct patterns of neuropathology observed among the FTLD-TDP spectrum of disorders, and may also lead to their associated clinical phenotypes.

POTENTIAL ROLE FOR WT SOD1 IN ALS PATHOGENESIS

Based on the similarities in disease phenotypes between SOD1-fALS and sALS, questions have been raised concerning the potential pathogenic role that WT SOD1 could play in sALS. If such a role were uncovered, it would have important implications in providing scientific investigators with a therapeutic target for treating the major proportion of all ALS that sALS comprises. In fact, there are currently a number of clinical trials under way to determine the efficacy of various treatments aimed at knocking down the levels of SOD1 to treat SOD1-fALS, which could therefore be proven useful for sALS patients. This idea materialized from several in vitro studies, described above, that displayed the ability for WT SOD1 to adopt a misfolded conformation under mild destabilizing conditions (Chattopadhyay et al., 2008; Chia et al., 2010).

In addition, when this misfolded isoform of WT SOD1 was added to cultured motor neurons it displayed a dose-dependent toxicity, revealing the acquisition of toxic properties for this misfolded species (Ezzi et al., 2007). Notably, misfolded WT SOD1 has been found to serially transmit between HEK293 cell cultures via conditioned media, containing seeding aggregates or misfolded SOD1-loaded exosomes (Grad et al., 2014). There have also been several in vivo studies that have indirectly examined the effects of WT SOD1 on disease pathogenesis by breeding mutant SOD1 transgenic mice to human WT SOD1-overexpressing lines of mice. When bred to homozygosity, WT SOD1-overexpressing mice express the transgene at similar levels as mutant SOD1 mice and accumulate SOD1 pathologic inclusions similar to the mutant SOD1 mice, yet they never develop MND (Jaarsma et al., 2000; Jonsson et al., 2006). When human SOD1 mutants are bred to human WT transgenic mice, an acceleration of disease onset is observed, demonstrating the ability for WT SOD1 to augment disease pathogenesis (Jaarsma et al., 2000; Deng et al., 2006; Prudencio et al., 2009a, 2010; L. Wang et al., 2009).

How WT SOD1 is able to modulate disease has not been solved, but several hypotheses have been brought forward, including stabilization of the mutant protein by interactions with WT SOD1 (Fukada et al., 2001; Prudencio et al., 2010) or the direct interaction and seeding of WT SOD1 by mutant SOD1 through redox processes or templated misfolding (Deng et al., 2008; Prudencio et al., 2010). The latter possibility is supported by the observation that WT SOD1 is converted into an insoluble aggregated species in these bigenic mice (Deng et al., 2008; Prudencio et al., 2009a). Additionally, human WT SOD1 did not accelerate MND in transgenic mice expressing murine SOD1 containing a G86R mutation, suggesting an SOD1 species barrier, thought to occur due to the conformational differences among the two proteins (Dickinson, 1976; Audet et al., 2010). Moreover, the finding that conversion of human SOD1 is at least partially dependent on tryptophan 32 (Grad et al., 2011) may explain why mouse SOD1, which lacks tryptophan, cannot interact with human WT SOD1 in these cross-breeding experiments.

A mouse model was also developed to study the effect of extreme overexpression of WT SOD1 at levels similar to those observed for some of the more commonly used mutant SOD1 transgenic mouse models, which express the protein up to 25-fold over endogenous SOD1 expression levels. These extreme WT SOD1 overexpressing mice were found to develop MND with pathologic hallmarks similar to those found following expression of mutant SOD1 transgenes (Graffmo et al., 2012). Together, these data highlight the experimental evidence revealing the potential for WT SOD1 to adopt a misfolded, potentially toxic, conformer in vivo.

Since it was shown that WT SOD1 can misfold, studies have been undertaken to determine whether there exists a misfolded conformer in postmortem spinal cord tissue from sALS patients. To accomplish this, researchers utilized various conformation-specific antibodies to misfolded forms of SOD1. One of these antibodies, C4F6, was raised against the G93A mutation of SOD1 and is believed to recognize a loop structure around the 93rd amino acid of SOD1 that becomes destabilized when SOD1 misfolds, allowing the antibody to bind (Ayers et al., 2014b; Urushitani et al., 2007).

The immunoreactivity of the antibody was first tested in tissue from sALS cases by Bosco et al. (2010), who found neuronal inclusions in ~50% (4 of 9) of the cases they examined. Subsequent studies using separate sources of sALS tissue revealed no C4F6-positive immunoreactivity to misfolded SOD1 species in the 50 samples examined (Brotherton et al., 2012; Ayers et al., 2014b). A similar antibody, B8H10, which was also raised against G93A-SOD1, was unable to detect misfolded SOD1 in transformed lymphoblastoid cell lines derived from 10 sALS patients (Gros-Louis et al., 2010; Pickles et al., 2013).

Grad et al. (2011) also produced monoclonal antibodies to two disease-specific epitopes that are buried in natively structured WT SOD1; amino acids 145–151 (at the dimer interface (Rakhit et al., 2007) and with a sulfonic acid derivative of cysteine at position 146) and 125–142 (at the electrostatic loop). The authors tested these antibodies against tissue from sALS cases and discovered immunoreactive neuronal inclusions in all of the 20 cases they examined (Grad et al., 2014). Two rabbit polyclonal antibodies raised against amino acids 145–151 lacking oxidation of cysteine 146, termed SEDI and residues 42–48, termed USOD, were tested against the spinal cords from 10 additional cases with no immunoreactivity detected (Kerman et al., 2010). A study from Forsberg et al. (2010) tested antibodies raised against residues 4–20 and 131–153 were capable of detecting immunoreactive inclusions in all 29 of their sALS cases. Lastly, a recent publication took a comprehensive approach and tested a panel of conformational antibodies against sALS cases. Using immunoprecipitation and immunohistochemistry, they displayed no immunoreactivity in the samples they tested (Da Cruz et al., 2017).

Taken together, these data highlight the contradictory reports with respect to detecting misfolded conformers of WT SOD1 in tissue from sALS patients. Some important variables that could account for these discrepancies include the source of tissue and levels of fixation, the amount of neurodegeneration within the spinal cord, and the immunohistochemical and antigen retrieval methods used, and other issues. One alternative strategy that was used to test for the presence of misfolded WT SOD1 in sALS cases was by testing the seeding activity of spinal cord homogenates prepared from postmortem tissue. Using an organotypic slice culture assay prepared from the spinal cords of the MND permissive G85R-SOD1:YFP mouse line, Ayers et al. (2016a) added homogenates from more than 30 sALS cases and controls. Although homogenates prepared from patients carrying the A4V-SOD1 mutation were capable of inducing a robust G85R-SOD1:YFP inclusion pathology in the spinal cord slices, homogenates from the sALS and various controls failed to induce any pathology (Ayers et al., 2016a). There is obviously much work still required to fully understand the role of WT SOD1 in sALS cases, potentially by eliminating as many of the confounding variables as possible.

As mentioned, greater than 95% of all ALS cases, both sALS and fALS, involve the accumulation of cytoplasmic, insoluble, and aggregated inclusions of TDP-43 (Arai et al., 2006; Neumann et al., 2006). Therefore, if WT SOD1 is in fact involved in the pathogenesis of sALS, there is the potential for these two proteins to interact and affect their disease-specific properties. To address this, Pokrishevsky et al. (2012) used their disease-specific epitope antibodies specific for misfolded SOD1 and revealed SOD1 immunoreactive inclusions in motor neurons of postmortem tissue from sALS patients with cytoplasmic TDP-43 inclusions, along with from patients with a mutation in the gene encoding FUS (Fig. 18.3). They also demonstrated that the in vitro overexpression of mutant FUS and TDP-43 in human cell lines induced the misfolding of endogenous WT SOD1; however, co-localization of the proteins was not observed, suggesting an indirect effect on SOD1 (Pokrishevsky et al., 2012).

In a subsequent study, the same authors demonstrated that conditioned media from cells overexpressing mutated FUS or TDP-43 were capable of inducing the misfolding of endogenous WT SOD1 in cell culture experiments (Pokrishevsky et al., 2016). Furthermore, it was found that the induced misfolded species of WT SOD1 was able to propagate intercellularly and induce the induction of endogenous WT SOD1 misfolding in recipient cells (Pokrishevsky et al., 2016), accompanied by a small but statistically significant decrease in cell viability. Interestingly, there was no propagation of TDP43 or FUS pathology observed in the recipient cells. These two studies suggest that misfolded TDP-43 and FUS, once re-localized to the cytoplasm, are able to induce the misfolding of WT SOD1, thereby causing a prion-like cascade of SOD1 misfolding throughout the CNS.

CONCLUSIONS

At the time of its discovery, the concept of a protein conformation capable of replicating and inducing a heritable conformational change without the need for a nucleic acid genome was heretical. However, the characteristics of the disease-misfolded prion protein and its ability to transmit disease, replicate, and spread are now widely accepted throughout the scientific community. In fact, in the last decade a wealth of evidence has emerged supporting similar properties observed for many of the misfolded proteins implicated in other neurodegenerative

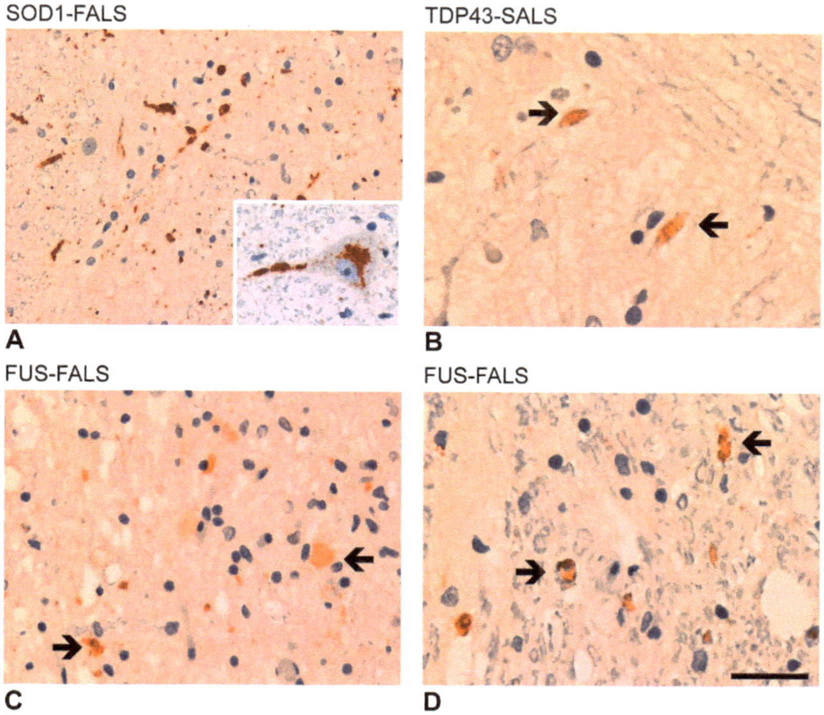

Fig. 18.3. Misfolded SOD1 immunohistochemistry in ventral gray matter and corticospinal tracts of cervical spinal cord of amyotrophic lateral sclerosis (ALS) patients. (**A**) Cases of familial ALS with SOD1 mutations show extensive accumulation of misfolded SOD1 in swollen and normal-sized axons as well as in the perikarya of some lower motor neurons (inset). (**B**) Cases of sporadic ALS with TDP43 pathology had misfolded SOD1 accumulation only in small numbers of normal-sized axons (arrows). (**C**, **D**) In the case of familial ALS with FUS mutation, misfolded SOD1 accumulated in some swollen axons in the ventral gray matter (**C**, arrows) and a moderate number of normal-sized axons in corticospinal tract (**D**, arrows). Scale bar, 60 μm (**A**, **C**); 30 μm (**B**, **D**). (Reproduced from Pokrishevsky E, Grad LI, Yousefi M, et al. (2012) Aberrant localization of FUS and TDP43 is associated with misfolding of SOD1 in amyotrophic lateral sclerosis. PLoS ONE 7: e35050.)

diseases, such as Alzheimer disease, Parkinson disease, tauopathies, and, as described in this chapter, ALS. Multiple studies have now demonstrated the ability for SOD1, TDP-43, FUS, and, most recently, C9orf72-encoded polypeptides to display properties similar to those of prions. The majority of these are cell-free and in vitro assays, while SOD1 remains the only ALS-linked protein to demonstrate several prion-like properties in vivo. One of the more important findings was the demonstration that pre-fibrilized recombinant SOD1 was capable of inducing disease in a permissive transgenic mouse model (Ayers et al., 2016a) – a finding which eluded the prion field for some time and that strongly implicates a protein-only mechanism for the induced pathology and phenotypes observed in experimental models and human fALS disease.

The role of WT SOD1 in sALS cases remains unresolved and could have important therapeutic implications, as it could highlight a therapeutic target for the ~90% of cases that sALS comprises. As outlined above, there are a wide range of estimates as to the percentage of sALS cases that contain a misfolded species of SOD1, the majority of them based upon immunoreactivity to antibodies specific to an abnormal conformation of SOD1. One potential variable that may be contributing to these discrepancies is the level and forms of misfolded SOD1 that accumulates in the CNS. It remains to be seen how abundant misfolded species of WT SOD1 are in sALS cases in comparison to the abundance of misfolded SOD1 in fALS cases. Additionally, the abundant fibrillar SOD1 inclusions observed in SOD1 fALS suggest that, if WT SOD1 seeding exists, it comprises a more evasive species, such as oligomers. Perhaps the only way to unequivocally determine whether misfolded forms of WT SOD1 have a role in the pathogenesis of sALS is to test whether an effective SOD1-targeted therapy for SOD1-linked fALS patients is also effective in sALS patients.

One of the most important implications of the prion-like properties being ascribed to ALS-causing proteins, such as cell-to-cell transmission, is that it should, theoretically, create an extracellular pool of misfolded proteins that could be targeted by immune therapies to prevent the spread of the disease. This hypothesis has been applied to tau and has resulted in clinical testing of monoclonal antibodies aimed at blocking the spreading of tau in

Alzheimer disease and other tauopathies (Yanamandra et al., 2015). Both passive and active immunization approaches have been employed in transgenic SOD1 mouse lined to target the misfolded, toxic species of SOD1, with varying degrees of success (Urushitani et al., 2007; Gros-Louis et al., 2010; Takeuchi et al., 2010; Liu et al., 2012). Although these studies produced a lengthening of the disease course, the increased survival was modest. This is most likely due to the extreme overexpression of SOD1 in the models used and the ubiquitous expression of the protein, which results in an aggressive disease course, making it difficult to assess the antibody's effect on disease pathogenesis. Therefore, a more suitable model to test these therapies may be one of the recent in vivo seeding models, which appear to closely mimic the natural disease course observed in ALS cases.

Although the proteins discussed in this chapter, as well as those implicated in other neurodegenerative disorders, have displayed many of the same properties observed for prions, there still exists a major difference in the virulence between these proteins. With the lone exception being a study suggesting the human transmission of amyloid-β from the injection of pituitary-derived growth hormone (Jaunmuktane et al., 2015), the propensity for PrP^{TSE} to transmit between individuals and between species has not been observed for toxic proteins implicated in other neurodegenerative diseases. There are many factors that may contribute to this, including the extreme stability of PrP^{TSE}, the ubiquitous expression of the cellular form of the protein throughout the body, and the ability for PrP^{TSE} to accumulate to high levels in the CNS and peripheral tissues. Although these differences do exist, the greater commonality of characteristics they exhibit allows researchers to better understand their biology, and hopefully find therapies whose mechanisms can be shared among these many debilitating disorders.

References

Alberti S, Halfmann R, King O et al. (2009). A systematic survey identifies prions and illuminates sequence features of prionogenic proteins. Cell 137: 146–158.

Al-Chalabi A, Hardiman O (2013). The epidemiology of ALS: a conspiracy of genes, environment and time. Nat Rev Neurol 9: 617–628.

Arai T, Hasegawa M, Akiyama H et al. (2006). TDP-43 is a component of ubiquitin-positive tau-negative inclusions in frontotemporal lobar degeneration and amyotrophic lateral sclerosis. Biochem Biophys Res Commun 351: 602–611.

Atarashi R, Wilham JM, Christensen L et al. (2008). Simplified ultrasensitive prion detection by recombinant PrP conversion with shaking. Nat Methods 5: 211–212.

Atkin JD, Farg MA, Walker AK et al. (2008). Endoplasmic reticulum stress and induction of the unfolded protein response in human sporadic amyotrophic lateral sclerosis. Neurobiol Dis 30: 400–407.

Audet J-N, Gowing G, Julien J-P (2010). Wild-type human SOD1 overexpression does not accelerate motor neuron disease in mice expressing murine Sod1 G86R. Neurobiol Dis 40: 245–250.

Ayers J, Kincaid AE, Bartz JC (2009). Prion strain targeting independent of strain-specific neuronal tropism. J Virol 83: 81–87.

Ayers J, Fromholt S, Koch M et al. (2014a). Experimental transmissibility of mutant SOD1 motor neuron disease. Acta Neuropathol 128: 791–803.

Ayers J, Xu G, Pletnikova O et al. (2014b). Conformational specificity of the C4F6 SOD1 antibody; low frequency of reactivity in sporadic ALS cases. Acta Neuropathol Commun 2: 55.

Ayers J, Diamond J, Sari A et al. (2016a). Distinct conformers of transmissible misfolded SOD1 distinguish human SOD1-FALS from other forms of familial and sporadic ALS. Acta Neuropathol 132: 827–840.

Ayers J, Fromholt SE, O'Neal VM et al. (2016b). Prion-like propagation of mutant SOD1 misfolding and motor neuron disease spread along neuroanatomical pathways. Acta Neuropathol 131: 103–114.

Bartz JC, Kincaid AE, Bessen RA (2002). Retrograde transport of transmissible mink encephalopathy within descending motor tracts. J Virol 76: 5759–5768.

Bartz JC, Kramer ML, Sheehan MH et al. (2007). Prion interference is due to a reduction in strain-specific PrPSc levels. J Virol 81: 689–697.

Basso M, Pozzi S, Tortarolo M et al. (2013). Mutant copper-zinc superoxide dismutase (SOD1) induces protein secretion pathway alterations and exosome release in astrocytes: implications for disease spreading and motor neuron pathology in amyotrophic lateral sclerosis. J Biol Chem 288: 15699–15711.

Bergh J, Zetterström P, Andersen PM et al. (2015). Structural and kinetic analysis of protein-aggregate strains in vivo using binary epitope mapping. Proc Natl Acad Sci U S A 112: 4489–4494.

Bessen RA, Marsh RF (1994). Distinct PrP properties suggest the molecular basis of strain variation in transmissible mink encephalopathy. J Virol 68: 7859–7868.

Bidhendi EE, Bergh J, Zetterström P et al. (2016). Two superoxide dismutase prion strains transmit amyotrophic lateral sclerosis–like disease. J Clin Invest 126: 2249–2253.

Boillée S, Vande Velde C, Cleveland DW (2006a). ALS: a disease of motor neurons and their nonneuronal neighbors. Neuron 52: 39–59.

Boillée S, Yamanaka K, Lobsiger CS et al. (2006b). Onset and progression in inherited ALS determined by motor neurons and microglia. Science 312: 1389–1392.

Borchelt DR, Lee MK, Slunt HS et al. (1994). Superoxide dismutase 1 with mutations linked to familial amyotrophic lateral sclerosis possesses significant activity. Proc Natl Acad Sci U S A 91: 8292–8296.

Bosco DA, Morfini G, Karabacak NM et al. (2010). Wild-type and mutant SOD1 share an aberrant conformation and a common pathogenic pathway in ALS. Nat Neurosci 13: 1396–1403.

Brotherton TE, Li Y, Cooper D et al. (2012). Localization of a toxic form of superoxide dismutase 1 protein to pathologically affected tissues in familial ALS. Proc Natl Acad Sci U S A 109: 5505–5510.

Bruce M, Chree A, McConnell I et al. (1994). Transmission of bovine spongiform encephalopathy and scrapie to mice: strain variation and the species barrier. Philos Trans R Soc Lond Ser B Biol Sci 343: 405–411.

Bruijn LI, Houseweart MK, Kato S et al. (1998). Aggregation and motor neuron toxicity of an ALS-linked SOD1 mutant independent from wild-type SOD1. Science 281: 1851–1854.

Caughey B, Raymond GJ, Bessen RA (1998). Strain-dependent differences in beta-sheet conformations of abnormal prion protein. J Biol Chem 273: 32230–32235.

Chan PK, Chattopadhyay M, Sharma S et al. (2013). Structural similarity of wild-type and ALS-mutant superoxide dismutase-1 fibrils using limited proteolysis and atomic force microscopy. Proc Natl Acad Sci U S A 110: 10934–10939.

Chattopadhyay M, Durazo A, Sohn SH et al. (2008). Initiation and elongation in fibrillation of ALS-linked superoxide dismutase. Proc Natl Acad Sci U S A 105: 18663–18668.

Chia R, Tattum MH, Jones S et al. (2010). Superoxide dismutase 1 and tgSOD1 mouse spinal cord seed fibrils, suggesting a propagative cell death mechanism in amyotrophic lateral sclerosis. PLoS ONE 5: e10627.

Clavaguera F, Bolmont T, Crowther RA et al. (2009). Transmission and spreading of tauopathy in transgenic mouse brain. Nat Cell Biol 11: 909–913.

Cleveland DW, Laing N, Hurse PV et al. (1995). Toxic mutants in Charcot's sclerosis. Nature 378: 342–343.

Crapo JD, Oury T, Rabouille C et al. (1992). Copper,zinc superoxide dismutase is primarily a cytosolic protein in human cells. Proc Natl Acad Sci U S A 89: 10405–10409.

Cushman M, Johnson BS, King OD et al. (2010). Prion-like disorders: blurring the divide between transmissibility and infectivity. J Cell Sci 123: 1191–1201.

Da Cruz S, Bui A, Saberi S et al. (2017). Misfolded SOD1 is not a primary component of sporadic ALS. Acta Neuropathol 351: 602.

DeJesus-Hernandez M, Mackenzie IR, Boeve BF et al. (2011). Expanded GGGGCC hexanucleotide repeat in noncoding region of C9ORF72 causes chromosome 9p-linked FTD and ALS. Neuron 72: 245–256.

Deng H-X, Shi Y-Z, Furukawa Y et al. (2006). Conversion to the amyotrophic lateral sclerosis phenotype is associated with intermolecular linked insoluble aggregates of SOD1 in mitochondria. Proc Natl Acad Sci U S A 103: 7142–7147.

Deng H-X, Han-Xiang D, Jiang H et al. (2008). Molecular dissection of ALS-associated toxicity of SOD1 in transgenic mice using an exon-fusion approach. Hum Mol Genet 17: 2310–2319.

Dickinson AG (1976). Scrapie in sheep and goats. Front Biol 44: 209–241.

Ding X, Ma M, Teng J et al. (2015). Exposure to ALS-FTD-CSF generates TDP-43 aggregates in glioblastoma cells through exosomes and TNTs-like structure. Oncotarget 6: 24178–24191.

Engelender S, Isacson O (2017). The threshold theory for Parkinson's disease. Trends Neurosci 40: 4–14.

Ezzi SA, Urushitani M, Julien J-P (2007). Wild-type superoxide dismutase acquires binding and toxic properties of ALS-linked mutant forms through oxidation. J Neurochem 102: 170–178.

Farg MA, Sundaramoorthy V, Sultana JM et al. (2014). C9ORF72, implicated in amytrophic lateral sclerosis and frontotemporal dementia, regulates endosomal trafficking. Hum Mol Genet 23: 3579–3595.

Feiler MS, Strobel B, Freischmidt A et al. (2015). TDP-43 is intercellularly transmitted across axon terminals. J Cell Biol 211: 897–911.

Fevrier B, Vilette D, Archer F et al. (2004). Cells release prions in association with exosomes. Proc Natl Acad Sci U S A 101: 9683–9688.

Field LS, Furukawa Y, O'Halloran TV et al. (2003). Factors controlling the uptake of yeast copper/zinc superoxide dismutase into mitochondria. J Biol Chem 278: 28052–28059.

Forsberg K, Jonsson PA, Andersen PM et al. (2010). Novel antibodies reveal inclusions containing non-native SOD1 in sporadic ALS patients. PLoS ONE 5: e11552.

Fraser H (1982). Neuronal spread of scrapie agent and targeting of lesions within the retino-tectal pathway. Nature 295: 149–150.

Fukada K, Nagano S, Satoh M et al. (2001). Stabilization of mutant Cu/Zn superoxide dismutase (SOD1) protein by coexpressed wild SOD1 protein accelerates the disease progression in familial amyotrophic lateral sclerosis mice. Eur J Neurosci 14: 2032–2036.

Furukawa Y, Kaneko K, Yamanaka K et al. (2008). Complete loss of post-translational modifications triggers fibrillar aggregation of SOD1 in the familial form of amyotrophic lateral sclerosis. J Biol Chem 283: 24167–24176.

Furukawa Y, Kaneko K, Yamanaka K et al. (2010). Mutation-dependent polymorphism of Cu,Zn-superoxide dismutase aggregates in the familial form of amyotrophic lateral sclerosis. J Biol Chem 285: 22221–22231.

Furukawa Y, Kaneko K, Watanabe S et al. (2011). A seeding reaction recapitulates intracellular formation of Sarkosyl-insoluble transactivation response element (TAR) DNA-binding protein-43 inclusions. J Biol Chem 286: 18664–18672.

Gajdusek DC (1977). Unconventional viruses and the origin and disappearance of kuru. Science 197: 943–960.

Gendron TF, Belzil VV, Zhang Y-J et al. (2014). Mechanisms of toxicity in C9FTLD/ALS. Acta Neuropathol 127: 359–376.

Giordana MT, Piccinini M, Grifoni S et al. (2010). TDP-43 redistribution is an early event in sporadic amyotrophic lateral sclerosis. Brain Pathol 20: 351–360.

Goldfarb LG, Petersen RB, Tabaton M et al. (1992). Fatal familial insomnia and familial Creutzfeldt-Jakob disease: disease phenotype determined by a DNA polymorphism. Science 258: 806–808.

Goldstein LH, Abrahams S (2013). Changes in cognition and behaviour in amyotrophic lateral sclerosis: nature of impairment and implications for assessment. Lancet Neurol 12: 368–380.

Gomes C, Keller S, Altevogt P et al. (2007). Evidence for secretion of Cu,Zn superoxide dismutase via exosomes from a cell model of amyotrophic lateral sclerosis. Neurosci Lett 428: 43–46.

Grad LI, Guest WC, Yanai A et al. (2011). Intermolecular transmission of superoxide dismutase 1 misfolding in living cells. Proc Natl Acad Sci U S A 108: 16398–16403.

Grad LI, Yerbury JJ, Turner BJ et al. (2014). Intercellular propagated misfolding of wild-type Cu/Zn superoxide dismutase occurs via exosome-dependent and -independent mechanisms. Proc Natl Acad Sci U S A 111: 3620–3625.

Grad LI, Rouleau GA, Ravits J et al. (2016). Clinical spectrum of amyotrophic lateral sclerosis (ALS). In: Cold Spring Harb Perspect Med doi: 10.1101/cshperspect.a024117.

Graffmo KS, Forsberg K, Bergh J et al. (2012). Expression of wild-type human superoxide dismutase-1 in mice causes amyotrophic lateral sclerosis. Hum Mol Genet 22: 51–60.

Griffith JS (1967). Self-replication and scrapie. Nature 215: 1043–1044.

Gros-Louis F, Soucy G, Larivière R et al. (2010). Intracerebroventricular infusion of monoclonal antibody or its derived Fab fragment against misfolded forms of SOD1 mutant delays mortality in a mouse model of ALS. J Neurochem 113: 1188–1199.

Guo W, Chen Y, Zhou X et al. (2011). An ALS-associated mutation affecting TDP-43 enhances protein aggregation, fibril formation and neurotoxicity. Nat Struct Mol Biol 18: 822–830.

Gurney ME, Pu H, Chiu AY et al. (1994). Motor neuron degeneration in mice that express a human Cu,Zn superoxide dismutase mutation. Science 264: 1772–1775.

Hanspal MA, Dobson CM, Yerbury JJ et al. (2017). The relevance of contact-independent cell-to-cell transfer of TDP-43 and SOD1 in amyotrophic lateral sclerosis. Biochim Biophys Acta 1863: 2762–2771.

Hasegawa M, Nonaka T, Tsuji H et al. (2011). Molecular dissection of TDP-43 proteinopathies. J Mol Neurosci 45: 480–485.

Howland DS, Liu J, She Y et al. (2002). Focal loss of the glutamate transporter EAAT2 in a transgenic rat model of SOD1 mutant-mediated amyotrophic lateral sclerosis (ALS). Proc Natl Acad Sci U S A 99: 1604–1609.

Hsiao KK, Groth D, Scott M et al. (1994). Serial transmission in rodents of neurodegeneration from transgenic mice expressing mutant prion protein. Proc Natl Acad Sci U S A 91: 9126–9130.

Igaz LM, Kwong LK, Xu Y et al. (2008). Enrichment of C-terminal fragments in TAR DNA-binding protein-43 cytoplasmic inclusions in brain but not in spinal cord of frontotemporal lobar degeneration and amyotrophic lateral sclerosis. Am J Pathol 173: 182–194.

Iko Y, Kodama TS, Kasai N et al. (2004). Domain architectures and characterization of an RNA-binding protein, TLS. J Biol Chem 279: 44834–44840.

Ilieva H, Polymenidou M, Cleveland DW (2009). Non-cell autonomous toxicity in neurodegenerative disorders: ALS and beyond. J Cell Biol 187: 761–772.

Jaarsma D, Haasdijk ED, Grashorn JA et al. (2000). Human Cu/Zn superoxide dismutase (SOD1) overexpression in mice causes mitochondrial vacuolization, axonal degeneration, and premature motoneuron death and accelerates motoneuron disease in mice expressing a familial amyotrophic lateral sclerosis mutant SOD1. Neurobiol Dis 7: 623–643.

Jaunmuktane Z, Mead S, Ellis M et al. (2015). Evidence for human transmission of amyloid-β pathology and cerebral amyloid angiopathy. Nature 525: 247–250.

Johnson BS, Snead D, Lee JJ et al. (2009). TDP-43 is intrinsically aggregation-prone, and amyotrophic lateral sclerosis-linked mutations accelerate aggregation and increase toxicity. J Biol Chem 284: 20329–20339.

Johnston JA, Dalton MJ, Gurney ME et al. (2000). Formation of high molecular weight complexes of mutant Cu, Zn-superoxide dismutase in a mouse model for familial amyotrophic lateral sclerosis. Proc Natl Acad Sci U S A 97: 12571–12576.

Jonsson PA, Graffmo KS, Andersen PM et al. (2006). Disulphide-reduced superoxide dismutase-1 in CNS of transgenic amyotrophic lateral sclerosis models. Brain 129: 451–464.

Jucker M, Walker LC (2013). Self-propagation of pathogenic protein aggregates in neurodegenerative diseases. Nature 501: 45–51.

Kabashi E, Durham HD (2006). Failure of protein quality control in amyotrophic lateral sclerosis. Biochim Biophys Acta 1762: 1038–1050.

Kang SH, Li Y, Fukaya M et al. (2013). Degeneration and impaired regeneration of gray matter oligodendrocytes in amyotrophic lateral sclerosis. Nat Neurosci 16: 571–579.

Kanouchi T, Ohkubo T, Yokota T (2012). Can regional spreading of amyotrophic lateral sclerosis motor symptoms be explained by prion-like propagation? Journal of Neurology. Neurosurgery & Psychiatry 83: 739–745.

Karch CM, Prudencio M, Winkler DD et al. (2009). Role of mutant SOD1 disulfide oxidation and aggregation in the pathogenesis of familial ALS. Proc Natl Acad Sci U S A 106: 7774–7779.

Kerman A, Liu H-N, Croul S et al. (2010). Amyotrophic lateral sclerosis is a non-amyloid disease in which extensive misfolding of SOD1 is unique to the familial form. Acta Neuropathol 119: 335–344.

Kim D-K, Kang B, Kim OY et al. (2013). EVpedia: an integrated database of high-throughput data for systemic analyses of extracellular vesicles. J Extracell Vesicles 2: 20384.

Kocisko DA, Come JH, Priola SA et al. (1994). Cell-free formation of protease-resistant prion protein. NeuroReport 370: 471–474.

Kovács GG, Trabattoni G, Hainfellner JA et al. (2002). Mutations of the prion protein gene phenotypic spectrum. J Neurol 249: 1567–1582.

Kwiatkowski TJ, Bosco DA, Leclerc AL et al. (2009). Mutations in the FUS/TLS gene on chromosome 16 cause familial amyotrophic lateral sclerosis. Science 323: 1205–1208.

Lagier-Tourenne C, Polymenidou M, Cleveland DW (2010). TDP-43 and FUS/TLS: emerging roles in RNA processing and neurodegeneration. Hum Mol Genet 19: R46–R64.

Levine TP, Daniels RD, Gatta AT et al. (2013). The product of C9orf72, a gene strongly implicated in neurodegeneration, is structurally related to DENN Rab-GEFs. Bioinformatics 29: 499–503.

Ling S-C, Polymenidou M, Cleveland DW (2013). Converging mechanisms in ALS and FTD: disrupted RNA and protein homeostasis. Neuron 79: 416–438.

Liu H-N, Tjostheim S, DaSilva K et al. (2012). Targeting of monomer/misfolded SOD1 as a therapeutic strategy for amyotrophic lateral sclerosis. J Neurosci 32: 8791–8799.

Mackenzie IRA, Neumann M, Baborie A et al. (2011). A harmonized classification system for FTLD-TDP pathology. Acta Neuropathol 122: 111–113.

Mackenzie IRA, Frick P, Grässer FA et al. (2015). Quantitative analysis and clinico-pathological correlations of different dipeptide repeat protein pathologies in C9ORF72 mutation carriers. Acta Neuropathol 130: 845–861.

Münch C, Bertolotti A (2011). Self-propagation and transmission of misfolded mutant SOD1: prion or prion-like phenomenon? Cell Cycle 10.

Münch C, O'Brien J, Bertolotti A (2011). Prion-like propagation of mutant superoxide dismutase-1 misfolding in neuronal cells. Proc Natl Acad Sci U S A 108: 3548–3553.

Neumann M, Sampathu DM, Kwong LK et al. (2006). Ubiquitinated TDP-43 in frontotemporal lobar degeneration and amyotrophic lateral sclerosis. Science 314: 130–133.

Nomura T, Watanabe S, Kaneko K et al. (2014). Intranuclear aggregation of mutant FUS/TLS as a molecular pathomechanism of amyotrophic lateral sclerosis. J Biol Chem 289: 1192–1202.

Nonaka T, Masuda-Suzukake M, Arai T et al. (2013). Prion-like properties of pathological TDP-43 aggregates from diseased brains. Cell Rep 4: 124–134.

Ogihara NL, Parge HE, Hart PJ et al. (1996). Unusual trigonal-planar copper configuration revealed in the atomic structure of yeast copper-zinc superoxide dismutase. Biochemistry 35: 2316–2321.

Olney RK, Murphy J, Forshew D et al. (2005). The effects of executive and behavioral dysfunction on the course of ALS. Neurology 65: 1774–1777.

Parge HE, Hallewell RA, Tainer JA (1992). Atomic structures of wild-type and thermostable mutant recombinant human Cu,Zn superoxide dismutase. Proc Natl Acad Sci U S A 89: 6109–6113.

Peelaerts W, Bousset L, Van der Perren A et al. (2015). α-Synuclein strains cause distinct synucleinopathies after local and systemic administration. Nature 522: 340–344.

Peretz D, Scott MR, Groth D et al. (2001). Strain-specified relative conformational stability of the scrapie prion protein. Protein Sci 10: 854–863.

Perez-Gonzalez R, Gauthier SA, Kumar A et al. (2012). The exosome secretory pathway transports amyloid precursor protein carboxyl-terminal fragments from the cell into the brain extracellular space. J Biol Chem 287: 43108–43115.

Pickles S, Destroismaisons L, Peyrard SL et al. (2013). Mitochondrial damage revealed by immunoselection for ALS-linked misfolded SOD1. Hum Mol Genet 22: 3947–3959.

Pokrishevsky E, Grad LI, Yousefi M et al. (2012). Aberrant localization of FUS and TDP43 is associated with misfolding of SOD1 in amyotrophic lateral sclerosis. PLoS ONE 7: e35050.

Pokrishevsky E, Grad LI, Cashman NR (2016). TDP-43 or FUS-induced misfolded human wild-type SOD1 can propagate intercellularly in a prion-like fashion. Sci Rep 6: 22155.

Prudencio M, Durazo A, Whitelegge JP et al. (2009a). Modulation of mutant superoxide dismutase 1 aggregation by co-expression of wild-type enzyme. J Neurochem 108: 1009–1018.

Prudencio M, Hart PJ, Borchelt DR et al. (2009b). Variation in aggregation propensities among ALS-associated variants of SOD1: Correlation to human disease. Hum Mol Genet 18: 3217–3226.

Prudencio M, Durazo A, Whitelegge JP et al. (2010). An examination of wild-type SOD1 in modulating the toxicity and aggregation of ALS-associated mutant SOD1. Hum Mol Genet 19: 4774–4789.

Prusiner SB (1982). Novel proteinaceous infectious particles cause scrapie. Science 216: 136–144.

Rakhit R, Robertson J, Vande Velde C et al. (2007). An immunological epitope selective for pathological monomer-misfolded SOD1 in ALS. Nat Med 13: 754–759.

Raposo G, Stoorvogel W (2013). Extracellular vesicles: exosomes, microvesicles, and friends. J Cell Biol 200: 373–383.

Ravits J (2014). Focality, stochasticity and neuroanatomic propagation in ALS pathogenesis. Exp Neurol 262: 121–126.

Reisin R (2012). Frequency of the C9orf72 hexanucleotide repeat expansion in patients with amyotrophic lateral sclerosis and frontotemporal dementia: a cross-sectional study. Yearbook of Neurology and Neurosurgery 2012: 170–172.

Renton AE, Majounie E, Waite A et al. (2011). A hexanucleotide repeat expansion in C9ORF72 is the cause of chromosome 9p21-linked ALS-FTD. Neuron 72: 257–268.

Rosen DR, Siddique T, Patterson D et al. (1993). Mutations in Cu/Zn superoxide dismutase gene are associated with familial amyotrophic lateral sclerosis. Nature 362: 59–62.

Rothstein JD, Van Kammen M, Levey AI et al. (1995). Selective loss of glial glutamate transporter GLT-1 in amyotrophic lateral sclerosis. Ann Neurol 38: 73–84.

Saborio GP, Permanne B, Soto C (2001). Sensitive detection of pathological prion protein by cyclic amplification of protein misfolding. Nature 411: 810–813.

Sacino AN, Thomas MA, Ceballos-Diaz C et al. (2013). Conformational templating of α-synuclein aggregates in neuronal-glial cultures. Mol Neurodegener 8: 17.

Sacino AN, Brooks M, Thomas MA et al. (2014). Intramuscular injection of α-synuclein induces CNS α-synuclein pathology and a rapid-onset motor phenotype in transgenic mice. Proc Natl Acad Sci U S A 111: 10732–10737.

Sanders DW, Kaufman SK, DeVos SL et al. (2014). Distinct tau prion strains propagate in cells and mice and define different tauopathies. Neuron 82: 1271–1288.

Saxena S, Cabuy E, Caroni P (2009). A role for motoneuron subtype-selective ER stress in disease manifestations of FALS mice. Nat Neurosci 12: 627–636.

Silverman JM, Fernando SM, Grad LI et al. (2016). Disease mechanisms in ALS: misfolded SOD1 transferred through exosome-dependent and exosome-independent pathways. Cell Mol Neurobiol 36: 377–381.

Stathopulos PB, Rumfeldt JAO, Scholz GA et al. (2003). Cu/Zn superoxide dismutase mutants associated with amyotrophic lateral sclerosis show enhanced formation of aggregates in vitro. Proc Natl Acad Sci U S A 100: 7021–7026.

Suh E, Lee EB, Neal D et al. (2015). Semi-automated quantification of C9orf72 expansion size reveals inverse correlation between hexanucleotide repeat number and disease duration in frontotemporal degeneration. Acta Neuropathol 130: 363–372.

Sun S, Ling S-C, Qiu J et al. (2015). ALS-causative mutations in FUS/TLS confer gain and loss of function by altered association with SMN and U1-snRNP. Nat Commun 6: 6171.

Surmeier DJ, Obeso JA, Halliday GM (2017). Selective neuronal vulnerability in Parkinson disease. Nat Rev Neurosci 18: 101–113.

Takeuchi S, Fujiwara N, Ido A et al. (2010). Induction of protective immunity by vaccination with wild-type apo superoxide dismutase 1 in mutant SOD1 transgenic mice. J Neuropathol Exp Neurol 69: 1044–1056.

Telling GC, Parchi P, Dearmond SJ et al. (1996). Evidence for the conformation of the pathologic isoform of the prion protein enciphering and propagating prion diversity. Science 274: 2079–2082.

Tsuji H, Arai T, Kametani F et al. (2012). Molecular analysis and biochemical classification of TDP-43 proteinopathy. Brain 135: 3380–3391.

Turner B, Atkin J, Farg M et al. (2005). Impaired extracellular secretion of mutant superoxide dismutase 1 associates with neurotoxicity in familial amyotrophic lateral sclerosis. J Neurosci 25: 108.

Urushitani M, Kurisu J, Tsukita K et al. (2002). Proteasomal inhibition by misfolded mutant superoxide dismutase 1 induces selective motor neuron death in familial amyotrophic lateral sclerosis. J Neurochem 83: 1030–1042.

Urushitani M, Ezzi SA, Julien J-P (2007). Therapeutic effects of immunization with mutant superoxide dismutase in mice models of amyotrophic lateral sclerosis. Proc Natl Acad Sci U S A 104: 2495–2500.

Vance C, Rogelj B, Hortobágyi T et al. (2009). Mutations in FUS, an RNA processing protein, cause familial amyotrophic lateral sclerosis type 6. Science 323: 1208–1211.

Wang J, Slunt H, Gonzales V et al. (2003). Copper-binding-site-null SOD1 causes ALS in transgenic mice: aggregates of non-native SOD1 delineate a common feature. Hum Mol Genet 12: 2753–2764.

Wang J, Farr GW, Zeiss CJ et al. (2009). Progressive aggregation despite chaperone associations of a mutant SOD1-YFP in transgenic mice that develop ALS. Proc Natl Acad Sci U S A 106: 1392–1397.

Wang L, Sharma K, Grisotti G et al. (2009). The effect of mutant SOD1 dismutase activity on non-cell autonomous degeneration in familial amyotrophic lateral sclerosis. Neurobiol Dis 35: 234–240.

Watts JC, Condello C, Stöhr J et al. (2014). Serial propagation of distinct strains of Aβ prions from Alzheimer's disease patients. Proc Natl Acad Sci U S A 111: 10323–10328.

Weissmann C (1991). A "unified theory" of prion propagation. Nature 352: 679–683.

Westergard T, Jensen BK, Wen X et al. (2016). Cell-to-cell transmission of dipeptide repeat proteins linked to C9orf72-ALS/FTD. Cell Rep 17: 645–652.

Williamson TL, Cleveland DW (1999). Slowing of axonal transport is a very early event in the toxicity of ALS-linked SOD1 mutants to motor neurons. Nat Neurosci 2: 50–56.

Yamanaka K, Chun SJ, Boillée S et al. (2008). Astrocytes as determinants of disease progression in inherited amyotrophic lateral sclerosis. Nat Neurosci 11: 251–253.

Yanamandra K, Jiang H, Mahan TE et al. (2015). Anti-tau antibody reduces insoluble tau and decreases brain atrophy. Ann Clin Transl Neurol 2: 278–288.

Zu T, Liu Y, Bañez-Coronel M et al. (2013). RAN proteins and RNA foci from antisense transcripts in C9ORF72 ALS and frontotemporal dementia. Proc Natl Acad Sci U S A 110: E4968–E4977.

Section V

Diagnosis and treatment

Handbook of Clinical Neurology, Vol. 153 (3rd series)
Human Prion Diseases
M. Pocchiari and J. Manson, Editors
https://doi.org/10.1016/B978-0-444-63945-5.00019-2

Chapter 19

Prion protein amplification techniques

ALISON J.E. GREEN[1]* AND GIANLUIGI ZANUSSO[2]

[1]*National CJD Research and Surveillance Unit, University of Edinburgh, Edinburgh, United Kingdom*

[2]*Department of Neurosciences, Biomedicine and Movement Sciences, University of Verona, Verona, Italy*

Abstract

Protein amplification techniques exploit the ability of PrP^{TSE} to induce a conformational change in prion protein (PrP) in a continuous fashion, so that the small amount of PrP^{TSE} found in tissues and biologic fluids in prion diseases can be amplified to a point where they are detectable by conventional laboratory techniques. The most widely used protein aggregation assays are protein misfolding cyclic amplification assay (PMCA) and real-time quaking-induced conversion (RT-QuIC). These assays have been used extensively in both animal and human prion disease in studies ranging from the development of diagnostics, understanding disease transmission potential, to investigating mechanisms underlying neurodegeneration. In human prion disease, cerebrospinal fluid (CSF) RT-QuIC analysis has been shown to be a highly sensitive and specific test for sporadic Creutzfeldt–Jakob disease (sCJD) and has now been included in the diagnostic criteria. It is also a useful investigation for some genetic forms of prion disease where other cerebrospinal fluid tests may be negative. PMCA shows great potential for the diagnosis of variant CJD (vCJD) and has the ability to distinguish vCJD from sCJD, which may become increasingly important with emergence of a patient with neuropathologically confirmed vCJD associated with *PRNP* codon129MV, which indicates that a new wave of vCJD cases is likely and that these may be difficult to distinguish from sCJD.

INTRODUCTION

The definitive diagnosis of Creutzfeldt–Jakob disease (CJD) and other prion diseases can only be made by the neuropathologic examination of brain tissue, taken either at postmortem or at biopsy, and the demonstration of the disease-associated form of prion protein (PrP^{TSE}). However, early clinical diagnosis of these diseases is needed not only for the patient and families but also to ensure that treatable diseases are not missed and to prevent the potential for secondary transmission of disease by blood transfusion or the reuse of contaminated surgical instruments.

The diagnosis of CJD and other prions diseases can be difficult in the early stages of disease as the initial presenting symptoms may be variable and nonspecific. Clinical diagnosis is based on the presence of a series of clinical neurologic features and of distinct abnormalities of supportive diagnostic investigations such as magnetic resonance imaging, electroencephalogram and cerebrospinal fluid (CSF) biomarkers such as CSF 14-3-3 (Budka et al., 1995; World Health Organization Communicable Disease Surveillance and Response, 2003; Zerr et al., 2009). These tests are useful but none have the necessary degree of sensitivity (Collins et al., 2006; Wieser et al. 2006; Chohan et al., 2010) or are not entirely specific for prion diseases and therefore lack diagnostic accuracy (Zerr et al., 2000; Geschwind et al., 2003; Sanchez-Juan et al., 2006; Meissner et al., 2009; Vitali et al., 2011; Zanusso et al., 2011, 2016; Hamlin et al., 2012; Puoti et al., 2012).

The unique feature of prion disease is the presence of abnormal disease-associated PrP (PrP^{TSE}), which is a protease-resistant, misfolded form of a normal constitutive

*Correspondence to: Alison Green, PhD FRCPath, The National CHD Research and Surveillance Unit, Western General Hospital, Crewe Road, Edinburgh EH4 2XU, United Kingdom. Tel: +44-131-537-1980, E-mail: Alison.Green@ed.ac.uk

protein, prion protein (PrP). Traditional laboratory techniques such as immunoassays are not able to distinguish between PrP and PrP^{TSE} due to the lack of available antibodies that can distinguish between PrP and PrP^{TSE}. The use of Western blotting techniques, which are able to identify PrP^{TSE} after removing PrP by protease digestion, are too insensitive to be used routinely to detect PrP^{TSE} in biologic fluids.

The development of protein aggregation has resulted in techniques that have sufficient sensitivity to enable the detection of PrP^{TSE} in biologic fluids and tissues such as CSF, blood, urine and olfactory mucosa (OM) in individuals infected with prion diseases.

AMPLIFICATION TECHNIQUES

Protein amplification techniques exploit the ability of PrP^{TSE} to induce a conformational change in PrP in a continuous fashion, so that the minute amount of PrP^{TSE} found in biologic fluids such as blood and CSF can be amplified to a threshold of detection by conventional laboratory techniques.

The most widely used protein aggregation assays include protein misfolding cyclic amplification assay (PMCA) (Soto et al., 2002) with Western blotting detection (Soto and Saborio, 2001) or using surround optical fiber immunoassay (SOFIA) (Rubenstein and Chang, 2013) and real-time quaking-induced conversion (RT-QuIC) which uses thioflavin-T fluorescence to detect PrP^{TSE} or Western blotting (Atarashi et al., 2007; Wilham et al., 2010).

Protein misfolding amplification assay

PMCA was first described in 2001 (Saborio et al., 2001) and in this technique brain homogenates (Soto et al., 2002) or cell extracts (Yokoyama et al., 2011; Imamura et al., 2016) are the source of PrP^{C} and the conversion to PrP^{TSE} can be seeded by the addition of PrP^{TSE} found in brain and peripheral tissues, such as spleen and tonsil (Rubenstein and Chang, 2013) and biologic fluids such as blood (Bougard et al., 2016; Concha-Marambio et al., 2016) and urine (Moda et al., 2014).

To increase the sensitivity of PMCA a series of sonication/rest cycles have been included to break up the aggregated PrP^{TSE} into smaller fragments which can induce further aggregation. A further improvement in the sensitivity of PMCA has been the development of serial PMCA, where small amounts of the PMCA reaction products are seeded into fresh sources of substrate (Castilla et al., 2005). The combination of serial PMCA and Western blotting has increased the detection of brain PrP^{TSE} from 6–12 pg to down to 1 ag, whilst the use of PMCA and SOFIA has been shown to have the same magnitude of sensitivity as animal bioassays (Rubenstein and Chang, 2013). However the use of multiple cycles of sonication can lead to the generation of spontaneous aggregation of substrate in the absence of any seed (Barria et al., 2009; Cosseddu et al., 2011).

The widespread use of PMCA has been hampered by a number of difficulties, such as requirement of brain material as a substrate, the difficulty in standardizing the procedure, the number of cycles required to achieve the necessary sensitivity, and the need for a separate detection system. In addition there is a lack of consistency between laboratories using the same protocols, although the recent adaptations may go some way towards alleviating this issue (Saá et al., 2006; Moudjou et al., 2016).

The first descriptions of PMCA used brain material from Syrian hamster as substrate; however, this is not available in all laboratories and large numbers of animals are needed to ensure the continuity and consistency of the substrate supply. This is true of other animal brain PrP substrates (Brandner et al., 1996; Fischer et al., 1996; Cronier et al., 2004; Tixador et al., 2010; Langevin et al., 2011; Béringue et al., 2012).

The use of human brain material has been suggested as a single human brain contains a large amount of PrP; however, for PMCA to work optimally a match between the codon 129 genotype of the prion protein gene (*PRNP*) of the PrP^{TSE} of the seed and the substrate is needed. This limits the usefulness of human brain material.

Alternative nonbrain sources of PrP^{C}, such as human platelets (Jones et al., 2007), cultured cells (Yokoyama et al., 2011; Imamura et al., 2016), and recombinant PrP (rPrP) (Atarashi et al., 2007), have been proposed. Human platelets are impractical due to the lack of regular supply and other health and safety implications of blood-borne human viruses such as hepatitis C and human immunodeficiency virus; cultured cells are promising as this has the potential to be a widely used source of substrate which avoids many of the pitfalls of using human material; and rPrP can be produced in large amounts and can be standardized for use across laboratories.

In PMCA, Western blotting after proteinase K treatment is a labor-intensive and time-consuming detection system, but it allows the identification of PrP glycotype, which is important in investigating the biochemical nature of the PrP^{TSE} within the seeding material. SOFIA is a more rapid detection system but does not yield any information regarding PrP^{TSE} isotype.

The need for multiple rounds of sonication cycles to achieve the necessary sensitivity is a major drawback; however, the introduction of accelerants such as beads (Gonzalez-Montalban et al., 2011; Moda et al., 2014; Bougard et al., 2016; Moudjou et al., 2016), RNA and poly (A), and lipids (Deleault et al., 2007, 2012; Wang et al., 2011) has improved the sensitivity and reduced the overall reaction time. A recent PMCA adaptation, which includes the use of ceramic beads and either polymerase chain reaction tubes or conventional 96-well microtiter plates, has removed the need for multiple sonication cycles, reduced the amplification time to 48 hours, and has the potential to be adapted for a high-throughput assay (Moudjou et al., 2016).

The reaction products generated by PMCA are infectious and many studies have shown that these products retain similar biochemical and structural properties to the PrP^{TSE} found inthe seeding material (Saá et al., 2006; Weber et al., 2007; Castilla et al., 2008a; Klingeborn et al., 2011; Shikiya and Bartz, 2011) (Fig. 19.1).

Amyloid seeding assay (ASA)

ASA had been the first assay using a recombinant protein as substrate of replication and 96-well plates with continuous shaking on a plate reader at 37°C and a simple fluorescence readout which measures the kinetics of fibril formation. Although this system was innovative and the limit of detection was 1 fg of prions, a positive reaction was determined by the lag phases between normal controls and pathologic samples, limiting the specificity of this assay.

Real-time quaking-induced conversion

The development of RT-QuIC (Wilham et al., 2010; Atarashi et al., 2011) has been a major advance in the use of protein aggregation assays, since it combined the protein aggregation assay with an integral detection system. RT-QuIC uses rPrP as a substrate and the reaction is seeded with PrP^{TSE} from brain tissue or peripheral tissues. It is set up in a 96-well microtiter plate, which facilitates its use as a high-throughput assay. The PrP aggregates that are formed are broken up using intermittent shaking rather than the sonication of PMCA. The inclusion of Thioflavin-T, a dye that binds to amyloid aggregates, means that the kinetics of fibril formation can be monitored in real time using standard fluorescent spectrophotometers. After an initial lag phase of 5–10 hours for reactions seeded with sporadic CJD (sCJD) brain tissue and 30–40 hours for CSF samples, there is a rapid increase in the fluorescent signal until it reaches a maximum at 40 hours for brain tissue and 90 hours for CSF (McGuire et al., 2012) (Fig. 19.2).

The first generation of RT-QuIC assays were undertaken using full-length hamster rPrP (rPrP)

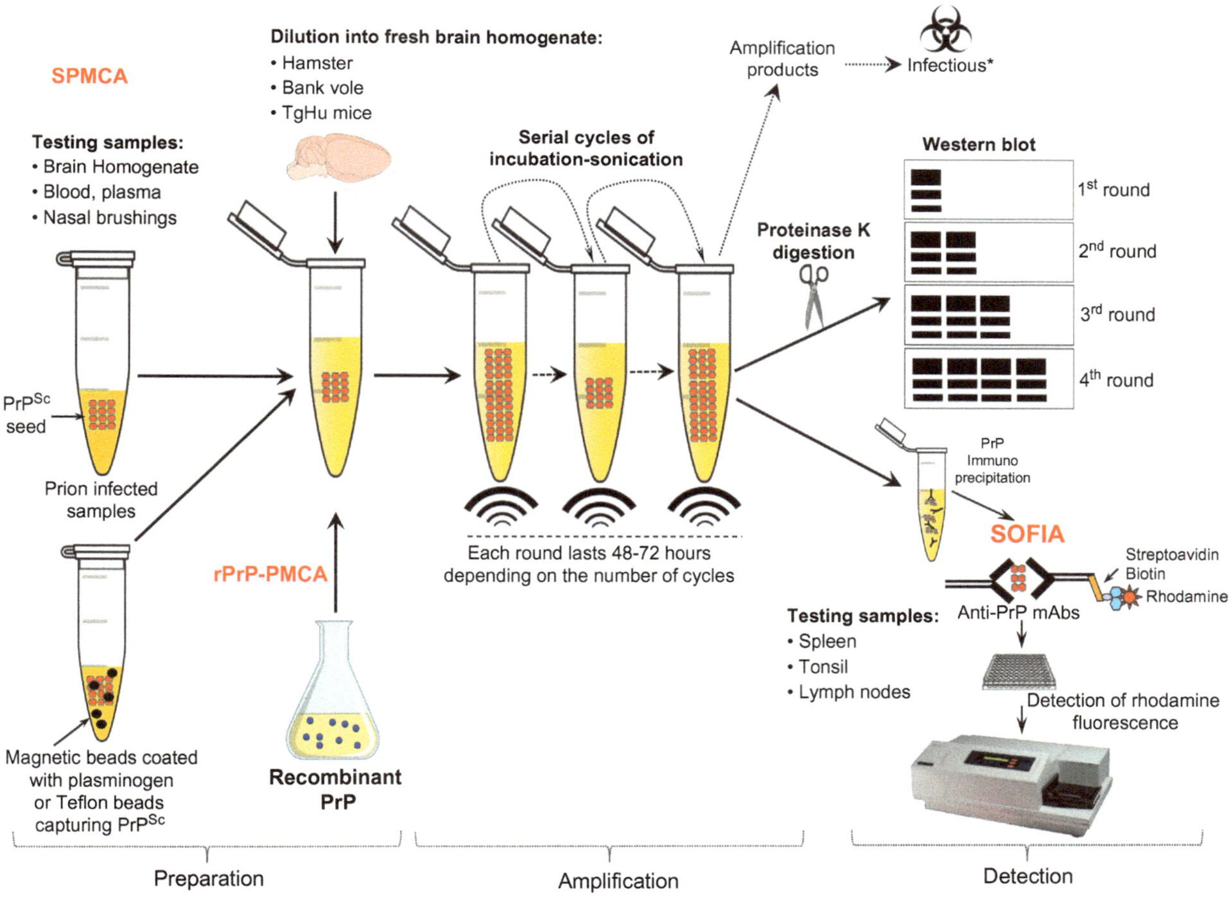

Fig. 19.1. Amplification assays based on seeded conversion of brain PrP^C or recombinant prion protein (rPrP) to PrP^{TSE} by sample sonication and detection of PrP^{TSE} by Western blot or by optical laser immunoassay (SOFIA: surround optical fiber immunoassay). *Not determined in rPrP-PMCA. *PMCA*, protein misfolding cyclic amplification assay; *SPMCA*, serial protein misfolding cyclic amplification.

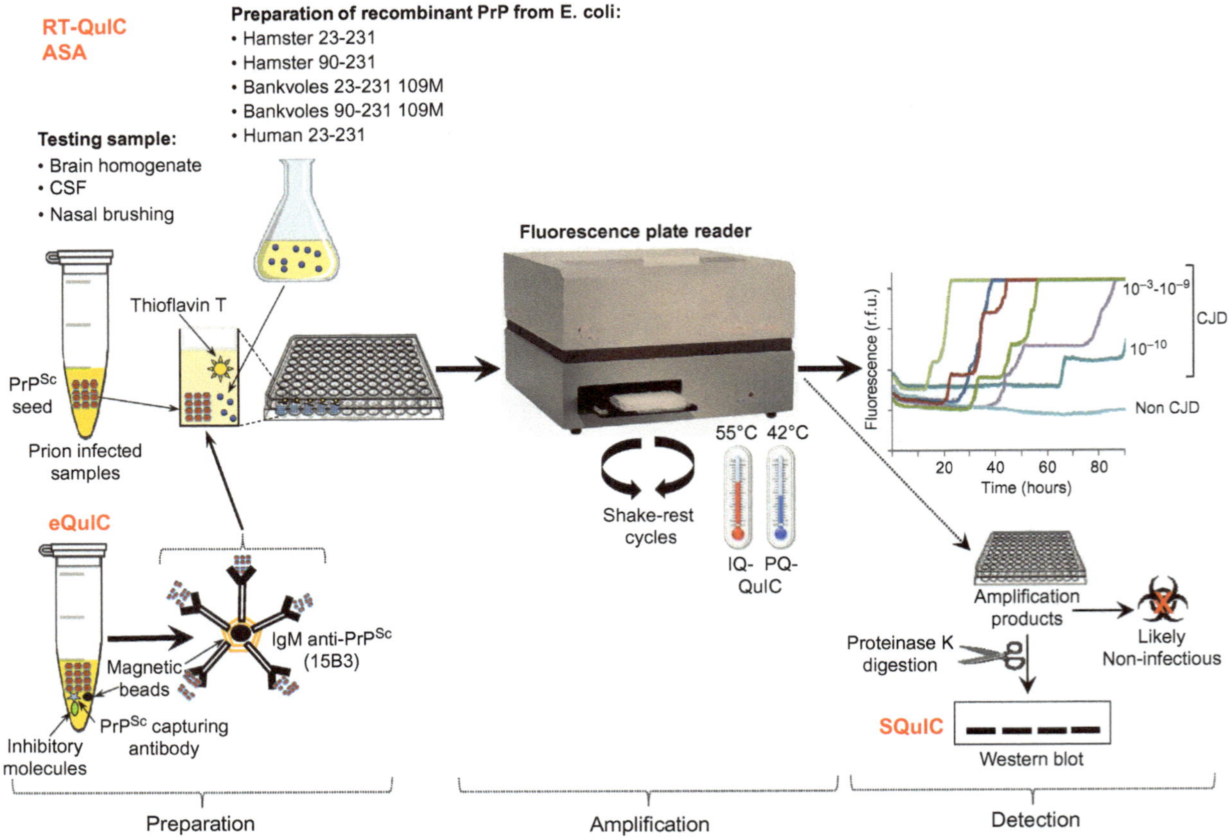

Fig. 19.2. PrP^{TSE} amplification assays based on seeded fibrillation of recombinant prion protein (rPrP) by automated tube shaking and detection of PrP amplification products by ThT fluorecescence or Western blot analysis. *ASA*, amyloid seeding assay; *CJD*, Creutzfeldt–Jakob disease; *CSF*, cerebrospinal fluid; *eQuIC*, enhanced quaking-induced conversion; *PrP*, prion protein; *RT-QuiC*, real-time quaking-induced conversion; *SQuIC*, standard quaking-induced conversion.

(SHarPrP[23-231]) (Wilham et al., 2010) or full-length human rPrP-codon 129 methionine (Atarashi et al., 2011) as substrates. These substrates work very well when seeded with brain or CSF samples from sCJD but not with those from variant CJD (vCJD) samples (Peden et al., 2012). To improve the sensitivity and ability of RT-QuIC to detect vCJD PrP^{TSE}, an adaptation of RT-QuIC, known as e-QuIC was developed. This introduced an initial immunoprecipitation step using magnetic beads coated with a monoclonal immunoglobulin M antibody 15B3, which is selective for PrP^{TSE} and other abnormal PrP oligomers but not for PrP monomers, with a subsequent improved RT-QuIC method which used a sheep-hamster chimeric rPrP and substrate replenishment at 24 hours (Orru and Caughey, 2011). The e-QuIC assay was able to detect 1 ag of vCJD PrP^{TSE} in brain material diluted in plasma. However, the assay was difficult to standardize and less reproducible than the standard RT-QuIC.

The use of bank vole (a rodent) rPrP has been postulated as the universal substrate as it is able to support aggregation seeded by many infectious tissues. However, rPrP is prone to self-aggregation and needs stringent analytic conditions to ensure that false-positive reactions are not obtained. Studies using truncated Syrian hamster rPrP (SHarPrP[90-231]) and modified reaction conditions (second-generation RT-QuIC) have demonstrated that this substrate enables RT-QuIC reactions seeded with sCJD samples to occur more rapidly than those using full-length hamster rPrP, with increased sensitivity and no reduction in specificity (Orru et al., 2015).

Finally, the reaction products of RT-QuIC using full-length hamster rPrP have not demonstrated the ability to transmit disease when inoculated into a 263K hamster scrapie model (Byron Caughey, personal communication).

DIFFERENCES BETWEEN PMCA AND RT-QUIC

Whilst PMCA and RT-QuIC are similar in their basic underlying methodology, there are some major differences in terms of their amplification and detection

Table 19.1

Real-time quaking-induced conversion (RT-QuIC) and protein misfolding cyclic amplification assay (PMCA) prion amplification assays

Assay variants	Principle	Pros	Cons
RT-QuIC ASA sQuIC eQuIC	• Seeded fibrillation of rPrP • Shaking • Multiwell ThT detection or Western blot (sQuIC)	• Rapid, low-cost, multiwell ThT detection • A short training is requested • Highly sensitive and specific • Amplification products are not infectious • Highly efficient in sCJD and gCJD prion amplification • Applicable to biologic fluid in humans and animals • Humans: CSF, olfactory mucosa	• Inefficient in vCJD (except eQuIC) • Not ready for a wide screening blood test
PMCA rPrP-PMCA PMCA-SOFIA	• Seeded conversion of brain PrP^C or seeded fibrillation (rPrP-PMCA) • Sonication • Western blot or SOFIA	• High sensitivity (0.1 ag) and specificity • Highly efficient in detecting vCJD prions • Brain, spleen, liver, blood, plasma, urine	• Long duration (four-round assay takes around 10 days) • Sonication difficult to standardize • Amplification products are infectious • Inefficient in detecting sCJD and gCJD prions

ASA, amyloid seeding assay; CSF, cerebrospinal fluid; eQuIC, enhanced quaking-induced conversion; gCJD, genetic Creutzfeldt–Jakob disease; rPrP: recombinant prion protein; sCJD, sporadic Creutzfeldt–Jakob disease; SOFIA, surround optical fiber immunoassay; sQuIC, standard quaking-induced conversion; vCJD, variant Creutzfeldt–Jakob disease.

systems, ease of use, and throughput and clinical applications (Table 19.1).

Amplification and detection systems

One crucial step in the amplification processes of both PMCA and RT-QuIC is the use of mechanical forces to break up the initially formed aggregates of PrP^{TSE} into smaller units that can then go on to induce further aggregation. PMCA uses sonication and this has been found to be difficult to standardize, not only between laboratories but sometimes within laboratories themselves. This is mainly due to the mechanics of the sonicator horn which can result in noneven sonication throughout the tubes of a single assay, with the position and distance from the sonicator horn influencing the number of effective sonication cycles (Castilla et al., 2005; Gonzalez-Montalban et al., 2011; Morales et al., 2012). However, in contrast, RT-QuIC uses intermittent shaking rather than sonication to break up the initially formed aggregates and this is much more easily standardized and replicated between laboratories.

PMCA is a two-step process with an initial amplification step followed by a separate detection system, whether this is Western blotting or an enzyme-linked immunosorbent assay (ELISA)-based technique such as SOFIA. This not only adds time to the overall process but adds in another labor-intensive step. In addition the detection systems used are the limiting steps in the overall sensitivity of the assay. However, RT-QuIC combines an amplification and detection system, which decreases the analytic hands-on time, and improves sensitivity and standardization.

Although RT-QuiC is as sensitive as PMCA in being able to detect as little as 1 fg PrP^{TSE} in the brain of sCJD patients (Atarashi et al., 2011; Peden et al., 2012), it is much quicker than PMCA, with results being obtained within 2 days rather than 4–5 days (Wilham et al., 2010).

Sources and properties of the substrate

Both PMCA and RT-QuIC use PrP as a substrate. However, PMCA works better with native intact mammalian PrP which contains the glycosylphosphatidylinositol anchor and the attached glycans. Finding a cheap, reliable, and consistent source of mammalian PrP has been one of the major drawbacks of PMCA. In addition, many PMCA assays require a match between the *PRNP* codon 129 genotype of the substrate and the seed. This is particularly difficult when using the assay for diagnostic purposes, where the *PRNP* codon 129 genotype of the seed is unknown. RT-QuIC, however, uses rPrP which does not have a glycosylphosphatidylinositol anchor or any glycan side chains. The rPrP most commonly used is of either hamster or human origin and does not require matching of the substrate and seed *PRNP* codon 129 genotype (Atarashi et al., 2011; McGuire et al., 2012; Cramm et al., 2015; Foutz et al., 2017; Lattanzio et al., 2017).

Throughput and ease of use

RT-QuIC is better adapted to being used as a high-throughput diagnostic assay than PMCA. It is generally quicker with a combined amplification and detection system, it is easy to perform, and has been adapted to a 96-well microtiter plate to enable a more rapid throughput of samples. The use of rPrP as a source of substrate ensures that there is a reliable and reproducible supply. In addition, the reaction products of RT-QuIC are not infectious and therefore specialized containment laboratories are not required to perform the assay. This is in contrast to PMCA, where small amounts of infectious PrP^{TSE} can be amplified between 6000-fold and a million-fold (Barria et al., 2012), and as such PMCA must be undertaken in specialized containment laboratories by highly trained laboratory staff. It should also be mentioned that, in the absence of PrP^{TSE}, prolonged PMCA reactions might generate de novo prion strains, with unpredictable infectivity, and this option dictates caution when handling PMCA reaction products (Cosseddu et al., 2011). RT-QuIC is a highly reproducible assay, as has been shown by a number of studies demonstrating a high degree of intralaboratory agreement after analyzing CSF samples blind to the diagnosis (Cramm et al., 2016; McGuire et al., 2016).

Differences in seeding amplification efficiencies

One of the major differences between PMCA and RT-QuIC is their differing abilities to amplify PrP^{TSE} from sporadic, variant, and genetic forms of CJD. Whilst PMCA readily amplifies PrP^{TSE} from vCJD brain tissue (Jones et al., 2007), blood (Bougard et al., 2016; Concha-Marambio et al., 2016), and urine (Moda et al., 2014), it is considerably less efficient at seeding brain tissue from sCJD and genetic CJD (gCJD) patients. Recent studies have failed to amplify PrP^{TSE} from blood (Bougard et al., 2016; Concha-Marambio et al., 2016) or urine from sCJD or gCJD cases (Moda et al., 2014). However, it is unclear whether this is due to the lack of efficiency of PMCA or the absence of PrP^{TSE} in these body fluids in sCJD and gCJD (Table 19.2 and Fig. 19.3).

Reflecting what is going on in vivo

Because the end-product of the PMCA reaction retains infectivity (Saá et al., 2006; Weber et al., 2007; Castilla et al., 2008b; Klingeborn et al., 2011; Shikiya and Bartz, 2011) and maintains the structural and biochemical properties of the seed (Castilla et al., 2008b), this technique is valuable for investigating the mechanisms of different patterns of PrP^{TSE} misfolding and their relation with infectivity.

USE OF RT-QUIC AND PMCA IN THE DIAGNOSIS OF HUMAN PRION DISEASES

Sporadic CJD

Cerebrospinal fluid

The first generation of RT-QuIC assays used full-length rPrP of either human (Atarashi et al., 2011; Sano et al., 2013; Park et al., 2016) or Syrian hamster (Wilham et al., 2010; McGuire et al., 2012; Peden et al., 2012; Orru et al., 2014; Lattanzio et al., 2017) origin, a detergent-free buffer, and reaction temperatures of 37 or 42°C. A variety of orbital shakers and fluorescent readers have been used: the most common are the FLUOstar Omega or Optima for assays using hamster rPrP and the Tecan Infinite M200 or F200 for those using human rPrP. Using these first-generation assays, RT-QuIC was shown to have a sensitivity ranging from 77% to 89% and a specificity of 99–100% (Atarashi et al., 2011; McGuire et al., 2012; Orru et al., 2014; Park et al., 2016; Bongianni et al., 2017; Lattanzio et al., 2017) (Table 19.3).

The sensitivity of first-generation RT-QuIC was not found to be significantly influenced by the *PRNP* codon 129 genotype (Atarashi et al., 2011; McGuire et al., 2012; Lattanzio et al., 2017). However when the *PRNP* codon 129 was combined with the PrP^{Res} glycotype, the sensitivity of first-generation RT-QuIC was found to be lower in the MM2 and VV2 subtypes (Lattanzio et al., 2017). However this study found that the kinetics of the RT-QuIC reaction, as assessed by the lag phase and the final fluorescent values, was not influenced by the sCJD subtype (Lattanzio et al., 2017). These results support those of a previous study (Cramm et al., 2015), which found no difference in the RT-QuIC kinetics between MM1 and MM2, MV1 and MV2, or VV1 and VV2; however it was noted that the

Table 19.2

Real-time quaking-induced conversion (RT-QuIC) and protein misfolding cyclic amplification assay (PMCA) diagnostic application in human prion disease

	Sporadic CJD	Genetic CJD	Gerstmann–Sträussler–Scheinker	Fatal familial insomnia	Variant CJD
RT-QuIC	CSF, OM	CSF • V180I • E200K • V203I • V210I • OM • E200K • V210I • V180I	CSF • P102L OM • P102L	CSF	Brain tissue Spiked plasma[a]
PMCA	Brain tissue Spleen[b] Tonsil[b] Lymph nodes[b]	Brain tissue	Brain tissue A117V F198S H187R	OM	Brain tissue Blood Plasma Urine Spleen[b] Tonsil[b] Lymph nodes[b]

[a]Enhanced quaking-induced conversion.
[b]Surround optical fiber immunoassay (SOFIA).
CJD, Creutzfeldt–Jakob disease; CSF, cerebrospinal fluid; OM, olfactory mucosa.

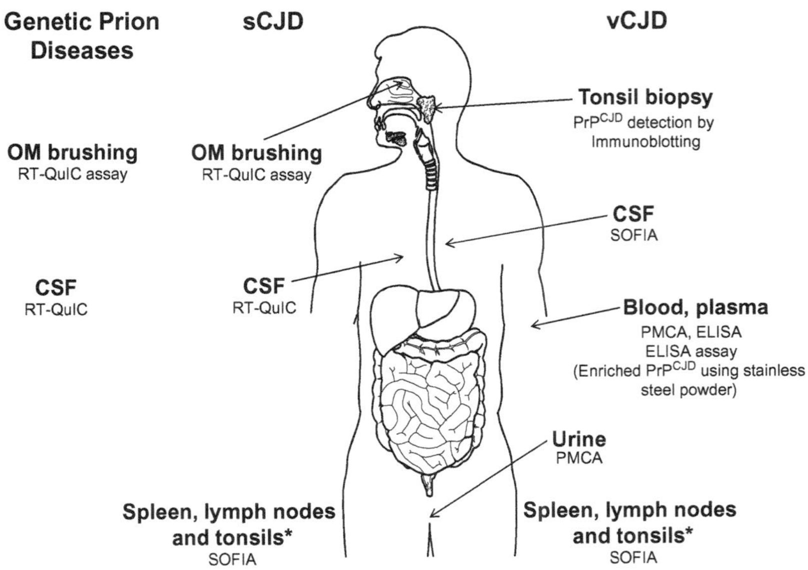

Fig. 19.3. Practical application of amplification techniques in human prion disease diagnostics. *Postmortem samples. *CSF*, cerebrospinal fluid; *ELISA*, enzyme-linked immunosorbent assay; *OM*, olfactory mucosa; *PMCA*, protein misfolding cyclic amplification assay; *RT-QuiC*, real-time quaking-induced conversion; *sCJD*, sporadic Creutzfeldt–Jakob disease; *SOFIA*, surround optical fiber immunoassay; *vCJD*, variant Creutzfeldt–Jakob disease.

Table 19.3

Sensitivity and specificity of first- and second-generation real-time quaking-induced conversion (RT-QuIC) assays for sporadic Creutzfeldt–Jakob disease (CJD) and genetic prion diseasesa

RT-QuIC	Human prion disease	Recombinant PrP	Biologic fluid/tissue	Sensivitity (%)	Specificity (%)	Reference
First generation	Definite sCJD	Full-length human	CSF	All (85)	100	Atarashi et al. (2011)
First generation	Definite sCJD	Full-length hamster	CSF	All (89)	99	McGuire et al. (2012)
				MM (90); MV (88); VV (95)		
First generation	Genetic prion disease	Full-length human	CSF	GSS: P102L (90); FFI (83.3); E200K (82); V203I (100)	100	Sano et al. (2013)
First generation	Definite and probable sCJD	Full-length human	CSF	All (77)	100	Park et al. (2016)
First generation	Definite and probable sCJD	Full-length hamster	CSF	Definite: MM(V)1 (89); VV2 (78); MV2 (81); MM2 (23)[a]		Lattanzio et al. (2017)
	Genetic			Probable: MM (84); MV (72); VV (91)	94	
	prion diseases			E200K (95) V210I (100); insertions (100); D178N-129V (50); R208H (0); V203I (50)		
	Variable protease-sensitive prionopathy			VPSPr (0)		
First generation	Definite and probable sCJD	Full-length hamster	CSF	All (77)	100	Orru et al. (2014)
			OM	MM (79); MV (75); VV (100)	100	
				All (97)		
				MM (100); MV (89); VV (100)		
First generation	Definite and probable	Full-length hamster	CSF	All (72)	100	
Second generation	sCJD	Truncated hamster	OM	Definite (79); probable (65);	100	Bongianni et al. (2017)
			CSF	all (97)	100	
				Definite (100); probable (94);		
				all (86)		
				Definite (70); probable (100)		
	Definite sCJD	Full-length hamster	CSF	All (64)	100	Orru et al. (2015)
First generation		Truncated hamster		All (91)	100	
Second generation				MM1 (94) MV1 (100) MV2 (100) VV2 (100)		
Second generation	Definite sCJD	Truncated hamster		All (94)	99	Foutz et al. (2017)
	genetic CJD		CSF	MM1 (96) MV1 (93) MV2 (89) VV1 (75) VV2 (100) MM2-Cortical (78)		
First generation		Full-length hamster		36 Definite; 68 probable; 3 gCJD and 1 GSS (73)		Groveman et al. (2016)
Second generation	Definite and probable sCJD	Truncated hamster	CSF	36 Definite, 68 probable, MM (98) MV (96) VV (90);	100	
	genetic CJD			3 gCJD and 1 GSS	100	

[a]Includes both cortical and thalamic variants.

CSF, cerebrospinal fluid; gCJD, genetic Creutzfeldt–Jakob disease; GSS, Gerstmann–Straussler–Scheinker; M, methionine; OM. olfactory mucosa brushings; PrP, prion protein; sCJD, sporadic Creutzeldt-Jakob disease; V, valine.

RT-QuIC reaction was quicker in MM1 than MV1 or VV1 (Table 19.3).

A number of studies in sCJD have shown that there is no relationship between the RT-QuIC kinetics and age at onset of disease, disease duration of CSF sampling, or timing of the lumbar puncture expressed as a percentage of the total disease duration (McGuire et al., 2012; Lattanzio et al., 2017), although Cramm et al. (2015) demonstrated that patients with a longer disease duration has a longer lag phase and a lower final fluorescent value.

Over 1000 non-CJD CSF samples have been analyzed in these studies and only three have demonstrated a positive RT-QuIC result (McGuire et al., 2012; Lattanzio et al., 2017). One patient had a diagnosis of vascular dementia but died without postmortem confirmation of disease (McGuire et al., 2012). The second patient had a clinical diagnosis at the time of CSF analysis of frontotemporal dementia and was lost to follow-up. The third patient had a diagnosis of paraneoplastic syndrome accompanying breast carcinoma; however it is unclear whether diagnosis was confirmed at postmortem. The specificity of first-generation Rt-QuIC assays is close to 100% and is significantly better than surrogate markers such as CSF 14-3-3 or tau protein (Lattanzio et al., 2017).

Despite the significant advance these first-generation RT-QuIC assays have made to the antemortem diagnosis of sCJD, there has been a need to improve their sensitivity and speed. A major advance has been the development of the second-generation RT-QuIC assay which utilizes an N-terminally truncated Syrian hamster rPrP (SHarPrP[90-231]) and includes the addition of 0.002% sodium dodecyl sulfate to the reaction buffer and an increase in the reaction temperature to 55°C (Orru et al., 2015). A small initial study of 11 CSF samples from neuropathologically confirmed sCJD compared both RT-QuIC assays and demonstrated that the second-generation RT-QuIC assay was considerably faster, being complete within 24–48 hours, and more sensitive, as it detected 91% of sCJD compared to 64% using the traditional RT-QuIC technique, without any loss of specificity. These results have been confirmed in a larger study (Groveman et al., 2016), which also demonstrated that the second-generation RT-QuIC assay had better reproducibility.

A large combined retrospective and prospective study of sCJD CSF samples has shown that this second-generation RT-QuIC has an overall sensitivity of 94% (Foutz et al., 2017). This study also showed that the sensitivity was dependent on the sCJD subtype, with the typical subtypes of MM1 and MV1 having a sensitivity of 96% and 93% respectively, whereas those rarer subtypes such as VV1 and MM2-cortical had lower sensitivities of 75% and 78%, respectively. Interestingly, this study found that the kinetics of the RT-QuIC reaction could distinguish between the MM1 and MM2 and the VV1 and VV2 subtypes. However, more data are required before firm conclusions can be made. This study also found a positive result in a patient with neuropathologically confirmed Lewy body dementia (LBD); however subsequent phosphotungstic acid precipitation followed by Western blotting and conformational-dependent immunoassay detected low but significant amounts of PrP^{TSE} that were not observable by immunohistochemistry. It is unclear whether this patient would have developed sCJD if the individual had not died of LBD.

If on one hand the above studies have shown CSF RT-QuIC is a sensitive and specific test for sCJD, on the other hand, two international studies have demonstrated that the assay is robust and reproducible among laboratories (Cramm et al., 2016; McGuire et al., 2016). One study showed that laboratories in different countries using a range of rPrP sources and instrumentation produced identical results when analyzing the same set of CSF samples (McGuire et al., 2016). As a result of these studies RT-QuIC has been included in the diagnostic criteria for sCJD (www.cjd.ed.ac.uk).

Olfactory mucosa

The presence of PrP^{TSE} in the olfactory pathway, including the olfactory neuroepithelium, in both postmortem and biopsy tissue of sCJD patients has been well documented (Zanusso et al., 2003; Tabaton et al., 2004). Olfactory epithelium nasal brushings have been used as a means of improving the premortem diagnosis of sCJD using RT-QuIC (Orru et al., 2014). OM brushings and CSF samples were collected from 31 patients with CJD and from 43 patients with other neurodegenerative diseases. The OM and CSF samples were analyzed using a first-generation RT-QuIC assay. Positive RT-QuIC results were obtained in 30 of 31 of the OM samples and in 23 of 30 CSF cases of CJD. The RT-QuIC responses seen with OM samples were quicker and showed higher final fluorescent readings than those seen with CSF. None of the OM or CSF samples from patients with other neurologic diseases were positive (Orru et al., 2014; Zanusso et al., 2014).

In a recent study (Bongianni et al., 2017), the diagnostic sensitivity of RT-QuIC analyses in CSF and OM samples from 86 patients with a clinical diagnosis of probable, possible, or suspected sCJD was evaluated. CSF samples were tested by standard and improved RT-QuIC conditions while OM samples were tested with standard RT-QuIC. RT-QuIC assay resulted in 95% sensitivity in CSF samples and 97% in OM and 100%

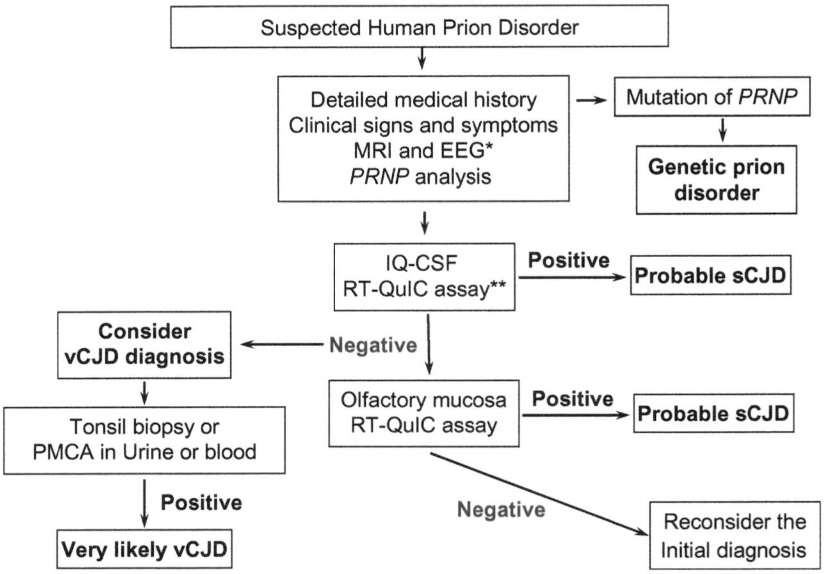

Fig. 19.4. Algorithm for in vivo diagnosis of human prion diseases.*Referring to established diagnostic criteria; **using hamster recombinant prion protein (rPrP) as conventional conditions. *EEG*, electroencephalogram; *IQ-CSF*, Improved quaking-induced conversion-cerebrospinal fluid; *MRI*, magnetic resonance imaging; *PMCA*, protein misfolding cyclic amplification assay; *RT-QuiC*, real-time quaking-induced conversion; *sCJD*, sporadic Creutzfeldt–Jakob disease; *vCJD*, variant Creutzfeldt–Jakob disease.

specific. However, if both samples were considered the overall specificity and sensitivity were 100%. Based on these findings, a diagnostic algorithm for sCJD was proposed which combines CSF and OM RT-QuIC testing (Bongianni et al., 2017) (Fig. 19.4).

Genetic CJD

Cerebrospinal fluid and olfactory mucosa

Although the diagnosis of genetic prion diseases is obtained by *PRNP* gene sequencing, there are fewer data available regarding the clinical utility of RT-QuIC in gCJD and prion disease than for sCJD. The largest single study was undertaken by Sano et al. (2013), looking at 56 cases of genetic forms of prion disease. CSF RT-QuIC assay was positive in 90% of patients with Gerstmann–Sträussler–Scheinker due to a *PRNP* P102L mutation. This was in marked contrast to other CSF biomarkers such as CSF 14-3-3 and tau protein, which were only positive in 20% of these cases. This study also found that CSF RT-QuIC was positive in 83.3% of patients with fatal familial insomnia (*PRNP* D178N-M) and in 100% of patients with *PRNP* V203I mutations. In these groups of patients elevated CSF 14-3-3 and tau protein were not detected or only detected in 50%, respectively. Therefore CSF RT-QuiC is a major advance in the premortem diagnosis of these conditions. CSF RT-QuIC has a sensitivity of 82–100% in patients with gCJD associated with *PRNP* E200K mutations (Sano et al., 2013; Foutz et al., 2017; Lattanzio et al., 2017). There are reports of CSF RT-QuIC results in a small number of cases of other mutations and these are listed in Table 19.3.

RT-QuIC seeding activity has also been detected in OM samples from 8 patients with genetic prion diseases carrying E200K, V210I, V180I, and P102L *PRNP* mutations. However, the small number of patients did not permit any conclusions about relative sensitivity (Bongianni et al., 2017).

A recent study has shown that OM samples from 2 patients with fatal familial insomnia (*PRNP* D178N-M) were positive for both RT-QuIC and PMCA but no such positivity was found in OM samples from patients with Alzheimer disease, Parkinson disease, or other neurodegenerative conditions (Redaelli et al., 2017).

Iatrogenic CJD

There is very little available information regarding the use of protein aggregation assays in the diagnosis of iatrogenic CJD. However, CJD instrument contamination events continue to occur. In 2013, a patient who had undergone neurosurgery in New Hampshire later developed sCJD. Before the patient's disease was diagnosed, the same surgical equipment used on the CJD patient was used on 13 subsequent patients, putting those patients at risk for prion infection. Brown and Farrell (2015a, b) suggested that RT-QuIC testing of nasal brushings and

CSF should be applicable to all patients with dementia or cerebellar signs as a means of preventing the risk of iatrogenic CJD transmission.

A recent study investigated dura mater graft-associated CJD (dCJD) by PMCA (Takeuchi et al., 2016). There are two distinct neuropathologic phenotypes of dura mater graft-associated CJD. The most prevalent is represented by a nonplaque-type (np-dCJD), which resembles sCJD (MM1 and MV1 subtypes) and the other is a rarer form called plaque-type CJD (p-dCJD) which is associated with kuru plaques and a PrP^{res} glycotype with an electrophoretic mobility between type 1 and type 2. The p-dCJD is linked to the V2 strain of CJD, which is associated with sCJD MV2 and VV2 subtypes. The amplification of brain PrP^{TSE} from these dCJD cases has shown that PMCA can preferentially amplify PrP^{TSE} from p-dCJD cases but not from np-dCJD cases.

A small study of 22 cases of iatrogenic CJD secondary to human cadaveric growth hormone administration showed that CSF RT-QuIC was positive in 14 cases, giving a sensitivity of 64% (Green, unpublished data).

Variant CJD

The use of RT-QuIC to amplify PrP^{TSE} from vCJD brain tissue using full-length Syrian hamster rPrP ($SHarPrP^{Sen}$[23-231]) has been less than promising (Peden et al., 2012). Alternative techniques, such as e-QuiC (Orru and Caughey, 2011), have been tried but with little success; however, the use of full-length bank vole $rPrP^{Sen}$ (23–230) has been shown to be able to support amplification of vCJD brain tissue (Orru et al., 2015). In contrast, PMCA readily amplifies PrP^{TSE} from vCJD brain tissue from both patients (Jones et al., 2007) and animal models (Saborio et al., 2001).

Cerebrospinal fluid

RT-QuIC using full-length Syrian hamster rPrP (SHarPrP[23-231]) has failed to amplify PrP^{TSE} from vCJD CSF (Mok et al., 2017; Green, personal communication). However, the use of full-length bank vole rPrP (23-230) has shown to be able to support amplification of vCJD brain tissue (Orru et al., 2015). Recent modifications of the PMCA assay have enabled amplification and detection of PrP^{TSE} from urine and plasma from vCJD patients (Moda et al., 2014; Bougard et al., 2016; Concha-Marambio et al., 2016), therefore there is a good possibility that these techniques could detect PrP^{TSE} in the CSF from vCJD.

Urine

The first report of the use of PMCA to detect vCJD PrP^{TSE} in biologic fluids came in 2014, when Moda et al. detected PrP^{TSE} in the urine of patients with vCJD. This study analyzed a total of 238 urine samples from vCJD, sCJD, genetic prion disease, control patients, and healthy controls in a blinded study. Of the 14 vCJD patients, PrP^{TSE} was detected in 13, whilst none of the 68 sCJD or 4 genetic prion diseases had detectable PrP^{TSE}. None of the 100 urine samples from patients with either neurodegenerative or nonneurodegenerative diseases or the 52 healthy subjects had detectable PrP^{TSE}. Multiple rounds of sonication were required to amplify the PrP^{TSE} to detectable amounts by Western blotting, suggesting that the amount of PrP^{TSE} present in the urine is small and is thought to be around 40–100 oligomeric PrP^{TSE} units/mL. The sensitivity of this PMCA assay is 93% with a specificity of 100% and is able to clearly distinguish between vCJD and sCJD (Moda et al., 2014). The latter is very important as the emergence of a patient with neuropathologically confirmed vCJD associated with *PRNP* codon129MV, and indicates that a new wave of vCJD cases is likely and that these may be difficult to distinguish from sCJD (Mok et al., 2017).

Plasma

The detection of PrP^{TSE} in the blood of vCJD has been a major priority, not only to improve the diagnosis of vCJD in life but also to ensure the safety of blood and blood products. Two recent adaptations of the PMCA assay have made it possible to detect PrP^{TSE} in blood from clinical vCJD patients (Bougard et al., 2016; Concha-Marambio et al., 2016) and also in preclinical blood samples taken from two vCJD (Bougard et al., 2016).

Both of these studies have used a preanalytic treatment step. One used a sarkosyl precipitation of whole blood, plasma, or white blood cells or prior to amplification using brain homogenate from transgenic mice expressing human PrP-*PRNP* codon 129MM (TgHuPrP[129MM]) (Concha-Marambio et al., 2016). The second study incubated plasma samples with magnetic nanobeads coated with plasminogen for 90 minutes at 25°C, prior to PMCA amplification using Teflon beads and brain homogenate from transgenic mice overexpressing by sixfold human PrP-129M (tg650 line) (Bougard et al., 2016). These preanalytic steps are necessary to remove factors from blood and its components that inhibit the PMCA reaction.

Concha-Marambio and coworkers (2016) detected PrP^{TSE} after two to three rounds of PMCA in all 14 vCJD blood samples analyzed. They found comparable amounts of PrP^{TSE} in whole blood, plasma, and white cells. No PrP^{TSE} was detected in any of the 16 sCJD blood samples analyzed, even after six rounds of PMCA. None of the 88 patients with other neurodegenerative diseases, including other protein misfolding disorders such as Alzheimer disease, LBD, frontotemporal dementia and Parkinson disease, were positive.

Similar results were obtained by Bougard et al. (2016), who detected PrP^{TSE} in all 18 vCJD patients and in none of 134 patients with other neurodegenerative disorders, including Alzheimer disease, LBD, Parkinson disease, or any of the 104 healthy subjects. This study investigated 40 patients with neuropathologically confirmed sCJD and 27 with probable sCJD. Of these sCJD patients, 1 patient with neuropathologically confirmed sCJD (MM2 subtype) was positive. There was no evidence of vCJD at postmortem or any clinical suspicion of vCJD during life.

Two of the vCJD patients investigated were regular blood donors and as such had aliquots of blood stored prior to the onset of symptoms. One patient had seven preclinical blood samples taken, ranging from 55 to 7 months prior to onset of symptoms. The second patient had four preclinical blood samples stored, ranging from 30 to 2 months prior to the onset of symptoms. Both of these patients had detectable blood PrP^{TSE} preclinically: 1 patient had detectable PrP^{TSE} from 31 months prior to the onset of symptoms and the other from 16 months.

These studies suggest that PMCA analysis of blood can be used as an accurate diagnostic test for vCJD, can distinguish vCJD from sCJD, and can detect preclinical vCJD disease at least 16 months prior to the onset of symptoms.

CONCLUSIONS

Protein aggregation assays such as RT-QuIC and PMCA have a very important role in the diagnosis of and research into prion diseases. CSF RT-QuIC analysis has been shown to be a highly sensitive and specific test for sCJD and has now been included in the diagnostic criteria. It is also a useful investigation for some genetic forms of prion disease, such as Gerstmann–Sträussler–Scheinker and fatal familial insomnia, where other CSF tests may be negative. PMCA shows great potential for the diagnosis of vCJD and has the ability to distinguish vCJD from sCJD, which may become increasingly important. In addition the ability of PMCA to replicate infectivity as well as the biochemical and structural properties of PrP^{TSE} means this is a valuable tool for understanding the underlying pathologic processes involved in prion protein misfolding.

References

Atarashi R, Moore RA, Sim VL et al. (2007). Ultrasensitive detection of scrapie prion protein using seeded conversion of recombinant prion protein. Nat Methods 4: 645–650.

Atarashi R, Satoh K, Sano K et al. (2011). Ultrasensitive human prion detection in cerebrospinal fluid by real-time quaking-induced conversion. Nat Med 17: 175–178.

Barria MA, Mukherjee A, Gonzalez-Romero D et al. (2009). De novo generation of infectious prions in vitro produces a new disease phenotype. PLoS Pathog 5: e1000421.

Barria MA, Gonzalez-Romero D, Soto C (2012). Cyclic amplification of prion protein misfolding. Methods Mol Biol 849: 199–212.

Béringue V, Herzog L, Jaumain E et al. (2012). Facilitated cross-species transmission of prions in extraneural tissue. Science 335: 472–475.

Bongianni M, Orrù C, Groveman BR et al. (2017). Diagnosis of human prion disease using real-time quaking-induced conversion testing of olfactory mucosa and cerebrospinal fluid samples. JAMA Neurol 74: 155–162.

Bougard D, Brandel JP, Bélondrade M et al. (2016). Detection of prions in the plasma of presymptomatic and symptomatic patients with variant Creutzfeldt–Jakob disease. Sci Transl Med 8: 370.

Brandner S, Raeber A, Sailer A et al. (1996). Normal host prion protein (PrPC) is required for scrapie spread within the central nervous system. Proc Natl Acad Sci U S A 93: 13148–13151.

Brown P, Farrell M (2015a). A practical approach to avoiding iatrogenic Creutzfeldt–Jakob disease (CJD) from invasive instruments. Infect Control Hosp Epidemiol 36: 844–848.

Brown P, Farrell M (2015b). A new practical diagnostic test for Creutzfeldt–Jakob disease. Infect Control Hosp Epidemiol 36: 849.

Budka H, Aguzzi A, Brown P et al. (1995). Neuropathological diagnostic criteria for Creutzfeldt–Jakob disease (CJD) and other human spongiform encephalopathies (prion diseases). Brain Pathol 5: 459–466.

Castilla J, Saá P, Soto C (2005). Detection of prions in blood. Nat Med 11: 982–985.

Castilla J, Gonzalez-Romero D, Saá P et al. (2008a). Crossing the species barrier by PrP(Sc) replication in vitro generates unique infectious prions. Cell 134: 757–768.

Castilla J, Morales R, Saá P et al. (2008b). Cell-free propagation of prion strains. EMBO J 27: 2557–2566.

Chohan G, Pennington C, Mackenzie JM et al. (2010). The role of cerebrospinal fluid 14-3-3 and other proteins in the diagnosis of sporadic Creutzfeldt–Jakob disease in the UK: a 10-year review. J Neurol Neurosurg Psychiatry 81: 1243–1248.

Collins SJ, Sanchez-Juan P, Masters CL et al. (2006). Determinants of diagnostic investigation sensitivities across the clinical spectrum of sporadic Creutzfeldt–Jakob disease. Brain 129: 2278–2287.

Concha-Marambio L, Pritzkow S, Moda F et al. (2016). Detection of prions in blood from patients with variant Creutzfeldt–Jakob disease. In: Sci Transl Med 8:370ra183.

Cosseddu GM, Nonno R, Vaccari G et al. (2011). Ultra-efficient PrP(Sc) amplification highlights potentialities and pitfalls of PMCA technology. PLoS Pathog 7: e1002370.

Cramm M, Schmitz M, Karch A et al. (2015). Characteristic CSF prion seeding efficiency in humans with prion diseases. Mol Neurobiol 51: 396–405.

Cramm M, Schmitz M, Karch A et al. (2016). Stability and reproducibility underscore utility of RT-QuIC for diagnosis of Creutzfeldt–Jakob disease. Mol Neurobiol 53: 1896–1904.

Cronier S, Laude H, Peyrin JM (2004). Prions can infect primary cultured neurons and astrocytes and promote neuronal cell death. Proc Natl Acad Sci U S A 101: 12271–12276.

Deleault NR, Harris BT, Rees JR et al. (2007). Formation of native prions from minimal components in vitro. Proc Natl Acad Sci U S A 104: 9741–9746.

Deleault NR, Walsh DJ, Piro JR et al. (2012). Cofactor molecules maintain infectious conformation and restrict strain properties in purified prions. Proc Natl Acad Sci U S A 109: E1938–E1946.

Fischer M, Rulicke T, Raeber A et al. (1996). Prion protein (PrP) with amino-proximal deletions restoring susceptibility of PrP knockout mice to scrapie. EMBO J 15 (6): 1255–1264.

Foutz A, Appleby BS, Hamlin C et al. (2017). Diagnostic and prognostic value of human prion detection in cerebrospinal fluid. Ann Neurol 81: 79–92.

Geschwind MD, Martindale J, Miller D et al. (2003). Challenging the clinical utility of the 14-3-3 protein for the diagnosis of sporadic Creutzfeldt–Jakob disease. Arch Neurol 60: 813–816.

Gonzalez-Montalban N, Makarava N, Savtchenko R et al. (2011). Relationship between conformational stability and amplification efficiency of prions. Biochemistry 50: 7933–7940.

Groveman BR, Orrú CD, Hughson AG et al. (2016). Extended and direct evaluation of RT-QuIC assays for Creutzfeldt–Jakob disease diagnosis. Ann Clin Transl Neurol 4: 139–144.

Hamlin C, Puoti G, Berri S et al. (2012). A comparison of tau and 14-3-3 protein in the diagnosis of Creutzfeldt–Jakob disease. Neurology 79: 547–552.

Imamura M, Tabeta N, Kato N et al. (2016). Heparan sulfate and heparin promote faithful prion replication in vitro by binding to normal and abnormal prion proteins in protein misfolding cyclic amplification. J Biol Chem 291: 26478–26486.

Jones M, Peden AH, Prowse CV et al. (2007). In vitro amplification and detection of variant Creutzfeldt–Jakob disease PrPSc. J Pathol 213: 21–26.

Klingeborn M1, Race B, Meade-White KD et al. (2011). Lower specific infectivity of protease-resistant prion protein generated in cell-free reactions. Proc Natl Acad Sci U S A 108: E1244–E1253.

Langevin C, Andreoletti O, Le Dur A et al. (2011). Marked influence of the route of infection on prion strain apparent phenotype in a scrapie transgenic mouse model. Neurobiol Dis 41 (1): 219–225.

Lattanzio F, Abu-Rumeileh S, Franceschini A et al. (2017). Prion-specific and surrogate CSF biomarkers in Creutzfeldt–Jakob disease: diagnostic accuracy in relation to molecular subtypes and analysis of neuropathological correlates of p-tau and Aβ42 levels. Acta Neuropathol 133: 559–578.

McGuire LI, Peden AH, Orru CD et al. (2012). RT-QuIC analysis of cerebrospinal fluid in sporadic Creutzfeldt–Jakob disease. Ann Neurol 72: 278–285.

McGuire LI, Poleggi A, Poggiolini I et al. (2016). Cerebrospinal fluid real-time quaking-induced conversion is a robust and reliable test for sporadic Creutzfeldt–Jakob disease: An international study. Ann Neurol 80: 160–165.

Meissner B, Kallenberg K, Sanchez-Juan P et al. (2009). MRI lesion profiles in sporadic Creutzfeldt–Jakob disease. Neurology 72: 1994–2001.

Moda F, Gambetti P, Notari S et al. (2014). Prions in the urine of patients with variant Creutzfeldt–Jakob disease. N Engl J Med 371: 530–539.

Mok T, Jaunmuktane Z, Joiner S et al. (2017). Variant Creutzfeldt–Jakob disease in a patient with heterozygosity at PRNP codon 129. N Engl J Med 376: 292–294.

Morales R, Duran-Aniotz C, Diaz-Espinoza R et al. (2012). Protein misfolding cyclic amplification of infectious prions. Nat Protoc 7: 1397–1409.

Moudjou M, Chapuis J, Mekrouti M et al. (2016). Glycoform-independent prion conversion by highly efficient, cell-based, protein misfolding cyclic amplification. Sci Rep 6: 29116.

Orru CD, Caughey B (2011). Prion seeded conversion and amplification assays. Top CurrChem 305: 121–133.

Orru CD, Bongianni M, Tonoli G et al. (2014). A test for Creutzfeldt–Jakob disease using nasal brushings. N Engl J Med 371: 519–529.

Orru CD, Groveman BR, Hughson AG et al. (2015). Rapid and sensitive RT-QuIC detection of human Creutzfeldt–Jakob disease using cerebrospinal fluid. MBio: 6.

Park JH, Choi YG, Lee YJ et al. (2016). Real-time quaking-induced conversion analysis for the diagnosis of sporadic Creutzfeldt–Jakob disease in Korea. J Clin Neurol 12: 101–106.

Peden AH, McGuire LI, Appleford NE et al. (2012). Sensitive and specific detection of sporadic Creutzfeldt–Jakob disease brain prion protein using real-time quaking induced conversion. J Gen Virol 93: 438–449.

Puoti G, Bizzi A, Forloni G et al. (2012). Sporadic human prion diseases: molecular insights and diagnosis. Lancet Neurol 11: 618–628.

Redaelli V, Bistaffa E, Zanusso G et al. (2017). Detection of prion seeding activity in the olfactory mucosa of patients with fatal familial insomnia. Sci Rep 7: 46269.

Rubenstein R, Chang B (2013). Re-assessment of PrP(Sc) distribution in sporadic and variant CJD. PLoS One 8: e66352.

Saá P, Castilla J, Soto C (2006). Ultra-efficient replication of infectious prions by automated protein misfolding cyclic amplification. J Biol Chem 281: 35245–35252.

Saborio GP, Permanne B, Soto C (2001). Sensitive detection of pathological prion protein by cyclic amplification of protein misfolding. Nature 411: 810–813.

Sanchez-Juan P, Green A, Ladogana A et al. (2006). CSF tests in the differential diagnosis of Creutzfeldt–Jakob disease. Neurology 67: 637–643.

Sano K, Satoh K, Atarashi R et al. (2013). Early detection of abnormal prion protein in genetic human prion diseases now possible using real-time QUIC assay. PLoS One 8: e54915.

Shikiya RA, Bartz JC (2011). In vitro generation of high-titer prions. J Virol 85: 13439–13442.

Soto C, Saborío GP (2001). Prions: disease propagation and disease therapy by conformational transmission. Trends Mol Med 7: 109–114.

Soto C, Saborio GP, Anderes L (2002). Cyclic amplification of protein misfolding: application to prion-related disorders and beyond. Trends Neurosci 25: 390–394.

Tabaton M, Monaco S, Cordone MP et al. (2004). Prion deposition in olfactory biopsy of sporadic Creutzfeldt–Jakob disease. Ann Neurol 55: 294–296.

Takeuchi A, Kobayashi A, Parchi P et al. (2016). Distinctive properties of plaque-type dura mater graft-associated Creutzfeldt–Jakob disease in cell-protein misfolding cyclic amplification. Lab Investig 96: 581–587.

Tixador P, Herzog L, Reine F et al. (2010). The physical relationship between infectivity and prion protein aggregates is strain-dependent. PLoS Pathog 6: e1000859.

Vitali P, Maccagnano E (2011). Caverzasi E, et al. Diffusion-weighted MRI hyperintensity patterns differentiate CJD from other rapid dementias Neurology 76: 1711–1719.

Wang F, Wang X, Ma J (2011). Conversion of bacterially expressed recombinant prion protein. Methods 53: 208–213.

Weber P, Giese A, Piening N et al. (2007). Generation of genuine prion infectivity by serial PMCA. Vet Microbiol 123: 346–357.

Wieser HG, Schindler K, Zumsteg D (2006). EEG in Creutzfeldt-Jakob disease. Clin Neurophysiol 117 (5): 935–951.

Wilham JM, Orrú CD, Bessen RA et al. (2010). Rapid end-point quantitation of prion seeding activity with sensitivity comparable to bioassays. PLoS Pathog 6: e1001217.

World Health Organization Communicable Disease Surveillance and Response (2003). WHO manual for surveillance of human transmissible spongiform encephalopathies including variant Creutzfeldt–Jakob disease, WHO, Geneva.

Yokoyama T, Takeuchi A, Yamamoto M et al. (2011). Heparin enhances the cell-protein misfolding cyclic amplification efficiency of variant Creutzfeldt–Jakob disease. Neurosci Lett 498: 119–123.

Zanusso G, Ferrari S, Cardone F et al. (2003). Detection of pathologic prion protein in the olfactory epithelium in sporadic Creutzfeldt–Jakob disease. N Engl J Med 348: 711–719.

Zanusso G, Fiorini M, Ferrari S et al. (2011). Cerebrospinal fluid markers in sporadic Creutzfeldt–Jakob disease. Int J Mol Sci 12: 6281–6292.

Zanusso G, Bongianni M, Caughey B (2014). A test for Creutzfeldt–Jakob disease using nasal brushings. N Engl J Med 371: 1842–1843.

Zanusso G, Monaco S, Pocchiari M et al. (2016). Advanced tests for early and accurate diagnosis of Creutzfeldt–Jakob disease. Nat Rev Neurol 12: 325–333.

Zerr I, Pocchiari M, Collins S et al. (2000). Analysis of EEG and CSF 14-3-3 proteins as aids to the diagnosis of Creutzfeldt–Jakob disease. Neurology 55: 811–815.

Zerr I, Kallenberg K (2009). Summers DM, et al. Updated clinical diagnostic criteria for sporadic Creutzfeldt–Jakob disease Brain 132: 2659–2668.

Handbook of Clinical Neurology, Vol. 153 (3rd series)
Human Prion Diseases
M. Pocchiari and J. Manson, Editors
https://doi.org/10.1016/B978-0-444-63945-5.00020-9

Chapter 20

Differential diagnosis with other rapid progressive dementias

MICHAEL D. GESCHWIND[1]* AND KATY MURRAY[2]
[1]*Memory and Aging Center, Department of Neurology, University of California, San Francisco, CA, United States*
[2]*Anne Rowling Regenerative Neurology Clinic, University of Edinburgh, Edinburgh, United Kingdom*

Abstract

Prion diseases are unique in medicine as in humans they occur in sporadic, genetic, and acquired forms. The most common human prion disease is sporadic Creutzfeldt–Jakob disease (CJD), which commonly presents as a rapidly progressive dementia (RPD) with behavioral, cerebellar, extrapyramidal, and some pyramidal features, with the median survival from symptom onset to death of just a few months. Because human prion diseases, as well as other RPDs, are relatively rare, they can be difficult to diagnose, as most clinicians have seen few, if any, cases. Not only can prion diseases mimic many other conditions that present as RPD, but some of those conditions can present similarly to prion disease. In this article, the authors discuss the different etiologic categories of conditions that often present as RPD and also present RPDs that had been misdiagnosed clinically as CJD. Etiologic categories of conditions are presented in order of the mnemonic used for remembering the various categories of RPDs: VITAMINS-D, for vascular, infectious, toxic-metabolic, autoimmune, mitochondrial/metastases, iatrogenic, neurodegenerative, system/seizures/sarcoid, and demyelinating. When relevant, clinical, imaging, or other features of an RPD that overlap with those of CJD are presented.

INTRODUCTION

As presented in other chapters in this volume, human prion diseases have varied presentations, from rapidly progressive dementias (RPDs) that lead to death in just weeks or months from onset, to more slowly progressive syndromes, with durations of a few years, that could easily be confused for more typical neurodegenerative syndromes, such as Alzheimer disease (AD), frontotemporal dementia (FTD), Parkinson disease (PD), multiple system atrophy, and others. Depending on the specific prion protein gene (*PRNP*) mutation, genetic prion diseases, in particular, can present more slowly, with durations of a few years to more than a decade (Kim et al., 2017), making them even more difficult to differentiate clinically from typical, slowly progressive nonprion neurodegenerative diseases. This chapter presents disorders that might mimic prion diseases, with a focus on RPDs that lead from onset to dementia in usually less than 1–2 years but often in just weeks to months (Geschwind, 2015). It does not cover RPDs that typically progress to dementia in extremely short timeframes – i.e., hours or days – such as those resulting from infectious meningitis or acute strokes. It chapter also does not attempt to present a diagnostic decision tree or work-up for RPD, for which several articles have been published elsewhere (Woodruff, 2007; Rosenbloom and Atri, 2011; Geschwind, 2016).

Sporadic Creutzfeldt–Jakob disease (sCJD) is often referred to as "the great mimicker" because it can initially present similarly to so many other conditions (Paterson et al., 2012). Conversely, other conditions might mimic sCJD in terms of the type and rate of progression of neurologic symptoms, the elevation of cerebrospinal fluid (CSF) biomarkers of neuronal cell injury, and the presence of

*Correspondence to: Michael D. Geschwind, MD, PhD, University of California, San Francisco (UCSF), Memory and Aging Center, 675 Nelson Rising Lane, Suite 190, San Francisco CA 94158, United States. Tel: +1-415-476-2900, Fax: +1-415-476-0213, E-mail: michael.geschwind@ucsf.edu

periodic sharp-wave complexes on electroencephalogram (EEG) and/or cortical or deep nuclei hyperintensities on T2-weighted or diffusion-weighted imaging (DWI) magnetic resonance imaging (MRI) abnormalities (Chapman et al., 2000; Tschampa et al., 2001; Geschwind et al., 2003; Schmidt et al., 2012; Geschwind, 2015; Rosenbloom et al., 2015). We start by providing an overview of disorders that often present as RPDs, reviewing RPD referrals to several tertiary medical centers as well as cases referred to three major prion referral centers as CJD but that ultimately had nonprion diagnoses.

Findings from CJD and RPD referral centers

Three retrospective studies examined the causes of RPD patients admitted to three tertiary medical centers, two in Europe (Athens and Barcelona) and one in Brazil (Rio de Janeiro) (Table 20.1). The Athens study (Papageorgiou et al., 2009) reviewed the diagnoses of RPD cases referred to an inpatient unit in a tertiary referral center over 3 years, from 2004 to 2006. The authors defined RPD as progression from first symptom onset to dementia in less than 1 year. That study, however, excluded cases with acute cognitive impairment in the setting of a confusional state, caused by acute infectious, metabolic, or toxic causes such as acute viral encephalitis, acute hyponatremia, hypoglycemia, and recent use of anticholinergic drugs. The researchers identified 68 RPD subjects, with the single largest category being nonprion neurodegenerative diseases (60.3%; discussed more in the section below on neurodegenerative causes of RPD), followed by CJD (13.2%), autoimmune (8.8%), and equally represented infection, normal-pressure hydrocephalus and "other" (5.9% each). The autoimmune cases included

Table 20.1

Causes of rapid progressive dementia (RPD) in three tertiary care hospitals[a]

Athens cohort[b] (Papageorgiou et al., 2009) (*n* = 68)			Barcelona cohort[b] (Sala et al., 2012) (*n* = 49)			Rio cohort[b] (Neto et al., 2016) (*n* = 61)		
Diagnosis	*n*	%	*Diagnosis*	*n*	%	*Diagnosis*	*n*	%
Nonprion NDD	41	60.3	Nonprion NDD	18	36.7	Autoimmune[c]	28	45.9
AD	12		DLB	5		Infection	13	21.3
FTD	11		AD+CVD	4		CJD	7	11.5
DLB	4		FTD	4		Other[d]	6	9.8
MSA	2		AD	3		Metabolic	4	6.6
PSP	1		FTD-MND	2		Nonprion NDD	3	4.9
CJD	9	13.2	CJD	15	30.6	FTD	2	
Autoimmune[$]	6	8.8	Other^	5	10.2	DLB	1	
Infection	4	5.9	VaD	4	8.2			
NPH	4	5.9	Toxic-metabolic	4	8.2			
Other^	4	5.9	Unknown	3	6.2			
Total	68	100		49	100			

[a]See text.

[b]Athens cohort: patients hospitalized from January 2004 through December 2006 for dementia diagnosis with RPD defined as patient demented < 1 year after first cognitive symptom. Excluded: causes of acute cognitive impairment in context of confusional state from acute infectious, metabolic, or toxic causes (e.g., acute viral encephalitis, acute hyponatremia, hypoglycemia, and recent use of anticholinergic drugs). Barcelona cohort: patients admitted to hospital from October 1994 through March 2009 and were selected from a cerebrospinal fluid 14-3-3 registry. RPD was defined as a dementia occurring <1 year after the onset of the first cognitive symptom. Excluded: cases with acute cognitive impairment (<1 month), usually in the context of an acute confusional state, or cases with pre-existing dementia (>1 year from the first cognitive symptom). Rio cohort: patients admitted to inpatient neurologic unit from March 2012 through February 2015. RPD defined as progressing from initial symptoms to moderate (Mini Mental Status Exam (MMSE) <20) or severe (MMSE <10) within a few months to 2 years. Excluded: acute confusional states (delirium) secondary to metabolic or toxic encephalopathies.

[c]Athens autoimmune: 1 each scleroderma, sarcoidosis, systemic lupus erythematosus, primary central nervous system (CNS) vasculitis, limbic encephalitis, multiple sclerosis. Rio autoimmune: 10 anti-*N*-methyl-D-aspartate receptor (anti-NMDAR) encephalitis, 5 unknown, 3 sarcoidosis, 3 primary CNS vasculitis, 2 paraneoplastic encephalopathies, 2 Hashimoto encephalopathy, 1 each unidentified neuronal surface antibodies, Behçet, relapsing polychondritis with encephalopathy.

[d]Other. Athens cohort: CNS tumor, vitamin B_{12} deficiency, drug-induced, chronic psychosis; Barcelona cohort: paraneoplastic (syndrome of inappropriate antidiuretic hormone in the setting of cancer), CNS infection, autoimmune encephalopathy, nonconvulsive status epilepticus, chronic hydrocephalus; Rio cohort: vascular dementia, recurrent stupor, CNS lymphoma, adrenoleukodystrophy, posterior reversible encephalopathy syndrome.

AD, Alzheimer disease; CJD, Creutzfeldt–Jakob disease; CVD, cardiovascular disease; DLB, dementia with Lewy bodies; FTD, frontotemporal dementia; MND, motor neuron disease; MSA = multiple system atrophy; NDD = neurodegenerative disease; NPH, normal-pressure hydrocephalus; PSP, progressive supranuclear palsy; VaD, vascular dementia.

antibody-mediated limbic encephalopathies (LEs) as well as systemic rheumatologic or autoimmune conditions, including scleroderma ($n = 2$), sarcoidosis, systematic lupus erythematosus, central nervous system (CNS) primary vasculitis, and multiple sclerosis (MS). Infections included neurosyphilis, human immunodeficiency virus (HIV), encephalitis, and Q fever. Other conditions included CNS tumor, vitamin B_{12} deficiency, drug-induced dementia, and dementia in the setting of chronic psychosis. For the entire cohort, the mean age at onset was 65.5 ± 10.0 SD years (median: 66.7; range: 35.3–82.8), with the age of onset for the CJD cases being very close to the non-CJD cohort. The time to dementia, however, was much shorter for CJD than for non-CJD causes (mean of ~3 months vs. ~8 months), although there was great overlap in the ranges (Papageorgiou et al., 2009). One issue with this study is that the authors excluded some toxic-metabolic conditions (unclear what type), which potentially could have included conditions that sometimes can present as RPD or even mimic CJD (Geschwind, 2016).

A second retrospective study reviewed all RPD admissions over 16 years (from 1994 to 2009) at a major Barcelona hospital (Table 20.1) (Sala et al., 2012). Hospitalized patients were selected from a CSF 14-3-3 registry, with dementia occurring less than 1 year after the onset of the first cognitive symptom. Researchers excluded cases with acute cognitive impairment of durations less than 1 month or cases with pre-existing dementia (greater than 1 year from first cognitive symptom). The largest group of the 49 RPD subjects was – similar to the Athens study – nonprion neurodegenerative diseases (36.7%), followed by CJD (30.6%), and then vascular dementia and toxic-metabolic conditions (8.2% each). There were single cases of nonautoimmune paraneoplastic syndrome, infection, antibody-mediated encephalopathy, nonconvulsive status epilepticus and hydrocephalus, as well as three undiagnosed cases. The mean age of onset was 72.4 ± 11.6 SD (range 41–86), with time from onset to evaluation of 4.6 ± 3.8 (1–12) months. Among the 19 cases followed until death, mean survival was 8.6 ± 9.5 months, but the prion subset had significantly shorter survival (3.3 ± 2.4 (1–8) vs. 14 ± 11.1 (5–34), $p = 0.04$) (Sala et al., 2012).

In the Rio de Janeiro study, researchers reviewed cases referred to an inpatient neurologic unit over 3 years, from 2012 to 2015, with RPD defined as progressing to moderate or severe dementia in a timeframe ranging from months to less than 2 years (Table 20.1). They excluded acute confusional states (e.g., delirium) from toxic or metabolic causes. Their findings were quite different from those of the two older studies, as they found autoimmune and infectious etiologies to be much more common (Neto et al., 2016). CJD accounted for 11.5% of cases, similar to the rate identified in the Athens study. The higher infectious etiology of RPDs in Brazil is not unexpected, as there is a high prevalence of infectious agents in this region. The higher percentage of autoimmune cases, however, is probably attributable to increasing awareness and the expanding ability to test for antibody-mediated encephalopathies (Graus et al., 2016; Neto et al., 2016).

Another way to ascertain mimickers of CJD is to review cases referred to CJD referral centers that turn out not to have CJD. Table 20.2 shows the breakdown of nonprion/CJD diagnoses (misdiagnoses) referred to the German CJD Surveillance Center, the US National Prion Disease Pathology Surveillance Center (NPDPSC) and the University of California, San Francisco (UCSF) Memory and Aging Center (MAC) (Poser et al., 1999; Chitravas et al., 2011; Geschwind, 2015). In the German study, slightly more than one-third of patients referred for CJD evaluation by outside physicians were ultimately found by pathology or clinical follow-up to have nonprion diagnoses. Importantly, although about half had a nonprion neurodegenerative disease, many patients had conditions that were not only treatable, but potentially reversible (Poser et al., 1999).

The UCSF MAC is a major clinical prion referral center in the United States. Approximately one-quarter of the UCSF RPD cohort had an in-person inpatient or outpatient evaluation; for the remainder, the researchers conducted detailed reviews of records and communications with the patients, families, and/or their physicians. About one-quarter of all referrals to, and about 45% of those evaluated in person at, UCSF ultimately received non-CJD/ nonprion diagnoses. Table 20.2 shows the breakdown of nonprion diagnoses over an approximately 8-year period from 2002 to 2010 (Geschwind et al., 2008; Geschwind, 2016).

The most common nonprion RPD diagnostic category was nonprion neurodegenerative diseases, followed by undiagnosed dementias and vascular dementia. Antibody-mediated encephalopathies and related autoimmune neurologic conditions were also common, even in some of these cohorts. As some of these studies are one to two decades old, however, it is likely that antibody-mediated encephalopathies today are an even larger percentage of nonprion RPDs than shown in Table 20.2. At UCSF, several patients had adult-onset leukoencephalopathies/ leukodystrophies of unclear cause. Several patients with meningoencephalitis were referred as suspected CJD despite pleiocytosis being extremely rare in prion disease (Green et al., 2007; Geschwind et al., 2008).

To help monitor for potential new forms of human prion disease in the United States, the Centers for Disease Control and Prevention funds the US NPDPSC (Cleveland, OH) to perform brain autopsies on all referred suspected prion cases. Of the 1106 autopsies performed over about a 10-year period, 32% ($n = 352$) of the subjects did not have prion disease. Among the 304 in whom the

Table 20.2

Diagnostic breakdown of non-Creutzfeldt–Jakob disease rapidly progressive dementia referrals to three Creutzfeldt–Jakob disease centers[a]

German cohort (Poser et al., 1999) ($n = 124$) (37)[b]	%	National Prion Disease Pathology Surveillance Center (NPDPSC) cohort (Chitravas et al., 2011) ($n = 304$) (304)[b]	%	University of California, San Francisco (UCSF) cohort (Geschwind, 2016) ($n = 104$) (21)[b]	%
Alzheimer disease	27	Alzheimer disease	51	Antibody-mediated or autoimmune[c]	13
Unclassified dementia	16	Vascular disease	12	Unclassified dementia	13
Cerebrovascular (vascular dementia, cerebrovascular accident)	9	Immune-mediated	9	Psychiatric	12
Encephalitis – unknown	8	Neoplasia	8	Dementia with Lewy bodies	8
Parkinson disease	5	Infections	5	Encephalitis not otherwise specified	8
Psychiatric	5	Unspecified degenerative disease	3	Neoplasm	8
Motor neuron disease	2	Frontal lobe degeneration	3	Frontotemporal dementia with or without motor neuron disease	7
Multiple sclerosis	2	Metabolic	2	Corticobasal syndrome or degeneration	6
Paraneoplastic	2	Hippocampal sclerosis	2	Alzheimer disease[d]	5
Toxicity	2	Dementia with Lewy bodies	1	Central nervous system vasculitis	3
Alcohol-induced	2	Taupathy, not otherwise specified	1	Encephalopathy not otherwise specified	3
Brain tumor	2	Hereditary diffuse leukoencephalopathy with spheroids	1	Leukoencephalopathy	3
Chronic epilepsy	2	Progressive supranuclear palsy	1	Progressive supranuclear palsy	3
Corticostriatonigral degeneration	2	Other[e]	2	Vascular dementia	2
Familial spastic paraplegia	2			Other[e]	8
Hashimoto encephalopathy	2				
Hereditary ataxia	2				
Huntington disease	2				
Metabolic disorder	2				
Primary central nervous system lymphoma	2				
Other[e]	4				
Total	100	Total	100	Total	100

Reproduced with permission from Geschwind (2016).

[a]Numbers in parentheses indicate the number of pathology-proven cases.

[b]If a single case in cohort, placed under "Other."

[c]Includes antivoltage-gated potassium channel complex, glutamic acid decarboxylase (GAD65), Yu, Hu, CV2, adenylate kinase5, α-amino-3-hydroxy-5-methylisoxazole-4-proprionic acid (AMPA) receptor, glial, neuropil, and other antibodies as well as Hashimoto encephalopathy.

[d]Includes 2 mixed Alzheimer with Lewy bodies.

[e]Other UCSF cohort cases include hydrocephalus, mesial temporal sclerosis, vertigo, germinoma, methylmalonic acidemia, multiple sclerosis, methotrexate toxicity, and pathology-proven sarcoid. Other German cohort cases include leukoencephalopathy, amyloid angiopathy, fatal familial insomnia, hypoxia, and Niemann–Pick lipoid histiocytosis. Other NPDPSC cohort cases include corticobasal degeneration, adult polyglucosan body disease, Huntington disease, Marchiafava–Bignami disease, and superficial siderosis.

Table 20.3

Differential for possible rapid progressive dementia mimickers of Creutzfeldt–Jakob disease by etiologic category

Vascular/ischemic
Vascular dementia
Multi-infarct dementia
Thalamic, callosal, or other strategic infarcts
Sinus venous thrombosis
Dural arteriovenous fistulas
Subdural hematoma
Cerebral amyloid angiopathy-related inflammation
Abeta-amyloid-related angiopathy
Primary central nervous system (CNS) vasculitis
Primary angiitis of the CNS
Posterior reversible encephalopathy syndrome
Cerebroretinal microangiopathy with calcifications and cysts
Subacute diencephalic angioencephalopathy
Infectious
Viral encephalitis, including herpes simplex virus
Human immunodeficiency virus dementia
Fungal infections (e.g., CNS aspergillosis, coccidioidomycosis)
Spirochete infection/syphilis
Subacute sclerosing panencephalitis (young adults)
Progressive multifocal leukoencephalopathy
Amebic infection (e.g., balamuthia)
Lyme disease (rarely encephalopathy)
Whipple disease (rarely rapid)
Urinary tract infection or pneumonia in elderly or mild-dementia patient
Toxic-metabolic
Electrolyte disturbances (Na, Ca, Mg, P)
Endocrine abnormalities (thyroid, parathyroid, adrenal)
Extrapontine myelinolysis
Vitamin B_{12} (cyanocobalmin) deficiency
Vitamin B_1 (thiamine) deficiency (Wernicke)
Hepatic encephalopathy
Portosystemic shunt encephalopathy
Acquired hepatocerebral degeneration
Uremic encephalopathy
Hypoxia/hypercarbia
Hyper/hypoglycemia
Niacin deficiency (not usually rapid)
Folate deficiency (dementia rare)
Poikilothermia
Phenylketonuria
Porphyria
Metal toxicity (bismuth, Li, Hg, Mg (parkinsonism))
Methylmalonic academia
Autoimmune
Antibody-mediated dementia/encephalopathy
Lupus cerebritis
Other central nervous system vasculitides
Hashimoto encephalopathy
Acute disseminated encephalomyelitis (also under demyelinating)
Metastases/neoplasm-related/mitochondrial
Paraneoplastic diseases – limbic encephalopathy
Metastases to CNS
Primary CNS lymphoma
Intravascular lymphoma
Lymphomatoid granulomatosis
Lymphomatosis cerebri
Gliomatosis cerebri
Metastatic encephalopathy
Carcinomatous meningitis
Mitochondrial encephalopathies (e.g., mitochondrial encephalopathy lactic acidosis, strokes, and leukoencephalopathy)
Iatrogenic
Medication toxicity (e.g. lithium, bismuth, methotrexate, chemotherapy)
Illicit drug use
Neurodegenerative
Prion disease
Alzheimer disease
Dementia with Lewy bodies
Frontotemporal dementia
Corticobasal degeneration
Progressive supranuclear palsy
Neurofilament inclusion body disease
Progressive subcortical gliosis
Systemic/seizures/sarcoid/structural
Sarcoidosis
Epilepsy
Nonconvulsive status epilepticus
Spontaneous intracranial hypotension
Demyelinating
Multiple sclerosis
Acute demyelinating encephalomyelitis
Extrapontine myelinolysis (also under metabolic)

NPDPSC confirmed a specific nonprion pathologic diagnosis, 77% had incurable conditions, but 23% ($n = 71$) had treatable or reversible dementias (Chitravas et al., 2011). Of these 71 treatable cases, 37% were immune-mediated, 35% were neoplasia, 20% were infections, and 8% were metabolic disorders (Chitravas et al., 2011). Although one positive aspect of this NPDPSC study was that all cases were pathology-proven, this is also a shortcoming, as it does not include RPD patients who did not die or come to autopsy. Thus, many conditions that were treatable or reversible if caught early enough would not have been included, whereas they would have been included in the German and UCSF studies, which included nonpathology-proven cases.

Table 20.3 presents the major etiologic categories of RPDs as illustrated by the mnemonic VITAMINS-D, for vascular, infectious, toxic-metabolic, autoimmune, mitochondrial/metastases, iatrogenic, neurodegenerative, systemic/seizures/sarcoid, and demyelinating. The table also includes many examples of conditions in each etiologic category that can present as RPD, some of which might mimic CJD. Some conditions could be represented in more than one category. In the rest of this chapter, we discuss various RPDs based on etiologic category, with a focus on those that are more likely to mimic CJD.

VASCULAR

Numerous vascular etiologies – including strategic strokes or multiple infarcts, cerebral amyloid angiopathy-related inflammation (CAA-ri), dural arteriovenous fistulas (DAVFs), sinus thrombosis, and hypertensive encephalopathy – can cause RPD, sometimes having clinical overlap with CJD (Harkness et al., 2004; Geraldes et al., 2012; Mendonca et al., 2012; Labeyrie et al., 2014; Pasi et al., 2014; Geschwind, 2016). Other secondary vascular insults that also can present as RPD, such as CNS vasculitis and intravascular lymphoma, are discussed in other sections.

Multiple infarcts can cause RPD with restricted diffusion on MRI, although the pattern would have a vascular distribution and usually would not be the pattern of cortical ribboning, basal ganglia, or thalamic hyperintensity seen in CJD (Vitali et al., 2011). Strategic strokes – particularly those affecting the basal ganglia or thalamus – might have a DWI/apparent diffusion coefficient (ADC) MRI pattern overlapping with those seen in prion disease. Ischemia in each of the four primary arterial territories in the thalamus causes a different syndrome, which can include behavioral, amnestic, and other cortical symptoms, some of which could overlap with conditions with limbic or diffuse brain involvement (Auchus et al., 2002; Carrera and Bogousslavsky, 2006; Stretz and Finelli, 2015), as often occurs in CJD. CJD can also have acute, stroke-like onset, but in CJD the restricted diffusion pattern of changes will persist and spread over weeks to months (Cataldi et al., 2000; Hohler and Flynn, 2006). Other imaging modalities – such as hemosiderin-sensitive MRI sequences, MR angiography, MR venography, CT angiography, and conventional angiography – can aid in diagnosis of vascular RPD etiologies.

Several cases of DAVFs causing RPD have been published. Most cases present with headache, progressive confusion, and amnesia progressing over the course of weeks to months; some cases also have presented with seizures, gait instability, and/or focal neurologic deficits, including aphasia, facial palsy, or hemiparesis. If a DAVF is suspected, it is important to auscultate the skull in the region of MRI abnormality, as a bruit often can be heard, which helps to confirm the diagnosis. Among 20 published cases we reviewed, diagnosis was made by angiogram. Treatments (usually embolization alone, but sometimes surgery or both) improved cognitive function in most cases (mean age was 60 years (range 55–77years). The time from onset to development of dementia ranged from approximately 2 to 12 months (Zeidman et al., 1995; Hurst et al., 1998; Geraldes et al., 2012; Mendonca et al., 2012; Abe et al., 2014; Labeyrie et al., 2014; Pasi et al., 2014; Imazeki et al., 2015).

On brain MRI, the most common abnormalities are diffuse high-signal intensities in the cerebral or cerebellar white matter with enlarged vessels over the hemispheric surface on T2-weighted imaging. There has been at least one report of a case with basal ganglia T2-weighted hyperintensity (Fig. 20.1) (Geraldes et al., 2012), although this was in the globus pallidus – an area not commonly involved radiologically in CJD (Vitali et al., 2011). As DAVFs are readily treatable, they are important to consider in an RPD patient with patchy diffuse white-matter MRI hyperintensities.

Sinus venous thrombosis can present as RPD; depending on the location of the thrombus, it might present with headaches, papilledema, visual loss or other focal neurologic deficits, seizures, altered mental status, or even coma. Brain MRI typically shows cerebral edema and venous infarction – although MRI findings can be subtle, with mild white-matter hyperintensity, and therefore easily missed – and CT or MR venogram is helpful for identifying the thrombus. MRI findings might overlap somewhat with CJD; thrombosis of deep veins might cause unilateral or symmetric basal ganglia and/or thalamic T2-weighted hyperintensity as well as T2-weighted cortical hyperintensity with or without restricted diffusion (Fig. 20.2) (Wasay and Azeemuddin, 2005; Geraldes et al., 2012). These findings might raise concern for CJD, but concomitant edema and/or contrast enhancement as well as a venous drainage distribution of the abnormalities found in sinus venous thrombosis should suggest against a prion diagnosis.

Cerebral amyloid angiopathy (CAA) can cause an RPD, particularly when there is CAA-ri. Patients with CAA-ri often present with subacute cognitive decline or encephalopathy, headache, seizures, and/or focal neurologic deficits. Age of onset is around 67, about a decade younger than in CAA (Eng et al., 2004; Kirshner and Bradshaw, 2015; Miller-Thomas et al., 2016). Hemosiderin-sensitive sequences typically reveal multiple large or small hemorrhages, often in areas in which there are T2-weighted white-matter hyperintensities and edema (Sarazin et al., 2002; Crosta et al., 2015; Yamada, 2015). Vasogenic, confluent edema, superficial siderosis, and leptomeningeal enhancement may also be seen (Crosta et al., 2015). Elevated erythrocyte sedimentation rate, CSF pleiocytosis, and/or protein are present in a minority of patients. Although the majority of cases have poor outcome, many cases improve with steroids (Eng et al., 2004; Kirshner and Bradshaw, 2015; Miller-Thomas et al., 2016).

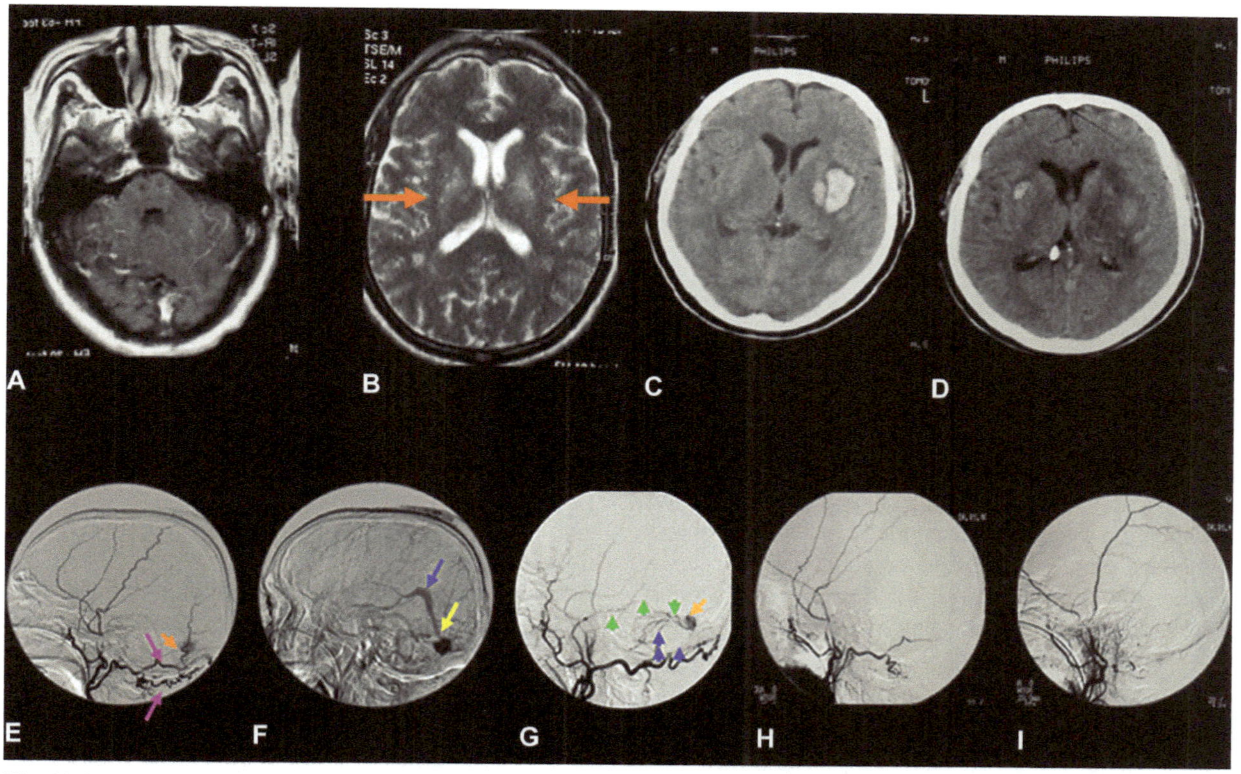

Fig. 20.1. Imaging in a dural arteriovenous fistula. (**A** and **B**) T1-weighted brain magnetic resonance imaging (MRI) scan with gadolinium and T2-weighted brain MRI scan performed on admission for a 64-year-old hypertensive, diabetic man, who was admitted for a 3-month history of progressive cognitive decline, gait disturbance, and myoclonus. Engorged cerebellar veins (**A**) and basal ganglia hypersignal on T2-weighted brain MRI (red arrows) without white-matter involvement (**B**). (**C**) Computed tomographic (CT) scan performed 2 days after admission showing a left capsulolenticular hematoma. (**D**) CT scan performed 9 days after admission showing a recurrent right lenticular hemorrhage. Left (**E**, **F**, and **G**) and right (**E** and **I**) external carotid angiography before (**E**, **F**, and **G**) and after (**H** and **I**) embolization. Pre-embolization angiography (**E**, **F**, and **G**) depicts a type IIb (Djindjian and Merland classification) dural fistula. The occipital artery afferents can be seen (purple arrows), the fistula point (orange arrow), and the early appearance of the veins, such as the torculla (yellow), proximal lateral sinus, and engorged straight sinus (blue), with stasis in the deep venous system. Postembolization images (**H** and **I**) show total angiographic exclusion of the fistula. (Reproduced with permission from Geraldes R, Albuquerque L, Ferro JM, et al. (2012) Rapidly progressive cognitive impairment, ataxia, and myoclonus: an unusual presentation of a dural arteriovenous fistula. J Stroke Cerebrovasc Dis 21: 619 e613–615.)

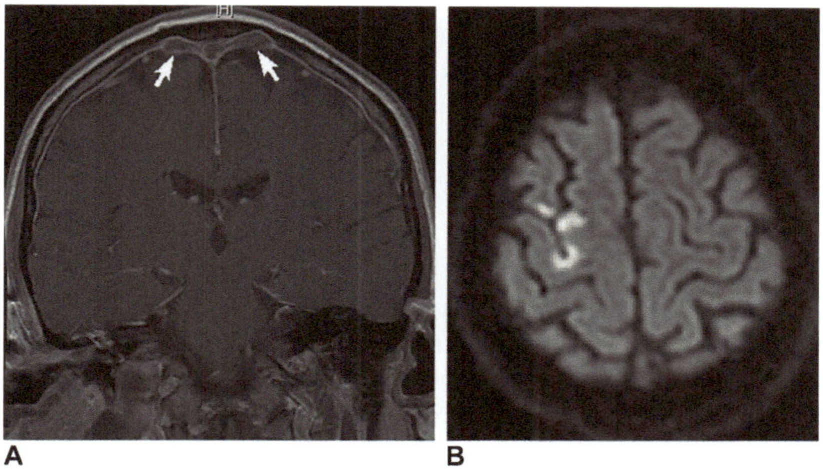

Fig. 20.2. Sinus venous thrombosis with cortical ribboning. Brain magnetic resonance imaging in sinus venous thrombosis. Cortical venous infarction in a 58-year-old man, secondary to a superior sagittal sinus thrombosis. (**A**) Coronal, contrast-enhanced, T1-weighted image demonstrates superior sagittal sinus thrombosis. There is propagation of thrombus into cortical veins (arrows). (**B**) The diffusion-weighted image ($b = 1000\ s/mm^2$) demonstrates cortical restricted diffusion in the right posterior frontal region. (Reproduced with permission from Sheerin F, Pretorius PM, Briley D, et al. (2008) Differential diagnosis of restricted diffusion confined to the cerebral cortex. Clin Radiol 63: 1245–1253.)

Primary angiitis of the CNS, although a vasculitis, can present clinically and radiologically very similarly to CAA-ri, whereas CAA-ri has amyloid deposition in blood vessels and is a perivasculitis (Moussaddy et al., 2015). The mean age of onset of primary angiitis of the CNS is about 45 years, much younger than for CAA-ri (Kirshner and Bradshaw, 2015).

Two rare angiopathies that have been reported to manifest as RPDs with clinical overlap with CJD are cerebroretinal microangiopathy with calcifications and cysts and subacute diencephalic angioencephalopathy. Although cerebroretinal microangiopathy with calcifications and cysts is a very rare condition that more commonly occurs in children, a case has been reported of a 62-year-old with 2 months' rapidly progressive cognitive decline, ataxia, spasticity, and seizures with calcifications and contrast enhancement on neuroimaging (Cachia et al., 2014). Subacute diencephalic angioencephalopathy, an RPD that some authors consider a severe form of posterior reversible encephalopathy syndrome, is characterized by acute cognitive changes, sometimes with seizures, and often rapid progression to death, with imaging showing bilateral thalamic involvement. Pathology usually has shown a profound vasculopathy with noninflammatory parenchymal necrosis and gliosis. Brain MRI typically shows nonenhancing confluent fluid-attenuated inversion recovery (FLAIR)/T2 hyperintensities in the thalamus and sometimes other regions, such as the occipital and temporal lobes and the pons (Fig. 20.3) (Graffeo et al., 2016).

INFECTIONS

A wide variety of infections can present with subacute encephalitis or RPD, which might mimic prion disease.

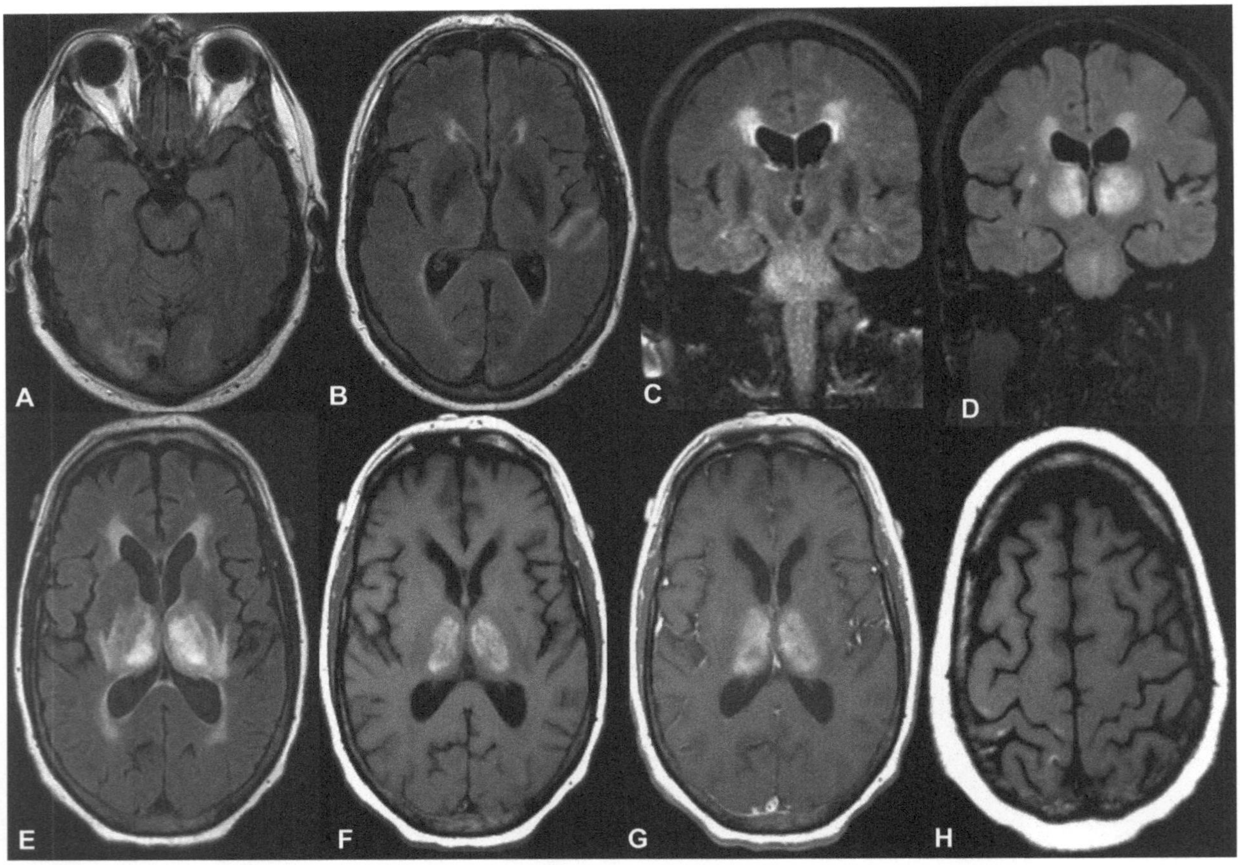

Fig. 20.3. Brain magnetic resonance imaging of a 68-year-old patient with subacute diencephalic angioencephalopathy. Nonenhancing, confluent subcortical axial fluid-attenuated inversion recovery (FLAIR) hyperintensities in the occipital lobes (**A**) and left temporal lobe (**B**) in the early phases with nasal dysarthria. Confluent nonenhancing abnormal coronal T2-weighted signal symmetrically in the pons, as well as confluent periventricular T2-weighted signal, about 17 months later when he had parieto-occipital headaches, confusion, and speech and language deficits. (**C**). One month later, when he developed an encephalopathy with tremor, dystonia, postural instability, and a shuffling gait, FLAIR images demonstrated bilaterally symmetric T1- and T2-weighted hyperintense, abnormal signal in the thalami (**D**, coronal; **E**, axial). Thalamic abnormalities enhanced minimally following gadolinium administration on axial T1-weighted images (**F**, unenhanced; **G**, enhanced). (**H**) Small T1- and T2-weighted hyperintense cortical foci on axial T1-weighted images. (Reproduced with permission from Graffeo CS, Dawson ET, Murphy ME, et al. (2016) Expanding the spectrum of subacute diencephalic angioencephalopathy. J Clin Neurosci 23: 8–13.)

It is important to identify these prion mimics, because many are treatable and early recognition and treatment are typically associated with better long-term outcomes. There is significant geographic variability in the prevalence of many of these infections, although this is constantly evolving due to climate change and the increase in world travel. This is especially relevant with tick- and mosquito-borne viruses. For example, Japanese encephalitis has now spread from Asia to northern territories of Australia; there have been rapid increases in West Nile virus infection in North America and Toscana virus in southern Europe; and the chikungunya virus has emerged in the tropics and subtropics. Clinicians need to be alert to not only local and indigenous infections, but also to those potentially affecting returning travelers. The immune status of an individual is vital in determining which infections the person might be at risk of acquiring and how these infections present. Therefore, we recommend HIV testing for all individuals presenting with a rapid dementia, even in the absence of conventional risk factors.

Most infectious encephalitides typically present acutely or subacutely over a few days, and the time course is readily distinguishable from even the most rapid case of prion disease. A proportion of infections, however, have a more insidious course, which can add to diagnostic confusion. Other clues to look for include clinical features of fever, myalgia, meningism; clues from the history, such as returning travelers, infectious contacts, or immunocompromised state (including from medication); and investigation results such as elevated serum inflammatory markers, eosinophilia (for parasitic infections) and CSF pleiocytosis. Infectious encephalitides can be subdivided into viral, bacterial, fungal, parasitic, and amebic etiologies, plus all opportunistic infections infecting immunosuppressed individuals (Geschwind, 2016). Despite best efforts, the etiologic agent often cannot be identified; in one large US study, the California Encephalitis Project, more than 60% of cases went undiagnosed (Glaser et al., 2003), although eventually some of them were ultimately identified not as infections, but rather as autoimmune encephalitis, such as *N*-methyl-D-aspartate receptor (NMDAR) encephalitis. The application of metagenomic next-generation sequencing of human CSF to identify nonhuman DNA of potentially harmful infectious agents is changing the field of infectious disease (Berger and Wilson, 2016; Schlaberg et al., 2017). This technology is becoming available clinically and has already improved our ability to identify causative infectious organisms in diagnostically difficult neurologic cases (Wilson et al., 2014, 2015, 2017; Chiu et al., 2017).

Viral infections

Herpes simplex virus (HSV) type 1 is a relatively common cause of viral encephalitis worldwide and potentially treatable if identified early. If HSV encephalitis is a possible diagnosis, it is important to start empiric early treatment with acyclovir while awaiting CSF viral polymerase chain reaction (PCR) results. As false negatives do occur, if there is a high suspicion for HSV infection, two or three serial lumbar punctures with HSV PCR might be required or next-generation sequencing might be considered (Berger and Wilson, 2016). HSV encephalitis has an acute to subacute time course of a few days, but more insidious onset is well recognized. Brain MRI in HSV encephalitis typically shows T2-weighted hyperintensities in the medial temporal lobes, edema, and/or hemorrhage. Cortical ribboning, often with restricted diffusion, particularly in the setting of seizures, has also been reported, which might be confused with CJD (Fig. 20.4) (Sheerin et al., 2008; McGinnis, 2011). Other herpesviruses to consider include HSV-2, enterovirus, Epstein–Barr virus, cytomegalovirus, and human herpesvirus types 6A and 6B (Agut et al., 2017). These are ubiquitous viruses that rarely cause significant neurologic disease but occasionally can cause encephalitis, particularly in immunocompromised individuals such as those with acquired immunodeficiency syndrome (AIDS) or in the posttransplant setting.

Japanese encephalitis, caused by a mosquito-borne flavivirus, is the most significant cause of viral encephalitis worldwide. Most infections are asymptomatic, but a very small number – less than 1% – develop potentially fatal encephalitis, often with extrapyramidal manifestations. Treatment is aimed at prevention through mosquito and pig control and through vaccination, as there is no specific antiviral therapy (Misra and Kalita, 2010). Other flaviviruses that usually cause minimal, if any, symptoms but in rare instances can cause severe encephalitis include West Nile virus and Toscana virus. Diagnosis is based on positive serology, and treatment is largely supportive.

Subacute sclerosing panencephalitis is caused by a mutated and slow, but persistent, form of the wild-type measles virus. Although rare and usually a pediatric illness, it can present in young (Chakor and Santosh, 2013) and even early middle-aged adults (Gascon and Frosch, 1998; Prashanth et al., 2006; Anuja et al., 2018). The clinical phenotype of prominent myoclonus, progressive cognitive decline, visual disturbance, and pyramidal and extrapyramidal signs can be easily mistaken for CJD (though the age of onset is typically younger than with sporadic prion disease). The typical EEG in subacute sclerosing panencephalitis is periodic triphasic complexes similar to those seen in sCJD, but at a lower frequency. The diagnosis is confirmed by raised antimeasles antibody titer in the CSF. It is invariably fatal, usually within 1–3 years of onset (Prashanth et al., 2006).

Bacterial infections, including spirochetes

Syphilis, caused by the spirochete *Treponema pallidum*, if untreated may cause dementia in its tertiary stage.

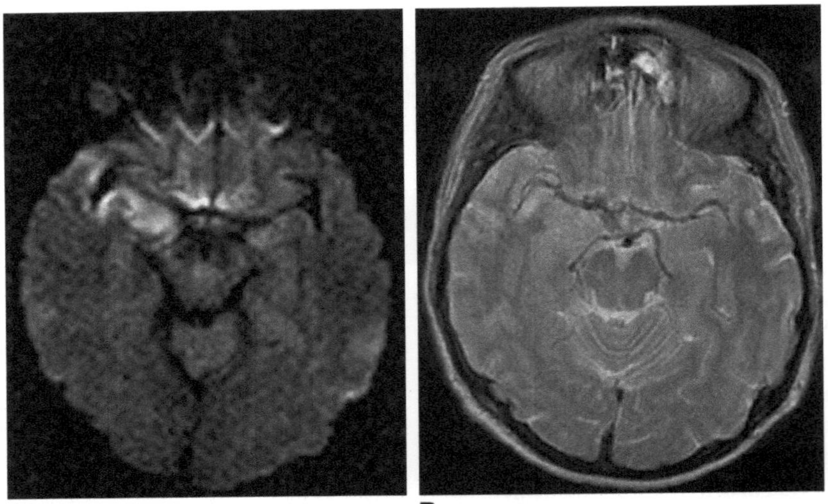

Fig. 20.4. Brain magnetic resonance imaging in herpes simplex encephalitis. Herpes simplex encephalitis in a 65-year-old woman. (**A**) The diffusion-weighted images ($b = 1000\ s/mm^2$) show cortical high signal in the right temporal pole. This extended into the cingulate gyrus (not shown). (**B**) T2-weighted images demonstrate only subtle changes in the same location. The apparent diffusion coefficient map (not shown) confirmed restricted diffusion in the areas involved. (Reproduced with permission from Sheerin F, Pretorius PM, Briley D, et al. (2008) Differential diagnosis of restricted diffusion confined to the cerebral cortex. Clin Radiol 63: 1245–1253.)

Other neuropsychiatric symptoms of neurosyphilis include mood disturbance, psychosis, ataxia, and movement disorders. RPD attributable to neurosyphilis has been reported (Lee et al., 2009; Marra, 2015; Anuja et al., 2018). Diagnosis of tertiary syphilis is based on the clinical phenotype supported by CSF lymphocytosis and positive treponemal and nontreponemal tests in CSF and serum (Janier et al., 2014). In many developed countries, including the United States, the incidence of syphilis has been increasing since 2000 (Marra, 2016). Tertiary syphilis is potentially treatable with intravenous long-acting penicillin.

Lyme disease, caused by the *Borrelia burgdorferi* spirochete, can also manifest as an encephalomyelitis in addition to the more common skin, joint, and peripheral nervous system manifestations. Again, it is diagnosed by serology and supportive CSF and imaging and is treatable (Dandashi et al., 2016). Unfortunately, many patients referred to our dementia clinic at UCSF with cognitive problems attributed to Lyme disease have had false-positive Lyme antibody tests and likely do not have Lyme disease. Accepted algorithms for Lyme antibody testing should be followed to avoid such false-positive cases (Moore et al., 2016).

Whipple disease is a rare, systemic disease caused by the bacteria *Tropheryma whipplei*. It characteristically causes a malabsorption syndrome with weight loss, abdominal pain, diarrhea, and arthralgia. Up to 45% of cases can have neuropsychiatric manifestations preceding the gastrointestinal features, including behavioral change, cerebellar signs, and seizures; although rare, a small number of cases can also present with severe RPD (Christidi et al., 2014). In addition, a few cases presenting as RPD have been published (Hurth et al., 2015; Hale et al., 2016). Diagnosis is based on identification of *T. whipplei* by PCR from serum, CSF, jejunal biopsy or brain biopsy, or positive periodic acid–Schiff staining on small-bowel biopsy. It is treatable with prolonged antibiotic therapy.

Bartonella henselae is the etiologic agent for cat scratch disease, which is usually a benign, self-limiting illness of childhood with lymphadenopathy. In rare cases it can cause a subacute encephalopathy, often with seizures, in adults and children, as well as in immunocompetent and immunocompromised patients (Yamashita et al., 2012). Mycoplasma infections can also, in rare instances, cause encephalitis, and serologic testing should be considered (Glaser et al., 2003). We are aware of two reports of cases with restricted diffusion in the bilateral pulvinar and also T2-weighted cortical ribboning in adults with encephalopathy, although both cases had prolonged seizures (Singhal et al., 2003).

Opportunistic CNS infections

It is vital to know a patient's HIV status because rare infectious and noninfectious diseases enter the differential diagnosis, largely reflecting the degree of T-cell-mediated immunosuppression. Although improved availability and efficacy of modern antiretroviral therapy mean that opportunistic CNS infections are diminishing in treated HIV patients, a large proportion of HIV-infected individuals are unaware of their diagnosis and therefore remain untreated and vulnerable to infection.

Treatment of CNS opportunistic infections can be particularly challenging in HIV patients because antiretroviral therapy can result in immune reconstitution inflammatory syndrome, causing paradoxic worsening of infection-related symptoms (Bowen et al., 2016). Infections that cause disease in both immunocompetent and immunosuppressed individuals often demonstrate different clinical and radiographic features depending on immune status. For example, tuberculosis (TB) is one of the most prevalent worldwide infections, affecting individuals regardless of their immune state, but in those with underlying HIV, TB is more likely to be disseminated throughout the body and TB meningitis is more common. Additionally, diagnosis can be hindered by negative tuberculin skin tests and less dramatic CSF findings compared with immunocompetent individuals, with lower levels of CSF lymphocytosis. TB meningitis characteristically presents with nonspecific features of malaise, fever, headache, and confusion / reduced conscious level, but it can also present with focal signs of lower cranial nerve dysfunction and limb weakness.

Toxoplasmosis in the HIV setting typically manifests as multiple cerebral abscesses presenting with focal neurologic signs, sometimes preceded by a nonspecific prodrome of cognitive decline or personality change (Hegde et al., 2011; Basavaraju, 2016). Such cases usually should not be confused with CJD; however, on rare occasions toxoplasmosis encephalitis occurs with no focal lesions and a corresponding diffuse presentation of confusion and cognitive impairment. Toxoplasmosis might be suspected by the presence of typical ring-enhancing lesions on MRI and can usually be diagnosed by CSF PCR for *Toxoplasma gondii*, but occasionally brain biopsy is required. It is treatable with first-line sulfadiazine and pyrimethamine (Basavaraju, 2016).

Cryptococcal meningitis is a fungal infection with *Cryptococcus neoformans*, or, less frequently, *C. gattii*, occurring with severe immunosuppression (CD4 count less than 50 cells/μL). A leading cause of HIV-associated fatal opportunistic infections worldwide, it has an insidious presentation over weeks, with headache, malaise, fever, and altered cognition occurring in at least 25% of cases. Those with altered mental state are most likely to mimic prion disease and also to have the worst prognosis (Jarvis et al., 2014). Treatment is with amphotericin B-based regimes, followed by antiretroviral therapy.

Progressive multifocal leukoencephalopathy (PML) is a demyelinating CNS disease caused by reactivation of the ubiquitous JC polyomavirus (John Cunningham virus) in immunosuppressed patients. It occurs in AIDS but is increasingly recognized in people receiving long-term immunomodulatory therapy for diverse conditions, such as MS, inflammatory bowel disease, systemic lupus erythematosus, and posttransplant (Bloomgren et al., 2012; Molloy et al., 2017).

The JC virus infects astrocytes and oligodendrocytes, causing a progressive white-matter syndrome. This can manifest as isolated behavioral cognitive decline, seizures, and focal signs such as cortical visual impairment or hemiparesis. It is usually fatal if the cause of the immunosuppression cannot be reversed, and survivors are typically severely disabled, as there is no specific antiviral therapy available. Withdrawal of the immunosuppressive drug aids survival, but recovery can be complicated by immune reconstitution inflammatory syndrome (N'Gbo N'gbo Ikazabo et al., 2016). Early diagnosis of PML improves the outcome but relies on a high level of clinical suspicion, identification of JC virus DNA in CSF or brain biopsy, and appreciation of the characteristic white-matter hyperintensities on MRI (and distinguishing these from alternatives such as toxoplasmosis or cryptococcal lesions, or multiple sclerosis plaques when PML occurs in the context of immunotherapy for MS).

HIV-associated neurocognitive disorder is a term encompassing varying severities of cognitive impairment seen in HIV, independent of opportunistic infection, and most likely attributable to direct HIV infection within the brain with secondary neurodegeneration. Historically there were many cases of AIDS dementia complex, now termed HIV-associated dementia, with a severe, rapid, subcortical dementia causing death within a year and easily mistaken for prion disease if HIV status was not known. With the advent of highly active retroviral therapy, however, these RPDs are now rare, at least in the western world. Unfortunately, more than 50% of individuals with HIV continue to experience cognitive impairment, but this is milder, cortical rather than subcortical phenotype, more slowly progressive over many years, and seemingly independent of antiretroviral therapy, viral load, or CD4 count (Clifford and Ances, 2013).

TOXIC-METABOLIC

Toxic-metabolic etiologies of RPDs should always be considered, as many are treatable and even reversible. Identification of such conditions requires a thorough review of medications – including over-the-counter, herbals, and supplements – and a detailed exposure history, such as reviewing the work and home environments. Although all patients with dementia should be screened for vitamin B_{12} and thyroid deficiency, as the clinical deficits are often or potentially reversible, these generally do not present as an RPD. Other endocrine dysfunction might also be considered, depending on the clinical presentation. Any dementia screen should include basic electrolytes (including serum calcium, magnesium, and phosphorus levels).

Elevated lithium, often iatrogenic, can cause encephalopathy or RPD. In addition to confusion, patients might have myoclonus, gait disturbance, parkinsonism, visual disturbances, and other neurologic abnormalities (Kikyo and Furukawa, 1999).

Lead exposure from environmental and occupational sources continues to be an issue in many communities and homes. Inorganic lead poisoning in adults typically leads to peripheral neuropathy, whereas lead poisoning in children often leads to cognitive impairment and encephalopathy, particularly with acute exposure. Organic lead is a gasoline additive and much more toxic than inorganic lead; even minimal exposure can cause psychiatric and behavioral symptoms, including agitation, disturbed sleep patterns, and hallucinations (Bolla, 1999), with a predilection for adversely affecting the limbic system (Verity, 1990).

Similarly to lead toxicity, inorganic and organic mercury can lead to neurotoxicity and encephalopathy. A prime example of this is the "mad as a hatter" syndrome, with tremor and neurobehavioral disorder caused by inorganic mercury exposure in industrial settings (Bolla, 1999).

Organic mercury toxicity usually results in a triad of concentric visual field loss, paresthesias, and cerebellar ataxia, without tremor. It has also occurred, sometimes in large numbers, from grain contamination as well as industrial exposure. Acute arsenic toxicity, although typically tested for in serum and urine heavy-metal screens, causes early gastrointestinal and circulatory problems, followed weeks later by a length-dependent sensorimotor polyneuropathy and desquamation of palms and soles; it generally does not cause an RPD (Bolla, 1999). Testing for heavy-metal exposure requires a 24-hour urine test, not a spot urine, and possibly hair and/or nail analysis. Bismuth toxicity is discussed under iatrogenic exposure, below.

Many metabolic disorders, from hypercalcemia to poikilothermia, can result in RPD (Bouwman et al., 2009; Rosche et al., 2015); thus, such etiologies are addressed here briefly, including some that may have overlapping findings, particularly radiologically, with CJD.

Thiamine deficiency should always be considered, as there can be substantial clinical and radiographic overlap between Wernicke encephalopathy and CJD. Unlike CJD, however, Wernicke encephalopathy is treatable and even reversible if caught early enough. Thiamine (vitamin B_1) deficiency classically presents as an acute/subacute dementia/confusion (including memory loss) with ophthalmoparesis (often with vertical and/or horizontal nystagmus), and ataxia. Not all of these features may be present, however. If these symptoms arise acutely (days to weeks), it is commonly called Wernicke encephalopathy. If the deficiency is not recognized and treated soon enough, some cognitive symptoms, such as memory difficulties, can become irreversible. Persistent memory difficulties are referred to as Korsakoff syndrome (Scalzo et al., 2015). These syndromes, Wernicke and Korsakoff, are typically described together, since it is unknown if the person's symptoms will resolve during their initial presentation.

Although Wernicke–Korsakoff syndrome was historically associated with alcoholic patients, it is now more common in persons without alcoholism, with a 3.5:1 ratio of females to males. It is often seen in persons who have insufficient nutrition or cannot absorb certain nutrients, such as through gastric bypass surgery, or from repeated vomiting (hyperemesis gravidarum) (Scalzo et al., 2015). Brain MRI can show T2-weighted hyperintensities and sometimes restricted diffusion (DWI hyperintensities and ADC map hypointensities) in various brain regions, including mammillary bodies, dorsomedial nucleus of the thalamus, midbrain tectum, periaqueductal gray and, less commonly, even the cortex (Kinoshita et al., 2001; Halavaara et al., 2003; Geschwind, 2016). These imaging features can overlap with those seen in CJD (Fig. 20.5). An RPD case referred to our center as sCJD had T2-weighted and DWI hyperintensity in the dorsomedial thalami, periaqueductal gray, and cortex (cortical ribboning), some of which showed restricted diffusion. Because the cortical ribboning was along the primary motor strip, symmetrically, an area usually spared radiologically (and pathologically) in prion disease (Young et al., 2005; Vitali et al., 2011), we considered Wernicke encephalopathy and recommended urgent treatment. Unfortunately, the patient died prior to initiation of treatment and Wernicke encephalopathy was confirmed at autopsy (Geschwind, 2016).

Hypoglycemia, with or without seizures, can result in neurologic syndromes consistent with an RPD, sometimes even with imaging features suggestive of CJD (Cubo et al., 1998; Lo et al., 2006; Milligan et al., 2009; Sharma et al., 2009; Rosenbloom et al., 2015). Sustained hypoglycemia may result in confusion, weakness, seizures, and even coma, with T2-weighted and DWI hyperintensities with restricted diffusion in the cortex (insular, temporal, and occipital), basal ganglia, and hippocampus and relative sparing of the thalamus (Cubo et al., 1998; Lo et al., 2006; Sharma et al., 2009). MRI can show both cortical and subcortical FLAIR and DWI hyperintensities with restricted diffusion in a pattern suggestive of CJD (Fig. 20.6) (Rosenbloom et al., 2015). Persistent cerebral cortex, caudate, lenticular nucleus, substantia nigra, and hippocampus MRI abnormalities lasting days to months or longer have been described in patients in a persistent vegetative state from hypoglycemia (Fujioka et al., 1997). In addition, white-matter abnormalities can be found in structures such as the internal capsule and corpus callosum (Rosenbloom et al., 2015).

Wilson disease (also known as progressive lenticular degeneration or hepatolenticular degeneration) is an autosomal-recessive disorder due to mutations in ATP7B, causing copper accumulation, particularly in the liver,

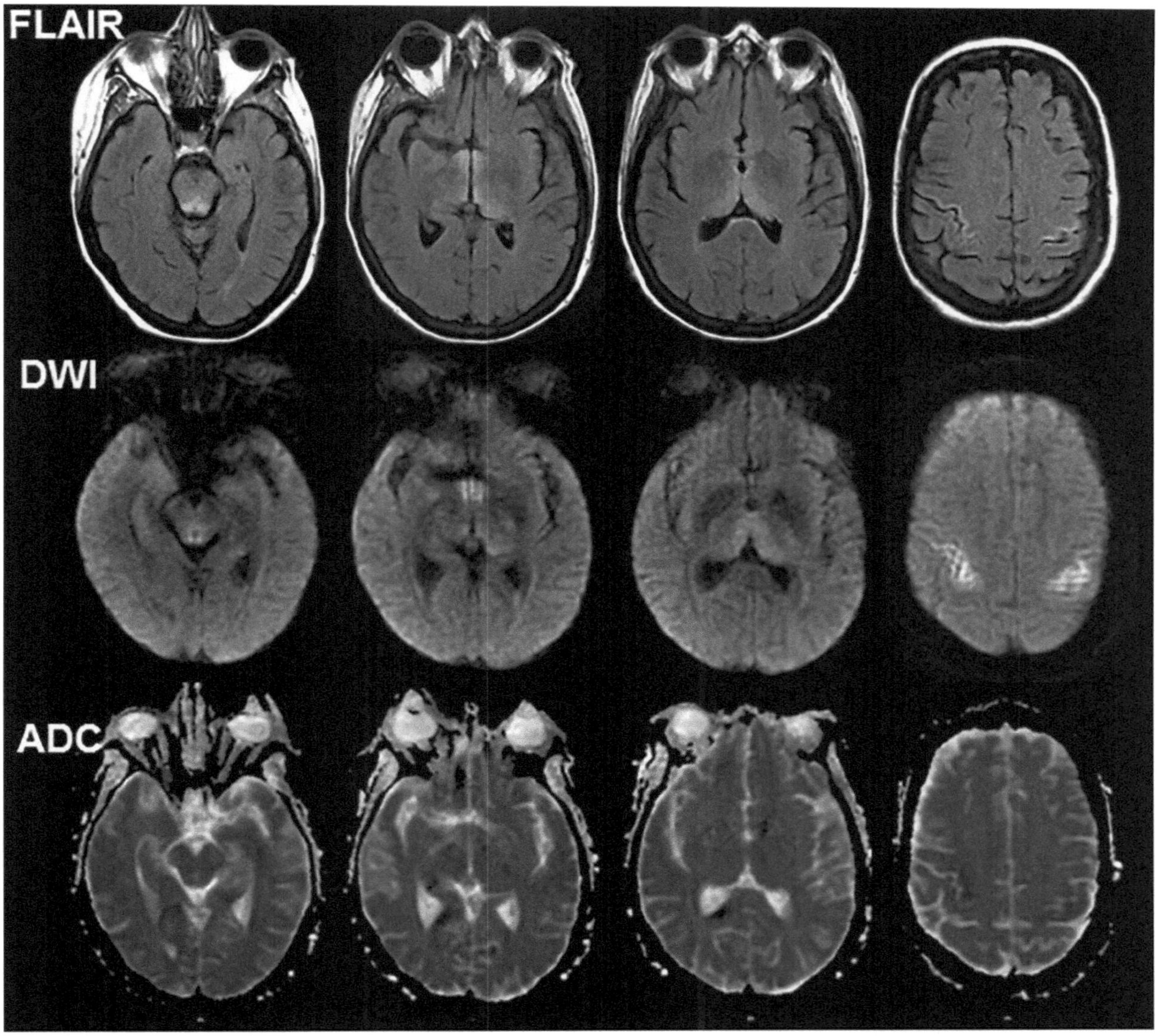

Fig. 20.5. Brain magnetic resonance imaging (MRI) in Wernicke encephalopathy with features overlapping with Creutzfeldt–Jakob disease. MRI, axial fluid-attenuated inversion recovery (FLAIR), diffusion-weighted imaging (DWI), and apparent diffusion coefficient (ADC) map sequences showing T2-weighted and DWI hyperintensities in the periaqueductal gray and midbrain tectum, medial thalamus, and perirolandic cortex with relative sparing of the mammillary bodies. The ADC map sequences primarily show cortical ribboning hypointensity in the perirolandic cortex, corresponding to hyperintensities on FLAIR and DWI. The preferential involvement of the perirolandic cortex is the opposite to the cortical pattern typically seen in sporadic Creutzfeldt–Jakob disease, in which there is generally sparing of the perirolandic region, particularly the primary motor cortex (Vitali et al., 2011).

brain, and cornea. It typically presents before age 50, usually in childhood or young adulthood, with an extrapyramidal movement disorder, dysexecutive function, amnesia, and neuropsychiatric symptoms; the latter may be the earliest features. If not diagnosed and treated soon enough, Wilson disease can lead to hepatic injury, including cirrhosis (Pfeiffer, 2011). Although neurologic symptoms usually progress slowly from the gradual accumulation of copper in the CNS, MRI can mimic CJD with T2-weighted and DWI striatal or thalamic hyperintensities (Sener, 2003; Favrole et al., 2006; Pfeiffer, 2011). One study with 13 symptomatic patients found that FLAIR hyperintensity was slightly more common than DWI, and diffusion was increased in these areas and in the white matter. Interestingly, there was restricted diffusion in the putamen in five presymptomatic subjects (Favrole et al., 2006). Thus, in some ways similar to sCJD (Caverzasi et al., 2014), the disease may begin with restricted diffusion.

When neurologic symptoms are present, slit-lamp examination usually reveals Kayser–Fleischer rings (Demirkiran et al., 1996). Diagnosis usually is confirmed by identifying elevated 24-hour urinary excretion of copper and low levels of serum ceruloplasmin. If the

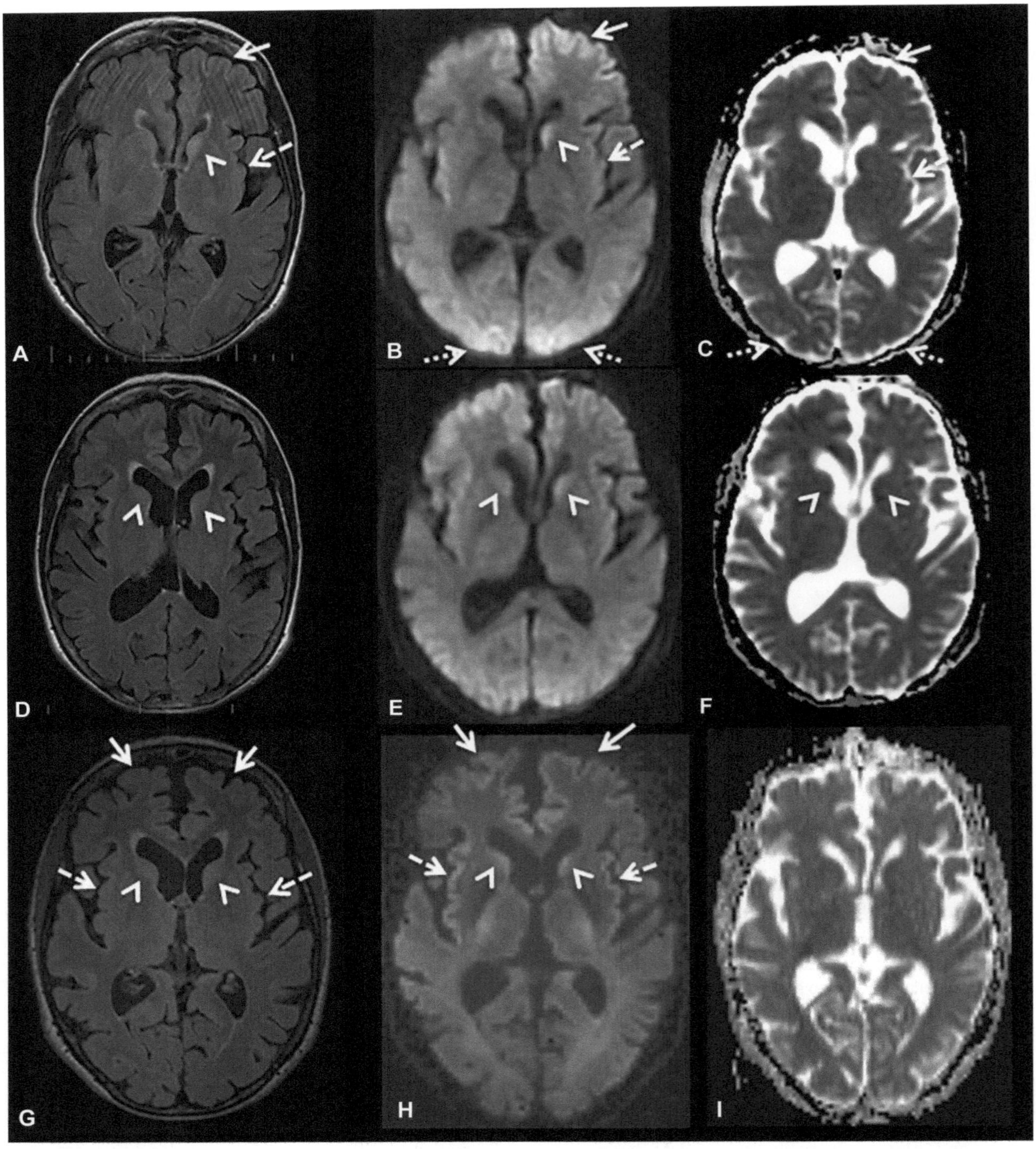

Fig. 20.6. Serial magnetic resonance imaging (MRI) in a 66-year-old woman with hypoxic/hypoglycemic encephalopathy. Fluid-attenuated inversion recovery (FLAIR) (**A**, **D**, **G**), diffusion-weighted imaging (DWI) (**B**, **E**, **H**), and apparent diffusion coefficient (ADC) map (**C**, **F**, **I**) sequences, in radiologic orientation, 2 days (**A–C**), 3 weeks (**D–F**), and 1 month (**G–I**) after onset. Initial MRI (**A–C**) shows left frontal (solid arrows), left insular (dashed arrows), bilateral medial occipital (dotted arrows), and left caudate (arrowhead) FLAIR/DWI hyperintensity with restricted diffusion. Repeat MRI about 3 weeks later (**D–F**) showed possible reduced FLAIR/DWI hyperintensity in the bilateral caudate heads (**D–F**; arrowhead) and medial occipital regions, and possible increased right caudate FLAIR hyperintensity and restricted diffusion (**D–F**; solid arrow). A third MRI 1 week later, 1 month after onset (**G–I**), revealed more intense FLAIR/DWI insular (**G**, **H**; dashed arrows) and frontal cortical hyperintensities (**G**, **H**; solid arrows) and possible restricted diffusion and FLAIR hyperintensity still present in the caudate heads (**G**, **H**; arrowheads). (Reproduced with permission from Rosenbloom MH, Tartaglia MC, Forner SA, et al. (2015) Metabolic disorders with clinical and radiologic features of sporadic Creutzfeldt–Jakob disease. Neurol Clin Pract 5: 108–115.)

diagnosis is still unclear, liver biopsy to identify elevated copper levels might be necessary. Liver function testing should also be performed (Pfeiffer, 2011).

Hepatic encephalopathy, often divided into acute and chronic forms, refers to a spectrum of neuropsychiatric abnormalities occurring in patients with liver dysfunction. Although most cases are caused by cirrhosis and portal hypertension or from portal-systemic shunts (Paul et al., 2015), the condition can also occur in patients with acute liver failure. Neurologic symptoms are thought to result from either cerebral edema (Rovira et al., 2008) or a shift in the balance between inhibitory and excitatory neurotransmission with a net increase of inhibitor transmission (Sharma et al., 2009). Other clinical features can vary widely, but the condition can mimic prion disease both clinically and radiologically. Brain MRI may show T1-weighted hyperintensity in the globus pallidus (which is sometimes also seen in CJD: de Priester et al., 1999), subthalamic region, and midbrain; it can also show diffuse cortical edema and T2-weighted hyperintensity, usually with sparing of the perirolandic and occipital regions (Rovira et al., 2008; Sharma et al., 2009). Hepatic encephalopathy, particularly acute forms, can also show FLAIR and DWI cortical ribboning (hyperintensities), often with restricted diffusion (ADC map hypointensity) with features similar to CJD (Sharma et al., 2009; McKinney et al., 2010), although, unlike CJD, there are also often white-matter hyperintensity (internal capsule and cortical white matter) and specific magnetic resonance spectroscopy (MRS) abnormalities (Sharma et al., 2009), the latter of which often improve with reversal or treatment of the hepatic encephalopathy (McKinney et al., 2010).

Another metabolic condition that can present as an RPD and mimic sCJD clinically and sometimes radiologically is extrapontine myelinolysis, caused by rapid shifts in sodium, often from iatrogenic inappropriately fast correction of hyponatremia. This most frequently presents as encephalopathy, often in combination with extrapyramidal features (de Souza, 2013). T2-weighted and DWI hyperintensities (sometimes with restricted diffusion on ADC map) in the deep nuclei can overlap with those seen in CJD. Unlike CJD, the deep nuclei diffusion abnormalities often disappear over weeks to months (Fig. 20.7) (Rosenbloom et al., 2015). Management is largely supportive, and although symptoms are usually refractory to medical therapy, reasonable functional recovery is seen with time in approximately 50% of individuals (Singh et al., 2014). Prevention of the initial osmotic demyelination is key.

AUTOIMMUNE

As shown in Tables 20.1 and 20.2, autoimmune conditions, particularly antibody-mediated encephalopathies, are now one of the most commonly identified causes of RPD and in some cases might mimic CJD clinically and radiologically (Geschwind et al., 2007; Fermo et al., 2014; Hoftberger, 2015). Although many autoimmune disorders, including rheumatologic illnesses, can cause RPD (Vernino et al., 2007), this section will focus on antibody-mediated disorders.

The field of antibody-mediated encephalopathies has grown dramatically over the past decade. As recently as 15–20 years ago, most antibody-mediated causes of RPD were paraneoplastic conditions, in which antibodies produced in reaction to an underlying cancer were directed against intracellular antigen targets. These intracellular antibodies were often named after the initials of the first patients in whom they were identified (e.g., anti-Hu, Ri, Yo, CV2 Tr, Ma1, Ma2, amphiphysin), and the syndromes often responded poorly to immunosuppression.

Over the past 10–15 years, a few key laboratories around the world have been instrumental in identifying novel antibodies against cell surface or synaptic targets that cause LEs or other forms of RPD, many of which respond very well to immunosuppression (Graus et al., 2004; Thieben et al., 2004; Vincent et al., 2004, 2009; Vitaliani et al., 2005; Bataller et al., 2007; Dalmau et al., 2007; Graus and Dalmau, 2007; Geschwind et al., 2008; Irani et al., 2010; Vincent et al., 2011). Some of the newly identified cell surface antibodies that can cause RPD are against the following proteins: leucine-rich, glioma inactivated 1 protein (LGI1) and contactin-associated protein-2 (CASPR2) (both formerly reported as voltage-gated potassium channel (VGKC) antibodies (Vincent et al., 2004; Irani et al., 2010; Lai et al., 2010), alpha-amino-3-hydroxy-5-methyl-4-isoxazolepropionic acid receptor (AMPAR) (Lai et al., 2009), NMDAR, dipeptidyl-peptidase-like protein-6, a subunit of Kv4.2 potassium channels (Boronat et al., 2013), glutamic acid decarboxylase (GAD65), gamma-aminobutyric acid B-receptor and A-receptor, and aquaporin-4 (McKeon, 2016; McKeon and Pittock, 2016). Currently, this group of antibody-mediated RPDs associated with cell surface and synaptic antigens is far more common than the more traditional classic onconeural antibodies. A few of these are discussed below, focusing on cases that might overlap with or even mimic CJD.

Many of these antibodies, including LGI1 and AMPAR, present predominantly as a LE. Some antibodies are associated with other features that may help distinguish them from other antibody-mediated causes of RPD and from CJD.

LGI1 typically presents with LE, temporal lobe seizures, hyponatremia, and facial brachial dystonic spells/seizures (FBDS), the latter of which are virtually pathognomonic

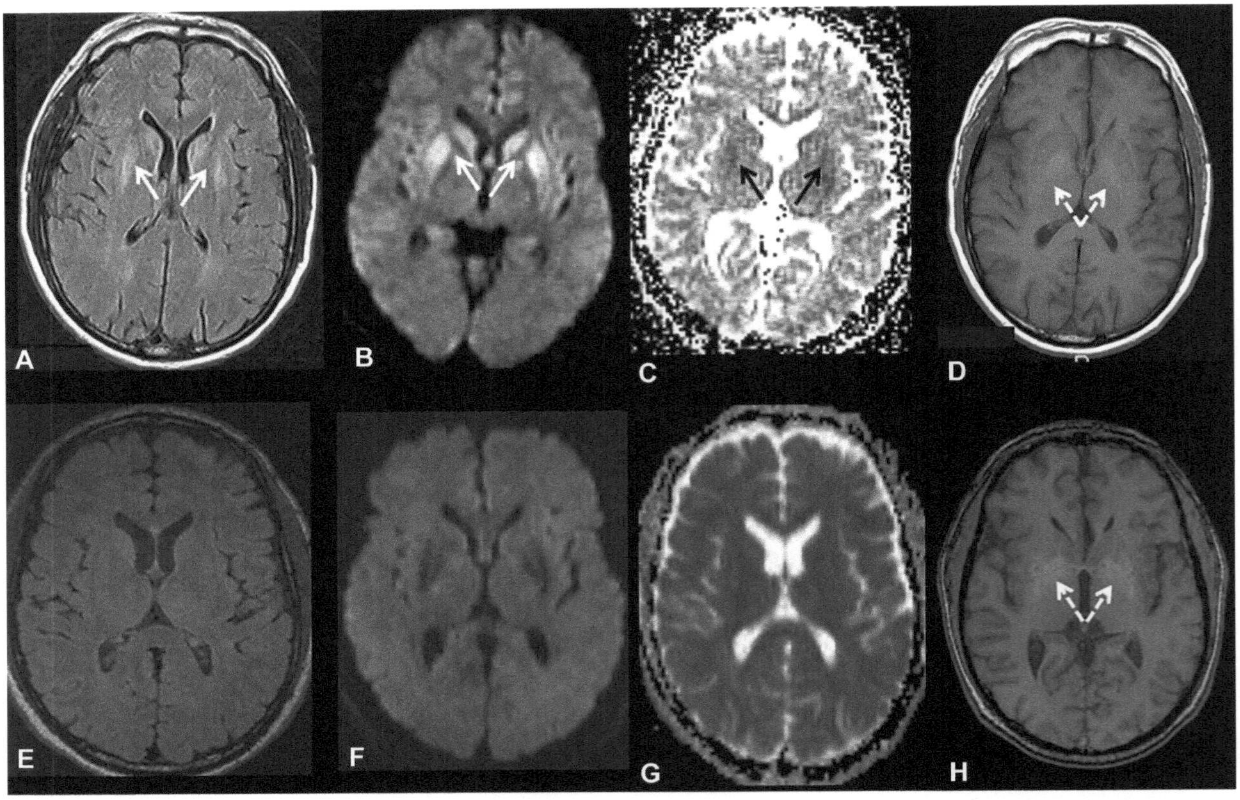

Fig. 20.7. Serial brain magnetic resonance imaging (MRI) in a 50-year-old man with extrapontine myelinolysis. Fluid-attenuated inversion recovery (FLAIR) (**A**, **E**), diffusion-weighted imaging (DWI) (**B**, **F**), apparent diffusion coefficient (ADC) map (**C**, **G**) and T1 (**D**, **H**) sequences, in radiologic orientation, 2 months (**A–D**) and 3 months (**E–H**) after onset. Initial MRI, 2 months after onset (**A–D**), shows symmetric bilateral striatal FLAIR/DWI hyperintensities (**A**, **B**; solid white arrows) with corresponding hypointensities on the ADC map suggesting restricted diffusion (**C**; solid black arrows). Bilateral globus pallidus hyperintensities were present on T1-weighted imaging (**D**; dashed arrows). MRI 1 month later (**E–H**), 3 months after onset, shows resolution of the prior FLAIR, DWI, and ADC map abnormalities, although no change in the globus pallidus T1 hyperintensities (**H**; dashed arrows). (Reproduced with permission from Rosenbloom MH, Tartaglia MC, Forner SA, et al. (2015) Metabolic disorders with clinical and radiologic features of sporadic Creutzfeldt–Jakob disease. Neurol Clin Pract 5: 108–115.)

for LGI1. FBDS often can be an early feature, prior to the onset of LE and seizures. If treated at this stage of illness, patients usually will not progress to develop other features of the syndrome (Irani et al., 2011). Many cases show T2-weighted hyperintensities in the medial temporal lobes, consistent with LE, although there have been a few reports of cases with some FLAIR with or without DWI cortical hyperintensity (Geschwind et al., 2008; Savard et al., 2016) or asymmetric T2/FLAIR striatal hyperintensity (Irani et al., 2011; Yoo and Hirsch, 2014). In these cases, however, FBDS usually was present to suggest LGI1 encephalitis, and even though there might have been some DWI hyperintensity, there was no corresponding ADC hypointensity, indicating restricted diffusion suggestive of CJD.

Compared with myoclonus, FBDS is slower, longer, more sustained, and has a dystonic component; patients usually are aware of FBDS and have no memory lapses, although sometimes they have brief amnesia for the episode (Irani et al., 2011). We reported a case of VGKC (LGI1 and CASPR2 not tested) with CJD-like periodic sharp-wave complexes on EEG, as well as FLAIR and DWI anterior cingulate cortical ribboning (Savard et al., 2016). There been several reported cases of sCJD and other conditions with positive VGKC antibodies, usually in the absence of LGI1 and CASPR2 antibodies, sometimes referred to as "VGKC+ double-negative" cases (Angus-Leppan et al., 2013a, b; Newey et al., 2013; Celicanin et al., 2017). The prevailing evidence suggests that most of these are false-positive VGKC cases, as the VGKC antibodies and the radioimmunoassay methods for detecting them are not as specific as those for LGI1 and CASPR2 and the syndromes are usually not consistent with an autoimmune neurologic disorder (Graus and Gorman, 2016; van Sonderen et al., 2016; Lang et al., 2017).

A poignant case report is of a 72-year-old male who presented with an RPD over 3 weeks and met probable sCJD criteria (Geschwind et al., 2007; Zerr et al., 2009; Staffaroni et al., 2017). He had an RPD with aphasia, myoclonus, cerebellar, extrapyramidal signs, focal higher cortical signs, MRI with subtle DWI cortical ribboning hyperintensity, with possible corresponding hypointensity on ADC map (i.e., restricted diffusion), positive CSF 14-3-3, and elevated CSF total tau. Antibody panels revealed slightly elevated VGKC and voltage-gated calcium channel and high antithryoperoxidase antibodies. High-dose steroids provided quick, dramatic, and full recovery. Although the precise cause of the patient's RPD was not really identified, the combination of his dramatic response to steroids, mild hyponatremia, and elevated serum autoantibodies suggested an autoimmune etiology (Fermo et al., 2014). It is also important to note that rarely diseases can co-occur, exemplified by a case report of a 77-year-old man with classic LGI1 encephalitis who recovered with immunosuppression, only to develop 4 months later symptoms of CJD. His total course for the two illnesses was only 17 months, with autopsy confirming sCJD (Kim et al., 2017).

AMPAR encephalitis typically presents as LE with prominent short-term memory loss, behavioral changes, and, in some instances, other neurologic symptoms (Lai et al., 2009; Hoftberger, 2015). Brain MRI can show extensive hyperintense FLAIR and/or DWI cortical ribboning, overlapping somewhat with CJD, although it was not mentioned in the reports whether these cases showed reduced diffusion as is seen in CJD. About two-thirds of AMPAR cases have CSF pleiocytosis, helping to further differentiate it from CJD (Lai et al., 2009; Hoftberger, 2015).

NMDAR encephalitis usually presents as a multistage illness, starting with a flu-like illness and then progressing from psychosis, memory problems, seizures, and aphasia into a nonresponsive state with catatonic features often associated with atypical hyperkinetic movements and body posturing. Occurring predominantly in children and young adults, with or without tumor association, NMDAR encephalitis responds to treatment but can relapse. Although it usually does not mimic CJD clinically, it is a form of RPD. Rare cases with T2-weighted basal ganglia hyperintensities have been reported (Urbach et al., 2015), which might raise diagnostic concern for CJD.

Several excellent reviews of antibody-mediated RPDs have been published and cover other syndromes that are not, or only briefly, discussed here (Linnoila et al., 2014; Ramanathan et al., 2014; Leypoldt et al., 2015; Graus et al., 2016; McKeon, 2016; McKeon and Pittock, 2016). In general, unless a syndrome is highly pathognomonic, we recommend testing for antibody-mediated causes of RPD by sending for comprehensive panels of antibodies. This is because some patients have more than one potentially causative antibody and some antibodies might predict the syndrome whereas others might predict the cancer and thus facilitate the oncologic work-up (Pittock et al., 2004). For most of these syndromes, serum is equally as sensitive as, or more sensitive than, CSF, but in some syndromes, such as NMDAR encephalitis, CSF has higher sensitivity for antibody detection (Dalmau et al., 2011; Geschwind, 2016). Therefore, when possible, we recommend sending both the serum and CSF for antibody panels. If a paraneoplastic or antibody-mediated etiology is suspected for an RPD syndrome in a patient who is negative for comprehensive panels of known commercially available antibodies, physicians should consider sending blood and/or CSF to a research laboratory that specializes in identifying novel antibodies (Lancaster and Dalmau, 2012).

MITOCHONDRIAL

Mitochondrial disease – particularly mitochondrial encephalopathy, lactic acidosis, strokes, and leukoencephalopathy (MELAS) – can present not only as an RPD (Kelley et al., 2009), but sometimes also with imaging findings, such as T2-weighted and DWI cortical hyperintensities, overlapping with CJD (Carroll, 2007). Various mitochondrial disorders are sometimes recognizable by the family history, typically with maternal inheritance, and other characteristic clinical features, both neurologic (myopathy, neuropathy, ophthalmoplegia, ptosis, seizures, ataxia) and nonneurologic (short stature, diabetes, cardiomyopathy, cardiac conduction defects, deafness). Diagnosis of mitochondrial disease can be difficult because of its pleomorphic clinical manifestations and because maternal mutation carriers may be asymptomatic or oligosymptomatic. In a patient with unexplained neurologic symptoms, one should consider mitochondrial disease, particularly if there are gray- and white-matter T2-weighted MRI abnormalities or clinical features consistent with mitochondrial disease (Finsterer, 2004; Marques-Matos et al., 2016).

Classic MELAS symptoms include headache, partial seizures, short stature, muscle weakness, exercise intolerance, deafness, diabetes, and slowly progressive dementia, but symptoms can occur acutely or subacutely (Saneto et al., 2008). Patients with RPD caused by MELAS might have a history of recurrent neurologic episodes, often with some recovery. MRI often shows regions of edema on T1, T1 hyperintensities in deep nuclei, T2-weighted gray-matter hyperintensities in the cortex, deep nuclei, and white matter, and even cortical ribboning and/or even restricted diffusion, the latter of which mistakenly might be confused with CJD (Sheerin et al., 2008; Vitali et al., 2011; Weiss et al.,

2011; Mizrachi et al., 2006). Unlike with CJD, however, MELAS often includes not just gray-matter involvement but also vasogenic edema causing adjacent white-matter involvement, and often the T2-weighted and DWI lesions regress and even disappear over weeks to a few months (Yoneda et al., 1999; Mizrachi et al., 2006; Marques-Matos et al., 2016). Although some literature suggests that MELAS can be differentiated from stroke because MELAS shows increased diffusion and stroke-restricted diffusion, this is probably incorrect, as diffusion in MELAS varies depending on when during the time course of lesions the MRI is performed (Yoneda et al., 1999; Mizrachi et al., 2006).

Other mitochondrial disorders have been reported to present as RPD, sometimes with features of CJD (Kelley et al., 2009). MRS in mitochondrial encephalopathies often shows a strong lactate signal, and CSF can show elevated lactate and/or pyruvate (Yoneda et al., 1999; Saneto et al., 2008; Weiss et al., 2011, but the specimens must be kept on ice and handled appropriately for these tests.

Malignancy

Although multiple metastases or glioblastoma multiforme are usually easy to identify as a cause of rapid cognitive decline, perhaps the greatest diagnostic challenge comes from primary CNS lymphoma and intravascular lymphoma. Primary CNS lymphoma comprises high-grade diffuse B-cell non-Hodgkin lymphoma (Weaver et al., 2007). Immunosuppression is a significant risk factor, but incidence is rising in all populations (Sierra del Rio et al., 2009). Immunocompromised individuals have more lesions, less homogeneous diffusion restriction/enhancement on MRI, and shorter survival, even with aggressive therapy. Diagnosis can be challenging, relying on a combination of MRI showing focal or multifocal enhancing lesions, sometimes with leptomeningeal involvement; slit-lamp assessment looking for vitreal involvement; large-volume CSF, including flow cytometry for immunophenotyping; MRS demonstrating choline and lipid/lactate peaks (Taillibert et al., 2008); and the gold standard of tissue pathology from brain/leptomeningeal/vitreous biopsy (Giannini et al., 2014). Steroids cause necrosis of the cancerous cells, transiently shrinking CNS lymphoma lesions and thereby often delaying pathologic diagnosis. Prognosis remains poor, usually measured in months, but survival can be prolonged through aggressive treatment, including whole-brain radiotherapy; chemotherapy, such as high-dose methotrexate; and potentially stem cell transplantation.

Lymphomatosis cerebri is a rare variant of primary CNS lymphoma in which there is diffuse infiltration of tissue without the formation of discrete masses. It often presents as an RPD with bilateral lesions in the deep nuclei or lobar regions, often without contrast enhancement (Bakshi et al., 1999; Leschziner et al., 2011; Yu et al., 2017). There can be bright regions on DWI, including in the deep nuclei, but often there is vasogenic edema with increased diffusion (Bakshi et al., 1999; Yu et al., 2017). As in many conditions that cause rapid neuronal injury, particularly CNS-infiltrative cancers, CSF biomarkers of such injury, such as 14-3-3, can be positive (Weaver et al., 2007).

Intravascular lymphoma is an even rarer manifestation of non-Hodgkin lymphoma in which the lymphocytes are restricted to the lumen of small and medium-sized blood vessels. It typically presents with symptoms secondary to CNS or skin involvement, or with pyrexia of unknown origin, but can involve virtually any organ. Relapsing stroke-like presentations are classic, but a recent meta-analysis found that 42% of published intravascular lymphoma cases had CNS symptoms, the most common of which was dementia/cognitive impairment, affecting 60% of this group (Fonkem et al., 2016). Intravascular lymphoma can present as an RPD, sometimes mimicking CJD. There are often multiple areas of restricted diffusion and T2-weighted hyperintensities on MRI, but in a vascular distribution and not in a pattern found in CJD (Heinrich et al., 2005). Diagnosis relies on biopsy of affected organs, especially the skin, but is particularly challenging if the only symptoms relate to the CNS. It is frequently an autopsy diagnosis, though clues can be gleaned from raised serum lactate dehydrogenase, bone marrow immunophenotype, whole-body CT, and brain MRI. Treatment is with chemotherapy (Garcia-Munoz et al., 2015).

IATROGENIC

The armory of illegal drugs is ever expanding, particularly with increasing manufacture of so-called "legal highs." Although new legislation has rendered many of these illegal in the United Kingdom, continental Europe, and the United States, they are still readily obtainable on the black market. History of recent illicit drug use should always be sought, as it may be concealed. When in doubt, a toxicology screen should be performed, even though it can only detect a portion of the street drugs in use (Welch, 2011). Likewise, alcohol abuse also can be hidden; it can cause Wernicke encephalopathy, necessitating urgent B-vitamin replacement with intravenous Pabrinex or its equivalent (B-vitamins such as thiamine hydrochloride, riboflavin, pyridoxine hydrochloride and nicotinamide, as well as vitamin C and glucose), and always prior to giving isolated parenteral glucose, which would otherwise exacerbate the problem. Cognitive impairment secondary to prescribed medication occurs, and common culprits (sometimes in combination) include opiates, anticholinergic drugs, antidepressants, and anticonvulsants (Shinohara and Yamada, 2016). Several cases of lithium toxicity mimicking prion disease with rapid dementia, ataxia, and myoclonic jerks have been reported (Finelli, 1992; Mouldi et al., 2006). Physicians need to be alert to the cognitive adverse effects of the medications they prescribe and be prepared to withdraw medication in the face of encephalopathy of uncertain etiology.

Over-the-counter supplements can also be potential neurotoxins, especially with chronic ingestion. Bismuth is a good example of this, having long been recognized as a cause of reversible subacute encephalopathy, often with additional features such as multifocal myoclonus, which can mimic CJD (Burns et al., 1974; Sampognaro et al., 2017). The increased availability of such supplements via the internet, and the common misperception that all nonprescribed, "natural" remedies are safe, means that physicians need to actively enquire about supplement use rather than relying on patients to volunteer this information. Extrapontine myelinolysis, often an iatrogenic cause of RPD, is discussed above under toxic-metabolic causes of RPD.

NEURODEGENERATIVE

The most common misdiagnoses for CJD are the much more common nonprion neurodegenerative diseases, as shown in Table 20.2. Nonprion neurodegenerative diseases also are among the most common causes of RPD (Table 20.1); this is not surprising given the prevalence of neurodegenerative diseases. In many cases of nonprion neurodegenerative disease, there is often a slow, gradual decline over several years, with family and friends missing the early signs of dementia until symptoms reach a threshold. At that point the signs and symptoms become clear, with a resulting misconception that the patient had a rapid decline. Another common scenario is a sudden worsening of an elderly patient, or a patient with an underlying undiagnosed dementia, from a metabolic perturbation or infection (e.g., urinary tract infection, pneumonia) (Geschwind et al., 2008; Geschwind, 2016).

As noted in Tables 20.1 and 20.2, in rare cases nonprion neurodegenerative dementias progress rapidly, with dementia occurring within 1 year from the onset of the first symptom or death occurring within 1–3 years from first-symptom onset (Josephs et al., 2009; Schmidt et al., 2012). These neurodegenerative dementias include corticobasal degeneration, FTD, FTD and motor neuron disease (FTD-MND) and atypical, rare cases of AD and dementia with Lewy bodies (Poser et al., 1999; Geschwind et al., 2007, 2008; Cohen et al., 2015). Just over 40% of the Athens RPD cohort (Table 20.1) were nonprion neurodegenerative dementias, with AD and FTD the most common, followed by various other neurodegenerative diseases, including multiple system atrophy, dementia with Lewy bodies, PD dementia, progressive supranuclear palsy, and corticobasal syndrome (Papageorgiou et al., 2009). Similarly, the most common cause of RPD in the Barcelona cohort was nonprion neurodegenerative diseases, accounting for more than one-third of their cases, with AD, FTD, and dementia with Lewy bodies the most common (Sala et al., 2012). It is not clear why only 5% of the inpatient RPD cases in the Rio cohort were diagnosed as nonprion neurodegenerative disorders (Neto et al., 2016). In the Catalan brain bank, not shown in Table 20.1, nonprion neurodegenerative diseases were the second most common cause of RPD, behind only CJD (Grau-Rivera et al., 2015b).

Some genetic forms of neurodegenerative diseases can also present as RPD; these include those caused by mutations in the microtubule-associated tau protein (*MAPT*) and the chromosome 9 open reading frame 72 (C9orf72) genes. One patient with FTD-MND due to a C9orf72 mutation died within 1 year of disease onset (Grau-Rivera et al., 2015a). FTD-MND cases, whether genetic or sporadic, can progress quite rapidly in general. Particularly with young-onset RPDs, it is important to consider genetic neurodegenerative diseases, such as NCL or Niemann–Pick type C, depending on the clinical presentation. Although patients typically live for many years with these disorders, some cases can progress rapidly to dementia (Sevin et al., 2007; Kelley et al., 2009).

Many of the rapidly progressive subtype of AD (rpAD) cases referred to European CJD surveillance centers as CJD had significant clinical overlap with prion disease, including RPD presentations and elevated CSF biomarkers. Forty-two percent of rpAD cases had elevated CSF 14-3-3. Interestingly, rpAD cases were less likely to have an apolipoprotein E4 (ApoE4) allele than typical AD cases (Schmidt et al., 2012). In an older study from the German CJD Surveillance Center, among pathology-proven AD and dementia with Lewy bodies cases referred to the center clinically as CJD, about one-half fulfilled World Health Organization symptom criteria for CJD (WHO, 1998). Twenty-five percent of the AD cases had periodic sharp-wave complexes on EEG and 10% had positive 14-3-3 (Tschampa et al., 2001). A study of rpAD cases in the United States found a connection between rapid progression and levels of abeta42-amyloid with distinct structural characteristics and suggested prion-like conformational abeta42-amyloid strains in AD (Cohen et al., 2015). Another study with some of the same authors comparing rapidly versus typically progressive AD cases found differences in the types of other proteins present in AD plaques, suggesting that rpAD might be a different subtype of AD (Drummond et al., 2017).

There is a growing body of literature supporting the notion that some of these nonprion neurodegenerative disorders might spread in the brain in a prion-like manner. The misfolded proteins associated with nonprion-related protein disorders might even cause disease when directly inoculated from one animal into another (Watts et al., 2013; Walker and Jucker, 2015; Watts and Prusiner, 2017). Thus, it is perhaps not surprising that some of these other neurodegenerative diseases might have clinical overlap with CJD.

SYSTEMIC DISORDERS, SARCOID, AND SEIZURES

Numerous systemic illnesses can mimic RPD, often in older individuals with an already vulnerable brain susceptible to delirium, but also – although less frequently – in younger adults with rare diseases. These include mitochondrial diseases, which can have systemic involvement because of the varied distribution of mitochondria throughout the body; RPDs resulting from these disorders are discussed above in the mitochondrial section.

Neurosarcoidosis most frequently manifests as a cranial nerve palsy, but it often also includes headache, ataxia, weakness, mild cognitive impairment, and/or seizures (Oksanen, 1986). In rare cases it can present as a dementia with prominent and occasionally rapid cognitive decline (Schielke et al., 2001). The vast majority (more than 95%) of individuals with neurosarcoid also have evidence of systemic sarcoid (Smith et al., 2004), resulting in abnormalities on chest X-ray/CT and serum (elevated angiotensin-converting enzyme, high calcium, deranged liver function tests), but these are nonspecific findings. CSF lymphocytes and protein are usually mildly elevated but can be normal. Likewise, brain MRI can be normal or show a wide range of abnormalities, including leptomeningeal enhancement (diffuse or nodular), hydrocephalus, a single tumor-like mass, or diffuse, nonspecific white-matter lesions (Spencer et al., 2005). Imaging results usually do not mimic CJD. The gold-standard diagnostic test, however, is demonstration of noncaseating granulomas on biopsy, usually most easily obtained from a lymph node, although brain and meningeal biopsy might be required. Treatment is immunosuppressive, with steroids usually the first option, accompanied by a longer-term agent such as methotrexate, azathioprine, or infliximab.

sCJD can cause nonconvulsive status epilepticus (Espinosa et al., 2010), but the presence of cortical ribboning or deep nuclei hyperintensity on T2-weighted and/or DWI MRI could mistakenly lead to a diagnosis of prion disease in instances in which the patient actually has reversible nonconvulsive status alone (Wada et al., 2003). As with CJD, seizures, particularly when prolonged, can also result in restricted diffusion (Fig. 20.8). With seizures, however, the DWI abnormalities should disappear within days to weeks once the seizures stop (Chu et al., 2001; Hufnagel et al., 2003; Chatzikonstantinou et al., 2011). The clinical picture in

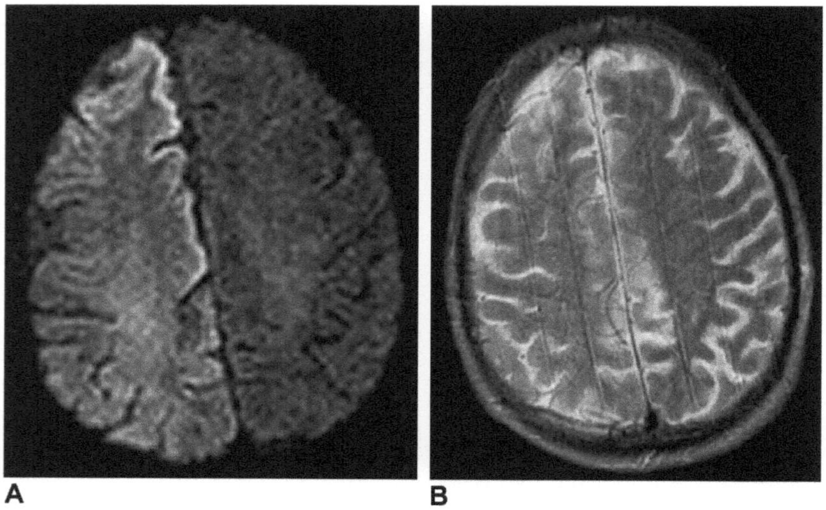

Fig. 20.8. Postictal cortical diffusion restriction. A 56-year-old man with a past history of intractable seizures was admitted with focal motor status epilepticus. (**A**) There is increased cortical signal on diffusion-weighted images (b =1000 s/mm2) throughout the entire right cerebral hemisphere confirmed on the apparent diffusion coefficient map (not shown) to be diffusion restriction. (**B**) The T2 images are slightly marred by movement artefact but show subtle cortical swelling and high signal as well as increased white-matter signal intensity. These areas do not conform to the boundaries of any arterial territory. (Reproduced with permission from Sheerin F, Pretorius PM, Briley D, et al. (2008) Differential diagnosis of restricted diffusion confined to the cerebral cortex. Clin Radiol 63: 1245–1253.)

nonconvulsive status can be one of a progressive encephalopathy with myoclonic-type jerks, and the rhythmic epileptiform EEG changes can compound diagnostic confusion, occasionally resembling CJD EEG changes of periodic complexes (Murray, 2008).

Structural causes of encephalopathy need to be considered, such as subdural hematoma or normal-pressure hydrocephalus, but can usually be readily identified by brain imaging with either CT or MRI. Spontaneous intracranial hypotension usually results from CSF hypovolemia from a CSF spinal leak. Typical symptoms include orthostatic headache, daytime somnolence, cognitive dysfunction, and personality changes. Several cases of an FTD-like presentation have been reported (Wicklund et al., 2011). Although most cases have insidious onset and slow progression, RPD cases have also been reported (Agarwal et al., 2009; Capizzano et al., 2016). Imaging usually shows a sagging brain with compression of the diencephalon and brainstem, which might be mistaken for a tumor or other mass. Identifying the location of a CSF leak and treatment with a blood patch can often lead to dramatic recovery and even reversal of the syndrome (Wicklund et al., 2011; Capizzano et al., 2016). If a blood patch is unsuccessful, it might be necessary to look for an arachnoid cyst or other fistulas (Fishman and Dillon, 2002). For unclear reasons, some cases resolve with steroids (Hong et al., 2002).

DEMYELINATING DISEASE

MS is the archetypal demyelinating disease of the CNS, and cognitive impairment is a major, though often overlooked, symptom. Cognitive impairment in MS is thought to reflect a combination of gray-matter damage, white-matter lesion load, and overall brain atrophy. Studies estimate that 40–70% of MS sufferers have cognitive dysfunction, depending on the neuropsychologic tests used and population studied (Rocca et al., 2015). MS only rarely causes diagnostic confusion, such as when it develops rapidly, affects multiple cognitive domains, and/or occurs at disease onset. This is particularly recognized in the rarer and more aggressive subtypes of tumefactive MS, Marburg's variant, and Balo concentric sclerosis (Karaarslan et al., 2001; Rahmlow and Kantarci, 2013; Hamed, 2015). Treatment for acute cognitive decline in the context of a relapse is similar to that of any MS relapse, with high-dose steroids, followed by disease-modifying therapy for those with a relapsing remitting MS course. Many of the cognitive problems, however, occur in the context of progressive disease without defined inflammatory relapses, and there currently is no specific treatment for this phase or even successful symptomatic therapy for MS cognitive impairment.

Neuromyelitis optica is an autoimmune demyelinating CNS disease distinct from MS by virtue of its primarily astrocyte-driven pathology and its pathogenic antibody, aquaporin 4. Optic nerves and spinal cord are preferentially affected, but symptomatic cerebral syndromes can occur, and subacute encephalopathy is reported in this context (Hervas-Garcia et al., 2014). The diagnosis can usually be made by a combination of MRI changes, positive aquaporin 4 antibody or MOG antibody, and often prior clinical events suggestive of neuromyelitis optica (Wingerchuk et al., 2015).

Acute disseminated encephalomyelitis is another immune-mediated demyelinating CNS disease that predominantly affects children but also occurs in adults with a similar, though possibly more severe, clinical phenotype, when diagnosis can be more challenging (Ketelslegers et al., 2011). Acute disseminated encephalomyelitis is classically monophasic but multiphasic relapsing forms exist, overlapping with both MS and NMO. As the name suggests, encephalopathy is characteristic, with behavioral change and alteration in conscious level being the most common presenting features, often coexisting with motor deficits, fever, and seizures plus antecedent infection (Yang et al., 2016). The evolution is rapid, typically over 2–5 days, thus distinguishing it from even the most aggressive neurodegenerative dementias. The diagnosis is largely one of exclusion, supported by CSF lymphocytic pleiocytosis and characteristic MRI changes of multifocal white-matter hyperintensities and frequent involvement of basal ganglia and thalami, plus hopefully a positive response to treatment with high-dose steroids. Numerous rarities, however, have been reported to mimic acute disseminated encephalomyelitis, including mitochondrial disorders, hemophagocytic syndromes, gliomatosis cerebri, and infectious and autoimmune encephalitis (Pohl et al., 2016).

Systemic lupus erythematosus has neuropsychiatric manifestations ranging in severity from mild behavioral change to reduced conscious level, and in time can progress from an acute encephalopathy to a dementia-like illness over months (Joseph and Scolding, 2010). Patients can also experience headaches, seizures, aseptic meningitis, and arterial and venous strokes. The pathogenesis of the cognitive problems are multifactorial and can include autoimmune antibody-mediated disease, a small-vessel vasculopathy, venous or arterial thrombosis, and cases of posterior reversible encephalopathy syndrome due either to the lupus itself or related to its complications (hypertension) or treatment (cytotoxic drugs) (Hanly, 2014; Ferreira et al., 2016). There has been long-term debate as to whether demyelination is part of the pathogenesis of neurolupus. Although many pathologic studies of CNS lupus show no evidence of primary demyelination (Scolding and Joseph, 2002), there are rare cases of tumefactive demyelination in lupus (Verma and Arya, 2012), plus the increased incidence of neuromyelitis optica-associated demyelination in individuals with systemic lupus erythematosus (Wingerchuk and Weinshenker, 2012), suggesting that the situation is complex and that demyelination is a likely factor in at least some cases of neurolupus.

CONCLUSION

The work-up of a patient with an RPD, including CJD, can be challenging. Many disorders can mimic CJD in clinical presentation and on ancillary laboratory testing with CSF biomarkers and brain MRI. Accurate diagnosis of CJD, and differentiating it from other RPDs, has improved over the past decade because of the increasing use of diffusion MRI (DWI and ADC) as well as more specific prion detection methods in the CSF, such as with protein cyclic multiplication assay and real-time quaking-induced conversion assay (Geschwind, 2015). T2-weighted and DWI hyperintensities in the cortex and/or deep nuclei, which are very helpful for CJD diagnosis, are sometimes seen in similar patterns in other disorders. It is important to have an organized, thorough approach to the diagnostic assessment and to consider other disorders, particularly treatable ones, before concluding a diagnosis of CJD.

References

Abe K, Okuda O, Ohishi H et al. (2014). Multiple dural arteriovenous fistulas causing rapid progressive dementia successfully treated by endovascular surgery: case report. Neurol Med Chir (Tokyo) 54: 145–149.

Agarwal P, Menon S, Shah R et al. (2009). Spontaneous intracranial hypotension: two cases including one treated with epidural blood patch. Ann Indian Acad Neurol 12: 179–182.

Agut H, Bonnafous P, Gautheret-Dejean A (2017). Update on infections with human herpesviruses 6A, 6B, and 7. Med Mal Infect 47: 83–91.

Angus-Leppan H, Rudge P, Mead S et al. (2013a). Autoantibodies in sporadic Creutzfeldt-Jakob disease. JAMA Neurol 70: 919–922.

Angus-Leppan H, Rudge P, Mead S et al. (2013b). Creutzfeld-Jakob disease–reply. JAMA Neurol 70: 1589.

Anuja P, Venugopalan V, Darakhshan N et al. (2018). Rapidly progressive dementia: an eight year (2008-2016) retrospective study. PLoS One 13: e0189832.

Auchus AP, Chen CP, Sodagar SN et al. (2002). Single stroke dementia: insights from 12 cases in Singapore. J Neurol Sci 203–204: 85–89.

Bakshi R, Mazziotta JC, Mischel PS et al. (1999). Lymphomatosis cerebri presenting as rapidly progressive dementia: clinical, neuroimaging and pathologic findings. Dement Geriatr Cogn Disord 10 (2): 152–157.

Basavaraju A (2016). Toxoplasmosis in HIV infection: an overview. Trop Parasitol 6: 129–135.

Bataller L, Kleopa KA, Wu GF et al. (2007). Autoimmune limbic encephalitis in 39 patients: immunophenotypes and outcomes. J Neurol Neurosurg Psychiatry 78: 381–385.

Berger JR, Wilson MR (2016). Next-generation sequencing of tissue: a logical extension. Neurol Neuroimmunol Neuroinflamm 3: e261.

Bloomgren G, Richman S, Hotermans C et al. (2012). Risk of natalizumab-associated progressive multifocal leukoencephalopathy. N Engl J Med 366: 1870–1880.

Bolla K (1999). In: C Goetz, E Pappaert (Eds.), Chapter 39. Exogenous acquired metabolic disorders of the nervous system: toxins and illicit drugs. Textbook of Clinical Neurology. W.B. Saunders, Philadelphia.

Boronat A, Gelfand JM, Gresa-Arribas N et al. (2013). Encephalitis and antibodies to dipeptidyl-peptidase-like protein-6, a subunit of Kv4.2 potassium channels. Ann Neurol 73: 120–128.

Bouwman NA, Verhagen WI, Meulstee J (2009). EEG abnormalities in poikilothermia suggesting Creutzfeldt–Jakob disease. Clin EEG Neurosci 40: 196–199.

Bowen LN, Smith B, Reich D et al. (2016). HIV-associated opportunistic CNS infections: pathophysiology, diagnosis and treatment. Nat Rev Neurol 12: 662–674.

Burns R, Thomas DW, Barron VJ (1974). Reversible encephalopathy possibly associated with bismuth subgallate ingestion. Br Med J 1 (5901): 220–223.

Cachia D, Smith T, Paydarfar D et al. (2014). A case of early-onset rapidly progressive dementia. JAMA Neurol 71: 1445–1449.

Capizzano AA, Lai L, Kim J et al. (2016). Atypical presentations of intracranial hypotension: comparison with classic spontaneous intracranial hypotension. AJNR Am J Neuroradiol 37: 1256–1261.

Carrera E, Bogousslavsky J (2006). The thalamus and behavior: effects of anatomically distinct strokes. Neurology 66: 1817–1823.

Carroll MB (2007). MELAS masquerading as a systemic vasculitis. J Clin Rheumatol 13: 334–337.

Cataldi ML, Restivo O, Reggio E et al. (2000). Deafness: an unusual onset of genetic Creutzfeldt–Jakob disease. Neurol Sci 21: 53–55.

Caverzasi E, Henry RG, Vitali P et al. (2014). Application of quantitative DTI metrics in sporadic CJD. Neuroimage Clin 4: 426–435.

Celicanin M, Blaabjerg M, Maersk-Moller C et al. (2017). Autoimmune encephalitis associated with voltage-gated potassium channels-complex and leucine-rich glioma-inactivated 1 antibodies - a national cohort study. Eur J Neurol 24: 999–1005.

Chakor RT, Santosh NS (2013). Subacute sclerosing panencephalitis presenting as rapidly progressive young-onset dementia. J Pak Med Assoc 63: 921–924.

Chapman T, McKeel Jr DW, Morris JC (2000). Misleading results with the 14-3-3 assay for the diagnosis of Creutzfeldt–Jakob disease. Neurology 55: 1396–1397.

Chatzikonstantinou A, Gass A, Forster A et al. (2011). Features of acute DWI abnormalities related to status epilepticus. Epilepsy Res 97: 45–51.

Chitravas N, Jung RS, Kofskey DM et al. (2011). Treatable neurological disorders misdiagnosed as Creutzfeldt–Jakob disease. Ann Neurol 70: 437–444.

Chiu CY, Coffey LL, Murkey J et al. (2017). Diagnosis of fatal human case of St. Louis encephalitis virus infection by metagenomic sequencing, California, 2016. Emerg Infect Dis 23: 1964–1968.

Christidi F, Kararizou E, Potagas C et al. (2014). Neurocognitive impairment in Whipple disease with central nervous system involvement. Cogn Behav Neurol 27: 51–56.

Chu K, Kang DW, Kim JY et al. (2001). Diffusion-weighted magnetic resonance imaging in nonconvulsive status epilepticus. Arch Neurol 58: 993–998.

Clifford DB, Ances BM (2013). HIV-associated neurocognitive disorder. Lancet Infect Dis 13: 976–986.

Cohen ML, Kim C, Haldiman T et al. (2015). Rapidly progressive Alzheimer's disease features distinct structures of amyloid-beta. Brain 138: 1009–1022.

Crosta F, Orlandi B, De Santis F et al. (2015). Cerebral amyloid angiopathy-related inflammation: report of a case with very difficult therapeutic management. Case Rep Neurol Med 2015 (483020).

Cubo E, Andres MT, Rojo A et al. (1998). Neuroimaging of hypoglycemia. Rev Neurol 26: 774–776.

Dalmau J, Lancaster E, Martinez-Hernandez E et al. (2011). Clinical experience and laboratory investigations in patients with anti-NMDAR encephalitis. Lancet Neurol 10: 63–74.

Dalmau J, Tuzun E, Wu HY et al. (2007). Paraneoplastic anti-N-methyl-D-aspartate receptor encephalitis associated with ovarian teratoma. Ann Neurol 61: 25–36.

Dandashi JA, Nizamutdinov D, Dayawansa S et al. (2016). Texas occurrence of Lyme disease and its neurological manifestations. J Neuroinfect Dis 7.

de Priester JA, Jansen GH, de Krijk JR et al. (1999). New MRI findings in Creutzfeldt Jacob disease; high signal in the globus pallidus on T1 weighted images. Neuroradiology 41: 265–268.

de Souza A (2013). Movement disorders and the osmotic demyelination syndrome. Parkinsonism Relat Disord 19: 709–716.

Demirkiran M, Jankovic J, Lewis RA et al. (1996). Neurologic presentation of Wilson disease without Kayser-Fleischer rings. Neurology 46: 1040–1043.

Drummond E, Nayak S, Faustin A et al. (2017). Proteomic differences in amyloid plaques in rapidly progressive and sporadic Alzheimer's disease. Acta Neuropathol 133: 933–954.

Eng JA, Frosch MP, Choi K et al. (2004). Clinical manifestations of cerebral amyloid angiopathy-related inflammation. Ann Neurol 55: 250–256.

Espinosa PS, Bensalem-Owen MK, Fee DB (2010). Sporadic Creutzfeldt–Jakob disease presenting as nonconvulsive status epilepticus case report and review of the literature. Clin Neurol Neurosurg 112: 537–540.

Favrole P, Chabriat H, Guichard JP et al. (2006). Clinical correlates of cerebral water diffusion in Wilson disease. Neurology 66: 384–389.

Fermo OP, Izbudak I, Sutter R et al. (2014). Autoimmune encephalitis mimicking Creutzfeldt Jacob disease. Neurol Clin Pract 4: 493–495.

Ferreira TS, Reis F, Appenzeller S (2016). Posterior reversible encephalopathy syndrome and association with systemic lupus erythematosus. Lupus 25: 1369–1376.

Finsterer J (2004). Mitochondriopathies. Eur J Neurol 11: 163–186.

Finelli PF (1992). Drug induced Creutzfeldt-Jakob like syndrome. J Psychiatr Neurosci 17 (3): 103–105.

Fishman RA, Dillon WP (2002). Spontaneous intracranial hypotension causing reversible frontotemporal dementia. Neurology 59: 787. author reply 787.

Fonkem E, Dayawansa S, Stroberg E et al. (2016). Neurological presentation of intravascular lymphoma (IVL): meta-analysis of 654 patients. BMC Neurol 16: 9.

Fujioka M, Okuchi K, Hiramatsu KI et al. (1997). Specific changes in human brain after hypoglycemic injury. Stroke 28: 584–587.

Garcia-Munoz R, Rubio-Mediavilla S, Robles-de-Castro D et al. (2015). Intravascular large B cell lymphoma. Leuk Res Rep 3 (1): 21–23.

Gascon GG, Frosch MP (1998). Case records of the Massachusetts General Hospital. Weekly clinicopathological exercises. Case 15-1998. A 34-year-old woman with confusion and visual loss during pregnancy. N Engl J Med 338: 1448–1456.

Geraldes R, Albuquerque L, Ferro JM et al. (2012). Rapidly progressive cognitive impairment, ataxia, and myoclonus: an unusual presentation of a dural arteriovenous fistula. J Stroke Cerebrovasc Dis 21 (619): e613–615.

Geschwind MD (2015). Prion diseases. Continuum (Minneap Minn) 21: 1612–1638.

Geschwind MD (2016). Rapidly progressive dementia. Continuum (Minneap Minn) 22: 510–537.

Geschwind MD, Martindale J, Miller D et al. (2003). Challenging the clinical utility of the 14-3-3 protein for the diagnosis of sporadic Creutzfeldt–Jakob disease. Arch Neurol 60: 813–816.

Geschwind MD, Haman A, Miller BL (2007). Rapidly progressive dementia. Neurol Clin 25: 783–807.

Geschwind MD, Shu H, Haman A et al. (2008). Rapidly progressive dementia. Ann Neurol 64: 97–108.

Giannini C, Dogan A, Salomao DR (2014). CNS lymphoma: a practical diagnostic approach. J Neuropathol Exp Neurol 73 (6): 478–494.

Glaser CA, Gilliam S, Schnurr D et al. (2003). In search of encephalitis etiologies: diagnostic challenges in the California Encephalitis Project, 1998-2000. Clin Infect Dis 36: 731–742.

Graffeo CS, Dawson ET, Murphy ME et al. (2016). Expanding the spectrum of subacute diencephalic angioencephalopathy. J Clin Neurosci 23: 8–13.

Grau-Rivera O, Gelpi E, Carballido-Lopez E et al. (2015a). Rapidly progressive dementia with psychotic onset in a patient with the C9ORF72 mutation. Clin Neuropathol 34: 294–297.

Grau-Rivera O, Gelpi E, Nos C et al. (2015b). Clinicopathological correlations and concomitant pathologies in rapidly progressive dementia: a brain bank series. Neurodegener Dis 15: 350–360.

Graus F, Dalmau J (2007). Paraneoplastic neurological syndromes: diagnosis and treatment. Curr Opin Neurol 20: 732–737.

Graus F, Delattre JY, Antoine JC et al. (2004). Recommended diagnostic criteria for paraneoplastic neurological syndromes. J Neurol Neurosurg Psychiatry 75: 1135–1140.

Graus F, Gorman MP (2016). Voltage-gated potassium channel antibodies: Game over. Neurology 86: 1657–1658.

Graus F, Titulaer MJ, Balu R et al. (2016). A clinical approach to diagnosis of autoimmune encephalitis. Lancet Neurol 15: 391–404.

Green A, Sanchez-Juan P, Ladogana A et al. (2007). CSF analysis in patients with sporadic CJD and other transmissible spongiform encephalopathies. Eur J Neurol 14: 121–124.

Halavaara J, Brander A, Lyytinen J et al. (2003). Wernicke's encephalopathy: is diffusion-weighted MRI useful? Neuroradiology 45: 519–523.

Hale A, Geerling J, Schmolze D et al. (2016). A 63-year-old man with rapidly progressive dementia. Clinical Infectious Diseases 63: 138–139.

Hamed SA (2015). Variant of multiple sclerosis with dementia and tumefactive demyelinating brain lesions. World J Clin Cases 3: 525–532.

Hanly JG (2014). Diagnosis and management of neuropsychiatric SLE. Nat Rev Rheumatol 10: 338–347.

Harkness KA, Coles A, Pohl U et al. (2004). Rapidly reversible dementia in cerebral amyloid inflammatory vasculopathy. Eur J Neurol 11: 59–62.

Hegde AN, Mohan S, Lath N et al. (2011). Differential diagnosis for bilateral abnormalities of the basal ganglia and thalamus. Radiographics 31: 5–30.

Heinrich A, Vogelgesang S, Kirsch M et al. (2005). Intravascular lymphoma presenting as rapidly progressive dementia. Eur Neurol 54 (1): 55–58.

Hervas-Garcia JV, Grau-Lopez L, Domenech-Puigcerver S et al. (2014). Encephalopathy and neuromyelitis optica: the importance of recognising atypical symptoms. Rev Neurol 58: 20–24.

Hoftberger R (2015). Neuroimmunology: An expanding frontier in autoimmunity. Front Immunol 6: 206.

Hohler AD, Flynn FG (2006). Onset of Creutzfeldt–Jakob disease mimicking an acute cerebrovascular event. Neurology 67: 538–539.

Hong M, Shah GV, Adams KM et al. (2002). Spontaneous intracranial hypotension causing reversible frontotemporal dementia. Neurology 58: 1285–1287.

Hufnagel A, Weber J, Marks S et al. (2003). Brain diffusion after single seizures. Epilepsia 44: 54–63.

Hurst RW, Bagley LJ, Galetta S et al. (1998). Dementia resulting from dural arteriovenous fistulas: the pathologic findings of venous hypertensive encephalopathy. AJNR Am J Neuroradiol 19: 1267–1273.

Hurth K, Tarawneh R, Ghoshal N et al. (2015). Whipple's disease masquerades as dementia with Lewy bodies. Alzheimer Dis Assoc Disord 29: 85–89.

Imazeki R, Amari K, Sekiguchi T et al. (2015). Rapidly progressive dementia caused by a superior sagittal sinus dural arteriovenous fistula: a case report. Tokai J Exp Clin Med 40: 22–26.

Irani SR, Alexander S, Waters P et al. (2010). Antibodies to Kv1 potassium channel-complex proteins leucine-rich, glioma inactivated 1 protein and contactin-associated protein-2 in limbic encephalitis, Morvan's syndrome and acquired neuromyotonia. Brain 133: 2734–2748.

Irani SR, Michell AW, Lang B et al. (2011). Faciobrachial dystonic seizures precede Lgi1 antibody limbic encephalitis. Ann Neurol 69: 892–900.

Janier M, Hegyi V, Dupin N et al. (2014). 2014 European guideline on the management of syphilis. J Eur Acad Dermatol Venereol 28: 1581–1593.

Jarvis JN, Bicanic T, Loyse A et al. (2014). Determinants of mortality in a combined cohort of 501 patients with HIV-associated cryptococcal meningitis: implications for improving outcomes. Clin Infect Dis 58: 736–745.

Joseph FG, Scolding NJ (2010). Neurolupus. Pract Neurol 10: 4–15.

Josephs KA, Ahlskog JE, Parisi JE et al. (2009). Rapidly progressive neurodegenerative dementias. Arch Neurol 66: 201–207.

Karaarslan E, Altintas A, Senol U et al. (2001). Balo's concentric sclerosis: clinical and radiologic features of five cases. AJNR Am J Neuroradiol 22: 1362–1367.

Kelley BJ, Boeve BF, Josephs KA (2009). Rapidly progressive young-onset dementia. Cogn Behav Neurol 22: 22–27.

Ketelslegers IA, Visser IE, Neuteboom RF et al. (2011). Disease course and outcome of acute disseminated encephalomyelitis is more severe in adults than in children. Mult Scler 17: 441–448.

Kikyo H, Furukawa T (1999). Creutzfeldt–Jakob-like syndrome induced by lithium, levomepromazine, and phenobarbitone. J Neurol Neurosurg Psychiatry 66: 802–803.

Kim MO, Takada LT, Wong K et al. (2017). Genetic PrP prion diseases. Cold Spring Harb Perspect Biol. pii: a033134. https://doi.org/10.1101/ cshperspect.a033134.

Kinoshita Y, Inoue Y, Tsuru E et al. (2001). Unusual MR findings of Wernicke encephalopathy with cortical involvement. No To Shinkei 53: 65–68.

Kirshner HS, Bradshaw M (2015). The inflammatory form of cerebral amyloid angiopathy or "cerebral amyloid angiopathy-related inflammation" (CAARI). Curr Neurol Neurosci Rep 15: 54.

Labeyrie MA, Lenck S, Saint-Maurice JP et al. (2014). Dural arteriovenous fistulas presenting with reversible dementia are associated with a specific venous drainage. Eur J Neurol 21: 545–547.

Lai M, Hughes EG, Peng X et al. (2009). AMPA receptor antibodies in limbic encephalitis alter synaptic receptor location. Ann Neurol 65: 424–434.

Lai M, Huijbers MG, Lancaster E et al. (2010). Investigation of LGI1 as the antigen in limbic encephalitis previously attributed to potassium channels: a case series. Lancet Neurol 9: 776–785.

Lancaster E, Dalmau J (2012). Neuronal autoantigens–pathogenesis, associated disorders and antibody testing. Nat Rev Neurol 8: 380–390.

Lang B, Makuch M, Moloney T et al. (2017). Intracellular and non-neuronal targets of voltage-gated potassium channel complex antibodies. J Neurol Neurosurg Psychiatry 88: 353–361.

Lee CH, Lin WC, Lu CH et al. (2009). Initially unrecognized dementia in a young man with neurosyphilis. Neurologist 15: 95–97.

Leschziner G, Rudge P, Lucas S et al. (2011). Lymphomatosis cerebri presenting as a rapidly progressive dementia with a high methylmalonic acid. J Neurol 258 (8): 1489–1493.

Leypoldt F, Armangue T, Dalmau J (2015). Autoimmune encephalopathies. Ann N Y Acad Sci 1338: 94–114.

Linnoila JJ, Rosenfeld MR, Dalmau J (2014). Neuronal surface antibody-mediated autoimmune encephalitis. Semin Neurol 34: 458–466.

Lo L, Tan AC, Umapathi T et al. (2006). Diffusion-weighted MR imaging in early diagnosis and prognosis of hypoglycemia. AJNR Am J Neuroradiol 27: 1222–1224.

Marra CM (2015). Neurosyphilis. Continuum (Minneap Minn) 21: 1714–1728.

Marra CM (2016). Syphilis screening in neurology. JAMA Neurol 73: 926–927.

Marques-Matos C, Reis J, Reis C et al. (2016). Mitochondrial encephalomyopathy with lactic acidosis and strokelike episodes presenting before 50 years of age: When a stroke is not just a stroke. JAMA Neurol 73: 604–606.

McGinnis SM (2011). Infectious causes of rapidly progressive dementia. Semin Neurol 31: 266–285.

McKeon A (2016). Autoimmune encephalopathies and dementias. Continuum (Minneap Minn) 22: 538–558.

McKeon A, Pittock SJ (2016). Autoimmune dementias. Non-Alzheimer's and Atypical Dementia. John Wiley & Sons, Ltd.

McKinney AM, Lohman BD, Sarikaya B et al. (2010). Acute hepatic encephalopathy: diffusion-weighted and fluid-attenuated inversion recovery findings, and correlation with plasma ammonia level and clinical outcome. AJNR Am J Neuroradiol 31: 1471–1479.

Mendonca N, Santos G, Duro D et al. (2012). Multiple dural arteriovenous fistulas presenting as rapidly progressive dementia. Neurologist 18: 130–132.

Miller-Thomas MM, Sipe AL, Benzinger TL et al. (2016). Multimodality review of amyloid-related diseases of the central nervous system. Radiographics 36: 1147–1163.

Milligan TA, Zamani A, Bromfield E (2009). Frequency and patterns of MRI abnormalities due to status epilepticus. Seizure 18: 104–108.

Misra UK, Kalita J (2010). Overview: Japanese encephalitis. Prog Neurobiol 91: 108–120.

Mizrachi IB, Gomez-Hassan D, Blaivas M et al. (2006). Pitfalls in the diagnosis of mitochondrial encephalopathy with lactic acidosis and stroke-like episodes. J Neuroophthalmol 26: 38–43.

Molloy ES, Calabrese CM, Calabrese LH (2017). The risk of progressive multifocal leukoencephalopathy in the biologic era: prevention and management. Rheum Dis Clin North Am 43: 95–109.

Moore A, Nelson C, Molins C et al. (2016). Current guidelines, common clinical pitfalls, and future directions for laboratory diagnosis of Lyme disease, United States. Emerg Infect Dis 22.

Mouldi S, Le Rhun E, Gautier S et al. (2006). Lithium-induced encephalopathy mimicking Creutzfeldt-Jakob disease. Rev Neurol (Paris) 162 (11): 118–121.

Moussaddy A, Levy A, Strbian D et al. (2015). Inflammatory cerebral amyloid angiopathy, amyloid-beta-related angiitis, and primary angiitis of the central nervous system: similarities and differences. Stroke 46: e210–e213.

Murray K (2008). The phenotype of sporadic CJD in the UK between 1993-2004, and a review of the diagnostic criteria and differential diagnosis, University of Edinburgh, Edinburgh.

Neto AS, Soares Neto HR, Simabukuro MM et al. (2016). Rapidly progressive dementia: prevalence and causes in a neurologic unit of a tertiary hospital in Brazil. Alzheimer Dis Assoc Disord 31: 239–243.

Newey CR, Appleby BS, Shook S et al. (2013). Patient with voltage-gated potassium-channel (VGKC) limbic encephalitis found to have Creutzfeldt-Jakob disease (CJD) at autopsy. J Neuropsychiatry Clin Neurosci 25: E05–E07.

N'Gbo N'gbo Ikazabo R, Mostosi C, Quivron B et al. (2016). Immune-reconstitution inflammatory syndrome in multiple sclerosis patients treated with natalizumab: a series of 4 cases. Clin Ther 38: 670–675.

Oksanen V (1986). Neurosarcoidosis: clinical presentations and course in 50 patients. Acta Neurol Scand 73: 283–290.

Papageorgiou SG, Kontaxis T, Bonakis A et al. (2009). Rapidly progressive dementia: causes found in a Greek tertiary referral center in Athens. Alzheimer Dis Assoc Disord 23: 337–346.

Pasi M, Nappini S, Salvadori E et al. (2014). Rapidly progressive cognitive impairment in a patient with high flow dural arteriovenous fistulas, cerebral sinus thrombosis and protein S deficiency. J Clin Neurosci 21: 1654–1656.

Paterson RW, Torres-Chae CC, Kuo AL et al. (2012). Differential diagnosis of Jakob-Creutzfeldt disease. Arch Neurol 69: 1578–1582.

Paul WB, Aggarwall V, Kurian S et al. (2015). Portosystemic shunt presenting as rapidly progressive dementia. J Assoc Physicians India 63: 82–83.

Pfeiffer RF (2011). Wilson's disease. Handb Clin Neurol 100: 681–709.

Pittock SJ, Kryzer TJ, Lennon VA (2004). Paraneoplastic antibodies coexist and predict cancer, not neurological syndrome. Ann Neurol 56: 715–719.

Pohl D, Alper G, Van Haren K et al. (2016). Acute disseminated encephalomyelitis: updates on an inflammatory CNS syndrome. Neurology 87: S38–S45.

Poser S, Mollenhauer B, Kraubeta A et al. (1999). How to improve the clinical diagnosis of Creutzfeldt–Jakob disease. Brain 122: 2345–2351.

Prashanth LK, Taly AB, Ravi V et al. (2006). Adult onset subacute sclerosing panencephalitis: clinical profile of 39 patients from a tertiary care centre. J Neurol Neurosurg Psychiatry 77: 630–633.

Rahmlow MR, Kantarci O (2013). Fulminant demyelinating diseases. Neurohospitalist 3: 81–91.

Ramanathan S, Mohammad SS, Brilot F et al. (2014). Autoimmune encephalitis: recent updates and emerging challenges. J Clin Neurosci 21: 722–730.

Rocca MA, Amato MP, De Stefano N et al. (2015). Clinical and imaging assessment of cognitive dysfunction in multiple sclerosis. Lancet Neurol 14: 302–317.

Rosche J, Sieveking C, Kampf C et al. (2015). Creutzfeldt–Jakob-like syndrome due to hypercalcemic encephalopathy. Clin EEG Neurosci 46: 327–330.

Rosenbloom MH, Atri A (2011). The evaluation of rapidly progressive dementia. Neurologist 17: 67–74.

Rosenbloom MH, Tartaglia MC, Forner SA et al. (2015). Metabolic disorders with clinical and radiologic features of sporadic Creutzfeldt–Jakob disease. Neurol Clin Pract 5: 108–115.

Rovira A, Alonso J, Cordoba J (2008). MR imaging findings in hepatic encephalopathy. AJNR Am J Neuroradiol 29: 1612–1621.

Sala I, Marquie M, Sanchez-Saudinos MB et al. (2012). Rapidly progressive dementia: experience in a tertiary care medical center. Alzheimer Dis Assoc Disord 26: 267–271.

Sampognaro P, Vo KT, Richie M et al. (2017). Bismuth subgallate toxicity in the age of online supplement use. Neurologist 22 (6): 237–240.

Saneto RP, Friedman SD, Shaw DW (2008). Neuroimaging of mitochondrial disease. Mitochondrion 8: 396–413.

Sarazin M, Amarenco P, Mikol J et al. (2002). Reversible leukoencephalopathy in cerebral amyloid angiopathy presenting as subacute dementia. Eur J Neurol 9: 353–358.

Savard M, Irani SR, Guillemette A et al. (2016). Creutzfeldt-Jakob disease-like periodic sharp wave complexes in voltage-gated potassium channel-complex antibodies encephalitis: a case report. J Clin Neurophysiol 33: e1–e4.

Scalzo SJ, Bowden SC, Ambrose ML et al. (2015). Wernicke-Korsakoff syndrome not related to alcohol use: a systematic review. J Neurol Neurosurg Psychiatry 86: 1362–1368.

Schielke E, Nolte C, Muller W et al. (2001). Sarcoidosis presenting as rapidly progressive dementia: clinical and neuropathological evaluation. J Neurol 248: 522–524.

Schlaberg R, Chiu CY, Miller S et al. (2017). Validation of metagenomic next-generation sequencing tests for universal pathogen detection. Arch Pathol Lab Med 141: 776–786.

Schmidt C, Haik S, Satoh K et al. (2012). Rapidly progressive Alzheimer's disease: a multicenter update. Journal of Alzheimer's disease: JAD 30: 751–756.

Scolding NJ, Joseph FG (2002). The neuropathology and pathogenesis of systemic lupus erythematosus. Neuropathol Appl Neurobiol 28: 173–189.

Sener RN (2003). Diffusion MRI findings in Wilson's disease. Comput Med Imaging Graph 27: 17–21.

Sevin M, Lesca G, Baumann N et al. (2007). The adult form of Niemann-Pick disease type C. Brain 130: 120–133.

Sharma P, Eesa M, Scott JN (2009). Toxic and acquired metabolic encephalopathies: MRI appearance. AJR Am J Roentgenol 193: 879–886.

Sheerin F, Pretorius PM, Briley D et al. (2008). Differential diagnosis of restricted diffusion confined to the cerebral cortex. Clin Radiol 63: 1245–1253.

Shinohara M, Yamada M (2016). Drug induced cognitive impairment. Brain Nerve 68 (4): 421–428.

Sierra del Rio M, Rousseau A, Soussain C et al. (2009). Primary CNS lymphoma in immunocompetent patients. Oncologist 14 (5): 526–539.

Singh TD, Fugate JE, Rabinstein AA (2014). Central pontine and extrapontine myelinolysis: a systematic review. Eur J Neurol 21 (12): 1443–1450.

Singhal AB, Newstein MC, Budzik R et al. (2003). Diffusion-weighted magnetic resonance imaging abnormalities in *Bartonella* encephalopathy. J Neuroimaging 13: 79–82.

Smith JK, Matheus MG, Castillo M (2004). Imaging manifestations of neurosarcoidosis. AJR Am J Roentgenol 182: 289–295.

Spencer TS, Campellone JV, Maldonado I et al. (2005). Clinical and magnetic resonance imaging manifestations of neurosarcoidosis. Semin Arthritis Rheum 34: 649–661.

Staffaroni AM, Elahi FM, McDermott D et al. (2017). Neuroimaging in dementia. Semin Neurol 37: 510–537.

Stretz C, Finelli PF (2015). Differential diagnosis of restricted diffusion of the thalamus – focus on viral encephalitis. The Neurohospitalist 5: NP1–NP2.

Taillibert S, Guillevin R, Menuel C et al. (2008). Brain lymphoma: usefulness of the magnetic resonance spectroscopy. J Neurooncol 86: 225–229.

Thieben MJ, Lennon VA, Boeve BF et al. (2004). Potentially reversible autoimmune limbic encephalitis with neuronal potassium channel antibody. Neurology 62: 1177–1182.

Tschampa HJ, Neumann M, Zerr I et al. (2001). Patients with Alzheimer's disease and dementia with Lewy bodies mistaken for Creutzfeldt–Jakob disease. J Neurol Neurosurg Psychiatry 71: 33–39.

Urbach H, Rauer S, Mader I et al. (2015). Supratentorial white matter blurring associated with voltage-gated potassium channel-complex limbic encephalitis. Neuroradiology 57: 1203–1209.

van Sonderen A, Schreurs MW, de Bruijn MA et al. (2016). The relevance of VGKC positivity in the absence of LGI1 and Caspr2 antibodies. Neurology 86: 1692–1699.

Verity MA (1990). Comparative observations on inorganic and organic lead neurotoxicity. Environ Health Perspect 89: 43–48.

Verma R, Arya K (2012). Tumefactive demyelination associated with systemic lupus erythematosus. BMJ Case Rep 2012.

Vernino S, Geschwind M, Boeve B (2007). Autoimmune encephalopathies. Neurologist 13: 140–147.

Vincent A, Buckley C, Schott JM et al. (2004). Potassium channel antibody-associated encephalopathy: a potentially immunotherapy-responsive form of limbic encephalitis. Brain 127: 701–712.

Vincent A, Buckley C, Lang B et al. (2009). Clinical spectrum of voltage-gated potassium channel autoimmunity. Neurology 72: 99–100.

Vincent A, Bien CG, Irani SR et al. (2011). Autoantibodies associated with diseases of the CNS: new developments and future challenges. Lancet Neurol 10: 759–772.

Vitali P, Maccagnano E, Caverzasi E et al. (2011). Diffusion-weighted MRI hyperintensity patterns differentiate CJD from other rapid dementias. Neurology 76: 1711–1719.

Vitaliani R, Mason W, Ances B et al. (2005). Paraneoplastic encephalitis, psychiatric symptoms, and hypoventilation in ovarian teratoma. Ann Neurol 58: 594–604.

Wada Y, Yamamoto T, Kita Y et al. (2003). An autopsy case of encephalopathy associated with small cell carcinoma of the stomach with nonconvulsive status epilepticus resembling Creutzfeldt–Jakob disease. No To Shinkei 55: 423–428.

Walker LC, Jucker M (2015). Neurodegenerative diseases: expanding the prion concept. Annual Review of Neuroscience 38: 87–103.

Wasay M, Azeemuddin M (2005). Neuroimaging of cerebral venous thrombosis. Journal of neuroimaging : official journal of the American Society of Neuroimaging 15: 118–128.

Watts JC, Prusiner SB (2017). Beta-amyloid prions and the pathobiology of Alzheimer's disease. Cold Spring Harb Perspect Med. pii: a023507. https://doi.org/10.1101/cshperspect.a023507.

Watts JC, Giles K, Oehler A et al. (2013). Transmission of multiple system atrophy prions to transgenic mice. Proc Natl Acad Sci U S A 110: 19555–19560.

Weaver JD, Vinters HV, Koretz B et al. (2007). Lymphomatosis cerebri presenting as rapidly progressive dementia. Neurologist 13 (3): 150–153.

Weiss D, Brockmann K, Nagele T et al. (2011). Rapid emergence of temporal and pulvinar lesions in MELAS mimicking Creutzfeldt-Jakob disease. Neurology 77: 914.

Welch K (2011). Neurological complications of alcohol and misuse of drugs. Pract Neurol 11 (4): 206–219.

WHO (1998). Global surveillance, diagnosis and therapy of human transmissible spongiform encephalopathies: report of a WHO consultation Geneva, Switzerland 9–11 February 1998. World Health Organization: Emerging and other communicable diseases, surveillance and control, World Health Organization, Geneva, Switzerland.

Wicklund MR, Mokri B, Drubach DA et al. (2011). Frontotemporal brain sagging syndrome: an SIH-like presentation mimicking FTD. Neurology 76: 1377–1382.

Wilson MR, Naccache SN, Samayoa E et al. (2014). Actionable diagnosis of neuroleptospirosis by next-generation sequencing. N Engl J Med 370: 2408–2417.

Wilson MR, Shanbhag NM, Reid MJ et al. (2015). Diagnosing *Balamuthia mandrillaris* encephalitis with metagenomic deep sequencing. Ann Neurol 78: 722–730.

Wilson MR, Suan D, Duggins A et al. (2017). A novel cause of chronic viral meningoencephalitis: Cache Valley virus. Ann Neurol 82: 105–114.

Wingerchuk DM, Weinshenker BG (2012). The emerging relationship between neuromyelitis optica and systemic rheumatologic autoimmune disease. Mult Scler 18: 5–10.

Wingerchuk DM, Banwell B, Bennett JL et al. (2015). International consensus diagnostic criteria for neuromyelitis optica spectrum disorders. Neurology 85: 177–189.

Woodruff BK (2007). Evaluation of rapidly progressive dementia. Semin Neurol 27: 363–375.

Yamada M (2015). Cerebral amyloid angiopathy: emerging concepts. Journal of Stroke 17: 17–30.

Yamashita H, Ubano M, Uesaka Y et al. (2012). A 34-year-old woman with cat scratch disease who developed encephalopathy. Rinsho Shinkeigaku 52: 576–580.

Yang HQ, Zhao WC, Yang WM et al. (2016). Clinical profiles and short-term outcomes of acute disseminated encephalomyelitis in adult Chinese patients. J Clin Neurol 12: 282–288.

Yoneda M, Maeda M, Kimura H et al. (1999). Vasogenic edema on MELAS: a serial study with diffusion-weighted MR imaging. Neurology 53: 2182–2184.

Yoo JY, Hirsch LJ (2014). Limbic encephalitis associated with anti-voltage-gated potassium channel complex antibodies mimicking Creutzfeldt-Jakob disease. JAMA Neurol 71: 79–82.

Yu H, Gao B, Liu J et al. (2017). Lymphomatosis cerebri: a rare variant of primary cebtral nervous system lymphoma and MR imaging features. Cancer Imaging 17 (1): 26.

Young GS, Geschwind MD, Fischbein NJ et al. (2005). Diffusion-weighted and fluid-attenuated inversion recovery imaging in Creutzfeldt–Jakob disease: high sensitivity and specificity for diagnosis. AJNR Am J Neuroradiol 26: 1551–1562.

Zeidman SM, Monsein LH, Arosarena O et al. (1995). Reversibility of white matter changes and dementia after treatment of dural fistulas. AJNR Am J Neuroradiol 16: 1080–1083.

Zerr I, Kallenberg K, Summers DM et al. (2009). Updated clinical diagnostic criteria for sporadic Creutzfeldt-Jakob disease. Brain 132: 2659–2668.

Handbook of Clinical Neurology, Vol. 153 (3rd series)
Human Prion Diseases
M. Pocchiari and J. Manson, Editors
https://doi.org/10.1016/B978-0-444-63945-5.00021-0

Chapter 21

Symptomatic treatment, care, and support of CJD patients

BRIAN S. APPLEBY[1]* AND DEBORAH R. YOBS[2]

[1]*Departments of Pathology, Neurology, and Psychiatry and National Prion Disease Pathology Surveillance Center, Case Western Reserve University, Cleveland, OH, United States*

[2]*CJD Foundation, Akron, OH, United States*

Abstract

Prion diseases (e.g., Creutzfeldt–Jakob disease) are rapidly progressive neurodegenerative diseases that are invariably fatal. Diagnosing prion disease can be difficult and can lead to frustration. There is no currently available disease-altering treatment for prion diseases and the care and management of affected patients are directed towards symptomatic relief and quality of life. In this chapter, we highlight the many unique challenges of prion disease and how they affect care and management strategies. Symptomatic treatment follows many of the same principles observed in geriatric and/or hospice care, with some important differences due to disease-specific characteristics. We provide an overview of pharmacologic and nonpharmacologic strategies for managing symptoms of prion disease. Education and psychosocial support are also very important in managing patients and families affected by the illness and are discussed in detail. Readers of this chapter will understand the context of caring for a patient with prion disease and will be supplied with practical tools for managing symptoms and educating other healthcare personnel and caregivers. Additional resources for assistance in the care of prion disease patients are also discussed.

INTRODUCTION

Prion diseases are rapidly progressive neurodegenerative conditions that are invariably fatal. There are three etiologies of prion disease: sporadic, genetic, and acquired. Most prion diseases are of sporadic etiology (85%) and are comprised of sporadic Creutzfeldt–Jakob disease (sCJD), sporadic fatal insomnia (sFI), and variably protease-sensitive prionopathy (VPSPr). Genetic prion diseases account for 10–15% of cases and include genetic CJD (gCJD), Gerstmann–Sträussler–Scheinker syndrome (GSS), and fatal familial insomnia (FFI). Less than 1% of prion diseases are acquired via ritualistic cannibalism (kuru), medical transmission (iatrogenic CJD), or the ingestion of food contaminated with bovine spongiform encephalopathy (variant CJD).

Although definitive diagnosis of prion disease can only be achieved via neuropathologic examination, a probable diagnosis can be made by recognizing the clinical syndrome of prion disease and the use of several diagnostic tests (World Health Organization, 1998; Zerr et al., 2009). The clinical syndrome of sCJD includes the presence of two or more of the following symptoms with coexistent dementia: (1) cerebellar or visual impairments; (2) pyramidal or extrapyramidal signs; (3) myoclonus; and (4) akinetic mutism. The presence of periodic sharp-wave complexes on electroencephalogram is strongly suggestive of prion disease. Hyperintensity on diffusion-weighted imaging in the basal ganglia and/or two or more cortical areas (excluding the frontal cortex) is also highly suggestive, especially when there is restricted diffusion on apparent diffusion coefficient mapping (Vitali et al., 2011). Cerebrospinal fluid (CSF) 14-3-3 and tau proteins are markers of neuronal injury and are frequently used to help guide diagnosis (Hamlin et al., 2012). A disease-specific assay called real-time quaking-induced conversion (RT-QuIC) can also be used on CSF for diagnostic purposes

*Correspondence to: Brian S. Appleby, M.D., 3619 Park East Drive, Suite 206, Beachwood OH 44122, United States. Tel: +1-216-464-6412, E-mail: bsa35@case.edu

(Foutz et al., 2016). Genetic prion diseases can be diagnosed by sequencing the prion protein gene (*PRNP*).

Various challenges face patients, clinicians, and families dealing with prion diseases. Despite the advances made in diagnosing the disease within the last decade, there is still no treatment or cure for these conditions. Additionally, there are many unique features of prion disease that complicate clinical care. In this chapter, we will highlight the frequent challenges encountered in caring for a patient with prion disease and will offer a generalized approach to care as well as disease-specific interventions. The goal of this chapter is to help clinicians with the symptomatic care, management, and support of patients and families affected by prion diseases.

CHALLENGES

Diagnosis

Most prion diseases present as rapidly progressive dementias (RPD), which has an expansive differential diagnosis and necessitates multiple diagnostic studies. The extensive effort that is placed into correctly identifying the etiology of an RPD is largely to ensure that treatable diagnoses are not missed (Shrestha et al., 2015). The extensive work-up of RPD can be prolonged, especially with send-out laboratory studies that may not produce results for weeks. This often means that patients may not leave the hospital with a clear diagnosis. Additionally, physicians may not feel comfortable making a diagnosis of prion disease given its rarity and their lack of familiarity with the diagnosis. The advent of very specific diagnostic tests utilizing RT-QuIC will hopefully help ameliorate the uncertainty physicians may have in conveying the diagnosis of prion disease.

Using brain biopsies for diagnosis

Because the only way to definitely diagnosis prion disease is through neuropathologic examination, physicians may hesitate to give a diagnosis even though the patient meets criteria for probable prion disease and other treatable etiologies have been appropriately ruled out. For example, sometimes brain biopsies are unnecessarily performed on patients who had prior positive RT-QuIC CSF results. This tentative approach to diagnosis of prion disease is not only scientifically invalid, but unnecessarily contaminates instruments, is an unnecessary use of healthcare resources, and is also damaging to patients. Brain biopsies should not be performed in suspected cases of CJD, but rather cases in which a treatable diagnosis is being considered.

Communication

Providing quality medical care rests heavily on one's ability to communicate and it is the physician's responsibility to lead the patient and family through their journey to the best of the physician's ability. Many frustrations experienced by patients and families can be attributed to poor communication. Because making the diagnosis of prion disease involves excluding numerous other conditions, it is important to discuss with the patient and his/her family why tests are being conducted and their results. Frequently reviewing the diagnostic process with patients and families will help build a therapeutic relationship and avoid confusion. Once the diagnosis of a probable prion disease has been made, it should be quickly conveyed to the family so that appropriate services can be arranged. Family members have commented that sometimes they receive information that is "too little too late" (Biggs, 2003). Thus, when delivering news regarding prion disease diagnosis, it is also helpful to offer resources from which families can learn more about the condition. Examples of resources may include referral to a physician familiar with the condition, referral to a patient advocacy group (e.g., CJD Foundation), and distribution of vetted educational materials designed specifically for family members.

Medical teams have become large and sometimes families may get different information from different healthcare providers or may not get any information at all. For this reason, it is recommended that a key worker be designated as soon as the diagnosis of prion disease is made (Department of Health, 2000). The key worker is a healthcare provider who is a single point of communication with the family, which will ensure a consistent message. He/she may also be responsible for following up on any outstanding laboratory results, even after the patient has been discharged from hospital. If the family choses autopsy, it is imperative that someone who is in close contact with the family, such as the key worker, receives the results in order to expedite the disclosure of this information to the family.

One of the most helpful things that one can do for a patient is to enroll the use of social services. They can help coordinate care needs proactively (e.g., before discharge from hospital), arrange for hospice evaluation, help coordinate care from numerous healthcare professionals, counsel families on end-of-life and financial matters, and offer much-needed social support (Biggs, 2003).

How to give a diagnosis of prion disease

Notifying a patient or family member of an impending death is difficult but is one of the most important things a clinician does. Giving the diagnosis of prion disease is complicated and different from giving a diagnosis of other diseases. Receiving a diagnosis of prion disease is not like getting a diagnosis of cancer; people generally understand and have known people who have died from cancer. Receiving a diagnosis of prion disease is unlike receiving a diagnosis of Alzheimer disease, which is known to most people and likely has progressed gradually over years. Receiving a diagnosis of prion disease is perhaps most akin to learning of a sudden and unexpected tragedy that has resulted in the death of a loved one. It can be confusing and hard to contemplate.

Whenever delivering the diagnosis of prion disease, it is important to put yourself in the patient's shoes and to treat the individual as you would like to be treated. If you are not able to do this, it may be wise to ask someone to help you to convey the news. For example, if you are telling a spouse that his or her loved one has prion disease, imagine that you are that spouse. It is helpful to consider these things before you enter the room to help set the tone. We recommend that you have this conversation as soon as the patient's diagnosis is deemed to be probable prion disease. Families need as much time as possible to process the diagnosis and to spend time with their loved one.

We would suggest separating the family from the patient when you first disclose the diagnosis. A staff member may sit with the patient and perform an examination or question the person to help distract the patient from the absence of the family. Make sure the environment in which you meet with the family is comfortable. There should be enough chairs for everyone to sit and there should be no distractions or interruptions during the discussion. Tissues should be available. The clinician should also be seated close to the family members when the discussion occurs. Eye contact should be maintained at all times.

You should provide an overview of the clinical course and diagnostic test results to provide context as to why you are diagnosing their loved one with the disease. Once context has been provided, you should disclose the diagnosis directly and offer your condolences. Families may have conducted research and have some idea of what this diagnosis means before you tell them. It is most appropriate to remain silent once the diagnosis has been offered. Answer any and all questions that the family may have. We have been in a room with families for up to 2 hours discussing the diagnosis, prognosis, and management options. For this reason, it is recommended that these patients be seen at the end of the day so that you do not have to be concerned about your clinic schedule. It is advisable that you give them information from a support organization, such as the CJD Foundation, and offer a referral to them. We typically place this information and hospice orders in an unmarked envelope as many family members do not want their loved ones to see the information.

Many patients with prion disease have anosognosia and this impacts the manner in which you give the diagnosis. Before going back into the patient's room, it is recommended that you ask family members how they would like to proceed when reentering. We often inform the family about the likelihood of anosognosia and this may already be apparent to the family. We recommend to the family that we do not lie to the patient regarding the diagnosis, but that we only answer the questions the patient asks. When we go back into the room and ask the patient if s/he has any questions, the vast majority of patients will not ask anything. If they do ask questions, we directly answer the question that they ask and say nothing more unless they ask further questions. We often address hospice as "extra help" unless the patient is more cognizant and is able to understand his or her situation. It is helpful to remind the patient and family that you will be walking with them through their journey.

Family members and patients will respond to the diagnosis in a variety of ways. Some will be appreciative, some will be emotionally distraught, and some may be angry. Anger is sometimes directed against the diagnosing clinician. In our experience, the best way to handle this scenario is to say nothing, nod your head in agreement, and maintain eye contact. It is important to understand that typically the family member is angry at the diagnosis, not at the person delivering the news. Finally, when disclosing the diagnosis of prion disease, one must be sure to monitor one's own mood and emotions afterwards. Disclosing bad news is a tricky interplay of displaying empathy during the interaction, but knowing how to appropriately detach afterwards.

Education

A serious barrier in the clinical care of prion disease patients is education. The lack of education or misinformation regarding prion diseases pervades all sectors, including healthcare professionals, family members, media, funeral home directors and embalmers, and even certain support venues. There are multiple reasons why education about prion disease is difficult. The rarity of the illness results in many having never heard of the disease. The unique nature of a transmissible neurodegenerative disease that can be genetic may be quite confusing. Lastly, misinformation regarding transmissibility risks often forms a barrier to proper education regarding prion diseases.

Although healthcare professionals may be educated about prion disease, it is often with little and possibly outdated information. Additionally, there are precious few articles in the literature that focus on the care and management of prion disease patients compared to the amount of articles that discuss basic science or diagnostic aspects of the disease (Bailey et al., 2000; Rentz, 2003; D'Amour and Guimond, 2010). Families have commented that healthcare professionals tried to assist them but had very little knowledge and understanding of prion disease themselves (Biggs, 2003). This also impacts healthcare professionals, who may not feel prepared to care for someone with prion disease (D'Amour and Guimond, 2010).

In one study of nursing professionals, subjects received a score of 26% on an assessment regarding prion disease (D'Amour and Guimond, 2010). Some common misconceptions were that they did not know what the disease agent was or it was contracted from eating "contaminated beef." Eighty percent of respondents were misinformed regarding transmissibility risks and answered that biologic fluids could transmit infectious prions. Following the initial examination, respondents admitted to lack of knowledge of the disease and poor confidence in treating someone with prion disease. After an education session, participants scored an average of 91% on a second examination, which demonstrates that education can effectively combat these deficiencies. Educational resources for healthcare professionals are listed in Table 21.1.

Limited information is available for families to learn more about prion disease. Most of the literature in the public domain is for scientists or clinicians and is not written for the layperson. Media outlets may cover prion disease, but often do not provide a comprehensive assessment of the disease and often focus on a specific aspect such as transmissibility risk as it may pertain to a local hospital. Several internet sites focus on conspiracy theories involving prion disease and this further adds to family member distress (Bailey et al., 2000). Similar to education for healthcare professionals, the limited information provided for laypeople may be misleading or outdated. For example, family members may learn about the genetic aspects of prion disease but be lost to important subtle aspects like penetrance of specific mutations (Minikel et al., 2016). Therefore, it becomes the treating physician's responsibility to help educate families regarding the disease and be proactive about information that they may come across that may be misleading and/or distressing.

Dealing with families affected by genetic prion disease

Genetic prion disease carries unique challenges and heavily involves other family members. Genetic testing can be done via an antemortem blood test or on brain tissue at autopsy. It is important that the physician disclosing genetic results understands what s/he is reporting. The physician should understand the difference between polymorphisms and pathogenic genetic mutations and the importance of penetrance (Minikel et al., 2016). For this reason, the physician may want to work with a genetic counselor when disclosing genetic results (Bechtel and Geschwind, 2013).

Asymptomatic genetic testing

Some individuals with a family history of prion disease may want to be tested to see if they carry a genetic mutation. There are multiple reasons that individuals would want to know their genetic mutation status, including the feeling of needing to know, financial planning, family

Table 21.1

Resources for healthcare professionals

Name	Website
CJD Foundation (United States)	www.cjdfoundation.org
CJD International Support Alliance (international with links to support organizations in other countries)	http://cjdisa.com
National Prion Disease Pathology Surveillance Center	http://case.edu/med/pathology/centers/npdpsc/index.html
Centers for Disease Control and Prevention	https://www.cdc.gov/prions/cjd
Alzheimer's Association	www.alz.org
National Association for Homecare and Hospice, Homecare and Hospice Locator	http://www.nahc.org/resources-services/home-care-and-hospice-locator/
Social Security, Compassionate Allowances	https://www.ssa.gov/compassionateallowances
American Board of Genetic Counseling	http://www.abgc.net/ABGC/AmericanBoardofGeneticCounselors.asp

planning, or wanting to participate in research studies. Individuals who undergo asymptomatic genetic testing are strongly advised to see a genetic counselor first. Genetic counseling will help individuals understand what it means to have a genetic disease, evaluate how knowledge of the mutation may affect their life, and guide them in making important healthcare and financial decisions. Individuals may be counseled to purchase long-term care and/or life insurance policies prior to getting tested, which can be cancelled should they not carry a mutation.

Most asymptomatic testing will follow the Huntington disease protocol for genetic testing, which was initially developed for Huntington disease but is commonly used for other neurodegenerative disorders (Bechtel and Geschwind, 2013). An individual's mental state is examined on several occasions to ensure that they are of sound mind to receive the results. This psychiatric examination is important regardless of the test results, as a negative test result can also have severe consequences because of "survivor's guilt." Typically, asymptomatic testing is not done on minors.

We are increasingly seeing individuals who want to know their genetic status prior to having children because they are considering undergoing preimplantation genetic diagnosis (PGD) with in vitro fertilization (Uflacker et al., 2014). PGD is a technique that tests embryos for the genetic mutation and only implants embryos that do not have the mutation, essentially eliminating the disease from future generations. PGD can also be done even if the parent does not wish to know his or her genetic status. In some countries, PGD may be covered by insurance for those affected by prion disease.

END-OF-LIFE CONCERNS

Prion diseases are rapidly progressive and invariably fatal. With mean illness durations of 4–6 months, it is imperative that end-of-life concerns are addressed quickly. Below are some specific end-of-life issues that are pertinent to patients with prion disease.

Capacity and competence

Because prion diseases affect a patient's mental faculties, the issue of capacity as it relates to healthcare and financial matters needs to be quickly assessed. Capacity refers to a patient's ability to understand situations and make appropriate decisions and is usually evaluated by a licensed physician or psychologist. Importantly, capacity must be assessed with regard to the individual decision that is being made and is not all-encompassing. For example, a patient's capacity to consent to a lumbar puncture may not be equivalent to the decision of whom to designate as power of attorney (POA). Competency is assessed by a judge, who will usually use information from a medical professional's capacity assessment to make a legal designation of competence versus incompetence. There are several layers of advance directives that are affected by a patient's capacity/competence: healthcare POA, financial POA, living will, and guardianship.

Prior to losing decision-making capacity, a patient may designate someone as his/her POA. The role of a POA is to take over decision making if the patient is unable to express his or her wishes. There are two different types of POA: healthcare POA for medical decision making and financial POA for financial decision making. These two POAs do not need to be the same person and the legality of designating a POA differs by jurisdiction. A patient can only designate a POA if he/she holds the capacity at that time to make such a decision as determined by a healthcare professional.

A living will is a legal document that lays out what kind of medical care a patient would want to receive in certain scenarios (e.g., no life support in the setting of a terminal diagnosis with little chance of recovery). Living wills differ by jurisdiction and the patient must have the capacity to complete a living will as determined by a healthcare professional. In general, healthcare POAs are preferred over living wills as it allows the patient's wishes to be carried out by someone in situations that a living will may not properly address.

Guardianship is a legal status in which a court-appointed individual makes healthcare and financial decisions for an incapacitated patient. Guardianship procedures vary by jurisdiction but most will require an expert evaluation of capacity by a licensed healthcare professional that is used by a judge to ascertain competency and whether or not a guardian should be appointed.

Disability

Many patients are affected by prion disease when they are still working and financially supporting families. The acute loss of income with added care expenses can be financially disastrous for families. Following the diagnosis of prion disease, patients should be counseled to contact their employer's human resource department to receive guidance on their disability options. Some employers will offer private short-term and/or long-term disability policies. In the United States, long-term disability is also offered through the Social Security Administration (Social Security Disability Insurance: SSDI). Normally, there is a 2-year waiting period between SSDI approval and the receipt of benefits; however, certain diseases such as prion disease are placed on a "fast-track" (Compassionate Allowances, https://www.ssa.gov/compassionateallowances) in which benefits are immediately received upon approval of disability. If the patient qualifies for Medicaid, s/he will also receive this benefit immediately. Some countries offer specific programs for patients affected by prion disease. For example, the United Kingdom has a CJD care package that includes additional finances accessible by a care coordinator, social workers, physiotherapists, occupational and speech therapists, a general practitioner, and a district nurse that is aimed to help coordinate care of a patient with prion disease (Barnett, 2002; Barnett and McLean, 2005).

Life-prolonging measures

Choosing whether or not to pursue life-prolonging measures is often a struggle for family members. Because of this, it is important to understand what the patient's wishes are if possible. Life-prolonging measures include interventions such as artificial feeding tubes and artificial respiration. These interventions may prolong life in prion disease, as evidenced by differences observed in survival times between Japan, where life-prolonging interventions are common (mean survival time = 17 months), and Europe (mean survival time = 5 months) (Nagoshi et al., 2011). However, these measures do not affect the patient's overall condition or quality of life. The pursuit of life-prolonging measures is a personal one, but it is helpful to assist family members to understand that they can adversely affect quality of life.

Hospice

As soon as a diagnosis of prion disease is made, we strongly suggest that the patient be referred to hospice. Hospice can be a valuable resource for patients and families given its focus on the whole patient, family unit, and coordination of care. Depending on the hospice, the patient and family may receive access to specific services such as a visiting nurse, social worker, bereavement groups, and a volunteer pool that may help with home healthcare among other activities. A variety of therapies are often offered to the patient and include physical therapy, speech and language therapy, occupational therapy, art therapy, music therapy, and pet therapy. Hospice will help families maintain a safe and appropriate environment for the patient and can help by supplying hospital beds, shower chairs, and other items. Of note, not all therapies may be appropriate for patients with prion disease. For example, some patients with prion disease may be too sensitive to sound to engage in music therapy and may be frightened by pet therapy. In general, hospice will help tailor an individual treatment plan for each patient. If an autopsy is requested, they can also assist in communicating with autopsy and funeral home contacts.

SYMPTOM MANAGEMENT

Currently, there are no approved treatments for prion disease and treatment focuses on minimizing symptoms and maintaining quality of life. The basic tenets of geriatrics are often applicable to patients with prion disease:

- Only treat symptoms that are distressing to the patient or caregivers, or could potentially result in harm to either party.
- Make sure basic human needs are being assessed and met. Many symptoms such as agitation can be the result of a patient being hungry, tired, or needing to use the toilet. Agitation can also be caused by constipation, urinary tract infections, or urinary retention.
- Try nonpharmacologic interventions first.
- "Less is more" – always attempt to minimize the number and dose of medications given the susceptibility to adverse effects that these patients experience.
- When using medications "start low and go slow" – medications should be started at low doses and slowly increased as needed.
- Frequently re-evaluate for new or extinguished symptoms and the ongoing need for medications.

Nonpharmacologic management strategies

Nonpharmacologic treatment of symptoms is mainly aimed at alleviating basic human suffering and some disease-specific symptoms (Table 21.2). Some symptoms can exacerbate other more distressing symptoms and should be proactively treated. For example, pyrexia can often cause agitation or restlessness and nonpharmacologic strategies such as tepid sponging and the use of fans may be more effective than pharmacologic treatments (Bailey et al., 2000). Assessing the cause of distress can sometimes be difficult and will require the observation of nonverbal behaviors (e.g., holding one's stomach, facial grimaces) (Rentz, 2003). Below are some specific nonpharmacologic strategies for specific symptoms.

Sensory stimulation

Some patients with prion disease can be exceptionally affected by sensory stimuli.

Movement, touch, light, and noise can cause distress in those with visuospatial impairment and myoclonus and the environment can be readily adapted to prevent distress. If reflections seem to cause visual disturbance, reflective surfaces such as mirrors, windows, or glass tables or shiny appliances can be covered. A flickering or loud television can be disturbing. Soft lighting is ideal, as is quiet music if the patient tolerates it. It may be

Table 21.2

Nonpharmacologic interventions for prion disease (Rotkoff et al., 1997; Bailey et al., 2000; Gitlin et al., 2012)

Symptom	Interventions
Pyrexia	Tepid sponging, fans
Myoclonus/ hyperstartle	Minimize touching, quiet environment, soft lighting, soothing music, explain actions before touching. Limit visits and number of visitors. Remove telephone from patient's room. Tape over doorbell. Move patient away from nursing station
Visuospatial difficulties	Cover reflective surfaces such as mirrors, glass tables, and frames. Ensure patients are seeing items by moving around objects in front of them (e.g., rotating plate to insure they see all of the food)
Hemineglect	Place objects in easy reach of unaffected side
Incontinence	Condom catheters
Constipation	Daily bowel movement record, avoid rectal examination/suppository when possible, increase liquids
Skin breakdown	Preventive skin care, air mattress, absorbent diapers
Dysphagia/ rumination	Thickeners, cueing, trying food of different textures and temperature. Follow patient's lead on food preferences
Nausea/vomiting	Elevate bed, oral care, adjust feeding amount and content
Dementia	Assist with medication administration, cognitive aids (notes and calendars), supervision, use distraction in response to repetitive questioning, structured daily routine, offer simple choices, identify self and communicate your actions ahead of time
Psychosis/agitation	Art, music, and aroma therapy, make sure basic needs are being met, frequent toileting, assess for constipation, urinary tract infection, or urinary retention
Depression/anxiety	Counseling, pastoral care, art, music, and aroma therapy
Sleeping issues	Good sleep hygiene, routine schedule
Muscle contractures	Passive movement exercises, gentle massage

necessary to avoid loud sounds and large groups of people if they appear disruptive to the patient.

Nutrition

As prion disease progresses, the patient may have difficulty with appetite, chewing, focusing on a meal, and ultimately with swallowing. At early stages, ergonomic utensils may be helpful to enable self-feeding. As dysphagia progresses, it may be necessary to use puréed foods and thickener in fluids. Nourishment should be balanced with enticing foods. If the patient prefers less healthy foods such as milkshakes, or begins focusing on a very limited set of preferred foods, it is fine to move in that direction as long as the patient is obtaining adequate nourishment and is not encountering digestive difficulties. It may be difficult to keep patients hydrated due to cognitive concerns. Frequent reminders, prompts, and always having water nearby can help. Mouth care is important to keep the patient comfortable. Options include a washcloth, a child's toothbrush, and swabs.

Psychiatric symptoms

Prion disease patients frequently experience psychiatric symptoms. Remaining calm and not arguing when the patient expresses delusions and hallucinations is ideal. As long as patients are not a hazard to themselves or others, reassuring them and working through episodes with patience is best. If symptoms worsen or the patient is a danger to him/herself or others, then pharmacologic management may be needed.

Pharmacologic treatment

Symptoms may be severe enough or nonresponsive to nonpharmacologic treatment to the point of warranting pharmacologic intervention. Abiding by the principle of limiting medications, one can often choose a single medication that can treat more than one symptom (e.g., benzodiazepines for myoclonus, seizures, and agitation). The physician must also consider how certain medications will affect the disease course. For example, sedating medications that also affect mobility will likely shorten the disease course (e.g., benzodiazepines, neuroleptics). Moreover, side-effects of some medications may make caregiving more difficult. Giving benzodiazepines to a mobile patient with ataxia will increase the risk of falls and will require that caregivers take more precautions. Hence, these types of medications are generally used towards the later stages of the disease (Thompson et al., 2014). It is important to have discussions with the family about these potential side-effects prior to

Table 21.3

Pharmacologic treatments for prion disease (Bailey et al., 2000; Thompson et al., 2014; Shrestha et al., 2015)

Symptom	Intervention
Pain	Acetaminophen, opioids
Nausea/vomiting	Odansetron, try to avoid prochlorperazine due to extrapyramidal side-effects
Shortness of breath	Opioids
Depression/anxiety	SSRIs, SNRIs, mirtazapine, benzodiazepines
Insomnia	Melatonin, trazodone, benzodiazepines
Agitation	SSRIs, trazodone, low-potency neuroleptics (e.g., quetiapine), valproic acid, benzodiazepines
Psychosis	Low-potency neuroleptics (e.g., quetiapine), cholinesterase inhibitors, avoid typical neuroleptics when possible (e.g., haloperidol)
Seizures	Antiepileptic medications with benzodiazepines as needed
Myoclonus	Benzodiazepines (avoid short-acting benzodiazepines like alprazolam), antiepileptic medications

SNRIs, selective norepinephrine reuptake inhibitors; SSRIs, selective serotonin reuptake inhibitors.

starting new medications so as to temper expectations. Table 21.3 lists common symptoms of prion disease and their pharmacologic treatment options.

Pharmacologic treatment of neuropsychiatric symptoms

Pharmacologic treatment of neuropsychiatric symptoms can be particularly challenging for clinicians because the side-effects of psychiatric medications can be particularly troublesome for prion disease patients. Because many patients already experience gait imbalance, it may be prudent to initially treat agitation and anxiety with nonbenzodiazepine medications such as the various selective serotonin or norepinephrine reuptake inhibitors (SSRIs and SNRIs) and trazodone. Many patients also experience extrapyramidal symptoms as part of their illness, which may be exacerbated by antipsychotic medications. Typical antipsychotics, such as haloperidol, should be avoided to minimize extrapyramidal symptoms. It is important to note that most hospice order sets include haloperidol as a routine prn medication. There are some data that suggest cholinesterase inhibitors may be helpful in ameliorating psychotic symptoms in prion disease and thus may be used prior to an antipsychotic medication. If an antipsychotic is required, then an atypical antipsychotic with low D2 receptor potency (e.g., quetiapine) should be used at reduced doses initially to minimize extrapyramidal symptoms. As with any medication, the pros and cons of treatment should be weighed carefully. As such, only hallucinations that are distressing to the patient should be treated.

SUPPORT FOR CAREGIVERS

There is precious little scientific literature on caregiver burden in prion disease despite the voluminous amount of data on other neurodegenerative diseases like Alzheimer disease. The few studies on the subject demonstrate a tremendous amount of burden among caregivers, approaching that of other highly burdensome neurodegenerative disorders. Examining caregiver burden using the Zarit Burden Interview, Uflacker and colleagues (2015) found that caregiver burden in sCJD and behavioral variant frontotemporal dementia significantly exceeded that found in other young-onset dementias, including Alzheimer disease and language variants of frontotemporal dementia . These differences in caregiver burden were partially mediated by the number and severity of neuropsychiatric symptoms, as measured by the Neuropsychiatric Inventory, and, at least in this study, were not affected by cognitive or functional impairments. This important finding suggests that properly addressing distressing neuropsychiatric symptoms may positively impact caregiver burden and is an important management strategy to employ in patients with prion disease. However, in cases of variant CJD that were initially diagnosed with psychiatric illness, families were often angry about the initial psychiatric diagnosis, making it difficult to coordinate skilled psychiatric management later in the illness (Department of Health, 2000). As 16% of sCJD and genetic prion diseases were initially diagnosed with a primary psychiatric disorder in one study, this challenge may also occur in prion diseases other than vCJD (Appleby et al., 2014).

There are other aspects of care that likely contribute to caregiver burden but which have not been studied systematically. One might assume that the lack of education, poor familiarity with the disease of many healthcare professionals, difficulty in obtaining a diagnosis, aspects of transmissibility, and a possible genetic etiology contribute to caregiver burden. In one study, patients moved through an average of four different care settings before being admitted to hospice and the mean time from diagnosis to hospice admission was 9 days (range 1–21 days) (Bailey et al., 2000). Once in hospice the mean length of stay was 14 days (range 3–28 days), meaning that relationships had to be developed very quickly between hospice personnel and families. Family members often feel overburdened by the number of healthcare professionals involved in the patient's care or may be subject to unwanted media inquiries or questions from curious family members and healthcare professionals (Department of Health, 2000).

Relieving the caregiver's exhaustion and stress is crucial for both caregiver and patient. Family members have little time to care for themselves and to visit their own physicians while caring for a prion disease patient. They should be encouraged to self-care whenever possible. Exercising, getting adequate sleep, and eating healthfully will benefit the family members and enable them to continue caregiving for the patient. They may need encouragement to ask for help from professional caregivers or family and friends. The caregiver can also benefit from stress reduction through therapy, meditation, prayer, massage, and exercise.

In some cases, family members may pursue counseling, which can be helpful but needs to be approached in a manner that is sensitive to the situation. Traditional therapy in the context of prion disease may be inappropriate (Morris, 2010). When facing a terminal diagnosis, both the patient and/or family may not want to explore their feelings. The focus of counseling should be on brief encounters that focus on the family's needs, enabling them to make important decisions and arrive at solutions for their situation.

The role of the CJD Foundation and other patient support organizations

Family advocacy and support organizations, such as the CJD Foundation in the United States and others affiliated worldwide through the CJD International Support Alliance, offer valuable support for families and professionals at all stages of the disease through a variety of means. The CJD Foundation offers a 7-day helpline with trained staff and volunteers who accept calls from families, clinicians, hospice and healthcare providers, funeral professionals, and others. Families may contact the CJD Foundation at any stage of the disease. These support organizations are invaluable to clinicians as they can help answer many of the psychosocial questions that families ask when meeting with physicians.

Support groups and bereavement groups

Families affected by prion disease often benefit from peer support, whether during the caregiving phase or after the patient has died. Because of the disease's rarity, it can be difficult to find a support group that understands prion diseases. The CJD Foundation recommends families pursue both a prion disease-specific support group and a local support/bereavement group. Options include the following.

Teleconference support groups

The CJD Foundation conducts monthly teleconference support groups for caregivers at all stages, from diagnosis to bereavement. Some conferences are open question-and-answer discussions with a prion disease expert. Other calls feature a half-hour discussion on a specific topic followed by questions and answers. Teleconferences allow families to ask questions that they have not resolved with their physician, or at times raise issues that have concerned them for years after their loved one's passing – in an environment where others can benefit from hearing the response as well.

Conferences and workshops

The CJD Foundation hosts an annual conference for families and scientists, including family workshops and educational sessions. The program allows families to monitor scientific developments, lend support to other families, and participate in advocacy. Workshops are also hosted in regions around the United States each year. For information on workshops in other countries, consult the CJD International Support Alliance.

Dementia caregiver support groups

If local prion disease groups are not available, families can glean valuable advice from dementia caregiver groups, many of which are available at local Alzheimer's Association chapters (www.alz.org).

Local bereavement groups

The CJD Foundation recommends that families participate in bereavement groups in their communities. Referrals are available through hospice, religious organizations, and social workers. The CJD Foundation also offers periodic bereavement calls and workshops.

Social media

Peer discussions in private groups on social media can also be a source of support for families who are caregiving or grieving a loss. A number of CJD groups are available on Facebook.

CONCLUSION

Caring for and managing patients with prion disease can be challenging for clinicians. Many similar management strategies are employed in other geriatric or neuropsychiatric conditions and in a hospice setting. There are some disease-specific challenges of managing patients with prion disease, such as its rapid course, rarity, and misinformation regarding the illness. Despite these challenges, caring for patients with prion disease is very doable and there are multiple resources available to aid in their management.

ACKNOWLEDGMENTS

We would like to thank Suzanne Solvyns, Lauren Somple, and Beth Wachter for their valuable advice in preparing this manuscript. This manuscript was funded in part by the Stivison Fund for CJD Research.

References

Appleby BS, Rincon-Beardsley TD, Appleby KK et al. (2014). Initial diagnoses of patients ultimately diagnosed with prion disease. J Alzheimers Dis 42: 833–839.

Bailey B, Aranda S, Quinn K et al. (2000). Creutzfeldt–Jakob disease: extending palliative care nursing knowledge. Int J Palliat Nurs 6: 131–139.

Barnett F (2002). Nursing patients with variant Creutzfeldt–Jakob disease at home. Br J Community Nurs 7: 445–450.

Barnett F, McLean G (2005). Care management of Creutzfeldt–Jakob disease within the United Kingdom. J Nurs Manag 13: 111–118.

Bechtel K, Geschwind MD (2013). Ethics in prion disease. Prog Neurobiol 110: 29–44.

Biggs DA (2003). Creutzfeldt–Jakob disease: good practice guidelines for social services professionals. Available online at: http://www.prion.ucl.ac.uk/EasySiteWeb/GatewayLink.aspx?alId=745. Accessed 28 February 2017.

D'Amour R, Guimond P (2010). An experiential learning model applied to nurses working with patients with Creutzfeldt–Jakob disease. Can J Neurosci Nurs 32: 34–39.

Department of Health (2000). Creutzfeldt–Jakob disease: guidance for healthcare workers. Available online at: http://webarchive.nationalarchives.gov.uk/20130107105354/http:/www.dh.gov.uk/prod_consum_dh/groups/dh_digital assets/@dh/@en/documents/digitalasset/dh_4082370.pdf (accessed 02/28/2017).

Foutz A, Appleby BS, Hamlin C et al. (2016). Diagnostic and prognostic value of human prion detection in cerebrospinal fluid. Ann Neurol 81: 79–92.

Gitlin LN, Kales HC, Lyketsos CG (2012). Nonpharmacologic management of behavioral symptoms in dementia. JAMA 308: 2020–2029.

Hamlin C, Puoti G, Berri S et al. (2012). A comparison of tau and 14-3-3 protein in the diagnosis of Creutzfeldt–Jakob disease. Neurology 79: 547–552.

Minikel EV, Vallabh SM, Lek M et al. (2016). Quantifying prion disease penetrance using large population control cohorts. Sci Transl Med 8: 322ra9.

Morris C (2010). Counselling people with Creutzfeldt–Jakob disease (CJD) and their families. Dementia 9: 569–576.

Nagoshi K, Sadakane A, Nakamura Y et al. (2011). Duration of prion disease is longer in Japan than in other countries. J Epidemiol 21: 255–262.

Rentz CA (2003). Creutzfeldt–Jakob disease: two case studies. Am J Alzheimers Dis Other Demen 18: 171–180.

Rotkoff N, Labosky S, Dobson J et al. (1997). Nursing care of the resident with Creutzfeldt–Jakob disease. Geriatr Nurs 18: 155–159.

Shrestha R, Wuerz T, Appleby BS (2015). Rapidly progressive young-onset dementias: neuropsychiatric aspects. Psychiat Clin North Am 38: 221–232.

Thompson A, MacKay A, Rudge P et al. (2014). Behavioral and psychiatric symptoms in prion disease. Am J Psychiatry 171: 265–274.

Uflacker A, Doraiswamy PM, Rechitsky S et al. (2014). Preimplantation genetic diagnosis (PGD) for genetic prion disorder due to F198S mutation in the PRNP gene. JAMA Neurol 71: 484–486.

Uflacker A, Edmondson MC, Onyike CU et al. (2015). Caregiver burden in atypical dementias: comparing frontotemporal dementia, Creutzfeldt–Jakob disease, and Alzheimer's disease. Int Psychogeriatri 28: 269–273.

Vitali P, Maccagnano E, Caverzasi E et al. (2011). Diffusion-weighted MRI hyperintensity patterns differentiate CJD from other rapid dementias. Neurology 76: 1711–1719.

World Health Organization (1998). Global surveillance, diagnosis and therapy of human transmissible spongiform encephalopathies: report of a WHO consultation, WHO, Geneva, Switzerland.

Zerr I, Kallenberg K, Summers DM et al. (2009). Updated clinical diagnostic criteria for sporadic Creutzfeldt Jakob disease. Brain 132: 2659–2668.

Handbook of Clinical Neurology, Vol. 153 (3rd series)
Human Prion Diseases
M. Pocchiari and J. Manson, Editors
https://doi.org/10.1016/B978-0-444-63945-5.00022-2

Chapter 22

Identifying therapeutic targets and treatments in model systems

CORINNE LASMÉZAS[1]* AND RUTH GABIZON[2]

[1]*Departments of Immunology and Microbiology and Neuroscience, Scripps Florida, Jupiter, FL, United States*

[2]*Department of Neurology, The Agnes Ginges Center for Human Neurogenetics, Hadassah University Hospital, Jerusalem, Israel*

Abstract

In this chapter, we describe current therapeutic targets for prion diseases. We focus on targets that have been validated in vitro and in vivo, leaving out a plethora of theoretic targets that still require validation. We also show how the development of improved model systems for the study of prion infection and neurotoxic mechanisms has enabled target identification. Some therapeutic targets are prion-specific, such as PrP^{TSE}, while others are shared by other neurodegenerative diseases, for example, autophagy, cholesterol and energy metabolism, and neuroinflammation. In vivo models are discussed, and a genetic model of Creutzfeldt–Jakob disease particularly well suited for evaluation of prophylactic intervention is described in more detail.

INTRODUCTION

Prion diseases belong to the group of protein misfolding neurodegenerative diseases (PMNDs), like Alzheimer disease (AD), Parkinson disease, Huntington disease, amyotrophic lateral sclerosis, and frontotemporal dementia. The improper folding and aggregation of the prion protein (PrP) constitute the cause of the neurologic disease in prion diseases. This was postulated in 1982, when S. Prusiner found PrP aggregates in infectious brain fractions, and 25 years later amplification of misfolded and aggregated prion protein (PrP), along with the de novo production of infectivity, was achieved in the test tube (Deleault et al., 2007; Wang et al., 2010).

Prion diseases are infectious diseases, thereby revealing a fundamental concept, namely that protein aggregates can propagate from cell to cell and even organism to organism, and act as templates to the endogenous protein for the production of more of their misfolded selves. Meanwhile, in vitro models of "propagation" have also been developed for the proteins α-synuclein (Parkinson disease), tau (AD, frontotemporal dementia), and SOD1 (amyotrophic lateral sclerosis) (Luk et al., 2009; Grad et al., 2014; Sanders et al., 2014). Alpha-synuclein inoculation has been shown to induce Parkinson disease-like pathology at a minimum, or even a clinical disease, in transgenic mice expressing human α-synuclein (Desplats et al., 2009; Betemps et al., 2014; Ayers et al., 2017; Woerman et al., 2017). Tau (AD, frontotemporal dementia), Aβ 1–42 (AD), and SOD1 (amyotrophic lateral sclerosis) inoculations to transgenic mice expressing the human wild-type or disease-associated mutated proteins have been shown to trigger brain pathology mimicking that occurring in people affected by the respective disease (Epelbaum et al., 2015; Peeraer et al., 2015; Ayers et al., 2016).

It was therefore not surprising that prion diseases were first to offer in vitro and in vivo models to study protein misfolding-induced neurodegeneration and identify points of therapeutic intervention. Herein, we will describe therapeutic targets as well as some of these enabling models. Too many excellent models have been developed over the last 20 years to allow for an exhaustive review and we will not include PrP conversion assays, even though they constitute extremely valuable tools as front-line assays for therapeutic candidates focusing on PrP conversion, but are ill suited for probing

*Correspondence to: Corinne Lasmézas, DVM, PhD, Immunology and Microbiology, Neuroscience, Scripps Florida, 130 Scripps Way 2B2, 5500 Military Trail 22-119, Jupiter FL 33458, United States. Tel: +1-561-228-3456, E-mail: lasmezas@scripps.edu

the biology of cellular therapeutic targets and are discussed extensively elsewhere in this book.

From a therapeutic standpoint, prion pathogenesis is characterized by two mechanistically distinct phenomena, each of which needs to be targeted separately: the templated conversion of the protein PrP into its pathogenic, misfolded counterpart (PrP^{TSE}), leading to prion replication, and the toxicity of abnormal PrP for brain cells leading to neuronal dysfunction and death. Both phenomena will be discussed from both in vitro and in vivo investigations.

CELLULAR MODELS OF PRION INFECTION

PrP^{TSE} formation and propagation as a therapeutic target

Prion research in the 1970s and 1980s, including therapeutic studies (Pocchiari et al., 1987), involved inoculation of infectious prions to animal models, since no cell cultures were able to sustain prion replication. The first cell culture model was established in 1988 by Race et al. (1988), consisting of scrapie-infected murine neuroblastoma cells. Early studies allowed seminal discoveries on the cellular biology of prion replication, such as the finding that cell surface expression of endogenous PrP is necessary for productive infection and the half-lives of PrP (~4 hours) and PrP^{TSE} (>45 hours) (Caughey and Raymond, 1991). This discovery established cell surface expression of PrP as a potential therapeutic target for prion diseases, a target validated 2 years later when it was shown that PrP null mice are resistant to prion infection (Büeler et al., 1993; Manson et al., 1994). Based on this knowledge we developed a new high-throughput screening strategy to identify drugs reducing cell surface PrP levels. Using a library of compounds approved for human use, we identified two drugs preventing prion replication in cell culture, one of which delayed prion disease in a murine model of prion infection (Karapetyan et al., 2013). Another approach which was used was to target PrP based on the use of antibodies (Nicoll and Collinge, 2009).

It was also established early that, while individual cell clones exhibited robust infection, it was difficult to maintain infectivity in cell cultures without regular subcloning (Race et al., 1988). These technical difficulties slowed the development of in vitro models of prion infection. In 1997, a hypothalamic neuronal cell line, the GT1 cells, showed promise as the cells could be persistently infected with scrapie and exhibited apoptotic features (Schätzl et al., 1997).

Cellular models of prion propagation developed further in 2003, when the group of C. Weissmann isolated a subclone of murine neuroblastoma cells that were particularly susceptible to infection by RML prions (PK1 cells) and developed a quantitative in vitro assay to measure prion infectivity without having to inoculate mice with cell lysates (Kloehn et al., 2003). The assay was called the scrapie cell assay and has since been used by numerous laboratories with various modifications. The basic principle is that cells are grown in 96-well plates and exposed to serial dilutions of the prion material to be titrated; cells are cultured over several passages, to allow for wells that have received even single infectious units to become extensively infected as infection spreads between cells. The presence of PrP^{TSE} is then detected in each positive well using a PrP antibody, after proteinase K digestion of the normal PrP. The counting of positive cells is automated. At an appropriate dilution, only a fraction of the wells receive an infectious unit and score positive, and the infectious titer of the starting material can be determined by use of Poisson distribution and reference to standard curves. This assay allows researchers to measure, in a cellular system, the infectivity present in a given sample, but also to screen for drugs hampering the production of PrP^{TSE} in scrapie-infected cells with higher throughput than previously done.

The Weissmann group continued to perfect the assay, isolating various subclones of neuroblastoma cells exhibiting differential susceptibility to different strains of scrapie prions, enabling the study of prion strains in the cell system (Mahal et al., 2007; Karapetyan et al., 2009). The cellular model also allowed demonstration that prion strains are in fact populations that are present as quasi-species, thereby mimicking viral populations, and that these populations evolve as a result of the selection pressure of the environment (Li et al., 2010). Cell infection models revealed that pharmacologic treatments lead to strain-specific inhibition of prion replication and to the emergence of prion strains resistant to treatment (Ghaemmaghami et al., 2009; Browning et al., 2011). This important finding showed that antiprion treatments have to be evaluated using several prion strains in vitro and in vivo, whether they target PrP^{TSE} itself or a cellular factor, the modulation of which will lead to a change in the replicative environment of the prion, hence a change in the selection pressure, favoring a new, drug-resistant prion strain. However, the difficulty in targeting PrP^{TSE} is mitigated by the fact that multiple prion-susceptible cell lines susceptible to a wide range of prion strains have been developed in recent years. Examples are murine neuroblastoma cell-derived clones such as PK1 or CAD (Mahal et al., 2007), and the rabbit kidney epithelial cells RK13 that have been stably transfected with PrP from various species and extend the susceptibility range to murine, caprine, ovine, cervid, and bank vole prions (Arellano-Anaya et al., 2011; Kim et al., 2012; Dassanayake et al., 2016). Cell lines susceptible to human prions have been reported (Ladogana et al., 1995; Manuelidis et al., 2007), but sensitive and stable infection systems remain to be established. The reasons for this apparent resistance of cultured cells to human prions remain to be determined, but activation of lysosomal degradation has been suggested as a potential factor (Krejciova et al., 2014).

Cellular models of prion infection are now widely used as front-line assays to screen libraries of thousands of compounds or more for drugs preventing PrP^{TSE} formation, and to test the effect of potential therapeutics on prion replication and propagation (Kocisko et al., 2003; Kimata et al., 2007; Ghaemmaghami et al., 2010; Geissen et al., 2011; Karapetyan et al., 2013).

Autophagy and cholesterol metabolism as therapeutic targets

It was determined that altering cholesterol trafficking interfered with prion infection in cultured cells (Gilch et al., 2009; Hannaoui et al., 2014). In contrast, prion infection alters cellular cholesterol metabolism (Bate et al., 2008a, b; Bach et al., 2009; Vascellari et al., 2011; Montag et al., 2012; Cui et al., 2014). Thus, restoration of cholesterol homeostasis has emerged as a point of therapeutic intervention (Pani et al., 2010) and treatment with cholesterol-lowering statins has provided some benefit in murine models of prion disease (Mok et al., 2006; Kempster et al., 2007; Haviv et al., 2008; Vetrugno et al., 2009) (for details, see below).

Autophagy is a cellular mechanism by which cellular debris and protein aggregates are engulfed in a vesicle (the autophagosome) that then fuses with a lysosome, allowing degradation of the autophagic cargo. Stimulation of autophagy is able to reduce prion loads (Aguib et al., 2009; Heiseke et al., 2009a, b). For prion diseases as well as for other PMNDs, degradation of misfolded protein aggregates constitutes a therapeutic target under intense study (Ciechanover and Kwon, 2015).

Targeting neurotoxicity

A phenomenon which has confused, and is still confusing, the field, is that the "infectious" form of PrP responsible for cell-to-cell propagation and the "toxic" form of PrP leading to neuronal death may be distinct entities (Lasmézas et al., 1997; Sandberg et al., 2011). It is believed that higher-order aggregates of PrP constitute the infectious form, while low-molecular-weight PrP oligomers cause toxicity (Simoneau et al., 2007).

With the exception of GT1 cells (Schätzl et al., 1997), the prion-infected cell cultures mentioned previously continuously propagate and amplify prions without overt signs of neurotoxicity. This phenomenon has hampered the development of a simple cellular neurotoxicity assay mimicking prion-induced neuronal dysfunction and death occurring during prion infection in vivo (Brown et al., 2001; Liberski et al., 2004), as well as the discovery of therapeutic targets for neuroprotection.

A first step towards establishing in vitro models of neurotoxicity has been the discovery that the PrP peptide spanning residues 106–126 (PrP106–126) is neurotoxic to neurons (Forloni et al., 1993), a toxicity at least partially mediated by astrocytes (Forloni et al., 1994; Brown, 1999) and microglial cytokine release (Peyrin et al., 1999). PrP peptides of slightly different sizes were also neurotoxic (Tagliavini et al., 2001). Studies on PrP peptides have: (1) allowed demonstration of the involvement of glial cells in prion-linked neurotoxicity, a mechanism also referred to as gliosis, or neuroinflammation; and (2) shown that destabilization of the plasma membrane is a neurotoxic mechanism of the transmembrane domain of the prion protein (Haik et al., 2000; Mishra et al., 2002; Walsh et al., 2014). A recent study on the mechanism of membrane disruption by PrP106–126 showed similarity with the mechanism of toxicity of antimicrobial peptides (Pan et al., 2017). The involvement of microglial cells in the pathogenesis of prion diseases has been shown in murine models (Xie et al., 2013; Vincenti et al., 2015; Alibhai et al., 2016; Carroll et al., 2016) and in Creutzfeldt–Jakob disease (CJD) (Iaccarino et al., 2017). Modulation of neuroinflammation is thus a therapeutic target for prion diseases as much as it is for AD and Parkinson disease (Aguzzi and Zhu, 2017), even though a protective role of the microglial response has also been described (Zhu et al., 2016).

Establishment of a sensitive model of misfolded PrP-induced neurotoxicity and discovery of NAD as a therapeutic target

Evidence for the toxicity of full-length PrP was provided with the demonstration that murine and ovine PrP oligomers were toxic to primary neurons in vitro and after stereotaxic intracerebral injections in vivo (Simoneau et al., 2007). Mislocalized PrP, referred to as cytoplasmic PrP, was also shown to be toxic (Ma et al., 2002; Orsi et al., 2006). The Lasmézas lab then discovered that recombinant, monomeric misfolded PrP was highly toxic to neuronal cell types at nanomolar concentrations. We called this toxic PrP TPrP (Zhou et al., 2012). The monomeric, natively folded counterpart (NTPrP) was nontoxic over a large range of doses. This model of neurotoxicity is highly reproducible, sensitive, and portable in vivo as stereotaxic injection of TPrP above the hippocampus leads to acute neurotoxicity and death of hippocampal pyramidal neurons (Zhou et al., 2012). The TPrP model showed that protein conformation itself, rather than aggregation state, is the key determinant of neurotoxicity, and is being used in our laboratory to decipher molecular mechanisms of neurodegeneration. We discovered that TPrP induces depletion of the cellular metabolite nicotinamide adenine dinucleotide (NAD), causing severe energy deprivation and multiple pathway failures, and eventually neuronal death (Zhou et al., 2015). These studies identified NAD deprivation as a new therapeutic target for protein misfolding diseases.

Towards models of early neuronal dysfunction for therapeutic development

The field of antiprion therapeutics now is in need of additional cellular models able to report on early neuronal dysfunction, molecular markers, and morphologic changes that precede neuronal death (Belichenko et al., 2000). As a step forward, a recently described system allows the study of degeneration of dendritic spines on cultured hippocampal neurons after exposure to scrapie-infected mouse brain homogenates, well before chronic infection is established (Fang et al., 2016). It is to be expected that these models will emerge as our knowledge of mechanisms of neuronal dysfunction advances at the molecular and subcellular level, and will provide new tools for therapeutic development.

Drug screening using organotypic brain slices

The neuropathology of prion diseases involves not only neuronal damage and death, but also extensive microgliosis and astrocytosis (Fraser, 1976; Manuelidis et al., 1987; Lasmézas et al., 1996; Baker and Manuelidis, 2003; Vincenti et al., 2015). Early studies on the toxicity of PrP peptides replicated the involvement of both astrocytes and microglial cells in neurotoxic mechanisms (Forloni et al., 1994; Brown, 1999; Peyrin et al., 1999). A limitation of monocellular culture systems is that nonautologous mechanisms involved in disease pathogenesis cannot be replicated. The prion organotypic slice culture assay, described in 2008, addresses this limitation, allowing several readouts (PrP^{TSE} propagation, neuronal death, molecular markers) on prion-infected brain slices within a month (Falsig and Aguzzi, 2008; Sonati et al., 2013). A recent addition to the use of organotypic slice cultures in the therapeutic screening is real-time quaking-induced conversion (RT-QUIC) (OSCAR), combining prion infection of brain slices ex vivo with the sensitive detection of prions using the RT-QUIC in vitro amplification technique (Kondru et al., 2017).

However, notwithstanding the level of sophistication reached by the most recent systems developed in vitro/ex vivo, animal models of prion diseases are still indispensable to demonstrate therapeutic efficacy. A large choice of robust animal models are available, some of which are detailed below.

DISCOVERY AND VALIDATION OF THERAPEUTIC TARGETS USING *IN VIVO* MODELS OF PRION DISEASES

As of today, therapeutic intervention in human prion diseases has failed (Stewart et al., 2008; Geschwind, 2009). Indeed, some protocols suggested a reduction in the rate of patients' deterioration for short periods of time (Otto et al., 2004), and others were tested directly on humans after cell line experiments suggested they can reduce the accumulation of PrP^{TSE}, but none could reverse or even inhibit the advance of the severe neurologic deficits apparent at diagnosis, which makes it difficult to treat patients in the initial state. Therefore, development of treatments for prion diseases needs a new approach.

One possibility is that efforts should be mostly directed to develop preventive treatments for subjects at risk, as is the case for asymptomatic carriers of genetic prion diseases. In addition, such reagents could also be used on other subjects at risk of prion diseases; however, identification of these individuals depends on the development of early diagnostic tests, which will be sensitive, cheap, and simple enough to be applied to the general population. Such tests are being developed by several laboratories but whether they should be used extensively depends on many factors (Bongianni et al., 2017; Candelise et al., 2017; Orru et al., 2017). If indeed efforts are geared to develop preventive or prophylactic treatments, these should be safe enough to be administered for many years to healthy individuals, therefore candidate treatments should be screened for safety first.

Targeting PrP^{TSE} accumulation

In addition to the safety of candidate treatments, it is important to determine their biologic targets. In general, there are two major pathways to explore in the search for antiprion compounds. The first and obvious target in prion disease treatment would be the reduction of PrP^{TSE} accumulation. This can be done either by inhibiting the conversion of PrP^{C} to PrP^{TSE} or by reducing the expression of PrP^{C}. Candidate antiprion reagents that perform by one of these mechanisms can be screened for in cultured cells, as detailed previously, and after optimization tested for in animal experiments (Karapetyan et al., 2013; Silber et al., 2014; Imberdis et al., 2016).

Preventing neurodegeneration

The second family of targets for antiprion agents includes those that function against general neurodegenerative/oxidative damage. Oxidation of PrP^{TSE}, as for other key proteins in neurodegenerative diseases, and also of brain lipids, is part of the neurodegenerative process and such reduction may result in less neuronal death, even if the levels of disease-related PrP proteins are not reduced. While not impossible (see above), it is more difficult to establish a screening method for such targets in cells, therefore such candidate compounds should be tested directly in animal models. This of course is more expensive and time consuming, since the experiments should be done on a group of mice for each compound without previous screening. It is also more difficult to establish markers for treatment success, in addition to survival of the mice, which is obviously the ultimate goal.

An additional important point for all animal experiments, both the anti-PrP and neuroprotective ones, is the time point in disease advance in which treatment should commence. Preventive treatments in transgenic models of genetic prion diseases can be initiated from the day of birth or at the "adult" stage for mice, rather than waiting until the mice show signs of disease, since most genetic patients these days come from families which are aware of their situation as possible carriers. Many subjects from affected families are anxious to be enrolled in a prophylactic protocol, in particular if it is a nontoxic one that can be tolerated for many years. To this effect, mice would be treated from an early time point and until disease is well established or until the end point according to ethical considerations.

Protein translation inhibition: a target discovered in prion-infected mice

Protein translation inhibition provides an example where a novel mechanism of neurodegeneration for PMNDs was discovered in vivo in prion-infected mice. The group of G. Malluci initially noted a decline in synaptic protein levels to ~50% of control levels for several pre- (SNAP-25 and VAMP-2) and postsynaptic (PSD-95 and NMDAR1) proteins, then deciphered the pathway involved, namely activation of the PERK arm of the protein unfolding response leading to phosphorylation of eIF2a and translational repression (Moreno et al., 2012). Re-establishing translation rates by inhibiting eIF2α-P activity, genetically or pharmacologically, was found to restore memory, prevent neurodegeneration, and extend the survival of prion-infected mice (Moreno et al., 2013). Remarkably, the results originally established in prion-infected mice were also found to be directly translatable to murine models of tauopathies (Radford et al., 2015; Halliday et al., 2017).

Transgenic mice modeling for genetic prion diseases

Inherited prion diseases, such as genetic CJD (gCJD) and Gerstmann–Sträussler–Scheinker, are autosomal-dominant disorders linked to mutations in the gene encoding PrP, denominated *PRNP* (Hsiao and Prusiner, 1990; Kovacs et al., 2005). The largest focus of gCJD was identified among Libyan Jews carrying a missense mutation in codon 200 of *PRNP* (substituting lysine for glutamate, E200K) (Hsiao et al., 1991; Korczyn et al., 1991). This same mutation was also found in other communities around the world (Lee et al., 1999).

To be a model for the testing of preventive treatment, transgenic mice modeling for genetic prion disease should succumb spontaneously to neurologic disease in a high attack rate and a reasonable time frame, allowing for long-term treatments and measurable delay of onset well within the animals' lifespan. The model mice should also present prion-related biochemistry and pathology, as well as neurodegenerative features, such as neuronal loss.

Indeed, several animal models of genetic prion disease were generated in the past, thereby demonstrating that late onset and spontaneous genetic human prion diseases can be reconstructed in mice (Groschup and Buschmann, 2008; Solomon et al., 2010). However, while most were very useful in the study of prion disease pathogenesis, some do not present the properties required for testing antiprion compounds. The first transgenic mice imitating human genetic prion disease carried a P102L-PrP Gerstmann–Sträussler–Scheinker mutation on a mouse background and succumbed spontaneously to prion disease after about 4–6 months (Hsiao et al., 1990). However these mice presented poor PrP pathology (Hsiao et al., 1994; Telling et al., 1994). Transgenic lines mimicking the PrP insertional mutation (Harris et al., 2000), as well as both CJD (Dossena et al., 2008) and fatal familial insomnia D178N (Jackson et al., 2009) mutation presented prion-like clinical disease with low to marginal disease-related PrP, but no apparent disease transmission. Two transgenic lines mimicking the E200K PrP mutation, one on a human PrP gene and another on a mouse PrP gene, did not present disease or other prion-related properties (Telling et al., 1996; Asante et al., 2009). An additional line expressing an artificial mutant PrP form presented prion disease signs and pathology (Sigurdson et al., 2009), and could even transmit disease to mice over-expressing wild-type PrP; however, the great separation between age of disease onset in individual animals (145–637 days in a group of 47 mice) renders this line inappropriate for treatment experiments.

Use of TgMHu2ME199K mice, a chimeric human mice model of E200K CJD, to probe cholesterol metabolism and oxidative stress as therapeutic targets

In the Gabizon lab, we investigated a transgenic mouse model for E200K gCJD expressing a chimeric mouse/human PrP (Scott et al., 1992; Telling et al., 1994) both on a wild-type and a null PrP background, hereby denominated $TgMHu_2ME200K$/wt and $TgMHu_2ME200K$/ko respectively. The line on the wild-type background mimics most gCJD patients, who are heterozygous for the PrP mutation (Hsiao and Prusiner, 1990). Mice from both lines presented progressive neurodegenerative disease starting from 5–6 months of age, deteriorated, and died several months thereafter. Their brains showed age-related pathology characteristic of prion disease, such as gliosis and accumulated disease-related PrP, which was shown by immunoblots to be resistant to digestion by high concentrations of proteinase K (Friedman-Levi et al., 2014).

In addition, the neurodegenerative pathologic features of TgMHu2ME199K/KO mice as related to age and advance of clinical disease were studied (Fainstein et al., 2016). We found a facilitated progressive reduction in cortical neurons and synapses as compared to normal aging, starting at 4–6 months, and in accordance with neurologic disability. There was a significant decrease in neurogenesis at the subventricular / subependymal zone. A similar progressive loss of neurons in the CA1 and CA3 regions of the hippocampus was associated with impaired hippocampal-dependent memory function. Interestingly, there was increased hippocampal neurogenesis in TgMHu2ME199K/KO mice prior to decline in memory functions. Therefore, we believe the TgMHu2-ME199K/KO model can serve both to study the neurodegenerative pathways as well as to test neuroprotective drugs and regenerative therapies that may be relevant to other neurodegenerative conditions.

To this effect, we tested several compounds in these mice, to assess if previous agents tested on scrapie-infected mice as well as new agents developed by us can delay the aggravation of prion disease in this line (Forloni et al., 2002). This was the case for doxycycline, which delayed disease in scrapie-infected hamsters. When administered to patients doxycycline had no significant effect (Haik et al., 2014); however an important experiment was conducted to establish if it can have preventive properties when administered to carriers of pathogenic PrP mutations (Forloni et al., 2014). We also tested simvastatin, a cholesterol regulator with anti-inflammatory properties which was shown to delay scrapie advance in mice (Haviv et al., 2008).

The efficacy of cholesterol level modulation as an anti-prion approach has, however, been questioned recently by a study showing the lack of efficacy of three statins treatments in prolonging survival of scrapie-infected mice (Carroll et al., 2017). Most importantly, we tested our nanotechnology-based formulation of pomegranate seed oil (PSO), which works as a strong antioxidant and neuroprotective agent (Mizrahi et al., 2014). Figure 22.1 shows the effect of these reagents when administered from 70 to 180 days, a point in which these mice reach score 2, when disease is well established. Mice were scored for disease advance twice a week, as explained in previous publications (Ma et al., 2002). As can be seen, at least until this time, there were no significant effects for the administration of both doxycycline and simvastatin (unpublished results), while the results for PSO and nano-PSO were encouraging. It is important to stress that the doses of PSO in the nano-PSO treatment were 10 times less than in the PSO in food (Mizrahi et al., 2014). Therefore, future experiments were done with this formulation.

In a new study (Binyamin et al., 2017), we show that nano-PSO can be administered to an at-risk mouse from the day of birth continuously until death with a significant (5-month) increase in survival. Pathologic studies revealed that treatment with nano-PSO resulted in the reduction of GAG accumulation and lipid oxidation as well as a significant increase in stem cell neurogenesis, indicating a strong neuroprotective effect. In contrast, the clinical effect of nano-PSO did not correlate with

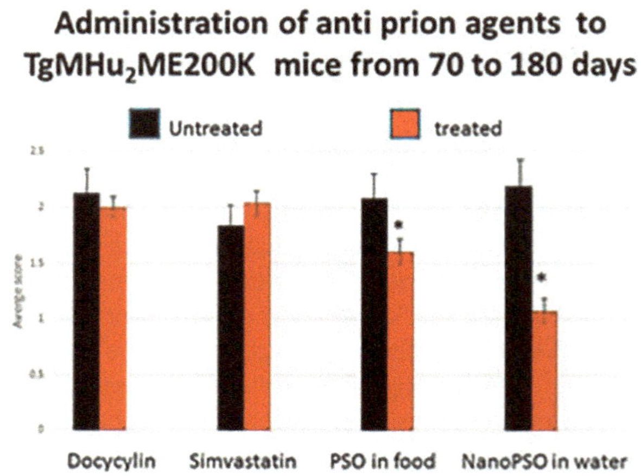

Fig. 22.1. TgMHu2ME199K mice were administrated several anti prion agents in their drinking water from 70 to 180 days. Doxycycline 10 mg/kg/day. Simvastatin: 20 mg/kg/day), Nano-PSO: 0.6 mg/kg/day/. Mice were followed periodically for clinical signs and scored as described (Scott et al., 1992; Telling et al., 1994).

reduction in the levels of disease-related PrP, the main prion marker. In the future, when specific, aggregated protein-related drugs are generated for patients suffering from neurodegenerative diseases, Nano-PSO may serve as a component for a treatment or prevention cocktail, in particular since its formulation is safe and comprises only approved food ingredients. We believe that transgenic models such as TgMHu2ME199K mice will play a significant role in the investigation of genetic prion disease pathogenesis and, most importantly, in the development of novel antiprion prophylactic treatments.

CONCLUSION

The last 10 years have witnessed major advances in our understanding of prion disease mechanisms and identification of multiple points of therapeutic intervention. This achievement is due in part to the development of new disease models, as well as relentless efforts by the prion disease scientific community to unravel the conundrum of a host protein being infectious and neurotoxic. A new murine model of genetic CJD allows evaluation of the prophylactic and therapeutic potential of drug candidates. The field of prion research seems to be starting a new chapter in the development of rationally designed treatments for these incurable diseases, with clinical trials on the horizon.

References

Aguib Y, Heiseke A, Gilch S et al. (2009). Autophagy induction by trehalose counteracts cellular prion infection. Autophagy 5: 361–369.

Aguzzi A, Zhu C (2017). Microglia in prion diseases. J Clin Invest 127: 3230–3239.

Alibhai J, Blanco RA, Barria MA et al. (2016). Distribution of misfolded prion protein seeding activity alone does not predict regions of neurodegeneration. PLoS Biol 14: e1002579.

Arellano-Anaya ZE, Savistchenko J, Mathey J et al. (2011). A simple, versatile and sensitive cell-based assay for prions from various species. PLoS One 6: e20563.

Asante EA, Gowland I, Grimshaw A et al. (2009). Absence of spontaneous disease and comparative prion susceptibility of transgenic mice expressing mutant human prion proteins. J Gen Virol 90: 546–558.

Ayers JI, Fromholt SE, O'Neal VM et al. (2016). Prion-like propagation of mutant SOD1 misfolding and motor neuron disease spread along neuroanatomical pathways. Acta Neuropathol 131: 103–114.

Ayers JI, Brooks MM, Rutherford NJ et al. (2017). Robust central nervous system pathology in transgenic mice following peripheral injection of alpha-synuclein fibrils. J Virol 91.

Bach C, Gilch S, Rost R et al. (2009). Prion-induced activation of cholesterogenic gene expression by Srebp2 in neuronal cells. J Biol Chem 284: 31260–31269.

Baker CA, Manuelidis L (2003). Unique inflammatory RNA profiles of microglia in Creutzfeldt–Jakob disease. Proc Natl Acad Sci U S A 100: 675–679.

Bate C, Tayebi M, Williams A (2008a). Cholesterol esterification reduces the neurotoxicity of prions. Neuropharmacology 54: 1247–1253.

Bate C, Tayebi M, Williams A (2008b). Sequestration of free cholesterol in cell membranes by prions correlates with cytoplasmic phospholipase A2 activation. BMC Biol 6: 8.

Belichenko PV, Brown D, Jeffrey M et al. (2000). Dendritic and synaptic alterations of hippocampal pyramidal neurones in scrapie-infected mice. Neuropathol Appl Neurobiol 26: 143–149.

Betemps D, Verchere J, Brot S et al. (2014). Alpha-synuclein spreading in M83 mice brain revealed by detection of pathological alpha-synuclein by enhanced ELISA. Acta Neuropathol Commun 2: 29.

Binyamin O, Keller G, Frid K et al. (2017). Continued administration of Nano-PSO significantly increased survival of genetic CJD mice. Neurobiol Dis 108: 140–147.

Bongianni M, Orru C, Groveman BR et al. (2017). Diagnosis of human prion disease using real-time quaking-induced conversion testing of olfactory mucosa and cerebrospinal fluid samples. JAMA Neurol 74: 155–162.

Brown DR (1999). Prion protein peptide neurotoxicity can be mediated by astrocytes. J Neurochem 73: 1105–1113.

Brown D, Belichenko P, Sales J et al. (2001). Early loss of dendritic spines in murine scrapie revealed by confocal analysis. Neuroreport 12: 179–183.

Browning S, Baker CA, Smith C et al. (2011). Abrogation of complex glycosylation by swainsonine results in strain- and cell-specific inhibition of prion replication. J Biol Chem 286: 40962–40973.

Büeler H, Aguzzi A, Sailer A et al. (1993). Mice devoid of PrP are resistant to scrapie. Cell 73: 1339–1347.

Candelise N, Schmitz M, Da Silva Correia SM et al. (2017). Applications of the real-time quaking-induced conversion assay in diagnosis, prion strain-typing, drug pre-screening and other amyloidopathies. Expert Rev Mol Diagn 17: 897–904.

Carroll JA, Striebel JF, Rangel A et al. (2016). Prion strain differences in accumulation of PrPSc on neurons and glia are associated with similar expression profiles of neuroinflammatory genes: comparison of three prion strains. PLoS Pathog 12: e1005551.

Carroll JA, Race B, Phillips K et al. (2017). Statins are ineffective at reducing neuroinflammation or prolonging survival in scrapie-infected mice. J Gen Virol 98: 2190–2199.

Caughey B, Raymond GJ (1991). The scrapie-associated form of PrP is made from a cell surface precursor that is both protease and phospholipase-sensitive. J Biol Chem 266: 18217–18223.

Ciechanover A, Kwon YT (2015). Degradation of misfolded proteins in neurodegenerative diseases: therapeutic targets and strategies. Exp Mol Med 47: e147.

Cui HL, Guo B, Scicluna B et al. (2014). Prion infection impairs cholesterol metabolism in neuronal cells. J Biol Chem 289: 789–802.

Dassanayake RP, Zhuang D, Truscott TC et al. (2016). A transfectant RK13 cell line permissive to classical caprine scrapie prion propagation. Prion 10: 153–164.

Deleault NR, Harris BT, Rees JR et al. (2007). Formation of native prions from minimal components in vitro. Proc Natl Acad Sci U S A 104: 9741–9746.

Desplats P, Lee HJ, Bae EJ et al. (2009). Inclusion formation and neuronal cell death through neuron-to-neuron transmission of alpha-synuclein. Proc Natl Acad Sci U S A 106: 13010–13015.

Dossena S, Imeri L, Mangieri M et al. (2008). Mutant prion protein expression causes motor and memory deficits and abnormal sleep patterns in a transgenic mouse model. Neuron 60: 598–609.

Epelbaum S, Youssef I, Lacor PN et al. (2015). Acute amnestic encephalopathy in amyloid-beta oligomer-injected mice is due to their widespread diffusion in vivo. Neurobiol Aging 36: 2043–2052.

Fainstein N, Dori D, Frid K et al. (2016). Chronic progressive neurodegeneration in a transgenic mouse model of prion disease. Front Neurosci 10: 510.

Falsig J, Aguzzi A (2008). The prion organotypic slice culture assay – POSCA. Nat Protoc 3: 555–562.

Fang C, Imberdis T, Garza MC et al. (2016). A neuronal culture system to detect prion synaptotoxicity. PLoS Pathog 12: e1005623.

Forloni G, Angeretti N, Chiesa A et al. (1993). Neurotoxicity of a prion protein fragment. Nature 362: 543–546.

Forloni G, Del Bo R, Angeretti N et al. (1994). A neurotoxic prion protein fragment induces rat astroglial proliferation and hypertrophy. Eur J Neurosci 6: 1415–1422.

Forloni G, Iussich S, Awari T et al. (2002). Tetracyclines affect prion infectivity. Proc Natl Acad Sci U S A 99: 10849–10854.

Forloni G, Tettamanti M, Lucca U et al. (2014). Preventive study in subjects at risk of fatal familial insomnia: Innovative approach to rare diseases. Prion 9: 75–79.

Fraser H (1976). The pathology of natural and experimental scrapie. In: RH Kimberlin (Ed.), Slow virus diseases of animals and man. North-Holland, New York, pp. 267–305.

Friedman-Levi Y, Mizrahi M, Frid K et al. (2014). PrP(ST), a soluble, protease resistant and truncated PrP form features in the pathogenesis of a genetic prion disease. PLoS One 8: e69583.

Geissen M, Leidel F, Eiden M et al. (2011). From high-throughput cell culture screening to mouse model: identification of new inhibitor classes against prion disease. ChemMedChem 6: 1928–1937.

Geschwind MD (2009). Clinical trials for prion disease: difficult challenges, but hope for the future. Lancet Neurol 8: 304–306.

Ghaemmaghami S, Ahn M, Lessard P et al. (2009). Continuous quinacrine treatment results in the formation of drug-resistant prions. PLoS Pathog 5: e1000673.

Ghaemmaghami S, May BCH, Renslo AR et al. (2010). Discovery of 2-aminothiazoles as potent antiprion compounds. J Virol 84: 3408–3412.

Gilch S, Bach C, Lutzny G et al. (2009). Inhibition of cholesterol recycling impairs cellular PrP(Sc) propagation. Cell Mol Life Sci 66: 3979–3991.

Grad LI, Yerbury JJ, Turner BJ et al. (2014). Intercellular propagated misfolding of wild-type Cu/Zn superoxide dismutase occurs via exosome-dependent and -independent mechanisms. Proc Natl Acad Sci U S A 111: 3620–3625.

Groschup MH, Buschmann A (2008). Rodent models for prion diseases. Vet Res 39: 32.

Haik S, Peyrin JM, Lins L et al. (2000). Neurotoxicity of the putative transmembrane domain of the prion protein. Neurobiol Dis 7: 644–656.

Haik S, Marcon G, Mallet A et al. (2014). Doxycycline in Creutzfeldt–Jakob disease: a phase 2, randomised, double-blind, placebo-controlled trial. Lancet Neurol 13: 150–158.

Halliday M, Radford H, Zents KAM et al. (2017). Repurposed drugs targeting eIF2α-P-mediated translational repression prevent neurodegeneration in mice. Brain 140: 1768–1783.

Hannaoui S, Shim SY, Cheng YC et al. (2014). Cholesterol balance in prion diseases and Alzheimer's disease. Virus 6: 4505–4535.

Harris DA et al. (2000). A transgenic model of a familial prion disease. Arch Virol Suppl 16: 103–112.

Haviv Y, Avrahami D, Ovadia H et al. (2008). Induced neuroprotection independently from PrPSc accumulation in a mouse model for prion disease treated with simvastatin. Arch Neurol 65: 762–775.

Heiseke A, Aguib Y, Riemer C et al. (2009a). Lithium induces clearance of protease resistant prion protein in prion-infected cells by induction of autophagy. J Neurochem 109: 25–34.

Heiseke A, Aguib Y, Schatzl HM (2009b). Autophagy, prion infection and their mutual interactions. Curr Issues Mol Biol 12: 87–98.

Hsiao K, Prusiner SB (1990). Inherited human prion diseases. Neurology 40: 1820–1827.

Hsiao KK, Scott M, Foster D et al. (1990). Spontaneous neurodegeneration in transgenic mice with mutant prion protein. Science 250: 1587–1590.

Hsiao K, Meiner Z, Kahana E et al. (1991). Mutation of the prion protein in Libyan Jews with Creutzfeldt–Jakob disease. N Engl J Med 324: 1091–1097.

Hsiao KK, Groth D, Scott M et al. (1994). Serial transmission in rodents of neurodegeneration from transgenic mice expressing mutant prion protein. Proc Natl Acad Sci U S A 91: 9126–9130.

Iaccarino L, Moresco RM, Presotto L et al. (2017). An in vivo 11C-(R)-PK11195 PET and in vitro pathology study of microglia activation in Creutzfeldt–Jakob disease. Mol Neurobiol 38: 445–457.

Imberdis T, Heeres JT, Yueh H et al. (2016). Identification of anti-prion compounds using a novel cellular assay. J Biol Chem 291: 26164–26176.

Jackson WS, Borkowski AW, Faas H et al. (2009). Spontaneous generation of prion infectivity in fatal familial insomnia knockin mice. Neuron 63: 438–450.

Karapetyan YE, Saa P, Mahal SP et al. (2009). Prion strain discrimination based on rapid in vivo amplification and analysis by the cell panel assay. PLoS One 4: e5730.

Karapetyan YE, Sferrazza GF, Zhou M et al. (2013). Unique drug screening approach for prion diseases identifies tacrolimus and astemizole as antiprion agents. Proc Natl Acad Sci U S A 110: 7044–7049.

Kempster S, Bate C, Williams A (2007). Simvastatin treatment prolongs the survival of scrapie-infected mice. Neuroreport 18: 479–482.

Kim HJ, Tark DS, Lee YH et al. (2012). Establishment of a cell line persistently infected with chronic wasting disease prions. J Vet Med Sci 74: 1377–1380.

Kimata A, Nakagawa H, Ohyama R et al. (2007). New series of antiprion compounds: pyrazolone derivatives have the potent activity of inhibiting protease-resistant prion protein accumulation. J Med Chem 50: 5053–5056.

Kloehn PC, Stoltze L, Flechsig E et al. (2003). A quantitative, highly sensitive cell-based infectivity assay for mouse scrapie prions. Proc Natl Acad Sci U S A 100: 11666–11671.

Kocisko DA, Baron GS, Rubenstein R et al. (2003). New inhibitors of scrapie-associated prion protein formation in a library of 2000 drugs and natural products. J Virol 77: 10288–10294.

Kondru N, Manne S, Greenlee J et al. (2017). Integrated organotypic slice cultures and RT-QuIC (OSCAR) assay: implications for translational discovery in protein misfolding diseases. Sci Rep 7: 43155.

Korczyn AD et al. (1991). A mutation in the prion protein gene in Creutzfeldt–Jakob disease in Jewish patients of Libyan, Greek, and Tunisian origin. Ann N Y Acad Sci 640: 171–176.

Kovacs GG, Puopolo M, Ladogana A et al. (2005). Genetic prion disease: the EUROCJD experience. Hum Genet 118: 166–174.

Krejciova Z, De Sousa P, Manson G et al. (2014). Human tonsil-derived follicular dendritic-like cells are refractory to human prion infection in vitro and traffic disease-associated prion protein to lysosomes. Am J Pathol 184: 64–70.

Ladogana A, Liu Q, Xi YG et al. (1995). Proteinase-resistant protein in human neuroblastoma cells infected with brain material from Creutzfeldt–Jakob patient. Lancet 345: 594–595.

Lasmézas CI, Deslys J-P, Demaimay R et al. (1996). Strain specific and common pathogenic events in murine models of scrapie and bovine spongiform encephalopathy. J Gen Virol 77: 1601–1609.

Lasmézas CI, Deslys JP, Robain O et al. (1997). Transmission of the BSE agent to mice in the absence of detectable abnormal prion protein. Science 275: 402–405.

Lee HS, Sambuughin N, Cervenakova L et al. (1999). Ancestral origins and worldwide distribution of the PRNP 200K mutation causing familial Creutzfeldt–Jakob disease. Am J Hum Genet 64: 1063–1070.

Li J, Browning S, Mahal SP et al. (2010). Darwinian evolution of prions in cell culture. Science 327: 869–872.

Liberski PP, Sikorska B, Bratosiewicz-Wasik J et al. (2004). Neuronal cell death in transmissible spongiform encephalopathies (prion diseases) revisited: from apoptosis to autophagy. Int J Biochem Cell Biol 36: 2473–2490.

Luk KC, Song C, O'Brien P et al. (2009). Exogenous alpha-synuclein fibrils seed the formation of Lewy body-like intracellular inclusions in cultured cells. Proc Natl Acad Sci U S A 106: 20051–20056.

Ma J, Wollmann R, Lindquist S (2002). Neurotoxicity and neurodegeneration when PrP accumulates in the cytosol. Science 298: 1781–1785.

Mahal SP, Baker CA, Demczyk CA et al. (2007). Prion strain discrimination in cell culture: the cell panel assay. Proc Natl Acad Sci U S A 104: 20908–20913.

Manson JC, Clarke AR, McBride PA et al. (1994). PrP gene dosage determines the timing but not the final intensity or distribution of lesions in scrapie pathology. Neurodegeneration 3: 331–340.

Manuelidis L, Tesin DM, Sklaviadis T et al. (1987). Astrocyte gene expression in Creutzfeldt–Jakob disease. Proc Natl Acad Sci U S A 84: 5937–5941.

Manuelidis L, Yu ZX, Barquero N et al. (2007). Cells infected with scrapie and Creutzfeldt–Jakob disease agents produce intracellular 25-nm virus-like particles. Proc Natl Acad Sci U S A 104: 1965–1970.

Mishra RS, Gu Y, Bose S et al. (2002). Cell surface accumulation of a truncated transmembrane prion protein in Gerstmann-Straussler-Scheinker disease P102L. J Biol Chem 277: 24554–24561.

Mizrahi M, Friedman-Levi Y, Larush L et al. (2014). Pomegranate seed oil nanoemulsions for the prevention and treatment of neurodegenerative diseases: the case of genetic CJD. Nanomedicine 10: 1353–1363.

Mok SW, Thielen KM, Riemer C et al. (2006). Simvastatin prolongs survival times in prion infections of the central nervous system. Biochem Biophys Res Commun 348: 697–702.

Montag J, Brameier M, Schmädicke AC et al. (2012). A genome-wide survey for prion-regulated miRNAs associated with cholesterol homeostasis. BMC Genomics 13: 486.

Moreno JA, Radford H, Peretti D et al. (2012). Sustained translational repression by eIF2alpha-P mediates prion neurodegeneration. Nature 485: 507–511.

Moreno JA, Halliday M, Molloy C et al. (2013). Oral treatment targeting the unfolded protein response prevents neurodegeneration and clinical disease in prion-infected mice. Sci Transl Med 5: 206ra138.

Nicoll AJ, Collinge J (2009). Preventing prion pathogenicity by targeting the cellular prion protein. Infect Disord Drug Targets 9: 48–57.

Orru CD, Wilham JM, Vascellari S et al. (2017). New generation QuIC assays for prion seeding activity. Prion 6: 147–152.

Orsi A, Fioriti L, Chiesa R et al. (2006). Conditions of endoplasmic reticulum stress favor the accumulation of cytosolic prion protein. J Biol Chem 281: 30431–30438.

Otto M, Cepek L, Ratzka P et al. (2004). Efficacy of flupirtine on cognitive function in patients with CJD: a double-blind study. Neurology 62: 714–718.

Pan J, Sahoo PK, Dalzini A et al. (2017). Membrane disruption mechanism of a prion peptide (106-126) investigated by atomic force microscopy, raman and electron paramagnetic resonance spectroscopy. J Phys Chem B 121: 5058–5071.

Pani A, Mandas A, Dessi S (2010). Cholesterol, Alzheimer's disease, prion disorders: a menage a trois? Curr Drug Targets 11: 1018–1031.

Peeraer E, Bottelbergs A, Van Kolen K et al. (2015). Intracerebral injection of preformed synthetic tau fibrils initiates widespread tauopathy and neuronal loss in the brains of tau transgenic mice. Neurobiol Dis 73: 83–95.

Peyrin JM, Lasmézas CI, Haïk S et al. (1999). Microglial cells respond to amyloidogenic PrP peptide by the production of inflammatory cytokines. Neuroreport 10: 723–729.

Pocchiari M, Schmittinger S, Masullo C (1987). Amphotericin B delays the incubation period of scrapie in intracerebrally inoculated hamsters. J Gen Virol 68: 219–223.

Prusiner SB (1982). Novel proteinaceous infectious particles cause scrapie. Science 216: 136–144.

Race RE, Caughey B, Graham K et al. (1988). Analysis of frequency of infection, specific infectivity, and prion protein biosynthesis in scrapie-infected neuroblastoma cell clones. J Virol 62: 2845–2849.

Radford H, Moreno JA, Verity N et al. (2015). PERK inhibition prevents tau-mediated neurodegeneration in a mouse model of frontotemporal dementia. Acta Neuropathol 130: 633–642.

Sandberg MK, Al-Doujaily H, Sharps B et al. (2011). Prion propagation and toxicity in vivo occur in two distinct mechanistic phases. Nature 470: 540–542.

Sanders DW, Kaufman SK, DeVos SL et al. (2014). Distinct tau prion strains propagate in cells and mice and define different tauopathies. Neuron 82: 1271–1288.

Schätzl H, Laszlo L, Holtzman DM et al. (1997). A hypothalamic neuronal cell line persistently infected with scrapie prions exhibits apoptosis. J Virol 71: 8821–8831.

Scott MR, Köhler R, Foster D et al. (1992). Chimeric prion protein expression in cultured cells and transgenic mice. Protein Sci 1: 986–997.

Sigurdson CJ, Nilsson KPR, Hornemann S et al. (2009). De novo generation of a transmissible spongiform encephalopathy by mouse transgenesis. Proc Natl Acad Sci U S A 106: 304–309.

Silber BM, Gever AR, Rao S et al. (2014). Novel compounds lowering the cellular isoform of the human prion protein in cultured human cells. Bioorg Med Chem 22: 1960–1972.

Simoneau S, Rezaei H, Sales N et al. (2007). In vitro and in vivo neurotoxicity of prion protein oligomers. PLoS Pathog 3: e125.

Solomon IH, Schepker JA, Harris DA (2010). Prion neurotoxicity: insights from prion protein mutants. Curr Issues Mol Biol 12: 51–61.

Sonati T, Reimann RR, Falsig J et al. (2013). The toxicity of antiprion antibodies is mediated by the flexible tail of the prion protein. Nature 501: 102–106.

Stewart LA, Rydzewska LH, Keogh GF et al. (2008). Systematic review of therapeutic interventions in human prion disease. Neurology 70: 1272–1281.

Tagliavini F, Forloni G, D'Ursi P et al. (2001). Studies on peptide fragments of prion proteins. Adv Protein Chem 57: 171–201.

Telling GC et al. (1994). Transmission of Creutzfeldt–Jakob disease from humans to transgenic mice expressing chimeric human-mouse prion protein. Proc Natl Acad Sci U S A 91 (21): 9936–9940.

Telling GC, Haga T, Torchia M et al. (1996). Interactions between wild-type and mutant prion proteins modulate neurodegeneration in transgenic mice. Genes Dev 10: 1736–1750.

Vascellari S, Banni S, Vacca C et al. (2011). Accumulation and aberrant composition of cholesteryl esters in Scrapie-infected N2a cells and C57BL/6 mouse brains. Lipids Health Dis 10: 132.

Vetrugno V, Di Bari MA, Nonno R et al. (2009). Oral pravastatin prolongs survival time of scrapie-infected mice. J Gen Virol 90: 1775–1780.

Vincenti JE, Murphy L, Grabert K et al. (2015). Defining the microglia response during the time course of chronic neurodegeneration. J Virol 90: 3003–3017.

Walsh P, Vanderlee G, Yau J et al. (2014). The mechanism of membrane disruption by cytotoxic amyloid oligomers formed by prion protein(106-126) is dependent on bilayer composition. J Biol Chem 289: 10419–10430.

Wang F, Wang X, Yuan C-G et al. (2010). Generating a prion with bacterially expressed recombinant prion protein. Science 327: 1132–1135.

Woerman AL, Watts JC, Aoyagi A et al. (2017). Alpha-synuclein: multiple system atrophy prions. In: Cold Spring Harb Perspect Med doi: 10.1101/cshperspect.a024588.

Xie WL, Shi Q, Zhang J et al. (2013). Abnormal activation of microglia accompanied with disrupted CX3CR1/CX3CL1 pathway in the brains of the hamsters infected with scrapie agent 263K. J Mol Neurosci 51: 919–932.

Zhou M, Ottenberg G, Sferrazza G-F et al. (2012). Highly neurotoxic monomeric alpha-helical prion protein. Proc Natl Acad Sci U S A 109: 3113–3118.

Zhou M, Ottenberg G, Sferrazza G-F et al. (2015). Neuronal death induced by misfolded prion protein is due to NAD+ depletion and can be relieved in vitro and in vivo by NAD+ replenishment. Brain 138: 992–1008.

Zhu C, Herrmann US, Falsig J et al. (2016). A neuroprotective role for microglia in prion diseases. J Exp Med 213: 1047–1059.

Handbook of Clinical Neurology, Vol. 153 (3rd series)
Human Prion Diseases
M. Pocchiari and J. Manson, Editors
https://doi.org/10.1016/B978-0-444-63945-5.00023-4

Chapter 23

Vaccination strategies

THOMAS WISNIEWSKI[1,2,3,4]* AND FERNANDO GOÑI[1,2]

[1] *Center for Cognitive Neurology, New York University School of Medicine, New York, NY, United States*

[2] *Department of Neurology, New York University School of Medicine, New York, NY, United States*

[3] *Department of Pathology, New York University School of Medicine, New York, NY, United States*

[4] *Department of Psychiatry, New York University School of Medicine, New York, NY, United States*

Abstract

Currently all prion diseases are without effective treatment and are universally fatal. It is increasingly being recognized that the pathogenesis of many neurodegenerative diseases, such as Alzheimer disease (AD), includes "prion-like" properties. Hence, any effective therapeutic intervention for prion disease could have significant implications for other neurodegenerative diseases. Conversely, therapies that are effective in AD might also be therapeutically beneficial for prion disease. AD-like prion disease has no effective therapy. However, various vaccine and immunomodulatory approaches have shown great success in animal models of AD, with numerous ongoing clinical trials of these potential immunotherapies. More limited evidence suggests that immunotherapies may be effective in prion models and in naturally occurring prion disease. In particular, experimental data suggest that mucosal vaccination against prions can be effective for protection against orally acquired prion infection. Many prion diseases, including natural sheep scrapie, bovine spongiform encephalopathy, chronic wasting disease, and variant Creutzfeldt–Jakob disease, are thought to be acquired peripherally, mainly by oral exposure. Mucosal vaccination would be most applicable to this form of transmission. In this chapter we review various immunologically based strategies which are under development for prion infection.

INTRODUCTION

Prion diseases are a large group of related neurodegenerative conditions which affect both animals and humans (Aguilar-Calvo et al., 2015; Greenlee and Greenlee, 2015; Wisniewski and Goni, 2015; Will and Ironside, 2017). These diseases all have long incubation periods but are typically rapidly progressive once clinical symptoms begin. All prion diseases are fatal, with no effective forms of treatment; however, increased understanding of their pathogenesis has recently led to the potential for effective therapeutic interventions in the future (Wisniewski and Goni, 2016; Giles et al., 2017; Teruya and Doh-Ura, 2017; Xanthopoulos et al., 2017).

Prion diseases are unique in that they can be inherited, they can occur sporadically, or they can be transmissible. The infectious agent in the prion disease is composed mainly or entirely of an abnormal conformation of a host-encoded glycoprotein called the prion protein, PrP^{C} (C for cellular). The replication of prions involves the recruitment of the normally expressed prion protein, which has mainly an alpha-helical structure, into a disease-specific conformation that is rich in beta-sheet structure (termed PrP^{TSE}, TSE for transmissible spongiform encephalopathy) and as a result is resistant to degradation with enzymes such as proteinase K, has reduced solubility, and is prone to form oligomeric assemblies and amyloid fibrils (Prusiner, 1982; Giles et al., 2017). The primary structure of PrP^{C} and PrP^{TSE} is identical,

*Correspondence to: Thomas Wisniewski, M.D., New York University School of Medicine, Alexandria ERSP, Rm 802, 450 East 29th Street, New York NY 10016, United States. Tel: +1-212-263-7993, Fax: +1-212-263-7528, E-mail: thomas.wisniewski@nyumc.org

with the only posttranslational modification difference identified so far being higher levels of oxidized methionine residues in PrP^{TSE} (Canello et al., 2008).

All prion diseases have commonality in their neuropathologic features. These illnesses tend to affect the gray matter of the central nervous system (CNS), producing neuronal loss, gliosis, and characteristic spongiform change (Head et al., 2015). The latter is a vacuolation of the neuropil, and to a variable degree, of the neurons. In addition, plaques with the typical staining properties of amyloid (e.g., apple-green birefringence after Congo red staining when viewed under polarized light) are observed in many of these conditions. In approximately 10% of patients with sporadic CJD, amyloid is present in the cerebellum or in the cerebral hemispheres. All cases of Gerstmann–Sträussler–Scheinker are associated with multicentric cerebellar plaques, while in kuru amyloid plaques are noted in about 70% of cases (Liberski et al., 2012). These amyloid plaques are immunoreactive with antibodies to the prion protein and do not immunoreact with antibodies to other amyloidogenic proteins, such as amyloid-beta (Aβ) (which is a key pathogenic protein deposited in Alzheimer disease (AD)) (Head et al., 2015).

NORMAL CELLULAR FUNCTION OF PrP^C

The human prion protein (PrP) gene (*PRNP*) is found on chromosome 20 and encodes a protein of 253 amino acids. PrP^C is a glycosylphosphatidylinositol-anchored cell surface glycoprotein; with numerous suggested roles, but its exact cellular functions remain unknown. PrP is found in most tissues of the body but is expressed at highest levels in the CNS, in particular in neurons. PrP is also expressed widely on cells of the immune system. Expression of PrP^C is a prerequisite for prion replication and the development of pathology (Brandner et al., 1996). The N-terminal region of PrP^C contains a segment of five repeats of an eight-amino-acid sequence (i.e., octapeptide repeat region) that contains a high-affinity binding site for metal ions; hence, PrP^C may have a role in copper and manganese transport or metabolism (Brown, 2011). Metal imbalance has been reported as an early change during prion infections (Thackray et al., 2002; Singh et al., 2013). Both copper and manganese chelation has been shown to prolong the incubation period of prion infection (Sigurdsson et al., 2003a; Brazier et al., 2010).

PrP^C has also been shown to have a potential role in a variety of functions, including cell proliferation, differentiation, and survival, neuroprotection, and synaptic function (Aguzzi et al., 2008; Onodera et al., 2014). In addition, PrP^C likely has a role in regulating immune function, as discussed below. At least some of these functions of PrP^C are likely to be important, since it is highly conserved among mammals and is found in all tetrapods and birds (Harris et al., 1993; Windl et al., 1995; Kretzschmar and Tatzelt, 2013). A more recently identified role for PrP^C is as a receptor for Aβ oligomers, in part mediating their toxicity via activating intracellular Fyn kinase to mediate synaptotoxicity (Chung et al., 2010; Um et al., 2012, 2013; Kostylev et al., 2015; Salazar and Strittmatter, 2016). Aβ oligomer-mediated toxicity is thought to be a key part of the pathogenesis of AD (Viola and Klein, 2015). Blocking this Aβ/PrP^C interaction is currently being tested in a phase I clinical trial as a therapeutic approach for AD (Nygaard et al., 2015). PrP^C may also be a receptor for other oligomeric species and may be involved in mediating other neurodegenerative disease-related pathology. A recent study has shown a relationship between PrP^C expression levels in the CNS and the degree of tau-related pathology following traumatic brain injury (Rubenstein et al., 2017). Hence the therapeutic targeting of PrP^C may have implications for other neurodegenerative disorders.

PATHOGENESIS OF PRION DISEASE AND RELATED CONFORMATIONAL NEURODEGENERATIVE DISORDERS

The most widely accepted hypothesis for the pathogenesis of prion diseases, initially described by Griffith (1967) and more explicitly detailed by Stanley Prusiner, is the protein-only hypothesis (Prusiner, 1982; Prusiner et al., 1998; Colby and Prusiner, 2011). Prusiner (Prusiner, 1982) introduced the term "prion" to indicate that scrapie is related to a proteinaceous infectious particle (PrP).This hypothesis suggests that prions contain no nucleic acid and are referred to as PrP^{TSE}. The latter represents a conformationally modified form of a normal cellular PrP^C, which is a normal host protein found on the surface of many cells, in particular neurons. PrP^{TSE}, when introduced into normal healthy cells, causes the conversion of PrP^C into PrP^{TSE}, initiating a self-perpetuating vicious cycle (Prusiner et al., 1998; Colby and Prusiner, 2011). The PrP^{TSE} originates from an exogenous source in acquired prion disease and from a spontaneous somatic conformational mutation in sporadic disease.

It is being increasingly recognized that the prion hypothesis as an epigenetic mechanism of transmitting information on protein conformation applies to numerous other biologic and pathologic situations, including very common disorders such as AD (Prusiner, 2012; Stopschinski and Diamond, 2017; Watts and Prusiner, 2017). If one defines a "prion" more broadly as a protein-based inheritance unit that confers a trait based on a posttranslational switch involving the acquisition of increased β-sheet structure, along with an increased propensity for aggregation, then "prion-like" spread of pathology can be used to describe the behavior of numerous proteins involved in a broad spectrum of "conformational" neurodegenerative disorders such as Aβ, tau, TDP-43, fused-in sarcoma (FUS), α-synuclein, and huntingtin (which are associated with AD (Aβ and tau), frontotemporal dementia (tau, TDP-43, or FUS), Parkinson disease (α-synuclein), and Huntington disease (huntingtin protein)) (Prusiner, 2012; Goedert, 2015; Stopschinski and Diamond, 2017; Watts and Prusiner, 2017). None of these neurodegenerative disorders have effective therapeutic approaches; however, numerous immunotherapeutic approaches, that in part target this prion-like spread of pathology, have been tested for AD with many ongoing clinical trials (Wisniewski and Goni, 2015; Stopschinski and Diamond, 2017; Wisniewski and Drummond, 2016).

It is interesting to note that, although the testing of immunomodulation is currently much more advanced for AD in comparison to vaccine therapies for prion disease, the first studies suggesting that this type of approach might be efficacious were conducted in prion disease models. It was first shown in 1988 that, when an anti-PrP^C polyclonal antibody was used ex vivo on a prion preparation prior to inoculation, a 2-log reduction in infectivity was noted, suggesting the potential of passive immunization to prevent prion infection (Gabizon et al., 1988).

That an active immunization approach might also be effective was suggested by experiments in 1998, showing that challenge with a slow strain of PrP^{TSE}, with a prolonged incubation, blocked the later expression of a more virulent, fast strain of PrP^{TSE}, mimicking vaccination with a live attenuated organism (Manuelidis, 1998). It was in 1999 that the seminal work of Dr. D. Schenk, showing that immunization with aggregated Aβ in an AD transgenic mouse model could reduce pathology, without apparent toxicity, ultimately led to a vast number of studies of immunotherapy for AD first in animal models and subsequently in clinical trials (Schenk et al., 1999; Wisniewski and Drummond, 2016). It is hoped that the current renewed interest in immunotherapeutic approaches for prion disease and the growing realization of the commonality in the pathogenesis of many neurodegenerative disorders may lead to more study in this area, which will ultimately produce effective treatments for prion infection.

THE IMMUNE SYSTEM AND PRION INFECTION

Although PrP^C is expressed predominantly in the central and peripheral nervous systems (Chesebro et al., 1985; Oesch et al., 1985), expression has also been reported in many cells of the immune system, including T and B lymphocytes, natural killer cells, monocytes, dendritic cells, and follicular dendritic cells (Aguzzi et al., 2013). Among lymphoid cells, PrP^C levels are lower in B cells compared to T cells, monocytes, and natural killer cells (Durig et al., 2000). PrP^C levels vary significantly between T-cell subtypes. For example, CD8+ cells have higher expression compared to CD4+ cells, and CD25+ cells express 4.5-fold higher PrP^C levels compared to CD25– cells (Isaacs et al., 2006). This diverse level of PrP^C expression in cells of the immune system suggests that PrP^C may have a regulatory role.

Although PrP knockout mice have no overt phenotype under normal conditions (Bueler et al., 1992; Manson et al., 1994), under immunologic stress there is evidence of immune dysregulation using models such as experimental autoimmune encephalomyelitis (Onodera et al., 2014). Experimental autoimmune encephalomyelitis is a widely used model for multiple sclerosis and acute disseminated encephalomyelitis that is considered the prototype for T-cell-mediated autoimmune disease in general (Lassmann and Bradl, 2017). A number of studies have shown that PrP knockout mice have a more aggressive disease with particularly reduced clinical improvement during the chronic phase of the disease (Tsutsui et al., 2008; Hu et al., 2010; Gourdain et al., 2012). These observations have led to the hypothesis that PrP^C may have a neuroprotective and anti-inflammatory role, involved in immune quiescence, specifically protecting immune-privileged organs such as the brain (Onodera et al., 2014; Bakkebo et al., 2015).

Due to the expression pattern of PrP^C in immune cells and the lack of an immune response to a self-antigen, the immune system is an active player very much involved in the peripheral, asymptomatic replication of prions and their eventual access to the CNS, which is associated with the clinical manifestations of prion infection (Aguzzi et al., 2013; Wisniewski and Goni, 2016). Numerous studies have shown that immune suppression with, for example, splenectomy or immunosuppressive drugs increases the incubation period (Aucouturier et al., 2000), while nonspecific immunostimulation has the opposite effect (Bremer et al., 2009). This asymptomatic incubation period, during which time the prion agent replicates peripherally, can be very long, lasting many months in experimental animals and up to 56 years in documented human cases associated with cannibalistic exposure to the prion agent (Collinge et al., 2006).

In humans it is not known how long peripheral prion replication occurs in the absence of significant neuroinvasion. This critical period would be the time when various antiprion therapeutic agents, which do not cross the blood–brain barrier, would have a chance of success. Lymphatic organs, including the spleen, tonsil, lymph nodes, and gut-associated lymphoid tissue, contain high concentrations of PrP^{TSE} long before PrP^{TSE} replication starts in the brain in peripherally acquired prion infections (Brown et al., 2000; Mabbott and MacPherson, 2006; Beekes and McBride, 2007).

Immune cells found to be particularly important for peripheral PrP^{TSE} replication include follicular dendritic cells and migratory bone marrow-derived dendritic cells (Kitamoto et al., 1991; Montrasio et al., 2000; Aucouturier et al., 2001; Mabbott and MacPherson, 2006; Beekes and McBride, 2007; Langevin et al., 2010). Dendritic cells from infected animals have been demonstrated to be capable of spreading the disease when passively transferred (Aucouturier et al., 2001; Langevin et al., 2010). It is hoped that immunotherapeutic approaches that overcome the self-tolerance of these immune cells will inhibit prion replication in the lymphorecticular system and ultimately prevent or delay significant neuroinvasion, particularly for peripherally acquired prion disease. However, a fine balance has to be achieved in order to produce an appropriate immune response, whilst avoiding potential autoimmune inflammatory toxicity (Mabbott, 2015; Burchell and Panegyres, 2016; Wisniewski and Goni, 2016).

An important consideration for the feasibility of such approaches is that peripheral infection and replication are much less important in some prion diseases, such as genetic forms, sporadic Creutzfeldt–Jakob disease, and in some types of scrapie (Bartz et al., 2005; Bessen et al., 2009; Siso et al., 2010; Friedman-Levi et al., 2014; Greenlee et al., 2014). Hence the potential beneficial effect of altering the immune response to PrP would have to be tailored to each particular PrP^{TSE} strain and route of infection. Success for some prion diseases may also require an immune response in the brain, something that is much more difficult to achieve, without the potential for toxicity.

That such a goal is achievable is suggested by data from studies in AD model animals and AD patients (Wisniewski and Goni, 2015; Selkoe and Hardy, 2016; Wisniewski and Drummond, 2016). AD is another conformational neurodegenerative disorder where the pathogenesis is related to the accumulation of self proteins in an abnormal conformation within the CNS; in the case of AD these proteins are Aβ and abnormally phosphorylated tau, which accumulate as toxic oligomers, as well as amyloid plaques and neurofibrillary tangles, respectively (Nelson et al., 2012; Selkoe and Hardy, 2016). A number of different immune-modulating approaches with effects within the CNS have been shown to ameliorate this pathology dramatically in animal models, with more limited success in human clinical trials (Wisniewski and Goni, 2015; Selkoe and Hardy, 2016; Sevigny et al., 2016; Wisniewski and Drummond, 2016; Drummond and Wisniewski, 2017).

IN VITRO STUDIES USING ANTI-PRP ANTIBODIES

A precise understanding of the molecular mechanisms and pathways involved in the PrP^{C} to PrP^{TSE} conversion remains to be elucidated; however, there is abundant evidence of the primal importance of "seeding" by aggregated PrP^{TSE} molecules acting as template for PrP^{C} binding and subsequent conversion to more PrP^{TSE} (Prusiner, 1982; Come et al., 1993). This interaction is critically dependent on the correct stereochemistry, as supported by the existence of a species barrier for prion infection, related to minor differences in the primary sequence of PrP^{C} in different species. Hence, it is not surprising that antibodies that may alter or mask the critical epitopes on PrP^{C} and/or PrP^{TSE}, involved during the mutual conformational complementarity required in prion propagation, will be inhibitory for prion replication.

This was first shown in 1988 when an anti-PrP^{C} polyclonal antibody was used ex vivo on a prion inoculum prior to injection and a significant reduction in the infectivity titer was noted (Gabizon et al., 1988). Using scrapie-infected cells it was later shown that an anti-PrP monoclonal antibody, 6H4 directed to residues 144–152, was able to clear infection in vitro (Enari et al., 2001). In the same year Peretz and col. used a number of different PrP-specific Fab fragments for scrapie clearance in chronically infected N2a cells. They found D13 (directed to residues 95–103) and D18 (directed to residues 132–156) to be the most effective at scrapie clearance (Peretz et al., 2001).

Kim and col. generated a large panel of antibodies raised to either recombinant mouse PrP or purified mouse PrP^{TSE} in PrP knockout mice, and tested them therapeutically in an N2a scrapie-infected cell line. They found that all anti-PrP antibodies that were able to bind to PrP^{C} on the cell surface, as judged by flow cytometry, were able to inhibit prion infection (Kim et al., 2004a, b).

Another study using a panel of anti-PrP monoclonal antibodies to different epitopes of PrP in scrapie-infected N2a cells found the most effective to be 6D11, which is directed to residues 95–105 (hence similar to D13); however, antibodies directed to residues 130–140 and 143–155 were also quite effective (Pankiewicz et al., 2006).

These various studies suggest that therapeutic antibodies need to have high affinities of binding to PrP^{C} and/or PrP^{TSE}, as well as targeting specific critical PrP domains. Proof of principle that passive immunization could be effective in vivo was first shown using transgenic mice that produced an anti-PrP monoclonal antibody. These mice were resistant to disease following challenge with a mouse-adapted scrapie strain (Heppner et al., 2001b).

THERAPEUTIC TARGETS AND THE POTENTIAL FOR TOXICITY

There are a number of different potential therapeutic targets for preventing/treating prion infection that include (Fig. 23.1): (1) blocking of entry of orally acquired PrP^{TSE} across the gut epithelial barrier by secretory anti-PrP immunoglobulin A (IgA); (2) enhanced clearance/elimination of PrP^{TSE} in the peripheral circulation/lymphoreticular tissue prior to passage across the blood–brain barrier into the CNS; (3) blocking the PrP^{C} to PrP^{TSE} conversion either in the periphery or in the CNS after neuroinvasion; (4) reducing available PrP^{C} levels so the substrate for PrP^{TSE} conversion is eliminated; (5) enhancing PrP^{TSE} clearance/elimination in the brain; and (6) blocking PrP^{TSE}-mediated toxicity and neuroinflammation in the CNS. Immune targeting of pathways 1 or 2 could be effective to prevent infection from a peripheral source and would not necessarily have to be PrP^{TSE}-specific, with a lower possibility of toxicity.

Targeting PrP^{TSE} in the CNS introduces the blood–brain barrier as a complication. Studies in AD models have shown that only about 0.1% of peripheral IgG crosses the blood–brain barrier (Wisniewski and Goni, 2015); hence, some means of enhancing CNS delivery might be required. Immune action within the CNS will likely be more effective in symptomatic disease (and may be required for prion disease where there is no significant peripheral replication phase); however, this carries a greater risk of toxicity.

Intracranial administration of anti-PrP monoclonal antibodies (that have no PrP^{C} or PrP^{TSE} specificity) was shown to induce neuronal apoptosis (Solforosi et al., 2004; Tayebi and Hawke, 2006). Other studies using different anti-PrP antibodies did not show significant toxicity (Klohn et al., 2012; Xanthopoulos et al., 2013). Using a panel of anti-PrP antibodies it was demonstrated that toxicity may be PrP epitope-dependent, with some antibodies showing no evidence of toxicity (Sonati et al., 2013). Hence, PrP^{C} can be a therapeutically viable therapeutic target, as also suggested by studies which have genetically ablated expression of PrP^{C} in the presence of early spongiform pathology, resulting in reversal of this pathology without toxicity (Mallucci et al., 2007; Verity and Mallucci, 2011). Nevertheless,

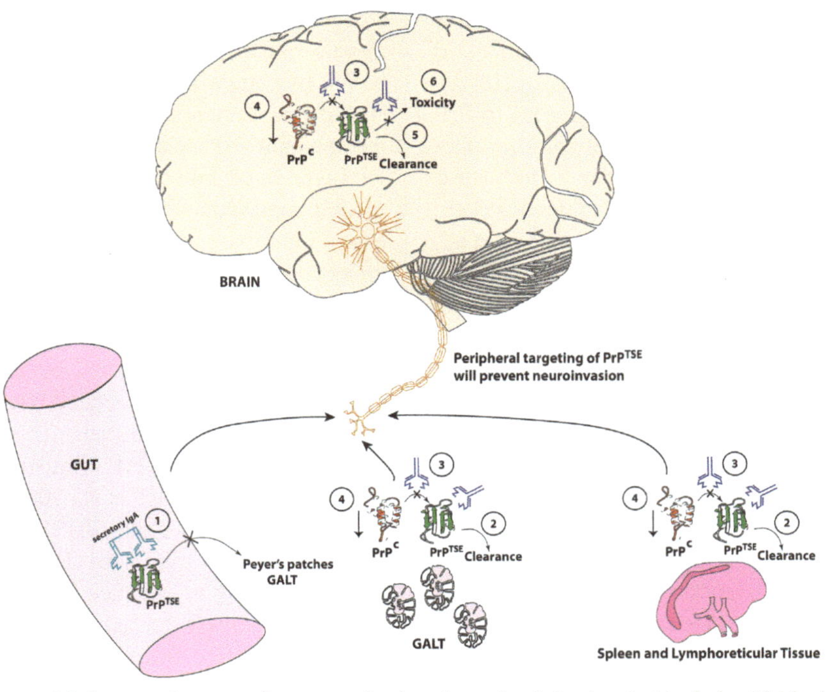

Fig. 23.1. Different potential therapeutic targets for preventing/treating prion infection that include: (1) blocking of entry of orally acquired PrP^{TSE} across the gut epithelial barrier by secretory anti-PrP^{Sc} immunoglobulin A (IgA); (2) enhancing clearance/elimination of PrP^{TSE} in gut-associated lymphatic tissue (GALT) and spleen/lymphoreticular tissue prior to crossing the blood–brain barrier into the central nervous system (CNS); (3) blocking conversion of PrP^{C} to PrP^{TSE} either in the periphery or in the CNS after neuroinvasion; (4) reducing available PrP^{C} levels so the substrate for PrP^{TSE} conversion is eliminated; (5) enhancing PrP^{TSE} clearance/elimination in the brain; (6) blocking PrP^{TSE}-mediated toxicity and neuroinflammation in the CNS.

it is likely that immunologic therapeutic targeting within the CNS will need to be PrP^{TSE}-specific to reduce the chances of toxicity.

PASSIVE IMMUNIZATION FOR PRION INFECTION

In an initial passive anti-PrP immunization study using a more classic approach where antibodies were injected systemically into nontransgenic, CD1 mice it was shown that monoclonal antibodies 8B4 (to mouse PrP residues 34–52) and 8H4 (to mouse PrP residues 175–185) given immediately after challenge with 139A scrapie by intraperitoneal (ip) injection (50 μg/week) resulted in a significant prolongation of the incubation period, with 10% of the 8B4 treated animals remaining disease-free in the group challenged with a lower dose of PrP^{TSE} (Sigurdsson et al., 2003b).

A similar study using higher doses (4000 μg/week ip) of either ICSM 18 (to mouse PrP residues 146–158) or ICSM 35 (to mouse residues 95 to 105) showed that prion infection from a peripheral source could be completely prevented if treatment was continued for 7 or 30 days immediately following PrP^{TSE} challenge or within 30 days (White et al., 2003). This approach could be used immediately following accidental exposure in humans to prevent future infection. Unfortunately, passive immunization was not found to be effective closer to the clinically symptomatic stages of prion infection (White et al., 2003).

Another study used 6D11, which is directed to PrP residues 95–105, immediately after ip challenge, producing a ~37% prolongation of the incubation period with a reduction in the severity of pathology (Pankiewicz et al., 2006; Sadowski et al., 2009). Song and col. (Song et al., 2008) demonstrated therapeutic efficacy with anti-PrP antibodies up to 120 days post inoculation, using direct intraventricular infusion, with a slight (~8%) prolongation of the incubation time, using the Chandler scrapie strain. The same group tested one of these monoclonal antibodies (31C6 to mouse PrP 143–149) by peripheral injection into the tail veins at 120 days post inoculation (at about the onset of clinical disease) and found no significant survival prolongation, but a slight reduction in pathology (Ohsawa et al., 2013).

The therapeutic effectiveness of passive immunization with monoclonal antibodies that specifically recognize PrP^{TSE} and not PrP^{C} remains to be tested. Our group has conducted studies generating antibodies that recognize the shared pathologic structure of Aβ oligomers, pathologic tau (in the form of paired helical filaments) and PrP^{TSE} (Wisniewski and Goni, 2015; Goni et al., 2016a, 2017). These antibodies were generated using a polymerized peptide derived from the carboxyl terminus of the British amyloidosis (ABri) peptide, oligomerized using glutaraldehyde as a cross-linker to form a stable population of oligomers, which we term pBri (Goni et al., 2010, 2013, 2017). This peptide lacks any sequence homology to Aβ, tau, or PrP (Vidal et al., 1999; Rostagno et al., 2005; Goni et al., 2010); however, when polymerized and used as an immunogen, it can produce monoclonal antibodies that recognize multiple pathologic conformers, including PrP^{TSE} (Goni et al., 2016a, 2017). Such antibodies, which have specificity for PrP^{TSE} and not PrP^{C}, might have therapeutic potential in prion disease; however, this remains to be evaluated.

ACTIVE VACCINATION FOR PRION INFECTION

A significant hurdle for the development of an active anti-PrP vaccine is overcoming T-cell tolerance to a self-antigen. For many years the dogma was that to generate anti-PrP antibodies it was required to use PrP knockout mice. However, more recent studies indicate an immune response can be mounted against PrP in animals expressing PrP. In fact, it has been documented that towards the clinical stages of prion infection some anti-PrP antibodies are generated (Sassa et al., 2010; Goni et al., 2015). The first in vivo studies of an active immunization-like approach showed that challenge with a slow strain of PrP^{TSE} blocked the later expression of a more virulent fast strain of PrP, mimicking vaccination with a live attenuated organism (Manuelidis, 1998).

We first demonstrated that active immunization with recombinant PrP delayed the onset of prion disease in wild-type mice; however, the therapeutic effect was very modest and eventually all the mice succumbed to the disease (Sigurdsson et al., 2002). The limited therapeutic effect could be explained by the observation that the antibodies generated against prokaryotic PrP often do not have a high affinity towards the cell surface, critical portions of PrP^{C} that are involved in binding and replication and that the anti-PrP titers generated were low (Polymenidou et al., 2004). Various investigators tried to increase the immunogenicity of the PrP immunogen, by using dimers or PrP aggregates (Gilch et al., 2003; Polymenidou et al., 2004; Xanthopoulos et al., 2013); alternatively, heterologous PrP peptides were used (Ishibashi et al., 2007).

Another way to enhance immunogenicity was with strong adjuvants such as CpG oligodeoxynucelotides that are Toll-like 9 receptor agonists and stimulate T- and B-cell repertoires against PrP (Rosset et al., 2004; Spinner et al., 2007). Interestingly, stimulation of immunity with CpG oligodeoxynucelotides alone has been shown to ameliorate all AD-related pathology (Scholtzova et al., 2014, 2017). Alternatively, repeated injections (biweekly) with PrP-absorbed Dynabeads, producing a multivalent immunogen, were able to induce an IgM PrP-specific humoral response that was associated with a slight (~11%) prolongation of incubation time after ip prion challenge (Tayebi et al., 2009).

In addition to these PrP peptide or recombinant protein-based approaches, DNA vaccines have been used to enhance an immune response. In these studies immunization with cDNA encoding for heterologous PrP fused to either a stimulatory T-cell stimulatory peptide (Alexandrenne et al., 2010) or a targeting protein that enhances antigen uptake and presentation via major histocompatibility complex class I has been used (Han et al., 2011). These DNA vaccines induce significant PrP-specific IgG but their ability to prevent prion infection has not been well studied.

Active immunization has also been examined using PrP displaying viral constructs. Virus-like particles are excellent immunogens that typically trigger a strong humoral immune response. Studies using this approach to immunize wild-type mice, rats, and/or rabbits have demonstrated that this can stimulate high titers of anti-PrP antibodies that recognize PrP^{C} and/or PrP^{TSE} (Nikles et al., 2005; Handisurya et al., 2007). In addition, this approach has been used to transduce dendritic cells with adenovirus expressing human PrP, which was subsequently utilized to immunize wild-type mice. The mice developed antimouse PrP antibodies associated with a reduction in PrP^{TSE} accumulation in the spleen and a prolongation of the incubation period (Rosset et al., 2009).

Induction of a more PrP^{TSE} active immune response has also been tried. It has been suggested that three epitopes that are more exposed in PrP^{TSE} include a YYR motif, a YML motif in β-sheet 1, and another YML within the rigid loop linking β-sheet 2 to α-helix 2. A vaccine based on these epitopes was able to induce a more PrP^{TSE}-specific antibody response in sheep (Marciniuk et al., 2014); however, whether this response is protective remains unknown.

MUCOSAL ACTIVE IMMUNIZATION

A potentially ideal means of using active immunization to prevent prion infection is by utilizing mucosal vaccination. The most obvious reason for using this approach is that the gut is the major route of entry for many prion diseases, such as chronic wasting disease (CWD), bovine spongiform encephalopathy, transmissible mink encephalopathy, and variant Creutzfeldt–Jakob disease. Mucosal immunization can be designed to induce primarily a humoral immune response with a secretory IgA response in the gut that can prevent or inhibit entry of the prion agent into the body.

We have developed prion vaccines that target gut-associated tissue, the main site of entry of the prion agent (Goni et al., 2005, 2008, 2015), which can be fully protective for peripheral prion infection. We have expressed PrP in attenuated *Salmonella* strains, where one or more genes responsible for virulence have been deleted, as a live vector for oral vaccination. Live attenuated strains of *Salmonella enterica* are very well characterized and have been used for many years as vaccines against salmonellosis in humans, as well as serving as a delivery system for the construction of multivalent vaccines with broad application in both human and veterinary medicine (Mastroeni et al., 2001; Moreno et al., 2010). A significant advantage for this system is that the safety of human administration of live attenuated *Salmonella* has been extensively confirmed in humans and animals, in whom it has been shown to be able to penetrate the gut mucosa and specifically deliver protein products to immune presenting cells in lymphoid follicles (Tacket et al., 2000; Kirkpatrick et al., 2006; Moreno et al., 2010; Roland and Brenneman, 2013). A variety of animals have been effectively immunized by an oral route using live *Salmonella*, to induce humoral mucosal responses (Villarreal-Ramos et al., 1998; Chabalgoity et al., 2000; Roland and Brenneman, 2013). *Salmonella* targets M cells, antigen sampling cells in the intestines, which importantly may also be critical for PrP^{TSE} uptake (Heppner et al., 2001a; Sigurdsson and Wisniewski, 2005; Mabbott and MacPherson, 2006; Goni et al., 2015). Therefore, this approach is more targeted than prior vaccination studies, providing a possible explanation for the improved efficacy (Goni et al., 2005, 2008, 2015).

The *Salmonella* vector can also express one or several repeating copies of PrP (which can be heterologous to enhance the immune response), producing and delivering a protein product that might simulate the three-dimensional sites critical for the PrP^{C} to PrP^{TSE} interaction (Goni et al., 2008, 2015). This approach takes into account that, if tolerance is broken, the majority of the B-cell response will be devoted to producing dimeric secretory IgA in the mucosa, with a more limited (in comparison to a conventional vaccination methodology) systemic IgG level, which will help to maintain an optimal level of anti-PrP systemic antibodies that can neutralize any PrP^{TSE} that breaches the gut barrier, with a low risk of autoimmune pathology.

With a mucosal immunization methodology the V regions selected for recombination, within the mesenteric lymphoid tissue, to produce neutralizing IgA are likely very distinct from a systemic humoral response. Our past data, using 139A scrapie prions in wild-type CD-1 mice, indicate that in animals which have a significant anti-PrP mucosal IgA response and a systemic anti-PrP IgG response, full protection against oral challenge with the PrP^{TSE} is possible (Goni et al., 2005, 2008).

Further refinement of mucosal immunization, aiming for greater specificity to critical epitopes expressed in PrP^{TSE} or that are involved in the conformational change to PrP^{TSE}, rather than high anti-PrP levels, is likely to lead to an effective means of preventing prion disease in animal and human populations at risk for prion exposure.

We have shown that mucosal immunization is able to partially protect from CWD in white-tailed deer (Goni et al., 2015). CWD appears to be the most infectious prionosis to date, affecting free-ranging and farmed ungulates (white-tailed deer, mule deer, elk, and moose), with significant zoonotic potential (Aguzzi and Sigurdson, 2004; Williams, 2005; Sigurdson, 2008; Gilch et al., 2011; Saunders et al., 2012; Aguilar-Calvo et al., 2015; Greenlee and Greenlee, 2015; Moreno and Telling, 2017; Waddell et al., 2018). CWD has been detected in 22 states of the United States, two Canadian provinces, South Korea, and, more recently, in Norway (Gilch et al., 2011; Robinson et al., 2012; Saunders et al., 2012; Greenlee and Greenlee, 2015; Moreno and Telling, 2017).

Mucosal immunization in deer was performed by numerous oral inoculations, along with tonsil and rectal vaccination that was supplemented with polymerized recombinant deer PrP, which was produced by cross-linking recombinant PrP as described for the ABri peptide (Goni et al., 2010, 2015). This vaccination strategy was able to break mucosal immunologic tolerance to PrP in deer, with production of gut and saliva IgA, as well as systemic IgM and IgG reactive to aggregated recombinant cervid PrP and also to PrP^{CWD}, which was associated with a significant prolongation of the incubation period and complete protection from clinical infection in one of the five vaccinated deer. These results indicated for the first time that specific antibody responses against the self-antigen PrP can be produced in the biologic fluids (gut and plasma) of large cervid mammals naturally at risk for prion infection, in association with at least partial protection from CWD infection.

CONCLUSION

Prion-like phenomena are increasingly being recognized to be part of the pathogenesis of numerous common human neurodegenerative diseases, including AD. Many encouraging experimental antiprion vaccine strategies have been reported. Passive immunization, immediately or shortly after exposure, has been successful in mouse models, preventing disease. In addition mucosal immunization has been shown to potentially prevent prion infection via an oral route in mouse models as well as in deer. The latter approach, with further refinement, would be potentially highly appropriate to stem the epidemic of CWD in North America and the recent emergence of CWD in Northern Europe. However, for effective immunotherapy near or at the time of clinical disease, methods to more specifically target PrP^{TSE}, that will be effective in the brain, are needed. Active and passive immunization approaches that specifically target pathology-associated conformers such as PrP^{TSE}, oligomeric Aβ, and paired helical filaments tau are currently under development and are being tested in both AD and prion models (Goni et al., 2013, 2015, 2016b, 2017; Marciniuk et al., 2014; Wisniewski and Goni, 2015; Drummond et al., 2018).

ACKNOWLEDGMENTS

This work was supported by National Institutes of Health grants NS073502 and AG008051. We thank Geoffrey Pires for help with producing the figure.

References

Aguilar-Calvo P, Garcia C, Espinosa JC et al. (2015). Prion and prion-like diseases in animals. Virus Res 207: 82–93.

Aguzzi A, Sigurdson CJ (2004). Antiprion immunotherapy: to suppress or to stimulate? Nat Rev Immunol 4: 725–736.

Aguzzi A, Baumann F, Bremer J (2008). The prion's elusive reason for being. Annu Rev Neurosci 31: 439–477.

Aguzzi A, Nuvolone M, Zhu C (2013). The immunobiology of prion diseases. Nat Rev Immunol 13: 888–902.

Alexandrenne C, Wijkhuisen A, Dkhissi F et al. (2010). Electrotransfer of cDNA coding for a heterologous prion protein generates autoantibodies against native murine prion protein in wild-type mice. DNA Cell Biol 29: 121–131.

Aucouturier P, Carp RI, Carnaud C et al. (2000). Prion diseases and the immune system. Clin Immunol 96: 79–85.

Aucouturier P, Geissmann F, Damotte D et al. (2001). Infected dendritic cells are sufficient for prion transmission to the CNS in mouse scrapie. J Clin Invest 108: 703–708.

Bakkebo MK, Mouillet-Richard S, Espenes A et al. (2015). The cellular prion protein: a player in immunological quiescence. Front Immunol 6: 450.

Bartz JC, DeJoia C, Tucker T et al. (2005). Extraneural prion neuroinvasion without lymphoreticular system infection. J Virol 79: 11858–11863.

Beekes M, McBride PA (2007). The spread of prions through the body in naturally acquired transmissible spongiform encephalopathies. FEBS J 274: 588–605.

Bessen RA, Martinka S, Kelly J et al. (2009). Role of the lymphoreticular system in prion neuroinvasion from the oral and nasal mucosa. J Virol 83: 6435–6445.

Brandner S, Raeber A, Sailer A et al. (1996). Normal host prion protein (PrP^{c}) is required for scrapie spread within the central nervous system. Proc Natl Acad Sci USA 93: 13148–13151.

Brazier MW, Volitakis I, Kvasnicka M et al. (2010). Manganese chelation therapy extends survival in a mouse model of M1000 prion disease. J Neurochem 114: 440–451.

Bremer J, Heikenwalder M, Haybaeck J et al. (2009). Repetitive immunization enhances the susceptibility of mice to peripherally administered prions. PLoS ONE 4: e7160.

Brown DR (2011). Prions and manganese: a maddening beast. Metallomics 3: 229–238.

Brown KL, Ritchie DL, McBride PA et al. (2000). Detection of PrP in extraneural tissues. Microsc Res Tech 50: 40–45.

Bueler H, Fischer M, Lang Y et al. (1992). Normal development and behaviour of mice lacking the neuronal cell-surface PrP protein. Nature 356: 577–582.

Burchell JT, Panegyres PK (2016). Prion diseases: immunotargets and therapy. Immunotargets Ther 5: 57–68.

Canello T, Engelstein R, Moshel O et al. (2008). Methionine sulfoxides on PrPSc: a prion-specific covalent signature. Biochemistry 47: 8866–8873.

Chabalgoity JA, Moreno M, Carol H et al. (2000). A dog-adapted *Salmonella typhimurium* strain as a basis for a live oral *Echinococcus granulosus* vaccine. Vaccine 19: 460–469.

Chesebro B, Race R, Wehrly K et al. (1985). Identification of scrapie prion protein-specific mRNA in scrapie infected and uninfected brain. Nature 315: 331–333.

Chung E, Ji Y, Sun Y et al. (2010). Anti-PrP^C monoclonal antibody infusion as a novel treatment for Aβ oligomer cognitive cognitive deficits. BMC Neuroscience 11: 130.

Colby DW, Prusiner SB (2011). Prions. Cold Spring Harb Perspect Biol 3: a006833.

Collinge J, Whitfield J, McKintosh E et al. (2006). Kuru in the 21st century – an acquired human prion disease with very long incubation periods. Lancet 367: 2068–2074.

Come JH, Fraser PE, Lansbury Jr PT (1993). A kinetic model for amyloid formation in the prion diseases: importance of seeding. Proc Natl Acad Sci USA 90: 5959–5963.

Drummond E, Wisniewski T (2017). Alzheimer's disease: experimental models and reality. Acta Neuropathol 133: 155–175.

Drummond E, Goni F, Liu S et al. (2018). Potential novel approaches to understand the pathogenesis and treat Alzheimer's disease. J Alzheimers Dis (in press). https://doi.org/10.3233/JAD-179909.

Durig J, Giese A, Schulz-Schaeffer W et al. (2000). Differential constitutive and activation-dependent expression of prion protein in human peripheral blood leucocytes. Br J Haematol 108: 488–495.

Enari M, Flechsig E, Weissmann C (2001). Scrapie prion protein accumulation by scrapie-infected neuroblastoma cells abrogated by exposure to a prion protein antibody. Proc Natl Acad Sci U S A 98: 9295–9299.

Friedman-Levi Y, Binyamin O, Frid K et al. (2014). Genetic prion disease: no role for the immune system in disease pathogenesis? Hum Mol Genet 23: 4134–4141.

Gabizon R, McKinley MP, Groth D et al. (1988). Immunoaffinity purification and neutralization of scrapie prion infectivity. Proc Natl Acad Sci U S A 85: 6617–6621.

Gilch S, Wopfner F, Renner-Muller I et al. (2003). Polyclonal anti-PrP auto-antibodies induced with dimeric PrP interfere efficiently with PrPSc propagation in prion-infected cells. J Biol Chem 278: 18524–18531.

Gilch S, Chitoor N, Taguchi Y et al. (2011). Chronic wasting disease. Top Curr Chem 305: 51–77.

Giles K, Olson SH, Prusiner SB (2017). Developing therapeutics for PrP prion diseases. Cold Spring Harb Perspect Med 7.

Goedert M (2015). Alzheimer's and Parkinson's diseases: the prion concept in relation to assembled Abeta, tau, and alpha-synuclein. Science 349: 1255555.

Goni F, Knudsen EL, Schreiber F et al. (2005). Mucosal vaccination delays or prevents prion infection via an oral route. Neurosci 133: 413–421.

Goni F, Prelli F, Schreiber F et al. (2008). High titers of mucosal and systemic anti-PrP antibodies abrogates oral prion infection in mucosal vaccinated mice. Neurosci 153: 679–686.

Goni F, Prelli F, Ji Y et al. (2010). Immunomodulation targeting abnormal protein conformation reduces pathology in a mouse model of Alzheimer's disease. PLoS ONE 5: e13391.

Goni F, Herline K, Peyser D et al. (2013). Immunomodulation targeting both Aβ and tau pathological conformers ameliorates Alzheimer's disease pathology in TgSwDI and 3xTg mouse models. J Neuroinflammation 10: 150.

Goni F, Mathiason CK, Yim L et al. (2015). Mucosal immunization with an attenuated *Salmonella* vaccine partially protects white-tailed deer from chronic wasting disease. Vaccine 33: 726–733.

Goni F, Herline K, Marta-Ariza M et al. (2016a). Disease modifying therapy by the infusion of an anti-conformational monoclonal antibody in an Abeta and tau 3xTg mouse model of Alzheimer's disease. Alzheimers Demen 12: p360.

Goni F, Marta-Ariza M, Herline K et al. (2016b). Anti-conformational monoclonal antibody effective in pre-clinical treatment of full Alzheimer's disease animal models by targeting pathological oligomeric forms of Abeta and modified tau. Eur J Immunol 46-S1: 1035.

Goni F, Marta-Ariza M, Peyser D et al. (2017). Production of monoclonals to pathologic β-sheet oligomeric conformers in neurodegenerative disease. Sci Rep 9881.

Gourdain P, Ballerini C, Nicot AB et al. (2012). Exacerbation of experimental autoimmune encephalomyelitis in prion protein (PrPc)-null mice: evidence for a critical role of the central nervous system. J Neuroinflammation 9: 25.

Greenlee JJ, Greenlee MH (2015). The transmissible spongiform encephalopathies of livestock. ILAR J 56: 7–25.

Greenlee JJ, Kunkle RA, Richt JA et al. (2014). Lack of prion accumulation in lymphoid tissues of PRNP ARQ/ARR sheep intracranially inoculated with the agent of scrapie. PLoS One 9: e108029.

Griffith JS (1967). Self-replication and scrapie. Nature 215: 1043–1044.

Han Y, Li Y, Song J et al. (2011). Immune responses in wild-type mice against prion proteins induced using a DNA prime-protein boost strategy. Biomed Environ Sci 24: 523–529.

Handisurya A, Gilch S, Winter D et al. (2007). Vaccination with prion peptide-displaying papillomavirus-like particles induces autoantibodies to normal prion protein that interfere with pathologic prion protein production in infected cells. FEBS J 274: 1747–1758.

Harris DA, Huber MT, Vankijken P et al. (1993). Processing of a cellular prion protein: identification of N-terminal and C-terminal cleavage sites. Biochem 32: 1009–1016.

Head MW, Ironside JW, Ghetti B et al. (2015). Prion disease. In: S Love, H Budka, JW Ironside et al. (Eds.), Greenfield's neuropathology, 9th edn. CRC Press, Boca Raton, FL.

Heppner FL, Christ AD, Klein MA et al. (2001a). Transepithelial prion transport by M cells. Nat Med 7: 976–977.

Heppner FL, Musahl C, Arrighi I et al. (2001b). Prevention of scrapie pathogenesis by transgenic expression of anti-prion protein antibodies. Science 294: 178–182.

Hu W, Nessler S, Hemmer B et al. (2010). Pharmacological prion protein silencing accelerates central nervous system autoimmune disease via T cell receptor signalling. Brain 133: 375–388.

Isaacs JD, Jackson GS, Altmann DM (2006). The role of the cellular prion protein in the immune system. Clin Exp Immunol 146: 1–8.

Ishibashi D, Yamanaka H, Yamaguchi N et al. (2007). Immunization with recombinant bovine but not mouse prion protein delays the onset of disease in mice inoculated with a mouse-adapted prion. Vaccine 25: 985–992.

Kim CL, Karino A, Ishiguro N et al. (2004a). Cell-surface retention of PrPC by anti-PrP antibody prevents protease-resistant PrP formation. J Gen Virol 85: 3473–3482.

Kim CL, Umetani A, Matsui T et al. (2004b). Antigenic characterization of an abnormal isoform of prion protein using a new diverse panel of monoclonal antibodies. Virology 320: 40–51.

Kirkpatrick BD, McKenzie R, O'Neill JP et al. (2006). Evaluation of *Salmonella enterica* serovar *typhi* (Ty2 aroC-ssaV-) M01ZH09, with a defined mutation in the *Salmonella* pathogenicity island 2, as a live, oral typhoid vaccine in human volunteers. Vaccine 24: 116–123.

Kitamoto T, Muramoto T, Mohri S et al. (1991). Abnormal isoform of prion protein accumulates in follicular dendritic cells in mice with Creutzfeldt–Jakob disease. J Virol 65: 6292–6295.

Klohn PC, Farmer M, Linehan JM et al. (2012). PrP antibodies do not trigger mouse hippocampal neuron apoptosis. Science 335: 52.

Kostylev MA, Kaufman AC, Nygaard HB et al. (2015). Prion-protein-interacting amyloid-beta oligomers of high molecular weight are tightly correlated with memory impairment in multiple Alzheimer mouse models. J Biol Chem 290: 17415–17438.

Kretzschmar H, Tatzelt J (2013). Prion disease: a tale of folds and strains. Brain Pathol 23: 321–332.

Langevin C, Gousset K, Costanzo M et al. (2010). Characterization of the role of dendritic cells in prion transfer to primary neurons. Biochem J 431: 189–198.

Lassmann H, Bradl M (2017). Multiple sclerosis: experimental models and reality. Acta Neuropathol 133: 223–244.

Liberski PP, Sikorska B, Lindenbaum S et al. (2012). Kuru: genes, cannibals and neuropathology. J Neuropathol Exp Neurol 71: 92–103.

Mabbott NA (2015). Prospects for safe and effective vaccines against prion diseases. Expert Rev Vaccines 14: 1–4.

Mabbott NA, MacPherson GG (2006). Prions and their lethal journey to the brain. Nat Rev Microbiol 4: 201–211.

Mallucci GR, White MD, Farmer M et al. (2007). Targeting cellular prion protein reverses early cognitive deficits and neurophysiological dysfunction in prion-infected mice. Neuron 53: 325–335.

Manson JC, Clarke AR, Hooper ML et al. (1994). 129/Ola mice carrying a null mutation in PrP that abolishes mRNA production are developmentally normal. Mol Neurobiol 8: 121–127.

Manuelidis L (1998). Vaccination with an attenuated Creutzfeldt–Jakob disease strain prevents expression of a virulent agent. Proc Natl Acad Sci U S A 95: 2520–2525.

Marciniuk K, Maattanen P, Taschuk R et al. (2014). Development of a multivalent, PrP(Sc)-specific prion vaccine through rational optimization of three disease-specific epitopes. Vaccine 32: 1988–1997.

Mastroeni P, Chabalgoity JA, Dunstan SJ et al. (2001). Salmonella: immune responses and vaccines. Vet J 161: 132–164.

Montrasio F, Frigg R, Glatzel M et al. (2000). Impaired prion replication in spleens of mice lacking functional follicular dendritic cells. Science 288: 1257–1259.

Moreno JA, Telling GC (2017). Molecular mechanisms of chronic wasting disease prion propagation. Cold Spring Harb Perspect Med pii: a024448. https://doi.org/10.1101/cshperspect.a024448.

Moreno M, Kramer MG, Yim L et al. (2010). Salmonella as live Trojan horse for vaccine development and cancer gene therapy. Curr Gene Ther 10: 56–76.

Nelson PT, Alafuzoff I, Bigio EH et al. (2012). Correlation of Alzheimer's disease neuropathologic changes with cognitive status: a review of the literature. JNEN 71: 362–381.

Nikles D, Bach P, Boller K et al. (2005). Circumventing tolerance to the prion protein (PrP): vaccination with PrP-displaying retrovirus particles induces humoral immune responses against the native form of cellular PrP. J Virol 79: 4033–4042.

Nygaard HB, Wagner AF, Bowen GS et al. (2015). A phase Ib multiple ascending dose study of the safety, tolerability, and central nervous system availability of AZD0530 (saracatinib) in Alzheimer's disease. Alzheimers Res Ther 7: 35.

Oesch B, Westaway D, Walchli M et al. (1985). A cellular gene encodes scrapie PrP 27-30 protein. Cell 40: 735–746.

Ohsawa N, Song CH, Suzuki A et al. (2013). Therapeutic effect of peripheral administration of an anti-prion protein antibody on mice infected with prions. Microbiol Immunol 57: 288–297.

Onodera T, Sakudo A, Tsubone H et al. (2014). Review of studies that have used knockout mice to assess normal function of prion protein under immunological or pathophysiological stress. Microbiol Immunol 58: 361–374.

Pankiewicz J, Prelli F, Sy MS et al. (2006). Clearance and prevention of prion infection in cell culture by anti-PrP antibodies. Eur J Neurosci 24: 2635–2647.

Peretz D, Williamson RA, Kaneko K et al. (2001). Antibodies inhibit prion propagation and clear cell cultures of prion infectivity. Nature 412: 739–743.

Polymenidou M, Heppner FL, Pellicioli EC et al. (2004). Humoral immune response to native eukaryotic prion protein correlates with anti-prion protection. Proc Natl Acad Sci 101: 14670–14676.

Prusiner SB (1982). Novel proteinaceous infectious particles cause scrapie. Science 216: 136–144.

Prusiner SB (2012). Cell biology. A unifying role for prions in neurodegenerative diseases. Science 336: 1511–1513.

Prusiner SB, Scott MR, DeArmond SJ et al. (1998). Prion protein biology. Cell 93: 337–348.

Robinson SJ, Samuel MD, O'Rourke KI et al. (2012). The role of genetics in chronic wasting disease of North American cervids. Prion 6: 153–162.

Roland KL, Brenneman KE (2013). Salmonella as a vaccine delivery vehicle. Expert Rev Vaccines 12: 1033–1045.

Rosset MB, Ballerini C, Gregoire S et al. (2004). Breaking immune tolerance to the prion protein using prion protein peptides plus oligodeoxynucleotide-CpG in mice. J Immunol 172: 5168–5174.

Rosset MB, Sacquin A, Lecollinet S et al. (2009). Dendritic cell-mediated-immunization with xenogenic PrP and adenoviral vectors breaks tolerance and prolongs mice survival against experimental scrapie. PLoS One 4: e4917.

Rostagno A, Tomidokoro Y, Lashley T et al. (2005). Chromosome 13 dementias. Cell Mol Life Sci 62: 1814–1825.

Rubenstein R, Chang B, Grinkina N et al. (2017). Tau phosphorylation induced by severe closed head traumatic brain injury is linked to the cellular prion protein. Acta Neuropathol Commun 5: 30.

Sadowski MJ, Pankiewicz J, Prelli F et al. (2009). Anti-PrP Mab 6D11 suppresses PrP^{Sc} replication in prion infected myeloid precursor line FDC-P1/22L and in the lymphoreticular system *in vivo*. Neurobiol Dis 34: 267–278.

Salazar SV, Strittmatter SM (2016). Cellular prion protein as a receptor for amyloid-beta oligomers in Alzheimer's disease. Biochem Biophys Res Commun 483: 1143–1147.

Sassa Y, Kataoka N, Inoshima Y et al. (2010). Anti-PrP antibodies detected at terminal stage of prion-affected mouse. Cell Immunol 263: 212–218.

Saunders SE, Bartelt-Hunt SL, Bartz JC (2012). Occurrence, transmission, and zoonotic potential of chronic wasting disease. Emerg Infect Dis 18: 369–376.

Schenk D, Barbour R, Dunn W et al. (1999). Immunization with amyloid-beta attenuates Alzheimer-disease-like pathology in the PDAPP mouse. Nature 400: 173–177.

Scholtzova H, Chianchiano P, Pan J et al. (2014). Toll-like receptor 9 stimulation for reduction of amyloid β and tau Alzheimer's disease related pathology. Acta Neuropathol Commun 2: 101.

Scholtzova H, Do E, Dhakal S et al. (2017). Innate immunity stimulation via Toll-like receptor 9 ameliorates vascular amyloid pathology in Tg-SwDI mice with associated cognitive benefits. J Neurosci 37: 936–959.

Selkoe DJ, Hardy J (2016). The amyloid hypothesis of Alzheimer's disease at 25 years. EMBO Mol Med 8: 595–608.

Sevigny J, Chiao P, Bussiere T et al. (2016). The antibody aducanumab reduces Abeta plaques in Alzheimer's disease. Nature 537: 50–56.

Sigurdson CJ (2008). A prion disease of cervids: chronic wasting disease. Vet Res 39: 41.

Sigurdsson EM, Wisniewski T (2005). Promising developments in prion immunotherapy. Exp. Review Vaccines 4: 607–610.

Sigurdsson EM, Brown DR, Daniels M et al. (2002). Vaccination delays the onset of prion disease in mice. AJP 161: 13–17.

Sigurdsson EM, Brown DR, Alim MA et al. (2003a). Copper chelation delays the onset of prion disease. JBC 278: 46199–46202.

Sigurdsson EM, Sy MS, Li R et al. (2003b). Anti-PrP antibodies for prophylaxis following prion exposure in mice. Neurosci Lett 336: 185–187.

Singh A, Haldar S, Horback K et al. (2013). Prion protein regulates iron transport by functioning as a ferrireductase. J Alzheimers Dis 35: 541–552.

Siso S, Gonzalez L, Jeffrey M (2010). Neuroinvasion in prion diseases: the roles of ascending neural infection and blood dissemination. Interdiscip Perspect Infect Dis: 747892.

Solforosi L, Criado JR, McGavern DB et al. (2004). Cross-linking cellular prion protein triggers neuronal apoptosis in vivo. Science 303: 1514–1516.

Sonati T, Reimann RR, Falsig J et al. (2013). The toxicity of antiprion antibodies is mediated by the flexible tail of the prion protein. Nature 501: 102–106.

Song CH, Furuoka H, Kim CL et al. (2008). Effect of intraventricular infusion of anti-prion protein monoclonal antibodies on disease progression in prion-infected mice. J Gen Virol 89: 1533–1544.

Spinner DS, Kascsak RB, LaFauci G et al. (2007). CpG oligodeoxynucleotide-enhanced humoral immune response and production of antibodies to prion protein PrPSc in mice immunized with 139A scrapie-associated fibrils. J Leukoc Biol 14: 36–43.

Stopschinski BE, Diamond MI (2017). The prion model for progression and diversity of neurodegenerative diseases. Lancet Neurol 16: 323–332.

Tacket CO, Sztein MB, Wasserman SS et al. (2000). Phase 2 clinical trial of attenuated Salmonella enterica serovar typhi oral live vector vaccine CVD 908-htrA in U.S. volunteers. Infect Immun 68: 1196–1201.

Tayebi M, Hawke S (2006). Antibody-mediated neuronal apoptosis: therapeutic implications for prion diseases. Immunol Lett 105: 123–126.

Tayebi M, Collinge J, Hawke S (2009). Unswitched immunoglobulin M response prolongs mouse survival in prion disease. J Gen Virol 90: 777–782.

Teruya K, Doh-Ura K (2017). Insights from therapeutic studies for PrP prion disease. Cold Spring Harb Perspect Med 7.

Thackray AM, Knight R, Haswell SJ et al. (2002). Metal imbalance and compromised antioxidant function are early changes in prion disease. Biochem J 362: 253–258.

Tsutsui S, Hahn JN, Johnson TA et al. (2008). Absence of the cellular prion protein exacerbates and prolongs neuroinflammation in experimental autoimmune encephalomyelitis. Am J Pathol 173: 1029–1041.

Um JW, Nygaard HB, Heiss JK et al. (2012). Alzheimer amyloid-β oligomer bound to post-synaptic prion protein activates Fyn to impair neurons. Nat Neurosci 15: 1227–1235.

Um JW, Kaufman AC, Kostylev MA et al. (2013). Metabotropic glutamate receptor 5 mediates signaling from Alzheimer Aβ oligomer bound to prion protein. Neuron 79: 887–902.

Verity NC, Mallucci GR (2011). Rescuing neurons in prion disease. Biochem J 433: 19–29.

Vidal R, Frangione B, Rostagno A et al. (1999). A stop-codon mutation in the BRI gene associated with familial British dementia. Nature 399: 776–781.

Villarreal-Ramos B, Manser J, Collins RA et al. (1998). Immune responses in calves immunised orally or subcutaneously with a live *Salmonella typhimurium* aro vaccine. Vaccine 16: 45–54.

Viola KL, Klein WL (2015). Amyloid beta oligomers in Alzheimer's disease pathogenesis, treatment, and diagnosis. Acta Neuropathol 129: 183–206.

Waddell L, Greig J, Mascarenhas M et al. (2018). Current evidence on the transmissibility of chronic wasting disease prions to humans – a systematic review. Transbound Emerg Dis 65: 37–49.

Watts JC, Prusiner SB (2017). Beta-amyloid prions and the pathobiology of Alzheimer's disease. Cold Spring Harb Perspect Med pii: a023507.

White AR, Enever P, Tayebl M et al. (2003). Monoclonal antibodies inhibit prion replication and delay the development of prion disease. Nature 422: 80–83.

Will RG, Ironside JW (2017). Sporadic and infectious human prion diseases. Cold Spring Harb Perspect Med 7.

Williams ES (2005). Chronic wasting disease. Vet Pathol 42: 530–549.

Windl O, Dempster M, Estibeiro P et al. (1995). A candidate marsupial PrP gene reveals two domains conserved in mammalian PrP proteins. Gene 159: 181–186.

Wisniewski T, Drummond E (2016). Developing therapeutic vaccines against Alzheimer's disease. Expert Rev Vaccines 15: 401–415.

Wisniewski T, Goni F (2015). Immunotherapeutic approaches for Alzheimer's disease. Neuron 85: 1162–1176.

Wisniewski T, Goni F (2016). Transmissible spongiform encephalopathies. In: CA Reiss (Ed.), Neurotophic viral infections, 2nd edn. Springer, New York, pp. 221–248.

Xanthopoulos K, Lagoudaki R, Kontana A et al. (2013). Immunization with recombinant prion protein leads to partial protection in a murine model of TSEs through a novel mechanism. PLoS One 8: e59143.

Xanthopoulos K, Dafou D, Kanata E et al. (2017). Immunobiology of prion diseases. In: Y Tutar (Ed.), Prion – an overview. InTech, Rijeka.

Handbook of Clinical Neurology, Vol. 153 (3rd series)
Human Prion Diseases
M. Pocchiari and J. Manson, Editors
https://doi.org/10.1016/B978-0-444-63945-5.00024-6

Chapter 24

Clinical trials

SIMON MEAD[1]* AND FABRIZIO TAGLIAVINI[2]

[1]*National Prion Clinic, National Hospital for Neurology and Neurosurgery, University College London Hospitals NHS Foundation Trust, and MRC Prion Unit at University College London Institute of Prion Diseases, London, United Kingdom*

[2]*Fondazione IRCCS Istituto Neurologico "Carlo Besta," Milan, Italy*

Abstract

Arguably the most important goal of prion research is the discovery of a safe and effective treatment for the human diseases. The final stages of the pathway to develop a treatment require clinical trials. Choices about how a trial is designed and conducted have a large impact on the chances of success. The gold-standard large randomized double-blind placebo-controlled study, which minimizes sources of bias and has been incredibly successful in other diseases, has been hard to achieve in Creutzfeldt–Jakob disease principally because of the rarity and rapidity of the clinical syndrome. To date, clinical trials have been restricted to repurposed compounds, doxycycline, quinacrine, pentosan polysulfate (PPS), and flupertine. In most cases, these trials have used survival as an endpoint, which, whilst clearcut, has limitations. Biomarkers have played a strong role in diagnosis and entry criteria, but only a limited role as secondary outcome measures. Recent developments suggest some possible improvements in trial design by use of new outcome measures that have more favorable properties, and biomarkers of neuronal damage and/or prion seeding activity. Alternative patient populations, including those at risk of genetic forms of prion disease, warrant more consideration. In the future, improved trial designs will be employed to test compounds designed specifically to treat prion diseases.

BACKGROUND

Clinical trials are research studies that prospectively seek to explore whether a medical intervention is safe and effective for humans. Interventions might include novel or repurposed drugs, surgery, physical or psychologic therapy, or alteration of diet and/or lifestyle. Clinical trials have a long history and some dramatic results. One of the earliest examples was conducted in 1747 by James Lind, who believed that scurvy could be treated by acids. He treated 12 seamen on the *Salisbury* diagnosed with scurvy, using six different interventions: "the consequence was that the most sudden and visible good effects were perceived from the use of the oranges and lemons; one of those who had taken them being at the end of six days fit for duty" (Lind, 1753). It would however be more than 50 years before the British Navy used lemon juice routinely to prevent scurvy. Some of these themes remain pertinent today: if the benefit of the intervention is strong, clinical trials need not recruit prohibitively large numbers of patients; the timeline of trials to change in medical practice can be very long and frustrating; and the precise mechanism of the intervention is commonly not understood or misunderstood.

Clinical trials are strongly regulated, although this aspect will not be covered here. The origins of special regulation are rooted in the initial responses to criminal medical experimentation by the Nazis, and similar scandals involving the involuntary and harmful experimentation on vulnerable or captive people, later extended as the Declaration of Helsinki by the World Health Organization (Rickham, 1964). Common elements of regulatory scrutiny are the documentation of informed

*Correspondence to: Professor Simon Mead, National Prion Clinic, National Hospital for Neurology and Neurosurgery, University College London Hospitals NHS Foundation Trust, Queen Square, London WC1N 3BG, United Kingdom. Tel: +44-203-448-4037, E-mail: s.mead@prion.ucl.ac.uk

consent and trial data, voluntary recruitment, confidentiality, and implementation of reasonable measures to assess the safety of the intervention.

Trials involve a comparison group, in the most rigorous circumstance through randomization of participants to receive either the intervention or a placebo treatment, or current best practice, but there are many alternative designs. A primary outcome measure is used as the key parameter to judge the effectiveness of an intervention which is commonly supplemented by related measures that might add more information about outcomes and mechanisms, including biomarkers (typically imaging and/or tissue or biofluid assays that inform about the disease process). Clinical trials are usually expensive, time consuming, mark the end result of a decade or more of laboratory research, and underline the success or failure of a translational medical program.

The design of a clinical trial seeks to minimize bias. Two of the key methods are randomization and blinding. Randomization seeks to diminish the effects of bias of confounding factors in the selection of participants. Blinding seeks to avoid the influence of knowledge of the treatment on the outcome measure itself, either through the patient or physicians. It is hard to eliminate bias completely, and so effective trial design should consider carefully the major potential sources of bias. Other major considerations are inclusion criteria, which must balance a desire for a homogenous study group with a need for the study results to be generalizable to the broader population. The sample size of a clinical trial is usually determined to ensure that the study has adequate (>80%) statistical power to address whether the intervention has a meaningful effect on the outcome measure ($p < 0.05$). All of these issues will be considered with respect to prion diseases in this chapter. We do not systematically review here the preclinical data for compounds that have yet to enter human studies.

CHALLENGES IN PRION DISEASE CLINICAL TRIALS

Despite intense scientific and clinical scrutiny, prion diseases have not been the focus of many clinical trials. No compound specifically developed for prion diseases has ever entered human study. There are several reasons for this unfortunate situation. Prion diseases are rare. Most countries with developed systems of surveillance document an annual incidence of 1–2 per million inhabitants, equating to a lifetime risk of approximately 1 in 5000 (Klug et al., 2013).

The problem of the rarity of the disorder is compounded by the rapidity of progression of the most common form, sporadic Creutzfeldt–Jakob disease (CJD). Whilst the median survival in most countries is in the order of 4–6 months (Pocchiari et al., 2004), diagnosis and referral to specialist centers are typically made late in the clinical course when patients have advanced disability, and the priority is palliative care. Transfer to a specialist center for an intervention is difficult in the later stages of disease. It is widely accepted in neurodegeneration, based on animal studies and the failure of many clinical trials in common dementias, that interventions are unlikely to show beneficial effects at advanced stages of disease. These practical aspects partly explain a lack of trial activity.

There are other challenges. Outcome measures and optimized clinical trial designs, until relatively recently, have not been specifically developed in CJD. Survival time has been the or a main outcome measure in all trials to date; however this choice is problematic, as discussed later. There is little commercial interest in drug development, and as a consequence only clinical academics have led studies and the only drugs tested are those which may be prescribed for other conditions. Participants in randomized studies have faced the option of seeking access to the study drug outside of the trial, potentially threatening its integrity. Understandably, patients and/or their family may feel that there is only one chance of a beneficial response to a treatment, and reject the possibility of a study that incorporates the possibility of receiving placebo treatment.

The situation is not completely futile, however; prion diseases have some aspects that make them amenable to potentially powerful studies. Trials rely on the assumption of clinical "equipoise," meaning that the physician and patient are uncertain because there is no good evidence to justify the choice of an intervention or none. A clinician facing this choice must consider the potential benefits of a novel treatment weighed against the risks of harm in the context of the severity of the disease. The length of the clinical trial phase of drug development has a lot to do with a need to put "safety first." The extreme severity of a universally terminal condition, usually rapidly, therefore puts in perspective the risks of an experimental treatment. Clinical equipoise arguably exists in prion disease for interventions that might have a low chance of benefit and serious and/or predictable risks.

Furthermore, prion diseases are relatively well understood from a disease pathogenesis point of view. Partly this has come about because of a fascination in their seemingly unique pathobiology, but also because of the investment consequent upon animal prion diseases and a notorious capacity for epidemics and iatrogenic incidents. Prion diseases have excellent animal and laboratory models, with unmodified mice and other rodents susceptible to mammalian prions, and cell and in vitro assays amenable to high-throughput screening studies and preclinical therapeutics. There is no question about the prime causal role of prions/prion protein (PrP) in the disease, as compared to other neurodegenerative diseases which either are immersed in debates about the right target or have heterogeneous disease etiology. For example, in Alzheimer disease, decades-long debates continue about the usefulness of the "amyloid hypothesis" and the relative merits of targeting amyloid beta (Aβ) and related multimeric assemblies, vs. tau and its assemblies, vs. completely novel targets. In frontotemporal dementia, the clinical syndrome is associated with multiple distinct protein pathologies, and causal mechanisms.

In neurodegenerative diseases there are broadly two types of intervention: those which aim to alter the underlying course of the disease, in the most optimistic situation, a "cure" or an intervention that halts progression, and those which aim to improve a specific symptom or overall disability whilst the drug continues to be administered, with no effect on underlying progression. In prion diseases, many interventions are currently used to manage symptoms, for example, antiepileptic drugs like clonazepam or levetiracetam for myoclonus, hypnotics for sleep disturbance, antipsychotics for psychosis. These are prescribed by physicians with only weak evidence for their benefit in prion disease, as a generalization from related disorders. Clinical trials might be considered for symptomatic therapies, but here our main consideration is of the development of treatments that modify the underlying course of prion diseases.

PUBLISHED TRIALS IN PRION DISEASE (TABLE 24.1)

Doxycycline

The therapeutic potential of tetracyclines in prion diseases was investigated due to their structural similarity with the anthracycline iododoxorubicin that was previously found to bind PrP amyloid and reduce the infectivity titer in prion-infected rodent brains (Tagliavini et al., 1997). Along with other biochemical properties, tetracycline was able to hinder assembly of PrP peptides into amyloid forms, decrease their toxicity in vitro, and revert the protease resistance of the disease-associated form of PrP (PrP^{Sc}) extracted from CJD brains (Tagliavini et al., 2000). Incubation of inoculate with tetracycline, prior to injection, reduced the detectable infectivity (Forloni et al., 2002), as had been seen for iododoxorubicin (Tagliavini et al., 1997); treatment of living animals at the same anatomic site, 1 hour after inoculation, resulted in an extension of survival time (De Luigi et al., 2008). As a result of these studies and because of the extensive clinical data on long-term tolerability and a favorable pharmacology, including blood–brain barrier penetration, doxycycline began to be prescribed compassionately for CJD at Carlo Besta Neurological Institute, Milan.

The first large clinical trial was a French–Italian randomized, double-blind, placebo-controlled study of doxycycline at an oral daily dose of 100 mg in patients with sporadic CJD and some inherited or acquired forms

Table 24.1

Clinical trial in human prion diseases

Drug	Country	Patient recruitment	Number	Design	Primary endpoint
Flupertine	Germany	Sporadic CJD and inherited prion disease	28	Randomized placebo-controlled	ADAS-cog
Pentosan polysulfate	United Kingdom	Variant and iatrogenic CJD and inherited prion disease	7	Observational	Survival
Pentosan polysulfate	Japan	Sporadic and iatrogenic CJD	11	Observational	Survival
Quinacrine	France	Sporadic CJD and inherited prion diseases	32	Observational	Survival
Quinacrine	United Kingdom	Sporadic CJD and inherited prion diseases	107	Observational	Survival and rating scales
Quinacrine	United States	Sporadic CJD	51	Randomized placebo-controlled (2 months)	Survival
Doxycycline	France/Italy	Sporadic CJD and inherited prion disease	121	Randomized placebo-controlled	Survival
Doxycycline	Germany	Sporadic CJD	100	Observational and randomized placebo-controlled	Survival

ADAS-cog, cognitive component of the Alzheimer's disease assessment scale; CJD, Creutzfeldt–Jakob disease.

of the disease (Haïk et al., 2014). The intention-to-treat population included 121 individuals and the main outcome measure was survival time from randomization. Secondary measures included clinical milestones based on feeding, continence, and onset of akinetic mutism. Several additional measures like analysis of cerebrospinal fluid (CSF) biomarkers, brain magnetic resonance imaging (MRI) and electrophysiologic studies were problematic because most patients could not participate at the trial centers due to disease progression. Efficacy was measured by hazard ratio (HR), which compares the rates of death over time (HR = 1.1 (0.8–1.7), $p = 0.5$), and the authors concluded that, although well tolerated, doxycycline did not significantly affect the course of CJD. Covariates in the statistical model included site, sex, age, etiology, disease duration prior to randomization, and the codon 129 genotype of the prion protein gene (*PRNP*). No significant effects were noted in a range of secondary tests, including subgroups based on the covariates listed and per-protocol analyses. Neuropathologic examination was performed in 39 out of the 121 (one-third of the treated population), and confirmed the diagnosis in all individuals. Analysis of doxycycline in the cerebral cortex showed that the compound reached a concentration in the low micromolar range and persisted in the brain for days (Haïk et al., 2014).

In discussion, the authors note the potential that higher doses of doxycycline or treatment at an earlier stage of disease might be beneficial (see later for discussion of future priorities and the treatment of presymptomatic at-risk individuals). A major achievement of the study was the demonstration that a rigorous placebo-controlled multicenter trial can be conducted in a disease as rare and rapidly progressive as prion disease.

The second trial was a German study with a complex design based on two substudies: a randomized double-blind placebo controlled study, and a compassionate use treatment group compared with matched untreated controls (Varges et al., 2017). A slight increase in survival time was seen when the results of the two groups were combined by meta-analysis (HR = 0.63 (0.402–0.999), $p = 0.049$). The authors concluded that doxycycline might be further studied in larger trials and earlier in the clinical course. Further, they found evidence of a differential effect in patients with different codon 129 genotypes, with the strongest effects in *PRNP* methionine homozygote individuals.

There are substantial differences between the French–Italian and German studies, with the latter demonstrating the recruitment of relatively early affected patients (median baseline Mini Mental State Examination (MMSE) was 20–21 in the German study, unreported in the French–Italian study), which could be relevant to a treatment response. However, compassionate use studies are vulnerable to selection bias. Even though correction was used for disease severity in the statistical model, questions remain about whether bias was fully adjusted for in the model. Aside from further clinical study of doxycycline, the German physicians recommend continued compassionate use, especially in methionine homozygous patients, and further development of trial design in prion disease given that they experienced difficulties in recruiting to the randomized study.

The doxycycline story illustrates some strong themes that run through prion disease therapeutics. A repurposed drug with a good safety record became used despite a not completely convincing preclinical story, because of a lack of alternatives and feasibility. Evidence from compassionate use justified more rigorous studies. Certainly, in sporadic CJD, we can conclude that there is no meaningful survival benefit for those in advanced stages. In the early stages of disease, a meaningful benefit remains possible, but further clinical studies would require a stronger preclinical portfolio of evidence.

Quinacrine

Quinacrine, described in early studies as a lysosomotrophic agent (a compound that penetrates and accumulates in lysosomes), has a tricyclic structure and was used in the 1930s and Second World War period as an antimalarial, shortly thereafter replaced by alternatives, and now is no longer commonly prescribed (Doh-ura et al., 2000; Korth et al., 2001). Quinacrine and related compounds were identified as possible prion therapeutics by studies that screened for the effectiveness of compounds in clearance of PrP^{Sc} in chronically prion-infected neuroblastoma cell cultures (Doh-ura et al., 2000; Korth et al., 2001). The crucial evidence of effectiveness in an in vivo rodent model of established prion infection was lacking, but because of a reasonable safety profile, and favorable tolerability and penetration of the blood–brain barrier, there was no strong reason not to proceed into compassionate use human studies. These experiences were widely reported in the international media and clinical trials were planned.

The first study to report treatment of CJD with quinacrine was a French open-label compassionate study in 2004. Thirty-two patients (2 with variant CJD) were treated with a 1g loading dose followed by 300 mg quinacrine daily. The authors reported survival time, Rankin score (a disability scale developed by stroke researchers), and brain lesion profiles stratified by codon 129 genotype (Haïk et al., 2004). The study did report a comparison group but no statistical analysis, being aware of the risk of bias selection of long-surviving patients for treatment. There was no strikingly strong treatment effect, such as reversal of symptoms or pathology, but more subtle effects could not be ruled out.

In 2009, the UK National Prion Clinic reported the results of the PRION-1 study (Collinge et al., 2009). Following a public consultation exercise, the study was designed as a patient preference trial, giving an option for open-label treatment, no treatment, or randomization. The study included a large proportion of patients with variant CJD or inherited prion disease over a wide range of disease severity at baseline. Only 2/107 patients chose randomization, therefore the study was essentially observational. Forty patients took quinacrine at some time in the study. Choice for quinacrine treatment was strongly linked to disease severity, in that the most severely affected chose no treatment, as there was no expectation that disability could be reversed. Once this bias was considered in the statistical analysis, no treatment effect was detectable using survival or rating scales.

PRION-1 employed mobile study teams to visit patients unable to travel to the trial center, to administer a wide range of neurologic, psychologic, and functional scales, including video recording (Mead et al., 2011; Carswell et al., 2012a). Four patients showed transient improvements in some rating scales. The study conclusions again emphasized the importance of recruiting patients with mild to moderate disease, acceptability of trial design to patients, the use of a single study team to minimize interobserver variation, and the importance of a randomization or other well-controlled designs.

In 2013, the US team at the University of California, San Francisco reported the results of a double-blind, placebo-controlled stratified randomization trial using quinacrine (Geschwind et al., 2013). The study design involved a 2-month second assessment at the trial center when all patients were offered open-label quinacrine. Sixty-nine patients were enrolled and 51 were included in the survival analysis. Survival at 2 months showed no treatment benefits (HR = 1.43, 0.58–3.53). In secondary analyses at 2 months, treated patients showed less decline measured by the Rankin scale and Clinical Dementia Rating – Sum of Boxes (CDR-SB), but not using several other scales.

In all studies, quinacrine was acceptably tolerated, resulting in a yellow skin discoloration and frequent liver enzyme elevation in serum, but psychiatric/behavioral disturbances were not a significant problem.

It remains debatable why quinacrine failed to show benefits in humans (Gayrard et al., 2005; Ghaemmaghami et al., 2009). Importantly, there was no convincing evidence that the intervention improved the survival time of rodents with established prion infection (Collins et al., 2002; Barret et al., 2003; Doh-ura et al., 2004). As the initiation of the clinical studies was based on the effects in vitro, evidence from rodent testing became available during recruitment. Drug levels were not measured in brain tissue in any of the studies.

Pentosan polysulfate

PPS is a semisynthetic penta-saccharide heparinoid derived from beechwood shavings. Relative to heparin it is a lower-molecular-weight, more sulfated, and more negatively charged compound. PPS resembles endogenous glycosaminoglycans with an average molecular weight of 4–5 kDa, the typical population is around 12–16 subunits, and it binds proteoglycans strongly.

PPS is indicated for the relief of bladder pain or discomfort associated with interstitial cystitis in the United States, and is widely used as a parenteral anticoagulant in continental Europe. The mechanism of action in insterstitial cystitis is unclear (Anderson and Perry, 2006). For anticoagulation PPS has 1/15th of the activity of heparin, acting predominantly by potentiation of thrombin inactivation by heparin cofactor II/factor VIII. PPS also has an anti-Xa activity in vivo which is more prolonged than its effect on activated partial thromboplastin time.

Prion therapeutic efficacy has been demonstrated repeatedly in vivo, including prolongation of incubation time following intraperitoneal (IP) inoculation of hamster models (scrapie 263K) and mouse models (scrapie 139A, ME7, C506M3, and bovine spongiform encephalopathy) and treatment before symptom onset. Diringer and Ehlers (1991) administered 3 × 10 mg PPS IP to mice around 2 months prior to IP inoculation with 139A scrapie at a range of dilutions. In the treated arm, animals either succumbed with 50% increased incubation times or did not develop clinical signs of disease. Four animals that did not develop clinical signs had no detectable brain PrP^{Sc}. Doh-ura et al. (2004) administered PPS by direct brain infusion in mice infected with 263K, RML, and Fukuoka-1 in Tg7 or Tga20 mice. PPS showed the greatest efficacy compared with amphotericin B (minor effect) and quinacrine, chloroquine, and E-64d cysteine protease inhibitor which showed no effect. PPS also had effects on PrP^{Sc} deposition in the treated cerebral hemisphere.

Farquhar and colleagues (1999) administered IP and orally single doses of 250 μg or 1 mg PPS to six mouse strains 7 hours after IP inoculation with ME7 or 22A. Incubation time was increased by up to 66% for the ME7 strain IP treatment. Oral dosing had no therapeutic effect. Kocisko et al. (2006) administered combination treatment of PPS and Fe(III)meso-tetra(4-sulfonatophenyl)porphine in Tg7 mice inoculated intracerebrally (IC) with the 263K hamster scrapie strain. Drug (50 μL of 0.05 mM PPS) was given IC at weekly intervals, 2, 4, or 5 weeks after inoculation. Both individual drugs prolonged incubation time, but in combination the difference was greater than additive. Ladogana et al. (1992) administered PPS at 50–100 mg/kg in hamsters inoculated IC or IP with 263K, either shortly before or after infection. In single doses 50 and 100 mg/kg were equally effective.

The pharmacokinetics of PPS is unusual, in part because it is a pharmaceutical product with a range of medium-molecular-weight compounds, and in part because these tightly bind serum proteins and proteoglycans on cell surfaces and connective tissue. PPS pharmacology is strongly influenced by length of dosing and route of administration. Oral bioavailability of PPS is very low after a single dose (Faaij et al., 1999). Pentosan at 300 mg/day orally is usually well tolerated. Importantly, the large molecular weight of PPS means that it does not cross the blood–brain barrier.

The major clinical studies of PPS are Japanese and from the United Kingdom; both are open-label. In Japan 11 patients were treated with intraventricular PPS at Fukuoka University from 2004 (Tsuboi et al., 2009), including 3 with inherited prion disease, 2 with iatrogenic CJD, and 6 with sporadic CJD. The authors' conclusion was that clinical features did not improve, but that the possibility of survival benefit remains. The treatment involved the placement of a right lateral ventricle catheter connected to a subcutaneous pump. One week later, if there were no complications, PPS infusion was started at 1 μg/kg/day and escalated to 120 μg/kg/day. Patients were assessed weekly and then monthly, and all deteriorated in their function. PPS treatment was associated with subdural fluid collection, although this did not appear to influence the clinical condition.

In the United Kingdom, 7 patients (2 with inherited prion disease, 2 with iatrogenic CJD, 3 with variant CJD) were treated at different clinical centers but all were reviewed by Dr. Bone for the Medical Research Council (MRC) Clinical Trials Unit, who incorporated the findings of previous case studies in his report (Bone et al., 2008). Several immediate complications of ventricular catheter insertion were noted, including stroke, pyrexia, and brain hemorrhage. Dose was escalated through a range 11–110 μg/kg/day. In terms of safety, 1 patient had an episode of tonic-clonic seizures, associated with raised inflammatory markers and sepsis, but these did not recur when the drug was restarted. No clearly PPS-specific toxicity was observed. Four patients were studied prospectively: 1 remained stable, 2 deteriorated minimally, and 1 substantially, based on assessments of major functional and neurologic milestones. Survival appeared to be longer in treated patients, but several sources of bias were discussed in the report, including selection, "lead-time" bias from attentive carers, or increased supportive end-of-life care.

Additional data on variant CJD reported recently from the UK group showed that 4 out of 5 individuals treated with PPS survived longer than the maximum survival in 171 patients not treated with PPS (Newman et al., 2014). Neuropathologic examination of 1 of these individuals, who received PPS for 8 years and lived for 105 months, showed severe but typical changes of prion disease. Neuropathology reports from Japan confirmed the typical findings of prion disease, with the possibility of some alterations in gliosis and abnormal prion protein (Terada et al., 2010; Honda et al., 2012).

Flupirtine

Flupirtine is a centrally acting nonopioid analgesic which is well tolerated and reduces the toxicity of a PrP peptide fragment following co-incubation (Perovic et al., 1995). The drug was studied in a German randomized double-blind study of oral dosing of up to 300–400 mg flupirtine (Otto et al., 2004). The study was notable for its use of a cognitive endpoint (cognitive component of the Alzheimer's Disease Assessment Scale, ADAS-Cog), and also managed to recruit relatively mildly affected patients with sporadic CJD (median MMSE was 19 in the treated group, 21.5 in the placebo). The ADAS-Cog score was reported as change between baseline and best score, which was typically obtained at the second or third assessment (2–4 weeks of treatment). Maximum mean difference in ADAS-Cog between treated and placebo was 12.2 in the intention-to-treat group, with similar changes in the per-protocol group and if imputation was not used for missing data; a change of four points in the score was predetermined to be a meaningful benefit. No survival benefit was seen.

Antimicrobials

In the 1970s and 1980s a number of antimicrobial agents were tested in single patients with CJD, or small case series, without any evidence of a beneficial response. These include acyclovir, amantadine, vidarabine, amphotericin, and interferons. They are reviewed elsewhere (Trevitt and Collinge, 2006; Stewart et al., 2008).

Symptomatic treatments

Through the clinical course of CJD, patients may be treated with a wide range of therapies directed against specific symptoms, including many centrally acting drugs like antidepressants, antipsychotics, and anticonvulsants. There is no doubt that many of these treatments are highly effective despite no formal clinical studies in CJD; for example, the use of clonazepam or levetiracetam for myoclonus (Striano et al., 2005). However, the management of other symptoms like sleep disturbances, psychiatric symptoms, or muscle rigidity is less straightforward. Some studies have attempted to systematically record treatments of symptoms and responses in systematic observational studies (Thompson et al., 2014).

OUTCOME MEASURES

Primary outcome measures

Choice of a primary outcome measure for a clinical trial is crucially important but until recently has seen very little attention in CJD. Most trials have used survival time alone, the exceptions being the flupirtine trial which used ADAS-Cog, and the PRION-1 trial which had co-primary outcome measures of survival time and lack of deterioration based on multiple assessments (Otto et al., 2004; Collinge et al., 2009). Death is a clearly defined and unambiguous event, but is problematic as an endpoint in CJD. The terminal events in CJD are typically respiratory failure related to deepening coma, brainstem dysfunction, or pneumonia. Anecdotally, survival can be strongly influenced by supportive end-of-life care, such as the use of enteral feeding, antibiotic treatment of infections, and aggressive treatment of respiratory failure, including by ventilation, and physical therapies. Choice of such measures is usually taken jointly with carers / family members and may be strongly associated with the use of experimental treatments. More systematic evidence about end-of-life choices and their influences on survival would be helpful.

Following the PRION-1 trial, the study research team analyzed the rating scales used towards the development of a designed prion disease outcome measure (Mead et al., 2011; Thompson et al., 2013). The choices were also influenced by the experiences of Dr. Bone and colleagues (2008) in their review of UK PPS-treated patients. The resulting 20-point MRC Prion Disease Rating Scale (shortened to MRC Scale) was based on the Barthel Activities of Daily Living Index, with contributions from the Clinical Dementia Rating – Sum of Boxes and the Glasgow Coma Scale (Lechi et al., 1983; Tiraboschi and Tagliavini, 2013; Thompson et al., 2013). The authors argued that the scale had advantages in that it covers a wide range of function, from independent living with minimal disability to advanced coma. The focus on patient functions avoids the problem of patient heterogeneity, in that everyday functions integrate visual, language, and other cognitive and motor abilities. The MRC Scale is simple to administer by doctors and other healthcare professionals, including over the telephone by carer interview, and has a high interobserver agreement (Thompson et al., 2013). Most importantly, the MRC Scale records abilities that are highly meaningful to patients and carers based on questionnaire and open-ended discussions (Thompson et al., 2013). The MRC Scale remains untested in a clinical trial.

Secondary outcomes measures (rating and assessment scales)

These might include choices from existing rating scales in related diseases or bespoke scores that measure elements of the neurologic or psychologic examination. Rating scales with some experience in trials of CJD include, for cognitive domains: MMSE, ADAS-Cog; psychiatric domains: Brief Psychiatric Rating Scale; global or physician judgement scales: Glasgow Coma Scale, Clinical Dementia Rating Scale – Sum of Boxes, Clinical Interview-Based Impression of Change plus carer input (CIBIC-P-plus), and Rankin scale; and functional scales: the Barthel Activities of Daily Living index. Each has its advantages and disadvantages (Table 24.2). The most significant problem for rating scales is floor effects for all but the Glasgow Coma Scale. Patients with CJD will often deteriorate from a state of mild to moderate disability to a comatose state in a matter of a few weeks. As a consequence a baseline rating scale is measured, which is then missing at all follow-up study times, making a meaningful statistical analysis very difficult.

There is also some experience from trials or observational studies of quantifying elements of the neurologic and/or psychologic examination. For example, in the US quinacrine trial, Animal and Phoneme Fluency, Forward and Backward Digit Span, and Symbol Digit Modalities were tested, although missingness was high (Geschwind et al., 2013). In a longitudinal clinical and imaging study focusing on inherited prion disease, an Israeli study team developed a rating scale based on a systematic neurologic assessment (Cohen et al., 2011). The UK National Prion Monitoring Cohort has studied the use of a Short Cognitive Assessment battery (Caine et al., 2015), although to date only cross-sectional data have been published. More work to develop secondary outcome measures, particularly those that attempt to quantify neurologic and psychologic assessments, towards measures that could be statistically analyzed in trials, would be of value. As above, the desirable qualities are simple, rapid assessment scales that work over a wide range of severity, correlate with progression, with high interobserver agreement, and minimal influence of indirect disease-related factors like concentration and fatigue.

Secondary outcome measures (imaging, neurophysiology, biofluids)

Biomarkers have had a massive influence on the conduct of trials of other neurodegenerative diseases. Diagnostic

Table 24.2

Outcome measures used in clinical trials or observational studies

Measure	Domain	Range	Advantages	Disadvantages
Survival	Clinical milestone	Time to event	Unambiguous, comparative to virtually all other CJD clinical trials	Survival per se not main objective of treatment Influenced by end-of-life supportive measures
MRC Prion Disease Rating Scale	Composite scale, functionally oriented	0–20	Functional and therefore meaningful to patients and carers, quick to administer including over the telephone, includes speech and cognitive components Rasch-modeled in CJD	Prion-specific rating scale Rasch model does not fit well in inherited prion disease
Mini Mental State Examination	Cognitive scale	0–30	Cognitive, important impairment in prion diseases, widely adopted around the world	Doesn't assess motor or psychiatric impairments, floor effects, not directed to cognitive profile of CJD patients
ADAS-cog	Cognitive scale	0–70	Cognitive, important impairment in prion diseases, widely adopted around the world	Doesn't assess motor or psychiatric impairments, floor effects, not directed to cognitive profile of CJD patients
Barthel ADL Index	Functional scale	0–20	Functional endpoint, meaningful to patients and carers, quick to administer over the telephone	Doesn't include direct measures of language or other cognitive functions
Glasgow Coma Scale	Clinical assessment	3–15	Quick, very wide range of disability assessed	Ceiling effects, insensitive to change in early stages of disease
Individual cognitive scales, e.g., phonemic and animal fluency, digit span	Neuropsychologic assessment	Variable	Focused and quick to administer, may be chosen to represent the cognitive profile of CJD patients	Only captures particular cognitive domains, only useful as secondary outcome measures
Rankin	Clinician-rated global scale	0–5	Global scale, quick to administer	Granular, might not be sensitive to clinically meaningful changes
CDR-SB	Clinician-rated cognitive scale	0–18	Quick to administer, carer reporting acceptable, only minor floor effects	Pure cognitive assessment
CIBIC-P-Plus	Clinician-rated global scale (with carer input)	1–7	Quick, global assessment that works at all levels of disease severity	Subjective assessment tool, uncertain consistency
Brief Psychiatric Rating Scale	Neuropsychiatric assessment scale	24–168	Specific tool for psychiatric features	Too focused to be a primary outcome measure, only relevant to early stages, and quite time consuming
Milestone-based assessments	Clinical assessments	Variable	Highly meaningful to patients and carers	Granular assessment tool, ad hoc tool
The CJD Neurological Status Scale	Range of assessments from the neurologic exam	(0–52) and (0–8)	Incorporates evidence of severity based on a systematic neurologic exam	May be difficult to score in advanced patients

ADAS-cog, cognitive component of the Alzheimer's Disease Assessment Scale; ADL, Activities of Daily Living; CDR-SB, Clinical Dementia Rating Scale Sum of Boxes; CIBIC-P-Plus, Clinical Interview-based Impression of Change plus carer input; CJD, Creutzfeldt–Jakob disease.

biomarkers are crucial to establish the correct diagnosis of CJD and have been a component of inclusion criteria in all trials (Fig. 24.1). Prion disease is fortunate in this circumstance, as we now have a wealth of tools that in the vast majority of cases can establish a confident disease diagnosis even in the very early stages, based on clinical features, exclusion of alternative diagnoses, and specifically, striatal, thalamic, and cortical hyperintensity on diffusion weighted or fluid-attenuated inversion recovery MRI of the brain, periodic sharp-wave complexes on electroencephalogram (EEG), CSF analysis using 14-3-3 protein, tau protein, and the real-time quaking-induced conversion assay (RT-QuIC). Early diagnosis for trials remains a crucial problem (see below), but diagnosis is not delayed because of the lack of specific diagnostic tests in sporadic CJD. As diagnostic biomarkers have now been added to epidemiologic criteria, it seems sensible to retain probable or definite CJD as key trial inclusion criteria. These criteria could be supplemented by an expert panel in complex cases or where there are necessarily missing data.

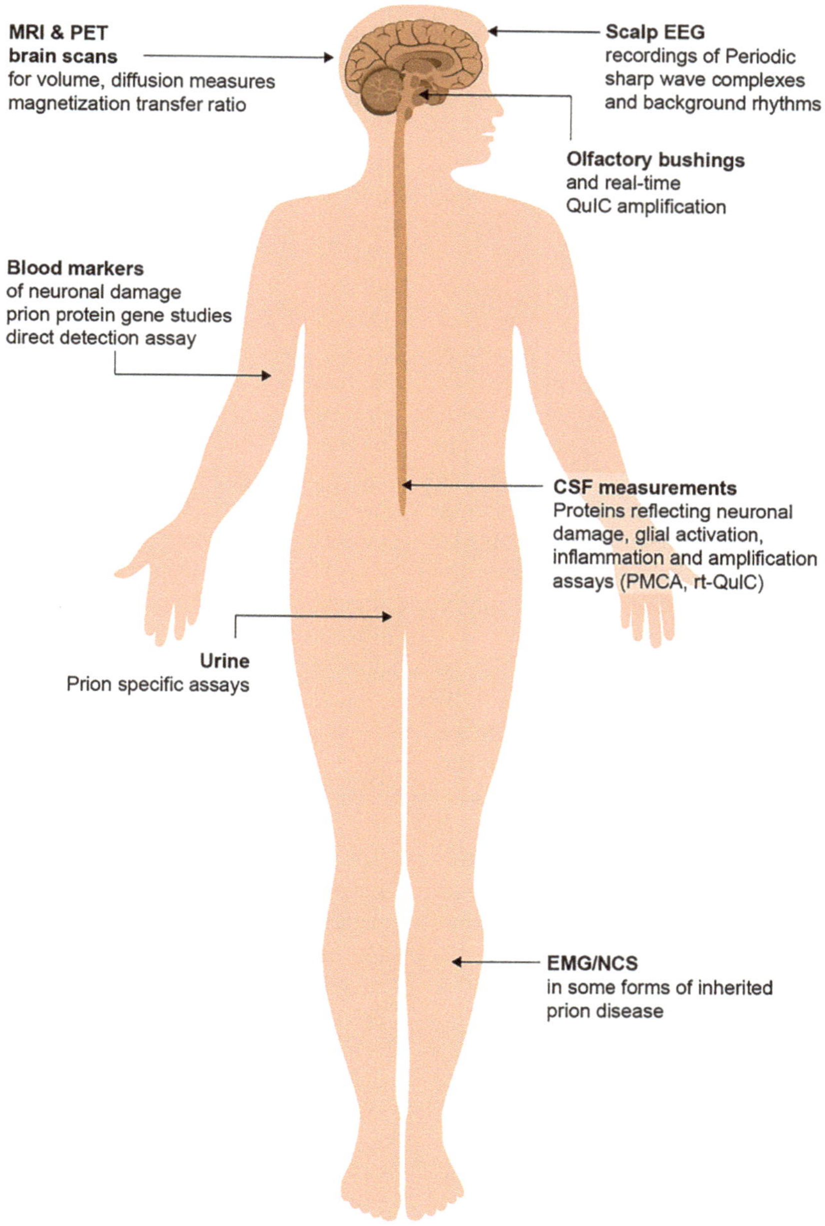

Fig. 24.1. Possible biomarkers in prion disease clinical trials. *CSF*, cerebrospinal fluid; *EEG*, electroencephalogram; *EMG*, electromyogram; *MRI*, magnetic resonance imaging; *NCS*, nerve conduction studies; *PET*, positron emission tomography; *PMC*; protein misfolding cyclic amplification; *rt-QuIC*, real-time quaking-induced conversion.

Biomarkers can serve many other purposes in trials, but such uses have been underemployed in prion diseases. Progression biomarkers show a strong correlation with disease severity and when studied longitudinally can provide confirmatory evidence that an intervention has altered the disease process. Such biomarkers measure downstream effects of an intervention. Examples might include imaged brain volume or hippocampal volume in Alzheimer disease (Scahill et al., 2002), caudate atrophy in Huntington disease (Novak et al., 2014), and atrophy of specific cortical brain regions in frontotemporal dementia (Rohrer et al., 2015). A small number of groups have attempted to develop imaging biomarkers in prion disease, with activity focused on MR parameters such as diffusion-based imaging, measurement of brain volume, and the magnetization transfer ratio (Siddique et al., 2010; Caverzasi et al., 2014; Cohen et al., 2015; Eisenmenger et al., 2016; De Vita et al., 2017; Grau-Rivera et al., 2017). No group has yet managed to get a high uptake of longitudinal imaging in a trial or observational study, and there is no suggestion that progression imaging biomarkers might have greater power than functional outcome measures. This is in marked contrast with more slowly progressive conditions, where functional outcome measures may require hundreds or thousands of participants in a trial for adequate power.

The release of neuronal, synaptic, or glial proteins into the cerebrospinal fluid or even (e.g. Neurofilament light, tau protein) might also reasonably provide an objective measure of ongoing disease activity downstream to the activity of a drug. Of course such measures are nonspecific to prion disease, but this is inconsequential, as diagnosis will already be established by entry criteria (Thompson et al., 2018).

Neurophysiologic methods may also have utility as progression biomarkers. The EEG recording in CJD changes dramatically through its clinical course, with a progressive loss of amplitude, slowing, and the appearance of periodic sharp-wave complexes in some patients. The synchronicity of the EEG recording can be used to measure the integrity of network function. EEG has some advantages in prion disease as it appears to be more acceptable to patients in advanced stages of disease when brain MRI may be difficult due to patient distress. One paper has looked at quantification of these changes in an observational study (Franko et al., 2016).

Ligand-positron emission tomography (PET) imaging has become very widely used in Alzheimer disease both as a diagnostic biomarker and as a marker of fibrillar Aβ, clearance of which is a key signal for an Aβ-targeting intervention. This kind of biomarker might be considered to be pharmacodynamic in that they are designed to look at the action of a drug in binding its target and having an effect on biologic processes. Unfortunately, in prion disease there is no specific ligand for abnormal forms of PrP, and in small studies, existing ligands do not seem to have good utility (Kepe et al., 2010; Hyare et al., 2012; Deters et al., 2016). As tau pathology is a strong pathologic feature in some forms of prion disease, tau ligand-PET might be explored as a biomarker in the future.

More promising as a pharmacodynamic biomarker would be to measure prions or prion seeding activity itself. We are now in a very fortunate position in prion disease that human in vitro assays of prion seeding are available, although specific development for clinical trial purposes would be welcome. Such assays involve elements of concentration of prions in a sample of biofluids and amplification through rounds of shaking (RT-QuIC) or sonication (protein misfolding cyclic amplification: PMCA) in an excess of biologically derived or recombinant prion protein. RT-QuIC has by far the greatest experience in the clinic, and works well in the cerebrospinal fluid and olfactory mucosa for sporadic CJD (Schmitz et al., 2016; Bongianni et al., 2017). On the other hand, PMCA enables PrP^{Sc} to be detected in peripheral tissues and body fluids such as urine and blood in variant CJD (Moda et al., 2014; Concha-Marambio et al., 2016). Some elements of cerebrospinal fluid RT-QuIC might be further developed, such as a linear quantification of the assay, and whether serial lumbar puncture would be acceptable to participants. For the purposes of translation of rodent therapeutics, it would be useful for cerebrospinal fluid RT-QuIC to be included in the preclinical development of interventions.

A key advance in prion disease clinical trials would be the greater use of biomarkers, particularly those which measure prion seeding activity and protein markers of downstream neuronal damage in biofluids.

TRIAL DESIGN

Sporadic CJD and other rapidly progressive prion diseases

The gold-standard trial design is a large randomized, placebo-controlled, double-blind study that recruits patients with CJD and only mild levels of disability. Our review of published studies reveals the challenges in achieving this trial design. Prion diseases are rare and are often diagnosed late in the clinical course. There are several reasons for this: early symptoms are nonspecific, and when a serious condition is apparent to patients and primary care, it progresses very rapidly. There are possibly some delays related to the recognition of imaging findings in secondary care (Carswell et al., 2012b). Consequently it is challenging to recruit large studies involving early, mildly affected patients. It is difficult to see major changes here, although education, trial publicity, systematic referral pathways, and automated imaging diagnostics may each have a role. Whether to include a disease severity criterion is an important issue, although it depends on the details of the intervention, trial procedures, and local practices about the referral of early CJD patients, which are likely to vary significantly around the world. It seems logical in most circumstances to exclude patients with very severe impairments, for example, a level of function equivalent to <5/20 on the MRC Scale, at which state patients would not be able to cooperate with cognitive or motor testing. There are several advantages of recruiting earlier affected patients: beyond an expectation of a better treatment response, patients themselves may be able to participate to a significant degree in the voluntary process of consenting for clinical study.

In several studies of repurposed drugs the trial design was challenged by the rejection of placebo as an option by participants who had alternative means to access the study drug. It should be envisaged that, in the future, the use of novel prion therapeutics would help the situation as there would only be access to the drug through the trial. Nevertheless, trial coordinators should involve patients and the public as much as possible in trial design and take into account their feelings. Reasonably, patients and their relatives may think that they have only one chance to access a treatment benefit, unlike trials of more slowly progressive conditions where sequential trial participation or posttrial compassionate phases are more realistic. In this respect, the delayed treatment option used in the US quinacrine trial was interesting (Geschwind et al., 2013).

In our opinion, the combination of a functional outcome measure (such as the MRC Scale) and survival has advantages. In simulations using natural history data from the National Prion Monitoring Cohort study, frequent measurement (several times weekly) over the telephone with the MRC Scale showed modest increases in power compared with survival alone, and is inherently a more meaningful outcome (Mead et al., 2016). These simulations used linear mixed modeling with age, gender, and codon 129 genotype as factors for baseline and decline.

In order to increase follow-up rates it seems logical to us to include an option for domiciliary visits, which necessitates use of a mobile study team. Opportunities for biomarker assessments, particularly cerebrospinal fluid, olfactory mucosa, urine, and blood sampling should be maximized.

There remains a role for small observational studies. As discussed above, these are vulnerable to bias in selection, but this can be corrected for in the statistical analysis as long as a reliable measure of baseline severity is recorded. The use of novel therapeutics will raise new questions in CJD trial design, as the "safety first" policy would normally necessitate a phase I study, often in healthy volunteers, to establish the human pharmacology, and initial safety and tolerability data. Depending on the predictable risks of the intervention, an open-label phase I study may be most appropriate, with pharmacologic and pharmacodynamic biomarkers. In a disease as rare as CJD it would be reasonable to expect that regulators might take the view that only a single, clearly successful large randomized placebo-controlled trial or well-conducted observational study with natural history comparison be required for approval.

Trial recruitment should also consider slowly progressive inherited prion diseases like those caused by the P102L mutation, or large octapeptide repeat insertions. The pool of symptomatic patients to recruit from at a point in time is surprisingly large compared with CJD, particularly at early stages of disease, because some inherited prion diseases can be more than 10 times less rapidly progressive than CJD (Mead, 2006). Unfortunately, the constraints on trial design are quite different for this group, making inclusion in the same study problematic. One consideration might be an open-label arm of a trial to study long-term safety in these patients running in parallel with a randomized design in CJD.

Adequately powered sample sizes are feasible in CJD either in a single large population country or by multicenter collaboration. Collaborative studies might more rapidly achieve recruitment targets, but have downsides of a less homogenous patient population and a greater need for study and outcome measure coordination. In order to decide on adequate power, a meaningful minimal effect size needs to be estimated. In simulation studies where slowing in rates of decline of the MRC Scale or survival time was the primary outcome, in order to achieve power to detect 50% slowing in decline, or equivalent benefits for survival, in a 1:1 randomized controlled trial, a sample of approximately 100 patients (50 per arm) was required. Smaller samples are required for similar power in observational studies compared to natural history data (~40 patients) (Mead et al., 2016).

Healthy individuals at risk of prion disease

A largely unconsidered trial design would be to recruit individuals at risk of prion disease because they carry highly penetrant gene mutations or have some high-risk iatrogenic exposures. One such trial, of individuals at risk of D178N/M129 inherited prion disease (i.e., fatal familial insomnia), is ongoing in Italy (Forloni et al., 2015). The obvious advantage of this trial design is the intervention prior to any neuronal damage, and the expectation of stronger treatment effects. A challenge of this trial design is low power because of the relatively low risk each year of an at-risk individual becoming symptomatic, although this question would benefit from rigorous statistical analysis. This type of trial would be particularly suitable for the use of biomarkers of disease activity, as discussed above. As yet, however, despite small reports of possibilities, there are no well-established biomarker abnormalities in the human presymptomatic phase. Again, this is an area that warrants further research development.

CONCLUSIONS AND FUTURE

Here we have reviewed some of the principles of clinical trials, the experiences in prion diseases and made some remarks about outcome measures and trial design. Relative to common neurodegenerative diseases, high-quality clinical trials have been challenging to organize and yet there are great opportunities. In prion disease we are clear about the pathogenic protein, and have laboratory methods that get close to directly measuring prion concentrations in biofluids. We study the actual neurodegenerative disease in rodent models, without resorting to the overexpression of multiple and mutant human proteins. However, as yet, despite decades of laboratory study and preclinical therapeutics, there has not been a single human study of an intervention designed specifically for prion disease. Those drugs which have entered trials have been safe drugs, repurposed from other uses, based on imperfect preclinical evidence of efficacy. Patient groups are calling for a treatment as a top priority and would welcome opportunities for more high-risk experimental therapeutic options directly derived from prion laboratory research.

A key priority moving forward is to test in humans compounds that show benefits in well-established rodent prion disease. Engagement of the pharmaceutical sector to support this costly activity would be welcome, of course, but in the context of high-profile multibillion-dollar trial failures in common neurodegenerative conditions a change in attitude cannot be expected. As an alternative, the continued interest of public sector funding and charitable sources is greatly welcome.

Avenues with potential promise from the commercial sector include the adaptation for prion disease of more generic technologies such as antisense oligonucleotide treatments, or alternatively the focus on downstream pathways that may have a role in multiple neurodegenerative diseases (Moreno et al., 2012; Radford et al., 2015). Further, the increasing parallels between prion and other neurodegenerative diseases, including the discovery and validation of PrP as a receptor for Aβ assemblies, might promote an increased focus on PrP as a therapeutic target (Lauren et al., 2009; Klyubin et al., 2014).

ACKNOWLEDGMENTS

Simon Mead is funded by the Medical Research Council (UK) and is a National Institute of Health Research Senior Investigator.

REFERENCES

Anderson VR, Perry CM (2006). Pentosan polysulfate – a review of its use in the relief of bladder pain or discomfort in interstitial cystitis. Drugs 66: 821–835.

Barret A, Tagliavini F, Forloni G et al. (2003). Evaluation of quinacrine treatment for prion diseases. J Virol 77: 8462–8469.

Bone I, Belton L, Walker AS et al. (2008). Intraventricular pentosan polysulphate in human prion disease: an observational study in the UK. Eur J Neurol 15: 458–464.

Bongianni M, Orrù C, Groveman BR et al. (2017). Diagnosis of human prion disease using real-time quaking-induced conversion testing of olfactory mucosa and cerebrospinal fluid samples. JAMA Neurol 74: 155–162.

Caine D, Tinelli RJ, Hyare H et al. (2015). The cognitive profile of prion disease: a prospective clinical and imaging study. Ann Clin Transl Neurol 2: 548–558.

Carswell C, Ranopa M, Pal S et al. (2012a). Video rating in neurodegenerative disease clinical trials: the experience of PRION-1. Dement Geriatr Cogn Dis Extra 2: 286–297.

Carswell C, Thompson A, Lukic A et al. (2012b). MRI findings are often missed in the diagnosis of Creutzfeldt–Jakob disease. BMC Neurol 12: 153.

Caverzasi E, Mandelli ML, DeArmond SJ et al. (2014). White matter involvement in sporadic Creutzfeldt–Jakob disease. Brain 137: 3339–3354.

Cohen OS, Prohovnik I, Korczyn AD et al. (2011). The Creutzfeldt–Jakob disease (CJD) neurological status scale: a new tool for evaluation of disease severity and progression. Acta Neurol Scand 124: 368–374.

Cohen OS, Chapman J, Korczyn AD et al. (2015). Familial Creutzfeldt–Jakob disease with the E200K mutation: longitudinal neuroimaging from asymptomatic to symptomatic CJD. J Neurol 262: 604–613.

Collinge J, Gorham M, Hudson F et al. (2009). Safety and efficacy of quinacrine in human prion disease (PRION-1 study): a patient-preference trial. Lancet Neurology 8: 334–344.

Collins SJ, Lewis V, Brazier M et al. (2002). Quinacrine does not prolong survival in a murine Creutzfeldt–Jakob disease model. Ann Neurol 52: 503–506.

Concha-Marambio L, Pritzkow S, Moda F et al. (2016). Detection of prions in blood from patients with variant Creutzfeldt–Jakob disease. Sci Transl Med 8: 370ra183.

De Luigi A, Colombo L, Diomede L et al. (2008). The efficacy of tetracyclines in peripheral and intracerebral prion infection. PLoS ONE 3: e1888.

Deters KD, Risacher SL, Yoder KK et al. (2016). [(11)C]PiB PET in Gerstmann-Sträussler-Scheinker disease. Am J Nucl Med Mol Imaging 6: 84–93.

De Vita E, Ridgway GR, White MJ et al. (2017). Neuroanatomical correlates of prion disease progression – a 3T longitudinal voxel-based morphometry study. Neuroimage Clin 13: 89–96.

Diringer H, Ehlers B (1991). Chemoprophylaxis of scrapie in mice. J Gen Virol 72: 457–460.

Doh-ura K, Iwaki T, Caughey B (2000). Lysosomotropic agents and cysteine protease inhibitors inhibit scrapie-associated prion protein accumulation. J Virol 74: 4894–4897.

Doh-ura K, Ishikawa K, Murakami-Kubo I et al. (2004). Treatment of transmissible spongiform encephalopathy by intraventricular drug infusion in animal models. J Virol 78: 4999–5006.

Eisenmenger L, Porter MC, Carswell CJ et al. (2016). Evolution of diffusion-weighted magnetic resonance imaging signal abnormality in sporadic Creutzfeldt–Jakob disease, with histopathological correlation. JAMA Neurol 73: 76–84.

Faaij RA, Srivastava N, van Griensven JMT et al. (1999). The oral bioavailability of pentosan polysulphate sodium in healthy volunteers. Eur J Clin Pharmacol 54: 929–935.

Farquhar C, Dickinson A, Bruce M (1999). Prophylactic potential of pentosan polysulphate in transmissible spongiform encephalopathies. Lancet 353: 117.

Forloni G, Iussich S, Awan T et al. (2002). Tetracyclines affect prion infectivity. Proc Natl Acad Sci U S A 99: 10849–10854.

Forloni G, Tettamanti M, Lucca U et al. (2015). Preventive study in subjects at risk of fatal familial insomnia: innovative approach to rare diseases. Prions 9: 75–79.

Franko E, Wehner T, Joly O et al. (2016). Quantitative EEG parameters correlate with the progression of human prion diseases. J Neurol Neurosurg Psychiatry 87: 1061–1067.

Gayrard V, Picard-Hagen N, Viguie C et al. (2005). A possible pharmacological explanation for quinacrine failure to treat prion diseases: pharmacokinetic investigations in an ovine model of scrapie. Br J Pharmacol 144: 386–393.

Geschwind MD, Kuo AL, Wong KS et al. (2013). Quinacrine treatment trial for sporadic Creutzfeldt–Jakob disease. Neurology 81: 2015–2023.

Ghaemmaghami S, Ahn M, Lessard P et al. (2009). Continuous quinacrine treatment results in the formation of drug-resistant prions. PLoS Pathog 5: e1000673.

Grau-Rivera O, Calvo A, Bargallo N et al. (2017). Quantitative magnetic resonance abnormalities in Creutzfeldt–Jakob disease and fatal insomnia. J Alzheimers Dis 55: 431–443.

Haïk S, Brandel JP, Salomon D et al. (2004). Compassionate use of quinacrine in Creutzfeldt–Jakob disease fails to show significant effects. Neurology 63: 2413–2415.

Haïk S, Marcon G, Mallet A et al. (2014). Doxycycline in Creutzfeldt–Jakob disease: a phase 2, randomised, double-blind, placebo-controlled trial. Lancet Neurol 13: 150–158.

Honda H, Sasaki K, Minaki H et al. (2012). Protease-resistant PrP and PrP oligomers in the brain in human prion diseases after intraventricular pentosan polysulfate infusion. Neuropathology 32: 124–132.

Hyare H, Ramlackhansingh A, Gelosa G et al. (2012). C-11-PiB PET does not detect PrP-amyloid in prion disease patients including variant Creutzfeldt–Jakob disease. J Neurol Neurosurg Psychiatry 83: 340–341.

Kepe V, Ghetti B, Farlow MR et al. (2010). PET of brain prion protein amyloid in Gerstmann-Straussler-Scheinker disease. Brain Pathol 20: 419–430.

Klug GM, Wand H, Simpson M et al. (2013). Intensity of human prion disease surveillance predicts observed disease incidence. J Neurol Neurosurg Psychiatry 84: 1372–1377.

Klyubin I, Nicoll AJ, Khalili-Shirazi A et al. (2014). Peripheral administration of a humanized Anti-PrP antibody blocks Alzheimer's disease Abeta synaptotoxicity. J Neurosci 34: 6140–6145.

Kocisko DA, Caughey B, Morrey JD et al. (2006). Enhanced antiscrapie effect using combination drug treatment. Antimicrob Agents Chemother 50: 3447–3449.

Korth C, May BC, Cohen FE et al. (2001). Acridine and phenothiazine derivatives as pharmacotherapeutics for prion disease. Proc Natl Acad Sci U S A 98: 9836–9841.

Ladogana A, Casaccia P, Ingrosso L et al. (1992). Sulphate polyanions prolong the incubation period of scrapie-infected hamsters. J Gen Virol 73: 661–665.

Lauren J, Gimbel DA, Nygaard HB et al. (2009). Cellular prion protein mediates impairment of synaptic plasticity by amyloid-beta oligomers. Nature 457: 1128–1132.

Lechi A, Tedeschi F, Mancia D (1983). Creutzfeld-Jakob disease: clinical, EEG and neuropathological findings in a cluster of eleven patients. Ital J Neurol Sci 4: 47–59.

Lind J (1753). A treatise on the scurvy. Pamphlet.

Mead S (2006). Prion disease genetics. Eur J Hum Genet 14: 273–281.

Mead S, Ranopa M, Gopalakrishnan GS et al. (2011). PRION-1 scales analysis supports use of functional outcome measures in prion disease. Neurology 77: 1674–1683.

Mead S, Burnell M, Lowe J et al. (2016). Clinical trial simulations based on genetic stratification and the natural history of a functional outcome measure in Creutzfeldt–Jakob disease. JAMA Neurol 73: 447–455.

Moda F, Gambetti P, Notari S et al. (2014). Prions in the urine of patients with variant Creutzfeldt–Jakob disease. N Engl J Med 371: 530–539.

Moreno JA, Radford H, Peretti D et al. (2012). Sustained translational repression by eIF2 alpha-P mediates prion neurodegeneration. Nature 485: 507–511.

Newman PK, Todd NV, Scoones D et al. (2014). Postmortem findings in a case of variant Creutzfeldt–Jakob disease treated with intraventricular pentosan polysulfate. J Neurol Neurosurg Psychiatry 85: 921–924.

Novak MJ, Seunarine KK, Gibbard CR et al. (2014). White matter integrity in premanifest and early Huntington's disease is related to caudate loss and disease progression. Cortex 52: 98–112.

Otto M, Cepek L, Ratzka P et al. (2004). Efficacy of flupirtine on cognitive function in patients with CJD: a double-blind study. Neurology 62: 714–718.

Perovic S, Pergande G, Ushijima H et al. (1995). Flupirtine partially prevents neuronal injury induced by prion protein fragment and lead acetate. Neurodegeneration 4: 369–374.

Pocchiari M, Puopolo M, Croes EA et al. (2004). Predictors of survival in sporadic Creutzfeldt–Jakob disease and other human transmissible spongiform encephalopathies. Brain 127: 2348–2359.

Radford H, Moreno JA, Verity N et al. (2015). PERK inhibition prevents tau-mediated neurodegeneration in a mouse model of frontotemporal dementia. Acta Neuropathol 130: 633–642.

Rickham PP (1964). Human experimentation. Code of ethics of the World Medical Association. Declaration of Helsinki. Br Med J 2: 177.

Rohrer JD, Nicholas JM, Cash DM et al. (2015). Presymptomatic cognitive and neuroanatomical changes in genetic frontotemporal dementia in the Genetic Frontotemporal dementia Initiative (GENFI) study: a cross-sectional analysis. Lancet Neurol 14: 253–262.

Scahill RI, Schott JM, Stevens JM et al. (2002). Mapping the evolution of regional atrophy in Alzheimer's disease: unbiased analysis of fluid-registered serial MRI. Proc Natl Acad Sci U S A 99: 4703–4707.

Schmitz M, Cramm M, Llorens F et al. (2016). The real-time quaking-induced conversion assay for detection of human prion disease and study of other protein misfolding diseases. Nat Protoc 11: 2233–2242.

Siddique D, Hyare H, Wroe S et al. (2010). Magnetization transfer ratio may be a surrogate of spongiform change in human prion diseases. Brain 133: 3058–3068.

Stewart LA, Rydzewska LH, Keogh GF et al. (2008). Systematic review of therapeutic interventions in human prion disease. Neurology 70: 1272–1281.

Striano P, Manganelli F, Boccella P et al. (2005). Levetiracetam in patients with cortical myoclonus: a clinical and electrophysiological study. Mov Disord 20: 1610–1614.

Tagliavini F, McArthur RA, Canciani B et al. (1997). Effectiveness of anthracycline against experimental prion disease in Syrian hamsters. Science 276: 1119–1122.

Tagliavini F, Forloni G, Colombo L et al. (2000). Tetracycline affects abnormal properties of synthetic PrP peptides and PrP(Sc) in vitro. J Mol Biol 300: 1309–1322.

Terada T, Tsuboi Y, Obi T, Doh-ura K et al. (2010). Less protease-resistant PrP in a patient with sporadic CJD treated with intraventricular pentosan polysulphate. Acta Neurol Scand 121: 127–130.

Thompson AG, Lowe J, Fox Z et al. (2013). The Medical Research Council Prion Disease Rating Scale: a new outcome measure for prion disease therapeutic trials developed and validated using systematic observational studies. Brain 136: 1116–1127.

Thompson A, Mackay A, Rudge P et al. (2014). Behavioral and psychiatric symptoms in prion disease. Am J Psychiatry 171: 265–274.

Thompson AGB, Luk C, Heslegrave AJ et al. (2018). Neurofilament light chain and tau concentrations are markedly increased in the serum of patients with sporadic Creutzfeldt-Jakob disease, and tau correlates with rate of disease progression. J Neurol Neurosurg Psychiatry. https://doi.org/10.1136/jnnp-2017-317793. pii: jnnp-2017-317793.

Tiraboschi P, Tagliavini F (2013). Prion disease: a promising rating scale for prion disease clinical research. Nat Rev Neurol 9: 366–367.

Trevitt CR, Collinge J (2006). A systematic review of prion therapeutics in experimental models. Brain 129: 2241–2265.

Tsuboi Y, Doh-ura K, Yamada T (2009). Continuous intraventricular infusion of pentosan polysulfate: clinical trial against prion diseases. Neuropathology 29: 632–636.

Varges D, Manthey H, Heinemann U et al. (2017). Doxycycline in early CJD: a double-blinded randomized phase II and observational study. J Neurol Neurosurg Psychiatry 88: 119–125.

Section VI

Public health issues

Handbook of Clinical Neurology, Vol. 153 (3rd series)
Human Prion Diseases
M. Pocchiari and J. Manson, Editors
https://doi.org/10.1016/B978-0-444-63945-5.00025-8

Chapter 25

The zoonotic potential of animal prion diseases

FIONA HOUSTON[1]* AND OLIVIER ANDRÉOLETTI[2]
[1]*Neurobiology Division, The Roslin Institute, Royal (Dick) School of Veterinary Studies, University of Edinburgh, Easter Bush, United Kingdom*
[2]*École Nationale Vétérinaire de Toulouse, Toulouse, France*

Abstract

Bovine spongiform encephalopathy (BSE) is the only animal prion disease that has been demonstrated to be zoonotic, causing variant Creutzfeldt–Jakob disease (vCJD) in humans. The link between BSE and vCJD was established by careful surveillance, epidemiologic investigations, and experimental studies using in vivo and in vitro models of cross-species transmission. Similar approaches have been used to assess the zoonotic potential of other animal prion diseases, including atypical forms identified through active surveillance. There is no epidemiologic evidence that classical or atypical scrapie, atypical forms of BSE, or chronic wasting disease (CWD) is associated with human prion disease, but the limitations of the epidemiologic data should be taken into account when interpreting these results. Transmission experiments in nonhuman primates and human PrP transgenic mice suggest that classic scrapie, L-type atypical BSE (L-BSE), and CWD may have zoonotic potential, which for L-BSE appears to be equal to or greater than that of classic BSE. The results of in vitro conversion assays to analyze the human transmission barrier correlate well with the in vivo data. However, it is still difficult to predict the likelihood that an animal prion disease will transmit to humans under conditions of field exposure from the results of in vivo or in vitro experiments. This emphasizes the importance of continuing systematic surveillance for both human and animal prion diseases in identifying zoonotic transmission of diseases other than classic BSE.

INTRODUCTION

Transmissible spongiform encephalopathies (TSEs) or prion diseases of animals include scrapie in sheep, chronic wasting disease (CWD) in cervids, bovine spongiform encephalopathy (BSE), and transmissible mink encephalopathy (TME), all of which are acquired through transmission of an infectious agent (prion). In humans, sporadic and genetic forms of TSE occur in addition to acquired diseases, the most common of which is sporadic Creutzfeldt–Jakob disease (sCJD). Concerns and speculation about cross-species transmission of TSEs, and particularly transmission of animal TSEs to humans, have existed since the infectious nature of these diseases was demonstrated, but there was no evidence of zoonotic transmission until the link between BSE and a novel human TSE (variant CJD or vCJD) was established in the late 1990s.

The evidence for transmission of BSE from cattle to humans came from a variety of sources, combining careful surveillance and epidemiologic studies with detailed experimental investigations, often involving the development of new techniques and animal models. The demonstration of zoonotic transmission of BSE also renewed concerns about risks to public health from other TSEs, leading to enhanced surveillance and efforts to control scrapie and CWD. In addition, the potential for human transmission of animal TSEs has been assessed experimentally using the same tools and models that were employed for BSE. In this chapter, we review the epidemiologic and in vivo and in vitro approaches used to

*Correspondence to: Fiona Houston, BSc, BVMS, PhD, Neurobiology Division, The Roslin Institute, R(D)SVS, University of Edinburgh, Easter Bush Campus, Edinburgh EH25 9RG, United Kingdom. Tel: +44-131-651-9100, E-mail: fiona.houston@roslin.ed.ac.uk

investigate the zoonotic potential of animal TSEs, along with their relative advantages and limitations, and assess the resulting evidence for associations between human TSEs and classic BSE, atypical BSE, classic scrapie, atypical scrapie, and CWD.

EPIDEMIOLOGIC ASSOCIATIONS BETWEEN HUMAN AND ANIMAL TSES

Comparative epidemiology

The comparison of the temporal and geographic distribution between TSE cases in humans and animals intuitively appears as a straightforward approach to identify a causative link between animal and human prion disease. In the United Kingdom, the development of a large BSE epidemic in the cattle population followed by the emergence of a new prion disease in humans (vCJD) facilitated identification of the zoonotic capacity of the BSE agent (Will et al., 1996). However, this success in the case of BSE should not lead to an underestimation of the limits of epidemiologic approaches for identifying a potential causative link between other animal and human prion diseases.

In humans, detection of cases of TSE disease relies exclusively on passive surveillance (clinical suspicion followed by postmortem confirmation). The true sensitivity of this monitoring system remains difficult to evaluate. Most countries only report anecdotally TSE in humans and assessing the epidemiologic situation in these geographic areas is impossible. Moreover, even in countries with specific and reliable TSE monitoring systems, the incidence of sCJD (the most common form of human TSE) ranges between 1 and 1.5 case per million population per year (Ladogana et al., 2005). Even when gathering data collected over decades, the relative rarity of cases limits the power of epidemiologic analysis (Barash, 2008).

In animals, the quality of historical epidemiologic data related to TSEs is very uncertain. The implementation in the early 2000s of active epidemiologic surveillance programs in the EU and North America demonstrated significant biases in our previous perception of the TSE prevalence in farmed animals (disease incidence and geographic distribution). Active surveillance also revealed the existence of atypical TSEs (atypical scrapie in small ruminants and BSE-H and BSE-L in cattle) that were totally unknown until this time (Biacabe et al., 2004; Benestad et al., 2008).

Whereas the strongest argument used to rule out the hypothesis of a link between the occurrence of certain TSE cases in human and animal TSEs was the presence of human prion disease in countries considered to be free of animal TSEs (like New Zealand and Australia), the discovery of atypical scrapie in these countries has invalidated this argument (Kittelberger et al., 2010; Cook et al., 2016).

In geographic areas where active surveillance programs were properly implemented (mainly within EU member states), the system certainly provides a reliable picture of the TSE epidemiologic situation in farmed livestock. However, these data still remain insufficient for assessing the existence of a link between animal TSEs and occurrence of human prion disease. Indeed, the potential incubation period of TSEs in humans (exceeding several decades) contrasts with the relatively short period (about a decade) over which the active surveillance programs have been established. This makes it very difficult to perform epidemiologic tracing for individual human TSE cases to identify potential sources of infection, when exposure is likely to have occurred many years in the past. In addition, the increase in international travel and trade (including food) implies that exposure to TSE agents in a particular country or geographic area cannot be solely inferred from the domestic prevalence of the disease.

CJD risk factors and etiology

Genetic forms of CJD are thought to be the consequence of spontaneous misfolding of normal prion protein (PrP) fostered by mutations in the PrP gene (Prusiner, 2001). Following the formation of an initial abnormal PrP nucleus, the prion propagates in the tissues of affected individuals who will develop the disease. In transgenic animals, the expression of mutated forms of PrP was reported to result in the occurrence of spontaneous prion disease (Jackson et al., 2009; Sigurdson et al., 2009). Although the final demonstration that an authentic prion (transmissible agent) can be spontaneously generated using a human PrP sequence is still lacking, these data considerably reinforced the plausibility of the concept.

sCJD is a relatively rare disease, occurring mainly in elderly people with an apparent random time and space distribution. Because these characteristics are inconsistent with a naturally transmitted infectious agent, it has been proposed that, as in familial CJD, the disease could be the consequence of a spontaneous nucleation of misfolded PrP. This phenomenon would be promoted by aging (somatic mutation or decrease in the efficacy of protein catabolism systems). While the idea of a spontaneous origin of sCJD cases is commonly accepted, this hypothesis is clearly not consistent with the well-established decline of sCJD incidence observed in people aged over 65 years. Moreover, several geographic clusters of sCJD cases have been identified, raising the possibility of an environmental origin of the disease (Arakawa et al., 1991; D'Aignaux et al., 2002; Linsell et al., 2004).

The search for a potential external cause (other than spontaneous disease occurrence) of human prion disease has been the subject of many epidemiologic studies. Among the potential risk factors for human TSE occurrence, exposure to animals and animal products was naturally considered. The seminal studies in the area were descriptive and based on the aggregation of historic data (Masters et al., 1979; Chatelain et al., 1981), while more recent investigations have relied on case–control studies. The most significant of them included several hundreds of sCJD cases identified in Europe ($n = 405$ affected patients) or the United States ($n = 663$ CJD patients) (van Duijn et al., 1998; Cocco et al., 2003). Several of these studies identified weak associations between sCJD occurrence and a number of risk factors like consumption of raw meat (odds ratio (OR): 1.63; 95% confidence interval (CI): 1.18–2.23), brain (OR: 1.68: 1.18–2.39), or exposure to fertilizers of animal origin (OR: 2.32; 95% CI: 1.38–2.91). However, the identified risk factors differed between the studies, and this lack of consistency supports the view that none of the investigated environmental factors is likely to explain the occurrence of sCJD in humans.

In conclusion, epidemiologic investigations carried out so far have failed to demonstrate any consistent correlation between sCJD occurrence in humans and exposure to environmental factors (including animals and animal-derived products). However, these epidemiologic studies cannot be regarded as definitive, and it remains a possibility that a proportion of sCJD cases result from an exposure to a particular animal prion disease.

THE HUMAN SPECIES BARRIER AND ITS MODELING

There are significant limitations to the sensitivity of epidemiologic investigations in establishing causal relationships between human and animal TSEs, not least because of the very variable extent of surveillance in animal and human populations worldwide. As a result, a variety of experimental approaches have been employed to assess the ability of animal TSEs to infect and cause disease in humans. It has long been recognized that attempts to transmit TSE agents from one species to another are limited by a "species barrier." Although some species appear totally refractory to infection, this often manifests as low/inconsistent attack rates and prolonged incubation periods or subclinical infection when the TSE agent is first injected into a new host species (primary transmission). However, upon continued subpassage and adaptation to the new host, attack rates increase and incubation periods become shorter, eventually becoming very predictable for a specific host with a defined dose and route of infection. The distribution of neuropathologic lesions (lesion profile) and disease-associated PrP (PrP^{TSE}) in the brain is also maintained on continued subpassage in the new host. The distinctive phenotypic characteristics (incubation period, clinical signs, lesion profile) that emerge following serial passage in a new host (often inbred laboratory mouse lines) have traditionally been the "gold standard" method for defining TSE strains (Bruce, 1993).

The potential for cross-species transmission of TSEs depends on a number of factors, including:

1. The host *PRNP* gene and PrP sequence: *PRNP* variation leading to minor changes in PrP amino acid sequence is known to have a major impact on susceptibility to TSE diseases in animals (Barron et al., 2001; Goldmann, 2008) and humans. In humans, variation at *PRNP* codon 129, leading to substitution of valine (V) for methionine (M), has the most significant impact on disease susceptibility, and appears to influence the clinical and pathologic phenotypes of TSE diseases (Palmer et al., 1991; Windl et al., 1996). The ability of a TSE agent to transmit to a new host is also related, in part, to differences in the primary sequence of PrP in donor and host species. Convincing evidence of this was first provided by experiments showing that transgenic mice expressing hamster PrP^{C} were susceptible to hamster-adapted scrapie, while wild-type mice were resistant (Scott et al., 1989). However, it is not possible to predict the potential for cross-species transmission through PrP sequence analysis alone.
2. TSE strain: different TSE strains show distinct differences in their abilities to infect different hosts. BSE appears to be unusual in having been naturally transmitted to diverse species, including goats, exotic ruminants, cats, and humans (Bruce et al., 1997), but most TSE strains appear to have a more restricted host range. For example, sCJD can readily be transmitted to bank voles but not to inbred wild-type mice (Nonno et al., 2006), while the reverse is true for vCJD (Bruce et al., 1997; Beringue et al., 2008c). The basis of strain selectivity for different hosts is not clear, but there is evidence that it is associated with the conformation of PrP^{TSE} molecules (Collinge and Clarke, 2007).
3. Route of infection and dose: experimental studies of cross-species transmission often use intracerebral (i.c.) injection of high-titer TSE inocula, which is the most efficient route of transmission (Kimberlin and Walker, 1988). However, natural TSE infections are thought to occur following peripheral exposure to low doses of infection, usually by the oral route (which is less efficient) (Hadlow et al., 1982).

It can therefore be difficult to predict the transmission risk under conditions of natural exposure on the basis of experimental transmission by i.c. injection.

4. Replication in lymphoid tissues: most experiments addressing cross-species transmission have focused on demonstration of infection and pathology in the brain and central nervous system, despite the fact that replication in lymphoid tissues is an important aspect of pathogenesis for many TSE strains. In a study in which transgenic mice expressing ovine or human PrP were inoculated with a range of TSEs from other hosts, including BSE and CWD, a much higher proportion of mice showed evidence of infection in spleen than in brain (Beringue et al., 2012). It is not clear how permissiveness of host lymphoid tissues to TSE replication contributes to cross-species transmission and adaptation, but this result does raise concerns over whether it is likely to result in silent carriers of infection.

A variety of in vivo and in vitro experimental models have been used to assess the zoonotic potential of animal TSEs, including nonhuman primates, inbred mouse lines and transgenic mice expressing human PrP, and cell-free molecular conversion systems.

In vivo models

Nonhuman primates

Nonhuman primates are considered as the most relevant animal model for assessing the risks of animal TSEs to human health. This follows from early experiments demonstrating that human TSEs, including kuru and sCJD, could be transmitted to nonhuman primates, producing diseases that were clinically and pathologically similar to the corresponding natural human diseases (Brown et al., 1994). In contrast, attempts to experimentally transmit human TSEs to many conventional laboratory species (mainly rodents) were largely unsuccessful (Gibbs and Gajdusek, 1973).

Chimpanzees (*Pan troglodytes*) are the species most closely related to humans, but their use in research is now very restricted. Old World monkeys, including rhesus and cynomolgus macaques, are also evolutionarily closely related to humans, and have been important species for TSE research. New World monkeys (e.g., squirrel monkeys) and prosimians (e.g., mouse lemurs) are less expensive and easier to work with, but are less closely related to humans. The degree of relatedness to humans may influence the interpretation of zoonotic risk following experimental transmission of animal TSEs to nonhuman primates.

The major drawbacks of using these species in TSE research are the ethical issues surrounding all experimental work involving nonhuman primates, as well as the long incubation periods following infection, and the expense of housing the animals in specialist containment facilities over protracted periods of time. However, the longevity of nonhuman primates can also allow detection of TSEs with longer incubation periods, in contrast to mice.

Transgenic mouse models

The demonstration that the species barrier preventing transmission of hamster scrapie to mice could be removed by expression of hamster PrP^C in transgenic mice (Scott et al., 1989) led to the development of many other transgenic mouse lines expressing PrP^C from different host species, including human, sheep, cattle, and cervid (Telling et al., 1995; Scott et al., 1997; Vilotte et al., 2001; Browning et al., 2004). Most of these lines were derived by standard transgenic techniques (microinjection of fertilized oocysts) in PrP null (PrP–/–) mice (to avoid interference from endogenous mouse PrP^C), and express variable levels of PrP^C depending on the number of copies of the transgene inserted into the host genome. There is usually an inverse relationship between the incubation period following TSE infection and the level of transgene expression in the brain. An alternative approach is used to produce gene-targeted transgenic mouse lines – in this technique, the transgene is injected into embryonic stem cells and replaces the host PrP^C sequence by homologous recombination, ensuring that the transgene is expressed under the same regulatory elements as the wild-type gene, and that PrP^C expression is at physiologic levels (Moore et al., 1998). Both overexpressing and gene-targeted transgenic mouse lines have been produced that express 129M and 129V human PrP^C variants (referred to as "humanized" transgenic models) (Telling et al., 1995; Asante et al., 2002; Kong et al., 2005; Bishop et al., 2006; Beringue et al., 2008b).

To assess the potential for an animal TSE to transmit to humans, groups of humanized transgenic mice and the parent wild-type mouse strain are experimentally infected with the TSE in question, usually by i.c. injection of infectious brain homogenate. Further groups of mice may be inoculated with defined human TSE isolates for comparison. The transmission barrier is assessed by comparing the attack rates (percentage of animals becoming infected and/or developing disease) and the incubation periods on primary transmission and subpassage in the same mouse lines. A high attack rate on primary transmission, accompanied by lack of significant shortening of the incubation period on continued subpassage, would be taken as evidence of a low transmission barrier, and therefore a significant risk of infection to humans. The distribution of neuropathologic lesions (lesion profile) and PrP^{TSE} in defined brain regions, as determined by histopathology, immunohistochemistry, and/or paraffin-embedded tissue blots, is also compared to that found following infection with human TSEs in the same mouse lines. Similarities in the disease phenotype (lesion profile, incubation time) of human and animal TSEs after propagation in the same animal model may indicate the involvement of a potentially common TSE agent.

In vitro models

Cell-free conversion assay (CFCA)

Although the nature of TSE infectious agents is still not precisely defined, it is generally accepted that it is mainly composed of a misfolded form (PrP^{TSE}) of a host encoded protein (PrP^{C}). PrP^{TSE} is distinguished from PrP^{C} on the basis of its altered biochemical properties (e.g., detergent insolubility, protease resistance). Within the host, TSE agents are thought to replicate by binding and conversion of normal PrP^{C} to the disease-associated conformation in a process of seeded nucleation and polymerization. This process can be replicated in vitro using cell-free systems in which PrP^{C} incubated with pre-existing PrP^{TSE} is converted to a protease-resistant form.

The CFCA was initially developed by Caughey and co-workers (Kocisko et al., 1994), and has been modified in other laboratories, but the basic principles remain the same. Radiolabeled PrP^{C} (termed "substrate") is expressed in mammalian cells or bacteria and purified, while PrP^{TSE} (termed "seed") is purified from infected tissues (usually brain). These highly purified components are mixed and incubated together, and the extent of conversion of PrP^{C} is estimated by measuring the amount of radiolabeled protease-resistant PrP following incubation. The method was used to examine cross-species transmission of scrapie in mice and hamsters, demonstrating that homologous reactions (e.g., hamster PrP^{C} seeded with hamster PrP^{TSE}) resulted in conversion of PrP^{C} to PrP^{TSE}, while nonhomologous reactions (e.g., mouse PrP^{C} with hamster PrP^{TSE}) were much less efficient, with low to negligible conversion of PrP^{C} (Kocisko et al., 1995). This critical experiment established the principle that in vitro techniques such as CFCA could produce results that correlate well with in vivo transmission experiments in transgenic mice (see above). Subsequently, the CFCA was used to assess the potential transmissibility of BSE, scrapie, and CWD to humans and other species, with results that were largely in agreement with available in vivo transmission data (Raymond et al., 1997).

The utility of the CFCA is limited by the low efficiency of the conversion reaction in vitro, requiring a large excess of input PrP^{TSE} as seed. For this reason, it has been largely superseded by in vitro techniques for cell-free amplification of PrP^{TSE}, such as protein misfolding cyclic amplification (PMCA) or quaking-induced conversion (QuIC).

Protein misfolding cyclic amplification

PMCA is based on the CFCA, and was developed to more closely mimic the replication of TSE agents in vitro (Saborio et al., 2001). Very small amounts of PrP^{TSE} are incubated in a large excess of PrP^{C} (usually provided by an uninfected brain homogenate or cell lysate), which induces conversion of a small proportion of PrP^{C} to PrP^{TSE}. The mixture is then sonicated, which breaks up aggregates of PrP^{TSE} into smaller fragments, thus increasing the number of potential sites (seeds) for subsequent binding and conversion of PrP^{C}. Alternating cycles of incubation and sonication can be applied until PrP^{TSE} has been amplified to a level at which it can be detected by conventional Western blot or enzyme-linked immunosorbent assay. The sensitivity of PMCA for PrP^{TSE} detection can be further increased by performing serial rounds of cyclic amplification, whilst replenishing the PrP^{C} substrate between each round. The newly generated PrP^{TSE} is infectious in vivo, and strain-specific properties of the PrP^{TSE} used to seed the reactions are conserved during in vitro amplification.

Amongst many other applications in TSE research, PMCA has been used to study transmission barriers. Castilla and colleagues (2008) showed that PMCA amplification of mouse PrP^{TSE} in hamster PrP^{C} substrate generated prions that were infectious for hamsters, and vice versa (for amplification of hamster PrP^{TSE} in mouse PrP^{C}), a process that mimics the adaptation occurring in vivo when a TSE agent or strain is subpassaged in a new host species. A number of studies from different laboratories have also used PMCA to assess and compare the zoonotic potential of animal prions, including BSE, scrapie, atypical TSEs, and CWD (Jones et al., 2009b; Kurt et al., 2009; Barria et al., 2011, 2014a). In addition, PMCA has been used to evaluate the effect of passage in intermediate hosts, as it can mimic the phenomenon of a TSE agent that will transmit between two species only after intermediate passage in a third species (Jones et al., 2009b; Krejciova et al., 2014).

The advantages of the PMCA technique are that it is rapid and inexpensive, producing results within days or weeks that would normally take months or years using in vivo transmission experiments. However, as yet it is not possible to correlate the ease of heterologous PrP^{C} conversion in vitro with the likelihood of transmission of TSEs between species in vivo.

Quaking-induced conversion

QuIC is a simplified version of PMCA in which recombinant PrP^{C} substrate (usually expressed in a bacterial expression system) is incubated with PrP^{TSE} in the absence of other cellular components, and subjected to periodic shaking rather than cycles of sonication and incubation (Atarashi et al., 2007). The conversion and fibrillization of PrP^{C} are followed in real time by the incorporation of thioflavin T, which emits a fluorescent signal when bound to PrP^{TSE} fibrils. The original QuIC assay used truncated recombinant hamster PrP (amino acids 90–231) as substrate, and demonstrated amplification of PrP^{TSE} from hamster, sheep, humans, and mice. This apparent lack of species specificity has limited the usefulness of QuIC in mechanistic assessment of species barriers. However, less promiscuous versions of the technique have been applied by a few groups to analyze the human species barrier to animal TSEs (Luers et al., 2013; Davenport et al., 2015).

ASSESSMENT OF THE EVIDENCE FOR AN ASSOCIATION BETWEEN ANIMAL AND HUMAN TSE DISEASES

Cattle TSE diseases

Classical BSE is the only animal TSE that has been recognized as a zoonotic agent, causing vCJD in humans. As such, the process by which this link was established provides an example of the types of evidence required to assess the zoonotic potential of other animal TSEs.

Classic BSE was first recognized in 1984–1985 as a novel TSE affecting cattle in the United Kingdom (Wells et al., 1987), causing an epidemic eventually involving over 180,000 animals. The origins of the disease have still not been clearly established, but the number of cases was amplified by the practice of recycling animal carcasses into cattle feed in the form of meat and bone meal (Wilesmith, 1996). Following legislation to ban the incorporation of meat and bone meal and animal protein in livestock feeds, the incidence of disease has declined to very low levels, with only occasional cases currently being identified in the United Kingdom.

BSE cases were subsequently identified in continental Europe and other countries worldwide, including Japan, Canada, the United States, and Israel, but the overall numbers of affected cattle were much lower than in the United Kingdom (total of 6193 recorded cases in EU countries between 1989 and 2016; http://www.oie.int/animal-health-in-the-world/bse-specific-data/). Reliable incidence figures are available only for EU member states since 2001, when widespread active surveillance involving mandatory testing of healthy slaughtered cattle and fallen stock was introduced.

BSE is unusual in that it has been shown to cross species barriers relatively readily, resulting in natural infection of humans, cats, and exotic ruminants, and efficient experimental transmission to mice, sheep, goats, and macaques. Transmission of various BSE isolates from infected cattle to a panel of inbred mouse lines produced very similar incubation periods and lesion profiles for each mouse line, depending on the mouse *PRNP* genotype (a or b) (Bruce et al., 1997). These results suggested that all cattle had been infected by a single strain of TSE agent, in contrast to the diversity of strains produced by passaging sheep scrapie in the same mouse lines. Consistent with this, all BSE cases examined displayed similar pathogenesis, with neuropathology characterized by gray-matter vacuolation predominantly in the brainstem, and infectivity restricted mainly to nervous tissues (Wells et al., 1989, 1998; Balkema-Buschmann et al., 2011), rather than showing widespread replication in lymphoid tissues, as seen in most cases of scrapie in sheep.

Following the implementation of active surveillance in the EU in 2001, a number of "atypical" cases of BSE were identified in aged asymptomatic cattle during slaughterhouse testing. Two major phenotypes with pathology and epidemiology distinct from classic BSE (C-BSE) were observed, termed bovine amyloidotic spongiform encephalopathy (BASE) or L-BSE (Casalone et al., 2004), and H-BSE (Biacabe et al., 2004) respectively. The biochemical properties of PrP^{TSE} isolated from these cases also differed from C-BSE in terms of the protease-resistant fragment size and ratio of glycoforms on Western blot. The prevalence of atypical BSE cases is low (1.9 cases H-BSE and 1.7 cases L-BSE per million cattle over 8 years old tested) (Biacabe et al., 2008), and it is unclear whether they result from exposure to an acquired TSE distinct from C-BSE, or arise spontaneously.

Epidemiologic association between BSE and human TSEs

The first cases of vCJD in individuals in the United Kingdom were reported in 1996 (Will et al., 1996). The age at onset was significantly younger than in sCJD, and the cases showed a novel clinical and neuropathologic phenotype, characterized by the presence of numerous "florid" plaques. Cases with a similar phenotype had not been identified prior to 1995, and were not observed in young patients in European countries undertaking a comparable level of active surveillance to the United Kingdom. This led to the hypothesis that the appearance of vCJD in the United Kingdom was linked to the risk of exposure to BSE.

To date, out of 231 vCJD cases identified worldwide, 178 cases have occurred in UK residents and 7 other cases had a reported period of residence in the United Kingdom of > 6 months between 1980 and 1996 (http://www.cjd.ed.ac.uk/surveillance/data-and-reports). The country with the second largest number of vCJD cases in the native population is France, with 27 confirmed cases. Thus, the observed geographic distribution of vCJD in the human population reflects the available data on the incidence of BSE in the cattle populations of the countries in question, but there are considerable uncertainties due to the very variable levels of surveillance for TSEs in human and animals worldwide.

All definite cases of vCJD that have undergone *PRNP* genetic analysis are homozygous for methionine at codon 129 (129MM), apart from the latest UK case, which was heterozygous (129MV) (Mok et al., 2017).

The true incidence and distribution of atypical L-BSE and H-BSE in cattle populations have not been determined, but the apparent rarity of these forms of BSE makes it very difficult to establish links with novel forms of human TSE disease through surveillance.

In vivo and in vitro transmission studies with BSE

Support for the hypothesis that BSE was linked to vCJD came initially from experiments in which BSE-infected cattle brain homogenate was injected intracerebrally into cynomolgus macaques (*Macaca fascicularis*) (Lasmezas et al., 1996). All three infected animals developed clinical signs reminiscent of those seen in vCJD patients and showed a similar distribution of neuropathology and PrP^{TSE} deposition, including florid plaques, in their brains. Subsequently, transmission of BSE to macaques by oral and intravenous routes (including blood transfusion) was demonstrated (Herzog et al., 2004; Lescoutra-Etchegaray et al., 2015), indicating that they were susceptible to infection by peripheral exposure routes similar to those predicted for humans. Experimental transmission of cattle BSE to nonhuman primates has also been demonstrated in marmosets, lemurs, and squirrel monkeys (Baker et al., 1993; Bons et al., 1999; Williams et al., 2007).

Additional evidence for the link between BSE and vCJD was provided by transmission studies in inbred mouse lines, in which mice injected with vCJD exhibited phenotypes (incubation periods and lesion profile) indistinguishable from those obtained following transmission of BSE or feline spongiform encephalopathy (also related to exposure to BSE), indicating that all three diseases were caused by the same TSE strain (Bruce et al., 1997). This was further reinforced by experiments in which transgenic mice expressing bovine PrP were injected with BSE, scrapie, and vCJD, which demonstrated that BSE and vCJD produced identical incubation times and neuropathology, distinct from those seen with scrapie (Scott et al., 1999).

Transmission of sCJD, vCJD, and BSE to transgenic mice expressing human 129V or 129M PrP revealed that, while sCJD transmitted efficiently, the humanized mice were relatively resistant to both vCJD and BSE, exhibiting low attack rates and long incubation times. In the mice expressing 129M, the low transmission efficiency of BSE was occasionally accompanied by a strain shift resulting in an alternative phenotype similar to sCJD in a proportion of mice (Asante et al., 2002), and vCJD in 129V-expressing mice produced a different molecular signature than the original inoculum on Western blot (Hill et al., 1997). Further evaluation of the potential transmissibility of BSE and vCJD to humans was carried out using gene-targeted transgenic mouse lines carrying the three human *PRNP* codon 129 genotypes, MM, MV, and VV, on an identical genetic background (Bishop et al., 2006). There was no evidence of transmission of BSE to any of the humanized lines after observation periods up to 700 days post infection, but it did transmit efficiently to a similar transgenic mouse line expressing bovine PrP. vCJD transmitted to all three humanized lines, producing different pathologic characteristics for each genotype, and a gradation in transmission efficiency from MM (most efficient) to VV (least efficient). Taken together, the results of experimental transmission of BSE to humanized transgenic mice suggest a large species barrier to cattle BSE in humans, which may explain the low numbers of vCJD cases to date, considering the high levels of exposure during the BSE crisis.

Sheep and goats are susceptible to BSE when experimentally infected by peripheral routes, including orally (Foster et al., 1993; Jeffrey et al., 2001). Since small ruminants would have been exposed to BSE-contaminated feed during the BSE epidemic, they may present an additional risk to humans, particularly if onward intraspecies transmission has maintained the infection, as for scrapie. However, there is little evidence that this has occurred on a large scale, as only two cases of natural BSE in goats (Eloit et al., 2005; Jeffrey et al., 2006) and none in sheep have been identified in EU countries. Human susceptibility to small ruminant-passaged BSE was assessed by injecting two different transgenic mouse lines expressing human 129M PrP with sheep, goat, and cattle BSE isolates (Padilla et al., 2011). Consistent with previous studies, the transmission efficiency of cattle BSE to the humanized mouse lines was low, but surprisingly, sheep- and goat-passaged BSE isolates produced high attack rates on primary transmission to the transgenic lines, and incubation times that were similar to those found after transmission of vCJD. Similar results were obtained when sheep-passaged BSE was injected into gene-targeted 129MM humanized transgenic mice (Plinston et al., 2011). This suggests that humans with the 129MM genotype may be more susceptible to small ruminant BSE agents than to cattle BSE. The failure to identify significant numbers of BSE cases in sheep and goats offers some reassurance, but underascertainment of the extent of disease may mean there is still a possibility of human exposure to small ruminant BSE.

In vitro experiments to model interspecies transmission barriers have produced results that are consistent with in vivo transmission studies. Using the CFCA, it was shown that PrP^{BSE} converted bovine PrP more efficiently than human PrP, and human 129M PrP more efficiently than 129V PrP (Raymond et al., 1997). Another study used PMCA to test the ability of BSE, scrapie, and vCJD to convert human PrP in brain homogenates from humanized transgenic mice with MM, MV, and VV codon 129 *PRNP* genotypes (Jones et al., 2009b). Cattle and sheep BSE isolates and vCJD were amplified in the humanized substrate with similar codon 129 genotype preferences (129MM > 129MV > 129VV), while scrapie failed to convert the human PrP. PMCA has also been used to model the effect of continued passage of BSE in sheep, with results that suggest that it may in time produce a scrapie-like molecular profile, but that when this occurs the ability to convert human PrP is lost (Krejciova et al., 2014).

Similar approaches have been used to assess the zoonotic potential of atypical BSE cases. Intracranial injection of L-BSE isolates from European and Japanese cattle in cynomolgus macaques produced a distinctive clinical and pathologic phenotype, and shorter survival times than in C-BSE-infected macaques (Comoy et al., 2008; Ono et al., 2011). Mouse lemurs (*Microcebus murinus*) were also shown to be susceptible to L-BSE following oral or i.c. inoculation (Mestre-Frances et al., 2012), while C-BSE could be transmitted only after a first passage in macaques. Inoculation of L-BSE, H-BSE, and C-BSE isolates into transgenic mice overexpressing human 129M PrP (tg650) demonstrated that, compared to C-BSE, L-BSE transmitted efficiently on primary transmission in the mice, with 100% attack rates and no shortening of incubation periods on subsequent subpassage (Beringue et al., 2008a). In contrast, H-BSE failed to transmit in the same mouse model. Another study using a different transgenic mouse model expressing wild-type levels of human 129M PrP also showed efficient primary transmission of L-BSE (Kong et al., 2008). In both studies, the L-BSE biochemical PrP^{TSE} signature was conserved following transmission to the mouse lines, and in tg650 mice it was indistinguishable from that produced by a human MM2 sCJD isolate. These results suggested that L-BSE is more virulent than C-BSE in primate and humanized transgenic mice, and may therefore pose a higher risk of zoonotic infection. However, in challenges of gene-targeted transgenic mice expressing human PrP, both L-BSE and H-BSE failed to produce any signs of clinical disease or PrP^{TSE} deposition (Wilson et al., 2012). In addition, biologic strain typing of L-BSE and a panel of sCJD subtypes in human PrP transgenic mice failed to find any evidence that L-BSE causes a recognized form of sCJD (Jaumain et al., 2016). This does not preclude the possibility that L-BSE may propagate in humans to cause a novel form of CJD.

An in vitro study compared the ability of a panel of animal TSEs, including L-BSE and H-BSE, to convert the human PrP by PMCA (Barria et al., 2014a). Neither L-BSE nor H-BSE was amplified in 129MM or 129VV substrates prepared from human brains or transgenic mice, while both C-BSE and vCJD converted the human PrP^{C}, as previously observed. These results suggest that atypical BSE cases present a lower risk of zoonotic disease than C-BSE.

Conclusions

The overwhelming weight of evidence from epidemiologic and experimental studies supports the view that vCJD resulted from transmission of classic BSE from cattle to humans. However, despite the fact that nonhuman primates are susceptible to BSE, results from experimental inoculation of a number of different humanized transgenic mouse lines suggest that there is a substantial transmission barrier to BSE in humans, which may explain the relatively small size of the vCJD epidemic. Of concern is the finding that BSE appears to increase in virulence for humans if it is first passaged in sheep, raising the possibility that small ruminants might present an additional reservoir of infection and risk to humans, although there is little evidence of widespread BSE infection in these species.

The epidemiologic data on atypical bovine TSEs (L-BSE and H-BSE) are limited, and although not all the results of experimental studies are in agreement, some transmission studies in nonhuman primates and humanized transgenic mice suggest that L-BSE may have zoonotic potential equal to or greater than C-BSE.

Small ruminant TSE diseases

Scrapie in small ruminants is a disease which has been described for several centuries. It was reported for the first time in sheep in the United Kingdom in 1732 and, a few years later, in 1759, in Germany. In the following centuries, scrapie endemically affected flocks in several countries (Detwiler, 1992). Goat scrapie was reported for the first time in a goat living in a sheep flock where the disease had been prevalent for several years (Detwiler and Baylis, 2003).

In 1998, the molecular and histopathologic spectrum of TSEs in sheep was extended by the discovery in Norway of an experimentally transmissible, PrP-related, neurologic disease of sheep (Nor98) that was clearly distinguishable from scrapie cases that had been previously reported (named classical scrapie), and was therefore considered to be an "atypical" form of scrapie (Benestad et al., 2008).

After 2001 and the implementation of active TSE surveillance plans, a number of similar cases were identified in most EU members states as well in many other countries, including the United States and Canada (Benestad et al., 2008). Atypical scrapie was also detected in Australia and New Zealand (Kittelberger et al., 2010; Cook et al., 2016), two countries that had been considered so far by the World Organisation for Animal Health (OIE) as TSE-free.

A retrospective study carried out in tissue banks identified atypical/Nor98 cases in sheep samples collected in the United Kingdom in 1987 (Webb et al., 2009). The analysis of data collected through the surveillance system in the United Kingdom between 2002 and 2006 suggested that atypical scrapie prevalence in this population could have remained stable over this period (McIntyre et al., 2008). Together these elements suggest that atypical/Nor98 might have been present but undetected in the small ruminant population for several decades.

Agent strains in sheep

Despite the relative uniformity of the clinical signs in the natural host, classic scrapie can be caused by TSE agents that harbor different biologic features. Historically, appreciation of potential scrapie diversity has relied on serial passaging of natural isolates to a panel of inbred mouse lines. The strains that preferentially replicated in the mice were isolated and biologic phenotype was compared. The considerable strain variation initially described (up to 20 strains:Dickinson, 1976) using this system might finally be restricted to a varying combination of three distinct strains (Bruce et al., 2002).

However the relationship between these mouse-adapted TSE agents and those initially present in the TSE isolates is a matter of debate. The propagation of natural TSE isolates into inbred mice lines implies the passage through a transmission barrier that can result in different outcome, including a radical and irreversible evolution of the biologic properties of the agent, a phenomenon called mutation. Moreover, wild-type mice have been described to be refractory to most TSE isolates prepared from sheep homozygous for the ARQ allele (Foster and Dickinson, 1988; Bruce et al., 2002) and to atypical/Nor98 (Le Dur et al., 2005; Bruce et al., 2007). In that context it is difficult to consider that the conventional mouse models provide a comprehensive and reliable picture of the diversity of the TSE agents in small ruminants.

Transgenic mice that overexpress the ovine, caprine, bovine, or even murine *PRNP* genes have been demonstrated to display a lower transmission barrier to scrapie agents than conventional mouse models (Scott et al., 1989; Groschup and Buschmann, 2008). As a striking example, atypical cases propagate without apparent barrier in transgenic mice overexpressing sheep VRQ allele (Le Dur et al., 2005).

Serial transmission of about 80 scrapie isolates from Europe in the same transgenic mouse line has so far permitted identification of at least four phenotypically distinct classes of agent (Beringue et al., 2007, 2008c; Thackray et al., 2007, 2012; Tixador et al., 2010). In contrast to classical scrapie, no strain variability has been observed among isolates of atypical scrapie (Le Dur et al., 2005; Arsac et al., 2007; Griffiths et al., 2010).

The transgenic mice are valuable models that will probably enable a more comprehensive view of strain diversity in small ruminants in the near future. In the meantime it still remains difficult to appreciate real diversity of TSE agents circulating in small ruminants or the potential relationships that might exist between agents causing scrapie in small ruminants and prion disease in other species.

Epidemiologic association between small ruminants and human TSEs

Several epidemiologic studies, generally based on case–control approaches, failed to identify exposure to small ruminants or small ruminant products as a risk factor for developing CJD (Brown et al., 1987; van Duijn et al., 1998). Countries considered to be TSE-free, like Australia and New Zealand, display a similar CJD prevalence as countries affected with scrapie. In addition, there is no apparent difference in the range of clinical and pathologic manifestations of human TSE cases between scrapie-affected countries and those supposed to be scrapie-free. This goes against the view that exposure to scrapie agents might be responsible for one or several particular TSE forms in humans. Together these elements led to the general opinion that small ruminant TSEs had no zoonotic potential.

For decades the identification of TSE in small ruminants relied on clinical suspicion (passive surveillance). In 2001–2002, in the EU, an active surveillance program for TSE in small ruminants was implemented, and has subsequently been adopted to some extent in a number of other countries, including the United States and Canada. Active surveillance relies on the systematic testing of a proportion of the slaughtered or found-dead animals for the detection of disease-associated PrP (PrP^{TSE}) in the posterior brainstem. The data collected through this surveillance system have clearly demonstrated that earlier evaluations of the prevalence of TSEs in small ruminants, and their geographic spread (on the basis of passive surveillance), were largely underestimated (Fediaevsky et al., 2008).

The fact that both Australia and New Zealand, two countries that had been considered for more than 50 years as TSE-free territories, were finally identified positive for atypical scrapie in their sheep flocks provides an example of how prion dogma can be reversed (Kittelberger et al., 2010; Cook et al., 2016).

Data collected through active surveillance programs will probably offer an opportunity to reassess the zoonotic potential of small ruminant TSE through informed and modern epidemiologic investigations. However, the incubation period for prion disease in humans after exposure to prions via the peripheral route, such as in iatrogenic CJD transmission and kuru, can exceed several decades (Collinge et al., 2006; Brown et al., 2012). In this context, it will be a challenge to combine epidemiologic data collected contemporarily in animal populations and humans to investigate the existence of a causative link between prion disease occurrences in these different hosts.

In vitro and in vivo transmission experiments with small ruminant TSEs

Seminal experiments failed to demonstrate the transmissibility of classical scrapie in nonhuman primates (chimpanzee) (Gibbs and Gajdusek, 1971). However, one natural sheep classic scrapie isolate transmitted in two out of two intracerebrally challenged marmosets. The incubation period observed with this scrapie isolate was slightly shorter than with a cattle BSE isolate, suggesting that the transmission barrier towards both isolates might not be different (Baker et al., 1993). However, because Old World monkey (chimpanzee and cynomolgus macaques) are evolutionary closer to humans than New World monkeys (marmosets), the significance of these results for the zoonotic potential of scrapie remains debated.

More recently, Comoy et al. (2015) described the successful transmission of a classic scrapie isolate (one of the panel of scrapie isolates described in Cassard et al., 2014) to a cynomolgus macaque. The incubation period in this animal was quite extended (> 10 years following intracerebral challenge) and the neuropathology observed was unique in comparison to other animal prion diseases (C-BSE, L-BSE) transmitted in this model (Comoy et al., 2015). To date there are no available results concerning the experimental transmission of atypical scrapie to nonhuman primates.

Besides bioassay in primates, the transmission of both atypical and classic scrapie isolates in mice expressing human PrP was tested in several studies. Gene-targeted transgenic mouse lines expressing physiologic levels of Met129, Val129, or MV129 human PrPs were challenged with two natural sheep scrapie isolates and two natural goat scrapie isolates (Plinston et al., 2011; Wilson et al., 2013). Primary transmissions of scrapie isolates were unable to cause disease in these mouse lines. The same mouse lines were also challenged with one atypical scrapie isolate but did not show any signs of disease pathology (Wilson et al., 2012). Serial passages in the same transgenic mouse lines, which could allow the identification of subclinical infection, were not performed. These results support the view that a substantial transmission barrier limits the propagation of both atypical and classic scrapie agents in human PrP-expressing hosts. However, these mice were also shown to be resistant to cattle BSE (Bishop et al., 2010). This strongly limits the value of the results obtained in these models which do not allow assessment of whether the zoonotic potential of classic or atypical scrapie is lower or higher than that of BSE.

Several transgenic mouse lines that overexpress human PrP have been developed over the last decade. Among them are the tg35 line that overexpresses human 129M PrP twofold, and the tg152 line that overexpresses human 129V PrP sixfold. Both lines were shown to have limited susceptibility to cattle BSE (Hill et al., 1997; Asante et al., 2002), but when challenged with five classic scrapie and five atypical scrapie isolates, there was no clinical disease or detectable accumulation of PrP^{TSE} in the inoculated mice (Wadsworth et al., 2013). However, in these experiments, subpassages of these isolates were not performed, and therefore it remains a possibility that subclinical propagation of prion disease could have occurred in some inoculated mice.

In a more recent study a panel of classic scrapie isolates was tested in different humanized transgenic mouse lines (Cassard et al., 2014). The mouse lines were homozygous for methionine (129MM/tg340) or valine (129VV/tg361) at codon 129 of human PrP, or were their F1 cross (129MV). All of these mouse lines expressed human PrP approximately fourfold more compared to that seen in normal human brain tissue. The three mouse lines were inoculated intracerebrally with a panel of six sheep scrapie isolates that had been collected between 1994 and 2002 from flocks naturally affected with the disease. Part of the isolates were also inoculated into tg650 mice, another mouse line that overexpresses (about sixfold) human 129M PrP. On first passage no clinical disease was observed in any of the scrapie-inoculated mice. However, one scrapie isolate produced subclinical infection in two out of six 129MV mice, while another caused a PrP^{TSE} accumulation in the brain of one out of six tg650 mice.

Serial blind passage of the isolates in the same mice lines led after second passage to positive transmission (clinical signs) in mice inoculated with three of six tested isolates. Interestingly, the sheep scrapie prions that propagated in humanized transgenic mouse models displayed a transmission efficacy (attack rate on first and second passage) that was comparable to that of cattle BSE. After third passage the propagated prions displayed a phenotype (incubation periods and PrP^{TSE} distribution in the brain) that was identical to those causing sCJD in humans. This last finding raised important questions about the possible link between TSE in small ruminants and occurrence of human TSE cases. These transmission experiments unambiguously showed that sheep scrapie prions propagate in mice that express variants of human PrP. While the efficiency of transmission at primary passage was low, subsequent passages resulted in a highly virulent prion disease in human PrP-expressing mice.

There are very few published studies in which the capacity of small ruminant TSE agents to propagate in human substrate was assessed using PMCA. None of them successfully amplified a small ruminant TSE agent using human brains and humanized transgenic mouse brains as substrate (Jones et al., 2009a; Barria et al., 2014b). However these experiments involved only a few classic scrapie (with unknown strain properties) and atypical scrapie isolates. These in vitro results reinforce the view that a substantial barrier limits the capacity of small ruminant TSE agents to propagate in humans. However they cannot be considered as reliable evidence of an absence of zoonotic potential of these prions.

Conclusions

The zoonotic potential of small ruminant TSE strains remains incompletely characterized. However results obtained recently in experimental models (primates and human PrP transgenic mice) demonstrated that at least some of these agents have the capacity to cross the human transmission barrier. While these findings do not automatically imply that small ruminant TSE agents have caused TSE disease in exposed humans, they clearly point out the need to reconsider this possibility. In the meanwhile, these data provide support for continuing the application of measures that were implemented to mitigate the exposure of human to small ruminant TSE agents.

Chronic wasting disease in cervids

CWD was first recognized in the 1960s, although it was not confirmed to be a prion disease until 1980 (Williams, 2005). Since its first identification in Colorado, the CWD-affected area has considerably expanded. The disease has now been identified in 20 US states and two Canadian provinces (Saskatchewan and Alberta) and it has become endemic in most of these regions. The prevalence of CWD in free-ranging cervids varies across North America, but can be as high as 30% in some areas (Williams, 2005).

Outside North America, CWD infection has been confirmed in captive cervids in South Korea as a result of importation of subclinically infected animals from Canada (Kim et al., 2005).

In April 2016, CWD was found in a free-ranging reindeer population in Norway and then later (June 2016) in two moose in a different region of Norway (Benestad et al., 2016). It is unclear at this stage if CWD presence in Norway has any relationship with the epidemics in North America.

CWD agent strains

There is clear evidence demonstrating that several prion strains are responsible for CWD in North American cervids. Bioassays in transgenic mice expressing cervid PrP of a panel of CWD isolates from various species and geographic locations in North America indicated the presence of two prevalent CWD prion strains (referred to as CWD1 and CWD2) that circulate either independently or as a strain mixture (Angers et al., 2010). Bioassays in heterologous PrP transgenic mice models or in conventional rodent models are consistent with these results (Tamguney et al., 2006; Crowell et al., 2015). However, it is difficult to consider that the strain-typing work carried out so far has provided us with a definitive picture of the diversity of CWD strains. In particular, there are currently no data concerning the nature of the prion(s) that caused the recent CWD outbreak in Norway, although transmission experiments in transgenic and conventional mouse lines are under way in several laboratories.

Finally, experimental transmission of BSE in cervids and bioassay in transgenic mice strongly support the contention that CWD agents are unrelated to classic BSE. However the potential relationships between CWD and other TSE agents that circulate in animal populations (TME, scrapie) are still uncertain.

Epidemiologic association between CWD and human TSEs

No new or unusual form of human TSE has been identified so far in countries where CWD epidemics have developed (Anderson et al., 2007). Comparison of the CJD prevalence rates between North America and other countries (Europe) does not suggest that CWD is responsible for a detectable increase in human prion disease prevalence.

A retrospective study carried out using state death registry data collected between 1979 and 2001 in Colorado failed to identify any statistical difference in CJD prevalence between CWD-endemic versus CWD-nonendemic counties (65 CJD cases / 506,335 deaths) (Mawhinney et al., 2006).

In the United States, retrospective investigations identified several sCJD cases that had a history of potential or demonstrated exposure to CWD prions through venison consumption or hunting cervids in affected areas (Belay et al., 2001). Longitudinal studies related to known dietary exposure to CWD failed to demonstrate an increased risk of developing a TSE in these individuals (Olszowy et al., 2014). Nevertheless, considering the limited duration of the observation period in these studies (in comparison with the potentially very long incubation periods for TSE in humans), the significance of these observations remains uncertain.

Collectively the epidemiological data suggest a lack of causative link between CWD epidemics in North America and the occurrence of human TSEs. However, because of the considerable limitations of the elements supporting this statement, it would probably be unwise at this stage to conclude on their sole basis an absence of zoonotic risk associated with CWD agents.

In vivo and in vitro transmission experiments with CWD

Although CWD was relatively recently identified, a number of studies specifically aiming at clarifying the capacity of CWD agent(s) to cross the human species barrier have already been carried out through experimental inoculation in human PrP-expressing transgenic mice and primates. A total of seven CWD isolates were bioassayed in different conventional and humanized transgenic mouse models, including models that expressed Met and/or Val at codon 129 of the *PRNP* gene. The lack of any disease transmission or PrP^{TSE} accumulation in the brains of the inoculated mice indicates the existence of a substantial transmission barrier (Kong et al., 2005; Tamguney et al., 2006; Wilson et al., 2012).

However, there are several limitations to these transmission experiments in humanized mouse models. The first one is the lack of secondary passage in human PrP transgenic mice models that was necessary for revealing the transmissibility of scrapie isolates and certain classic BSE isolates in similar models (Cassard et al., 2014). The second is the lack of information concerning the nature of the CWD agent(s) in the tested isolates.

In primates, successful transmission of CWD was reported in squirrel monkeys (*Saimiri sciureus*) following intracerebral (80% attack rate) and oral inoculation (15% attack rate). On secondary passage a reduction in the incubation period was observed, indicating the presence of a transmission barrier (Marsh et al., 2005; Race et al., 2009).

Macaques are evolutionarily closer to humans than squirrel monkeys. In two studies, cynomolgus macaques were challenged by intracerebral, oral, and intradermal routes with CWD isolates. These experiments are still ongoing, but after observation periods ranging from 1.5 to over 10 years there was no indication of prion disease transmission (Race et al., 2014). In contrast, cynomolgus macaques were shown to be susceptible to infection with classic BSE following intracerebral and oral inoculation (see above) (Lasmezas et al., 1996). These data suggest that macaques are more resistant to CWD than to BSE. However, challenge with scrapie in the macaque model resulted in disease after 10-year incubation periods (four times longer than with BSE), and it is certainly too early to draw conclusions on the final transmissibility of CWD in this model (Comoy et al., 2015).

Initial cell-free conversion studies suggested that the ability of CWD prions to convert human PrP^{C} into abnormal PrP^{TSE} was limited (Raymond et al., 2000). However, further experiments carried out using PMCA demonstrated that CWD prions can induce the conversion of human PrPC to protease-resistant PrP^{TSE} (Barria et al., 2011). In the earliest experiments, brain homogenates from transgenic mice expressing 129M or 129V human PrP could not support amplification of CWD isolates from white-tailed deer and mule deer (Kurt et al., 2009). However, after serial amplification rounds using cervid PrP-transgenic mouse brain as substrate, CWD prions from a naturally infected mule deer were then able to convert human PrP^{C} (Barria et al., 2011). In another study, an elk CWD isolate was also shown to convert human PrP^{C} from human brain, humanized mouse brain, and human-derived cell lines in PMCA reactions. Most interestingly, the resulting PrP^{TSE} resembled that of sCJD of the MM1 subtype, indicating a switch of the prion phenotype (Barria et al., 2014a).

Conclusions

CWD strains and their prevalence remain incompletely characterized. Currently available epidemiologic data indicate no clear association between the occurrence of TSEs in humans and exposure to CWD. Transmission experiments in animal models support the view that a substantial species barrier limits the transmissibility of CWD prions to humans. However in vitro conversion assays have demonstrated that at least certain CWD isolates have the capacity to propagate using human PrP as a substrate. Considering the uncertainties related to the zoonotic potential of CWD prions and the continuous expansion of its epidemics across North America, measures aiming at controlling this disease in animal populations and at limiting human exposure to these prions should be reinforced.

SUMMARY

Establishing the zoonotic potential of animal TSEs by epidemiologic approaches is extremely challenging, in view of factors including the low incidence of sCJD, the long incubation periods of acquired human TSEs, and the very variable levels of surveillance for animal TSEs in different countries/regions over time. A variety of in vivo and in vitro experimental models and techniques have been developed to assess the capacity of TSE agents to infect humans, but several different lines of evidence are required before zoonotic transmission can be confirmed. Nonhuman primates and humanized transgenic mice are currently the most representative in vivo models of the human species barrier. The results of in vitro conversion methods such as PMCA generally correlate well with in vivo data, presenting an attractive, inexpensive and rapid alternative to costly animal experiments for assessment of transmission barriers. Using a combination of these experimental approaches, there is now accumulating evidence that classic scrapie, L-BSE, and CWD may have zoonotic potential. However, it remains challenging to interpret the results of in vivo and in vitro experiments supporting a link between animal and human TSEs in the absence of epidemiologic evidence. This additional critical evidence is unlikely to be forthcoming unless there is continued systematic surveillance for both human and animal TSEs.

References

Anderson CA, Bosque P, Filley CM et al. (2007). Colorado surveillance program for chronic wasting disease transmission to humans: lessons from 2 highly suspicious but negative cases. Arch Neurol 64: 439–441.

Angers RC, Kang HE, Napier D et al. (2010). Prion strain mutation determined by prion protein conformational compatibility and primary structure. Science 328: 1154–1158.

Arakawa K, Nagara H, Itoyama Y et al. (1991). Clustering of three cases of Creutzfeldt–Jakob disease near Fukuoka City, Japan. Acta Neurol Scand 84: 445–447.

Arsac JN, Andreoletti O, Bilheude JM et al. (2007). Similar biochemical signatures and prion protein genotypes in atypical scrapie and Nor98 cases, France and Norway. Emerg Infect Dis 13: 58–65.

Asante EA, Linehan JM, Desbruslais M et al. (2002). BSE prions propagate as either variant CJD-like or sporadic CJD-like prion strains in transgenic mice expressing human prion protein. Embo J 21: 6358–6366.

Atarashi R, Moore RA, Sim VL et al. (2007). Ultrasensitive detection of scrapie prion protein using seeded conversion of recombinant prion protein. Nat Methods 4: 645–650.

Baker HF, Ridley RM, Wells GA (1993). Experimental transmission of BSE and scrapie to the common marmoset. Vet Rec 132: 403–406.

Balkema-Buschmann A, Fast C, Kaatz M et al. (2011). Pathogenesis of classical and atypical BSE in cattle. Prev Vet Med 102: 112–117.

Barash JA (2008). Do midlife hormonal changes play a role in the onset of sporadic Creutzfeldt–Jakob disease? An epidemiologic perspective. Med Hypotheses 71: 611–612.

Barria MA, Telling GC, Gambetti P et al. (2011). Generation of a new form of human PrP(Sc) in vitro by interspecies transmission from cervid prions. J Biol Chem 286: 7490–7495.

Barria MA, Balachandran A, Morita M et al. (2014a). Molecular barriers to zoonotic transmission of prions. Emerg Infect Dis 20: 88–97.

Barria MA, Ironside JW, Head MW (2014b). Exploring the zoonotic potential of animal prion diseases: in vivo and in vitro approaches. Prion 8: 85–91.

Barron RM, Thomson V, Jamieson E et al. (2001). Changing a single amino acid in the N-terminus of murine PrP alters TSE incubation time across three species barriers. Embo J 20: 5070–5078.

Belay ED, Gambetti P, Schonberger LB et al. (2001). Creutzfeldt–Jakob disease in unusually young patients who consumed venison. Arch Neurol 58: 1673–1678.

Benestad SL, Arsac JN, Goldmann W et al. (2008). Atypical/Nor98 scrapie: properties of the agent, genetics, and epidemiology. Vet Res 39: 19.

Benestad SL, Mitchell G, Simmons M et al. (2016). First case of chronic wasting disease in Europe in a Norwegian free-ranging reindeer. Vet Res 47: 88.

Beringue V, Andreoletti O, Le Dur A et al. (2007). A bovine prion acquires an epidemic bovine spongiform encephalopathy strain-like phenotype on interspecies transmission. J Neurosci 27: 6965–6971.

Beringue V, Herzog L, Reine F et al. (2008a). Transmission of atypical bovine prions to mice transgenic for human prion protein. Emerg Infect Dis 14: 1898–1901.

Beringue V, Le Dur A, Tixador P et al. (2008b). Prominent and persistent extraneural infection in human PrP transgenic mice infected with variant CJD. PLoS One 3: e1419.

Beringue V, Vilotte JL, Laude H (2008c). Prion agent diversity and species barrier. Vet Res 39: 47.

Beringue V, Herzog L, Jaumain E et al. (2012). Facilitated cross-species transmission of prions in extraneural tissue. Science 335: 472–475.

Biacabe AG, Laplanche JL, Ryder S et al. (2004). Distinct molecular phenotypes in bovine prion diseases. EMBO Rep 5: 110–115.

Biacabe AG, Morignat E, Vulin J et al. (2008). Atypical bovine spongiform encephalopathies, France, 2001-2007. Emerg Infect Dis 14: 298–300.

Bishop MT, Hart P, Aitchison L et al. (2006). Predicting susceptibility and incubation time of human-to-human transmission of vCJD. Lancet Neurol 5: 393–398.

Bishop MT, Will RG, Manson JC (2010). Defining sporadic Creutzfeldt–Jakob disease strains and their transmission properties. Proc Natl Acad Sci U S A 107: 12005–12010.

Bons N, Mestre-Frances N, Belli P et al. (1999). Natural and experimental oral infection of nonhuman primates by bovine spongiform encephalopathy agents. Proc Natl Acad Sci U S A 96: 4046–4051.

Brown P, Cathala F, Raubertas RF et al. (1987). The epidemiology of Creutzfeldt–Jakob disease: conclusion of a 15-year investigation in France and review of the world literature. Neurology 37: 895–904.

Brown P, Gibbs Jr CJ, Rodgers-Johnson P et al. (1994). Human spongiform encephalopathy: the National Institutes of Health series of 300 cases of experimentally transmitted disease. Ann Neurol 35: 513–529.

Brown P, Brandel JP, Sato T et al. (2012). Iatrogenic Creutzfeldt–Jakob disease, final assessment. Emerg Infect Dis 18: 901–907.

Browning SR, Mason GL, Seward T et al. (2004). Transmission of prions from mule deer and elk with chronic wasting disease to transgenic mice expressing cervid PrP. J Virol 78: 13345–13350.

Bruce ME (1993). Scrapie strain variation and mutation. Br Med Bull 49: 822–838.

Bruce ME, Will RG, Ironside JW et al. (1997). Transmissions to mice indicate that 'new variant' CJD is caused by the BSE agent. Nature 389: 498–501.

Bruce ME, Boyle A, Cousens S et al. (2002). Strain characterization of natural sheep scrapie and comparison with BSE. J Gen Virol 83: 695–704.

Bruce ME, Nonno R, Foster J et al. (2007). Nor98-like sheep scrapie in the United Kingdom in 1989. Vet Rec 160: 665–666.

Casalone C, Zanusso G, Acutis P et al. (2004). Identification of a second bovine amyloidotic spongiform encephalopathy: molecular similarities with sporadic Creutzfeldt–Jakob disease. Proc Natl Acad Sci U S A 101: 3065–3070.

Cassard H, Torres JM, Lacroux C et al. (2014). Evidence for zoonotic potential of ovine scrapie prions. Nat Commun 5: 5821.

Castilla J, Gonzalez-Romero D, Saa P et al. (2008). Crossing the species barrier by PrP(Sc) replication in vitro generates unique infectious prions. Cell 134: 757–768.

Chatelain J, Cathala F, Brown P et al. (1981). Epidemiologic comparisons between Creutzfeldt–Jakob disease and scrapie in France during the 12-year period 1968–1979. J Neurol Sci 51: 329–337.

Cocco PL, Caperna A, Vinci F (2003). Occupational risk factors for the sporadic form of Creutzfeldt–Jakob disease. Med Lav 94: 353–363.

Collinge J, Clarke AR (2007). A general model of prion strains and their pathogenicity. Science 318: 930–936.

Collinge J, Whitfield J, Mckintosh E et al. (2006). Kuru in the 21st century – an acquired human prion disease with very long incubation periods. Lancet 367: 2068–2074.

Comoy EE, Casalone C, Lescoutra-Etchegaray N et al. (2008). Atypical BSE (BASE) transmitted from asymptomatic aging cattle to a primate. PLoS One 3: e3017.

Comoy EE, Mikol J, Luccantoni-Freire S et al. (2015). Transmission of scrapie prions to primate after an extended silent incubation period. Sci Rep 5: 11573.

Cook RW, Bingham J, Besier AS et al. (2016). Atypical scrapie in Australia. Aust Vet J 94: 452–455.

Crowell J, Hughson A, Caughey B et al. (2015). Host Determinants of Prion Strain Diversity Independent of Prion Protein Genotype. J Virol 89: 10427–10441.

D'Aignaux JH, Cousens SN, Delasnerie-Laupretre N et al. (2002). Analysis of the geographical distribution of sporadic Creutzfeldt–Jakob disease in France between 1992 and 1998. Int J Epidemiol 31: 490–495.

Davenport KA, Henderson DM, Bian J et al. (2015). Insights into chronic wasting disease and bovine spongiform encephalopathy species barriers by use of real-time conversion. J Virol 89: 9524–9531.

Detwiler LA (1992). Scrapie. Rev Sci Tech 11: 491–537.

Detwiler LA, Baylis M (2003). The epidemiology of scrapie. Rev Sci Tech 22: 121–143.

Dickinson AG (1976). Scrapie in sheep and goats. Front Biol 44: 209–241.

Eloit M, Adjou K, Coulpier M et al. (2005). BSE agent signatures in a goat. Vet Rec 156: 523–524.

Fediaevsky A, Tongue SC, Noremark M et al. (2008). A descriptive study of the prevalence of atypical and classical scrapie in sheep in 20 European countries. BMC Vet Res 4: 19.

Foster JD, Dickinson AG (1988). The unusual properties of CH1641, a sheep-passaged isolate of scrapie. Vet Rec 123: 5–8.

Foster JD, Hope J, Fraser H (1993). Transmission of bovine spongiform encephalopathy to sheep and goats. Vet Rec 133: 339–341.

Gibbs Jr CJ, Gajdusek DC (1971). Transmission and characterization of the agents of spongiform virus encephalopathies: kuru, Creutzfeldt–Jakob disease, scrapie and mink encephalopathy. Res Publ Assoc Res Nerv Ment Dis 49: 383–410.

Gibbs Jr CJ, Gajdusek DC (1973). Experimental subacute spongiform virus encephalopathies in primates and other laboratory animals. Science 182: 67–68.

Goldmann W (2008). PrP genetics in ruminant transmissible spongiform encephalopathies. Vet Res 39: 30.

Griffiths PC, Spiropoulos J, Lockey R et al. (2010). Characterisation of atypical scrapie cases from Great Britain in transgenic ovine PrP mice. J Gen Virol 91: 2132–2138.

Groschup MH, Buschmann A (2008). Rodent models for prion diseases. Vet Res 39: 32.

Hadlow WJ, Kennedy RC, Race RE (1982). Natural infection of Suffolk sheep with scrapie virus. J Infect Dis 146: 657–664.

Herzog C, Sales N, Etchegaray N et al. (2004). Tissue distribution of bovine spongiform encephalopathy agent in primates after intravenous or oral infection. Lancet 363: 422–428.

Hill AF, Desbruslais M, Joiner S et al. (1997). The same prion strain causes vCJD and BSE. Nature 389 (448–450): 526.

Jackson WS, Borkowski AW, Faas H et al. (2009). Spontaneous generation of prion infectivity in fatal familial insomnia knockin mice. Neuron 63: 438–450.

Jaumain E, Quadrio I, Herzog L et al. (2016). Absence of evidence for a causal link between bovine spongiform encephalopathy strain variant L-BSE and known forms of sporadic Creutzfeldt–Jakob disease in human PrP transgenic mice. J Virol 90: 10867–10874.

Jeffrey M, Ryder S, Martin S et al. (2001). Oral inoculation of sheep with the agent of bovine spongiform encephalopathy (BSE). 1. Onset and distribution of disease-specific PrP accumulation in brain and viscera. J Comp Pathol 124: 280–289.

Jeffrey M, Martin S, Gonzalez L et al. (2006). Immunohistochemical features of PrP(d) accumulation in natural and experimental goat transmissible spongiform encephalopathies. J Comp Pathol 134: 171–181.

Jones M, Peden AH, Yull H et al. (2009a). Human platelets as a substrate source for the in vitro amplification of the abnormal prion protein (PrP) associated with variant Creutzfeldt–Jakob disease. Transfusion 49: 376–384.

Jones M, Wight D, Barron R et al. (2009b). Molecular model of prion transmission to humans. Emerg Infect Dis 15: 2013–2016.

Kim TY, Shon HJ, Joo YS et al. (2005). Additional cases of Chronic Wasting Disease in imported deer in Korea. J Vet Med Sci 67: 753–759.

Kimberlin RH, Walker CA (1988). Pathogenesis of experimental scrapie. Ciba Found Symp 135: 37–62.

Kittelberger R, Chaplin MJ, Simmons MM et al. (2010). Atypical scrapie/Nor98 in a sheep from New Zealand. J Vet Diagn Invest 22: 863–875.

Kocisko DA, Come JH, Priola SA et al. (1994). Cell-free formation of protease-resistant prion protein. Nature 370: 471–474.

Kocisko DA, Priola SA, Raymond GJ et al. (1995). Species specificity in the cell-free conversion of prion protein to protease-resistant forms: a model for the scrapie species barrier. Proc Natl Acad Sci U S A 92: 3923–3927.

Kong Q, Huang S, Zou W et al. (2005). Chronic wasting disease of elk: transmissibility to humans examined by transgenic mouse models. J Neurosci 25: 7944–7949.

Kong Q, Zheng M, Casalone C et al. (2008). Evaluation of the human transmission risk of an atypical bovine spongiform encephalopathy prion strain. J Virol 82: 3697–3701.

Krejciova Z, Barria MA, Jones M et al. (2014). Genotype-dependent molecular evolution of sheep bovine spongiform encephalopathy (BSE) prions in vitro affects their zoonotic potential. J Biol Chem 289: 26075–26088.

Kurt TD, Telling GC, Zabel MD et al. (2009). Trans-species amplification of PrP(CWD) and correlation with rigid loop 170N. Virology 387: 235–243.

Ladogana A, Puopolo M, Croes EA et al. (2005). Mortality from Creutzfeldt–Jakob disease and related disorders in Europe, Australia, and Canada. Neurology 64: 1586–1591.

Lasmezas CI, Deslys JP, Demaimay R et al. (1996). BSE transmission to macaques. Nature 381: 743–744.

Le Dur A, Beringue V, Andreoletti O et al. (2005). A newly identified type of scrapie agent can naturally infect sheep with resistant PrP genotypes. Proc Natl Acad Sci U S A 102: 16031–16036.

Lescoutra-Etchegaray N, Jaffre N, Sumian C et al. (2015). Evaluation of the protection of primates transfused with variant Creutzfeldt–Jakob disease-infected blood products filtered with prion removal devices: a 5-year update. Transfusion 55: 1231–1241.

Linsell L, Cousens SN, Smith PG et al. (2004). A case-control study of sporadic Creutzfeldt–Jakob disease in the United Kingdom: analysis of clustering. Neurology 63: 2077–2083.

Luers L, Bannach O, Stohr J et al. (2013). Seeded fibrillation as molecular basis of the species barrier in human prion diseases. PLoS One 8: e72623.

Marsh RF, Kincaid AE, Bessen RA et al. (2005). Interspecies transmission of chronic wasting disease prions to squirrel monkeys (*Saimiri sciureus*). J Virol 79: 13794–13796.

Masters CL, Harris JO, Gajdusek DC et al. (1979). Creutzfeldt–Jakob disease: patterns of worldwide occurrence and the significance of familial and sporadic clustering. Ann Neurol 5: 177–188.

Mawhinney S, Pape WJ, Forster JE et al. (2006). Human prion disease and relative risk associated with chronic wasting disease. Emerg Infect Dis 12: 1527–1535.

Mcintyre KM, Del Rio Vilas VJ, Gubbins S (2008). No temporal trends in the prevalence of atypical scrapie in British sheep, 2002-2006. BMC Vet Res 4: 13.

Mestre-Frances N, Nicot S, Rouland S et al. (2012). Oral transmission of L-type bovine spongiform encephalopathy in primate model. Emerg Infect Dis 18: 142–145.

Mok T, Jaunmuktane Z, Joiner S et al. (2017). Variant Creutzfeldt–Jakob disease in a patient with heterozygosity at PRNP codon 129. N Engl J Med 376: 292–294.

Moore RC, Hope J, McBride PA et al. (1998). Mice with gene targetted prion protein alterations show that Prnp, Sinc and Prni are congruent. Nat Genet 18: 118–125.

Nonno R, Di Bari MA, Cardone F et al. (2006). Efficient transmission and characterization of Creutzfeldt–Jakob disease strains in bank voles. PLoS Pathog 2: e12.

Olszowy KM, Lavelle J, Rachfal K et al. (2014). Six-year follow-up of a point-source exposure to CWD contaminated venison in an Upstate New York community: risk behaviours and health outcomes 2005-2011. Public Health 128: 860–868.

Ono F, Tase N, Kurosawa A et al. (2011). Atypical L-type bovine spongiform encephalopathy (L-BSE) transmission to cynomolgus macaques, a non-human primate. Jpn J Infect Dis 64: 81–84.

Padilla D, Beringue V, Espinosa JC et al. (2011). Sheep and goat BSE propagate more efficiently than cattle BSE in human PrP transgenic mice. PLoS Pathog 7: e1001319.

Palmer MS, Dryden AJ, Hughes JT et al. (1991). Homozygous prion protein genotype predisposes to sporadic Creutzfeldt–Jakob disease. Nature 352: 340–342.

Plinston C, Hart P, Chong A et al. (2011). Increased susceptibility of human-PrP transgenic mice to bovine spongiform encephalopathy infection following passage in sheep. J Virol 85: 1174–1181.

Prusiner SB (2001). Shattuck lecture–neurodegenerative diseases and prions. N Engl J Med 344: 1516–1526.

Race B, Meade-White KD, Miller MW et al. (2009). Susceptibilities of nonhuman primates to chronic wasting disease. Emerg Infect Dis 15: 1366–1376.

Race B, Meade-White KD, Phillips K et al. (2014). Chronic wasting disease agents in nonhuman primates. Emerg Infect Dis 20: 833–837.

Raymond GJ, Hope J, Kocisko DA et al. (1997). Molecular assessment of the potential transmissibilities of BSE and scrapie to humans. Nature 388: 285–288.

Raymond GJ, Bossers A, Raymond LD et al. (2000). Evidence of a molecular barrier limiting susceptibility of humans, cattle and sheep to chronic wasting disease. Embo J 19: 4425–4430.

Saborio GP, Permanne B, Soto C (2001). Sensitive detection of pathological prion protein by cyclic amplification of protein misfolding. Nature 411: 810–813.

Scott M, Foster D, Mirenda C et al. (1989). Transgenic mice expressing hamster prion protein produce species- specific scrapie infectivity and amyloid plaques. Cell 59: 847–857.

Scott MR, Safar J, Telling G et al. (1997). Identification of a prion protein epitope modulating transmission of bovine spongiform encephalopathy prions to transgenic mice. Proc Natl Acad Sci U S A 94: 14279–14284.

Scott MR, WILL R, IRONSIDE J et al. (1999). Compelling transgenetic evidence for transmission of bovine spongiform encephalopathy prions to humans. Proc Natl Acad Sci U S A 96: 15137–15142.

Sigurdson CJ, Nilsson KP, Hornemann S et al. (2009). De novo generation of a transmissible spongiform encephalopathy by mouse transgenesis. Proc Natl Acad Sci U S A 106: 304–309.

Tamguney G, Giles K, Bouzamondo-Bernstein E et al. (2006). Transmission of elk and deer prions to transgenic mice. J Virol 80: 9104–9114.

Telling GC, Scott M, Mastrianni J et al. (1995). Prion propagation in mice expressing human and chimeric PrP transgenes implicates the interaction of cellular PrP with another protein. Cell 83: 79–90.

Thackray AM, Hopkins L, Klein MA et al. (2007). Mouse-adapted ovine scrapie prion strains are characterized by different conformers of PrPSc. J Virol 81: 12119–12127.

Thackray AM, Lockey R, Beck KE et al. (2012). Evidence for co-infection of ovine prion strains in classical scrapie isolates. J Comp Pathol 147: 316–329.

Tixador P, Herzog L, Reine F et al. (2010). The physical relationship between infectivity and prion protein aggregates is strain-dependent. PLoS Pathog 6: e1000859.

Van Duijn CM, Delasnerie-Laupretre N, Masullo C et al. (1998). Case-control study of risk factors of Creutzfeldt–Jakob disease in Europe during 1993-95. European Union (EU) Collaborative Study Group of Creutzfeldt–Jakob disease (CJD). Lancet 351: 1081–1085.

Vilotte JL, Soulier S, Essalmani R et al. (2001). Markedly increased susceptibility to natural sheep scrapie of transgenic mice expressing ovine prp. J Virol 75: 5977–5984.

Wadsworth JD, Joiner S, Linehan JM et al. (2013). Atypical scrapie prions from sheep and lack of disease in transgenic mice overexpressing human prion protein. Emerg Infect Dis 19: 1731–1739.

Webb PR, Powell L, Denyer M et al. (2009). A retrospective immunohistochemical study reveals atypical scrapie has existed in the United Kingdom since at least 1987. J Vet Diagn Invest 21: 826–829.

Wells GA, Scott AC, Johnson CT et al. (1987). A novel progressive spongiform encephalopathy in cattle. Vet Rec 121: 419–420.

Wells GA, Hancock RD, Cooley WA et al. (1989). Bovine spongiform encephalopathy: diagnostic significance of vacuolar changes in selected nuclei of the medulla oblongata. Vet Rec 125: 521–524.

Wells GA, Hawkins SA, Green RB et al. (1998). Preliminary observations on the pathogenesis of experimental bovine spongiform encephalopathy (BSE): an update. Vet Rec 142: 103–106.

Wilesmith JW (1996). Recent observations on the epidemiology of bovine spongiform encephalopathy. In: CJ Gibbs JR (Ed.), Bovine spongiform encephalopathy: the BSE dilemma. Springer, New York.

Will RG, Ironside JW, Zeidler M et al. (1996). A new variant of Creutzfeldt–Jakob disease in the UK. Lancet 347: 921–925.

Williams ES (2005). Chronic wasting disease. Vet Pathol 42: 530–549.

Williams L, Brown P, Ironside J et al. (2007). Clinical, neuropathological and immunohistochemical features of sporadic and variant forms of Creutzfeldt–Jakob disease in the squirrel monkey (Saimiri sciureus). J Gen Virol 88: 688–695.

Wilson R, Plinston C, Hunter N et al. (2012). Chronic wasting disease and atypical forms of bovine spongiform encephalopathy and scrapie are not transmissible to mice expressing wild-type levels of human prion protein. J Gen Virol 93: 1624–1629.

Wilson R, King D, Hunter N et al. (2013). Characterization of an unusual transmissible spongiform encephalopathy in goat by transmission in knock-in transgenic mice. J Gen Virol 94: 1922–1932.

Windl O, Dempster M, Estibeiro JP et al. (1996). Genetic basis of Creutzfeldt–Jakob disease in the United Kingdom: a systematic analysis of predisposing mutations and allelic variation in the PRNP gene. Hum Genet 98: 259–264.

Handbook of Clinical Neurology, Vol. 153 (3rd series)
Human Prion Diseases
M. Pocchiari and J. Manson, Editors
https://doi.org/10.1016/B978-0-444-63945-5.00026-X

Chapter 26

Safety of blood, blood derivatives, and plasma-derived products

MARC L. TURNER*
Centre for Regenerative Medicine, University of Edinburgh and Scottish National Blood Transfusion Service, Edinburgh, United Kingdom

Abstract

There has been concern for several decades around the possibility that prion diseases may be transmissible by blood components and / or plasma products. Whilst the evidence in respect of transmission of sporadic Creutzfeldt–Jakob disease (CJD) is largely circumstantial, the identification of variant CJD gave rise to increased concern due to the evidence of prion accumulation in peripheral lymphoid tissue at the time of clinical disease. A series of studies of appendix tissues in the United Kingdom revealed prion accumulation in around 1 / 2000 of the individuals tested and raised further concern that there may be a significant proportion of the healthy population with subclinical infection posing an increased risk of transmission by substances of human origin (blood, plasma, tissues, organs) and interventional medical and surgical procedures. The former risk was realized with transmission of variant CJD infection to four individuals becoming evident between 2004 and 2006. These concerns precipitated significant changes to donor selection criteria internationally, to blood processing in the United Kingdom with the introduction of universal leucodepletion, and to the use of UK plasma for fractionation to plasma products. Considerable effort has also been invested in the development of peripheral blood assays for subclinical variant CJD and of prion reduction filters for blood components, though to date these technologies have not achieved routine clinical implementation. Whilst the variant CJD outbreak appears to be receding, continued vigilance is required in respect of the risks posed by all prion diseases to blood safety.

INTRODUCTION

Globally around 120 million blood components are used clinically each year, including red cell concentrates for patients with hemorrhage or anemia, platelet concentrates for patients with acute or chronic thrombocytopenia at risk of bleeding, and fresh frozen plasma and cryoprecipitate for patients with deficiencies of multiple coagulation factors. In addition, plasma from multiple donors is pooled in the manufacture of plasma products such as factor VIII and IX used in the management of hemophilia, immunoglobulins used in the management of immunodeficiencies, autoimmune conditions and passive immunization against some infections, and albumin used as a plasma expander. The possibility of the presence of infection in the peripheral blood of individuals with subclinical prion disease therefore raises concern that these diseases may be transmissible to, potentially, a large number of recipients.

Particular concern arose in the context of the outbreak of variant Creutzfeldt–Jakob disease (CJD) because of the known distribution of prions in peripheral lymphoid tissue prior to as well as during clinical disease (Ironside et al., 2000), and this risk materialized in the description of 4 cases of transmission of this prion infection by blood components described in 2004 and 2006 (Llewelyn et al., 2004; Peden et al., 2004; Wroe et al., 2006; Wilson and Ricketts, 2006). Although blood service organizations have taken several precautionary measures (Wilson and Ricketts, 2004), the persisting uncertainties surrounding the prevalence of subclinical prion infections, the nature, level, and distribution of infectivity in such individuals;

*Correspondence to: Marc L. Turner, MB, ChB, PhD, SNBTS Jack Copland Centre, 52 Research Avenue North, Heriot-Watt Research Park, Edinburgh EH14 4BE, United Kingdom. Tel: +44-752-525-3326, E-mail: marcturner@nhs.net

and the susceptibility of recipients to infection through this route continue to undermine our ability to accurately judge the magnitude of the risk and evaluate the impact of current and proposed risk management strategies.

CONSIDERATIONS IN RISK ASSESSMENT

The prevalence of subclinical infection

It is the prevalence and epidemiologic distribution of pre- or subclinical disease that drives the risk of secondary transmission, rather than the incidence of clinical disease. Although the incidence of sporadic CJD is known, the incubation period is uncertain and the prevalence of pre- or subclinical disease is unknown. Iatrogenic and familial forms of CJD are fortunately rare; however, it appears possible that preclinical infection may occur in some forms of disease. Those individuals in at-risk groups can often be identified by family or medical history and excluded as donors.

The prevalence and distribution of subclinical variant CJD are also unknown; however, the available data provide some important hints.

First, the median age of onset of disease has not altered over the past 2 decades in the way one would expect where a cohort of individuals has been exposed to the risk of infection over a discrete period (Will et al., 1996; Will, 2004; National CJD Surveillance Unit, 2016). These data suggest the existence of age-related susceptibility and/or exposure between the ages of 10 and 20 years (Cooper and Bird, 2003; Boelle et al., 2004; Clarke and Ghani, 2005), a cohort who would now be between 30 and 55 years old. The patients who have developed variant CJD in France have an older age profile than in those in the United Kingdom: the reason for this is unknown.

Mathematical modeling suggests a maximum likelihood of 3000 infected people (95% confidence interval (CI) 520–6810) in the United Kingdom, mainly in the 10–30-year age group (Clarke and Ghani, 2005). The data generated by study of tonsil and appendectomy samples have also been revealing (Ironside et al., 2000; Hilton et al., 2002; Frosh et al., 2004). The first of the studies revealed three out of 12,674 samples positive for abnormal prion protein (PrP) on Western blot (Hilton et al., 2004a) where the specificity is thought to be high but the sensitivity uncertain (Hilton et al., 2004b). A second study demonstrated 16 out of 32,441 appendectomy samples positive for abnormal PrP with similar prevalence across the 1941–1960 and 1961–1985 birth cohorts, gender, and geographic distribution (Gill et al., 2013). This is at variance with the number of individuals projected to develop clinical disease and suggests a probability of subclinical infection of 0.93 (95% CI 0.70–0.97) (Cooper et al., 2000; Clarke and Ghani, 2005). A third study of appendices removed before 1980 or from people born after January 1, 1996, cohorts who have been thought not to have been exposed to bovine spongiform encephalopathy (BSE) in the diet, has revealed that a similar proportion of appendices show abnormal PrP accumulation in both cohorts, leading to two possibilities: (1) that the BSE epidemic in the United Kingdom started earlier and lasted longer than previously thought; or (2) that the finding of abnormal PrP in peripheral lymphoid tissues is not specific for BSE / variant CJD. A combination of these two factors may be at play.

The potential existence of a cohort of individuals in the population with long-term subclinical infection (Hill and Collinge, 2003a, b) is consistent with experimental animal data (Wadsworth et al., 2004; Bishop et al., 2006), suggesting that methionine/valine heterozygosity or valine homozygosity at codon 129 of the *PRNP* gene predisposes to a prolonged period of subclinical infection. All clinical cases of variant CJD have been methionine homozygous at codon 129 (Head et al., 2004) until the recently described heterozygous patient (Mok et al., 2017). Moreover, the second reported case of transfusion-transmitted variant CJD prions was shown to be methionine/valine heterozygous at codon 129 (Peden et al., 2004). Two of the 3 patients who tested positive in the retrospective study of tonsils and appendices have also been shown to be valine homozygous at this locus (Ironside et al., 2006), suggesting that codon 129 genotype (among other things) may influence the propensity of an infected individual to develop clinical disease. Long-term studies on patients who developed kuru or iatrogenic CJD support this possibility. Individuals who were homozygous for methionine at codon 129 developed clinical disease sooner than those of other codon 129 genotypes, who have developed disease more sporadically and with longer incubation periods (in some cases, over 40 years from their likely infection).

A working assumption has therefore been made on the basis of these data that the underlying prevalence of subclinical infection in the United Kingdom may be around 1 in 2000 (95% CI 1 in 1250–1 in 3500) (Advisory Committee on Dangerous Pathogens (ACDP) TSE Risk Assessment Subgroup, 2012) and that there could be further cases of clinical disease in individuals with other codon 129 genotypes. There are no specific data on which to estimate the prevalence in other countries. However, from the relative incidence of clinical disease, one might expect prevalence in Ireland to be approximately 20% of that in the United Kingdom, that in France to be approximately 10%, and that in the Netherlands to be around 5%.

The nature, concentration, and distribution of infectivity

Our current understanding of the pathogenesis of prion diseases is largely predicated on animal studies. Biochemical and biologic assays point to the accumulation of high concentrations of PrP^{TSE} and infectivity in the central nervous system in all forms of prion disease; however, lower levels of PrP^{TSE} and infectivity have been demonstrated in a wide range of other tissues in human prion diseases and in naturally and experimentally infected animal prion diseases (World Health Organization, 2006).

Animal models of peripherally transmitted prion diseases (Mabbott and Turner, 2005; Aguzzi and Glatzel, 2006) point to follicular dendritic cells (Brown et al., 1999a; Bruce et al., 2000) in the germinal centers of lymphoid tissue as a key cell in the establishment of infection and not B lymphocytes, as initially suggested (Klein et al., 1998; Montrasio et al., 2001). The presence of prion accumulation in the follicular dendritic cells in tonsil, spleen, and lymph nodes of patients with variant CJD but not sporadic, familial, or centrally transmitted iatrogenic CJD (e.g., from dura mater or neurosurgical instrumentation) suggests a similar pathophysiology for CJD in humans following primary (e.g., cattle BSE to humans) or secondary and higher-order (human to human) peripheral transmission (Burthem and Roberts, 2003).

The exact nature of infectivity in peripheral blood and tissues is uncertain. Recent work suggests that, in brain homogenates, the maximum specific infectivity is associated with proteinase-resistant particles of 300–600 kDa (i.e., oligomers of 14–28 PrP molecules) (Silveira et al., 2005). There are also data suggesting that proteinase-sensitive forms of PrP^{TSE} are infectious. Further work in this area, particularly relating to the physicochemical characteristics of the infectious prion in plasma, is a priority.

Two sets of rodent studies are informative with regard to the likely concentration and distribution of infectivity in peripheral blood. The first studies were carried out in mice infected with the Fukuoka-1 strain of Gerstmann–Sträussler–Scheinker disease (Brown et al., 1998, 1999b) and provided the data on which the original risk assessments were based (Det Norske Veritas for the UK Department of Health, 2003). The second set of studies was carried out in hamsters infected with the 263K strain of scrapie and has led to a review of blood infectivity assumptions (Gregori et al., 2004; Spongiform Encephalopathy Advisory Committee, 2006). The transmission of prion infection by blood components drawn from donor sheep during both the incubation period and clinical phase of disease has been demonstrated in two different model systems using mice and sheep recipients (Houston et al., 2000, 2008; Hunter and Houston, 2002; Andreoletti et al., 2012).

In humans the data on peripheral blood infectivity in sporadic and familial CJD are open to interpretation (Brown et al., 1994), though recent data suggests that infectivity can be detected in the peripheral blood of patients with variant CJD using transgenic mice overexpressing bovine PrP (Douet et al., 2014).

The spatial distribution of infectivity also varies between models. Brown et al. (1998, 1999) mimicked to a certain extent clinical blood separation processes and demonstrated a four- to fivefold higher concentration of infectivity in the buffy coat (per unit volume) compared to plasma. Gregori et al. (2004) studied purified blood components and concluded that red cells and platelets have very little infectivity, and that approximately 40% of infectivity is associated with leukocytes, with most of the remainder residing within the plasma. In contrast, the studies in sheep (Houston et al., 2000, 2008; Hunter and Houston, 2002; Andreoletti et al., 2012) and in humans (Holada et al., 2002) described above suggest that infection can be transmitted by all blood components.

The temporal development of infectivity in peripheral tissues during the incubation period is similarly uncertain. In rodent models, a variety of patterns of change in infectivity and PrP^{TSE} concentration have been observed (Casaccia et al., 1989; Saa et al., 2006; Gregori et al., 2011). In humans, the pattern of development of infectivity in peripheral blood and tissues during CJD infection is unknown, although, as noted previously, abnormal PrP has been detected in an appendix sample removed 2 years before development of clinical variant CJD.

Clinical transmissibility of CJD by blood components and plasma products

Although there are a small number of reports of patients who have developed sporadic CJD following exposure to blood components (Klein and Dumble, 1993; Bennett and Daraktchiev, 2013), plasma derivatives (Creange et al., 1995, 1996; de Silva, 1996; Patry et al., 1998), or organ transplantation (Creange et al., 1995), these reports have not established a convincing link with sporadic CJD in the donors. To the contrary, a large number of epidemiologic case–control (Kondo and Kuroiwa, 1982; Davanipour et al., 1985; Harries-Jones et al., 1988; Esmonde et al., 1993; Wientjens et al., 1996; van Duijn et al., 1998; Will et al., 1998; Colins et al., 1999; Wilson et al., 2000; Zerr et al., 2000), look-back (Heye et al., 1994; Riggs et al., 2001), and surveillance (Brown, 1995; Operskalski and Mosley, 1995; Evatt, 1998; Evatt et al., 1998; Lee et al., 1998) studies over the past 35 years have demonstrated no clear evidence of transmission of sporadic CJD by blood transfusion or plasma derivatives. It should be borne in mind, however, that CJD is a rare disease and some cases of transmission by blood components or plasma products could have been missed if a detailed medical history and lookback to original donors were not undertaken.

In the United Kingdom, the Transfusion Medicine Epidemiology Review was established in 1996 in order to monitor potential linkage between CJD in donors and recipients (Hewitt et al., 2006). Individuals who develop CJD are reported to the UK Blood Services by the National CJD Research and Surveillance Unit (NCJD-RSU) to establish whether they have previously been blood donors. If they have been donors, the recipients are traced and notified. In the reverse arm, NCJD-RSU determines whether individuals who have developed CJD have themselves received blood. If they have been transfusion recipients, the UK Blood Services trace and notify the donors. Individuals identified in this way are considered to be "at risk for public health purposes" (Health Protection Agency, 2007). There are clear ethical and social tensions in adopting a notification strategy when the level of risk is uncertain, psychologic and social detriment may ensue, and no practical benefit accrues to the notified individuals (Boixiere et al., 2004; Hewitt, 2004). No direct linkage has been identified between donors and recipients with sporadic or familial CJD in this study; however, it has recently been reported that 2 patients with an extended history of treatment with clotting factors (one with hemophilia B and one with von Willebrand disease) developed sporadic CJD (Unwin et al., 2017). The authors comment that no causal link has been demonstrated between the treatment with plasma products and the occurrence of CJD, and this might reflect a chance event in the context for systematic surveillance in large populations.

Eighteen UK blood donors have gone on to develop variant CJD and, of their 66 traceable recipients (26 of whom are informative in the sense of having survived more than 5 years after transfusion), 3 have developed variant CJD and 1 showed evidence of subclinical infection at postmortem examination (having died of an unrelated condition) (Llewelyn et al., 2004; Peden et al., 2004; Wilson and Ricketts, 2006; Wroe et al., 2006). In France, 3 blood donors have developed variant CJD, although of their 18 traceable recipients, none has developed variant CJD at the time of writing.

Eleven of the above-noted UK blood donors also contributed 25 plasma donations to pools, from which a total of 178 plasma batches were manufactured before the United Kingdom began importing plasma in 1999. No recipients of implicated products have thus far developed clinical variant CJD – although 1 patient with hemophilia showed evidence of subclinical infection at postmortem, having died of other causes. Again, following risk assessment, many of these people are now regarded as "potentially at risk for public health purposes" (Bird, 2004).

APPROACHES TO RISK MANAGEMENT

In the face of the uncertainties in risk assessment, a precautionary set of assumptions is that, whilst there is little current evidence that sporadic CJD is transmitted by blood components or plasma products, it is likely that there exists a proportion of healthy people with subclinical variant CJD in the United Kingdom and other Western European countries, that infectivity is present in the peripheral blood of at least some of these individuals, and that transmission of disease is possible through blood and plasma products, though the precise magnitude of this risk is unclear. The best risk management approaches are those that are likely to have some benefit over the widest range of plausible scenarios. However, the effectiveness of such precautionary strategies may be partial or unknown and the potential for risk substitution and ethical dilemma needs to be considered.

Donor selection

Individuals with evidence of dementia or neurodegenerative disease should be excluded from blood and plasma donation on precautionary grounds. Similarly, potential donors should be excluded if they have been diagnosed as at risk of familial CJD by genetic testing, have two or more close relatives with CJD but have not themselves been genetically tested, or have undergone procedures known to pose a risk of iatrogenic transmission of CJD such as neurosurgery, or have received dura mater grafts or cadaveric pituitary hormones in the past.

Residence in the United Kingdom (and, to a lesser extent, Ireland and France) is clearly a risk factor for variant CJD and many countries exclude prospective blood donors who have lived in these countries (Ault, 1999). The stipulated period of residence varies widely, depending on the negative impact on the blood donor base and the perceived differential risk (Ponte, 2006). UK donors no longer donate plasma for manufacture of fractionated products. It has proved more difficult to delineate subpopulations who may be considered to be at higher risk of subclinical variant CJD than the general population. Individuals considered to be "presumed infected" or "at risk for public health purposes," due to exposure to an increased risk of variant CJD transmission through surgery, blood, or plasma products, are excluded from blood and plasma donation (Health Protection Agency, 2007).

Although blood transfusion in and of itself was thought unlikely to give rise to a self-sustaining outbreak, it was thought possible that transfusion in combination with other potential routes of transmission such as surgical or invasive medical procedures could result in such an event. Confirmation of clinical transmission of variant CJD via blood transfusion led to the introduction of deferral of donors in the United Kingdom who themselves have received blood components in order to reduce the risk of tertiary and higher-order transmissions, at the cost of a 5–10% loss in blood donations. However, surveys have documented considerable inconsistency in donor recall of blood transfusion, undermining confidence in the effectiveness of such measures. Donor exclusion criteria are blunt risk management tools that have the potential for significant negative impact on individual donors and on the blood and plasma supply for uncertain gain.

Donor screening assays

The development of peripheral blood assays aimed at the detection of subclinical CJD in donor populations is hampered by the absence of an antibody response or of detectable DNA associated with transmission of the infectious agent.

PrP^{TSE} detection remains the most promising route to development of a preclinical screening assay (Brown and Cervenakova, 2004; Cervenakova and Brown, 2004), despite caveats about the precise relationship with infectivity. Achieving the required levels of sensitivity and specificity has, however, proved to be a major challenge. It has been estimated that the threshold of detection may need to be as low as 10^6 molecules of PrP^{TSE}/mL in peripheral blood (Brown et al., 2001). Immunoblotting with proteinase K digestion and gel electrophoresis has been enhanced using phosphotungstic acid precipitation and chemiluminescence (Wadsworth et al., 2001), but is insufficiently sensitive to detect PrP^{TSE} in blood. Capillary immunoelectrophoresis following proteinase K digestion and competitive antibody binding was the first method to describe detection of PrP^{TSE} in blood (Schmerr et al., 1999), but proved complex and difficult to reproduce in other laboratories (Cervenakova et al., 2003). A number of attempts have now been made to move away from the use of proteinase K resistance as the defining principle (Minor and Brown, 2006).

Several assays use denaturation of PrP^{TSE} aggregates, the best characterized of which is the conformation-dependent immunoassay (Bellon et al., 2003)). A number of PrP^{TSE}-specific monoclonal antibodies have now been described, of which 15B3 is the best characterized (Korth et al., 1997). Several groups have developed assays predicated on differential binding of other ligands, including polyanionic compounds, synthetic polypeptides, streptomycin/calyx-6-arene, and palindromic peptides (Lane et al., 2003; Grosset et al., 2005). Some of these approaches have shown sufficient sensitivity to detect infectivity in the peripheral blood of prion-infected animals.

The Medical Research Council Prion Unit in London has developed a solid-state binding matrix to capture and concentrate PrP^{TSE} and coupled this to direct immunodetection of surface-bound material. The resultant assay has proved to be highly sensitive and capable of detecting PrP^{TSE} in the peripheral blood of just over 70% of patients with clinical variant CJD (Edgeworth et al., 2011), with acceptable specificity in normal controls (Jackson et al., 2014). Whether the failure to detect PrP^{TSE} in 30% of patients with clinical disease reflects insufficient sensitivity or an absence of abnormal prion in the blood and lymphoreticular tissue of some individuals is currently unclear (Mead et al., 2014).

Finally, three approaches appear to amplify PrP^{TSE} and/or infectivity. Protein folding cyclic amplification uses repeated cycles of incubation and sonication to amplify PrP^{TSE} up to 10^7-fold, whereas real-time quaking-induced conversion measures the rate of formation of amyloid fibrils (Henderson et al., 2014). In vitro cell culture has also proved capable of amplifying murine scrapie (Nishida et al., 2000). Protein folding cyclic amplification has proved particularly promising, with two recent papers demonstrating ability to detect PrP^{TSE} in the peripheral blood of patients in both the clinical and preclinical phases of variant CJD (Bougard et al., 2016; Concha-Marambio et al., 2016).

There is however a number of key concerns relating to the introduction of such assays to routine donor screening:

1. The specificity of an assay is dependent not only on its technical properties, but also on the population in which it is deployed. An assay with a satisfactory positive predictive value in the context of patients with suspect disease may have a very poor positive predictive value in the context of general population screening. There is therefore a clear need for a primary screening assay of high specificity, but also for confirmatory assays employing different analytical principles, to help sort the true from the false positives.
2. The validation of such assays is problematic (Minor, 2004a, b; Minor et al., 2004). The standard approach to validation of microbiologic screening assays uses large numbers of samples from patients known to have the disease in question. Patients with variant CJD in particular are fortunately now very rare, there being nobody alive with the disease at the time of writing. The development of peripheral blood screening assays has therefore had to be carried

out on spiked brain homogenates and endogenously infected animal models, with only final validation carried out on very small numbers of available human peripheral blood samples raising concerns around the generalization of the data to the broader population.

3. Consideration will need to be given to the impact of introduction of a screening assay on donors. There are likely to be difficulties in the discrimination of false from true positives and, indeed, in understanding the "meaning" of a true-positive result in terms of the implications for the donor. Donors will have to be informed that they will be screened and notified of any positive result. The psychologic and social impact on the individual is likely to be high and the negative impact on the blood supply could be profound (Blajchman et al., 2004; McCullough et al., 2004; Duncan et al., 2005).

Blood component processing

Whole blood is now rarely transfused, the majority of components being derived from whole-blood donation and processed into red cell concentrate (in additive solution), platelet concentrate, and fresh frozen plasma or in some cases collected via apheresis. In addition, in the United Kingdom, Ireland, France, and some other countries, all clinical blood components are subject to universal leukocyte reduction, which removes 3–4 $\log_{10}$ leukocytes (Kleinman, 1999; Murphy, 1999; St. Romaine et al., 2004). The rodent studies of Brown et al. (1998, 1999b) and Gregori et al. (2004) and the sheep studies of Houston et al. (2000, 2008) and Andreoletti et al. (2012) suggest that it is likely that component processing brings about some reduction in overall infectivity because of reduction in the amount of residual leukocytes and plasma. The four transmissions of variant CJD by blood components in the United Kingdom, described above, occurred prior to the introduction of universal leucodepletion and probably from an older form of red cell product containing more plasma. It is thought probable, therefore, that universal leucodepletion has had some mitigating impact on the risk of transmission of variant CJD by blood components.

Several companies have worked on the development of prion reduction filters for red cell components that offer the possibility of a further reduction in infectivity (Gregori et al., 2006; Sowemimo-Coker et al., 2006). There are concerns around the evaluation of the efficacy of these technologies given that they have been developed using spiked brain homogenates and endogenous infectivity animal models. Potential detrimental effects include additional blood loss in the dead volume of the filter and the possibility of alterations to red cell antigenicity or membrane properties. Cost-effectiveness of these technologies has also proved challenging and thus far no blood service has adopted them into routine practice.

Plasma product manufacture

It is unlikely that the virus inactivation steps used in the manufacture of plasma products will have a significant impact on prion infectivity (Taylor, 2003). However, work based on consideration of the likely physicochemical characteristics of the prion agent and the partitioning effects of the plasma fractionation process suggests that a significant reduction in infectivity may occur during manufacture, resulting in a relatively low risk of transmission by plasma products (Foster, 2004). Studies of spiked brain homogenates support this prediction, but are unlikely to accurately reflect the physicochemical nature of the infectious agent in plasma (Reichl et al., 2002; Stenland et al., 2002; Foster et al., 2004; Berardi et al., 2006). A smaller number of endogenous infectivity studies have been carried out in animal models that again support the general premise, but are unable to demonstrate more than a 1–2-log reduction because of low concentrations of infectivity in the starting material. Several manufacturers are using nanofiltration as a second virus reduction step, and these filters have, at least experimentally, demonstrated prion removal, mainly using brain homogenate spikes. One manufacturer has introduced a prion-binding affinity chromatography system as a risk reduction measure in solvent detergent-treated plasma. There has been no documented case of transmission of sporadic CJD by plasma derivatives. Surveillance of patients exposed to large volumes of plasma products has shown 1 patient with hemophilia who showed evidence of abnormal prion accumulation in the spleen on postmortem, having died of unrelated cause. Most individuals exposed to large volumes of plasma products are considered to be "potentially at risk for public health purposes" (Caulfield et al., 1997).

ETHICAL, LEGAL, AND SOCIETAL CONSIDERATIONS

Many of the issues raised above pose not only scientific and medical challenges, but also wider ethical, legal, and societal questions. Early uncertainty over the possibility of secondary transmission of CJD by blood transfusion or plasma derivatives led to the implementation of risk management strategies based on the precautionary principle, perhaps best articulated by the Krever Commission in Canada (Krever, 1997; Wilson et al., 2007):

> *Preventive action should be taken when there is evidence that a potentially disease-causing agent is or may be blood borne, even when there is no evidence that recipients have been affected.*

If harm can occur, it should be assumed that it will occur. If there are no measures that will entirely prevent the harm, measures that may only partially prevent transmission should be taken.

The evidence which emerged suggesting the existence of a cohort of individuals subclinically infected with variant CJD, along with the reports of clinical transmission by blood transfusion in 2004 and 2006, reinforced a precautionary stance at that time. However, the reduction in the number of new cases of BSE and variant CJD over the past few years, along with the absence to date of evidence of new cases of transmission of CJD by blood or plasma products, has led to a re-evaluation of the risk assessments in recent years. Important uncertainties persist around the prevalence and nature of subclinical infection in various forms of human prion disease and the effectiveness of current risk reduction measures, including donor selection procedures, component processing, and plasma fractionation.

Whilst the introduction of prion screening assays would help to clarify some aspects of the risk assessment and provide an added level of surety, such a measure would not be without potential countervailing risks and ethical problems (Childress and Beauchamp, 2001). The introduction of a donor screening assay could have a serious impact on the psychologic health of individuals who test positive, leading to difficulties in balancing nonmalfeasance with regard to the patient against nonmalfeasance with regard to the donor, and could have a serious negative impact on the sufficiency of blood and plasma supply (Sandler, 2006). Finally, the cost-effectiveness of additional measures such as donor screening will need to be evaluated in these times of constrained healthcare budgets.

As ever, the human prion diseases provide not just scientific and medical challenges, but profound ethical and policy dilemmas in the face of continuing uncertainty.

References

Advisory Committee on Dangerous Pathogens (ACDP) TSE Risk Assessment Subgroup (2012). Position statement on occurrence of vCJD and prevalence of infection in the UK population. http://media.dh.gov.uk/network/261/files/2012/08/ACDP-statement-vCJD-occurrence-and-prevalence-Jul-2012.pdf.

Aguzzi A, Glatzel M (2006). Prion infections, blood and transfusions. Nat Clin Pract Neurol 2: 321.

Andreoletti O, Litaise C, Simmons H et al. (2012). Highly efficient prion transmission by blood transfusion. PLoS Pathog 8: e1002782.

Ault A (1999). FDA bans UK blood donation. Nat Med 5: 720.

Bellon A, Seyfert-Brandt W, Lang W et al. (2003). Improved conformationdependent immunoassay: suitability for human prion detection with enhanced sensitivity. J Gen Virol 84: 1921–1925.

Bennett P, Daraktchiev M (2013). vCJD and transfusion of blood components: an updated risk assessment, Department of Health, London.

Berardi VA, Cardone F, Valanzano A et al. (2006). Preparation of soluble infectious samples from scrapie-infected brain: a new tool to study the clearance of transmissible spongiform encephalopathy agents during plasma fractionation. Transfusion 46: 652–658.

Bird SM (2004). Recipients of blood or blood products "at vCJD risk". Br Med J 328: 118–119.

Bishop MT, Hart P, Aitchison L et al. (2006). Predicting susceptibility and incubation time of human-to-human transmission of vCJD. Lancet Neurol 5: 393–398.

Blajchman MA, Goldman M, Webert KE et al. (2004). Proceedings of a consensus conference: the screening of blood donors for variant CJD. Transfus Med Rev 18: 73–92.

Boelle PY, Cesbron JY, Valleron AJ (2004). Epidemiological evidence of higher susceptibility to vCJD in the young. BMC Infect Dis 4: 26.

Boixiere A, Hergon E, Duchange N et al. (2004). Informing the transfused patient of the possible transmission of variant Creutzfeldt–Jakob disease by blood transfusion. Presse Med 33: 1533–1537.

Bougard D, Brandel J-P, Belondrade M et al. (2016). Detection of prions in the plasma of presymptomatic and symptomatic patients with variant Creutfeldt-Jakob disease. Sci Transl Med 8: 370ra182.

Brown P (1995). Can Creutzfeldt–Jakob disease be transmitted by transfusion? Curr Opin Hematol 2: 472–477.

Brown P, Cervenakova L (2004). The modern landscape of transfusion related iatrogenic Creutzfeldt–Jakob disease and blood screening tests. Curr Opin Hematol 11: 351–356.

Brown P, Gibbs Jr CJ, Rodgers-Johnson P et al. (1994). Human spongiform encephalopathy: the National Institutes of Health series of 300 cases of experimentally transmitted disease. Ann Neurol 35: 513–529.

Brown P, Rohwer RG, Dunstan BC et al. (1998). The distribution of infectivity in blood components and plasma derivatives in experimental models of transmissible spongiform encephalopathy. Transfusion 38: 810–816.

Brown KL, Stewart K, Ritchie DL et al. (1999a). Scrapie replication in lymphoid tissues depends on prion protein-expressing follicular dendritic cells. Nat Med 5: 1308–1312.

Brown P, Cervenakova L, McShane LM et al. (1999b). Further studies of blood infectivity in an experimental model of transmissible spongiform encephalopathy, with an explanation of why blood components do not transmit Creutzfeldt–Jakob disease in humans. Transfusion 39: 1169–1178.

Brown P, Cervenakova L, Diringer H (2001). Blood infectivity and the prospects for a diagnostic screening test in Creutzfeldt–Jakob disease. J Lab Clin Med 137: 5–13.

Bruce ME, Brown KL, Mabbott NA et al. (2000). Follicular dendritic cells in TSE pathogenesis. Immunol Today 21: 442–446.

Burthem J, Roberts DJ (2003). The pathophysiology of variant Creutzfeldt-Jacob disease: the hypotheses behind concerns for blood components and products. Br J Haematol 122: 3–9.

Casaccia P, Ladogana A, Xi YG et al. (1989). Levels of infectivity in the blood throughout the incubation period of hamsters peripherally injected with scrapie. Arch Virol 108: 145–149.

Caulfield T, Dossetor J, Boshkov L et al. (1997). Notifying patients exposed to blood products associated with Creutzfeldt–Jakob disease: integrating science, legal duties and ethical mandates. CMAJ 157: 1389–1392.

Cervenakova L, Brown P (2004). Advances in screening test development for transmissible spongiform encephalopathies. Expert Rev Anti-Infect Ther 2: 873–880.

Cervenakova L, Brown P, Soukharev S et al. (2003). Failure of immunocompetitive capillary electrophoresis assay to detect disease-specific prion protein in buffy coat from humans and chimpanzees with Creutzfeldt–Jakob disease. Electrophoresis 24: 853–859.

Childress JF, Beauchamp TL (2001). Principles of biomedical ethics, 5th edn. Oxford University Press, Oxford.

Clarke P, Ghani AC (2005). Projections of the future course of the primary vCJD epidemic in the UK: inclusion of subclinical infection and the possibility of wider genetic susceptibility. J R Soc Interface 2: 19–31.

Concha-Marambio L, Pritzkow S, Moda F et al. (2016). Detection of prions in blood from patients with variant Creutzfeldt–Jakob disease. Sci Transl Med 8: 370ra183.

Cooper JD, Bird SM (2003). Predicting the incidence of variant Creutzfeldt–Jakob disease from UK dietary exposure to bovine spongiform encephalopathy for the 1940 to 1969 and post-1969 birth cohorts. Int J Epidemiol 32: 784–791.

Cooper JD, Bird SM, de Angelis D (2000). Prevalence of detectable abnormal prion protein in persons incubating vCJD: Plausible incubation periods and cautious inference. J Epidemiol Biostat 5: 209–219.

Creange A, Gray F, Cesaro P et al. (1995). Creutzfeldt–Jakob disease after liver transplantation. Ann Neurol 38: 269–272.

Creange A, Gray F, Cesaro P et al. (1996). Pooled plasma derivatives and Creutzfeldt–Jakob disease (letter). Lancet 347: 482.

Davanipour Z, Alter M, Sobel E et al. (1985). A case-control study of Creutzfeldt–Jakob disease. Dietary risk factors. Am J Epidemiol 122: 443–451.

de Silva R (1996). Pooled plasma derivatives and Creutzfeldt–Jakob disease (letter). Lancet 347: 967.

Det Norske Veritas for the Department of Health (UK) (2003). Risk assessment of exposure to vCJD infectivity in blood and blood products, DNV Consulting, London. Available at http://www.dnv.com/binaries/vCJD_Update_Report_tcm4-74414.pdf.

Douet JY, Zafar S, Perret-Liaudet A et al. (2014). Detection of infecivity in the blood of persons with variant and sporadic Creutzfeldt–Jakob disease. Emerg Infect Dis 20 (1).

Duncan RE, Delatycki MB, Collins SJ et al. (2005). Ethical considerations in presymptomatic testing for variant CJD. J Med Ethics 31: 625–630.

Edgeworth JA, Farmer M, Sicilia A et al. (2011). Detection of prion infection in variant Cruetfeldt-Jakob disease: a blood based assay. Lancet 377: 487–493.

Esmonde TF, Will RG, Slattery JM et al. (1993). Creutzfeldt–Jakob disease and blood transfusion. Lancet 341: 205–207.

Evatt B (1998). Prions and haemophilia: assessment of risk. Haemophilia 4: 628–633.

Evatt B, Austin H, Barnhart E et al. (1998). Surveillance for Creutzfeldt–Jakob disease among persons with hemophilia. Transfusion 38: 817–820.

Foster PR (2004). Removal of TSE agents from blood products. Vox Sang 87 (suppl 2): 7–10.

Foster PR, Griffin BD, Bienek C et al. (2004). Distribution of a bovine spongiform encephalopathy-derived agent over ion-exchange chromatography used in the preparation of concentrates of fibrinogen and factor VIII. Vox Sang 86: 92–99.

Frosh A, Smith LC, Jackson CJ et al. (2004). Analysis of 2000 consecutive UK tonsillectomy specimens for disease-related prion protein. Lancet 364: 1260–1262.

Gill ON, Spencer Y, Richard-Loendt A et al. (2013). Prevalent abnormal prion protein in human appendixes after bovine spongiform encephalopathy epizootic: large scale survey. BMJ 347. https://doi.org/10.1136/bmj.f5675.

Gregori L, McCombie N, Palmer D et al. (2004). Effectiveness of leucoreduction for removal of infectivity of transmissible spongiform encephalopathies from blood. Lancet 364: 529–531.

Gregori L, Gurgel PV, Lathrop JT et al. (2006). Reduction in infectivity of endogenous transmissible spongiform encephalopathies present in blood by adsorption to selective affinity resins. Lancet 368: 2226–2230.

Gregori L, Yang H, Anderson S (2011). Estimation of variant Creutzfeldt–Jakob disease infectivity titres in human blood. Transfusion. https://doi.org/10.1111/j.1537-2995.2011.03199x.

Grosset A, Moskowitz K, Nelsen C et al. (2005). Rapid presymptomatic detection of PrP via conformationally responsive palindromic PrP peptides. Peptides 26: 2193–2200.

Harries-Jones R, Knight R, Will RG et al. (1988). Creutzfeldt–Jakob disease in England and Wales, 1980-1984: a case-control study of potential risk factors. J Neurol Neurosurg Psychiatry 51: 1113–1119.

Head MW, Bunn TJ, Bishop MT et al. (2004). Prion protein heterogeneity in sporadic but not variant Creutzfeldt–Jakob disease: UK cases 1991-2002. Ann Neurol 55: 851–859.

Health Protection Agency (2007). Creutzfeldt–Jakob disease (CJD), HPA, London. Available at http://www.hpa.org.uk.

Henderson DM, Davenport KA, Haley NJ et al. (2014). Quantitative assessment of prion infectivity in tissues and body fluids by RT-QuIC. J Gen Virol. https://doi.org/10.1099/vir.0069906-0.

Hewitt PE (2004). Implications of notifying donors and recipients. Vox Sang 87 (Suppl 2): 1–2.

Hewitt P, Llewelyn CA, Mackenzie J et al. (2006). Creutzfeldt–Jakob disease and blood transfusion: results of the UK Transfusion Medicine Epidemiology Review study. Vox Sang 91: 221–230.

Heye N, Hensen S, Muller N (1994). Creutzfeldt–Jakob disease and blood transfusion. Lancet 343: 298–299.

Hill AF, Collinge J (2003a). Subclinical prion infection in humans and animals. Br Med Bull 66: 161–170.

Hill AF, Collinge J (2003b). Subclinical prion infection. Trends Microbiol 11: 578–584.

Hilton DA, Ghani AC, Conyers L et al. (2002). Accumulation of prion protein in tonsil and appendix: review of tissue samples. Br Med J 325: 633–634.

Hilton DA, Ghani AC, Conyers L et al. (2004a). Prevalence of lymphoreticular prion protein accumulation in UK tissue samples. J Pathol 203: 733–739.

Hilton DA, Sutak J, Smith ME et al. (2004b). Specificity of lymphoreticular accumulation of prion protein for variant Creutzfeldt–Jakob disease. J Clin Pathol 57: 300–302.

Holada K, Vostal JG, Theisen PW et al. (2002). Scrapie infectivity in hamster blood is not associated with platelets. J Virol 76: 4649–4650.

Houston F, Foster JD, Chong A et al. (2000). Transmission of BSE by blood transfusion in sheep. Lancet 356: 999–1000.

Houston F, McCutcheon S, Goldman W et al. (2008). Prion diseases are efficiently transmitted by sheep. Blood 112: 4739–4745.

Hunter N, Houston F (2002). Can prion diseases be transmitted between individuals via blood transfusion? Evidence from sheep experiments. Dev Biol (Basel) 108: 93–98.

Ironside JW, Hilton DA, Ghani A et al. (2000). Retrospective study of prion-protein accumulation in tonsil and appendix tissues. Lancet 355: 1693–1694.

Ironside JW, Bishop MT, Connolly K et al. (2006). Variant Creutzfeldt–Jakob disease: prion protein genotype analysis of positive appendix tissue samples from a retrospective prevalence study. Br Med J 332: 1186–1188.

Jackson GS, Burk-Rafel J, Edgeworth JA et al. (2014). Population screening for variant Creutfeldt-Jakob disesae using a novel blood test: diagnostic accuracy and feasibility study. JAMA Neurol 71: 421–428.

Klein R, Dumble LJ (1993). Transmission of Creutzfeldt–Jakob disease by blood transfusion (letter). Lancet 341: 768.

Klein MA, Frigg R, Raeber AJ et al. (1998). PrP expression in B lymphocytes is not required for prion neuroinvasion. Nat Med 4: 1429–1433.

Kleinman S (1999). New variant Creutzfeldt–Jakob disease and white cell reduction: risk assessment and decision making in the absence of data. Transfusion 39: 920–924.

Kondo K, Kuroiwa Y (1982). A case control study of Creutzfeldt–Jakob disease: Association with physical injuries. Ann Neurol 11: 377–381.

Korth C, Stierli B, Streit P et al. (1997). Prion (PrPSc)-specific epitope defined by a monoclonal antibody. Nature 390: 74–77.

Krever H (1997). Commission of inquiry on the blood system in Canada, Health Canada, Ottawa, Ontario, Canada. 1997. Available at http://www.hc-sc.gc.ca/ahc-asc/activit/com.krever_e.html. Accessed 16 May 2008.

Lane A, Stanley CJ, Dealer S et al. (2003). Polymeric ligands with specificity for aggregated prion protein (abstract). Clin Chem 49: 1774–1775.

Lee CA, Ironside JW, Bell JE et al. (1998). Retrospective neuropathological review of prion disease in UK haemophilic patients. Thromb Haemost 80: 909–911.

Llewelyn CA, Hewitt PE, Knight RS et al. (2004). Possible transmission of variant Creutzfeldt–Jakob disease by blood transfusion. Lancet 363: 417–421.

Mabbott N, Turner M (2005). Prions and the blood and immune systems. Haematologica 90: 542–548.

McCullough J, Anderson D, Brookie D et al. (2004). Consensus conference on vCJD screening of blood donors: report of the panel. Transfusion 44: 675–683.

Mead S, Wadsworth JD, Porter MC et al. (2014). Variant Creutzfeldt–Jakob disease with extremely low lymphoreticular deposition of prion protein. JAMA Neurol 71: 340–343.

Minor PD (2004a). Technical aspects of the development and validation of tests for variant Creutzfeldt–Jakob disease in blood transfusion. Vox Sang 86: 164–170.

Minor PD (2004b). The challenge for the public health system. Contrib Microbiol 11: 208–215.

Minor P (2006). Brown P (2006) Diagnostic tests for antemortem screening of Creutzfeldt–Jakob disease. In: ML Turner (Ed.), Creutzfeldt–Jakob disease: managing the risk of transmission by blood, plasma, and tissues. AABB Press, Bethesda, MD, pp. 119–148.

Minor P, Newham J, Jones N et al. (2004). Standards for the assay of Creutzfeldt–Jakob disease specimens. J Gen Virol 85: 1777–1784.

Mok T, Jaunmuktane Z, Joiner S et al. (2017). Variant Creutzfeldt–Jakob disease in a patient with heterozygosity at PRNP codon 129. N Engl J Med 376: 292–294.

Montrasio F, Cozzio A, Flechsig E et al. (2001). B lymphocyte-restricted expression of prion protein does not enable prion replication in prion protein knockout mice. Proc Natl Acad Sci U S A 98: 4034–4037.

Murphy MF (1999). New variant Creutzfeldt–Jakob disease (nvCJD): the risk of transmission by blood transfusion and the potential benefit of leukocyte-reduction of blood components. Transfus Med Rev 13: 75–83.

Nishida N, Harris DA, Vilette D et al. (2000). Successful transmission of three mouse adapted scrapie strains to murine neuroblastoma cell lines over-expressing wild-type mouse prion protein. J Virol 74: 320–325.

Operskalski EA, Mosley JW (1995). Pooled plasma derivatives and Creutzfeldt–Jakob disease (letter). Lancet 346: 1224.

Patry D, Curry B, Easton D et al. (1998). Creutzfeldt–Jakob disease (CJD) after blood product transfusion from a donor with CJD. Neurology 50: 1872–1873.

Peden AH, Head MW, Ritchie DL et al. (2004). Preclinical vCJD after blood transfusion in a PRNP codon 129 heterozygous patient. Lancet 364: 527–529.

Ponte M (2006). Insights into the management of emerging infections: Regulating variant Creutzfeldt–Jakob disease transfusion risk in the UK and the US. PLoS Med 3: e342.

Reichl HE, Foster PR, Welch AG et al. (2002). Studies on the removal of a bovine spongiform encephalopathy-derived agent by processes used in the manufacture of human immunoglobulin. Vox Sang 83: 137–145.

Riggs JE, Moudgil SS, Hobbs GR (2001). Creutzfeldt–Jakob disease and blood transfusions: a meta-analysis of case-control studies. Mil Med 166: 1057–1058.

Saa P, Castilla J, Soto C (2006). Presymptomatic detection of prions in blood. Science 313: 92–94.

Sandler SG (2006). Variant Creutzfeldt–Jakob disease—the availability of a screening test will be the beginning, not the end, of difficult transfusion-related issues. Curr Opin Haematol 13: 445–446.

Schmerr MJ, Jenny AL, Bulgin MS et al. (1999). Use of capillary electrophoresis and fluorescent labeled peptides to detect the abnormal prion protein in the blood of animals that are infected with a transmissible spongiform encephalopathy. J Chromatogr A 853: 207–214.

Silveira JR, Raymond GJ, Hughson AG et al. (2005). The most infectious prion protein particles. Nature 437: 257–261.

Sowemimo-Coker SO, Pesci S, Andrade F et al. (2006). Pall leukotrap affinity prion-reduction filter removes exogenous infectious prions and endogenous infectivity from red cell concentrates. Vox Sang 90: 265–275.

Spongiform Encephalopathy Advisory Committee (SEAC) (2006). Position statement on TSE infectivity in blood, SEAC, London, UK, 2006. Available online at http://www.seac.gov.uk/statements/statement0806.htm.

St. Romaine C, Hazlehurst G, Jewell AP (2004). Leucodepletion for transmissible spongiform encephalopathies. Br J Biomed Sci 61: 48–54.

Stenland CJ, Lee DC, Brown P et al. (2002). Partitioning of human and sheep forms of the pathogenic prion protein during the purification of therapeutic proteins from human plasma. Transfusion 42: 1497–1500.

Taylor DM (2003). Inactivation of TSE agents: safety of blood and blood derived products. Transfus Clin Biol 10: 23–25.

National CJD Research and Surveillance Unit. 25th Annual Report (2016). Available online at: http://www.cjd.ed.ac.uk/documents/worldfigs.pdf.

Unwin P, Thaniqaikumar K, Molesworth A et al. (2017). Sporadic Creutzfeldt–Jakob disease in 2 plasma produce recipients, United Kingdom. Emerg Infect Dis 23: 893–897.

van Duijn CM, Delasnerie-Laupretre N, Masullo C et al. (1998). Casecontrol study of risk factors of Creutzfeldt–Jakob disease in Europe during 1993-95. European Union (EU) Collaborative Study Group of Creutzfeldt–Jakob disease (CJD). Lancet 351: 1081–1085.

Wadsworth JD, Joiner S, Hill AF et al. (2001). Tissue distribution of protease resistant prion protein in variant Creutzfeldt–Jakob disease using a highly sensitive immunoblotting assay. Lancet 358: 171–180.

Wadsworth JD, Asante EA, Desbruslais M et al. (2004). Human prion protein with valine 129 prevents expression of variant CJD phenotype. Science 306: 1793–1796.

Wientjens DP, Davanipour Z, Hofman A et al. (1996). Risk factors for Creutzfeldt–Jakob disease: a reanalysis of case-control studies. Neurology 46: 1287–1291.

Will R (2004). Variant Creutzfeldt–Jakob disease. Folia Neuropathol 42 (Suppl A): 77–83.

Will RG, Ironside JW, Zeidler M et al. (1996). A new variant of Creutzfeldt–Jakob disease in the UK. Lancet 347: 921–925.

Will RG, Alperovitch A, Poser S et al. (1998). Descriptive epidemiology of Creutzfeldt–Jakob disease in six European countries, 1993-1995. EU Collaborative Study Group for CJD. Ann Neurol 43: 763–767.

Wilson K, Ricketts MN (2004). Transfusion transmission of vCJD: a crisis avoided? Lancet 364: 477–479.

Wilson K, Ricketts MN (2006). A third episode of transfusion-derived vCJD. Lancet 368: 2037–2039.

Wilson K, Code C, Ricketts MN (2000). Risk of acquiring Creutzfeldt–Jakob disease from blood transfusions: systematic review of case-control studies. Br Med J 321: 17–19.

Wilson K, Graham I, Ricketts N et al. (2007). Variant Creutzfeldt–Jakob disease and the Canadian blood system after the tainted blood tragedy. Soc Sci Med 64: 174–185.

World Health Organization (2006). WHO guidelines on tissue infectivity distribution in transmissible spongiform encephalopathies, WHO, Geneva, Switzerland. Available online at http://www.who.int/bloodproducts/CS/TSEPUBLISHEDREPORT.pdf. Accessed 16 May 2008.

Wroe SJ, Pal S, Siddique D et al. (2006). Clinical presentation and pre-mortem diagnosis of variant Creutzfeldt–Jakob disease associated with blood transfusion: a case report. Lancet 368: 2061–2067.

Zerr I, Brandel JP, Masullo C et al. (2000). European surveillance on Creutzfeldt–Jakob disease: a case-control study for medical risk factors. J Clin Epidemiol 53: 747–754.

Handbook of Clinical Neurology, Vol. 153 (3rd series)
Human Prion Diseases
M. Pocchiari and J. Manson, Editors
https://doi.org/10.1016/B978-0-444-63945-5.00027-1

Chapter 27

Public health: surveillance, infection prevention, and control

HESTER WARD[1,2]*, ANNA MOLESWORTH[3], SULISTI HOLMES[1], AND KATY SINKA[4]

[1]*NHS National Services Scotland, Edinburgh, United Kingdom*

[2]*Usher Institute of Population Health Sciences and Informatics, University of Edinburgh, Edinburgh, United Kingdom*

[3]*National CJD Research and Surveillance Unit, Western General Hospital, Edinburgh, United Kingdom*

[4]*Centre for Infectious Disease Surveillance and Control, National Infection Service, Public Health England, London, United Kingdom*

Abstract

Human prion diseases, though relatively rare, remain an ongoing public health problem. They are fatal diseases, with unconventional host responses and no early diagnostic tests or robust treatments. Public health measures were put in place to protect the food chain in the United Kingdom from the late 1980s, with similar measures following elsewhere. However, human prion diseases are transmissible through other routes, including through blood transfusion and surgery. As a result, the public health threat remains for all forms of human prion diseases and makes continued surveillance and infection prevention and control imperative.

INTRODUCTION

In 1986 a new form of animal prion disease, bovine spongiform encephalopathy (BSE), was identified in the United Kingdom. This was the start of the BSE epidemic in which millions of cattle were slaughtered and over 400,000 infected cattle were estimated to have entered the human food chain, causing considerable concern regarding the risk of transmission to humans (Wilesmith et al., 1988; Anderson et al., 1996). Ten years later this concern was realized when variant Creutzfeldt–Jakob disease (vCJD) was first identified (Will et al., 1996) and subsequently linked to the zoonotic transmission of BSE (Collinge et al., 1996; Bruce et al., 1997; Hill et al., 1997; Scott et al., 1999), most likely through dietary consumption of contaminated beef products (Ward et al., 2006).

Human prion diseases, though relatively rare, remain an ongoing public health problem, even after the decline of the vCJD epidemic. They remain fatal diseases, with no known treatments or vaccinations. The results of UK prevalence studies have suggested asymptomatic carriage of the vCJD abnormal prion protein in the general population (Gill et al., 2013). Moreover, the host response is not conventional and to date there are no early diagnostic tests for prion diseases. Public health measures were put in place to protect the food chain in the United Kingdom from the late 1980s and similar measures followed for the rest of Europe. However, human prion diseases are transmissible through other routes, including through blood transfusion and surgery, with each of the different forms of the disease in humans having specific risk factors and degree of spread though the body, influencing the potential for onward transmission. As a result, the public health threat remains for all forms of human prion diseases and makes continued surveillance and infection prevention and control an imperative.

SURVEILLANCE OF HUMAN PRION DISEASE

The public health response to human prion disease requires timely and complete ascertainment of cases and a mechanism to mitigate against the risk of further

*Correspondence to: Hester J.T. Ward, BSc, MBBS, MRCP, FFPH, Information Services Division (ISD), NHS National Services Scotland, 1 South Gyle Crescent, Edinburgh EH12 9EB, United Kingdom. Tel: +44-131-275-6832, E-mail: hester.ward@nhs.net

spread. Key to this is surveillance of cases, in all their different forms, together with their risk factors, assessment of public health risk at the individual and population level, and the subsequent management of this risk.

Worldwide, a number of national and international initiatives undertake surveillance of prion disease. While systems vary in sophistication and accuracy between countries, case reporting to the European Centre for Disease Prevention and Control (ECDC) from national registers across Europe has enabled European-wide monitoring of prion disease and the EuroCJD Network has also facilitated international projects looking at risk factors for prion disease (http://www.eurocjd.ed.ac.uk/). Guidance is also available from the World Health Organization on the minimal requirements of an effective surveillance system (World Health Organization, 2003).

Case ascertainment

Surveillance of human prion disease requires clear definitions of the different forms of disease. The standard diagnosis of both variant and sporadic forms of CJD relies on a clinical diagnosis of a relatively rapidly progressing dementia with other neurologic features, supplemented by a range of investigations, principally cerebrospinal fluid-based tests and brain magnetic resonance imaging. The diagnosis is confirmed through postmortem pathologic investigations using standard histologic, immunohistochemical, and biochemical approaches to detect morphologic changes and the presence of abnormal prion protein in the brain and other body tissues peripheral to the central nervous system (http://www.cjd.ed.ac.uk/sites/default/files/criteria.pdf; World Health Organization, 2010). Genetic and iatrogenic forms of CJD also require a known genetic mutation or iatrogenic exposure, respectively. The identification of these may not be straightforward: genetic testing raises ethical concerns and issues for individuals and their families and as a result families frequently do not consent to be tested. Additionally, because of the rarity of the diseases and their long incubation periods, it can be difficult to determine if iatrogenic transmission has occurred.

From the clinician's perspective, it is important to distinguish between prion disease and other types of dementia, particularly because the latter may respond positively to treatment (Geschwind, 2016; Mead and Rudge, 2016). In the United Kingdom and a number of other countries, clinicians and pathologists are asked to refer patients with any suspicion of prion disease to the national surveillance center, which can provide a source of expertise in the diagnosis of a disease that is encountered infrequently at the local level, by offering further diagnostic advice and scrutiny.

From a surveillance perspective, the opportunity for clinicians to informally discuss any and all suspected cases helps case ascertainment and potentially the detection of new forms of disease that are atypical. This was how the first cases of vCJD were identified following the BSE epidemic, since they presented differently to the sporadic form of disease (Will et al., 1996). More recently, the identification of a new form of prion disease, variably proteinase-sensitive prionopathy, has been described, amongst cases previously considered to be sporadic, but with atypical clinical and pathologic characteristics (Head et al., 2009). Surveillance may also enable the future identification of atypical vCJD cases arising as a result of secondary transmission through blood (Davidson et al., 2014) or with different genotypic susceptibility to the BSE agent (d'Aignaux et al., 2001; Mok et al., 2017), as well as other atypical forms of prion disease linked to animal disease, such as chronic wasting disease, atypical BSE, or scrapie, should these diseases prove to be zoonotic (Barria et al., 2014).

In all forms of human prion disease, the diagnosis is principally neurologic and/or neuropathologic. However, the involvement of other specialties, particularly old age psychiatry and elderly (geriatric) medicine, may also be considered as a means of enhancing surveillance of prion disease. In these specialties older patients presenting with a dementing illness are common. Some may have features shared with prion disease, but clinicians' indepth knowledge of prion disease may be lacking or the diagnosis compounded by atypical presentation. Therefore, a diagnosis of prion disease may be delayed or missed (Bradford et al., 2009; Josephs et al., 2009; Karch et al., 2014; El Tawil et al., 2015; Staekenborg et al., 2016).

Case referrals may also be supplemented from other sources, for example, a retrospective review of death certificates in order to detect cases that might not otherwise have been reported.

Epidemiologic risk

Another function of surveillance is the identification and monitoring of epidemiologic risk factors. Not only is this important in order to understand the disease better, but it informs public health measures to prevent onward transmission. This involves the collection and scrutiny of detailed epidemiologic information about each case and then analysis and interpretation of risk at a population level. Although patients themselves are usually too unwell to answer questions, their relatives may be able to assist and further information can be obtained through reviewing medical notes, electronic health and imaging records, and death certificates.

A number of different approaches to epidemiologic investigation may be involved to ascertain risk factors.

Firstly, the space–time aggregation of cases can provide powerful circumstantial evidence that cases are linked through transmission of abnormal prion protein. This has been implicated for sporadic CJD (sCJD), for example, in those undergoing similar surgical procedures in the same hospital relatively close in time (Brown et al., 2012; Bonda et al., 2016). Even if the number of cases involved might be expected by chance alone, consideration may still be given to the further investigation of these associations in order to allay local concerns or identify an underlying public health risk (Monk and Bryant, 2001; Molesworth et al., 2010). Another approach taken involves lookback and tracing, where the contacts of an index case are identified and then investigated themselves, retrospectively or prospectively, for evidence of prion disease. In this way, for example, the reporting of prion disease to the UK national blood services has enabled the identification of links between those cases, who had been blood donors and the recipients of the associated products, and so the probable transmission of vCJD through blood transfusion (Llewelyn et al., 2004; Peden et al., 2004). In the United Kingdom, donors of blood to and recipients of blood from cases of prion disease continue to be investigated for evidence of prion disease (Hewitt et al., 2006; Urwin et al., 2016). Case–control studies have also been used to determine whole-population risk. While they have supported a dietary hypothesis for vCJD (Ward et al., 2006), a history of surgery or blood transfusion has been associated with risk for sCJD in some studies, but not all (de Pedro Cuesta et al., 2012).

PRION DISEASE AND PUBLIC HEALTH

Variant CJD

The occurrence of vCJD is linked primarily to the consumption of BSE-infected beef (Ward et al., 2006). At the time of writing, 231 cases of vCJD have been diagnosed in 12 countries worldwide since the disease was first reported in 1996. About 80% of these have occurred in the United Kingdom or in individuals who had a history of residing in the United Kingdom. France, which received beef exports from the United Kingdom during the BSE epidemic, is the next most affected country, with 12% of cases. No other country has reported more than 5 cases. Three diagnoses of vCJD, all from the United Kingdom, have been attributed to secondary transmission through blood transfusion.

Prevalence studies measuring the occurrence of abnormal prion deposition in archived appendix tissues from the age group most exposed to BSE in the United Kingdom (born 1941–1985) estimate the prevalence of abnormal prion deposition at 1:2000 (Gill et al., 2013). If this deposition is indeed linked to vCJD it is likely to be a consequence predominantly of dietary exposure to BSE, but also potentially from secondary exposure through blood transfusion or surgery. Transmission through blood transfusion or surgery may also be possible, including from individuals without clinical symptoms of vCJD, that is, asymptomatic carries of infection (Peden et al., 2004; Department of Health, 2005). Although recent cases of clinical vCJD have declined to low levels, there may yet be further cases in those with a long incubation period in genotypes other than MM at codon 129 (d'Aignaux et al., 2001; Mok et al., 2017).

Sporadic CJD

The most common clinical form of human prion disease is sCJD, sometimes referred to as classic CJD. Worldwide it occurs with an incidence of 1–2 cases per million population per year, affecting mostly older people aged 65 years and above. Idiopathic in origin, by definition, its occurrence is unpredictable; however, there is evidence that exposure to sCJD in medical settings has resulted in transmission from person to person due to accidental inoculation of prion-contaminated tissue (Brown et al., 2012; Bonda et al., 2016).

Genetic CJD

Overall 10–15% of human prion diseases can be attributed to a disease-specific mutation in the prion protein gene (*PRNP*). There are several different forms of genetic CJD and over 30 different mutations have been identified in families in several countries worldwide (Lee et al., 1999; World Health Organization, 2003; Mead, 2006). The inheritance is autosomal-dominant, resulting in children of an individual with the abnormal gene having a 50% chance of inheriting the abnormality. The age of onset and duration of disease vary depending on which mutation has been inherited. Although it has not been proven to date, it is assumed on a precautionary basis that exposure to abnormal prions in tissues of a patient with genetic CJD in the medical setting can result in transmission risk. Therefore, public health precautions are relevant for patients with diagnosed genetic CJD and extend to those individuals with no clinical symptoms who have a recognized risk of developing inherited prion disease later in life. This includes where genetic testing indicates the presence of a *PRNP* mutation, or a non-tested individual has a blood relative with a genetic mutation indicative of genetic CJD. In addition, because not everyone who carries a mutation will have undergone genetic testing, individuals will also be considered at risk of inherited prion disease if they have two or more blood relatives, diagnosed with CJD or other prion disease.

Iatrogenic CJD

Iatrogenic transmission of prion disease has been documented through several routes. More than 230 individuals worldwide have developed prion disease from treatment with pooled cadaveric pituitary-derived human growth hormone. Most cases occurred in France, the United Kingdom, and the United States, followed by New Zealand, but there have also been small numbers reported from five other countries (Brown et al., 2012; Bonda et al., 2016). The use of human growth hormone was stopped after the first cases of prion disease were recognized in 1985. The average incubation period observed is 17 years, but deaths from prion disease are still occurring among this group of individuals; the longest incubation period is reported to be 42 years. A small number of women, all treated in Australia, developed prion disease after treatment with pituitary-derived gonadotropin used for fertility treatment, the most recent occurring in 1995. The use of this product was discontinued during the 1970s and 1980s.

Individuals who have had certain kinds of surgery are at increased risk of developing prion disease. Those most affected have been recipients of contaminated dura mater grafts between 1969 and 1993. To date over 230 individuals from 19 different countries are known to have developed prion disease as a consequence (Brown et al., 2012; Bonda et al., 2016). The peak years of onset were during the 1990s; however, small numbers of cases continue to occur. More than 60% of affected patients were diagnosed in Japan (Brown et al., 2012; Hamaguchi et al., 2013), where both use of dura grafts in general and the use of the most implicated product, Lyodura, were more frequent than in other countries. The use of Lyodura reduced substantially after 1991, but may not have ceased completely until 1997.

Several instances of surgical transmission from an index patient with prion disease undiagnosed at time of surgery, either through transplantation of contaminated corneal tissues or reuse of contaminated neurosurgical instruments or stereotactic electroencephalogram electrodes, have been documented in the past (Brown et al., 2012). At the time of writing, there have been no new reports of surgical transmission through these routes for over 20 years.

RISK MANAGEMENT OF TRANSMISSION OF PRION DISEASE

Although iatrogenic transmission is unlikely to account for a high proportion of cases of human prion disease, the possibility of person-to-person spread requires control measures to mitigate against risk at the population level and in respect of any ongoing risk posed by an individual or his or her contacts. Underlying these issues is the current absence in routine practice of both an effective means of decontamination that can fully remove the prion agent from surgical instruments and a validated blood test suitable for the diagnosis of preclinical stages of disease or of subclinical carriage of abnormal prion protein in the general population.

Those at increased risk of prion disease

In some countries patients who are considered at increased risk of prion disease – genetic prion disease or through healthcare exposure, for example, treatment with human pituitary-derived growth hormone – are informed of this increased at-risk status and asked to carry out certain precautions for public health purposes to prevent potential onward transmission of prion disease.

In the United Kingdom people are notified of being "at increased risk for public health purposes" because of their family or medical history (Public Health England and Health Protection Scotland, 2015). The consideration to notify someone that s/he is at increased risk of prion disease is not taken lightly because of the ethical and practical issues surrounding it. The aim of notification is to inform the person of public health precautions that are required and to offer support. In the United Kingdom, those notified as at increased risk of prion disease are asked to not donate blood, cells, tissues, or organs, although individual assessment is recommended for life-saving hematopoietic stem cell and solid-organ transplantation/donation (SABTO, 2011). They are also asked to inform their family of their status and to notify their medical carers if undergoing medical or dental procedures (Public Health England and Health Protection Scotland, 2015). Usually, the risk of being infected is uncertain, but it is likely to be low. The primary (or secondary) care physician, in conjunction with public health colleagues, is usually best placed to inform the patient. The physician informing the patient is asked to record the at-risk status in the patient's medical records and to pass on this information if or when the person is referred for medical care.

Follow-up of those at increased risk of prion disease varies between countries in extent and methods used. The purpose is to increase epidemiologic understanding of prion disease and to ensure public health precautions are implemented. At-risk individuals are followed up through a combination of their care providers, national prion disease surveillance, or death registers. This helps to ascertain any surgical or other procedures they have undergone (to ensure appropriate controls were put in place), the occurrence of prion disease and, where available, the detection of abnormal prion at postmortem in peripheral tissues of patients with no neurologic features (asymptomatic carriers). Surgical instruments removed from use should either be destroyed or retained for exclusive use for that at-risk patient (following decontamination according to national standards) (see below).

Specific methods of follow-up include registers of patients who were treated with human growth hormone (US growth hormone register: https://www.niddk.nih.gov/health-information/health-topics/endocrine/national-hormone-pituitary-program/Pages/national-hormone-pituitary-program-comprehensive-report.aspx; Huillard d'Aignaux et al., 1999; Swerdlow et al., 2003), patients who have had surgical exposures to potentially contaminated instruments (Hamaguchi et al., 2009; Public Health England and Health Protection Scotland, 2015) and, in the United Kingdom, patients who have been treated with blood or blood products linked to a donor who later died from vCJD or pooled plasma products sourced from UK plasma during the 1990s (Hewitt et al., 2006; Zaman et al., 2011).

Public health organizations globally have developed guidelines and regulations for the management of patients with a clinical diagnosis of prion disease and for certain patients with an increased risk of developing prion disease, in order to prevent onward transmission in community and healthcare settings. The World Health Organization provides public health guidance (www.who.int/mediacentre/factsheets/fs180/en/) and there are risk reduction measures in the majority of European Economic Area countries (http://ecdc.europa.eu/en/publications/Publications/1106_TER_Review_of_guidelines_for_prevention_of%20CJD.pdf).

In the United Kingdom, a national CJD Incidents Panel was established to provide expert advice on public health risk prevention. Between 2000 and 2013 this panel developed UK guidance and set precedents for risk management decisions, which are still used today. Other countries have developed guidance on prevention of onward transmission of prion disease through health and other care, which are similar to the United Kingdom, but differ in detail, such as which patient groups are included and tissue classification of risk (Australia: http://www.health.gov.au/internet/main/publishing.nsf/content/3A968399995CFCE5CA257BF000211E32/$File/CJDInfectionControlGuidelinesJan2013.pdf; Canada: http://www.phac-aspc.gc.ca/nois-sinp/pdf/cjd-eng.pdf; United States: http://www.cdc.gov/prions/cjd/infection-control.html).

Preventing onward transmission of prion disease during clinical care

It is important that people diagnosed with prion diseases and those who have been notified that they are at increased risk of prion disease (see above) are able to live full lives and that the risk of transmission to others is minimized. Given the many uncertainties surrounding the potential risk of transmission, guidance to prevent transmission is based on an estimation of the risk and then a balance of that risk against the actions and processes required to prevent transmission (Advisory Committee on Dangerous Pathogens, 2015). In practice, decision making regarding what action to undertake requires a balance of probabilities, risks, and benefits.

Prospective management of surgical procedures

In the United Kingdom a precautionary approach is taken in relation to the risk management of prion disease in relation to surgery (Advisory Committee on Dangerous Pathogens, 2015). When individuals are due to undergo any elective or emergency surgical or endoscopic procedure, they should be asked whether they have ever been notified that they are at increased risk of prion disease for public health purposes. Additional screening questions to detect possible unrecognized prion disease risks are asked if the person is undergoing surgery known to involve tissue which is considered particularly (high-risk) infective for prion disease, for example, neurosurgery or posterior eye surgery (Advisory Committee on Dangerous Pathogens, 2015). The distribution of infectivity in tissues has been categorized based on observations of naturally occurring disease or experimental transmissions (World Health Organization, 2010). The patient's medical notes and referral letter should also be examined for any mention of prion disease and consideration given to early clinical history or signs of the disease, for example, cognitive impairment and/or ataxia.

If the patient is unable to respond, for instance if the patient is unconscious or a child, and it is not possible to obtain this information by proxy from the family or primary care physician, the surgery should not be delayed and should go ahead using normal infection control procedures (Advisory Committee on Dangerous Pathogens, 2015). However, following the precautionary principle, if the surgery involves potentially infective tissue, then any reusable instruments that have been in contact with relevant tissues should be quarantined until the patient's risk status for prion disease has been confirmed.

If the patient has been diagnosed with prion disease, or following the above screening process the patient is identified as being at increased risk of prion disease, guidance is followed to reduce the risk of transmitting infection through use of surgical instruments (World Health Organization, 1999; Advisory Committee on

Dangerous Pathogens, 2015). Single-use instruments should be used where possible. The handling of reusable instruments will depend on the type of prion disease involved and the tissue exposure risk, with the instruments retained and decontaminated in line with national prion disease guidance, or removed from general use (destroyed or quarantined for exclusive use on the same patient). For retained instruments, a tracking system should be in place.

Retrospective management of surgical incidents

In the United Kingdom, a surgical incident occurs when a patient with or at increased risk of prion disease has previously had an invasive procedure involving potentially infective tissue for prion diseases and precautions were not taken to prevent instruments being used on other patients. In most cases incidents relate to invasive procedures that were carried out before the patient was diagnosed or identified as at increased risk. Incidents can occur when a person with the disease is preclinical and has no symptoms, or has an atypical presentation of prion disease, which is subsequently recognized, or when an emergency procedure is carried out and a preclinical risk assessment was, therefore, unable to be performed.

Surgical incidents have implications for the patients subsequently exposed to the potentially contaminated instruments (the "contacts") and for the instruments themselves. Guidance for incidents involving prion disease is published in the United Kingdom (Public Health England and Health Protection Scotland, 2015). Again, the precautionary principle applies and the necessary actions depend on the type of prion disease, the type of surgery (tissue infectivity), and the number of cycles of decontamination that the instruments have undergone. Typically, the infection control team in the hospital (or other secondary care unit) are required to notify the incident to the local/national public health team. They will work together to undertake a lookback exercise and risk assessment, identify instruments which pose an onward transmission risk and remove them from use, and identify and inform patients who may be at increased risk of prion disease following the incident. If the specific instruments used on the index patient are unable to be traced, the risk of transmission from the incident should be considered and whether specific control mechanisms, such as decontamination measures, might be implemented. However, the risk of removal of surgical instruments from use should be considered in addition to the risk of transmission of prion disease. Prion disease-specific infection control guidelines (Advisory Committee on Dangerous Pathogens, 2015; see above) should be followed when surgery is undertaken in the future on the index case and identified surgical contacts at increased risk of prion disease.

Hospital and community care

There is no evidence that normal social interaction or routine clinical care poses a risk to relatives, friends, or carers, including healthcare workers. Patients with prion disease can be nursed in open wards using standard infection prevention and control precautions (Advisory Committee on Dangerous Pathogens, 2015). An assessment of the infectivity of tissues involved needs to be undertaken before any procedure is performed and appropriate precautions put in place. Body secretions and body fluids are low risk for prion disease; therefore, most procedures will be low risk. Those at increased risk of prion disease should be treated like any other patient, using universal precautions (Advisory Committee on Dangerous Pathogens, 2015).

Spillages of any bodily fluid from someone with or at risk of prion disease should be treated by removal of contaminated material and cleaning as per national prion disease guidance. Clinical waste should be assessed in relation to risk: higher-risk materials should be incinerated and low-risk materials (low-risk tissues and body fluids such as urine, saliva, sputum, blood, and feces) should be disposed of as per usual local clinical waste disposal mechanisms. Bed linen should be cleaned and processed according to local guidelines, unless contaminated with higher-risk tissue, in which case they should be incinerated (Advisory Committee on Dangerous Pathogens, 2015).

Dental treatment is considered low-risk and people with prion disease or those at increased risk should be treated like any other person according to local guidance. Dental instruments that are destined for reuse should be processed according to local practice and retained for use (World Health Organization, 1999; Advisory Committee on Dangerous Pathogens, 2015; Australian Government Department of Health, 2013).

Occupational exposure

Although links to occupation have not been proven, there have been cases of prion disease in healthcare and laboratory workers and a transmission risk is theoretically plausible. The highest risk of occupational exposure is from inoculation of high-risk tissues, for example, through puncture wounds or exposure through broken skin or mucous membranes. Healthcare and laboratory workers who work with potentially prion-infected tissues should be trained in good handling and health safety procedures. Local occupational health and laboratory safety guidance should be followed in relation to infection

Table 27.1

Prion resistance to chemical and physical processes

Chemical disinfectants	Gaseous disinfectants	Physical processes
Ineffective	**Ineffective**	**Ineffective**
Alcohol	Ethylene oxide	Boiling
Ammonia	Formaldehyde	Dry heat (<300°C)
β-Propiolactone		Ionizing, ultraviolet, or microwave
Formalin		
Hydrochloric acid		
Peracetic acid		
Phenolics		
Sodium dodecyl sulfate (5%)		
Variably or partially effective		**Variably or partially effective**
Chlorine dioxide		Autoclaving at 121°C for 15 minutes
Glutaraldehyde		Boiling at 3% sodium dodecyl sulfate
Guanidinium thiocyanate (4M)		
Iodophores		
Sodium dichloroisocyanurate		
Sodium metaperiodate		
Urea (6M)		

Reproduced from: World Health Organization (1999) WHO infection control guidelines for transmissible spongiform encephalopathies. Report of a WHO consultation, Geneva, Switzerland, 23–26 March 1999. Available online at: http://www.who.int/csr/resources/publications/bse/WHO_CDS_CSR_APH_2000_3/en/ (accessed December 21, 2016).

prevention and control procedures (Advisory Committee on Dangerous Pathogens, 2015). Wounds should be encouraged to bleed, and washed and dressed, while splashes into eyes/mouths should be irrigated (World Health Organization, 1999; Advisory Committee on Dangerous Pathogens, 2015). Surveillance of those who have had a documented potential occupational exposure is undertaken in the United Kingdom and elsewhere in Europe (Alcalde-Cabero et al., 2012).

Decontamination and prion agents

Challenges

Effective decontamination is key to reducing the overall risk of transmission of prion diseases (World Health Organization, 1999, Lumley, 2008; Rutala and Weber, 2010; European Centre for Disease Prevention and Control, 2013). Consequently, the World Health Organization and many countries take special precautions for decontamination of medical instruments (World Health Organization, 1999; Public Health Agency of Canada (PHAC), 2007; Australian Government Department of Health, 2013; European Centre for Disease Prevention and Control, 2013; Advisory Committee on Dangerous Pathogens, 2015; Centers for Disease Control and Prevention (CDC), 2015).

However, prion agents are particularly resistant to current physical and chemical methods of decontamination. The prion glycoprotein is resistant to protease (the enzyme degrading protein) and insoluble in nondenaturing detergent (Yuan et al., 2006). Although a number of research studies on prion deactivation technologies have been conducted, it remains that the misfolded prion agent cannot be completely inactivated by commonly used disinfection and sterilization processes, as summarized in Table 27.1 (Dickinson and Taylor, 1978; Rohwer, 1984; Taylor et al., 1998; Weinstein et al., 2001; Fichet et al., 2004; Baxter et al., 2005; Jackson, 2005; Sutton et al., 2006; Rutala and Weber, 2010). The use of alkaline hydrolysis has practical constraints, may cause damage to the instruments, and may increase occupational risks to staff undertaking the decontamination process (World Health Organization, 1999; Brown and Merritt, 2003).

Current practice

Medical instruments come in various materials, shapes, and sizes. The materials and design affect their cleanability. Instruments with long, narrow lumens, hinges, and crevices present a greater challenge to the cleaning process than solid planar instruments (Lipscomb et al., 2006a). Material incompatibility with cleaning agents and high temperatures may restrict the choice of decontamination process. For example, flexible endoscopes and robotic instruments require nonthermal inactivation processes. Due to the uncertainty that instruments with intricate design can be adequately cleaned, the complete removal of protein from these types of instruments cannot be assured. For this reason, in some countries, certain instruments are recommended as single-use, such as dental burrs and broaches.

The general standard and recommendations of decontamination guidance tend to concentrate on improving, controlling, and monitoring the decontamination process, including tracking instruments throughout the decontamination process and use in patients (Advisory Committee on Dangerous Pathogens, 2015; Department of Health, 2016). The focus of attention has been the cleaning process due to the limited impact of the disinfection/sterilization process on prion protein removal. The cleaning process includes chemical, mechanical, and thermal processes. An effective cleaning process requires the optimization of all three processes, including a validation step to confirm consistency in reaching the acceptable limit set in the standards or in national guidelines.

Surgical instruments are preferably cleaned in an automated validated washer disinfector (International Organization for Standardization (ISO) 2006a, b; Department of Health, 2016), or, under special circumstances, they are cleaned using other methods instructed by the manufacturer, such as manual or ultrasonic cleaning. Thermolabile flexible endoscopes are precleaned manually before being processed in an automated validated endoscope washer disinfector (International Organization for Standardization (ISO) 2006a, 2008). An endoscope washer disinfector is equipped with connectors designed to allow flushing of all internal channels of the endoscopes. During validation for cleaning efficacy, artificial test soil is applied to the instruments, or their surrogates, before they are placed in the machines (International Organization for Standardization (ISO), 2005). After the completion of the process, residual contaminants are measured against the limit set in the standards or by national guidelines. Protein testing has been widely used as one of the cleaning indicators by the ISO 15883 standard and in national guidelines (International Organization for Standardization (ISO), 2006a, b, 2008; Advisory Committee on Dangerous Pathogens, 2015; Department of Health, 2016).

Visual inspection of the surface of each instrument is a universal method used for routine monitoring of all instruments after the cleaning process. In addition, the UK guidance promotes quantitative residual protein monitoring on a regular basis as well as visual inspection (Department of Health, 2016).

Addition precautions in higher-risk situations

The risk of transmission of prion disease through medical instruments depends on the infectivity of the tissues in contact with the instruments, the prion disease type or at-risk status of the patient, and the degree of invasiveness of the instruments (Rutala and Weber, 2010). Depending on these parameters, the current practice of reducing risks of prion transmission through contaminated medical instruments ranges from incineration to various decontamination processes. The World Health Organization specified the recommended level of decontamination based on patient and tissue categories in relation to prion disease risk. Multiple reprocessing possibly would reduce the infectivity; however, complete removal of prion protein could not be assured and is, therefore, not recommended in the United Kigndom (Thomas et al., 2013).

Single use of instruments for patients with certain prion disease risks and for difficult-to-clean instruments is recommended as the preferable option by the World Health Organization and most countries (World Health Organization, 1999; Public Health Agency of Canada (PHAC), 2007; Australian Government Department of Health, 2013; European Centre for Disease Prevention and Control, 2013; Advisory Committee on Dangerous Pathogens, 2015; Centers for Disease Control and Prevention (CDC), 2015). For example in the United Kingdom, the National Institute for Health and Care Excellence guidelines IP 196 (National Institute for Health and Care Excellence (NICE), 2006) recommended the use of high-quality, single-use alternatives for supplementary instruments in contact with high-risk prion disease tissues. It is acknowledged that there is a financial burden and environmental cost associated with the disposal of single-use instruments, thus recycling material from instruments and the introduction of procurement strategies should be considered. Indeed, although single-use instruments are manufactured to be used once then discarded, the reuse and reprocessing of single-use instruments have been implemented or considered in a few countries (Food and Drug Administration, 2006; Eucomed, 2014).

The range of single-use instruments may be limited; therefore, in certain circumstances, reusable alternatives might be used. The recommendations on decontamination of reusable medical instruments to inactivate prion from high-risk tissues vary between countries. The survey carried out by the ECDC observed variation in the decontamination guidance among 15 European Union countries (European Centre for Disease Prevention and Control, 2013). The guidance produced by the World Health Organization and countries such as the United States and Canada recommends that alkaline hydrolysis (using sodium hydroxide or sodium hydrochloride) followed by thermal sterilization is a valid method of decontamination. However, it is widely recognized that not all instruments and equipment are compatible with this thermal and chemical process (Public Health Agency of Canada (PHAC), 2007; Australian Government Department of Health, 2013). Furthermore, the process raised occupational health concerns for staff undertaking decontamination processes (Brown and Merritt, 2003). The United Kingdom has removed its recommendation of using an alkaline hydrolysis process, and recommends disposal and incineration for high-risk tissues (Advisory Committee on Dangerous Pathogens, 2015). Similarly, Australia removed alkaline hydrolysis as an option and introduced additional decontamination procedures to the routine process (Australian Government Department of Health, 2013).

Most countries also include recommendations on the management aspects of instruments, including traceability systems, handling, labeling, packaging, quarantining, segregation, and transport (World Health Organization, 1999; Public Health Agency of Canada (PHAC), 2007; Australian Government Department of Health, 2013; European Centre for Disease Prevention and Control, 2013; Advisory Committee on Dangerous Pathogens, 2015; Centers for Disease Control and Prevention (CDC), 2015).

The future

Although in practice a combination of decontamination approaches may be used, because of the limitations of current chemical and physical decontamination practices, the emphasis has shifted towards improving the effectiveness of the cleaning process. Due to its hydrophobic properties, the abnormal prion protein adheres strongly to stainless steel surfaces, making it more difficult to remove when left to dry on the instrument surface (Lipscomb et al., 2007). Immediate cleaning or keeping instruments moist facilitates the removal of protein and makes the cleaning process easier. Various methods or products are available to keep instruments moist, for example, humidified bags, chemical-containing moistening agents, or cloths moistened with sterile water. The selected method or product should be tested on site, prior to use, to ensure its effectiveness and determine any possible undesirable effects on instruments, equipment, and the overall process. When chemical moistening agents are used, the compatibility with the devices and equipment should be assessed to avoid adverse impacts on the quality of the devices and the cleaning process. For example, inadequate rinsing of moistening chemical agents left on medical instruments might cause build-up of foam in the washer disinfector, affecting its cleaning performance.

Attempts to reduce the adherence of protein to instruments and to improve its removal have included the development of coatings (Secker et al., 2012), and the use of new technologies such as plasma and enzymes for removal. However, none of these has yet been widely adopted. Research into finding more sensitive protein detection methods for use with surgical instruments and endoscopes has been carried out (Baxter et al., 2005, 2006; Lipscomb et al., 2006b; Cloutman-Green et al., 2015), but so far commercialization of these products has been limited. Research on the indicator for washer disinfector cleaning performance has also been undertaken (Ungurs et al., 2010). Clearly, there is room for further development and improvement in prion-specific decontamination methods that can be applied and used in current healthcare settings.

CONCLUSION

While our knowledge of prion diseases, which have been recognized in animals and humans for hundreds of years, has increased over the last 30 years following the BSE and vCJD epidemics, many uncertainties remain. The emergence of chronic wasting disease in Europe is an example of the potential threat of these diseases to animal and human health (Benestad et al., 2016).

The long incubation periods, the lack of easy diagnostic tests in life, the potential for asymptomatic infection, the transmission through medical practice, and the difficulty in decontamination of medical instruments mean that public health measures to reduce transmission of prion diseases in the community and in healthcare remain imperative.

References

Advisory Committee on Dangerous Pathogens (ACDP), Department of Health (2015). Minimise transmission risk of CJD and vCJD in healthcare settings. Available at: https://www.gov.uk/government/publications/guidance-from-the-acdp-tse-risk-management-subgroup-formerly-tse-working-group [accessed 21 Dec. 2016].

Alcalde-Cabero E, Almazán-Isla J, Brandel JP et al. (2012). Health professions and risk of sporadic Creutzfeldt–Jakob disease, 1965 to 2010. In: Eurosurveillance 17: pii20144.

Anderson RM, Donnelly CA, Ferguson NM et al. (1996). Transmission dynamics and epidemiology of BSE in British cattle. Nature 382: 779–788.

Australian Government Department of Health (2013). Infection control guidelines. [online] Available at: http://www.health.gov.au/internet/main/publishing.nsf/content/icg-guidelines-index.htm [accessed 22 Dec. 2016].

Barria MA, Balachandran A, Morita M et al. (2014). Molecular barriers to zoonotic transmission of prions. Emerg Infect Dis 20: 88–97.

Baxter HC, Campbell GA, Whittaker AG et al. (2005). Elimination of transmissible spongiform encephalopathy infectivity and decontamination of surgical instruments by using radio-frequency gas-plasma treatment. J Gen Virol 86: 2393–2399.

Baxter R, Baxter H, Campbell G et al. (2006). Quantitative analysis of residual protein contamination on reprocessed surgical instruments. J Hosp Infect 63: 439–444.

Benestad SL, Mitchell G, Simmons M et al. (2016). First case of chronic wasting disease in Europe in a Norwegian free-ranging reindeer. Vet Res 47: 88.

Bonda DJ, Manjila S, Mehndiratta P et al. (2016). Human prion diseases: surgical lessons learned from iatrogenic prion transmission. Neurosurg Focus 41: E10.

Bradford A, Kunik ME, Schulz P et al. (2009). Missed and delayed diagnosis of dementia in primary care: prevalence and contributing factors. Alzheimer Dis Assoc Disord 23: 306–314.

Brown SA, Merritt K (2003). Use of containment pans and lids for autoclaving caustic solutions. Am J Infect Control 31: 257–260.

Brown P, Brandel J-P, Sato T et al. (2012). Iatrogenic Creutzfeldt–Jakob disease, final assessment. Emerg Infect Dis 18: 901–907.

Bruce ME, Will RG, Ironside JW et al. (1997). Transmissions to mice indicate that /'new variant/' CJD is caused by the BSE agent. Nature 389: 498–501.

Centers for Disease Control and Prevention (CDC) (2015). Infection control Creutzfeldt–Jakob Disease, classic (CJD) prion disease. Available at: https://www.cdc.gov/prions/cjd/infection-control.html [accessed 21 Dec. 2016].

Cloutman-Green E, Canales M, Zhou Q et al. (2015). Biochemical and microbial contamination of surgical devices: a quantitative analysis. Am J Infect Control 43: 659–661.

Collinge J, Sidle KCL, Meads J et al. (1996). Molecular analysis of prion strain variation and the aetiology of 'new variant' CJD. Nature 383: 685–690.

d'Aignaux JN, Cousens SN, Smith PG (2001). Predictability of the UK variant Creutzfeldt–Jakob disease epidemic. Science 294: 1729–1731.

Davidson LR, Llewelyn CA, Mackenzie JM et al. (2014). Variant CJD and blood transfusion: are there additional cases? Vox Sang 107: 220–225.

Department of Health (2016). Health technical memorandum (HTM) 01-01: management and decontamination of surgical instruments (medical devices) used in acute care. Available at: https://www.gov.uk/government/publications/management-and-decontamination-of-surgical-instruments-used-in-acute-care [accessed 22 Dec. 2016].

de Pedro Cuesta J, Ruiz Tovar M, Ward H et al. (2012). Sensitivity to biases of case-control studies on medical procedures, particularly surgery and blood transfusion, and risk of Creutzfeldt–Jakob disease. Neuroepidemiology 39: 1–18.

Dickinson AG, Taylor DM (1978). Resistance of scrapie agent to decontamination. N Engl J Med 299: 1413–1414.

El Tawil S, Mackay G (2015). Variant Creutzfeldt–Jakob disease in older patients. J Neurol Neurosurg Psychiatry 86: 1279–1280.

European Centre for Disease Prevention and Control (ECDC) (2013). Technical report: review of guidelines for prevention of Creutzfeldt–Jakob disease transmission in medical settings in EU Member States and Norway. Available at: http://ecdc.europa.eu/en/publications/Publications/1106_TER_Review_of_guidelines_for_prevention_of%20CJD.pdf [accessed 22 Dec. 2016].

Eucomed (2014). The revision of the EU Medical Devices Directives. Available at: http://www.medtecheurope.org/sites/default/files/01042014_MTE_The%20Revision%20of%20the%20EU%20medical%20devices%20directive_PositionPaper.pdf.

Fichet G, Comoy E, Duval C et al. (2004). Novel methods for disinfection of prion-contaminated medical devices. Lancet 364: 521–526. https://doi.org/10.1016/S0140-6736(04)16810-4.

Food and Drug Administration (2006). Reprocessing of single-use devices. Available at: www.fda.gov/MedicalDevices/DeviceRegulationandGuidance/ReprocessingofSingle-UseDevices/default.htm [accessed 26 Dec. 2016].

Geschwind MD (2016). Rapidly progressive dementia. Continuum (Minneap Minn) 22: 510–537.

Gill ON, Spencer Y, Richard-Loendt A et al. (2013). Prevalent abnormal prion protein in human appendixes after bovine spongiform encephalopathy epizootic: large scale survey. BMJ 15: 347. Oct.

Hamaguchi T, Noguchi-Shinohara M, Nozaki I et al. (2009). Medical procedures and risk for sporadic Creutzfeldt–Jakob disease, Japan, 1999–2008. Emerg Infect Dis 15: 265–271.

Hamaguchi T, Sakai K, Noguchi-Shinohara M et al. (2013). Insight into the frequent occurrence of dura mater graft-associated Creuzfeldt–Jakob disease in Japan. J Neurol Neurosurg Psychiatry 84: 1171–1175.

Head MW, Knight R, Zeidler M et al. (2009). A case of protease sensitive prionopathy in a patient in the UK. Neuropathol Appl Neurobiol 35: 628–632.

Hewitt PE, Llewelyn CA, Mackenzie J et al. (2006). Creutzfeldt–Jakob disease and blood transfusion: results of the UK Transfusion Medicine Epidemiological Review study. Vox Sang 91: 221–230.

Hill AF, Desbruslais M, Joiner S et al. (1997). The same prion strain causes vCJD and BSE. Nature 389: 448–450.

Huillard d'Aignaux J, Costagliola D, Maccario J et al. (1999). Incubation period of Creutzfeldt–Jakob disease in human growth hormone recipients in France. Neurology 53: 1197–1201.

International Organization for Standardization (ISO) (2005). ISO/TS 15883-5:2005 Washer-disinfectors – part 5: test soils and methods for demonstrating cleaning efficacy. Available at: http://www.iso.org/iso/iso_catalogue/catalogue_tc/catalogue_detail.htm?csnumber=41175 [accessed 26 Dec. 2016].

International Organization for Standardization (ISO) (2006a). ISO 15883-1:2006 Washer-disinfectors – part 1: general requirements, terms and definitions and tests. Available at: http://www.iso.org/iso/iso_catalogue/catalogue_tc/catalogue_detail.htm?csnumber=41076 [accessed 26 Dec. 2016].

International Organization for Standardization (ISO) (2006b). ISO 15883-2 (2006)Washer-disinfectors- part 2: requirements and tests for washer-disinfectors employing thermal disinfection for surgical instruments, anaesthetic equipment, bowls, dishes, receivers, utensils, glassware, etc. [online] available at: https://www.iso.org/obp/ui/#iso:std:iso:15883:-2:ed-1:v1:en [accessed 21 Dec. 2016].

International Organization for Standardization (ISO) (2008) ISO 15883-4:2008 Washer-disinfectors – part 4: requirements and tests for washer-disinfectors employing chemical disinfection for thermolabile endoscopes. Available at: http://www.iso.org/iso/iso_catalogue/catalogue_tc/catalogue_detail.htm?csnumber=42060 [accessed 26 Dec. 2016].

Jackson G (2005). An enzyme-detergent method for effective prion decontamination of surgical steel. J Gen Virol 86: 869–878.

Josephs KA, Ahlskog JE, Parisi JE et al. (2009). Rapidly progressive neurodegenerative dementias. Arch Neurol 66: 201–207.

Karch A, Raddatz LM, Ponto C et al. (2014). Diagnostic profiles of patients with late-onset Creutzfeldt–Jakob disease differ from those of younger Creutzfeldt–Jakob patients: a historical cohort study using data from the German National Reference Center. J Neurol 261: 877–883.

Lee HS, Sambuughin N, Cervenakova L et al. (1999). Ancestral origins and worldwide distribution of the PRNP 200K mutation causing familial Creutzfeldt–Jakob disease. Am J Hum Genet 64: 1063–1070.

Llewelyn CA, Hewitt PE, Knight RS et al. (2004). Possible transmission of variant Creutzfeldt–Jakob disease by blood transfusion. Lancet 363: 417–421.

Lipscomb I, Sihota A, Keevil CW (2006a). Comparative study of surgical instruments from sterile-service departments for presence of residual gram negative endotoxin and proteinaceous deposits. J Clin Microbiol 44: 3728–3733.

Lipscomb I, Sihota A, Botham M et al. (2006b). Rapid method for the sensitive detection of protein contamination on surgical instruments. J Hosp Infect 62: 141–148.

Lipscomb I, Pinchin H, Collin R et al. (2007). Effect of drying time, ambient temperature and pre-soaks on prion-infected tissue contamination levels on surgical stainless steel: concerns over prolonged transportation of instruments from theatre to central sterile service departments. J Hosp Infect 65: 72–77.

Lumley J (2008). The impact of Creutzfeldt–Jakob disease on surgical practice. Ann R Coll Surg Engl 90: 91–94.

Mead S (2006). Prion disease genetics. Eur J Hum Genet 14: 273–281.

Mead S, Rudge P (2016). CJD mimics and chameleons. Pract Neurol 0: 1–9.

Mok T, Jaunmuktane Z, Joiner S et al. (2017). Variant Creutzfeldt–Jakob disease in a patient with heterozygosity at PRNP codon 129. N Engl J Med 376: 292–294.

Molesworth AM, Cousens SN, Noel GO et al. (2010). Variant Creutzfeldt–Jakob disease in the United Kingdom: a countrywide or local risk? J Epidemiol Community Health 64: 616–621.

Monk P, Bryant G (2001). Final report of the investigation into the North Leicestershire cluster of variant Creutzfeldt–Jakob disease. Leicester 2001. In: Leicestershire NHS Health Authority, http://webarchive.nationalarchives.gov.uk/20140714084352/http://www.hpa.org.uk/web/HPAwebFile/HPAweb_C/1194947321932.

National Institute for Health and Care Excellence (NICE) (2006). Patient safety and reduction of risk of transmission of Creutzfeldt–Jakob disease (CJD) via interventional procedures. Available at: https://www.nice.org.uk/guidance/ipg196 [accessed 26 Dec. 2016].

Peden AH, Head MW, Ritchie DL et al. (2004). Preclinical vCJD after blood transfusion in a PRNP codon 129 heterozygous patient. Lancet 364: 527–529.

Public Health England and Health Protection Scotland (2015). Public health action following a report of a new case of CJD or a person at increased risk of CJD, https://www.gov.uk/government/uploads/system/uploads/attachment_data/file/474338/CJD_public_health_action_new_case_301015.pdf.

Public Health Agency of Canada (PHAC) (2007). Nosocomial and occupational infections. Available at: http://www.phac-aspc.gc.ca/nois-sinp/cjd/cjd-eng.php [accessed 22 Dec. 2016].

Rohwer RG (1984). Virus like sensitivity of the scrapie agent to heat inactivation. Science 10: 600–602.

Rutala W, Weber D (2010). Guideline for disinfection and sterilization of prion-contaminated medical instruments. Infect Control Hosp Epidemiol 31: 107–117.

SABTO (2011) (Advisory Committee on the Safety of Blood, Tissues and Organs, UK). Guidance on the microbiological safety of human organs, tissues and cells used for transplantation. Available at https://www.gov.uk/government/uploads/system/uploads/attachment_data/file/215959/dh_130515.pdf [accessed 7th March 2017].

Scott MR, Will R, Ironside J et al. (1999). Compelling transgenetic evidence for transmission of bovine spongiform encephalopathy prions to humans. Proc Natl Acad Sci 96: 15137–15142.

Secker T, Hervé R, Zhao Q et al. (2012). Doped diamond-like carbon coatings for surgical instruments reduce protein and prion-amyloid biofouling and improve subsequent cleaning. Biofouling 28: 563–569.

Staekenborg SS, Pijnenburg YA, Lemstra AW et al. (2016). Dementia and rapid mortality: who is at risk? J Alzheimers Dis 53: 135–142.

Sutton JM, Dickinson J, Walker JT et al. (2006). Methods to minimize the risks of Creutzfeldt–Jakob disease transmission by surgical procedures: where to set the standard? Clin Infect Dis 43: 757–764.

Swerdlow AJ, Higgins CD, Adlard P et al. (2003). Creutzfeldt–Jakob disease in United Kingdom patients treated with human pituitary growth hormone. Neurology 61: 783–791.

Taylor DM, Fernie K, McConnell I et al. (1998). Observations on thermostable subpopulations of the unconventional agents that cause transmissible degenerative encephalopathies. Vet Microbiol 64: 33–38.

Thomas J, Chenoweth C, Sullivan S (2013). Iatrogenic Creutzfeldt–Jakob disease via surgical instruments. J Clin Neurosci 20: 1207–1212.

Ungurs M, Hesp J, Poolman T et al. (2010). Quantitative measurement of the efficacy of protein removal by cleaning formulations; comparative evaluation of prion-directed cleaning chemistries. J Hosp Infect 74: 144–151.

Urwin PJM, Mackenzie JM, Llewelyn CA et al. (2016). Creutzfeldt–Jakob disease and blood transfusion: updated results of the UK Transfusion Medicine Epidemiology Review Study. Vox Sang 110: 310–316.

Ward HJ, Everington D, Cousens SN et al. (2006). Risk factors for variant Creutzfeldt–Jakob disease: a case-control study. Ann Neurol 59: 111–120.

Weinstein R, Rutala W, Weber D (2001). Creutzfeldt–Jakob Disease: recommendations for disinfection and sterilization. Clin Infect Dis 32: 1348–1356.

Wilesmith JW, Wells GA, Cranwell MP et al. (1988). Bovine spongiform encephalopathy: epidemiological studies. Vet Rec 123: 638–644.

Will RG, Ironside JW, Zeidler M et al. (1996). A new variant of Creutzfeldt–Jakob disease in the UK. Lancet 347: 921–925.

World Health Organization (1999) WHO infection control guidelines for transmissible spongiform encephalopathies. Report of a WHO consultation, Geneva, Switzerland, 23–26 March 1999. Available online at: http://www.who.int/csr/resources/publications/bse/WHO_CDS_CSR_APH_2000_3/en/ (accessed December 21, 2016).

World Health Organization (2003). WHO manual for surveillance of human transmissible spongiform encephalopathies, World Health Organization, Geneva.

World Health Organization (2010). WHO table on tissue infectivity distribution in transmissible spongiform encephalopathies, World Health Organization, Geneva.

Yuan J, Xiao X, McGeehan J et al. (2006). Insoluble aggregates and protease-resistant conformers of prion protein in uninfected human brains. J Biol Chem 281: 34848–34858.

Zaman SM, Hill FG, Palmer B et al. (2011). The risk of variant Creutzfeldt–Jakob disease among UK patients with bleeding disorders, known to have received potentially contaminated plasma products. Haemophilia 17: 931–937.

Handbook of Clinical Neurology, Vol. 153 (3rd series)
Human Prion Diseases
M. Pocchiari and J. Manson, Editors
https://doi.org/10.1016/B978-0-444-63945-5.00028-3

Chapter 28

Concluding remarks

MAURIZIO POCCHIARI[1]* AND JEAN MANSON[2]
[1]*Department of Neuroscience, Istituto Superiore di Sanità, Rome, Italy*
[2]*Centre for Clinical Brain Sciences, University of Edinburgh, Edinburgh, United Kingdom*

Abstract

This is the first volume of the *Handbook of Clinical Neurology* totally devoted to prion diseases. The reason for this choice is to inform neurologists and neuroscientists about the remarkable advances that this field has made in the diagnosis of human and animal prion diseases, understanding the pathogenesis of disease, and in the development of novel in vivo and in vitro models. In recent years, the knowledge of prion replication and mechanisms of prion spreading within the brain and peripheral organs of infected people has also become important for understanding other protein misfolded diseases of the brain, such as Alzheimer disease, Parkinson disease, and amyotrophic lateral sclerosis. Researchers in these diseases have recognized that the process within an individual leading to the deposition of misfolded proteins within the central nervous system shares remarkable common mechanisms with prion diseases, leading to the terminology of "prion-like diseases."

The commonality between prion and other neurodegenerative diseases is perhaps one of the most important developments of the last decade and advances in understanding pathogenic mechanisms or possible routes to treatments in one of them may also provide solutions for the other diseases. It is now clear that, similarly to prions, other seeds of misfolded proteins (e.g., A-beta, alfa-synuclein, tau, SOD1, TDP-43, FUS) are able to induce pathologic conformational changes in their respective naïve proteins and through this mechanism their spreading within the central nervous system and occasionally from the periphery to the brain (Walker, 2016). This effect, originally revealed in animal models of Alzheimer and Parkinson disease, amyotrophic lateral sclerosis, and tauopathies (Walker and Jucker, 2015), has been recently confirmed in subjects who underwent dura mater grafts or treatment with human growth hormone extracted from cadaveric human pituitaries where pathologists found foci of misfolded tau and A-beta proteins, other than the prion protein, in their brains (Jaunmuktane et al., 2015; Frontzek et al., 2016; Hamaguchi et al., 2016; Ritchie et al., 2017; Cali et al., 2018; Duyckaerts et al., 2018).

These data indicate that the accidental injection of each disease-specific misfolded protein might induce its de novo formation. However, these subjects did not develop any clinical or instrumental signs related to the type of misfolded protein accumulating in their brains, leaving uncertainties about the pathologic significance of these findings. Epidemiologic investigations should specifically address the possible iatrogenic risks of neurodegenerative diseases other than Creutzfeldt–Jakob disease (CJD) for exploring whether prion-like diseases might occasionally be transmitted by medical or surgical procedures, as has occurred for CJD (iatrogenic CJD).

A discrepancy between the formation and accumulation of misfolded proteins in the brain and clinical disease occasionally occurs in prion diseases as well (Piccardo et al., 2007; Barron et al., 2016), arguing that the occurrence of disease might involve other factors. This remarkable feature continues to challenge us and may

*Correspondence to: Maurizio Pocchiari, Department of Neuroscience, Istituto Superiore di Sanità, Viale Regina Elena 299, Rome, Italy. Tel: +39-064-9903203, E-mail: maurizio.pocchiari@iss.it

have deep implications for future development of therapeutic compounds. We have gained a greater understanding on the replication of the misfolded protein both in vitro and in vivo, but the exact relationship between misfolded protein, infection, and neurotoxicity is not yet defined.

New and sensitive techniques such as real-time quaking-induced conversion, protein misfolding cyclic amplification, and a few other assays have been developed to detect the only valid and specific biomarker, the pathologic prion protein (PrP^{TSE}), in blood, cerebrospinal fluid, and other tissues, with a remarkably high level of sensitivity and specificity (Zanusso et al., 2016). These assays provide an early and accurate diagnosis in living patients and animals but they are still available only in specialized laboratories. Moreover, these techniques might, under certain conditions, amplify prion infectivity as well (Morales et al., 2012), requiring biosafety laboratories of class 3 and experienced personnel (Bistaffa et al., 2017). Finally, it is still uncertain whether these tests might identify preclinical or subclinical infected individuals and they are therefore still of little value for the screening of blood and organ donors or for determining the prevalence of transmissible spongiform encephalopathy (TSE) diseases in animal and human populations. Thus, the true prevalence of TSE diseases in animal and human populations remains unknown.

The number of bovine spongiform encephalopathy (BSE) cases has consistently declined throughout the world, but there are still occasional cases in animals born after the stringent enforcement of the ban on the use of animal proteins (OIE, 2018), questioning either the real compliance with the feed ban or the presence of other sources of infection. Scrapie in sheep and goats is also declining in countries that have adopted genetic selective breeding for resistant animals (Hagenaars et al., 2010), but this procedure has its own risks in the long term because it might favor the replication of rare scrapie strains with higher zoonotic potential than more common strains, usually present in the sheep population.

A new challenging epidemic is also emerging in the form of chronic wasting disease (CWD) in wild and captive populations of members of the deer family. CWD has been identified in the United States since the mid-1960s (recognized as a prion disease in 1980) (Williams and Young, 1980), and continues to spread throughout the United States and Canada, with so far no successful strategy for halting the epidemic (US National Wildlife Health Center, 2018). In 2016–2017, a few cases of CWD were identified in wild moose, reindeer, and red deer in Norway and new cases continue to be reported in 2016–2018 (Benestad et al., 2016). The origin of the disease in Norway remains unknown but it is likely that it will soon spread to other nearby countries despite the great efforts put in place to avoid a novel epidemic of animal prion disease in Europe (Stokstad, 2017). CWD-infected deer have infection in a wide variety of peripheral tissues in addition to the central nervous system and this prion agent appears to be the most highly infectious so far encountered, with the ability to spread readily between individuals (Hannaoui et al., 2017).

Although it is not currently known whether CWD has zoonotic potential, some assay systems suggest that CWD PrP^{TSE} is able to convert the human PrP protein into a misfolded form (Davenport et al., 2015). A number of different strains of CWD are present in the deer population (Duque Velásquez et al., 2015; Herbst et al., 2017) and each strain may have a different zoonotic potential, but whether this would indeed occur naturally is difficult to predict. There is no evidence at this stage of a human prion disease associated with CWD (Waddell et al., 2018), although if it were to present as sporadic CJD, any such association would prove difficult.

A similar difficulty applies in determining the zoonotic potential of typical and atypical scrapie in sheep and goats and atypical forms of BSE. Indeed, the association between classic BSE and human disease (variant CJD) was possible only because the BSE agent infection caused a striking different phenotype from classic forms of human prion diseases. The early age at onset, psychiatric or persistent painful sensory symptoms at onset, bilateral brain pulvinar sign at the MRI, the extensive PrP^{TSE} deposition with florid plaques throughout the brain (Heath et al., 2011; Ritchie and Ironside, 2017), and the concentration of these atypical cases in the United Kingdom, with the largest number of BSE cases in the cattle population, were essential features for realizing that a novel form of CJD distinguished from sporadic CJD had emerged.

Continuing the surveillance of all forms of animal and human prion diseases is therefore necessary to readily identify possible changes in the number of cases but, more importantly, to promptly recognize novel emerging phenotypes. In the last years, great advances have been made in the identification of novel forms of CJD, such as variably protease-sensitive prionopathy (Zou et al., 2010) or in the subclassification of sporadic CJD based on clinical, instrumental, neuropathology, and PrP^{TSE} Western blot signature (Meissner et al., 2009; Parchi et al., 2012; Puoti et al., 2012). Epidemiologic studies based on the identification of all subtypes of sporadic CJD would be important for understanding the distribution of each subtype in different geographic regions and monitoring eventual changes that might give evidence of possible novel or not yet recognized risk factors.

There are still many unanswered questions on the source of infection, if any, in sporadic CJD. A part from a few hundred cases of proven intrahuman transmission through medical or surgical procedures (iatrogenic CJD) (Brown et al., 2012), in most cases it is not yet possible to trace or prove any eventual cause relation between past events (e.g., surgery, organ transplant, blood transfusion, other potential source of infection) and disease, mostly because of the long and unpredictable incubation period (Puopolo et al., 2011; López et al., 2017). Onset and duration of disease in sporadic and genetic TSE diseases are also largely unpredictable (Pocchiari et al., 2004; Heinemann et al., 2007) and these uncertainties influence the design of clinical trials for testing antiprion drugs or for choosing the time to start preventive therapy in healthy people carrying one of the several point or insert mutations of the PrP gene (*PRNP*) (Pocchiari and Ladogana, 2015).

Amino acid changes in the sequence of PrP facilitate the misfolding of the protein and the formation of PrP^{TSE}, but the timing of this process is unpredictable and might eventually occur very late in life or does not occur at all. Depending upon the type of mutation of the *PRNP* gene, some carriers develop disease at a young age, others in advanced age, and some remain disease-free for all their life (Ladogana et al., 2005). This variability occurs even in carriers belonging to the same family, suggesting that some other endogenous or exogenous factors are involved in the timing of disease onset (Pocchiari et al., 2013). Searching for these factors is becoming a great priority for better understanding the pathogenesis of prion diseases and for giving more relevant information to family members in relation to their risk of developing the disease.

Finally, much focus has been placed on the early events of the disease process as a route to identifying intervention strategies. The importance of the immune system in modulating the disease process has now become clear in all prion-like diseases and this has provided new avenues for therapeutic intervention (Alibhai et al., 2016; Mabbott, 2017). The challenge is now to understand the response of multiple cell types in the brain not only during the neurodegenerative process but also during aging, as the aging brain is clearly an important factor in these diseases. Another area for intervention has been the clearance of the misfolded protein and strategies such as enhanced autophagy are being examined as routes to clearing the brain of the misfolded protein (Cortes et al., 2012; Barmada et al., 2014).

Therapy for prion diseases is still in its infancy and it is premature to forecast when a valid antiprion drug will be available for testing in humans. There are excellent animal models for prion diseases that recapitulate biochemical, pathologic, and clinical features of human diseases and preclinical studies on a variety of animal/prion strain combinations have shown that so far the only valid strategy to delay or, in some occasions, prevent onset of disease is to give antiprion drugs before the appearance of clinical signs (Vetrugno et al., 2015). There are so far no drugs that are able to substantially modify the disease course when given in the clinical phase of disease, even if given at a very early stage. Based on these experimental data, the only rational approach today is to prevent the disease rather than attempt a curative therapy. In line with these data is the ongoing trial with doxycycline in carriers of the D178N/129M mutation of the *PRNP* gene belonging to a large Italian family with fatal familial insomnia (Forloni et al., 2015).

In the last 10 years, there have been great scientific advances in the field of prion disease and here we have aimed to give an insight into these advances, but there are still many unanswered questions that deserve further research and public health attention. However, despite the gaps in our knowledge, our growing understanding of the protein misfolding diseases is now yielding new targets and opening new avenues for intervention for this group of devastating diseases.

References

Alibhai J, Blanco RA, Barria MA et al. (2016). Distribution of misfolded prion protein seeding activity alone does not predict regions of neurodegeneration. PLoS Biol 14: e1002579.

Barmada SJ, Serio A, Arjun A et al. (2014). Autophagy induction enhances TDP43 turnover and survival in neuronal ALS models. Nat Chem Biol 10: 677–685.

Barron RM, King D, Jeffrey M et al. (2016). PrP aggregation can be seeded by pre-formed recombinant PrP amyloid fibrils without the replication of infectious prions. Acta Neuropathol 132: 611–624.

Benestad SL, Mitchell G, Simmons M et al. (2016). First case of chronic wasting disease in Europe in a Norwegian free-ranging reindeer. Vet Res 47: 88.

Bistaffa E, Rossi M, De Luca CMG et al. (2017). Biosafety of prions. Prog Mol Biol Transl Sci 150: 455–485.

Brown P, Brandel JP, Sato T et al. (2012). Iatrogenic Creutzfeldt–Jakob disease, final assessment. Emerg Infect Dis 18: 901–907.

Cali I, Cohen ML, Hak S et al. (2018). Iatrogenic Creutzfeldt–Jakob disease with amyloid-β pathology: an international study. Acta Neuropathol Commun 6: 5.

Cortes CJ, Qin K, Cook J et al. (2012). Rapamycin delays disease onset and prevents PrP plaque deposition in a mouse model of Gerstmann-Straussler-Scheinker disease. J Neurosci 32: 12396–12405.

Davenport KA, Henderson DM, Bian J et al. (2015). Insights into chronic wasting disease and bovine spongiform encephalopathy species barriers by use of real-time conversion. J Virol 89: 9524–9531.

Duque Velásquez C, Kim C, Herbst A et al. (2015). Deer prion proteins modulate the emergence and adaptation of chronic wasting disease strains. J Virol 89: 12362–12373.

Duyckaerts C, Sazdovitch V, Ando K, Seilhean D et al. (2018). Neuropathology of iatrogenic Creutzfeldt–Jakob disease and immunoassay of French cadaver-sourced growth hormone batches suggest possible transmission of tauopathy and long incubation periods for the transmission of Abeta pathology. Acta Neuropathol 135: 201–212.

Forloni G, Tettamanti M, Lucca U et al. (2015). Preventive study in subjects at risk of fatal familial insomnia: innovative approach to rare diseases. Prion 9: 75–79.

Frontzek K, Lutz MI, Aguzzi A et al. (2016). Amyloid-β pathology and cerebral amyloid angiopathy are frequent in iatrogenic Creutzfeldt–Jakob disease after dural grafting. Swiss Med Wkly 146: w14287.

Hagenaars TJ, Melchior MB, Bossers A et al. (2010). Scrapie prevalence in sheep of susceptible genotype is declining in a population subject to breeding for resistance. BMC Vet Res 6: 25.

Hamaguchi T, Taniguchi Y, Sakai K et al. (2016). Significant association of cadaveric dura mater grafting with subpial Aβ deposition and meningeal amyloid angiopathy. Acta Neuropathol 132: 313–315.

Hannaoui S, Schatzl HM, Gilch S (2017). Chronic wasting disease: emerging prions and their potential risk. PLoS Pathog 13: e1006619.

Heath CA, Cooper SA, Murray K et al. (2011). Diagnosing variant Creutzfeldt–Jakob disease: a retrospective analysis of the first 150 cases in the UK. J Neurol Neurosurg Psychiatry 82: 646–651.

Heinemann U, Krasnianski A, Meissner B et al. (2007). Creutzfeldt–Jakob disease in Germany: a prospective 12-year surveillance. Brain 130: 1350–1359.

Herbst A, Velásquez C, Triscott E et al. (2017). Chronic wasting disease prion strain emergence and host range expansion. Emerg Infect Dis 23: 1598–1600.

Jaunmuktane Z, Mead S, Ellis M et al. (2015). Evidence for human transmission of amyloid-β pathology and cerebral amyloid angiopathy. Nature 525: 247–250.

Ladogana A, Puopolo M, Poleggi A et al. (2005). High incidence of genetic human transmissible spongiform encephalopathies in Italy. Neurology 64: 1592–1597.

López FJG, Ruiz-Tovar M, Almazán-Isla J et al. (2017). Risk of transmission of sporadic Creutzfeldt–Jakob disease by surgical procedures: systematic reviews and quality of evidence. Euro Surveill 22 (43): 16–00806.

Mabbott NA (2017). Immunology of prion protein and prions. Prog Mol Biol Transl Sci 150: 203–240.

Meissner B, Kallenberg K, Sanchez-Juan P et al. (2009). MRI lesion profiles in sporadic Creutzfeldt–Jakob disease. Neurology 72: 1994–2001.

Morales R, Duran-Aniotz C, Diaz-Espinoza R et al. (2012). Protein misfolding cyclic amplification of infectious prions. Nat Protoc 7: 1397–1409.

OIE (2018). BSE situation in the world and annual incidence rate. Available online at http://www.oie.int/en/animal-health-in-the-world/bse-specific-data/. Accessed 23 January 2018.

Parchi P, de Boni L, Saverioni D et al. (2012). Consensus classification of human prion disease histotypes allows reliable identification of molecular subtypes: an inter-rater study among surveillance centres in Europe and USA. Acta Neuropathol 124: 517–529.

Piccardo P, Manson JC, King D et al. (2007). Accumulation of prion protein in the brain that is not associated with transmissible disease. Proc Natl Acad Sci U S A 104: 4712–4717.

Pocchiari M, Ladogana A (2015). Rethinking of doxycycline therapy in Creutzfeldt–Jakob disease. J Neurol Neurosurg Psychiatry 86: 705.

Pocchiari M, Puopolo M, Croes EA et al. (2004). Predictors of survival in sporadic Creutzfeldt–Jakob disease and other human transmissible spongiform encephalopathies. Brain 127: 2348–2359.

Pocchiari M, Poleggi A, Puopolo M et al. (2013). Age at death of Creutzfeldt–Jakob disease in subsequent family generation carrying the E200K mutation of the prion protein gene. PLoS One 8: e60376.

Puopolo M, Ladogana A, Vetrugno V et al. (2011). Transmission of sporadic Creutzfeldt–Jakob disease by blood transfusion: risk factor or possible biases. Transfusion 51: 1556–1566.

Puoti G, Bizzi A, Forloni G et al. (2012). Sporadic human prion diseases: molecular insights and diagnosis. Lancet Neurol 11: 618–628.

Ritchie DL, Ironside JW (2017). Neuropathology of human prion diseases. Prog Mol Biol Transl Sci 150: 319–339.

Ritchie DL, Adlard P, Peden AH et al. (2017). Amyloid-β accumulation in the CNS in human growth hormone recipients in the UK. Acta Neuropathol 134: 221–240.

Stokstad E (2017). Norway seeks to stamp out prion disease. Science 356: 12–13.

US National Wildlife Health Center (2018). https://www.nwhc.usgs.gov/disease_information/chronic_wasting_disease/. Accessed 23 January 2018.

Vetrugno V, Puopolo M, Cardone F et al. (2015). The future for treating Creutzfeldt–Jakob disease. Expert Opin Orphan Drugs 3: 57–74.

Waddell L, Greig J, Mascarenhas M et al. (2018). Current evidence on the transmissibility of chronic wasting disease prions to humans – a systematic review. Transbound Emerg Dis 65: 37–49.

Walker LC (2016). Proteopathic strains and the heterogeneity of neurodegenerative diseases. Annu Rev Genet 50: 329–346.

Walker LC, Jucker M (2015). Neurodegenerative diseases: expanding the prion concept. Annu Rev Neurosci 38: 87–103.

Williams ES, Young S (1980). Chronic wasting disease of captive mule deer: a spongiform encephalopathy. J Wildl Dis 16: 89–98.

Zanusso G, Monaco S, Pocchiari M et al. (2016). Advanced tests for early and accurate diagnosis of Creutzfeldt–Jakob disease. Nat Rev Neurol 12: 325–333.

Zou WQ, Puoti G, Xiao X et al. (2010). Variably protease-sensitive prionopathy: a new sporadic disease of the prion protein. Ann Neurol 68: 162–172.

Index

NB: Page numbers in *italics* refer to figures and tables.

A

Acquired prion disease 207, 420, 422
Active vaccination 424–425
Acute disseminated encephalomyelitis 391
Acute prion infection 52
  cell biology *54*
  cellular binding and uptake of PrP^{TSE} 52–55, *53*
AD. *see* Alzheimer disease
Aggregated amyloid-beta
  immunoreactive deposits of *312*
  prion-like properties of 307–309
Agitation 404
Alpers, Michael P. 4–5
Alpha-amino-3-hydroxy-5-methyl-4-isoxazolepropionic acid receptor (AMPAR) 385
  encephalitis 387
ALS. *see* Amyotrophic lateral sclerosis
Alzheimer disease (AD) 21, 243–244, 322, 389–390
  biomarkers 304
  differential diagnosis 304
  epidemiology 303–304
  genetics 304–305
  incidence and prevalence of 303
  ligand-positron emission tomography imaging 440
  neuritic plaques of 257–260
  neuropathology *305*, 306–307
    amyloid 305–306
  pathology in humans 311–312
  prion-like properties of aggregated amyloid-beta (Aβ) 307–309
  risk factors 305
  signs and symptoms 303
Amino acid
  changes in prion protein *114*
  polymorphism in sheep and goats *113*
Amplification. *see specific types of amplification*
Amyloid *33*, 34–35, 305–306
  cascade hypothesis 306
  deposits 244
    prion protein 245
  fibrils 21, 33
    of α-synuclein 323
  particles 30–31
  plaques 21, 29
Amyloid-beta (Aβ)
  aggregation 309
    immunoreactive deposits *312*
  prion-like properties 307–310
  proteopathy 309–312
  seeds 307–309, *308*
Amyloid-beta precursor protein (APP) 304
Amyloid-beta-type cerebral amyloid angiopathy (Aβ-CAA) 306
Amyloidogenic protein misfolding pathway *33*
Amyloidosis, prion protein 244, *246*
  cerebral 248–261
Amyloid plaques 136, 158, 244
  PrP^{TSE} 209
Amyloid seeding assay (ASA) 359
Amyotrophic lateral sclerosis (ALS)
  bulbar-onset 343
  incidence 337
  misfolded proteins in
    C9orf72 *339*, 340–341
    fused-in sarcoma *339*, 340, 342–343
    superoxide dismutase-1 338, *339*, 341–342
    TDP-43 338–340, *339*, 342–343
    translocated in liposarcoma *339*, 340
  pathology 343–345
  protein strains 345–347, *346*
  symptoms 337, 343–345
  WT SOD1 347–348
Animal prion disease *86*
  scanning surveillance 130–131
  statutory surveillance 129–130
  surveillance and detection 130–131
  targeted surveillance 130
Anosognosia 401
Antibodies, α-synuclein 322
Antimicrobials 436
Anti-prion protein monoclonal antibodies 422–424
Antipsychotics 406
Antisense oligonucleotides (ASOs) 331
Apolipoprotein E (ApoE) 304–305
APP. *see* Amyloid-beta precursor protein
ASOs. *see* Antisense oligonucleotides
Astrocytic gliosis 158
Astrocytosis 195
Asymptomatic genetic testing 402–403
Ataxic gait 208
Atrophy
  cerebellar 195
  cerebral cortical 195
Atrophy *(Continued)*
  multiple systems 324–325
  thalamic 271, 285, 289
Atypical dementia 179–180
Atypical scrapie 112, 455
Autophagy 32, 411
  chaperone-mediated 326–327
  lysosomal-autophagy system 326
  mTOR-dependent 61

B

Baby hamster kidney cells (BHK) 55
Ballooned neurons 182–183
Bartonella henselae 380
Basal ganglia 195
B-cells 87, 94
  follicles 92
Benzodiazepines 405–406
Biomarker 166–167, 437–440, *439*
  Creutzfeldt–Jakob disease 213–214
Blood component processing 468
Blood transfusion 466–467
Born after the real ban (BARB) cases 123
Borrelia burgdorferi spirochete 380
Bovine amyloidotic spongiform encephalopathy (BASE) 72, 452
Bovine spongiform encephalopathy (BSE) 46–47, 52, 72, 86–87, 121–122, 191–192, 425, 464, 473, 486
  agents, heat stability *130*
  atypical forms of 123–124
  classic 122–123, *125*
  clinical signs of 122
  diagnosis 126
    amplification techniques 128–129
    confirmatory tests 126–128, *127–128*
    sampling and rapid tests 126
  epidemiology 122–124
  genome 125–126
  vs. human transmissible spongiform encephalopathy 452–453
  in vivo and in vitro transmission 453–454
  laboratory testing for 131
  mouse-adapted 47, 50
  pathogenesis 125
  prions 90
    and risk assessment, inactivation 129
  in sheep 115
  statutory surveillance for 129–130

Bovine spongiform encephalopathy (BSE) *(Continued)*
survival times and attack rates of ovine *124*
transmission of 73–74
Brain
biopsies 400
cell culture 46–47
lesions, immunohistochemistry and histopathology *186*
magnetic resonance imaging (MRI) 180
Brownell–Oppenheimer variant 157
BSE. *see* Bovine spongiform encephalopathy
Bulbar-onset amyotrophic lateral sclerosis 343

C

Cadaver-derived human growth hormone (c-hGH) 311
Capillary immunoelectrophoresis 467
Caregivers
burden 406
support for 406–408
Case ascertainment 474
C-BSE. *see* Classic bovine spongiform encephalopathy
Celiac mesenteric ganglion complex (CMGC) *125*
Cell culture
brain 46–47
models of infection, in vitro 45
multicellular three-dimensional 50
primary 50
prion spread in 61–63
Cell-free conversion assay (CFCA) 32–34
transmissible spongiform encephalopathies 451
Cell-free prion 93
Cell lines establishment 47–49, *48–49*
Cell models of prion infection 45–46
brain cell culture 46–47
cell lines establishment 47–49, *48–49*
multicellular three-dimensional cell culture 50
primary cell culture 50
Cell-painting technique 29
Cell surface receptor molecule 26
Cellular binding and uptake of PrP^{TSE} 52–55
Cellular mechanisms of propagation 329–330
Cellular model, therapeutic targets
autophagy 411
cholesterol metabolism 411
drug screening using organotypic brain slices 412
neurotoxicity 411–412
PrP^{TSE} formation and propagation 410–411
Cellular prion protein (PrP^C) 21, 45–46
amino acid sequence of human *23*
biochemistry, effect of sequence variations 27–28
cellular function of 420
Cellular prion protein (PrP^C) *(Continued)*
conversion to PrP^{TSE} 32–33
molecular mechanism 32–33, *33*
dimers of 25
expression 47, 50–51
and regulation 21–22
functions 25–27, *26*
gene encoding 21–22
glycophosphatidylinositol membrane anchor of 24
glycoprotein 85
glycosylation on 24, 29
immune system 86, 421
primary structure, sequence motifs and process 22–24
protective effect of 26
RK13 cells of 47
role 59
secondary, tertiary, and quaternary structure 24–25
shedding of 117
synaptic loss 158
targeted ablation of 25–26
variations and importance of posttranslational modifications in 24
Central nervous system (CNS) 22, 47
cellular prion protein 86
immune system 96–99
Cerebellar atrophy 195
Cerebral amyloid angiopathy (CAA) 376
Cerebral amyloidose, prion protein 248–261
Cerebral cortical atrophy 195
Cerebroretinal microangiopathy 378
Cerebrospinal fluid (CSF) 166–168, *167*, 179–180
markers 277
fatal familial insomnia 277
sporadic fatal insomnia 289
Cervids
chronic wasting disease in 86–87
histologic lesions in 136
Chandler scrapie 46
Chemokine 92
Chimpanzees *(Pan troglodytes)* 450
Chinese hamster ovary (CHO) cells 52–54
Cholesterol metabolism 411
Chronic inflammation 95
Chronic wasting disease (CWD) 74–75, 486
in cervids 86–87
agent strains 457–458
vs. human transmissible spongiform encephalopathy 458
in vivo and in vitro transmission 458–459
clinical signs of 135–136
effects of host genetic variability in transgenic mice 141–143
experimental transmission
to natural hosts 138
to noncervid species 139
histopathology 136
Chronic wasting disease (CWD) *(Continued)*
mucosal immunization 425–426
natural transmission 137–138
pathogenesis 136
prions
detection 138
in saliva, blood, urine, and feces 138
in vitro amplification 139–140
role of host genetics in 140–143
strains 143–145
strains of 72
transgenic mouse models of 139
zoonotic potential of 145–146
CJD. *see* Creutzfeldt–Jakob disease
Classic bovine spongiform encephalopathy (C-BSE) 122–123, *125*
Clathrin-mediated endocytosis 55
Clinical trials
antimicrobials 436
biomarkers 437–440, *439*
challenges in prion disease 432–433
doxycycline 433–434, *433*
flupirtine *433*, 436
outcome measures
primary 437, *438*
secondary 437–440, *438*
pentosan polysulfate *433*, 435–436
quinacrine *433*, 434–435
symptomatic treatments 436–437
trial design
healthy individuals at risk of prion disease 441–442
rapidly progressive prion diseases 440–441
sporadic Creutzfeldt–Jakob disease 440–441
Clonazepam 436–437
Cluster plaques 195–196
CMGC. *see* Celiac mesenteric ganglion complex
Codon 129
genotypes *159*, 163
polymorphism 163–164, 176, 179
of *PRNP* 158–159
Cofactors 34
conversion of PrP^C to PrP^{TSE} 33–34, *33*
Confluent spongiform changes 195
Conformational neurodegenerative disorders 420–421
Contactin-associated protein-2 (CASPR2) 385
Conventional dendritic cells 92–93
Conventional transgenic mouse model 73
C9orf72 protein 340–341
Cortical ribboning 379, 382
Cortical variant *76*
CpG oligodeoxynucelotides 424–425
Creutzfeldt–Jakob disease (CJD) 2–3, 5–6, 31, 46–47, 50, 207, 272, 357, 485. *see also specific types of Creutzfeldt–Jakob disease*
bereavement groups 407–408

Creutzfeldt–Jakob disease (CJD) *(Continued)*
challenges
asymptomatic genetic testing 402–403
brain biopsies 400
communication 400
diagnosis 400–401
education 401–402, *402*
genetic prion disease 402
clinical transmissibility, blood components and plasma products 465–466
dementia caregiver support groups 407
end-of-life concerns
capacity 403
competence 403
disability 403–404
hospice 404
life-prolonging measures 404
foundation 407
human pituitary-derived growth hormone-associated 208–209
nonpharmacologic treatment 404–405, *405*
pharmacologic treatment 405–406, *406*
risk assessment
clinical transmissibility 465–466
infectivity 465
prevalence of subclinical infection 464
risk management
blood component processing 468
donor screening assays 467–468
donor selection 466–467
plasma product manufacture 468
social media 408
support groups 407–408
symptom management
nonpharmacologic management 404–405, *405*
nutrition 405
pharmacologic treatment 405–406, *406*
psychiatric symptoms 405
sensory stimulation 404–405
teleconference support groups 407
Cryptococcal meningitis 381
Cryptococcus neoformans 381
CWD. *see* Chronic wasting disease

D

Decontamination, and prion agents 479–481
Degradation
protein 61
PrP^{TSE} 57, 61
Dementia 161–162, 166–167, 303
see also Rapidly progressive dementia (RPD)
atypical 179–180
caregiver support groups 407
defined 304
frontotemporal 389
Parkinson disease 327
thalamic 271–272
Dementia with Lewy bodies (DLB) 322, 365
Demyelinating disease 391–392
Demyelination, peripheral nervous system (PNS) 27
Dendrites 90
Dendritic cells (DC) 87, 422
dendritic cells propagate prions towards 92–93
follicular 87–89
Dense prion protein synaptic accumulation 195–196
Diffusion-weighted imaging (DWI) 180
Disease-associated prion protein 183–185
proteinase K titration of *184*
DMNV. *see* Dorsal motor nucleus of the vagus
DNA vaccines 425
D178N mutation 272–273, 281–282, 284–285
D178N-129M 276–277, 280, 283
mutant protein 284–285
prion protein 284–285
Donor screening assays 467–468
Donor selection 466–467
Dorsal motor nucleus of the vagus nerve (DMNV) *94*, *125*
Doxycycline 414, 433–434, *433*
Drug screening, organotypic slice cultures 412
Dural arteriovenous fistulas (DAVFs) 376, *377*
Dura mater graft-associated Creutzfeldt–Jakob disease (dCJD)
biochemical features 212–213, *213*
clinical features 208, *209*
genotype 214
neuropathologic features 209–212, *210*
Dysautonomia 273–275

E

Early endosomes (EE) *54*
ECM. *see* Extra cellular matrix
E200K-129M haplotype 77–78
Electroencephalogram (EEG) 165
periodic sharp-wave complexes on 179
variant Creutzfeldt–Jakob disease 201
Electroencephalography (EEG)
fatal familial insomnia 277
sporadic fatal insomnia 289
Encephalitis
AMPAR 387
Japanese 379
subacute sclerosing panencephalitis 379
Encephalomyelitis
acute disseminated 391
experimental autoimmune 421
Encephalopathy. *see also* Bovine spongiform encephalopathy (BSE); Transmissible spongiform encephalopathy (TSE)
bovine amyloidotic spongiform 72, 452
feline spongiform 139
hepatic 385
Encephalopathy *(Continued)*
progressive multifocal leukoencephalopathy 381
subacute diencephalic angioencephalopathy 378, *378*
transmissible mink 425
Wernicke 382, *383*
Endocytosis 330
clathrin-mediated 55
Endososomal sorting complex required for transport (ESCRT) system 62–63
Enteritis 95
European Centre for Disease Prevention and Control (ECDC) 474
Exogenous PrP^{TSE} *53–54*, 57
Experimental autoimmune encephalomyelitis 421
Experimental models of human prion disease
conventional transgenic mouse model 73
familial Creutzfeldt–Jakob disease 77–78
fatal familial insomnia 78–79
gene-targeted models 73
Gerstmann–Sträussler–Scheinker disease 78
human mouse model 72–73
inherited/genetic forms of prion disease 77–79
intraspecies transmission in humans 75–77
species barrier in acquired diseases 73–75
sporadic disease 77
Extra cellular matrix (ECM) 51–52
Extrapontine myelinolysis 385, *386*

F

Facial brachial dystonic spells/seizures (FBDS) 386
Familial Creutzfeldt–Jakob disease (fCJD) 6, 77–78, 272
Familial transmissible spongiform encephalopathy 6–7
Fatal familial insomnia (FFI) 7–8, 73, 78–79
animal models 283–284
cell models 283
cerebral cortex *280*
clinical characteristics *275*
clinical disease progression of *276*
clinical phenomenology 273
definition 272–273
demographics 273
diagnostic criteria *276*
diagnostic tests 276–279
cerebrospinal fluid markers 277
electroencephalography 277
neuroimaging 277–278
polysomnography 277
therapeutics 278–279
differential diagnosis 276

Fatal familial insomnia (FFI) *(Continued)*
disease-associated prion protein
general characteristics 281
$_{res}PrP^{TSE}$ amount and distribution 281, *282*
structure 281–282
epidemiology 273
etiology and pathogenesis 284–285
experimental animal transmission 282–283
history 271–272
mediodorsal thalamic nucleus in *279*
neuropathology 279–280
signs and symptoms 273–276
in vitro amplification 283
FDC. *see* Follicular dendritic cells
Feline spongiform encephalopathy (FSE) 139
FFI. *see* Fatal familial insomnia
Fibrillar α-synuclein 323, 329
Florid plaques, in variant Creutzfeldt–Jakob disease brain 195–196, *195*
FLUOstar Omega 362
Flupirtine *433*, 436
Follicles
associated epithelium 90–91
B-cell 92
Follicular dendritic cells (FDC) 87–89, *88–89*
acquire prions as complement-opsonized complexes 90
independent prion accumulation and neuroinvasion 90
within Peyer's patches 93
Food contamination 192
Fourier transform infrared (FT-IR) spectroscopy 30
Fowler, Malcolm 2–3
Frontotemporal dementia (FTD) 389
Frontotemporal lobar degeneration with ubiquitin-positive inclusions (FTLD-U) 340
FSE. *see* Feline spongiform encephalopathy
Fused-in sarcoma/translocated in liposarcoma (FUS/TLS) *339*, 340

G

GAG. *see* Glycosaminoglycan
Gajdusek, Daniel Carleton 2, *2*, 4
GALT. *see* Gut-associated lymphoid tissues
Genetic counseling 402–403
Genetic Creutzfeldt–Jakob disease
demographic and laboratory characteristics of *221–222*
diagnostic approach 220
genotypes and phenotypes associated with
A224V-129V 234
D178N-129V 226–227
E196A-129M 229
E200G-129V 231
E196K-129M 229
Genetic Creutzfeldt–Jakob disease *(Continued)*
E200K-129M 229–231
E196K-129V 229
E200K-129V 229–231
E211Q-129M 233–234
G114V-129M 224–226
I215V-129M 234
M232R-129M 234–235
octapeptide repeat deletions 236
octapeptide repeat insertions 235
5–7 OPRI 236
1–4 OPRI-129M 235–236
1–4 OPRI-129V 235–236
P105T-129V 223–224
R148H-129M 226
R208H 129M 232–233
R208H-129V 232–233
T183A-129M 227–228
T188K-R-A 228–229
V180I-129M 227
V203I-129M 231–232
V210I-129 M 233
V180I-129V 227
V203I-129V 231–232
V210I-129V 233
neuropathologic alterations in *225*
prion protein mutations linked to *220*
public health 475
RT-QUIC and PMCA in
cerebrospinal fluid 366
olfactory mucosa 366
surveillance 220
Genetic prion disease 77, 219–220, 402
Genotype
dura mater graft-associated Creutzfeldt–Jakob disease 214
human growth hormone Creutzfeldt–Jakob disease 214–215
Gerstmann–Sträussler–Scheinker (GSS) disease 7, 73, 78, *97–98*, 243–244
cerebral cortex of patient with *252–253*, *255*, *258–259*, *262*
cerebral hemisphere of patient with *252*, *255*, *258*
dominantly inherited prion protein cerebral amyloidoses 248–261, 263–265
A133V-129M-219K 256
A117V-129V 254
178DEL2BP-129M 263–264
differential diagnosis 264–265
D202N-129V 260
E211D-129V 260
F198S-129V 257–260, *257*
G131V-129M 255–256
H187R-129V 256–257
INS 168BP-129M 263–264
INS 216BP-129M 263–264
INS 288BP-120M 263–264
INS 24BP-129V 264
INS 144BP-120V 263–264
INS 192BP-129V 263–264
M232T-129M 261
P102L-129M 250–252
Gerstmann–Sträussler–Scheinker (GSS) disease *(Continued)*
P102L-129V 252–253
P105L-129V 253–261
P84S-129V 250
P105S-129V 253–254
P105T-129V 254
Q212P-129M 260
Q217R-129V 260–261
Q160X-129M 262–263
Q227X-129V 261
R136S-129M 256
S132I-129M 256
V176G-129V 256
Y218N-129V 261
Y145X-129M 261–262
Y163X-129V 263
Y226X-129V 263
epidemiology
age and gender distribution 245
incidence and prevalence 245
genetics 245–247, *246*, *246*
insertional mutation between codon 129 and 130 264
MRI scans of patient with *251*, *255*
Gibbs, Clarence J. Jr. *4*, 5
Gliosis 411
astrocytic 158
Glutamine/asparganine (Q/N) residues 342–343
Glycophosphatidylinositol (GPI) membrane anchor 22, *23*, 24
Glycoprotein 21
cellular prion protein 85
Glycosaminoglycan (GAG) 52–54
inhibitors 55
as receptors 52–53
sulfation 51–52
Glycosylation
cellular prion protein 24, 29
N-linked 22, 24, 28–29
prion protein 70
Goat
amino acid polymorphisms in *113*
prion protein amino acid variation in *113*
PRNP gene in 117
G-protein-coupled receptor 126 (GPR126) 27
GT1 cells 47
Guardianship 403
Gut-associated lymphoid tissues (GALT) 87, 91
follicular dendritic cells within 90–91
prions accumulation in 93–94, *94*

H

HaB cells 46–47
Hadlow, William J. 3–4, *3*
Haloperidol 406
Hazard ratio (HR) 433–434
Healthcare professionals 401–402, *402*
Hemophilia 193
variant Creutzfeldt–Jakob disease infection 9
Heparin sulfate proteoglycans (HSPG) *54*

Hepatic encephalopathy 385
Herpes simplex virus (HSV) type 1 379, *380*
hGH. *see* Human growth hormone
Hospice 404
Host genetic variability, in transgenic mice 141–143
Human embryonic kidney cells (HEK293)
  misfolded WT SOD1 347
  TDP-43 343
Human growth hormone (hGH) Creutzfeldt–Jakob disease *209*
  biochemical features 213
  genotype 214–215
  neuropathologic features 211–212
Human pituitary-derived growth hormone-associated Creutzfeldt–Jakob disease 208–209
Human prion strain 72
Human species barrier 449–452
Huntington disease 21, 403
Hypoglycemia 382

I

Iatrogenic Creutzfeldt–Jakob disease (iCJD) 8–10
  biomarkers 213–214
  experimental animal models *211*
  history 207–208
  public health 476
  RT-QUIC and PMCA in 366–367
Iatrogenic disease 388–389
iCJD. *see* Iatrogenic Creutzfeldt–Jakob disease
ICSM 18 424
ICSM 35 424
Immune system
  cellular prion protein 86
  in central nervous system 96–99
  and prion infection 421–422
Immunization
  mucosal 425–426
  passive 424
Immunoblotting 467
Immunomodulation 421
Immunosenescence 96
Immunotherapy 330
Infectivity 465
Inflammation, chronic 95
Inflammatory stromal cells 90
Inhibitors
  glycosaminoglycan 55
  lysosomal 57
Intermediolateral cell column (IML) *94*
Internal fragment
  7-kDa 183, *183*, 256–257, 260
  8 kDa 262
  9 kDa 256
  11 kDa 260
  14 kDa 257
Intracranial hypotension 391
Intravascular lymphoma 388
In vitro amplification
  of chronic wasting disease prions 139–140
  fatal familial insomnia 283
  variably protease-sensitive prionopathy 187
In vitro cell based system 45
In vitro models 45, 323
  transmissible spongiform encephalopathy
    cell-free conversion assay 451
    protein misfolding cyclic amplification 451–452
    quaking-induced conversion 452
In vitro prion titration assay 47
In vivo models
  diagnostic algorithm for sporadic Creutzfeldt–Jakob disease *366*
  of prion infection 45, 47
  therapeutic targets
    neurodegeneration 413
    protein translation inhibition 413
    PrP^{TSE} accumulation 412
    $TgMHu_2ME199K$ mice 414–415, *414*
    transgenic mice modeling 413–414
  transmissible spongiform encephalopathy
    nonhuman primates 450
    transgenic mouse models 450–451

J

Japanese encephalitis 379
Jellison, William 3
John Cunningham virus 381

K

Klatzo, Igor 2–3, *3*
Knock-in mouse models 75
Korsakoff syndrome 382
Kuru 2, 5–6
  plaques variant *76*

L

Late endosomes/multivesicular bodies (LE/MVB) *54*
LCPs. *see* Luminescent conjugated polythiophenes
LDL. *see* Low-density lipoprotein
Leucine-rich, glioma inactivated 1 protein (LGI1) 385–386
Levetiracetam 436–437
Lewy body 321–322
Lewy body dementia (LBD) 365
Lewy body disease 322
Lewy neurites 321–322
Lewy pathology 322–323
Limb-onset amyotrophic lateral sclerosis 343
Lipoprotein receptor-related protein (LRP1) 52, *54*, 55
Low-density lipoprotein (LDL) 56–57
Luminescent conjugated polythiophenes (LCPs) 69–70
Lyme disease 380
Lymph nodes *88–89*
  endothelial venules in 90
  mesenteric 92–94, *94*
Lymphocyte-activation gene 3 (LAG3) 329
Lymphoid tissues, in variant Creutzfeldt–Jakob disease 194–195
Lymphomatosis cerebri 388
Lymphotoxins (LT) 89
Lysosomal inhibitors 57

M

Macrophages
  depletion of 93
  destruction of prions by 93
Macropinocytosis 56
Madin-Darby bovine kidney cell clones 47
Magnetic resonance imaging (MRI) 165–166, *166*
  brain 180
  Gerstmann–Sträussler–Scheinker disease *251*, *255*
  variably protease-sensitive prionopathy 180
Mammalian prion protein *23*, 45–46
MBM. *see* Meat and bone meal
M cells 90–91
  abundance of 95
  density in gut epithelium 91
  differentiation 91
  expression 91
  maturation 96
  role 91
Meat and bone meal (MBM) 122–123
Membrane anchor, glycophosphatidylinositol 22, *23*, 24
Metabolism
  cholesterol 411
  thalamic hypometabolism 277–278, *278*
Methionine heterozygosity 464
Microglia 96–98
  activation 98
  in brain 99
  response *97–98*, 98–99
Microspheres, restriction of internalization of 55
Miniplaques immunostain *182*
Misfolding, protein 21, 24, 31, 33
  amyloidogenic protein *33*
  cellular prion protein 32
  prion protein 31, 34
  of recombinant protein 24–25
  in vitro 28–29
Missense mutation 325
Mitochondrial disease 387–388
Mitogen stimulation 95
Mononuclear phagocytes 92–93
MRC Scale 437, 440–441
MRI. *see* Magnetic resonance imaging (MRI)
MSA. *see* Multiple systems atrophy
M1 strain 209–211
Mucosal immunization 425–426

Multiple sclerosis (MS) 391
Multiple systems atrophy (MSA) 324–325
Multivesicular body (MVB) 60, 62, 329–330
Murine CAD5 cells 47
Murine neuroblastoma cells 47
Murine PrP^{TSE} 56–57
Mutant gene expression 73
Mutation
  D178N 272–273, 281–282, 284–285
  human prion protein 73
  missense 325
  PRNP 219–220, *223*, 226, 245
    molecular diagnosis of 248
    neuropathologic phenotypes and *247–248*
  α-synuclein 325–326
MVB. *see* Multivesicular body
Myelinolysis, extrapontine 385, *386*

N

Nano-pomegranate seed oil (PSO) 414–415, *414*
Necropsy 135–136
Nestin-positive neural stem cells 50
Neuritic plaque 257–260, 263
  of Alzheimer disease 257–260
Neurodegeneration 96, *97–98*, 306, 413
Neurodegenerative disease 389–390
Neurofibrillary tangle 244, 253–254, 256–261
  atomic structure of 265
  tau 245
Neuroinvasion, prion 90, 94–95, *94*
Neuromyelitis optica 391
Neuronal cell 50
  cell lines 47
Neuronal dysfunction 412
Neuron-intrinsic mechanism 322–323
Neuropsychiatric symptoms, pharmacologic treatment of 406
Neurosarcoidosis 390
Neurospheres, prion infection of 50
Neurotoxicity 411–412
Neurotropic virus 322
Neurovegetative test 272
N-glycans *23*, 24–25
Nicotinamide adenine dinucleotide (NAD) 411–412
NIH 3T3 fibroblast cells 47
N-linked glycosylation, on cellular prion protein 24
N-methyl-D-aspartate receptors (NMDARs) encephalitis 387
Nocturnal sleep 271–272
Nonhuman primates, transmissible spongiform encephalopathy 450
Nonphagocytic cells 55
Nonplaque-type dCJD 208, *209*
Nonsense polymorphisms 115
Normal-pressure hydrocephalus 180
Nor98 scrapie 112
Nosology of human transmissible spongiform encephalopathy 12
Novel prion disease 77
Nutrition 405

O

Octapeptide repeat deletions (OPRDs) 236
Octapeptide repeat region, insertional mutations in 263–264
Olfactory model 324
Oligomeric proteins 32
OPRDs. *see* Octapeptide repeat deletions
Organotypic slice cultures 50
  drug screening 412
Ovine prion protein, VRQ allele of *124*

P

Parkinson disease (PD) 21, 321
  as prion-like disease 322–323
Parkinson disease dementia (PDD) 327
Passive immunization 424
PD. *see* Parkinson disease
Pentosan polysulfate (PPS) *433*, 435–436
  dose 436
  oral bioavailability 436
  pharmacokinetics 436
Periodic sharp-wave complexes (PSWCs) 165, 208, 277
Peripheral nervous system (PNS) 22
  demyelination 27
Persistent prion infection
  cellular location of PrP^{TSE} formation 59–60
  establishment of
    adaptation 58–59
    cell-specific factors 59
    role of cellular prion protein 59
  prion spread in cell culture 61–63
  PrP^{TSE} degradation 61
PET. *see* Positron emission tomography
Peyer's patches 87, *88–89*, 90, 93, *94*
  follicular dendritic cells within 93
  infection within, after oral exposure 90–91
  maturation of M cells in 96
Phagocytic cells, PrP^{TSE} degradation in 57
Phagocytosis 93
Phosphatidylethanolamine (PE) 70
Plaque-type dCJD 208, *209*
Plasma fractionation 468
Plasma products, manufacture of 468
PMCA. *see* Protein misfolding cyclic amplification
PMDs. *see* Protein misfolding diseases
Polydipsia 135–136
Polymorphic codon 129 220
Polymorphism
  at codon 129 176, 179, *276*
    of *PRNP* gene 193
  human prion protein 73
  methionine (M)-valine (V) 272
  M129V 281–282
  nonsense 115
  single-nucleotide 112, 326
Polysomnography (PSG) 162
  fatal familial insomnia 277
  sporadic fatal insomnia 289
Polyuria 135–136
Pomegranate seed oil (PSO) 414, *414*
Positron emission tomography (PET) 272–273, 278–279
Postictal cortical diffusion restriction 390–391, *390*
Power of attorney (POA) 403
Preimplantation genetic diagnosis (PGD) 403
Primary angiitis, central nervous system 378
Primary cerebellar granular neurons 50
Prion 11–12, 45–46
  accumulation 87–90, *88–89*
    FDC-independent 90
    within GALT *94*
    GALT of upper gastrointestinal tract 93–94
  agents, replication 47
  destruction by macrophages 93
  infected cells 46
  infected cerebellar slices 50
  infected murine neuroblastoma cells 47
  mouse model 72–73
  neuroinvasion 90, 94–95
    initial pathways *94*
    from intestine *94*
  physical heterogeneity of 129
  propagation 90, 285, 292
  replication 46
  susceptible cell lines *48–49*
  transmission
    sporadic Creutzfeldt–Jakob disease *76*, 77
    variably proteasesensitive prionopathy *76*
    variant Creutzfeldt–Jakob disease *76*
Prion disease
  diagnosis 400–401
  pathogenesis 21, 420–421
    effects of host age 96
    effects of inflammation and pathogen co-infection 95
    immune system in CNS 96–99
Prion hypothesis 32
Prion infection
  acute (*see* Acute prion infection)
  cell-based determinants of susceptibility to 51–52
Prion-like process, potential for therapeutics 330–331
Prion-like seeding 311–312
Prion protein (PrP) 21, 85–99, 338
  see also specific types of prion protein
  amino acid
    changes *114*
    variation in sheep and goats *113*
  amyloid
    aggregation assays 167–168
    deposits 245
    miniplaques 182
    seeding assay 359
  amyloidosis 244, *246*
  bands, Western blot analysis *249*
  cell surface expression of 410

Prion protein (PrP) *(Continued)*
- cerebral amyloid angiopathy variant 261–263
- cerebral amyloidoses 248–261
- in cerebrospinal fluid 232
- deposition in transgenic mice *75*
- disease-specific 85–86
- gene 111–112, 219
- histopathology and *182*
- immunoblot of abnormal *186*
- immunohistochemistry *181–182*, 279–280
- immunoreactivity 228
- immunostaining 181–182
- impact of disease-specific *97–98*
- mislocalized 411–412
- molecules 46
- mutations linked to genetic Creutzfeldt–Jakob disease *220*
- N-linked glycosylation 70
- N-terminus of 114
- peptides 411–412
- peptide spanning residues 106–126 (PrP106–126) 411
- polymorphisms and mutations of human 73
- potential forms of 24–25
- production of 73
- protein misfolding amplification assay 358–359, *359*
  - in human prion diseases 362–368, *363*, *363*
  - *vs.* real-time quaking-induced conversion 360–362, *361*
- real-time quaking-induced conversion 359–360, *360*
  - in human prion diseases 362–368, *363*, *363*
- spongiform degeneration and *181*

Prion protein gene (PRNP) 371, 475

Prion strain 281–283, 290–292, 410–411
- accumulate in secondary lymphoid organs 86–87
- biology 69–71
- defined 69, 163–164
- in humans 72
- in natural prion diseases of livestock and cervids 71–72
- tropism 71
- variation in 69

PRION-1 trial 435, 437

PRND gene 21–22

PRNP gene 21–22, 26–27, 31, 50, 73, 112
- alleles 115
  - determination 140–141
  - highly susceptible 115–116
  - neutral 116
  - reduced susceptibility/resistance 116
- amino acid polymorphisms with scrapie susceptibility/resistance 115
- codon 129 of 158–159, 361–365
- genotypes 115
- in goats 117
- haplotypes 114–115

PRNP gene *(Continued)*
- mutation 219–220, *223*, 226, 245
  - molecular diagnosis of 248
  - neuropathologic phenotypes and *247–248*
- polymorphism at codon 129 of 193
- in sheep 117

Progressive multifocal leukoencephalopathy (PML) 381

Propagation, prion 285, 292

Protease-sensitive prionopathy (PSPr) 175–176, *177*

Proteasome, role in PrP^{TSE} degradation 61

Protein
- degradation 61
- DNA-binding study 117
- translation inhibition in prion-infected mice 413

Proteinase K (PK) 175
- resistant prion protein *188*
- resistant PrP (PrP^{res}) 224
- sensitive 184–185
- titration of disease-associated prion protein *184*
- treated prion protein *183*

Protein misfolding amplification assay (PMCA) 486
- accelerants 358–359
- cultured cells 358
- genetic Creutzfeldt–Jakob disease
  - cerebrospinal fluid 366
  - olfactory mucosa 366
- human brain 358
- human platelets 358
- iatrogenic Creutzfeldt–Jakob disease 366–367
- *vs.* real-time quaking-induced conversion 360–362, *361*
- recombinant prion protein 358, *359*
- sensitivity 358
- sonication/rest cycles 358
- sporadic Creutzfeldt–Jakob disease
  - cerebrospinal fluid 362–365, *364*
  - olfactory mucosa 365–366
- transmissible spongiform encephalopathies 451–452
- variant Creutzfeldt–Jakob disease
  - cerebrospinal fluid 367
  - plasma 367–368
  - urine 367
- western blotting 358

Protein misfolding cyclic amplification (PMCA) 11–12, 70, 128, 136, 139–140, 187, 195

Protein misfolding diseases (PMDs) 21, 31

Protein misfolding neurodegenerative diseases (PMNDs) 409

Protein-only hypothesis 420

Proteopathy 304–306
- amyloid-beta (Aβ) 309–312
- strains 310–311

PrP. *see* Prion protein

PrP^{TSE} 21, 24, 28–35, 45–46, 136, 420
- accumulation *88–89*, 194–195
  - therapeutic targets 412

PrP^{TSE} *(Continued)*
- amyloid plaques 209
- biochemical properties 34–35
- cellular binding and uptake of 52–55
- conformation-dependent immunoassay 69–70
- degradation 57, 61
- depositions 157–158
- disease-specific 85–86
- exogenous *53–54*
  - localization of 57
- formation 57–58
  - cellular location 59–60
  - efficiency 69–70
  - strain-specific rates 69–70
- function 31–32
- heterogeneity in population of 61
- hydrogen/deuterium exchange rates in 30
- molecular mechanisms of conversion of PrP^{C} to 32–33, *33*
- oxidation of 413
- peripheral localization of 194–195
- primary structure and posttranslational modifications 28–30
- role for cofactors in conversion 33–34
- secondary, tertiary, and quaternary structure 30–31
- sequence variations 31
- trafficking 56–57
- uptake 55–56
- western blotting analysis *29*, *128*

PSG. *see* Polysomnography

PSPr. *see* Protease-sensitive prionopathy

PSWCs. *see* Periodic sharp-wave complexes

Psychiatric abnormalities 176

Psychiatric symptoms 405

Public health
- genetic Creutzfeldt–Jakob disease 475
- iatrogenic Creutzfeldt–Jakob disease 476
- prion resistance to chemical and physical process *479*
- risk management
  - decontamination and prion agents 479–481
  - hospital and community care 478
  - increased risk of prion disease 476–477
  - occupational exposure 478–479
  - surgical incidents 478
  - surgical procedures 477–478
- sporadic Creutzfeldt–Jakob disease 475
- surveillance
  - case ascertainment 474
  - epidemiologic risk 474–475
- variant Creutzfeldt–Jakob disease 475

Pyrexia 404

Q

Quaking-induced conversion (QuIC), transmissible spongiform encephalopathy 452

Quantitative polymerase chain reaction (qPCR) 51
Quetiapine 406
Quinacrine *433*, 434–435

R

Rabbit kidney epithelial (RK13) cells 47, 52
RAMALT biopsy 93
Rapid eye movement (REM) stage 272
Rapidly progressive dementia (RPD) 400
  autoimmune 385–387
  demyelinating disease 391–392
  iatrogenic 388–389
  infections
    bacterial 379–380
    central nervous system 380–381
    viral *378*, 379, *380*
  mimickers 375–376, *375*
  mitochondrial disease 387–388
  neurodegenerative 389–390
  neurosarcoidosis 390
  referral centers *377*, 389
  seizures 390–391, *390*
  systemic disorders 390–391
  in tertiary care hospitals 372–373, *372*
  toxic-metabolic etiologies 381–385, *383*
  vascular etiologies 376–378
Real-time quaking-induced conversion (RT-QUIC) 11–12, 128, 136, 140, 167–168, 467, 486
  bank vole recombinant prion protein 360
  genetic Creutzfeldt–Jakob disease
    cerebrospinal fluid 366
    olfactory mucosa 366
  iatrogenic Creutzfeldt–Jakob disease 366–367
  immunoprecipitation 359–360
  intermittent shaking 361
  organotypic slice cultures 412
  vs. protein misfolding amplification assay 360–362, *361*
  recombinant prion protein 359, *360*
  sporadic Creutzfeldt–Jakob disease 359
    cerebrospinal fluid 362–365, *364*
    olfactory mucosa 365–366
  Syrian hamster recombinant prion protein 360
  thioflavin-T 359, *360*
  variant Creutzfeldt–Jakob disease 359–360
    cerebrospinal fluid 367
    plasma 367–368
    urine 367
Recombinant prion protein (recPrP) 24–25, 358, *359*
Recycling endosomes (RE) *54*
Regional brain distribution of protease-resistant prion protein (resPrPTSE) 184–185
  in fatal familial insomnia *282*
Regional cerebral metabolism of glucose (rCMRglu), serial fluorodeoxyglucose positron emission tomography of *278*
Risk management
  decontamination and prion agents 479–481
  hospital and community care 478
  increased risk of prion disease 476–477
  occupational exposure 478–479
  surgical incidents 478
  surgical procedures 477–478
RK13 cells. *see* Rabbit kidney epithelial cells
Robertson, E. Graeme 2–3
Rocky Mountain Laboratory (RML) prions 90
RPD. *see* Rapidly progressive dementia
RT-QUIC. *see* Real-time quaking-induced conversion

S

Salmonella enterica 425
Salmonella typhimurium 95
Schwann cells 47
sCJD. *see* Sporadic Creutzfeldt–Jakob disease
sCJDMM2 279–280, *282*, 285, 289–292, *291*
Scrapie 3
  agent 46
  atypical 112
  cell assay 410
  classic 111–112
  forms of 111
  infected cells 51
  resistance 112
  in sheep 111–112
  in small ruminants
    agent strains in sheep 455
    vs. human TSEs 455–456
    in vitro and in vivo transmission 456–457
  susceptibility, genetic study 112–117
Scrapie mouse brain (SMB) cells 46
Scrapie-negative cells 51
Scrapie-positive cells 51
Secondary lymphoid organs (SLO) 86
  dendritic cells propagate prions towards FDC in 92–93
  prion strains accumulate in 86–87
  propagation of prions within 90
Secondary tauopathy 158–159
Seeded polymerization 45–46
Seeding, prion-like 311–312
Seizures 390–391
Sensory stimulation 404–405
Serial fluorodeoxyglucose positron emission tomography *278*
sFI. *see* Sporadic fatal insomnia
Sheep
  amino acid polymorphisms in *113*
  bovine spongiform encephalopathy in 115
Sheep *(Continued)*
  prion protein amino acid variation in *113*
  PRNP gene in 117
Sheep scrapie brain pool 1 (SSBP/1) 71–72
Single-nucleotide polymorphisms 112, 326
Sinus venous thrombosis 376, *377*
Sleep spindle 277, 289
Slow infections 2–5
Smadel, Joseph E. 4
SMB cells. *see* Scrapie mouse brain cells
Speech impairment 176, 179
Spleen 87, *88–89*, 93–94, *94*
Spongiform encephalopathy 244
  see also specific types of spongiform encephalopathy
  familial transmissible 6–7
Sporadic Creutzfeldt–Jakob disease (sCJD) 46, 72, 155, 208, 371–372, 448–449
  Brownell–Oppenheimer variant of 157
  cerebrospinal fluid analysis 166, *167*
    prion protein-amyloid aggregation assays 167–168
    routine cerebrospinal fluid parameters 166
    surrogate markers 166–167
  clinical diagnosis 168–169, *168*
    electroencephalogram 165
    magnetic resonance imaging 165–166, *166*
  clinical features 156–157
    advanced stages 157
    disease evolution 157
    early stage 157
  clinical findings *156*
  clinical syndrome 399–400
  clinicopathologic features 159–160, *160*
  distinctive histopathologic features *161*
  epidemiology 156, *156*
  general features 160–165
  genetic aspects 156
  Heidenhain variant of 157
  molecular and pathologic features 163
  molecular basis of phenotypic variability in *159*
  neuropathologic features 157
    amyloid plaques 158
    astrocytic gliosis 158
    microglial activation 158
    neuronal loss 158
    PrP^{TSE} depositions 157–158
    secondary tauopathy 158–159
    spongiform change 158
    synaptic loss 158
  neuropsychiatric symptoms and signs *157*
  phenotypic heterogeneity of 163–164
  phenotypic variability and prion strains 163–165
  prions, iatrogenic transmission *211*
  public health 475

Sporadic Creutzfeldt–Jakob disease (sCJD) *(Continued)*
- RT-QUIC and PMCA in
  - cerebrospinal fluid 362–365, *364*
  - olfactory mucosa 365–366
- subtypes 159, 163, *168*
  - MM(V)1 161
  - MM2C 162
  - MM(V)1 + 2C 163
  - MM2T 162
  - MV2K 162
  - P-MM1 163
  - VV1 162
  - VV2 161–162
  - VV2+1 163
- transmission *76*, 77

Sporadic diseases 77
Sporadic familial insomnia 162
Sporadic fatal insomnia (sFI) 285, *286–287*
- cerebral cortex *290*
- clinical characteristics *288*
- clinical criteria *288*
- diagnostic tests
  - cerebrospinal fluid markers 289
  - electroencephalography 289
  - neuroimaging 289
  - polysomnography 289
- differential diagnosis 288
- disease-associated prion protein
  - distinctive features 290–291
  - general characteristics 290
- epidemiology 285–288
- experimental animal transmission 291–292
- neuropathology 289–290
- pathogenetic hypothesis 292
- signs and symptoms 288

Sporadic prion disease 175–176, 185, *186*, 187
SPRN gene 21–22
Strain
- cofactors 70
- prion 281–283, 290–292
- sCJDMM2 291

Stromal cells 46–47
Subacute diencephalic angioencephalopathy 378, *378*
Subacute sclerosing panencephalitis 379
Superoxide dismutase-1 (SOD1) protein *339*
- in amyotrophic lateral sclerosis 338
- exosomes 344–345
- G85R mutation 342
- in vitro cell-free assay 341
- in vivo assay 341–342
- misfolding
  - cervical spinal cord of amyotrophic lateral sclerosis patients 348, *349*
  - intercellular transmission 343–344, *344*
- motor neurons 338
- mutations 338

Superoxide dismutase-1 (SOD1) protein *(Continued)*
- prion protein 341
- propagation and seeding 341–342
- protein-only hypothesis 341
- WT SOD1 341–342

Symptom management
- nonpharmacologic management 404–405, *405*
- nutrition 405
- psychiatric symptoms 405
- sensory stimulation 404–405

α-Synuclein 321–322, 409
- accumulation of 327
- aggregation of 322
- amyloid fibrils of 323
- animal models of cell-to-cell transfer of 323–324
- antibodies 322
- fibrillar 323, 329
- fibrils 328
- formation of 323–324, *326*
- levels of 326
- misfolding and permissive templating 325–327
- mutations of 325–326
- pathogenic strains 327–329
- pathology 324, *325*
- redistribution of *324*

α-Synucleinopathies 328, 330
Syphilis 379–380
Systemic lupus erythematosus 391–392

T

Tau
- in brain 304
- prion-like properties of aggregated 310–311
- protein 264, 306–307
- seeds 310–311
- strains, bioactivity 310–311

Tauopathy 306
- secondary 158–159

T cells 87
Teleconference support groups 407
Tetracycline 433
$TgMHu_2ME199K$ mice 414–415, *414*
$TgMHu_2ME200K$ mice 414–415
Thalamic atrophy 271, 285, 289
Thalamic dementia 271–272
Thalamic hypometabolism 277–278, *278*
Thalamic nuclei 271–272, 279–280
Therapeutic targets
- cellular models
  - autophagy 411
  - cholesterol metabolism 411
  - drug screening using organotypic brain slices 412
  - neurotoxicity 411–412
  - PrP^{TSE} formation and propagation 410–411
- identification and assessment of 79
- in vivo models
  - neurodegeneration 413
  - protein translation inhibition 413

Therapeutic targets *(Continued)*
  - PrP^{TSE} accumulation 412
  - $TgMHu_2ME199K$ mice 414–415, *414*
  - $TgMHu_2ME200K$ mice 414–415
  - transgenic mice modeling 413–414
- for prion infection 423–424, *423*

Thiamine (vitamin B_1) deficiency 382
Thioflavin T 452
Tingible body macrophages 93
TMER. *see* Transfusion Medicine Epidemiology Review
Tonsil biopsy 201
Toxicity
- arsenic 382
- cellular 32
- glutamate-related excitotoxicity 26
- lead 382
- lithium 382
- mercury 382
- neuronal 29, 31
- proteo-toxicity 31–32

Toxoplasma gondii 381
Toxoplasmosis 381
TPrP model 411–412
43-kDa Transactive response (TAR) DNA-binding protein (TDP-43) 338–340, *339*, 342–343
Transcription factors 21–22
Transfusion Medicine Epidemiology Review (TMER) 9, 466
Transgenic mouse, effects of host genetic variability in 141–143
Transgenic mouse model 73–74
- of chronic wasting disease 139
- conventional 73
- for genetic prion disease 413–414
- transmissible spongiform encephalopathies 450–451

Trans-Golgi network (TGN) pathway *54*
Transmissible mink encephalopathy (TME) 425
Transmissible spongiform encephalopathy (TSE) 2–3, 21, 46, 85, 191, 486
- agents, unconventional nature 10–12
- bovine spongiform encephalopathy
  - *vs.* human 452–453
  - in vivo and in vitro transmission 453–454
- chronic wasting disease in cervids
  - agent strains 457–458
  - *vs.* human 458
  - in vivo and in vitro transmission 458–459
- human species barrier 449–452
- human *vs.* animal
  - comparative epidemiology 448
  - Creutzfeldt–Jakob disease risk factors and etiology 457–458
- in vitro models
  - cell-free conversion assay 451
  - protein misfolding cyclic amplification 451–452
  - quaking-induced conversion 452

Transmissible spongiform encephalopathy (TSE) *(Continued)*
- in vivo models
  - nonhuman primates 450
  - transgenic mouse models 450–451
- nosology of human 12
- prion protein sequence 449
- *PRNP* gene 449
- replication in lymphoid tissues 450
- route of infection and dose 449
- scrapie in small ruminant
  - agent strains in sheep 455
  - *vs.* human 455–456
  - in vitro and in vivo transmission 456–457
- statutory surveillance for 129–130
- strains 449
- transmission
  - of animal *74*
  - by blood components 8–9
  - by contaminated neurosurgical instruments and human derived hormones and tissues 8

Treponema pallidum 379–380
Tropheryma whipplei 380
TSE. *see* Transmissible spongiform encephalopathy
Tuberculosis (TB) 380–381
Tumor necrosis factor-α (TNF-α) 89
Tunneling nanotubes (TNT) 63, 95

U
Upper gastrointestinal tract, prion accumulation GALT of 93–94

V
Vaccination, active 424–425
Valine heterozygosity 464
Valine homozygosity 464
Variably protease-sensitive prionopathy (VPSPr) 77, 175
- animal models 187–188
- clinical characteristics *178*
- clinical course 179, *179*
- clinical features, demographics 176–179
- clinical tests
  - cerebrospinal fluid 179–180
  - diagnostic workup 179
  - electroencephalogram 179
  - neuroimaging 180
- definition 176
- differential diagnosis 180
- disease-associated prion protein 183–185
- epidemiology 176
- etiology and pathogenesis 188
- experimental transmission 185–187
- neuropathology 180–183
- transmission *76*
- in vitro amplification 187

Variant Creutzfeldt–Jakob disease (vCJD) 8, 72, 75–77, *75*, 94–96
- blood-contaminated cases of 193–194
- blood tests 200–201
- bovine spongiform encephalopathy 191–192, 452–453
- cerebellar features 198
- cerebral MR 199–200, *200*
- cerebrospinal fluid examination 200
- clinical features
  - age 196
  - duration 196
  - general illness profile 196–197
  - sex 196
- cognitive impairment 198
- diagnosis 198–201, *199*
- electroencephalogram 201
- epidemiology aspects 191–194
- hallmarks of 195
- infections 9–10
  - in asymptomatic UK patient with hemophilia 9
- involuntary movements 198
- lymphoid tissues in 194–195
- management 201–202
- mucosal immunization 425
- nasal brushing 201
- pain/sensory features 197–198
- pathologic aspects
  - neuropathology 195–196
  - peripheral localization of PrP^{TSE} 194–195
- psychiatric features 197
- public health 475
- RT-QUIC and PMCA in
  - cerebrospinal fluid 367
  - plasma 367–368
  - urine 367
- tonsil biopsy 201
- transmission *76*
- treatment 201
- in United Kingdom 192–193
- urine tests 201

vCJD. *see* Variant Creutzfeldt–Jakob disease (vCJD)
VPSPr. *see* Variably protease-sensitive prionopathy
VRQ 115–116
V2 strain 209–211

W
Wernicke encephalopathy 382, *383*
Whipple disease 380
Wilson disease 382–383
WT SOD1 protein 341–342
- in amyotrophic lateral sclerosis pathogenesis 347–348
- in sporadic amyotrophic lateral sclerosis 349

Z
Zigas, Vincent 2, *2*
Zoonotic potential, of chronic wasting disease 145–146

Erratum

In: Pocchiari & Manson / Human Prion Diseases, Volume 153 of the Handbook of Clinical Neurology Series

Correction in Chapter 1 Human transmissible spongiform encephalopathies: historic view. On pages 3 and 4 in Chapter 1, the photos of William Hadlow and Clarence J. Gibbs, Jr. were inadvertently switched. Please see the correct photographs and identifying names below:

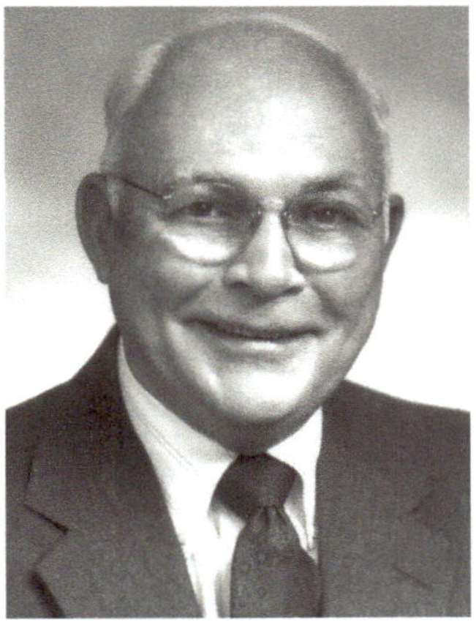

Fig. 1.4. Clarence J. Gibbs, Jr. in the late 1990s. (Courtesy of National Institute of Neurological Diseases and Stroke.)

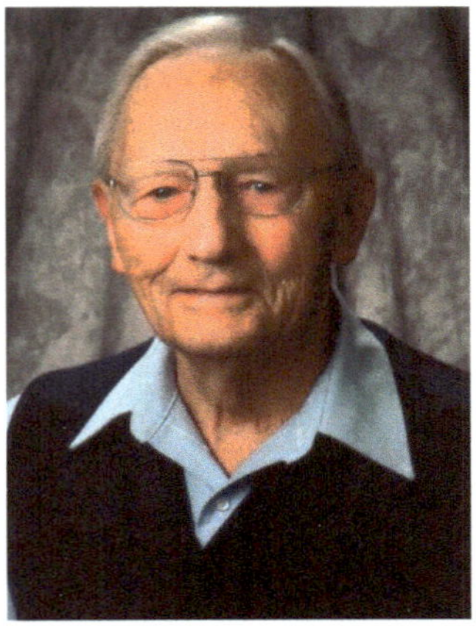

Fig. 1.5. William Hadlow at age 90. (Courtesy of Rocky Mountain Laboratory, National Institute of Allergy and Infectious Diseases, National Institutes of Health.)

FSC
www.fsc.org
MIX
Papier | Fördert gute Waldnutzung
FSC® C083411

Kolibri 360 GmbH
Ferdinand-Jühlke-Straße 7
99095 Erfurt, Deutschland
produktsicherheit@kolibri360.de